Modern Pharmacology

Modern Pharmacology

Fourth Edition

Edited by

Charles R. Craig, Ph.D.

Professor of Pharmacology and Toxicology,
West Virginia University School of Medicine, Morgantown, West Virginia

Robert E. Stitzel, Ph.D.

Professor and Associate Chairman of Pharmacology and Toxicology,
West Virginia University School of Medicine, Morgantown, West Virginia

Little, Brown and Company
Boston/New York/Toronto/London

Library of Congress Cataloging-in-Publication Data
Modern pharmacology / edited by Charles R. Craig, Robert E. Stitzel.
   —4th ed.
     p.   cm.
   Includes bibliographical references and index.
   ISBN 0-316-15932-8
   1. Pharmacology.   I. Craig, Charles R.   II. Stitzel, Robert E.
RM300.M58   1994
615'.1—dc20   93-35535
                                                   CIP

Printed in the United States of America

RRD-OH

Editorial: Evan R. Schnittman, Rebecca Marnhout
Production Editor: Karen Feeney
Copyeditor: Libby Dabrowski
Indexer: Nancy Weaver
Production Supervisor/Designer: Louis C. Bruno, Jr.
Cover Designer: Hannus Design Associates

Contents

Preface   **ix**

Contributing Authors   **xi**

I. General Principles of Pharmacology

1. Development of Pharmacological Thought   **3**
   Robert E. Stitzel

2. Mechanisms of Drug Action   **9**
   William W. Fleming

3. Drug Absorption and Distribution   **19**
   Theodore E. Gram

4. Metabolism of Drugs   **33**
   Theodore E. Gram

5. Excretion of Drugs   **47**
   William O. Berndt and Robert E. Stitzel

6. Pharmacokinetics   **55**
   Peter R. Gwilt

7. Drug Delivery Systems   **65**
   Peter R. Gwilt

8. Principles of Toxicology   **73**
   Mark J. Reasor and Mary E. Davis

9. Drug Testing in Humans   **85**
   Joseph J. McPhillips

10. Ethics in Pharmacology   **93**
    Janet Fleetwood

II. Drugs Affecting the Autonomic Nervous System

11. Introduction to the Autonomic Nervous System   **101**
    William W. Fleming

12. Adrenomimetic Drugs   **115**
    Tony J.-F. Lee and Robert E. Stitzel

13. Adrenoceptor Antagonists   **129**
    David P. Westfall

14. Directly Acting Cholinomimetics   **145**
    Brenda K. Colasanti

15. Muscarinic Blocking Drugs   **151**
    Donald B. Hoover

16. Cholinesterases and Cholinesterase Inhibitors **161**
    Donald B. Hoover

17. Ganglionic Blocking Agents **169**
    Thomas C. Westfall

18. Drugs Affecting Neuromuscular Transmission **177**
    Robert L. Volle and Michael D. Miyamoto

III. Drugs Affecting the Cardiovascular System

19. Vasoactive Substances: Renin, Angiotensin, and Kinins **187**
    Lisa A. Cassis and Michael J. Peach

20. Cholesterol and Hypocholesterolemic Drugs **197**
    Richard J. Cenedella

21. Water, Electrolyte Metabolism, and Diuretic Drugs **211**
    William O. Berndt and Robert E. Stitzel

22. Antihypertensive Drugs **229**
    David P. Westfall

23. Calcium Channel Blockers **249**
    Vijay C. Swamy and David J. Triggle

24. Cardiac Glycosides and Other Drugs Used in Myocardial Insufficiency **255**
    Ernst Seifen

25. Antianginal Drugs **265**
    Garrett J. Gross

26. Antiarrhythmic Drugs **275**
    Shawn C. Black and Benedict R. Lucchesi

27. Anticoagulant, Antiplatelet, and Fibrinolytic (Thrombolytic) Drugs **313**
    Jeffrey S. Fedan

IV. Drugs Affecting the Central Nervous System

28. Introduction to Central Nervous System Pharmacology **327**
    Charles R. Craig

29. Inhalational Anesthetics **337**
    David J. Smith

30. General Anesthetics: Gases and Volatile Liquids **345**
    Frank G. Zavisca

31. General Anesthetics: Intravenous Drugs **353**
    Michael B. Howie and David J. Smith

32. Local Anesthetics **361**
    J. David Haddox and Patricia L. Baumann

33. Sedative-Hypnotic and Anxiolytic Drugs **369**
    John W. Dailey

34. Central Nervous System Stimulants **379**
    David A. Taylor

35. Antipsychotic Drugs **387**
    Brenda K. Colasanti

36. Drugs Used in Mood Disorders **397**
    Albert J. Azzaro and Herbert E. Ward

37. Anticonvulsant Drugs 413
    Charles R. Craig

38. Drugs Used in Parkinsonism and Other Basal Ganglia Disorders 425
    Charles O. Rutledge

39. Opioid and Nonopioid Analgesics 431
    Billy Martin

40. Ethanol and Other Aliphatic Alcohols 451
    Walter A. Hunt

41. Contemporary Drug Abuse 459
    Brenda K. Colasanti and Billy Martin

V. Drugs Used to Treat Inflammatory Disorders

42. Lipid Mediators of Homeostasis and Inflammation 477
    Eric P. Brestel and Knox Van Dyke

43. Antiinflammatory and Antirheumatic Drugs 485
    Donald C. Kvam

44. Drugs Used in Gout 501
    Knox Van Dyke

45. Drugs Used in Asthma 509
    Theodore J. Torphy and Douglas W.P. Hay

46. Drugs Used in Dermatological Disorders 523
    Mary-Margaret Chren and David R. Bickers

VI. Chemotherapy

47. Introduction to Chemotherapy 537
    Irvin S. Snyder and Roger G. Finch

48. Synthetic Organic Antimicrobials (Sulfonamides, Trimethoprim, Nitrofurans, Quinolones, Methenamine) 545
    Roger G. Finch and Irvin S. Snyder

49. β-Lactam Antibiotics 555
    Irvin S. Snyder and Roger G. Finch

50. Aminoglycoside-Aminocyclitol Antibiotics 569
    Roger G. Finch and Irvin S. Snyder

51. Tetracyclines, Chloramphenicol, Macrolides, and Lincosamides 575
    Irvin S. Snyder and Roger G. Finch

52. Bacitracin, Glycopeptide Antibiotics, and the Polymyxins 583
    Roger G. Finch and Irvin S. Snyder

53. Drugs Used in Tuberculosis and Leprosy 587
    Irvin S. Snyder and Roger G. Finch

54. Antiviral Drugs 599
    Knox Van Dyke

55. Drugs Used in Acquired Immunodeficiency Syndrome 607
    Knox Van Dyke

56. Antiprotozoal Drugs 617
    Roger G. Finch and Irvin S. Snyder

57. Antimalarial Drugs 627
    Knox Van Dyke and Zuguang Ye

58. Anthelmintic Drugs **637**
    Irvin S. Snyder and Roger G. Finch

59. Antifungal Drugs **647**
    Roger G. Finch and Irvin S. Snyder

60. Antiseptics, Disinfectants, and Sterilization **657**
    Irvin S. Snyder and Roger G. Finch

61. The Rational Basis for Cancer Chemotherapy
    663
    Branimir I. Sikic

62. Antineoplastic Agents **673**
    Branimir I. Sikic

63. Immunomodulating Drugs **705**
    Daniel Wierda and Leonard J. Sauers

VII. Drugs Affecting the Endocrine System

64. Introduction to Endocrine Pharmacology **719**
    John A. Thomas

65. Hypothalamic and Pituitary Gland Hormones
    723
    Priscilla S. Dannies

66. Adrenocortical Hormones and Drugs Affecting the
    Adrenal Cortex **731**
    Ronald P. Rubin

67. Estrogens, Progestins, and Antiestrogens **747**
    Jeannine S. Strobl

68. Androgens and Anabolic Steroids **761**
    Frank L. Schwartz and Roman J. Miller

69. Thyroid and Antithyroid Drugs **775**
    John M. Connors

70. Parathyroid Hormone, Calcitonin, and Vitamin D
    787
    Frank L. Schwartz

71. Insulin, Glucagon, Somatostatin, and Orally
    Effective Hypoglycemic Drugs **797**
    John A. Thomas and Michael J. Thomas

VIII. Additional Important Drugs

72. Histamine and Histamine Antagonists **811**
    Richard J. Head and Knox Van Dyke

73. Drugs Used in Gastrointestinal Disorders **823**
    Donald G. Seibert

74. Vitamins **839**
    Suzanne Barone

75. Drugs for the Control of Supragingival Plaque
    847
    Angelo Mariotti and Arthur F. Hefti

Index **855**

Preface

It has been interesting for us as pharmacologists to look back to 1976 when we first began to accumulate the information necessary to begin a textbook in pharmacology. At that time there were virtually no books available to fill the niche between the large compendia of pharmacological information and the several smaller, almost outline, forms of drug information that were also available.

From our own years of teaching experience and from the comments of many of our colleagues at institutions both in the United States and abroad, it was increasingly clear that students taking upper level pharmacology courses needed a comprehensive, but not exhaustive, text to help them understand the complexities of pharmacology in the time frame of a single semester. This need was reflected in the increasing and almost universal use of extensive faculty-generated notes, handouts, and study guides. We hoped to satisfy this need when we began the first edition of *Modern Pharmacology*.

In the intervening 20 years between beginning the first edition and the publication of this fourth edition we have noted many important therapeutic changes. For example, the sedative-hypnotic barbiturates and several classes of diuretics are no longer widely used. Many new classes of drugs, such as the calcium channel blocking agents, immunomodulating drugs, and the benzodiazepines, have now come into prominent use. In addition to new drugs becoming available, new ways of using existing compounds, and even new diseases (e.g., AIDS and Alzheimer's) have been identified. We now include chapters on bioethics and dental therapeutics in this fourth edition.

It is clear that the discipline of pharmacology, as well as the practice of medicine, has undergone major intellectual changes in recent years. We have attempted to reflect these changes by adding new material while eliminating information of lesser importance. We also have reoriented the way in which material is presented both from drug mechanistic and clinical management points of view. We sincerely trust that this latest edition will assist students and address what is truly modern in *Modern Pharmacology*.

C.R.C.
R.E.S.

Contributing Authors

Albert J. Azzaro, Ph.D.
Professor of Neurology, Pharmacology and Toxicology, Behavioral Medicine, and Psychiatry, West Virginia University School of Medicine, Morgantown, West Virginia
36. Drugs Used in Mood Disorders

Suzanne Barone, Ph.D.
74. Vitamins

Patricia L. Baumann, M.D.
Assistant Professor of Anesthesiology, Emory University School of Medicine; Clinical Director, Pain Consultation Service, The Emory Clinic Center for Pain Medicine, Crawford W. Long Memorial Hospital, Atlanta
32. Local Anesthetics

William O. Berndt, Ph.D.
Professor of Pharmacology, University of Nebraska College of Medicine, Omaha, Nebraska
5. Excretion of Drugs
21. Water, Electrolyte Metabolism, and Diuretic Drugs

David R. Bickers, M.D.
Professor and Chairman of Dermatology, Case Western Reserve University School of Medicine; Director, Department of Dermatology, University Hospitals of Cleveland, Cleveland
46. Drugs Used in Dermatological Disorders

Shawn C. Black, Ph.D.
Lecturer, Department of Pharmacology, University of Michigan Medical School, Ann Arbor, Michigan
26. Antiarrhythmic Drugs

Eric P. Brestel, M.D.
Associate Professor of Medicine, East Carolina University School of Medicine, Greenville, North Carolina
42. Lipid Mediators of Homeostasis and Inflammation

Lisa A. Cassis, Ph.D.
Assistant Professor, University of Kentucky College of Pharmacy, Lexington, Kentucky
19. Vasoactive Substances: Renin, Angiotensin, and Kinins

Richard J. Cenedella, Ph.D.
Professor and Chairman, Department of Biochemistry, Kirksville College of Osteopathic Medicine, Kirksville, Missouri
20. Cholesterol and Hypocholesterolemic Drugs

Mary-Margaret Chren, M.D.
Assistant Professor of Dermatology, Case Western Reserve University School of Medicine; Assistant Professor of Dermatology, University Hospitals of Cleveland and Cleveland Veterans Affairs Medical Center, Cleveland
46. Drugs Used in Dermatological Disorders

Brenda K. Colasanti, Ph.D.
Adjunct Professor of Pharmacology and Toxicology, West Virginia University School of Medicine, Morgantown, West Virginia
14. Directly Acting Cholinomimetics
35. Antipsychotic Drugs
41. Contemporary Drug Abuse

John M. Connors, Ph.D.
Associate Professor of Physiology, West Virginia University School of Medicine, Morgantown, West Virginia
69. Thyroid and Antithyroid Drugs

Charles R. Craig, Ph.D.
Professor of Pharmacology and Toxicology, West Virginia University School of Medicine, Morgantown, West Virginia
28. Introduction to Central Nervous System Pharmacology
37. Anticonvulsant Drugs

John W. Dailey, Ph.D.
Associate Professor of Pharmacology, Department of
Basic Sciences, University of Illinois College of
Medicine at Peoria, Peoria, Illinois
33. Sedative-Hypnotic and Anxiolytic Drugs

Priscilla S. Dannies, Ph.D.
Professor of Pharmacology, Yale University School of
Medicine, New Haven, Connecticut
65. Hypothalamic and Pituitary Gland Hormones

Mary E. Davis, Ph.D.
Professor of Pharmacology and Toxicology, West
Virginia University School of Medicine, Morgantown,
West Virginia
8. Principles of Toxicology

Jeffrey S. Fedan, Ph.D.
Professor of Pharmacology and Toxicology, West
Virginia University School of Medicine; Research
Pharmacologist, National Institute for Occupational
Safety and Health, Morgantown, West Virginia
*27. Anticoagulant, Antiplatelet, and Fibrinolytic
(Thrombolytic) Drugs*

Roger G. Finch, F.R.C.P., F.R.C.Path.
Professor of Infectious Diseases, The University of
Nottingham; Consultant Physician, The City Hospital,
Nottingham, United Kingdom
47. Introduction to Chemotherapy
*48. Synthetic Organic Antimicrobials (Sulfonamides,
Trimethoprim, Nitrofurans, Quinolones, Methenamine)*
49. β-Lactam Antibiotics
50. Aminoglycoside-Aminocyclitol Antibiotics
*51. Tetracyclines, Chloramphenical, Macrolides, and
Lincosamides*
52. Bacitracin, Glycopeptide Antibiotics, and the Polymyxins
53. Drugs Used in Tuberculosis and Leprosy
56. Antiprotozoal Drugs
58. Anthelmintic Drugs
59. Antifungal Drugs
60. Antiseptics, Disinfectants, and Sterilization

Janet Fleetwood, Ph.D.
Director, Medical Humanities Program, and Assistant
Professor, Department of Community and Preventive
Medicine, Medical College of Pennsylvania,
Philadelphia
10. Ethics in Pharmacology

William W. Fleming, Ph.D.
Professor and Mylan Chairman of Pharmacology and
Toxicology, West Virginia University School of
Medicine, Morgantown, West Virginia
2. Mechanisms of Drug Action
11. Introduction to the Autonomic Nervous System

Theodore E. Gram, Ph.D.
Head (retired), Section on Drug Interactions, Laboratory
of Biology, National Cancer Institute, Bethesda,
Maryland
3. Drug Absorption and Distribution
4. Metabolism of Drugs

Garrett J. Gross, Ph.D.
Professor of Pharmacology and Toxicology, Medical
College of Wisconsin, Milwaukee
25. Antianginal Drugs

Peter R. Gwilt, Ph.D.
Associate Professor of Pharmaceutical Sciences,
University of Nebraska College of Medicine, Omaha,
Nebraska
6. Pharmacokinetics
7. Drug Delivery Systems

J. David Haddox, D.D.S., M.D.
Associate Professor and Director, Division of Pain
Medicine, Department of Anesthesiology, Emory
University School of Medicine; Director, The Emory
Clinic Center for Pain Medicine, Crawford W. Long
Memorial Hospital, Atlanta
32. Local Anesthetics

Douglas W.P. Hay, Ph.D.
Associate Fellow of Inflammation and Respiratory
Pharmacology, SmithKline Beecham Pharmaceuticals,
King of Prussia, Pennsylvania
45. Drugs Used in Asthma

Richard J. Head, Ph.D.
Assistant Chief of CSIRO Division of Human
Nutrition, CSIRO, Adelaide, South Australia
72. Histamine and Histamine Antagonists

Arthur F. Hefti, D.M.D., P.D.
Professor of Periodontology, University of Florida
College of Dentistry, Gainesville, Florida
75. Drugs for the Control of Supragingival Plaque

Donald B. Hoover, Ph.D.
Professor of Pharmacology, East Tennessee State
University, James H. Quillen College of Medicine,
Johnson City, Tennessee
15. Muscarinic Blocking Drugs
16. Cholinesterases and Cholinesterase Inhibitors

Michael B. Howie, M.D.
Professor of Anesthesiology, Ohio State University
College of Medicine; Vice Chairperson of
Anesthesiology, The Ohio State University Hospitals,
Columbus, Ohio
31. General Anesthetics: Intravenous Drugs

Walter A. Hunt, Ph.D.
Chief, Neurosciences and Behavioral Research Branch, National Institute on Alcohol Abuse and Alcoholism, Rockville, Maryland
40. Ethanol and Other Aliphatic Alcohols

Donald C. Kvam, Ph.D.
Associate Director for Clinical Pharmacology, 3M Pharmaceuticals, St. Paul, Minnesota
43. Antiinflammatory and Antirheumatic Drugs

Tony J.-F. Lee, Ph.D.
Professor of Pharmacology, Southern Illinois University School of Medicine, Springfield, Illinois
12. Adrenomimetic Drugs

Benedict R. Lucchesi, M.D., Ph.D.
Professor of Pharmacology, University of Michigan Medical School, Ann Arbor, Michigan
26. Antiarrhythmic Drugs

Joseph J. McPhillips, Ph.D.
Director of Clinical Research, Boehringer Mannheim Pharmaceuticals, Rockville, Maryland
9. Drug Testing in Humans

Angelo Mariotti, D.D.S., Ph.D.
Assitant Professor of Periodontology, Department of Pharmacology and Therapeutics, University of Florida College of Medicine, Gainesville, Florida
75. Drugs for the Control of Supragingival Plaque

Billy Martin, Ph.D.
Professor of Pharmacology and Toxicology, Virginia Commonwealth University, Medical College of Virginia, Richmond, Virginia
39. Opioid and Nonopioid Analgesics
41. Contemporary Drug Abuse

Roman J. Miller, Ph.D.
Professor of Biology, Eastern Mennonite College, Harrisonburg, Virginia
68. Androgens and Anabolic Steroids

Michael D. Miyamoto, Ph.D.
Professor of Pharmacology, East Tennessee State University, James H. Quillen College of Medicine, Johnson City, Tennessee
18. Drugs Affecting Neuromuscular Transmission

Michael J. Peach*
Associate Dean for Research, Professor of Pharmacology, University of Virginia School of Medicine, Charlottesville, Virginia
19. Vasoactive Substances: Renin, Angiotensin, and Kinins

---

*Deceased

Mark J. Reasor, Ph.D.
Professor of Pharmacology and Toxicology, West Virginia University School of Medicine, Morgantown, West Virginia
8. Principles of Toxicology

Ronald P. Rubin, Ph.D.
Professor and Chairman, Department of Pharmacology and Therapeutics, State University of New York at Buffalo School of Medicine and Biomedical Sciences, Buffalo, New York
66. Adrenocortical Hormones and Drugs Affecting the Adrenal Cortex

Charles O. Rutledge, Ph.D.
Dean and Professor of Pharmacology, Purdue University School of Pharmacy and Pharmacological Sciences, West Lafayette, Indiana
38. Drugs Used in Parkinsonism and Other Basal Ganglia Disorders

Leonard J. Sauers, Ph.D.
Section Head, Human Safety Department, The Procter and Gamble Company, Cincinnati
63. Immunomodulating Drugs

Frank L. Schwartz, M.D.
Clinical Associate Professor of Medicine, West Virginia University School of Medicine, Morgantown; Medical Director, Diabetes Center, Camden Clark Memorial Hospital, Parkersburg, West Virginia
68. Androgens and Anabolic Steroids
70. Parathyroid Hormone, Calcitonin, and Vitamin D

Donald G. Seibert, M.D.
Assistant Professor of Medicine, West Virginia University School of Medicine; Attending Physician, Gastrointestinal Section, Department of Medicine, Ruby Memorial Hospital, Morgantown, West Virginia
73. Drugs Used in Gastrointestinal Disorders

Ernst Seifen, M.D., Ph.D.
Professor of Anesthesiology and Pharmacology and Toxicology, University of Arkansas College of Medicine, Little Rock, Arkansas
24. Cardiac Glycosides and Other Drugs Used in Myocardial Insufficiency

Branimir I. Sikic, M.D.
Associate Professor of Oncology, Stanford University School of Medicine, Stanford, California
61. The Rational Basis for Cancer Chemotherapy
62. Antineoplastic Agents

David J. Smith, Ph.D.
Professor of Anesthesiology and Pharmacology and Toxicology, West Virginia University School of Medicine, Morgantown, West Virginia
29. Inhalational Anesthetics
31. General Anesthetics: Intravenous Drugs

Irvin S. Snyder, Ph.D.
Professor of Microbiology and Immunology, West Virginia University School of Medicine, Morgantown, West Virginia
47. Introduction to Chemotherapy
48. Synthetic Organic Antimicrobials (Sulfonamides, Trimethoprim, Nitrofurans, Quinolones, Methenamine)
49. β-Lactam Antibiotics
50. Aminoglycoside-Aminocyclitol Antibiotics
51. Tetracyclines, Chloramphenicol, Macrolides, and Lincosamides
52. Bacitracin, Glycopeptide Antibiotics, and the Polymyxins
53. Drugs Used in Tuberculosis and Leprosy
56. Antiprotozoal Drugs
58. Anthelmintic Drugs
59. Antifungal Drugs
60. Antiseptics, Disinfectants, and Sterilization

Robert E. Stitzel, Ph.D.
Professor and Associate Chairman of Pharmacology and Toxicology, West Virginia University School of Medicine, Morgantown, West Virginia
1. Development of Pharmacological Thought
5. Excretion of Drugs
12. Adrenomimetic Drugs
21. Water, Electrolyte Metabolism, and Diuretic Drugs

Jeannine S. Strobl, Ph.D.
Professor of Pharmacology and Toxicology, West Virginia University School of Medicine, Morgantown, West Virginia
67. Estrogens, Progestins, and Antiestrogens

Vijay C. Swamy, Ph.D.
Associate Professor of Biochemical Pharmacology, State University of New York at Buffalo School of Pharmacy, Buffalo, New York
23. Calcium Channel Blockers

David A. Taylor, Ph.D.
Professor of Pharmacology and Toxicology, West Virginia University School of Medicine, Morgantown, West Virginia
34. Central Nervous System Stimulants

John A. Thomas, Ph.D.
Professor of Pharmacology, University of Texas Health Science Center at San Antonio, San Antonio
64. Introduction to Endocrine Pharmacology
71. Insulin, Glucagon, Somatostatin, and Orally Effective Hypoglycemic Drugs

Michael J. Thomas, M.D., Ph.D.
Clinical Fellow of Medicine, Division of Endocrinology, Washington University School of Medicine, St. Louis
71. Insulin, Glucagon, Somatostatin, and Orally Effective Hypoglycemic Drugs

Theodore J. Torphy, Ph.D.
Director of Inflammation and Respiratory Pharmacology, SmithKline Beecham Pharmaceuticals, King of Prussia, Pennsylvania
45. Drugs Used in Asthma

David J. Triggle, Ph.D.
Distinguished Professor, Dean's Office, State University of New York at Buffalo School of Pharmacy, Buffalo, New York
23. Calcium Channel Blockers

Knox Van Dyke, Ph.D.
Professor of Pharmacology and Toxicology, West Virginia University School of Medicine, Morgantown, West Virginia
42. Lipid Mediators of Homeostasis and Inflammation
44. Drugs Used in Gout
54. Antiviral Drugs
55. Drugs Used in Acquired Immunodeficiency Syndrome
57. Antimalarial Drugs
72. Histamine and Histamine Antagonists

Robert L. Volle, Ph.D.
President Emeritus, National Board of Medical Examiners, Philadelphia
18. Drugs Affecting Neuromuscular Transmission

Herbert E. Ward, M.D.
Assistant Professor of Psychiatry, West Virginia University School of Medicine, Morgantown, West Virginia
36. Drugs Used in Mood Disorders

David P. Westfall, Ph.D.
Professor and Chairman, Department of Pharmacology, University of Nevada School of Medicine, Reno, Nevada
13. Adrenoceptor Antagonists
22. Antihypertensive Drugs

Thomas C. Westfall, Ph.D.
William Beaumont Professor and Chairman, Department of Pharmacological and Physiological Science, Saint Louis University School of Medicine, St. Louis
17. Ganglionic Blocking Agents

Daniel Wierda, Ph.D.
Research Scientist, Biochemical Toxicology, Lilly Research Laboratories, Eli Lilly and Company, Greenfield, Illinois
63. Immunomodulating Drugs

Zuguang Ye, M.S.
Associate Professor and Vice Chairman of
Pharmacology, Institute of Chinesa Materia Medica,
China Academy of Traditional Chinese Medicine,
Beijing, People's Republic of China
57. Antimalarial Drugs

Frank G. Zavisca, M.D., Ph.D.
Staff Anesthesiologist, University of Texas
Southwestern Medical Center at Dallas, Southwestern
Medical School; Staff Anesthesiologist, Department of
Anesthesiology, Parkland Memorial Medical Center,
Dallas
30. General Anesthetics: Gases and Volatile Liquids

General Principles of Pharmacology

1

Development of Pharmacological Thought

Robert E. Stitzel

To understand a science, one has to know its history and development. It should be useful, then, and we hope entertaining, for students to understand the background and underlying assumptions of *pharmacology,* a discipline that defines itself in simple yet all-encompassing terms: the study of the interaction of chemicals with biological systems.

One of the earliest concerns of humankind was a desire for protection against the evils of disease and suffering. Since the conquering of these afflictions often determined survival and since the current state of knowledge did not permit the rational use of *drugs* (chemical entities, both endogenous and foreign, that are capable of reacting with biological systems), it should not be surprising that additional help was sought from supernatural powers. This was especially true of the ancient Greeks, who believed that it was by whim that the gods dispensed prosperity or pestilence. Thus, early in human history a natural bond was formed between religion and the use of drugs. Those who became most proficient in the use of drugs to treat disease were the "mediators" between this world and the spirit world, namely, the priests, shamans, holy persons, witches, and soothsayers. Much of their power within the community was derived from the cures that they could effect with drugs. It was believed that the sick were possessed by demons and that health could be restored by identifying the demon and finding a way to cast it out.

Originally, religion dominated its partnership with *therapeutics* (the application of chemical substances in the diagnosis, prevention, and treatment of disease, or, additionally, the use of drugs for the intentional modification of normal physiological and biochemical function), and divine intervention was called upon for every treatment. However, the use of drugs to effect cures led to a profound and drastic change in both religious thought and structure. As more became known about the effects of drugs, the importance of divine intervention began to recede, and the treatment of patients effectively became a province of the priest rather than the gods whom the priest served. This process of cultural evolution, brought about at least in part by the growing understanding of the curative powers of natural products and decreasing reliance on supernatural intervention, forever altered the relationship between humanity and its gods. Furthermore, when the priests began to apply the information learned from treating one patient to the treatment of other patients, the religious approach began to lose most of its remaining proponents: There was at last a recognition that a regularity prevailed in the natural world that was independent of supernatural whim or will. Therapeutics thus evolved from its roots in magic to a foundation in experience. This was the cornerstone for the formulation of a scientifically based practice of medicine.

People began to believe that nature alone could provide the means to remove pain and disease, and thus they sought remedies in nature, that is, in plants, minerals, and animals. A variety of medicinal agents were collected on the basis of their symbolic qualities as well as their relation to astrological signs and portents. For example, since the sword symbolized strength and power, the early Greek physicians attempted to use iron therapy against weakness and anemia. The observation that the horn of the rhinoceros is powerful led Chinese physicians to propose it as a potent aphrodisiac (with subsequent intensive hunting and near extinction of rhinoceroses).

While it is often tempting to dwell on the more bizarre, and seemingly absurd, therapeutic practices of the ancients, it should always be kept in mind that these practitioners brought forth their explanations in good faith. Furthermore, many of their "drugs" were added to the therapeutic armamentarium only after considerable trial and error and application of clinical judgment. We should not automatically brand their explanations as silly and as having no basis by today's "rational" standards. We must assume that these early drug users were just as intelligent as we are and that they had good reasons, *in light of the facts then available,* for what they said and did. The answer to the question, What did they consider good reasons?, is not a simple one: It must take into consideration their entire intellectual, ethical, and cultural background.

Contributions of Many Cultures

The ancient Chinese wrote extensively on medical subjects. The *Pen Tsao,* for instance, was written about 2700 B.C. and contained classifications of individual medicinal plants as well as compilations of plant mixtures to be used for medical purposes. The Chinese *doctrine of signatures* (like used to treat like) enables us to understand why medicines of animal origin were of such great importance in the Chinese pharmacopoeia.

Ancient Egyptian medical papyri contain numerous prescriptions. The largest and perhaps the most important of these, the *Ebers Papyrus* (1550 B.C.), contains about 800 prescriptions quite similar to those written today in that they have one or more active substances (e.g., cathartic, purgative) as well as vehicles (animal fats for ointments; and water, milk, wine, beer, or honey for liquids) for suspending or dissolving the active drug. These prescriptions also commonly offer a brief statement of how the preparation is to be prepared (mixed, pounded, boiled, strained, left overnight in the dew) and how it is to be used (swallowed, inhaled, gargled, applied externally, or given as an enema). Cathartics and purgatives were particularly in vogue since both the patients and the physician could tell almost immediately whether or not the "end" result had been achieved. It was reasoned that, in causing the contents of the gastrointestinal tract to be forcibly ejected, one simultaneously drove out the disease-producing evil spirits that had taken hold of the unfortunate patient. Whether the cure was worse than the disease was a subject of active debate.

At a very early stage in the history of pharmacology there were attempts to codify and standardize remedies. The records that have come down to us from China, India, Sumeria, Egypt, and Greece are frequently concerned with the accumulation, development, and recording of local drug lore; this was an integral part of each culture. Many of these writings, some dating as far back as 4000 B.C., contain numerous dietary suggestions and recipes extolling the benefits of virtually every known variety of fruit, vegetable, grain, grass, or bulb. This codification of drug lore was based on information that had accumulated during earlier centuries.

The level of drug usage achieved by the Egyptians undoubtedly had a great influence on Greek medicine and literature. Observations on the medical effects of various natural substances can be found in both the *Iliad* and the *Odyssey.* Battle wounds were frequently covered with powdered plant leaves or bark; their astringent and pain-reducing actions derived from the tannins they contained. It may have been mandrake root (containing atropine-like

substances that induce a "twilight sleep") that protected Ulysses from Circe. The oriental hellebore, which contains the cardiotoxic *Veratrum* alkaloids, was smeared on arrow tips to increase their killing effects. The fascination of the Greeks with the toxic effects of various plant extracts led to an increasing body of knowledge concerned primarily with the poisonous aspects of drugs (the science of *toxicology*). We could cite Plato's description of the death of Socrates as one of the principal early toxicological accounts, since he gave a very accurate, albeit rather personal, description of the toxicological properties of the juice of the hemlock fruit. His description of the paralysis of sensory and motor nerves, followed eventually by central nervous system depression and respiratory paralysis, precisely matches the known actions of the potent hemlock alkaloid, coniine.

The Indian cultures of Central and South America, although totally isolated from the Old World, developed drug lore and usage in a fashion almost parallel to that of the older civilization. The use of drugs played an intimate part in the rites, religions, history, and knowledge of the South American Indians. The knowledge of medicinal remedies possessed by the Aztecs probably accumulated both during their migration into the valley of Mexico and through their commerce with the Mayans to the southeast, the Zapotecs to the south, and the Tarascans to the west. These contacts greatly expanded their knowledge of the abundant flora of these regions, much of which was believed to be of medicinal value. As we have already seen for European medicines, New World medicine was also closely tied to religious thought. All the Indian cultures treated their patients with a blend of religious rituals and herbal remedies. Incantations, charms, and appeals to various deities were as important as the appropriate application of poultices, decoctions, and infusions.

Early drug practitioners both in Europe and South America gathered herbs, plants, animals, and minerals and often blended them into a variety of foul-smelling and ill-flavored concoctions. The fact that many of these preparations were so distasteful led to an attempt to improve on the "cosmetic" properties of these mixtures to ensure patient use. Individuals who began to search for improved product formulation were largely responsible for the founding of the disciplines of *pharmacy* (the science of preparing, compounding, and dispensing medicines) and *pharmacognosy* (the identification and preparation of crude drugs from natural sources).

A problem that has remained with us over the centuries is the tendency of some physicians to prescribe large numbers of drugs where one or two would be sufficient. The patient often suffers more from the side effects of the drugs than from the illness being treated. We can trace the history of this polypharmaceutical approach to Galen (A.D. 131–201), who was considered the greatest European physician after Hippocrates. He believed that drugs had certain essential properties, such as warmth, coldness, dryness, or humidity, and that by using several drugs he could combine these properties to adjust for deficiencies in the patient. Galen's major error was one that is only slightly less common today: He formulated general rules and laws before sufficient factual information was available to justify their formulation.

By the first century A.D. it was clear to both physician and "protopharmacologist" alike that there was much variation to be found from one biological extract to another, even when these were prepared by the same individual. It was reasoned that to fashion a rational and reproducible system of therapeutics and to study pharmacological activity one had to obtain standardized and uniform medicinal agents. Nero's surgeon, Dioscorides, was among the first to write extensively on the careful preparation of drugs, and he also identified an increasing problem—adulteration of drugs by unscrupulous profiteers. Human nature evidently has not changed much in the last two millennia, since we still require a "watchdog" to protect us from ineffective or adulterated medicinals.

Development of Pharmacological Thought

Religion dominated the world both politically and intellectually from the time of Galen to the Renaissance. It was believed that absolute truths existed and that these were not to be questioned. This same reasoning was applied to scientific thought during this period. It was felt that one could not improve on the knowledge handed down by the ancient Greeks, and in particular that the therapeutic knowledge of Galen should not be questioned. It was only when religious ideas came into question during the Reformation that people felt free to criticize and cast doubt on the infallibility of the present state of knowledge, and it was only when people began to challenge the formerly irrefutable power of authority that modern science could be said to have begun. Such a change in attitude occurred in the sixteenth century, a period of political and intellectual unrest. No longer was anything considered as settled. Both new lands and new ideas were being explored. In science, Copernicus (1473–1543) and Vesalius (1514–1564) typified the period in their emphasis on direct observation.

Perhaps the greatest notion of the period was the absolute conviction that every occurrence or event had a cause that could be discovered and examined. This was the real origin and driving force behind scientific inquiry. It was soon accepted that the secrets of nature could be unraveled through careful observation and that the facts discovered would eventually lead to the formulation of general principles or hypotheses. This was in great contrast to previous beliefs, which held that laws preceded observa-

tions. Such an approach to the examination of natural phenomena singled out science from among all other European movements of the sixteenth and seventeenth centuries. Although scientific inquiry was born in Europe, owing to the universality and applicability of its ideas, it quickly found its home to be the entire world. It was soon discovered that the scientific outlook, in contrast to many other beliefs, was readily transferable from country to country and from one ethnic group to another.

Although we have been talking about science and scientific thought in general, pharmacology, as a part of science, did not escape this revolution in thought. What Copernicus was doing for science as a whole, a young itinerant physician named Philippus Aureolus Theophrastus Bombastus von Hohenheim (1493–1541), who called himself Paracelsus, was beginning to do for pharmacology. Perhaps his two primary contributions were his vigorous attacks on the previously untouchable galenical polypharmaceutical system (e.g., one fifteenth-century prescription contains 110 different ingredients) and his insistence that drugs should be subjected to critical investigation.

At the end of the eighteenth and the beginning of the nineteenth centuries, methods became available for the isolation of active principles from crude drugs. The simultaneous development of the discipline of chemistry made it possible to isolate and synthesize chemically pure compounds that would give reproducible biological results. In 1806, Serturner (1783–1841) isolated the first pure active principle when he purified morphine from the opium poppy. Many other chemically pure active compounds were soon obtained from crude drug preparations, including emetine by Pelletier (1788–1844) from ipecacuanha root; quinine by Carentou (1795–1877) from cinchona bark; strychnine by Magendie (1783–1855) from nux vomica; and, in 1856, cocaine by Wöhler (1800–1882) from coca.

The isolation and use of pure substances allowed for an analysis of what was soon to become one of the basic concerns of pharmacology, that is, the quantitative study of drug action. It was soon realized that drug action is produced along a continuum of effects with low doses producing less, but essentially similar, effects on organs and tissues as do high doses. It was also noted that the appearance of toxic effects of drugs was frequently a function of the dose-response relationship.

Pharmacology and the Experimental Method

Clearly, the primary advances in pharmacological thought at this time were due to the progress of chemistry, but these centuries also saw serious attempts to establish the physiological basis of drug action. Although "ex-

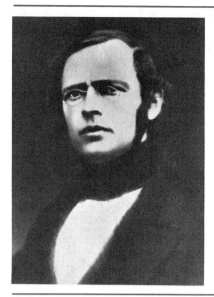 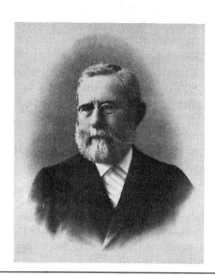 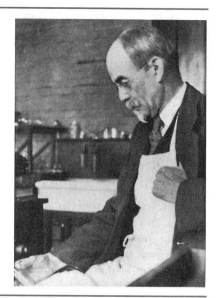

Figure 1-1. The three important figures in the early history of pharmacology are Rudolf Bucheim, Oswald Schmiedeberg, and John Jacob Abel *(left to right)*. They not only created new laboratories devoted to the laboratory investigation of drugs, but also firmly established the new discipline through the training of future faculty, the writing of textbooks, and the founding of scientific journals and societies.

periments" had been performed in medicine for centuries, they were quite isolated occurrences. In medical thought the turning point is best marked by William Harvey's famous experiments (1628) demonstrating the motion of the heart and the circulation of blood. This not only made clear a fundamental function of the body but also demonstrated the use one could make of a new and powerful tool, the *experimental method.*

In pharmacology the experiments of the seventeenth and eighteenth centuries were primarily concerned with examining the toxicity of different drugs, studying the general symptoms elicited by them, and searching for antidotes to them. A closer analysis of drug mechanism of action, however, was impossible since the understanding of normal body function was still quite limited. By the beginning of the nineteenth century this situation had changed, and the first experiments to bring about some understanding of drug action could be made.

In the realm of scientific thought, the name of Claude Bernard (1813–1878) must be at the forefront. His contributions go far beyond those specific discoveries that he made in the fields of physiology and pharmacology. He is a pivotal figure in the physiological sciences, and his approach to the understanding of biological phenomena has had a profound influence on the way diagnosticians and scientists confront medical problems. It was Bernard, perhaps more than any other individual, who was associated with the application of the experimental method to medicine. He believed that scientists must ask significant questions, design appropriate experiments to test the questions

posed, analyze the resulting data, and finally, formulate a testable hypothesis or conclusion. His work and experience culminated in the writing of one of the seminal monographs in science, which surely must rank with the writings of Darwin as far as its importance in setting new directions and standards of inquiry is concerned. In *Introduction to the Study of Experimental Medicine*, Bernard offered a criterion for measuring the importance of future scientific discoveries from which we still profit. He stated, "We usually give the name of discovery to recognition of a new fact: But I think that the idea connected with the discovered fact is what really constitutes discovery. . . . A great discovery is a fact whose appearance in science gives rise to ideas shedding a bright light which dispels many obscurities and shows us new paths."

Until the nineteenth century, the rapid development of pharmacology as a distinct discipline was hindered by the lack of the sophisticated chemical methodology needed to extract pure, active principles from crude plant and animal sources. Development also was impaired by limited knowledge of physiological mechanisms. The significant advances made through laboratory studies of animal physiology, accomplished by investigators such as Françoise Magendie and Claude Bernard, provided an environment conducive to the creation of similar laboratories for the study of pharmacological phenomena.

One of the first laboratories devoted almost exclusively to drug research was established in Dorpat, Estonia in the late 1840s by Rudolph Bucheim (1820–1879) (Fig. 1-1). The laboratory, built in Bucheim's home, was devoted to studying the actions of agents such as cathartics, alcohol, chloroform, anthelmintics, and heavy metals. Bucheim believed that "the investigation of drugs . . . is a task for a pharmacologist and not for a chemist or pharmacist, who until now have been expected to do this. . . . [It is] perhaps necessary . . . to rouse pharmacology from its sleep. [However,] the sleep is not a natural one since pharmacology, as judged by its past accomplishments, has no reason for being tired."

Although the availability of a laboratory devoted to pharmacological investigations was important, much more was required to raise this discipline to the same prominent position occupied by other basic sciences; this included the creation of chairs in pharmacology at other academic institutions and the training of a sufficient number of talented investigators to occupy these positions. The latter task was largely accomplished by Bucheim's pupil and successor at Dorpat, Oswald Schmiedeberg (1838–1921), undoubtedly the most prominent pharmacologist of the nineteenth century (Fig. 1-1). In addition to conducting his own outstanding research on the pharmacology of diuretics, emetics, cardiac glycosides, and so forth, he wrote an important medical textbook and trained approximately 120 pupils from more than 20 countries. Many of these new investigators either started or developed laboratories devoted to experimental pharmacology in their own countries.

One of Schmiedeberg's most outstanding students was John Jacob Abel, who has been called the Founder of American Pharmacology (Fig. 1-1). Abel occupied the chair of pharmacology first at the University of Michigan and then at Johns Hopkins University. Among his most important research accomplishments is an examination of the chemistry and subsequent isolation of the active principles from the adrenal medulla (a monobenzoyl derivative of epinephrine) and the pancreas (crystallization of insulin). He also examined mushroom poisons, investigated the chemotherapeutic actions of the arsenicals and antimonials, conducted studies on tetanus toxin, and designed a model for an artificial kidney. In addition, Professor Abel founded the *Journal of Experimental Medicine,* the *Journal of Biological Chemistry,* and the *Journal of Pharmacology and Experimental Therapeutics.* He continued his active research career even after his formal retirement from the university. His devotion to pharmacological research, his enthusiasm for the training of students in this new discipline, and his establishment of journals and scientific societies proved critical in the rise of experimental pharmacology in the United States.

Pharmacology, as a separate and vital discipline, has interests that distinguish it from the other basic sciences and pharmacy. Its primary concern is not the cataloguing of all the biological effects that result from the administration of chemical substances but rather the dual aims of (1) providing an understanding of normal and abnormal body physiology and biochemistry through the application of drugs as experimental tools, and (2) applying to clinical medicine the information gained from fundamental investigation and observation.

A report in the *Status of Research in Pharmacology* has described some of the founding principles on which the discipline is based and which distinguish pharmacology from other fields of study. These principles include the study of

- The relationship between drug concentration and biological response
- Drug action over time
- Factors affecting absorption, distribution, binding, metabolism, and elimination of chemicals
- Structure-activity relationships
- Biological changes that result from repeated drug use—tolerance, addiction, adverse reactions, altered rates of drug metabolism, and so forth
- Antagonism of the effects of one drug by another
- The process of drug interaction with cellular macromolecules (receptors) to alter physiological function (that is, receptor theory)

In the last 100 years there has been an extraordinary growth in medical knowledge. This expansion of information has come about largely through the contributions that the biological sciences have made to medicine by a systematic approach to the understanding and treatment of disease. The experimental method and technological advances are the foundations upon which modern medicine is built. The question we must now face is: Can we reasonably expect that all future methodological advances will eventually permit an understanding of all disease processes?

The information we are accumulating, especially from the fields of psychiatry and psychopharmacology, suggests that measuring and adjusting body chemicals alone will not invariably lead to cures. Today physician and pharmacologist alike must recognize that a thorough understanding of drug action will not guarantee the patient's return to health. The behavioral and psychosocial components of disease and the manifestations of that disease in an individual patient cannot be ignored. Clinical tests, laboratory data, and appropriate pharmacotherapy must be blended with an understanding of the social system and the social and psychological pressures that impinge on each patient. Giving primacy solely to biological factors and ignoring or downgrading the psychobiological unity of humans and the importance of nonbiological variables on biological processes must eventually lead to an "unscientific" medicine.

Supplemental Reading

Bachman, C., and Bickel, M.H. History of drug metabolism: The first half of the 20th century. *Drug Metab. Rev.* 16:185, 1986.

Boussel, P., Bonnemain, H., and Bore, F. *History of Pharmacy and the Pharmaceutical Industry.* Lausanne: Asklepios, 1982.

Court, W.E. The doctrine of signatures or similitudes. *Tr. Pharmacol. Sci.* 6:225, 1985.

Fisher, J.W. Origins of American pharmacology. *Tr. Pharmacol. Sci.* 7:41, 1986.

De Pasquale, A. Pharmacognosy: The oldest modern science. *J. Ethnopharmacol.* 11:1, 1984.

Holmstead, B., and Liljestrand, G. (eds.). *Readings in Pharmacology.* New York: Macmillan, 1963.

Krantz, J. *Historical Medical Classics Involving New Drugs.* Baltimore: Williams & Wilkins, 1974.

Liu, C.X. Development of Chinese medicine based on pharmacology and therapeutics. *J. Ethnopharmacol.* 19:119, 1987.

Leake, C.D. *An Historical Account of Pharmacology to the Twentieth Century.* Springfield, Ill.: Thomas, 1975.

Mann, R.D. *Modern Drug Use: An Enquiry on Historical Principles.* Hingham, Mass.: Kluwer, 1984.

Olmstead, J., and Olmstead, E. *Claude Bernard and the Experimental Method in Medicine.* New York: Collier, 1961.

Paton, D.W.M. The Early Days of Pharmacology with Special Reference to the Nineteenth Century. In F.N.L. Poynter (ed.), *Chemistry in the Service of Medicine.* London: Pitman, 1963.

2

Mechanisms of Drug Action

William W. Fleming

Receptors

A fundamental concept of pharmacology is that, to initiate an effect in a cell, most drugs combine with some molecular structure on the surface of, or within, the cell. This molecular structure is called a *receptor*. The combination of the drug with the receptor results in a molecular change in the receptor, such as an altered configuration or charge distribution, and thereby triggers a chain of events leading to a *response*. This concept applies not only to the action of drugs but also to the action of naturally occurring substances such as hormones or neurotransmitters. Indeed, many drugs mimic the effects of hormones or transmitters because they combine with the same receptors as do these endogenous substances.

It is generally assumed that all receptors with which drugs combine exist to function as receptors for neurotransmitters, hormones, or other physiological substances. Thus, the discovery of a specific receptor for a group of drugs can lead to a search for previously unknown endogenous substances that combine with those same receptors. A classic example involves opioid receptors. In 1973, several research groups published evidence that morphine and related opioid drugs act on a specific receptor. This new knowledge led to the search for endogenous substances, the physiological function of which would depend on an interaction with the newly identified opiate receptors. Within 2 years, evidence was found for the existence of endogenous peptides with morphinelike activity. A series of these peptides have since been identified and are collectively termed *endorphins* and *enkephalins* (see Chap. 39). It is now clear that drugs such as morphine are merely mimicking endorphins or enkephalins by combining with the same receptors.

Drug Receptors and Biological Responses

The effects of a drug on a biological system must ultimately be reduced to a physicochemical interaction between the drug and the receptor. Although the term *receptor* is convenient, one should never lose sight of the fact that *receptors are, in actuality, molecular substances or macromolecules present in tissues that combine chemically with the drug.* Since most drugs have a considerable degree of *selectivity* in their actions, it follows that the receptors with which they interact must be equally unique. Thus, *receptors will interact with only a limited number of structurally related or complementary compounds.*

The drug-receptor interaction can be better appreciated through a specific example. The end-plate region of a skeletal muscle fiber contains large numbers of receptors having a high affinity for the transmitter acetylcholine (ACh). Each of these receptors, known as nicotinic receptors, is an integral part of a "channel" in the postsynaptic membrane that controls the inward movement of sodium ions (see Chap. 18, Fig. 18-1). At rest, the postsynaptic membrane is relatively impermeable to sodium. Stimulation of the nerve leading to the muscle results in the release of acetylcholine from the nerve fiber in the region of the end-plate. The acetylcholine combines with the receptors and changes them so that channels are opened and sodium flows inward. The more acetylcholine there is in the end-plate region, the more the receptors that are occupied and the more the channels that are opened. When the number of open channels reaches a critical value, sodium enters rapidly enough to disturb the ionic balance of the membrane, resulting in a localized depolarization. The localized depolarization (end-plate potential) triggers the activation of large numbers of voltage-dependent sodium channels, causing the conducted depolarization known as an action potential. The action potential leads to the release of calcium from intracellular binding sites. The calcium then interacts with the contractile proteins, resulting in shortening of the muscle cell. The sequence of events can be shown diagrammatically as follows:

$$\text{ACh} + \text{receptor} \rightarrow \text{Na}^+ \text{ influx} \rightarrow \text{action potential}$$
$$\rightarrow \text{increased free Ca}^{2+} \rightarrow \text{contraction}$$

The precise chain of events following drug-receptor interaction depends upon the particular receptor and the particular type of cell. The important concept at this stage of the discussion is that *specific receptive substances serve as triggers of cellular reactions.*

If we consider the sequence of events by which acetylcholine brings about muscle contraction through receptors, we can easily appreciate that foreign chemicals (drugs) can be designed to interact with the same process. A chemical with a molecular structure very similar to that of acetylcholine might be attracted to the receptor for acetylcholine and change the receptor's molecular orientation in a manner similar to that of acetylcholine, thereby initiating the chain of events that culminates in muscle contraction. Thus, the drug would *mimic* the actions of acetylcholine at the motor end-plate; nicotine and carbamylcholine are two drugs that have such an effect. *Chemicals that interact with a receptor and thereby initiate a cellular reaction are termed agonists.* Thus, acetylcholine itself, as well as the drugs nicotine and carbamylcholine, are agonists for the receptors in the skeletal muscle end-plate.

On the other hand, if a chemical is somewhat less similar to acetylcholine, it may interact with the receptor but be unable to induce the exact molecular change necessary to allow the inward movement of sodium. In this instance the chemical does not cause contraction but, because it occupies the receptor site, it inhibits the interaction of acetylcholine with its receptor. Such a drug is termed an *antagonist.* An example of such a compound is *d*-tubocurarine, an antagonist of acetylcholine at the end-plate receptors. Since it competes with acetylcholine for its receptor and prevents acetylcholine from producing its characteristic effects, administration of *d*-tubocurarine will result in muscle relaxation by interfering with acetylcholine's ability to induce and maintain the contractile state of the muscle cells.

Historically, receptors have been identified through a recognition of the relative selectivity by which certain exogenously administered drugs, neurotransmitters, or hormones exert their pharmacological effects. By applying mathematical principles to *dose-response relationships,* it became possible to estimate dissociation constants for the interaction between specific receptors and individual agonists or antagonists. Subsequently, methods were developed to measure the specific binding of radioactively labeled drugs to receptor sites in tissues and thereby determine not only the *affinity* of a drug for its receptor, but also the *density of receptors* per cell. For example, it has been estimated that there are approximately 85,000 β-adrenoceptors (a specific receptor for the neurotransmitter norepinephrine; see Chap. 11) per cell in dog ventricular muscle.

Much has been learned in recent years about the chemical structure of certain receptors. The nicotinic receptor on skeletal muscle, for example, is known to be composed of five subunits, each a glycoprotein weighing 40,000 to 65,000 daltons. These subunits are arranged as interacting helices that penetrate the cell membrane completely and surround a "central pit" that is a sodium ion channel. The binding sites for acetylcholine (see Chap. 14), and other agonists that mimic it, are located on one of the subunits that project extracellularly from the cell membrane. The binding of an agonist to these sites induces a conformational change in the glycoprotein whereby the side chains move away from the center of the channel, allowing sodium ions to enter the cell through the channel. The glycoproteins that make up the nicotinic receptor for acetylcholine serve as both the "walls" and the "gate" of the ion channel (see Chap. 18). This arrangement represents one of the simpler mechanisms by which a receptor may be "coupled" to a biological response.

Another receptor incorporated into an ion channel (chloride, in this instance) is the $GABA_a$ receptor (see Chap. 33 for details) for the amino acid neurotransmitter, gamma amino-butyric acid.

Many receptors are capable of initiating a chain of events involving "second messengers." Key factors in many of these second-messenger systems are very special proteins termed *G proteins,* short for guanine nucleotide-binding proteins. G proteins have the capacity to bind guanosine triphosphate (GTP) and hydrolyze it to guanosine diphosphate (GDP). At present, several different G proteins have been identified.

G proteins couple the activation of several different receptors to the next step in a chain of events. In a number of instances, the next step involves the enzyme adenylate cyclase. Many neurotransmitters, hormones, and drugs can either stimulate or inhibit adenylate cyclase through their interaction with different receptors; these receptors are coupled to adenylate cyclase through either a stimulatory (G_s) or an inhibitory (G_i) G protein. During the coupling process, the binding and subsequent hydrolysis of GTP to GDP provides the energy needed to terminate the coupling process.

The activation of adenylate cyclase enables it to catalyze the conversion of adenosine triphosphate (ATP) to 3' 5'-cyclic adenosine monophosphate (cAMP), which in turn can activate a number of enzymes known as *kinases.* Each kinase phosphorylates a specific protein or proteins.

Such phosphorylation reactions are known to be involved in the opening of some calcium channels as well as in the activation of other enzymes. In this system, the receptor is in the membrane with its binding site on the outer surface. The G protein is totally within the membrane while the adenylate cyclase is within the membrane but projects into the interior of the cell. The cAMP is generated intracellularly (see Fig. 12-4, Chap. 12).

Whether or not a particular agonist has any effect on a particular cell depends initially on the presence or absence of the appropriate receptor. However, the *nature* of the response depends on

- which G protein couples with the receptor,
- which kinase is activated
- which proteins are accessible for the kinase to phosphorylate.

The variety of possible responses is further increased by the fact that receptor-coupled G proteins can either activate enzymes other than adenylate cyclase or can directly influence ion channel functions.

A large family of receptors, including receptors for norepinephrine and epinephrine (α- and β-adrenoceptors), 5-hydroxytryptamine (serotonin or 5-HT receptors), and muscarinic acetylcholine receptors, are coupled to G proteins. Figure 2-1 presents the structure of one of these, the α_2-adrenoceptor from human kidney. All members of this family of G protein coupled receptors are characterized by seven membrane-enclosed domains plus extracellular and intracellular loops. *The specific binding sites*

for agonists occur at the extracellular surface while the interaction with G proteins occurs with the intracellular portions of the receptor.

The Chemistry of Drug-Receptor Binding

Biological receptors are capable of combining with drugs in a number of ways, and the forces that attract the drug to its receptor must be sufficiently strong and long-lasting to permit the initiation of the sequence of events that ends with the biological response. Those forces are *chemical bonds,* and a number of different types of bonds participate in the formation of the initial drug-receptor complex.

Covalent Bond

The bond formed when two atoms share a pair of electrons is called a *covalent bond.* It possesses a bond energy of approximately 100 kcal/mole and, therefore, is strong and stable, that is, it is essentially irreversible at body temperature. Covalent bonds are responsible for the stability of most organic molecules and can be broken only if sufficient energy is added or if a catalytic agent that can facilitate bond disruption, such as an enzyme, is present. Since bonds of this type are so stable at physiological temperatures, the binding of a drug to a receptor through covalent bond formation would result in the formation of a long-lasting complex.

Although most drug-receptor interactions are readily reversible, some compounds, such as the anticancer nitrogen mustards (see Chap. 62) and other alkylating agents form relatively irreversible complexes. Covalent bond formation is a desirable feature of an antineoplastic or antibiotic drug since long-lasting inhibition of cell replication is needed. However, covalent bond formation between environmental pollutants and cellular constituents may result in mutagenesis or carcinogenesis in normal, healthy cells. It should also be recognized that the very long duration of action associated with covalent bonding is not necessarily a desirable characteristic for most therapeutic agents.

If both of the shared electrons that form the covalent bond are derived from only one of the two atoms, the bond is called a *coordinate covalent bond.* Nitrogen, oxygen, and sulfur are the usual donor atoms in biological systems.

Coordinate covalent bond formation is important in drug ionization, certain types of drug-receptor interactions, and chelation reactions. An example of the pharmacological use of the last-named reaction is the formation of a *coordination complex* (e.g., a five- or six-member

Figure 2-1. Primary structure of the human kidney α_2-adrenoceptor. The amino acid sequence is represented by the one-letter code. (From J.W. Regan et al., Cloning and expression of a human kidney cDNA for *Proc. Natl. Acad. Sci. USA* 85:6301, 1988.)

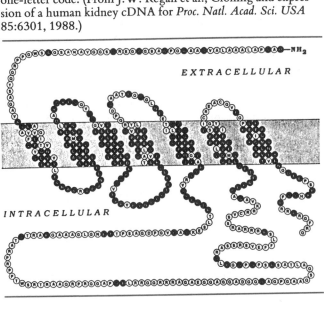

EXTRACELLULAR

INTRACELLULAR

ring) between a chelating agent and a metal cation. If the chelate complex formed is relatively stable, the result will be an effective reduction of the concentration of the cation in biological tissues.

Chelation reactions are often important in binding substrates to their enzymes and maintaining subcellular structure.

Ionic Bond

The formation of an *ionic bond* results from the electrostatic attraction that occurs between oppositely charged ions. The strength of this bond is considerably less (5 kcal/mole) than that of the covalent bond and will diminish in proportion to the square of the distance between the ionic species. Most macromolecular receptors have a number of ionizable groups at physiological pH (e.g., carboxyl, hydroxyl, phosphoryl, amino) that are available for interaction with an ionizable drug.

Hydrogen Bond

The *hydrogen bond* is, in a sense, a subspecies of the ionic bond. The hydrogen atom, with its strongly electropositive nucleus and single electron, can be bound to one strongly electronegative atom and still accept an electron from another electronegative donor atom such as nitrogen or oxygen and thereby form a bridge between these two donor atoms. Although individual hydrogen bonds have a strength of only 2 to 5 kcal/mole, the formation of several such bonds between two molecules (e.g., drug and receptor) can result in a relatively stable, yet still reversible, interaction. Such bonds serve to maintain the tertiary structure of proteins and nucleic acids and are thought to play a significant role in establishing the selectivity and specificity of drug-receptor interactions.

Van der Waal's Bond

Van der Waal's bonds are quite weak (0.5 kcal/mole) and become biologically important only when two atoms are brought into sufficiently close contact. They decrease inversely in proportion to the seventh power of the distance between the atoms.

Despite the relative weakness of the bond, van der Waal's forces play a significant part in determining drug-receptor specificity. Like the hydrogen bonds, several van der Waal's bonds may be established between two molecules, especially if the drug molecule and a receptor have complementary three-dimensional conformations and thus "fit" closely together. The closer the drug comes to the receptor, the stronger the possible binding forces that can be established. Slight differences in three-dimensional shape among a group of agonists and, therefore, slight differences in fit or strength of bonding forces that can be established between agonists and receptor form the basis for the *structure-activity relationships* that exist among related agonists.

Dynamics of Drug-Receptor Binding

The drug molecule, following its administration and passage to the area immediately adjacent to the receptor surface (sometimes called the *biophase*), must form bonds with the receptor before it can initiate a response. Resisting this bond formation is a random thermal agitation, which is inherent in every molecule and tends to keep the molecule in constant motion. Under normal circumstances, the electrostatic attraction of the ionic bond, which can be exerted over longer distances than can the attraction of either the hydrogen or van der Waal's bond, is the first force that draws the ionized molecule toward the oppositely charged receptor surface. This is a reasonably strong bond and will lend some stability to the drug-receptor complex.

Generally, the ionic bond must be reinforced through hydrogen or van der Waal's bond formation, or both, before significant receptor activation can occur. This is true because unreinforced bonds are too easily and quickly broken by the energy of thermal agitation to permit sufficient time for adequate drug-receptor interaction to take place. The better the structural congruity (i.e., fit) between drug and its receptor, the more secondary (i.e., hydrogen and van der Waal's) bond formation can occur.

Even if extensive binding has taken place, unless covalent bond formation has occurred, the drug-receptor complex can still dissociate. Once dissociation has occurred, drug action is terminated. For most drug-receptor interactions, there is a continual random association and dissociation. The frequencies of association and dissociation are a function of the affinity between the drug and the receptor, the density of receptors, and the concentration of drug in the biophase. *The magnitude of the response is generally considered to be a function of the concentration of the drug-receptor complexes formed at any moment in time.*

Dose-Response Relationship

To adequately understand drug-receptor interactions, it is necessary to quantify the relationship that exists between the drug and the biological effect it produces. Since the degree of effect produced by a drug is generally a func-

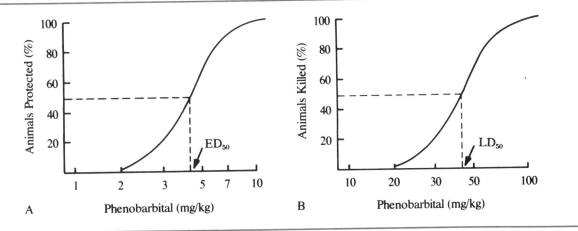

Figure 2-2. Quantal dose-response curves based on all-or-none responses. A. Relationship between the dose of phenobarbital and the protection of groups of rats against convulsions. B. Relationship between the dose of phenobarbital and the drug's lethal effects in groups of rats. ED_{50} = effective dose, 50 percent; LD_{50} = lethal dose, 50 percent.

tion of the amount of drug administered, we can express this relationship in terms of a *dose-response curve.* Because we cannot always quantify the concentration of drug in the biophase that is responsible for the particular effect produced, it is customary to correlate effect with dose administered.

In general, biological responses to drugs are *graded,* that is, the response continuously increases (up to the maximal responding capacity of the given responding system) as the administered dose is continuously increased. Expressed in receptor theory terminology, this means that *when a graded dose-response relationship exists, the response to the drug is directly related to the number of receptors with which the drug effectively interacts.* This is one of the basic tenets of pharmacology.

The principles derived from dose-response curves are the same in animals and humans. However, obtaining the data for complete dose-response curves in humans is generally very difficult or dangerous. We shall, therefore, use animal data to illustrate these principles.

Quantal Relationships

In addition to the responsiveness of a given patient, one may be interested in the relationship that exists between dose and some specified quantum of response among *all* individuals taking that drug. Such information is obtained by evaluating data obtained from a *quantal dose-response curve.*

Anticonvulsants are an example of drugs that can be suitably studied by use of quantal dose-response curves. For example, to assess the potential of new anticonvulsants to control epileptic seizures in humans, these drugs are initially tested for their ability to protect animals against experimentally induced seizures. In the presence of a given dose of the drug, the animal either exhibits the seizure or does not; that is, it either has or has not been "protected." Thus, in the design of this experiment, the effect of the drug (protection) is *all or none.* This type of response, *in contrast to a graded response,* must be described in a noncontinuous manner.

The construction of a quantal dose-response curve requires that data be obtained from many individuals. Although any given patient (or animal) either will or will not respond to a given dose, a comparison of individuals within a population shows that members of that population are not identical in their ability to respond to a particular dose. This variability can be expressed as a type of dose-response curve, sometimes termed a *quantal dose-response curve,* in which the dose (plotted on the horizontal axis) is evaluated against the percentage of animals in the experimental population that is protected by each dose (vertical axis). Such a dose-response curve for the anticonvulsant phenobarbital is illustrated in Fig. 2-2A. Five groups of 10 rats per group were used. The animals in any one group received a particular dose of phenobarbital of 2, 3, 5, 7, or 10 mg/kg body weight. The percentage of animals in each group protected against convulsions was plotted against the dose of phenobarbital. As can be seen from Fig. 2-2A, the lowest dose protected none of the 10 rats to which it was given, whereas 10 mg/kg protected 10 of 10. With the intermediate doses, some rats were protected and some were not; this indicates that the rats differ in their sensitivity to phenobarbital.

The quantal dose-response curve is actually a *cumulative plot* of the normal frequency distribution curve. The frequency distribution curve, in this case relating the minimum protective dose to the frequency with which it occurs in the population, generally is bell-shaped. If one graphs the cumulative frequency versus dose, one obtains the sigmoid-shaped curve of Fig. 2-2A. *The sigmoid shape is a characteristic of most dose-response curves when the dose is plotted on a geometric, or log, scale.*

Therapeutic Index

Effective Dose

The quantal dose-response curve represents estimates of the *frequency* with which each dose elicits the desired response in the population. In addition to this information, it also would be useful to have some way to express the average sensitivity of the entire population to phenobarbital. This is done through the calculation of an ED_{50} (effective dose, 50%; i.e., *the dose that would protect 50% of the animals*). This value can be obtained from the dose-response curve in Fig. 2-2A, as shown by the dashed lines. The ED_{50} for phenobarbital in this population is approximately 4 mg/kg.

Lethal Dose

Another important characteristic of a drug's activity is its *toxic effect.* Obviously, the ultimate toxic effect is death. A curve similar to that already discussed can be constructed by plotting percent of animals killed by phenobarbital against dose (Fig. 2-2B). From this curve, one can calculate the LD_{50} (lethal dose, 50%). Since *the degree of safety associated with drug administration depends on an adequate separation between doses producing a therapeutic effect (e.g., ED_{50}) and doses producing toxic effects (e.g., LD_{50}),* one can use a comparison of these two doses to estimate drug safety. Thus, one estimate of a drug's margin of safety is the ratio, LD_{50}/ED_{50}; this is referred to as the *therapeutic index.* The therapeutic index for phenobarbital used as an anticonvulsant is approximately 40/4, or 10.

As a general rule, a drug should have a high therapeutic index; however, some important therapeutic agents have low indices. For example, although the therapeutic index of the cardiac glycosides is only about 2 for the treatment and control of cardiac failure, these drugs are life-saving and are unequaled by any other class of drugs for many cases of cardiac failure. Therefore, in spite of a low margin of safety, they are the drugs of choice for this condition. The identification of a low margin of safety, however, dictates particular caution in their use; the appropriate dose for *each individual* must be determined separately.

It has been suggested that a more realistic estimate of drug safety would involve a comparison of the lowest dose that produces toxicity (e.g., LD_1) and the highest dose that produces a maximal therapeutic response (e.g., ED_{99}). A ratio less than unity would indicate that a dose effective in 99 percent of the population will be lethal in more than 1 percent of the individuals taking that dose. Figure 2-2 indicates that phenobarbital's ratio LD_1/ED_{99} is approximately 2.

Protective Index

The margin of safety is only *one* of several criteria to be used in determining a drug's clinical merit. Clearly, *the therapeutic index is a very rough measure of safety and generally represents only the starting point* in determining whether a drug is safe enough for human use. Usually, undesirable side effects occur in doses lower than the lethal doses. For example, phenobarbital induces drowsiness and an associated temporary neurological impairment. Since anticonvulsant drugs are intended to allow people suffering from epilepsy to live normal seizure-free lives, sedation is unacceptable. Thus, an important measure of safety for an anticonvulsant would be the ratio ED_{50} (neurological impairment)/ED_{50} (seizure protection). This ratio is called a *protective index.* The protective index for phenobarbital is approximately 3. It is easy to see that data derived from dose-response curves can be used in a variety of ways to compare the clinical usefulness of different drugs. For instance, a drug with a protective index of 1 is useless as an anticonvulsant, since the dose that protects against convulsion causes an unacceptable degree of drowsiness. A drug with a protective index of 5 would be a more promising anticonvulsant than one with an index of 2.

Graded Responses

More common than the quantal dose-response relationship is the situation in which a single animal (or patient) gives graded responses to graded doses; that is, as the dose is increased, the response increases. *With graded responses, one can obtain a complete dose-response curve in a single animal.* A good example is the effect of the drug, levarterenol (*l*-norepinephrine) on heart rate.

Results of experiments with levarterenol in guinea pigs are shown in Fig. 2-3. The data are typical of what one might obtain from constructing complete dose-response curves in each of five different guinea pigs (*a–e*). In animal *a*, a small increase in heart rate occurs at a dose of 0.001 μg/kg body weight. As the dose is increased, the response increases until, at 1.0 μg/kg, the maximum increase of 80 beats per minute occurs. Further increases in dose do not produce greater responses. At the other extreme, in guinea pig *e*, doses below 0.3 μg/kg have no effect at all and the maximum response occurs only at about 100 μg/kg.

Since an entire dose-response relationship is determined from one animal, the curve cannot tell us about the degree of biological variation inherent in a population of such animals. Rather, variability is reflected by a *family* of dose-response curves, such as those given in Fig. 2-3. The ED_{50} in this type of dose-response curve is the dose that produced 50 percent of the maximum response in one animal. In guinea pig *e*, the maximum response is an increase in heart rate of 80 beats per minute. Thus, 50 percent of

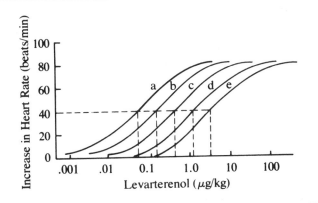

Figure 2-3. Dose-response curves illustrating the graded responses of five separate guinea pigs (a-e) to increasing doses of levarterenol. The responses are increases in heart rate above the rate measured before the administration of the drug. Dashed lines indicate 50 percent of maximum response (horizontal) and individual ED_{50} values (vertical).

the maximum is 40 beats per minute. From Fig. 2-3, it can be seen that the dose causing this effect in guinea pig *e* is about 3 μg/kg. The average sensitivity of all the animals to levarterenol can be estimated by combining the separate dose-response curves into a mean (average) dose-response curve and then calculating the mean ED_{50}. An estimate of the variation within the population can be indicated by calculating a statistical parameter such as a confidence interval.

It is also possible to construct quantal dose-response curves for drugs that produce graded responses. To do so, one chooses a quantum of effect—for example, an increase in heart rate of 20 to 30 beats per minute above the control or "resting" rate. Doses of the drug are then plotted against the frequency with which each dose produces this quantum of effect. The resulting graph has the same characteristics as the graph for the anticonvulsant activity of phenobarbital.

The reader may have noticed that the doses in Figs. 2-2 and 2-3 are not on an arithmetic but on a logarithmic, or geometric, scale (i.e., the doses are displayed as multiples). This is more apparent in Fig. 2-3 because of the greater range of doses involved. There are many reasons for the common practice of using geometric scales, some of which will become apparent later in this book. One important reason is that, in most instances, significant increases in response generally occur only when doses are increased in multiples. For example, in Fig. 2-3, curve *e*, if one increased the dose from 10 to 11 or 12 μg/kg, the change in response would hardly be measurable. However, if one increased it 3 times or 10 times (i.e., to 30 or 100 μg/kg), one could easily discern increased responses.

The concept of the therapeutic index as a measure of the margin of safety has already been discussed. In the

ratio LD_{50}/ED_{50}, the ED_{50} can be obtained from either quantal (see Fig. 2-2A) or graded (see Fig. 2-3) dose-response curves. In the latter case, it must be a *mean* ED_{50}, that is, the average ED_{50} obtained from several individuals.

Potency and Intrinsic Activity

Another drug characteristic that can be compared by use of ED_{50} values is *potency*. Figure 2-4 illustrates the mean dose-response curves of three hypothetical drugs that increase heart rate. Drugs *a* and *b* produce the same maximum response (an increase in heart rate of 80 beats per minute). However, the fact that the dose-response curve for drug *a* lies to the left of the curve for drug *b* indicates that drug *a* is more potent, that is, *less of drug a is needed to produce a given response*. The difference in potency is quantified by the ratio $ED_{50}b/ED_{50}a = 3/0.3 = 10$. Thus, drug *a* is 10 times as potent as drug *b*. In contrast, drug *c* has a lesser maximum effect than either drug *a* or drug *b*. Drug *c* is said to have a lower *intrinsic activity* than the other two drugs. Drugs *a* and *b* are full agonists with an intrinsic activity of 1; drug *c* is called a *partial agonist* and has an intrinsic activity of 0.5 because its maximum effect is half the maximum effect of *a* or *b*. The potency of drug *c*, however, is the same as that of drug *b*, because both drugs have the same ED_{50} (3 μg/kg). Note that the ED_{50} is the dose producing a response that is one-half of the maximal response to that *same* drug.

It is important not to equate greater potency of a drug with therapeutic superiority, since one might simply increase the dose of a less potent drug and thereby obtain an identical therapeutic response. Such factors as the severity and fre-

Figure 2-4. Idealized dose-response curves of three agonists (a, b, c) that increase heart rate but differ in potency, maximum effect, or both. Dashed lines are as in Fig. 2-3.

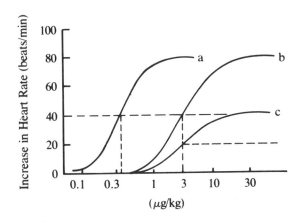

quency of undesirable effects associated with each drug and their cost to the patient are more relevant factors in the choice between two similar drugs.

Equations Derived from Drug-Receptor Interactions

It is important not to confuse the term *potency* with *affinity* or the term *intrinsic activity* with *efficacy*. The constants that relate an agonist A and its receptor R to the response may be represented as follows:

$$A + R \underset{k_2}{\overset{k_1}{\rightleftharpoons}} AR \overset{k_3}{\rightarrow} \text{response}$$

Affinity is k_1/k_2, and efficacy is represented by k_3. Thus, affinity and efficacy represent kinetic constants that relate the drug, the receptor, and the response at the molecular level. In contrast, potency and intrinsic activity are simple measurements, respectively, of the relative positions of dose-response curves on their horizontal axes and of their relative maxima. Affinity is *one* of the determinants of potency; efficacy contributes *both* to potency and to the maximum effect of the agonist. From Fig. 2-4 it would be correct to conclude that drug *c* has less efficacy (and less intrinsic activity) than either drug *a* or drug *b*. However, in contrast to intrinsic activity, no numerical value of efficacy can be calculated from the data presented. Unfortunately, the terms *potency* and *efficacy* are frequently used in a loose and misleading manner.

The mathematical relationship of response to efficacy and affinity is the following:

$$\frac{E_A}{E_m} = f\left\{ \frac{e[A]}{K_A + [A]} \right\}$$

This equation states that the ratio of the response (E_A) to a given concentration of an agonist to the maximum response (E_m) of the test system, such as an isolated strip of muscle, is a function (f) of efficacy (e) times the concentration of the agonist ([A]) divided by the dissociation constant (K_A) plus the concentration of the agonist. K_A is the reciprocal of the affinity constant and, under equilibrium conditions,

$$K_A = \frac{[R][A]}{[RA]}$$

[R] is the concentration of free receptors and [RA] is the concentration of receptors bound to agonist. Although the details are beyond the scope of a textbook of this nature, it should be noted that by the use of combinations of agonists and antagonists, dose-response curves, and mathematical relationships, it is possible to estimate the dissociation constants of agonists and antagonists for a given receptor and to estimate the relative efficacy of two agonists acting on the same receptor.

Drug Antagonism

The terms *agonist* and *antagonist* have already been introduced. There are several types of antagonism, which can be classified as follows:

1. Chemical antagonism
2. Functional antagonism
3. Competitive antagonism
   a. Equilibrium-competitive
   b. Nonequilibrium-competitive
4. Noncompetitive antagonism

Chemical Antagonism

Chemical antagonism involves a direct chemical interaction between the agonist and antagonist in such a way as to render the agonist pharmacologically inactive. A good example is the use of chelating agents to assist in the biological inactivation and removal from the body of toxic metals. *Chelation* involves a particular type of two-pronged attachment of the antagonist to a metal (the "agonist"). One chemical chelator, dimercaprol, is used in the treatment of toxicity from mercury, arsenic, and gold. After complexing with the dimercaprol, mercury is biologically inactive and the complex is excreted in the urine. The principle of chelation is illustrated with dimercaprol in Fig. 2-5 and is discussed earlier in the chapter.

Functional Antagonism

Functional antagonism is a term used to represent the interaction of two agonists that act independently of each other but happen to cause opposite effects. Thus, indirectly, each tends to cancel out or reduce the effect of the

Figure 2-5. Principle of chelation illustrated by interaction of mercury and dimercaprol.

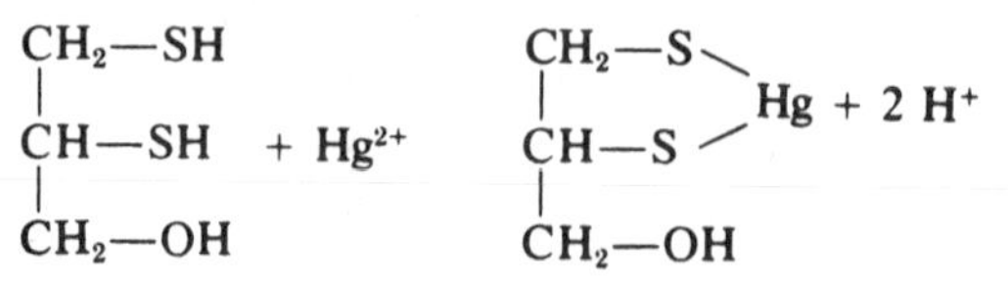

$$\begin{array}{l} CH_2{-}SH \\ | \\ CH{-}SH \\ | \\ CH_2{-}OH \end{array} + Hg^{2+} \quad \begin{array}{l} CH_2{-}S \\ | \qquad\quad\diagdown \\ \qquad\qquad Hg + 2\,H^+ \\ CH{-}S \diagup \\ | \\ CH_2{-}OH \end{array}$$

other. The classic example involves acetylcholine and epinephrine. These agonists have opposite effects on several different body functions. Acetylcholine slows the heart, and epinephrine accelerates it. Acetylcholine stimulates intestinal movement, and epinephrine inhibits it. Acetylcholine constricts the pupil, and epinephrine dilates it; and so on.

Competitive Antagonism

Competitive antagonism is the most frequently encountered type of drug antagonism in clinical practice. *The antagonist combines with the same site on the receptor as does the agonist but, unlike the agonist, does not induce a response;* that is, the antagonist has little or no *efficacy*. The antagonist competes with the agonist for its binding site on the receptor. Competitive antagonists can fall into either of two subtypes, depending on the type of bond formed between the antagonist and the receptor. If the bond is a loose one, the antagonism is called *equilibrium-competitive* or *reversible-competitive*. If the bond is covalent, however, the combination of the antagonist with the receptor is not readily reversible, and the antagonism is termed *nonequilibrium-competitive* or *irreversible-competitive*.

If the antagonism is of the equilibrium type, the antagonism increases as the concentration of the antagonist is increased. Conversely, the antagonism can be overcome (surmounted) if the concentration of the agonist in the *biophase* (the region where the receptors are located) is increased. This relationship can best be appreciated by examining dose-response curves, as in Fig. 2-6. Curve *a* is obtained in the absence of the antagonist. Curve *b* is obtained in the presence of a modest amount of the antagonist. The curves are parallel, and the maximum effects are equal. The antagonist has shifted the dose-response curve of the agonist to the right. Any level of response is still possible, but greater amounts of the agonist are required.

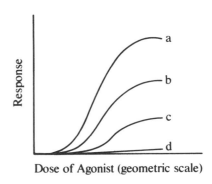

Figure 2-7. Idealized dose-response curves of an agonist in the absence (a) and the presence (b, c, d) of increasing doses of a nonequilibrium-competitive antagonist.

If the amount of the antagonist is increased, the dose-response curve is shifted farther to the right (curve *c*), still with no decrease in the maximum effect of the agonist. However, the amount of agonist required to achieve maximum response is greater with each increase in the amount of the antagonist present. Examples of equilibrium-competitive antagonists are atropine, *d*-tubocurarine, phentolamine, and naloxone.

It should be noted, of course, that this continual shift of the curve to the right, with no change in maximum as the dose of antagonist is increased, assumes that very large amounts of the agonist can be achieved in the biophase. This is generally true when the agonist is a drug being added from outside the biological system. However, if the agonist is a naturally occurring substance released from within the biological system (e.g., a neurotransmitter), the supply of the agonist may be quite limited. In that case, increasing the amount of antagonist ultimately abolishes all response.

The effect of a nonequilibrium antagonist on the dose-response curve of an agonist is quite different from the effect of an equilibrium antagonist, as illustrated in Fig. 2-7. As the dose of nonequilibrium antagonist is increased, the slope of the agonist curve and the maximum response achieved are progressively depressed. When the amount of antagonist is adequate (curve *d*), no amount of agonist can produce any response. The haloalkylamines, such as phenoxybenzamine, which form covalent bonds with receptors, are examples of nonequilibrium-competitive antagonists (see Chap. 13).

Noncompetitive Antagonism

In noncompetitive antagonism, the antagonist acts at a site beyond the receptor for the agonist. The difference between a competitive and a noncompetitive antagonist can be ap-

Figure 2-6. Idealized dose-response curves of an agonist in the absence (a) and the presence (b, c, d) of increasing doses of an equilibrium-competitive antagonist.

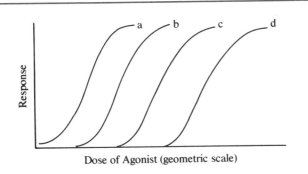

preciated from the following scheme, in which two agonists, A and B, interact with totally different receptor systems, R_A and R_B, to initiate a chain of events leading to contraction of a vascular smooth muscle cell. X is a competitive antagonist, and Y is a noncompetitive antagonist.

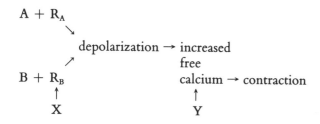

Antagonist X (competitive) has an affinity for R_B but not R_A. Thus, it specifically antagonizes agonist B. It does not antagonize agonist A. Antagonist Y acts on a receptor associated with the cellular translocation of calcium and inhibits the increase in intracellular free calcium. It will therefore antagonize the effects of both A and B, since they both ultimately depend on calcium movement to cause contraction.

The effect of a noncompetitive antagonist on the dose-response curve for an agonist would be the same as the effect of a nonequilibrium-competitive antagonist (see Fig. 2-7). The practical difference between a noncompetitive antagonist and a nonequilibrium-competitive antagonist is one of *specificity*. The former antagonizes agonists acting through more than one receptor system; the latter antagonizes only agonists acting through one receptor system. The antihypertensive drug diazoxide is one of the few examples of therapeutically useful noncompetitive antagonists (see Chap. 22).

Supplemental Reading

Black, J.W., Jenkinson, D.H., and Gerskowitch, V.P. (eds.). *Perspectives on Receptor Classification.* New York: Liss, 1987.

Kenakin, T.P. *Pharmacological Analysis of Drug-Receptor Interaction.* New York: Raven, 1987.

Levitzki, A. Beta-adrenergic receptors and their mode of coupling to adenylate cyclase. *Physiol. Rev.* 66:819, 1986.

Limbird, L.E. *Cell Surface Receptors: A Short Course on Theory and Methods.* Hingham, Mass.: Kluwer, 1985.

McCarthy, M.P., et al. The molecular neurobiology of the acetylcholine receptor. *Annu. Rev. Neurosci.* 9:383, 1986.

Ruffolo, R.R. Important concepts of receptor theory. *J. Auton. Pharmacol.* 2:277, 1982.

Ruffolo, R.R., Jr., et al. Structure and function of α-adrenoceptors. *Pharmacol. Rev.* 43:475, 1991.

Zifa, E., and Fillon, G. 5-Hydroxytryptamine receptors. *Pharmacol. Rev.* 44:401, 1992.

3

Drug Absorption and Distribution

Theodore E. Gram

In the preceding chapter it was stated that, for most drugs, the dose of drug administered determines the magnitude and duration of the response obtained. While this statement is accurate, it fails to tell us what proportion of the administered dose is actually responsible for producing the biological response; it also fails to inform us of the factors involved in determining the ultimate drug concentration achieved in the biophase.

Unless a drug acts topically (i.e., at its site of application), it first must enter the blood and then be distributed to its site of action. The mere presence of a drug in the blood, however, does not lead to a pharmacological response. To be effective, the drug must leave the vascular space and enter the intercellular or intracellular spaces, or both. The rate at which a drug reaches its site of action depends on two processes: its rate of absorption and its rate of distribution. *Absorption* involves the passage of the drug from its site of administration into the blood; *distribution* involves the delivery of the drug to the tissues. To reach its site of action after administration, a drug must cross a number of biological barriers and membranes, which are predominantly lipid in nature. Competing processes such as binding to plasma proteins, tissue storage, metabolism, and excretion (Fig. 3-1) determine the amount of drug finally available for interaction with specific receptors.

Properties of Biological Membranes that Influence Drug Passage

Much effort has been directed toward understanding the structural and functional characteristics of biomembranes that influence the passage of drugs. Although some substances are translocated by specialized transport mechanisms, and small polar compounds may filter through membrane pores, most foreign compounds penetrate cells by diffusing through lipid membranes.

A model of membrane structure, shown in Fig. 3-2, envisions the membrane as a mosaic structure composed of a discontinuous, *bimolecular,* lipid layer with fluidlike properties. A smaller component consists of glycoproteins or lipoproteins that are embedded in the lipid matrix and have ionic and polar groups protruding from one or both sides of the membrane. This membrane is thought to be capable of undergoing rapid localized shifts, whereby the relative geometry of specific adjacent proteins may change and form channels or pores. The presence of pores permits the membrane to be less restrictive to the passage of low-molecular-weight hydrophilic substances into cells. In addition to its role as a barrier to solutes, the cell membrane also has an important function in providing a structural matrix for a variety of enzymes and drug receptors. The model depicted is *not* thought to apply to capillaries.

Physicochemical Properties of Drugs and the Influence of pH

The ability of a drug to diffuse across membranes is frequently expressed in terms of its lipid-water partition coefficient rather than its lipid solubility per se. This coefficient is defined as the ratio of the concentration of the drug in two immiscible phases: a nonpolar liquid or organic solvent, representing the membrane; and an aqueous buffer, usually at pH 7.4, representing the plasma. The partition coefficient is a measure of the relative affinity of a drug for the lipid and aqueous phases. Increasing the polarity of a drug, either by increasing its degree of ionization or by adding a carboxyl, hydroxyl, or amino group to the molecule, decreases the lipid-water partition coefficient. Alternatively, reducing drug polarity through suppression of ionization, or the adding of lipophilic (e.g., phenyl-, t-butyl-) groups, results in an increase in the lipid-water partition coefficient.

Drugs, like most organic electrolytes, generally do not

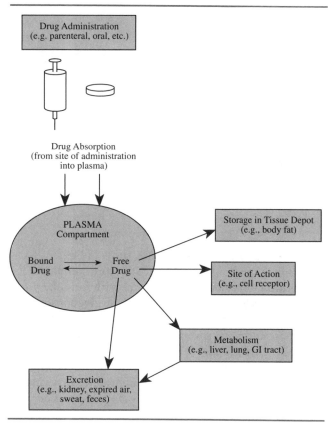

Figure 3-1. Factors that affect drug concentration at its site of action. Note that once a drug has been absorbed into the blood, it may be subjected to varying degrees of metabolism, storage in nontarget tissues, and excretion. The quantitative importance of each of these processes for a given drug will determine the ultimate drug concentration achieved at the site of action.

dissociate (i.e., form ions) completely in aqueous solution. Only a certain proportion of an organic drug molecule will ionize at a given pH. The smaller the fraction of total drug molecules ionized, the weaker the electrolyte. Since most drugs are either weak organic acids or bases (i.e., weak electrolytes), their degree of ionization will influence their lipid-water partition coefficient and hence their ability to diffuse through membranes.

The proportion of the total drug concentration that is present in either ionized or un-ionized form is dictated by the drug's dissociation or ionization constant (K) and the local pH of the solution in which the drug is dissolved.

The dissociation of a weak acid, RH, and a weak base, B, is described by the following equations:

$$RH \rightleftharpoons H^+ + R^- \text{ (acid)}$$
$$B + H^+ \rightleftharpoons BH^+ \text{ (base)}$$

If these equations are rewritten in terms of their dissociation constants (using K_a for both weak acids and weak

bases), we obtain

$$K_a = \frac{[R^-][H^+]}{[RH]} \text{ (acid)}$$

and

$$K_a = \frac{[H^+][B]}{[BH^+]} \text{ (base)}$$

By taking logarithms and then substituting the terms pK and pH for the negative logarithms of K_a and $[H^+]$, respectively, we arrive at the Henderson-Hasselbalch equations:

$$pH = pK_a + \log \frac{[R^-]}{[RH]} \text{ (acid)}$$

and

$$pH = pK_a + \log \frac{[B]}{[BH^+]} \text{ (base)}$$

It is customary to describe the dissociation constants of *both* acids and bases in terms of pK_a values. This is possible in aqueous biological systems because a simple mathematical relationship exists between pK_a, pK_b, and the dissociation constant of water pK_w.

$$pK_a + pK_b = pK_w = 14$$
$$pK_a = 14 - pK_b$$

The use of only pK_a values to describe the relative strengths of either weak bases or weak acids makes comparisons between drugs simpler. The lower the pK_a value ($pK_a < 6$) of an acidic drug, the stronger the acid (i.e., the larger the proportion of ionized molecules). The higher the pK_a value ($pK_a > 8$) of a basic drug, the stronger the base. Thus, knowing the pH of the aqueous medium in which the drug is dissolved and the pK_a of the drug, one can, using the Henderson-Hasselbalch equation, calculate the relative proportions of ionized and un-ionized drug present in solution. For example, when the pK_a of the drug (e.g., 7) is the same as the pH (e.g., 7) of the surrounding medium, there will be equal proportions of ionized $[R^-]$ and un-ionized $[RH]$ molecules (i.e., 50% of the drug is ionized).

The effect of pH on drug ionization is shown in Fig. 3-3. It should be noted that the relationship that exists between pH and degree of drug ionization is not linear but sigmoidal; that is, small changes in pH may greatly influence the degree of drug ionization, especially in those instances in which pH and pK_a values are initially similar.

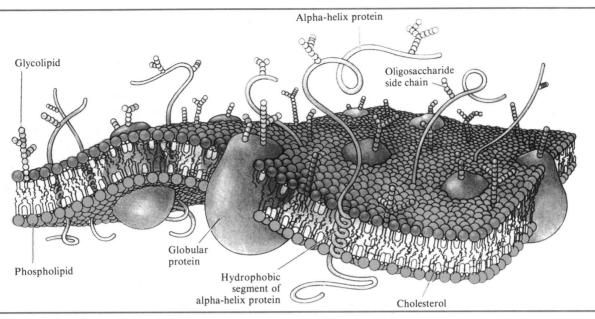

Figure 3-2. A diagrammatic representation of the plasma membrane. The plasma membrane is a phospholipid bilayer in which cholesterol and protein molecules are embedded. The bottom layer, which faces the cytoplasm, has a slightly different phospholipid composition than does the top layer, which faces the external medium. While phospholipid molecules can readily exchange laterally within their own layer, random exchange across the bilayer is rare. Both globular and helical kinds of protein traverse the bilayer. Cholesterol molecules tend to keep the tails of the phospholipids relatively fixed and orderly in the regions closest to the hydrophilic heads; the parts of the tails closer to the core of the membrane move about freely. This model is not believed to apply to blood or lymph capillaries. (From M.S. Bretscher, The molecules of the cell membrane. Sci. Am. 253:104, 1985. Copyright © 1985 by Scientific American, Inc. All rights reserved.)

Drug	Intestinal lumen pH 5.0	Membrane barriers	Plasma pH 7.4	Stomach pH 1.4
Weak acid— acetaminophen (pK_a 9.5)	[U] = 100 ⇅ [I] = 0.003 [Total] = 100.003	← ←	[U] = 100 ⇅ [I] = 0.79 [Total] = 100.79	[U] = 100 ⇅ [I] = 0.0 [Total] = 100.0
Weak base— diazepam (pK_a 3.3)	[U] = 100 ⇅ [I] = 2.0 [Total] = 102.0	← ←	[U] = 100 ⇅ [I] = 0.008 [Total] = 100.008	[U] = 100 ⇅ [I] = 7940.0 [Total] = 8040.0

Figure 3-3. Relative concentrations of the weak acid acetaminophen (pK_a 9.5) and a weak base, diazepam (pK_a 3.3), in some body fluid compartments. [ ] = concentration; U = un-ionized drug; I = ionized drug.

Mechanisms of Solute Transport Across Membranes

Except for intravenous administration, all routes of drug administration require that the drug be transported from the site of administration into the systemic circulation. A drug is said to be "absorbed" only when it has entered the blood or lymph capillaries. The transport of drugs across membranes involves one or more of the following processes: (1) passive diffusion, (2) filtration, (3) bulk flow, (4) active transport, (5) facilitated transport, (6) ion-pair transport, (7) endocytosis, and (8) exocytosis (see Fig. 3-4). These processes are also involved in the transport of substances necessary for cellular maintenance and growth.

Passive Diffusion

Most drugs pass through membranes by passive diffusion (down their concentration gradient) of the *un-ionized* moiety. The rate of diffusion is primarily dependent on the lipid-water partition coefficient rather than on lipid solubility per se. For example, the central nervous system depressant barbital is almost completely un-ionized at physiological pH and therefore should be able to cross membranes easily. However, barbital's lipid-water partition coefficient is sufficiently low that diffusion across membranes proceeds at an extremely slow rate. This slow rate of passage across CNS membranes largely explains why the time of onset of drug action after barbital administration (*latent period*) is delayed.

A drug will accumulate in the membrane until the ratio of its concentration in the membrane and its concentration in the extracellular fluid equals the partition coefficient. A concentration gradient is thereby established between the membrane and the intracellular space; this gradient is the driving force for the *passive transfer* of the drug into the cell. Thus, a drug that has a very high lipid-water partition coefficient will have a large concentration gradient, and this favors its rapid diffusion across the membrane and into the cell.

Filtration

The rate of filtration is dependent both on the existence of a pressure gradient as a driving force and on the size of the compound relative to the size of the pore through which it is to be filtered. In biological systems, the passage of many small water-soluble solutes through cylindrical pores or aqueous channels in the membrane is accomplished by filtration. The hypothetical diameter of these pores is about 7 Å, a size that generally limits passage to compounds of molecular weight less than 100 (e.g., urea, ethylene glycol). Substances of greater molecular weight (such as certain proteins that are known to be filtered) appear to be filtered through intercellular channels rather than through pores in cell membranes. A pore lined with cationic or anionic molecules will repel solutes of like charge but allow passage of oppositely charged compounds. To maintain osmolarity, water molecules generally accompany the compounds during membrane transport.

Bulk Flow

Most substances, lipid soluble or not, cross the capillary wall at rates that are extremely rapid in comparison with their rates of passage across other body membranes. In fact, the supply of most drugs to the various tissues is limited by blood flow rather than by restraint imposed by the capillary wall. This *bulk flow* of liquid occurs through intercellular pores and is the major mechanism of passage of drugs across most capillary endothelial membranes, with the exception of those in the CNS (see Chap. 28).

Active Transport

The energy-dependent movement of compounds across membranes, most often against their concentration gradient, is referred to as *active transport*. In general, drugs will not be actively transported unless they sufficiently resemble the endogenous substances (such as sugars, amino acids, nucleic acid precursors) that are the normal substrates for the particular carrier system involved. This transport involves the reversible binding of the molecule to be transferred to a membrane component (a "carrier") of complementary configuration.

Several mechanisms of active transport have been postulated. One transport model proposes that the drug molecule combines with a specific mobile carrier (Fig. 3-4), probably a protein, on one side of the membrane. The complex formed diffuses across the membrane to the opposite side, where the complex dissociates, thus releasing the drug into the aqueous compartment bordering the opposite membrane surface. The carrier protein can then return to its initial side to bind more drug. Another model involves a chainlike arrangement of sites in transport channels to which the drug can bind. The drug would be transferred from one site to another until it had traversed the membrane.

Type of transport		Membrane	Absorbed molecule

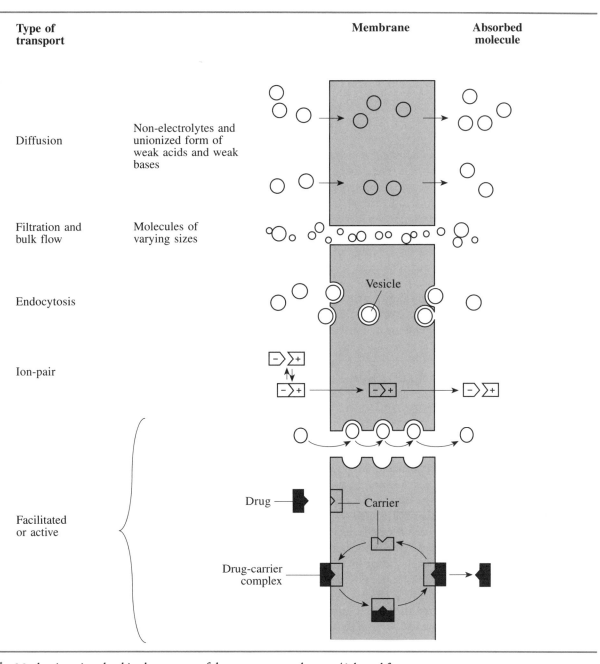

Diffusion — Non-electrolytes and unionized form of weak acids and weak bases

Filtration and bulk flow — Molecules of varying sizes

Endocytosis — Vesicle

Ion-pair

Facilitated or active — Drug — Carrier — Drug-carrier complex

Figure 3-4. Mechanisms involved in the passage of drugs across membranes. (Adapted from D.H. Smyth, *Absorption and Distribution of Drugs*. Baltimore: Williams & Wilkins, 1964; and W. Forth and W. Rummel (eds.), *Pharmacology of Intestinal Absorption: Gastrointestinal Absorption of Drugs*. Vols. 1 and 2. Oxford, England: Pergamon, 1975.)

Active transport of a particular substance occurs in one direction only. The number of molecules transported per unit time will reach a maximum (T_m) once the binding capacity of the carrier becomes saturated. Drugs such as levodopa (for parkinsonism), α-methyldopa (for hypertension), and the anticancer agents 5-fluorouracil and 5-bromouracil are actively transported. The herbicide paraquat accumulates in the lung against a concentration gradient and can ultimately result in pulmonary insufficiency and death.

Since active transport often requires energy in the form of adenosine triphosphate (ATP), compounds or conditions that inhibit energy production (e.g., iodoacetate, fluoride, cyanide, anaerobiosis) will impair active transport.

The transport of a given compound also can be inhibited competitively by the coadministration of other compounds that are of sufficient structural similarity that they can compete with the first substance for sites on the carrier protein.

Facilitated Diffusion

The transfer of drugs by *facilitated diffusion* has many of the characteristics associated with active transport, including being a protein carrier-mediated transport system that shows saturability and selectivity. It differs from active transport, however, in that no energy input is required beyond that necessary to maintain normal cellular function. Since, in facilitated transport, the movement of the transported molecule is from regions of higher to regions of lower concentrations, the driving force for facilitated transport is the concentration gradient. Although the initial rate of drug transfer will be proportional to the magnitude of the concentration gradient, eventually a point will be reached at which further increases in drug concentration no longer increase the transport rate, that is, T_m has been reached, since the binding sites on the carrier are now completely saturated.

Ion-Pair Transport

Absorption of some highly ionized compounds (e.g., sulfonic acids and quaternary ammonium compounds) from the gastrointestinal tract cannot be explained in terms of the transport mechanisms discussed above. These compounds are known to penetrate the lipid membrane despite their low lipid-water partition coefficients. It is postulated that these highly lipophobic drugs combine reversibly with such endogenous compounds as mucin in the gastrointestinal lumen, forming neutral *ion-pair complexes;* it is this neutral complex that penetrates the lipid membrane by passive diffusion.

Endocytosis

The mechanism of transport by *endocytosis* involves the cellular uptake of exogenous molecules or complexes inside plasma membrane-derived vesicles. This process can be divided into two major categories: (1) adsorptive or phagocytic uptake of particles that have been bound to the membrane surface, and (2) fluid or pinocytotic uptake, in which the particle enters the cell as part of the fluid phase. The solute contained within the vesicle is released intracellularly, possibly through lysosomal digestion of the vesicle membrane or by intermembrane fusion (Fig. 3-4).

Currently, use is being made of this endocytotic mechanism as a means of transporting drugs and enzymes into particular tissues that possess endocytotic activity. Compounds are linked to specific carriers, thereby increasing the cellular specificity of drug uptake. For example, some antitumor agents have been entrapped in liposomes or resealed erythrocytes, or formed into complexes with macromolecules such as DNA and antibodies, to be carried into specific tumor cells to which they are targeted. This approach not only improves the therapeutic effectiveness of the drugs but also reduces some of the acute and nonselective toxic effects commonly associated with their usual form of administration.

Absorption of Drugs from the Alimentary Tract

Oral Cavity and Sublingual Absorption

Direct absorption of drugs from the oral cavity or buccal mucosa, in contrast to absorption from the stomach and intestine, obviates the passage of the drug through the liver, with its subsequent metabolism to inactive metabolites ("first-pass" effect). Drugs absorbed from the oral cavity enter the general circulation directly. Although the surface area of the oral cavity is small, absorption can still be rapid if the drug has a high lipid-water partition coefficient and, therefore, can readily diffuse through lipid membranes. Since the diffusion process is very rapid for nonionized drugs, pK_a will be a major determinant of the lipid-water partition coefficient for a particular therapeutic agent. For instance, the weak base nicotine (pK_a 8.5) reaches peak blood levels four times faster when absorbed from the mouth (pH 6.0), where 40 to 50 percent of the drug is in the un-ionized form, than from the gastrointestinal tract (pH 1.0–5.0), where the drug exists mainly in its ionized (protonated) form.

Although the oral mucosa is highly vascularized and its epithelial lining is quite thin, the amount of drug absorption occurring from the oral cavity is limited. This is due in part to the relatively slow dissolution rate of most solid dosage forms and in part to the difficulty in keeping dissolved drug in contact with the oral mucosa for a sufficient length of time. These difficulties may be overcome if the drug is placed under the tongue (*sublingual* administration) in a formulation that allows rapid tablet dissolution in salivary secretions. The extensive network of blood vessels under the tongue facilitates rapid drug absorption. This is the route of choice for a drug like nitroglycerin (glyceryl trinitrate), whose coronary vasodilator effects are required quickly in cases of angina. Sublingual administration of nitroglycerin is preferred since, if swallowed, the drug would be absorbed from the gastrointestinal tract and carried to the liver, where it would be rapidly metabolized and inactivated.

Absorption from the Stomach

Although *the primary function of the stomach is not absorption,* its rich blood supply and the contact of its contents with the epithelial lining of the gastric mucosa provide a potential site for drug absorption. However, since stomach emptying time can be altered by many variables (e.g., volume of ingested material, type and viscosity of the ingested meal, body position, psychological state), the extent of gastric absorption will vary from patient to patient as well as at different times within a single individual.

The low pH of the gastric contents (pH 1.0–2.0) may have consequences for absorption because it can dramatically affect the degree of drug ionization. For example, the weak base diazepam (pK_a 3.3) will be highly protonated in the gastric juice, and, consequently, absorption across lipid membranes of the stomach will be particularly slow. On the other hand, the weak acid acetaminophen (pK_a 9.5) will exist mainly in its nonionized form and can more readily diffuse from the stomach into the systemic circulation (see Fig. 3-3).

Because of the influence of pH on ionization of weak bases, basic drugs may be trapped or lost in the stomach, even if they are administered intravenously. Since basic compounds exist primarily in their un-ionized form in the blood (pH 7.4), they readily diffuse from the blood into the gastric juice. Once in contact with the gastric contents (pH 1.0–2.0), they will ionize rapidly, thus restricting their diffusibility. At equilibrium, concentration of the un-ionized, lipid-soluble fraction will be identical on both sides of the gastric membranes, but there will be more *total* basic drug on the side where ionization is greatest (i.e., in gastric contents). This means of drug accumulation is called *ion trapping* (see Fig. 3-3).

Absorption from the Small Intestine

The epithelial lining of the small intestine is composed of a single layer of cells. It consists of many villi and microvilli and has a complex supply of blood and lymphatic vessels into which digested food and drugs are absorbed. The small intestine, with its large surface area and high blood perfusion rate, has a greater capacity for absorption than does the stomach. Most drug absorption occurs in the proximal jejunum (first 1–2 m in humans).

Although transfer of drugs across the intestinal wall can occur by facilitated transport, active transport, endocytosis, and filtration, the predominant process utilized for most drugs is diffusion. Thus, the pK_a of the drug and the pH of the intestinal fluid (pH 5.0) will strongly influence the rate of drug absorption. While weak acids like phenobarbital (pK_a 7.4) can be absorbed from the stomach, they are more readily absorbed from the small intestine because of the latter's extensive surface area.

Conditions that shorten intestinal transit time (e.g., diarrhea) decrease intestinal drug absorption, while increases in transit time will enhance intestinal absorption by permitting drugs to remain in contact with the intestinal mucosa longer. Although delays in gastric emptying time will increase gastric drug absorption, in general, *total* drug absorption may actually decrease since material will not be transferred to the large absorptive surface of the small intestine.

Absorption from the Large Intestine

Although the large intestine has a considerably smaller absorptive surface area than the small intestine, it may still serve as a site of drug absorption, especially for those compounds that have not been completely absorbed from the small intestine. However, little absorption occurs from this site since the relatively solid nature of the intestinal contents impedes diffusion of the *drug* from the contents to the mucosa.

The most distal portion of the large intestine, the rectum, can be used directly as a site of drug administration. This route is especially useful where the drug may cause gastric irritation, after gastrointestinal surgery, during protracted vomiting, and in uncooperative patients (e.g., children) or unconscious ones. Dosage forms may include solutions or suppositories. The processes involved in rectal absorption are similar to those described for other sites.

Although the surface area available for absorption is not large, absorption can still occur, owing to the extensive vascularity of the rectal mucosa. Drugs absorbed from the rectum largely escape the biotransformation process to which orally administered drugs are subject. Not only do rectally administered agents bypass the contents and enzymes of the stomach and intestine, but, in addition, *the blood that perfuses the rectum is not delivered directly to the liver and, therefore, rectally administered drugs escape hepatic first-pass metabolism.*

Factors Affecting Rate of Gastrointestinal Absorption

In addition to the lipid-water partition coefficient of drugs, local blood flow, and intestinal surface area, other factors may affect absorption from the gastrointestinal tract.

Gastric Emptying Time

The rate of gastric emptying markedly influences the rate at which drugs are absorbed, irrespective of whether

Table 3-1. Some Factors Influencing Gastric Emptying Time

Factor	Increased gastric emptying rate	Decreased gastric emptying rate
Physiological	Liquids, gastric distention	Solids, acids, fat
Pathological	Duodenal ulcers, gastroenterostomy, chronic pancreatitis	Acute abdomen trauma and pain, labor of childbirth, gastric juices, intestinal obstruction, pneumonia, diabetes mellitus
Pharmacological	Reserpine, anticholinesterases, guanethidine, cholinergic agents	Anticholinergic drugs, ganglionic blocking drugs, narcotic analgesics

Source: W. S. Nimmo, Drugs, disease and altered gastric emptying. *Clin. Pharmacokinet.* 1:189, 1976.

they are acids, bases, or neutral substances. In general, factors that accelerate gastric emptying time, thus permitting drugs to reach the large absorptive surface of the small intestine sooner, will increase drug absorption unless the drug is slow to dissolve. A list of physiological, pathological, and pharmacological factors that influence the rate of gastric emptying is provided in Table 3-1.

Intestinal Motility

Increased gastrointestinal motility may facilitate drug absorption by thoroughly mixing intestinal contents and thereby bringing the drug into more intimate contact with the mucosal surface. However, decreased gastrointestinal motility is not necessarily associated with a reduced rate of drug absorption.

Food

Absorption of most drugs from the gastrointestinal tract is reduced or delayed by the presence of food in the gut. Drugs such as decamethonium and tetracyclines, which are highly ionized, can complex with Ca^{2+} ions in membranes, food, or milk, leading to a reduction in their rate of absorption. For drugs that are ionized in the stomach and un-ionized in the intestine, overall absorption will be delayed by any factor that delays gastric emptying. Finally, increased splanchnic blood flow, as occurs during eating, will increase the rate of drug absorption.

Formulation Factors

The ability of solid dosage forms to dissolve, as well as the solubility characteristics of the individual drug in the highly acidic gastric juice, must be considered. For example, although the anticoagulant dicumarol has a very high lipid-water partition coefficient, it precipitates at the low pH of gastric juice, and the rate of its absorption is thereby reduced. This may be overcome by covering the tablets with an enteric coating that only dissolves in the relatively more alkaline secretions found in the small intestine. Drugs administered in aqueous solution are absorbed faster and more completely than are tablet or suspension forms. Suspensions of fine particles ("microcrystalline") are better absorbed than are those of larger particles.

Metabolism

Drugs may be inactivated in the gastrointestinal tract before they are absorbed. For example, orally administered oxytocin is inactivated by the proteolytic enzyme chymotrypsin, which is present in the gastrointestinal tract. Drugs may also be inactivated by metabolism during their passage through the intestinal wall and by the gut microflora.

Absorption of Drugs from the Lung

The lungs serve as a major site of administration for a number of agents given for both local and systemic effects. Such drugs can be inhaled as gases (e.g., volatile anesthetics) or as aerosols (suspended liquid droplets or solid particles). Absorption of agents from the lung is facilitated by the large surface area of the pulmonary alveolar membranes (50–100 sq m), the limited thickness of these membranes (approximately 0.2 μ), and the high blood flow to the alveolar region.

Pulmonary absorption of volatile anesthetics across the alveolar-capillary barrier is very rapid because of the relatively high lipid-water partition coefficients and small molecular radii of such agents. Many lipid-soluble drugs of diverse chemical structure and degree of ionization are absorbed by a process of facilitated diffusion at rates proportional to their lipid-water partition coefficients. The driving force for diffusion is a combination of the blood-air partition coefficient (which is a measure of the capacity of blood to dissolve drug) and the difference in partial pressure that exists between the alveoli and the arterial and venous blood. *Equilibration* occurs when the partial pressures of the drug in the gaseous phase and the plasma water become equal. Agents with high blood-air partition coefficients require more drug to be dissolved in the blood for equilibrium to be reached. Although the blood-air partition coefficient is the most important single factor in determining the equilibration curve, physiological factors also may alter the rate of equilibrium. (An expanded discussion of this topic is found in Chap. 29.)

Aerosolized solid or liquid particles are so small that they remain in suspension in a gaseous medium, which for the lung is air. Such aerosol particles may be deposited along the tracheobronchial tree or may penetrate as deeply as the alveolus. Solid particles in aerosols may be removed from the lung by direct absorption into the blood, by endocytosis, and by absorption through the lymphatic system. When the aerosol particle size is small (<1 μ), the amount of drug reaching the alveoli may be large, and therefore the systemic absorption of the drug may be appreciable.

Additional information relating to pulmonary drug administration is found in Chap. 45.

Absorption of Drugs Through the Skin

This topic is covered extensively in Chap. 46 and, therefore, is discussed only briefly at this point. Most drugs that have been incorporated into creams or ointments are applied to the skin for their local effect, especially on the superficial layers of the epidermis. As with other membranes, the diffusion rate of a drug through the skin is largely determined by the compound's lipid-water partition coefficient. However, the stratum corneum, or outer layer of the epidermis, forms a barrier against the rapid penetration of most drugs. This is due in large part to the relatively close-packed cellular arrangement and decreased amount of lipid in these cells. Thus, even highly lipid-soluble compounds will be absorbed much more slowly through the skin than from other sites. The dermis, on the other hand, is well supplied with blood and lymph capillaries and, therefore, is permeable to both lipid-soluble and water-soluble compounds. If penetration of the skin by lipid-insoluble compounds does occur, it is probably accomplished by diffusion through the hair follicles, sweat glands, or sebaceous glands.

Accidental absorption of toxic drugs through the skin may produce harmful systemic effects. Topical absorption of organic phosphates (e.g., parathion) and lipophilic insecticides such as DDT and chlordane by agricultural workers has proved fatal.

Absorption of Drugs After Parenteral Administration

Intramuscular and Subcutaneous Administration

Intramuscular and subcutaneous injections are by far the most common means of parenteral drug administration. Because of the high tissue blood flow and the ability of the injected solution to diffuse laterally, drug absorption generally is more rapid after intramuscular than after subcutaneous injection. Drug absorption from intramuscular and subcutaneous sites is dependent on the quantity and composition of the connective tissue, the capillary density, and the rate of vascular perfusion of the area. These factors can be influenced by the coinjection of agents that alter local blood flow (e.g., vasoconstrictors or vasodilators) or by substances that decrease tissue resistance to lateral diffusion (e.g., hyaluronidase).

Although the parenteral administration of aqueous drug solutions usually results in rapid drug absorption from intramuscular and subcutaneous sites, absorption can be delayed, to prolong systemic drug effects. This is accomplished by administering slowly dissolving forms of the drug, which serve as depots or drug reservoirs (see Chap. 7). Such procedures include the intramuscular injection of aqueous drug suspensions, subcutaneous implantation of compressed pellets, and injection of drugs in oil. A single intramuscular injection of an aqueous suspension of medroxyprogesterone acetate in humans elicits progestational effects for 30 days or more.

Advantages of the intramuscular and subcutaneous routes include an increased reliability and precision in the drug blood level finally achieved, reasonably rapid absorption and onset of drug action, and the ability to give large volumes of solution. There are, however, serious disadvantages as well. Pain, tenderness, local tissue necrosis (primarily with highly alkaline injections), microbial contamination, and nerve damage may be associated with these forms of parenteral administration.

Intravenous Administration

The intravenous method of drug administration ensures immediate pharmacological response; problems of absorption are circumvented because the entire quantity of drug enters the vasculature directly. Intravenous drug administration is widely employed in anesthesia (see Chap. 31) and in emergency medicine. This route is also useful for compounds that have a narrow therapeutic index, are poorly or erratically absorbed, are extremely irritating to tissues, or are rapidly metabolized before or during their absorption from other sites. The rate of injection should be slow enough, however, to prevent excessively high local drug concentrations and to allow for termination of the injection if undesired effects appear.

A serious disadvantage of intravenous drug administration becomes clearly apparent when an overdose is inadvertently given: The drug can neither be removed nor its absorption retarded. Other disadvantages include the possibilities of embolism (particularly if an insoluble drug is given), introduction of bacteria, and, when this route is used for prolonged periods, subcutaneous tissue infiltration. The possible introduction of the human immunodeficiency virus (HIV) is a well-known consequence of intravenous drug administration in addicts who use unsterile needles.

Factors Influencing Drug Distribution

Distribution involves the delivery of drug from the systemic circulation to tissues. Once a drug has entered the blood compartment, the *rate* at which it subsequently penetrates tissues and other body fluids depends on several factors. These include (1) capillary permeability, (2) blood flow—tissue mass ratio (i.e., perfusion rate), (3) extent of plasma protein and specific organ binding, (4) regional differences in pH, (5) transport mechanisms available, and (6) the permeability characteristics of specific tissue membranes.

The transfer of drugs from the capillary circulation to the interstitial spaces is faster than is the diffusion of drugs through biological membranes. The capillary walls in most tissues offer little resistance to permeation by nonprotein-bound dissolved materials, since capillary membranes are composed of an interlocking mosaic of endothelial cells whose junctions (*fenestrations*) function as

pores. Water-soluble compounds are carried through these junctions with the bulk flow of the liquid blood. Molecular size, rather than lipid solubility, is the major determinant of the rate of transcapillary movement. Larger molecules may be transported across capillary membranes by pinocytosis. Highly lipid-soluble drugs generally require only a single passage of blood through an organ to establish a blood-tissue equilibrium.

Drug delivery and eventual drug equilibration with intercellular tissue spaces are largely determined by the extent of organ blood flow. The composition of the capillary bed is usually not a limiting factor, except with the capillaries of the CNS. The renal and hepatic capillaries are especially permeable to the movement of most molecules, except those of particularly large size. The rate of passage of drugs across capillary walls can be influenced by agents that affect capillary permeability (e.g., histamine) or capillary blood flow rate (e.g., norepinephrine).

Volume of Distribution

The total volume of the fluid compartments of the body into which drugs may be distributed is approximately 40 liters (L) in a 70-kg adult. These compartments include plasma water (approximately 5 L), interstitial fluid (10 L), and the intracellular fluid (20 L). Total extracellular water comprises the sum of the plasma and the interstitial water. Factors such as sex, age, edema, and body fat can influence the volume of these various compartments.

The fluid volume in which a drug seems to distribute is referred to as the *apparent volume of distribution* (V_d). This mathematically arrived at value gives a rough indication of the overall distribution of a drug in the body (Table 3-2). For example, a drug with a V_d of approximately 12 L (i.e., interstitial fluid plus plasma water) is probably dis-

Table 3-2. Relationship Between Calculated Volume of Distribution (V_d) and the Tissue Compartments Involved

Calculated V_d (L)	Drugs	Tissue compartment in which drug is distributed
5	Heparin, spironolactone, clofibrate, warfarin, furosemide	Plasma water, vascular system
10–20	Aspirin, tolbutamide, gentamicin, streptomycin, ampicillin	Extracellular fluid (plasma water and interstitial fluid)
22—42	Methyldopa, amoxicillin, nitroglycerin, prednisolone	Whole body fluid (extracellular and intracellular fluids)
>70	Acetaminophen, propranolol, imipramine, desipramine, nortriptyline	Accumulation and binding in tissues

Sources: W. A. Ritschel, *Handbook of Basic Pharmacokinetics.* Hamilton, Ill.: Drug Intelligence, 1976. P. 194, and L. Z. Benet and L. B. Sheiner, Design and Optimization Dosage Regimens. In A. G. Gilman, L. S. Goodman, and A. Gilman (eds), *The Pharmacological Basis of Therapeutics* (6th ed.). New York: Macmillan, 1984. P. 1675.

Table 3-3. Blood Perfusion Rates in Adult Humans

Tissue	Percent of cardiac output	Blood flow (L/min)	Percent of body weight	Perfusion rate (ml/min/100 gm tissue)
Kidney	20	1.23	0.5	350
Brain	12	0.75	2.0	55
Lung	100	5.40	1.5	400
Liver	24	1.55	2.8	85
Heart	4	0.25	0.5	84
Muscle	23	0.80	40.0	5
Skin	6	0.40	10.0	5
Adipose tissue	10	0.25	19.0	3

tributed throughout extracellular fluid, but is unable to penetrate cells. Intravenously administered drugs with V_d values of 3 L (e.g., highly protein-bound or very high-molecular-weight substances) are likely to have their distribution restricted to the vascular compartment and hence will probably have limited systemic utility. In general, the greater the V_d, the greater the diffusibility of the drug. Some drugs have an apparent V_d greater than that of total body water. Such a value will result if the compound is bound or sequestered at some *extravascular* site. A highly lipid-soluble drug such as thiopental that can be extensively stored in fat depots may have a V_d considerably in excess of the entire fluid volume of the body.

The rate at which an equilibrium concentration of a drug is reached in the extracellular fluid of a particular tissue will depend on the tissue's perfusion rate; the greater the blood flow the more rapid the distribution of the drug from the plasma into the interstitial fluid. Thus, a drug will appear in the interstitial fluid of liver, kidney, and brain more rapidly than it will in muscle and skin (Table 3-3).

A detailed pharmacokinetic treatment of the concept of volume of distribution can be found in Chap. 6.

Binding of Drugs to Plasma Protein

Most drugs found in the vascular compartment will bind reversibly with one or more of the macromolecules in plasma. Although some drugs are simply dissolved in plasma water, most are associated with plasma components such as albumin, globulins, transferrin, ceruloplasmin, glycoproteins, and α- and β-lipoproteins. While many acidic drugs bind principally to albumin, basic drugs frequently bind to other plasma proteins, such as lipoproteins and α_1-acid glycoprotein (α_1-AGP), in addition to albumin. The extent of this binding will influence the drug's distribution and rate of elimination because *only the unbound drug can diffuse through the capillary wall, produce its systemic effects, be metabolized, and be excreted.*

Drugs ordinarily bind to protein in a reversible fashion and in dynamic equilibrium, according to the law of mass action. Since only the unbound (or free) drug diffuses through the capillary walls, extensive binding may decrease the intensity of drug action. The magnitude of this decrease is directly proportional to the fraction of drug bound to plasma protein. At low drug concentrations, the stronger the affinity between the drug and protein, the smaller the fraction that is free. As drug dosage is progressively increased, a point is reached at which the binding capacity of the protein becomes saturated and any additional drug will remain unbound.

The binding of a drug to plasma proteins will decrease its effective plasma to tissue concentration gradient, that is, the force that drives the drug out of the circulation, thereby slowing the rate of transfer across the capillary. As the free drug leaves the circulation, the protein-drug complex begins to dissociate and more free drug then becomes available for diffusion. Thus, binding does not prevent the drug from reaching its site of action but only retards the rate at which this occurs.

Extensive protein binding results in the blood's serving as a circulating drug reservoir. As free or unbound drug is eliminated from the body, more drug dissociates from the drug-plasma protein complex to replace free drug that was lost. Thus, extensive plasma protein binding may prolong drug availability and duration of action. This characteristic has been exploited therapeutically for drugs like suramin (used in treatment of trypanosomiasis), which are strongly bound to plasma protein. A single intravenous dose of suramin produces clinically effective plasma levels of the drug for up to 3 months.

Albumin

Of the plasma proteins, the most important contributor to drug binding is albumin. Although albumin has a *net* negative charge at serum pH, it can interact with both positive and negative charges on drugs. Many highly albumin-bound drugs are poorly soluble in water, and for such drugs binding to hydrophobic sites on albumin is often important. In general, only one or two molecules of an acidic drug are bound per albumin molecule, whereas basic, positively charged drugs are more weakly bound to a larger number of binding sites.

The binding of drugs to plasma proteins is usually nonspecific; that is, many drugs may interact with the same binding site. A drug with a higher affinity may displace a drug with weaker affinity. For example, administration of phenylbutazone can displace previously administered sulfonamides from their albumin-binding sites. Increases in the non-protein-bound drug fraction (i.e., free drug) can result in an increase in the drug's intensity of pharmacological response, side effects, and potential toxicity.

Drug displacement is of particular importance when compounds are highly bound to protein because a change in binding from 98 to 94 percent may increase the level of free, active drug threefold, that is, from 2 to 6 percent in this example. In general, however, displacement results only in a transient increase in the free plasma concentration of the displaced drug since the displaced drug rapidly becomes redistributed into other body water compartments. Thus, the concentration of unbound drug at the site of action may only increase slightly if at all.

Some disease states (e.g., hyperalbuminemia, hypoalbuminemia, uremia, hyperbilirubinemia) have been associated with changes in plasma protein binding of drugs. For example, in uremic patients the plasma protein binding of certain acidic drugs (e.g., penicillin, sulfonamides, salicylates, and barbiturates) is reduced.

Lipoproteins

Drugs that bind to lipoproteins do so by dissolving in the lipid portion of the lipoprotein core. The binding capacity of individual lipoproteins should be dependent on their lipid content, that is, very low-density lipoproteins (VLDL) > low-density lipoproteins (LDL) > high-density lipoproteins (HDL). It is also possible that the lipid and protein fractions may cooperate in the binding process, the drug first binding to a number of sites on the protein moiety and then dissolving in the lipid phase.

α_1-Acid Glycoprotein

The importance of α_1-AGP as a determinant of the plasma protein binding of basic drugs, including the psychotherapeutic drugs chlorpromazine, imipramine, spiroperidol, and nortriptyline, is becoming apparent. There is evidence of increased plasma α_1-AGP levels in certain physiological and pathological conditions, such as in injury, stress, surgery, trauma, rheumatoid arthritis, and celiac disease.

Selective Accumulation of Drugs

Drugs will not always be uniformly distributed to and retained by body tissues. The concentrations of some drugs will be either considerably higher or considerably lower in particular tissues than could be predicted on the basis of simple distribution assumptions. This observation is demonstrated in the following examples:

1. *Kidney.* Since the kidneys receive 20 to 25 percent of the cardiac output, they will be exposed to a relatively large amount of any systemically administered drug. The kidney also contains a protein (metallothionein) that has a high affinity for metals. This protein is responsible for the renal accumulation of cadmium, lead, and mercury.

2. *Eye.* Several drugs have an affinity for the retinal pigment melanin and thus may accumulate in the eye. Chlorpromazine and other phenothiazines bind to melanin and accumulate in the uveal tract, where they may cause retinotoxicity. Chloroquine concentration in the eye can be approximately 100 times that found in the liver.

3. *Fat.* Drugs with extremely high lipid-water partition coefficients have a tendency to accumulate in body fat. However, since blood flow to adipose tissue is low (about 3 ml/100 gm/min), distribution into body fat occurs slowly. Drug accumulation in body fat may result in either decreased therapeutic activity owing to the drug's removal from the circulation, or it may result in prolonged activity in those instances in which only low levels of the drug are needed to produce therapeutic effects. In the latter instance, fat depots provide a slow, sustained release of the active drug. Should body fat be seriously reduced, as occurs during starvation, stored compounds (e.g., DDT and chlordane) may be mobilized and toxic symptoms may ensue.

4. *Lung.* The lung receives the entire cardiac output, and therefore, drug distribution into this organ is very rapid. Compounds that accumulate in the lung are usually basic amines (e.g., antihistamines, imipramine, amphetamine, methadone, phentermine, chlorphentermine, and chlorpromazine) that possess large lipophilic groups and have pK_a values greater than 8.0. However, some nonbasic amines like the herbicide paraquat also can accumulate in the lung.

Carrier-mediated, sodium-dependent transport systems are known to remove 5-hydroxytryptamine and norepinephrine from the pulmonary circulation. These same carrier systems are thought to be responsible for the removal of some exogenous basic amines from the circulation, leading to their subsequent accumulation in the lung in concentrations far in excess of those found in the blood (e.g., tissue-to-blood ratio > 200 for imipramine, methadone, amphetamine, and chlorcyclizine). In addition to this carrier-mediated transport, some basic amines such as imipramine and methadone may enter the lung by diffusion and accumulate as a result of binding to pulmonary amphiphilic phospholipids.

5. *Bone.* Although bone is a relatively inert tissue, it can still accumulate such substances as tetracyclines, lead, strontium, and the antitumor agent cisplatin. These substances may accumulate in bone by adsorption onto the bone crystal surface and eventually be incorporated into the crystal lattice. The accumulation of large amounts of strontium may stimulate bone formation. Tetracycline deposition during odontogenesis may lead to a permanent yellow-brown discoloration of teeth, dysplasia, and poor bone development. Lead can substitute for calcium in the bone crystal lattice resulting in bone brittleness. Bone may become a reservoir for the slow release of toxic substances, such as lead and cisplatin.

Physiological Barriers to Drug Distribution

Blood-Brain Barrier

The capillary membrane that exists between the plasma and brain cells is much less permeable to water-soluble drugs than is the membrane between plasma and other tissues. Thus, the transfer of drugs into the brain is regulated by what has been called a *blood-brain barrier* (see Chap. 28). The blood-brain barrier consists of a single row of brain capillary endothelial cells that are joined by continuous *tight* intercellular junctions (see Fig. 28-5). Such an anatomical structure suggests that to gain access to the brain from the capillary circulation, drugs must pass through cells rather than between them. Only drugs that have a high lipid-water partition coefficient will be able to penetrate the tightly apposed capillary endothelial cells.

Drugs that are partially ionized and only moderately lipid soluble will penetrate at considerably slower rates. Lipid-insoluble or highly ionized drugs will fail to enter the brain in significant amounts. Because the pH of the cerebrospinal fluid is about 7.35, there is some tendency for weak organic bases to be more concentrated in the cerebrospinal fluid and for weak organic acids to be excluded. In addition, because only the unbound form of a drug is available for diffusion, extensive plasma protein binding also can have dramatic effects on the extent of drug transfer into the brain.

Inflammation, such as occurs in bacterial meningitis or encephalitis, may increase the permeability of the blood-brain barrier, thus permitting the passage of ionized lipid-insoluble compounds (e.g., penicillin and ampicillin) that would otherwise be restricted from penetrating into the brain extracellular fluid.

The flow of cerebrospinal fluid is essentially unidirectional; that is, it flows from its site of formation in the choroid plexus through the ventricles to its site of exit at the arachnoid villi. Drugs present in this fluid either can enter the brain tissue or be returned to the venous circulation in the *bulk flow* of cerebrospinal fluid carried through the arachnoid villi. Some drugs, such as penicillin, will not leave the cerebrospinal fluid compartment by bulk flow but will be actively transported by the choroid plexus out of the fluid and back into the blood. Finally, drugs may diffuse from brain tissue directly into blood capillaries.

An important consequence of all these routes of drug removal from the brain is that drugs that slowly penetrate the CNS may never achieve adequate therapeutic brain concentrations. Penicillin, for example, is a less effective antibiotic centrally than it is peripherally.

Placental Barrier

Embryologically, the placenta is derived from both fetal and maternal tissues and is perfused by both fetal and maternal blood. The blood vessels of the fetus and mother are separated by a number of tissue layers, which collectively constitute the *placental barrier.* Drugs that traverse this barrier will reach the fetal circulation. The placental barrier, like the blood-brain barrier, does not prevent transport of all drugs but is selective, and factors that regulate passage of drugs through any membrane (pK_a, lipid solubility, protein binding, etc.) are also applicable here.

Anatomically, the maternal vessels lead into and out of a reservoir of blood contained in the intervillous space in which the fetal blood vessels within the chorionic villi are bathed. In humans, the placental barrier has a mean thickness of 25 μ in early pregnancy but decreases to 2 μ at full term. This decrease in placental thickness does not, however, reduce the effectiveness of the barrier against nonpenetrating drug molecules.

The transfer of drugs across the placenta can be considered as a fairly typical case of transport across any biological membrane. In general, substances that are lipid soluble cross the placenta with relative ease in accordance with their lipid-water partition coefficient and degree of ionization. Highly polar or ionized drugs do not cross the placenta readily. However, most drugs used in labor and delivery are not highly ionized and will cross. They are generally weak bases with pK_a values of about 8.0 and tend to be more ionized in the fetal bloodstream since the pH of fetal blood is around 7.3 as compared to the maternal blood pH of 7.44. Differences in maternal and fetal blood pH could give rise to unequal concentrations of ionizable drugs in the mother and the fetus.

Molecular size also plays a part in placental transport, especially with water-soluble substances. Substances with molecular weights less than 600 cross the placenta with ease (e.g., warfarin). Those ranging between 600 and 1,000 cross with increasing difficulty (e.g., streptomycin), and those with values greater than 1,000 do not cross.

The concentration gradient across the placenta is a significant but poorly understood factor in transport. At the time of maternal drug administration there is a concentration gradient in favor of transfer. Generally, the higher the maternal dose the larger the concentration gradient in favor of transfer to the fetus. However, maternal, placental, and fetal drug metabolism will result in a decrease in the concentration gradient.

Most of the human uterine blood flow, averaging 500 ml/min, or 10 percent of the cardiac output, reaches the placenta. This allows a high concentration of diffusible drug to cross the placental barrier and reach the fetal circulation through the umbilical artery. Since most drugs are small and lipid soluble, the principal limiting factor in their placental transfer appears to be blood flow. Although about 90 percent of the fetally absorbed drug is immediately exposed to the fetal hepatic parenchyma, the fetal liver and extrahepatic organs are immature, and therefore most of the drug in the fetus usually remains unmetabolized and potentially toxic. The placenta is capable of metabolizing drugs, but its capacity is extremely limited.

There is a delay in the transfer of drugs to the fetus, such that onset of drug action in the mother is more rapid than in the fetus. For example, even a highly lipid-soluble anesthetic agent like thiopental, which rapidly equilibrates between maternal and fetal plasma, still requires about 15 min to attain full equilibrium. This elapsed time is short enough to allow delivery in anesthetized mothers without the babies showing signs of barbiturate-induced depression. Additional delays in the onset of drug action in the fetus may be due to drug binding by fetal plasma proteins.

As the level of drug decreases in the maternal blood, there is a reversal of diffusion through the placenta and the drug contained in the fetus passes back into the mother's blood. Hydrophilic drugs and their metabolites present in the fetus cannot readily cross back through the placenta into the maternal blood and therefore tend to remain in the fetal blood (e.g., thalidomide).

Steroids, which are highly lipid-soluble drugs, cross the placental barrier readily, whereas antibiotics (such as penicillin and streptomycin) penetrate the placenta slowly and require 10 to 20 hr for full equilibration to occur between maternal and fetal plasma. Ampicillin, however, is actively accumulated by the placenta in such a way that equilibrium is reached in about 90 min; ampicillin concentrations will continue to increase in the fetal plasma until, in about 5 hr, the fetal plasma concentration of the drug is seven times higher than that in maternal plasma.

Chronic maternal alcoholism may lead to congenital defects such as growth retardation and joint and cardiovascular malformations. The hypoxic effect of smoking on the fetus results from a saturation of fetal hemoglobin with carbon monoxide and may cause lower fetal weight, premature birth, and spontaneous abortion. Heroin and cocaine, self-administered by the mother, can cross the placenta and affect the fetus.

Blood-Testis Barrier

The existence of a barrier between the blood and testes is indicated by the absence of staining in testicular tissue after the intravascular injection of dyes. Morphological studies indicate that the barrier is located beyond the capillary endothelial cells and is most likely to be found at the specialized Sertoli-Sertoli cell junction.

The study of the blood-testis barrier has yielded a great deal of information relevant to spermatogenesis, infertility, and fertility control. The ability of this barrier to regulate the passage of steroids is of special interest due to the importance of steroids in the spermatogenic and sperm maturation process.

The blood-testis barrier is thought to play a role in the pathogenesis of several testicular neoplasms by preventing certain chemotherapeutic agents from reaching specific areas of the testis. Malignant cells, if protected by the barrier, could escape exposure to these chemotherapeutic agents.

Supplemental Reading

Baumann, P., et al. (eds.). *Alpha₁-Acid Glycoprotein: Genetics, Biochemistry, Physiological Functions, and Pharmacology.* New York: Liss, 1989.

Benet, L.S., Massoud, W., and Gambertoglio, J.G. (eds.). *Pharmacokinetic Basis for Drug Treatment.* New York: Raven, 1984.

Levine, R.R. *Pharmacology: Drug Actions and Reactions* (4th ed.). Boston: Little, Brown, 1990.

O'Malley, K., and Waddington, J.L. (eds.). *Therapeutics in the Elderly.* Amsterdam: Elsevier, 1985.

Neuwelt, E.A. (ed.). *Implications of the Blood-Brain Barrier and its Manipulation.* Vol. 1: *Basic Science Aspects.* Vol. 2: *Clinical Aspects.* New York: Plenum, 1989.

Oie, S. Drug distribution and binding. *J. Clin. Pharmacol.* 26:583, 1986.

Segal, M.B. *The Barriers and Fluids of the Eye and Brain.* Boca Raton, Fla.: CRC Press, 1989.

Tillement, J.-P., and Lindenlaub, E. (eds.). *Protein Binding and Drug Transport.* New York: Liss, 1987.

Wilkinson, G.R., and Rawlins, M.D.: *Drug Metabolism and Disposition: Considerations in Clinical Pharmacology.* Hingham, Mass.: Kluwer, 1985.

4

Metabolism of Drugs

Theodore E. Gram

Metabolism is a major mechanism by which drug action is terminated. In many instances, the rate of drug metabolism is the primary determinant of both duration and intensity of drug action. Almost all drugs that undergo metabolic transformation are converted to products (*metabolites*) that are more polar than the parent compound. This is of great significance in the overall biological handling of drugs. Not only does drug biotransformation generally diminish pharmacological activity by forming either inactive or less active products, but the increased polarity (reduced lipid solubility) of the metabolites results in a more rapid rate of renal drug clearance (see Chap. 5), since renal tubular reabsorption is diminished. In addition, the more highly ionized a compound becomes, the more likely that it will be excreted by one of the active anion or cation secretory mechanisms present in the cells of the renal proximal tubule (Fig. 4-1). It has been estimated that if renal excretion were the only means of terminating drug action, such highly lipophilic compounds as pentobarbital would exert their pharmacological effects for over 100 years.

It was formerly believed that all drug metabolites were pharmacologically inactive relative to the parent drug. Although this remains generally true, recent work has revealed exceptions. The term *prodrug* describes a compound that in itself has little or no biological activity but is metabolized to a pharmacologically active species. For example, the anticancer drug cyclophosphamide is biologically inert but is converted, predominantly in the liver, to an active cytotoxic drug. In addition, a number of compounds have been found to be converted by enzymes in the body to extremely toxic products. The commonly used analgesic acetaminophen and many chemical carcinogens such as benzo[a]pyrene, found in cigarette smoke, are examples of this group.

We may summarize by saying that drug metabolism *usually* results in the formation of products with markedly reduced pharmacological activity (e.g., hydroxylation of pentobarbital), *occasionally* in products with roughly equivalent activity (e.g., metabolism of methamphet-amine to amphetamine or the conversion of codeine to morphine), and *rarely* in products with markedly increased biological activity (e.g., activation of acetaminophen or benzo[a]pyrene to substances that bind covalently to tissue and cause necrosis).

The rate at which a drug disappears from the body is a function of both its rate of biotransformation and its rate of excretion (renal, biliary, pulmonary). If the combined effects of biotransformation and excretion result in a first-order kinetic (see Chap. 6) rate of drug elimination (as is true for most drugs), the decline in the concentration of the drug in the body can be mathematically described. This measure of drug disappearance is called the *biological half-life* ($t_{1/2}$), and it provides an estimate of the time required to reduce by one-half the quantity of drug present in a particular body compartment (e.g., plasma).

Not only is a knowledge of a drug's $t_{1/2}$ valuable in allowing a comparison between the elimination rates of several drugs, it is also useful in establishing dosage schedules within the therapeutic range.

Drug-Metabolizing Enzymes

The enzymes involved in the biotransformation of foreign compounds (xenobiotics) are distinct from those that participate in carbohydrate, protein, and lipid metabolism. Drugs and other xenobiotics undergo four general types of biotransformation reactions: (1) oxidation, (2) reduction, (3) hydrolysis, and (4) conjugation. The first three are referred to collectively as phase I reactions while conjugation is termed a phase II reaction. Oxidative enzymes are generally found in the endoplasmic reticulum; hydrolytic enzymes are most often located in the cell cytoplasm or in plasma, while conjugation enzymes can be found associated with cytoplasm and endoplasmic reticulum.

Enzymes catalyzing drug oxidation have been referred to as *drug-metabolizing enzymes*. It is realized now that this

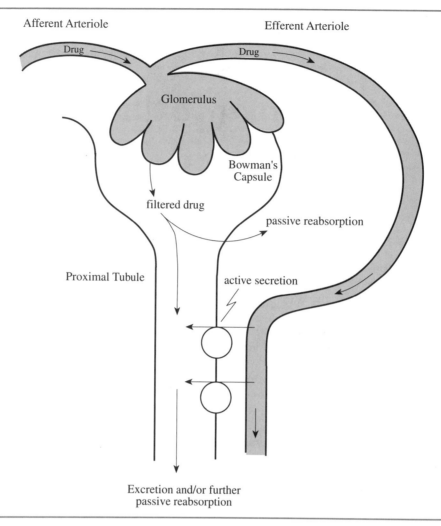

Figure 4-1. Renal excretion of drugs. Filtration of small, non–protein-bound drugs occurs through glomerular capillary pores. Lipid-soluble and un-ionized drugs are passively reabsorbed throughout the nephron. Active secretion of organic acids and bases occurs only in the proximal tubular segment.

term is too narrow since xenobiotic substrates other than drugs (e.g., pesticides, food additives) and some endogenous substances (e.g., steroid hormones, fatty acids, bilirubin, and thyroxine) are also acted upon by these enzymes. The enzymes found in the endoplasmic reticulum act upon a broad spectrum of chemically unrelated, mostly exogenous, lipid-soluble substrates. In addition to drugs, compounds subject to biotransformation include insecticides, herbicides, food additives (coloring agents or preservatives), industrial or automotive pollutants, and chemical carcinogens.

Because of its relative richness in enzymes (enzyme activity per gram of organ) and large mass, the *liver* is clearly the dominant organ in drug metabolism. However, many other tissues, including lung, kidney, intestinal mucosa, adrenal, skin, and placenta, also possess significant levels of drug-metabolizing activity (Table 4-1). Lower, but still measurable, activities are present in leukocytes, intestinal flora, gonads, spleen, eye, and brain. Regardless of where metabolism occurs, a single drug may undergo several biotransformation steps. A drug can be either excreted unchanged or converted to one or more metabolic products. Each of these metabolic products (metabolites) can, in turn, be excreted or further metabolized and then excreted.

In contrast to the oxidation-reduction reactions of intermediate metabolism, which involve transfer of hydrogen atoms, the oxidation of foreign compounds involves insertion of an oxygen atom into the substrate. This process is catalyzed by an enzyme system called a *monooxygenase* or *cytochrome P450 system.* The overall reaction requires both atoms of molecular oxygen: One atom is introduced

Table 4-1. Organ Distribution of Drug-Metabolizing Activity

Organ	Relative activity (%)
Liver	100
Lung	20
Kidney	8
Intestine	6
Placenta (term)	5
Adrenal	2
Skin	1
Brain	0.5

into the drug substrate; the other oxygen atom is reduced to water. Reduced nicotinamide-adenine dinucleotide phosphate (NADPH) is a source of reducing equivalents or electrons for these reactions.

The monooxygenase system has obligatory requirements for NADPH and O_2 and is almost exclusively associated with the endoplasmic reticulum of intact cells, where it is embedded in the phospholipid membranes of this organelle. Monooxygenase activity has also been found in the nuclear envelope.

The hepatic monooxygenase system is composed of an electron transfer chain consisting of three components, all of which have been isolated, purified, and studied in considerable detail. These are a flavoprotein, known as *NADPH cytochrome c (P450) reductase;* a hemoprotein called *cytochrome P450;* and a lipid component, *phosphatidylcholine.* The microsomal electron transfer chain may be presented schematically as shown in Fig. 4-2.

NADPH reduces NADPH cytochrome *c* (P450) reductase, which, in turn, reduces cytochrome P450. The reduced cytochrome P450-substrate-O_2 ternary complex then rearranges in some as yet unknown way to form hydroxylated substrate (product), oxidized cytochrome P450, and water. The requirement for phosphatidylcholine (PC) in microsomal hydroxylation reactions has been unequivocally established, but its precise physicochemical involvement is still unclear.

A most remarkable characteristic of the cytochrome P450-linked monooxygenase system is its *lack* of substrate specificity. It is now established that it is the cytochrome P450 component, or more correctly the cytochromes P450, a family of isozymes, that account for the broad substrate specificity of this enzyme system. Many different isozymes of P450 exist and are distinct in their molecular weight, catalytic activity, and immunochemical behavior. In addition, there are organ, species, and even sex differ-

Figure 4-2. The hepatic drug metabolizing cytochrome P450–dependent electron transfer chain found in the endoplasmic reticulum of many tissues, hepatic and extrahepatic. Cytochrome P450 is actually a family of hemoproteins that function as terminal oxidases in the oxidative metabolism of many drugs. Note that the drug substrate binds to the oxidized form of cytochrome P450, with the resulting complex then reduced by cytochrome P450 reductase. It is the reduced complex that is capable of interacting with molecular oxygen. Molecular rearrangement (second electron added) now takes place, ultimately generating an oxidized metabolite, water, and regenerating the oxidized form [Fe^{3+}] of cytochrome P450. The electron transport series of reactions appears to require a matrix containing phosphatidylcholine.

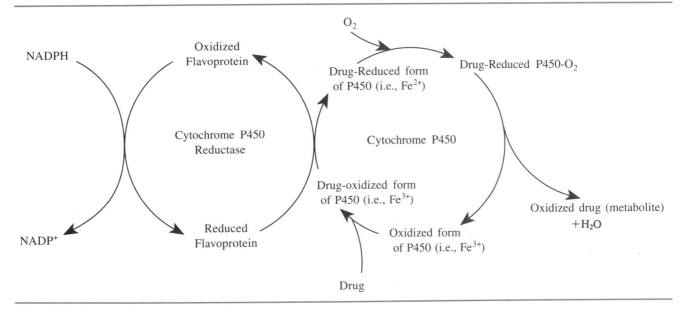

ences in the distribution of these structurally different proteins. At present, the cytochromes P450 consist of 100 distinct molecular species, each coded by different genes.

Chemical Pathways of Drug Metabolism

Oxidative Reactions

Oxidative (hydroxylation) reactions may be envisioned as involving a direct insertion of a hydroxyl functional group into the drug molecule. Hydroxylation may be followed by oxidation to form a ketone or, in the case of oxidative dealkylation, to form an unstable hydroxymethyl intermediate. The intermediate then undergoes carbon-oxygen bond cleavage. Examples of some types of oxidative reactions are given below and in Table 4-2.

Hydroxylation

Pentobarbital and amobarbital are converted to their respective pharmacologically inert alcohols.

Oxidative Dealkylation

Both N- and O-dealkylation reactions are known to occur. Morphine is converted to normorphine by N-de-

alkylation and codeine to morphine by O-dealkylation. Dealkylation reactions are not restricted to demethylation; alkyl groups of various lengths (e.g., ethyl, isopropyl, butyl) as well as aromatic groups are also cleaved from amines or ethers.

N-Oxidation

Drugs that contain amino groups such as imipramine and morphine can undergo N-oxidation.

Oxidation of Aliphatic Alcohols

The enzymatic oxidation of alcohols occurs almost exclusively in the liver. Alcohol dehydrogenase (ADH) has been known for some time and catalyzes ethanol → acetaldehyde → acetic acid.

Reductive Reactions

Reductases appear to be of only minor significance in humans. However, anaerobic microorganisms present in the ileum and colon are rich in reductive enzymes and undoubtedly contribute to the metabolism of xenobiotics in vivo following their excretion in bile.

Hydrolytic Reactions

In contrast to the enzymes involved in oxidative drug metabolism, most hydrolytic enzymes are found outside the endoplasmic reticulum. Although virtually all organs and tissues contain hydrolytic enzymes, they are found in especially high concentrations in liver, kidney, and plasma. Compounds that possess ester linkages (e.g., amides and esters) are the substrates for the enzymes involved.

The widely used analgesic drug meperidine undergoes both N-demethylation and hydrolysis in mammalian liver. N-demethylation is the predominant reaction in the rat, whereas hydrolysis, resulting in formation of the inactive metabolite meperidinic acid, is the major route of metabolism in humans.

The enzymology and even the classification of mammalian esterases is unclear. What is evident is that most mammalian tissues have a family of enzymes that cleave ester bonds. One simple classification distinguishes acetylcholinesterase ("true cholinesterase") from plasma or "pseudocholinesterase" (see Chap. 16). The exceedingly evanescent (about 5 min) action of the skeletal muscle relaxant succinylcholine is attributable to its rapid hydrolysis by plasma esterase. In some patients, however, succinylcholine has a prolonged effect (about 45–60 min) that can be attributed to the presence of a genetically de-

Table 4-2. Major Types of Chemical Reactions Involved in Drug Metabolism and Their Cellular Location

Endoplasmic reticulum	Other sites (primarily plasma and cytoplasmic enzymes)
Oxidation	Oxidation
Hydroxylation	Aldehyde oxidation
Dealkylation	Amine oxidation
Deamination	Deamination
N-Oxidation	Dehydrogenation
Dehalogenation	Dehydration
Reduction	Reduction
Nitroreduction	Aldehyde reduction
Azo reduction	Sulfoxide reduction
Hydrolysis	Hydrolysis
Ester hydrolysis	Ester hydrolysis
Amide hydrolysis	Amide hydrolysis
	Carbamate hydrolysis
	Ring scission
Conjugation (synthetic)	Conjugation (synthetic)
Glucuronide formation	Sulfation
	Acetylation
	Methylation
	Phosphorylation
	Amino acid conjugation
	Mercapturic acid formation

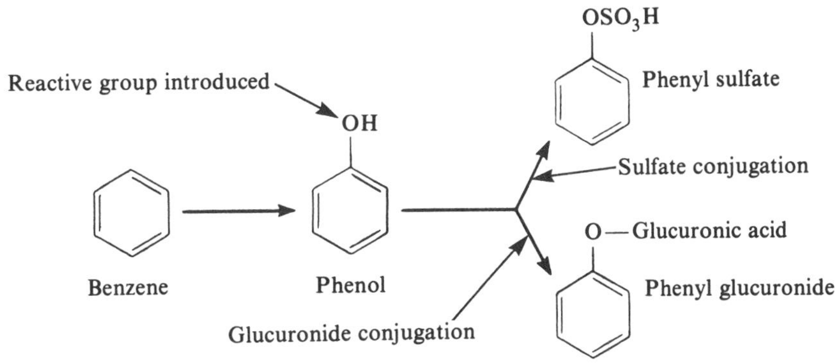

Figure 4-3. Two pathways of conjugation reactions.

termined "abnormal" plasma esterase that degrades the drug slowly and inefficiently. The incidence of this "abnormal" enzyme in an otherwise normal adult population is approximately 1 in 3,000.

Conjugation Reactions (Synthetic Reactions)

After xenobiotics are enzymatically oxidized, reduced, or hydrolyzed, the metabolites formed often contain one or more reactive chemical groups (e.g., hydroxyl, amino, or carboxylic acid). The reactive group has either been inserted directly into the drug, as occurs in the hydroxylation of benzene to form phenol (Fig. 4-3), or it may be "unmasked" following the oxidative reactions.

These reactive groups are amenable to *conjugation* reactions. This involves the chemical combination of the reactive group with a molecule provided by the body (e.g., glucuronic acid, sulfate, glycine, acetate). The resulting newly formed compound is, in general, pharmacologically inactive and more water soluble than the original parent drug. Thus, conjugation reactions not only decrease drug activity but also greatly increase the rate of drug excretion. In the metabolism of benzene (see Fig. 4-3), we find that phenol is eliminated twice as fast as benzene, while the sulfate and glucuronide conjugates are excreted 10 to 20 times as rapidly as benzene.

Glucuronide Conjugation

Glucuronide conjugation is probably the most common single metabolic reaction undergone by drugs and other xenobiotics; this results both from the frequent presence of reactive groups in drug molecules and from the ready availability of glucose, the carbohydrate from which glucuronic acid is derived. Substrates for glucuron-

idation include compounds possessing a hydroxyl (either phenolic or alcoholic), an amine, or a carboxylic acid group.

Glucuronide conjugation occurs in the liver; the metabolites are excreted in the bile and subsequently into the small intestine from which they may be reabsorbed. Glucuronidation reactions are catalyzed by a family of enzymes known as uridine diphosphate (UDP) glucuronyl-transferases. A required cofactor for these reactions is UDP–glucuronic acid (uridine 5′-diphosphate D-glucuronic acid, UDPGA). These enzymes are present in highest amounts in liver but are also found in kidney, intestine, lung, and other organs. Glucuronidation is nearly always a detoxication reaction.

As shown in Fig. 4-4, UDP-glucuronyltransferase activity is very low or absent during late fetal and early postnatal stages of life and later increases almost linearly to reach adult levels. (A similar ontogenic pattern occurs for the monooxygenase system.) This greatly reduced activity of UDP-glucuronyl transferase during the perinatal period has important clinical ramifications. Neonatal hyperbilirubinemia, which results from the inability of newborn, particularly premature, infants to convert bilirubin to the more water-soluble, readily excretable bilirubin glucuronide, can lead to *kernicterus,* a syndrome characterized by irreversible damage to the central nervous system. Normally, bilirubin in the plasma is either rapidly conjugated as the glucuronide and excreted in the bile or tightly bound to plasma proteins. When conjugation is extremely limited, the ability of plasma proteins to bind bilirubin is exceeded, and free bilirubin diffuses across the blood-brain barrier into the cerebral parenchyma.

Similarly, administration to newborn infants of drugs normally excreted as glucuronide conjugates can result in the achieving of toxic levels of the drug. For example, administration of the antibiotic chloramphenicol to infants deficient in UDP-glucuronyltransferase has resulted in excessive accumulation of the free drug in blood and tis-

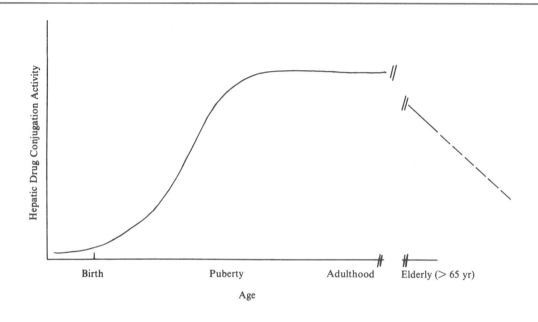

Figure 4-4. A schematic presentation of the ontogeny of hepatic drug metabolic activity.

sues and the appearance of a drug-associated toxicity known as the "gray baby" syndrome (see Chap. 52).

Patients who have a disease known as the Crigler-Najjar syndrome have been found to be almost totally deficient in hepatic UDP-glucuronyltransferase activity. These individuals excrete no bilirubin glucuronide. Patients with the Crigler-Najjar syndrome are highly jaundiced, frequently develop kernicterus, and usually die early in childhood.

An enzyme, β-glucuronidase, is capable of hydrolyzing glucuronide conjugates (see below); it is present in virtually all tissues but is particularly rich in the mucosa of the jejunum.

$$R-OH \xrightarrow{\text{UDP-glucuronyltransferase}} R-O-\text{glucuronide}$$

$$R-O-\text{glucuronide} \xrightarrow{\text{β-glucuronidase}} R-OH$$
$$+ \text{glucuronic acid}$$

The β-glucuronidase, present either in the intestinal mucosa or in the intestinal bacteria, can hydrolyze the newly formed conjugate, thereby reforming the compound that had previously undergone glucuronidation. If the now reformed parent drug is lipid soluble, it will be reabsorbed from the gastrointestinal tract. Such an *enterohepatic circulation* will prolong the retention time of the drug in the body.

Sulfate Conjugation

Sulfate conjugation is probably second only to glucuronidation as an important synthetic reaction (see Fig. 4-

3). Sulfate conjugation is catalyzed by a family of enzymes known as *sulfotransferases* that are present in the cell cytoplasm of liver and several other organs. The essential cofactor, that is, the sulfate donor, for this enzyme is 3'-phosphoadenosine 5'-phosphosulfate (PAPS). Sulfate conjugates are generally highly polar compounds and are readily excreted in the urine.

A characteristic of sulfate conjugation in vivo, not shared by the glucuronide pathway, is its saturability. For example, in humans acetylsalicylic acid (aspirin) is conjugated, in part, with sulfate. If the dose of the analgesic is increased progressively, the amount of sulfate conjugate excreted eventually reaches a maximum, after which further aspirin elimination occurs either as the glucuronide or as some other conjugate or as free drug. The saturability of sulfate conjugation is the result of depletion of endogenous amounts of the obligatory factor, PAPS.

N-Acetylation

A variety of primary amines undergo metabolic inactivation by *N*-acetylation. This reaction is catalyzed by enzymes (*N-acetyltransferases*) that utilize acetylcoenzyme A (acetyl-CoA) as a cofactor and are found in the cell cytoplasm of such organs as liver, intestine, kidney, and lung. Hepatic *N*-acetyltransferase catalyzes the acetylation of a number of commonly used drugs, such as isoniazid, sulfamethazine and other sulfonamides, *p*-aminosalicylic acid, and hydralazine.

Genetic studies in humans have shown individuals to be either rapid or slow acetylators; slow acetylators have low hepatic *N*-acetyltransferase activity and are homozygous for an autosomal recessive gene. Individuals who acetylate drugs slowly are especially susceptible to dose-dependent toxicity. Genetic influences on drug metabolism are discussed in greater detail later in this chapter under Pharmacogenetic Factors.

Methylation

Methyltransferases are found either in the cytoplasm or in the endoplasmic reticulum of many organs, including the liver, lung, and kidney; these enzymes generally use *S*-adenosylmethionine as a methyl donor. For example, the methylated metabolite, normetanephrine, has less than 1 percent of the biological activity of the parent compound norepinephrine.

Glutathione Conjugation

Some aromatic compounds, such as naphthalene, are excreted in the urine as *N*-acetylcysteine derivatives called *mercapturic acids*. Mercapturic acids originate through the conjugation of a xenobiotic with the tripeptide glutathione. Glutathione-conjugating reactions are catalyzed by enzymes present in the cytoplasm of the liver and, to a much lesser extent, the lung, kidney, and other organs. The commonly used analgesic, acetaminophen, is conjugated with glutathione, and sulfobromophthalein (BSP), a substance used in liver function tests, is excreted into the bile as the glutathione adduct. Glutathione conjugation is an extremely important pathway in the detoxication of a large variety of environmental toxicants and chemical carcinogens.

Amino Acid Conjugation

A wide variety of structurally unrelated carboxylic acids are conjugated with naturally occurring amino acids before excretion. Conjugation with glycine is most common, but other amino acids, including taurine and glutamine, are also used. In humans, a substantial portion (up to 50%) of salicylate, administered either as sodium salicylate or aspirin, is excreted in the urine as the glycine conjugate salicyluric acid.

Factors Affecting Drug Metabolism

Age

One of the most durable axioms in pharmacology is that the very young and very old (human or animal) tend to be more sensitive to the actions of drugs. Alterations in drug binding to plasma proteins, renal clearance, drug-receptor interactions, end-organ responsiveness, and drug metabolism all may contribute to this hyperresponsive-

ness. *Of these factors, a change in the rate of drug biotransformation is probably the most significant determinant.*

Of necessity, most of the direct information we have on drug metabolism as a function of age has been obtained in animals. However, indirect and inferential conclusions based on plasma half-lives, total body clearance, etc. suggest that extrapolations from animals to human perinates and neonates are valid. Early in fetal life drug-metabolizing enzyme activity is quite low, but begins to increase during the postnatal period. Rates of biotransformation often increase dramatically to adult levels at or about puberty (see Fig. 4-4).

Gerontological Considerations

In a society whose population is aging, increasing attention must be paid to a variety of special problems associated with drug therapy in the elderly. In the elderly, rates of drug metabolism generally tend to decline. Thus, these individuals gradually become more and more sensitive to a given drug dose as their ability to metabolize foreign compounds decreases. In addition, elderly individuals may have reductions in renal function that also contribute to a decrease in drug elimination.

Numerous physiological changes occur in aging animals or humans that may dramatically influence their responsiveness to drugs.

Absorption

Elderly patients may absorb drugs less completely or more slowly because of decreased splanchnic blood flow (resulting in large part from reduced cardiac output), or altered gastrointestinal motility. Cardiac output decreases by approximately 30 percent by age 65, and this results in a 45 to 50 percent decrease in gastrointestinal blood flow.

Distribution

Drug distribution in elderly patients may be altered by hypoalbuminemia, qualitative changes in drug-binding sites, reductions in relative muscle mass, increases in the proportion of body fat, and decreases in total body water. The plasma level of free, active drug is often a direct function of the extent of drug binding to plasma proteins. There is a well-documented age-dependent decline (~ 20%) in plasma albumin concentration in humans due to a reduced rate of hepatic albumin synthesis. These changes in serum albumin may affect the free drug concentration for a number of drugs, such as phenytoin, warfarin, and meperidine.

Metabolism

In addition to changes in metabolism that occur as a result of reduced hepatic enzyme activity, metabolism may be further impaired by a reduction in hepatic mass and blood flow (perfusion).

In a carefully controlled clinical study, the plasma half-

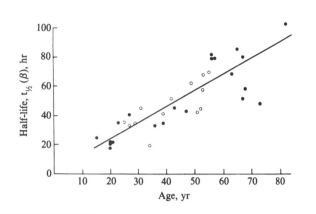

Figure 4-5. Correlation of diazepam plasma half-lives with age in humans. (From U. Klotz et al., The effects of age and liver disease on the disposition and elimination of diazepam in adult man. *J. Clin. Invest.* 55:347, 1975. Reproduced by copyright permission of the American Society for Clinical Investigation.)

Table 4-3. Plasma Half-Lives of Several Drugs in Young Adult and Elderly Patients

| Drug | Plasma or serum $t_{1/2}$ | |
	Young (20–30 yr)	Elderly (65–80 yr)
Penicillin G	20.7 min	39.1 min
Dihydrostreptomycin	5.2 hr	8.4 hr
Tetracycline	3.5 hr	4.5 hr
Kanamycin	107 min	282 min
Digoxin	51 hr	73 hr
Aminopyrine	3 hr	10 hr
Phenobarbital	71 hr	107 hr
Diazepam	20 hr	80 hr
Lidocaine	80.6 min	139.6 min
Chlordiazepoxide	8.9 hr	16.7 hr
Antipyrine	12.0 hr	17.4 hr
Phenylbutazone	81.2 hr	104.6 hr
Isoniazid	1.4 hr	1.5 hr
Warfarin	37 hr	44 hr

Source: Compiled from: J. G. Ouslander, Drug therapy in the elderly. *Ann. Intern. Med.* 95:711, 1981, and D. P. Richey and A. D. Bender, Pharmacokinetic consequences of aging. *Annu. Rev. Pharmacol. Toxicol.* 17:49, 1977, and references therein.

life of diazepam (*Valium*), a widely used antianxiety agent, exhibited a striking age dependency. At 20 years the $t_{1/2}$ was about 20 hr and this increased linearly with age to about 90 hr at 80 years (Fig. 4-5). Half-lives of other drugs in young and old patients are presented in Table 4-3. Oral administration of amobarbital, a drug metabolized almost exclusively in the liver, resulted in both higher plasma levels of unchanged drug and a significant reduction in the plasma concentration of its primary metabolite, 3'-hydroxy-amobarbital, in the urine of elderly patients (>65 years) compared to younger (20–30 years) individuals. These data, along with those taken from several other studies, demonstrate changes in drug half-life with increasing age, suggesting that, at least for some drugs, elderly patients have reduced metabolism or drug clearance, or both.

Excretion

Renal elimination of foreign compounds may be altered dramatically by reduced renal blood flow (again resulting from reduced cardiac output), reduced glomerular filtration rate, reduced tubular secretory activity, and a reduction in the number of functional nephrons with increasing age. It has been estimated that in humans from age 20 renal function declines by about 10 percent per decade of life. This is particularly important for drugs such as penicillin or digoxin, which are eliminated primarily by the kidney.

Receptor Sensitivity

Receptors may be reduced in number or in affinity or even in qualitative responsiveness.

Nutrition

Protein deficiency impairs drug metabolism. For example, sleeping time produced by barbiturates is increased as a result of prolonged protein malnutrition. Fat-free diets, or diets deficient in essential fatty acids, also impair drug metabolism. Although no specific requirement of the drug-metabolizing enzymes for dietary carbohydrate has been demonstrated, excessive intake of sucrose, glucose, or fructose will impair monooxygenase activity. The mechanism of this effect is unknown.

Rates of drug metabolism are impaired in vitamin A, riboflavin, ascorbic acid, and vitamin E deficiency states. Deficiencies of certain elements such as calcium and magnesium have a similar effect. It is interesting that severe iron deficiency, which can reduce hemoglobin and hematocrit levels to 25 percent of normal, has no effect on drug metabolism.

Feeding charcoal-broiled beef to volunteers markedly reduced the peak plasma concentration obtained after administration of phenacetin (Fig. 4-6). The reduction was completely reversible when the charcoal-broiled meat was replaced by a control diet. It was concluded that the charcoal-broiled beef stimulated the metabolism of phenacetin either by the intestinal epithelium or during its first pass through the liver. It is thought that Brussels sprouts, cabbage, cauliflower, or certain other vegetables also may stimulate the intestinal metabolism of certain drugs.

The effects of ethanol ingestion on hepatic drug me-

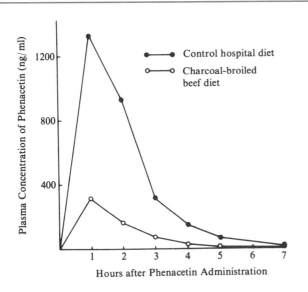

Figure 4-6. Plasma concentrations of phenacetin after the oral administration of 900 mg phenacetin to normal volunteers eating a control hospital diet for 7 days and then the charcoal-broiled beef diet for 4 days. Each value represents the mean of 9 subjects. (From A.P. Alvares, Interactions between environmental chemicals and drug biotransformation in man. *Clin. Pharmacokinet.* 3:462, 1978.)

Table 4-4. Plasma Half-Lives (hr) of Three Drugs in Chronic Alcoholics

Drug	Controls	Alcoholics
Tolbutamide	5.9	2.7*
Warfarin	41	27*
Phenytoin	24	16*

*Significantly different from controls at $P < .02$.
Source: R. M. Kater et al., Increased rate of clearance of drugs from the circulation of alcoholics. *Am. J. Med. Sci.* 258:35, 1969.

olism in the alcoholics. Chronic administration of ethanol can result in increased drug metabolism, increased hepatic cytochrome P450 content, and a proliferation of the smooth endoplasmic reticulum.

Enzyme Induction

Well over 200 chemically and pharmacologically unrelated drugs and other xenobiotics, when administered chronically to animals or humans, increase the activity of the monooxygenase enzymes and thus generally reduce the duration and intensity of drug action. This increase in enzyme activity results from a de novo synthesis of new enzyme (i.e., *induction*), and not from activation of latent or preexisting enzyme precursor. This enzyme induction can be blocked by the administration of protein synthesis inhibitors; this suggests the involvement of increased rates of protein and DNA-dependent RNA synthesis.

Phenobarbital and a number of polycyclic hydrocarbons, including the carcinogenic substance benzo[a]pyrene, are among the most thoroughly studied compounds capable of causing increases in the activity of the drug-metabolizing enzymes. Phenobarbital and benzo[a]pyrene administration each causes its own typical spectrum of enzyme stimulation. Phenobarbital, which stimulates the metabolism of a great many substrates, increases the amounts of smooth endoplasmic reticulum. Benzo[a]pyrene, which stimulates the metabolism of fewer substrates, does not. Phenobarbital also causes hepatomegaly (hyperplasia and hypertrophy), whereas benzo[a]pyrene does not.

Recent work has revealed the existence of many types of monooxygenase enzyme inducers based not only on their substrate spectrum, but more importantly, on the specific isozyme of cytochrome P450 that they induce. Among these are several isomers of the environmental pollutant group known as polychlorinated biphenyls (PCBs), several steroid hormones (estrogens, androgens, progestins, and adrenal corticoids), ethanol, and 2,3,7,8-tetrachlorodibenzo-1,4-dioxin (also known as TCDD), the notoriously toxic component found in Agent Orange, a defoliant used in Vietnam.

tabolism differ depending on whether the ingestion has been acute or chronic. *Chronic ethanol ingestion* increases the hepatic content of monooxygenase enzymes and cytochrome P450 and accelerates drug clearance from plasma. *Acute ethanol ingestion,* however, inhibits drug metabolism and prolongs and intensifies the effects of drugs, particularly central nervous system depressants. These observations account for the clinical finding that administration of a usually effective hypnotic dose of pentobarbital or secobarbital to a chronic alcoholic who has not been drinking for at least 24 hr is markedly less effective in these individuals, while the same dose administered immediately after ethanol ingestion produces an exaggerated ("additive") response. Studies performed in human volunteers have shown that acute ethanol intoxication results in at least a twofold increase in the plasma half-life of pentobarbital and meprobamate.

In the study shown in Table 4-4, drugs cleared from the plasma almost exclusively by hepatic metabolism were administered to alcoholic subjects and drug half-lives were determined. Alcoholics were defined as individuals who had a daily consumption of at least 250 gm ethanol for at least 3 months but were alcohol-free for several days before testing. Standard clinical liver function tests were normal in all patients. The data in Table 4-4 show that the plasma half-lives of tolbutamide, warfarin, and phenytoin were significantly shorter in chronic alcoholics than in control patients, and this reflects enhanced rates of metab-

The pharmacological significance of monooxygenase enzyme induction is nicely exemplified by data presented in Table 4-5. Zoxazolamine, an experimental drug that causes skeletal muscle relaxation or, in large doses, paralysis, is inactivated exclusively by metabolism; therefore, its duration of action (paralysis time) is largely a consequence of its rate of metabolism. Groups of animals were pretreated for about 4 days with either saline (controls) or various enzyme inducers. On the next day the animals were all injected with the same dose (mg/kg) of zoxazolamine and the paralysis time and enzyme activity were determined. It was clear from the results that the enzyme inducers both accelerated the rate of zoxazolamine metabolism and decreased the duration of its pharmacological effect.

Table 4-6 lists some of the compounds that act similarly to phenobarbital in their ability to stimulate human drug metabolism as well as some of the substrates whose metabolism is affected. The most common members of

the polycyclic hydrocarbon class of inducing agents are the well-known carcinogens found in coal tar, cigarette smoke, and charcoal-broiled meat: 3-methylcholanthrene and benzo[a]pyrene.

Considering that cigarette smoke is a rich source of benzo[a]pyrene, and that benzo[a]pyrene is a potent enzyme inducer, it might be inferred that tobacco smoke should induce drug metabolism. Exposure of pregnant rats to a cigarette smoke–air mixture for 5 hr daily for 3 days has been shown to produce a 12-fold increase in pulmonary monooxygenase activity, a fourfold increase in placental metabolism, and a doubling of activity in the liver. Data available on the effects of cigarette smoking on drug effects and pharmacokinetics in humans are found in Table 4-7.

The potential effects of enzyme induction on therapeutic drug effectiveness should encourage the physician to consider the consequences of *long-term therapy* with single or multiple drugs.

Table 4-5. Effect of Enzyme Inducers on the Duration of Action (in vivo) and the Metabolism (in vitro) of Zoxazolamine in Rats

Pretreatment	Paralysis time (min)	Metabolism (μmoles/gm liver/hr)
Control	730	0.53
Phenylbutazone	307	1.05
Barbital	181	1.64
Phenobarbital	102	2.02
Benzo[a]pyrene	17	2.63
3-Methylcholanthrene	12	—

Source: Taken in part from A. H. Cooney and J. J. Burns, Factors influencing drug metabolism. *Adv. Pharmacol.* 1:31, 1962.

Table 4-6. Phenobarbital-Type Agents that Stimulate Human Microsomal Enzyme Activity

Inducing agents	Substances whose metabolism is increased
Phenobarbital	Bilirubin
Chlorcyclizine	Chloramphenicol
Chlordane	Chlorpromazine
DDT	Codeine
Phenytoin	Cortisol
Glutethimide	Estradiol-17β
Meprobamate	Meperidine
Pentobarbital	Morphine
Phenylbutazone	Phenacetin
Tolbutamide	Phenylbutazone
	Testosterone
	Thyroxine
	Triamcinolone
	Zoxazolamine

Pharmacogenetic Factors

Large differences often exist among humans in their rates of plasma drug clearance. Recognition of the differences in drug metabolism and plasma half-lives among patients has raised the question of whether these differences were primarily the result of genetic or environmental influences.

Overall drug clearance (plasma half-life) has been stud-

Table 4-7. The Effect of Cigarette Smoking on Some Drug Parameters in Human Subjects

Drug	Parameter	Control	Smokers
Phenacetin	Peak plasma level (μg/ml)	2.2	0.4
Theophylline	Plasma $t_{1/2}$ (hr)	7.0	4.3
	Clearance (ml/min)	45	100
Warfarin	Plasma $t_{1/2}$ (hr)	51	38.1

Reports show lowered blood levels in smokers:
    Phenacetin
    Theophylline
    Imipramine
    Antipyrine
    Pentazocine
Reports of reduced pharmacological effect in smokers:
    Pentazocine
    Chlorpromazine
    Diazepam
    Chlordiazepoxide
    Propoxyphene

Source: Data compiled from A. P. Alvares, Interactions between chemicals and drug biotransformation in man. *Clin. Pharmacokinet.* 3:462, 1978, and G. W. Dawson and R. E. Vestal, Smoking and drug metabolism. *Pharmacol. Ther.* 15:207, 1982.

ied in identical (*monozygotic*) and fraternal (*dizygotic*) twins. In fraternal twins, the differences were sizable and approached those seen among unrelated individuals. In identical twins, there was virtually no intratwin difference in plasma half-lives of phenylbutazone, antipyrine, or dicumarol. That most of these adult identical twins lived in separate households, consumed different diets, and were exposed to different environments, but still exhibited striking similarities in plasma drug half-lives, would tend to minimize the influence of environmental factors and imply a predominantly genetic control over drug metabolism in human subjects.

A Swedish study demonstrated differences exceeding 100-fold in the plasma half-life of the psychotropic agent nortriptyline in a large group of patients. This observation is of considerable clinical importance since drugs are ordinarily administered on a fixed-dosage schedule. Obviously, patients who metabolize and clear nortriptyline rapidly may be "undermedicated" and will not receive its full therapeutic benefit, whereas slow metabolizers may experience mild to severe drug toxicity resulting from progressive drug accumulation.

As mentioned earlier (see under *N*-Acetylation), two distinct populations have been identified on the basis of their ability to *N*-acetylate the antitubercular drug isoniazid: rapid and slow acetylators (Fig. 4-7). Isoniazid is metabolized exclusively by *N*-acetylation, and the metabolite formed, acetylisoniazid, is rapidly excreted in the urine. Thus, the major determinant in whole-body clearance of isoniazid is the rate of *N*-acetylation. Obviously, slow acetylators are more subject to isoniazid toxicity. It is interesting to note that the acetylation rate seems to have an ethnic component. Thus, the slowest acetylators were Eskimos, Japanese, and Chinese, while rapid acetylators were Egyptians, Israelis, Scandinavians, and Finns. The pharmacogenetic considerations of succinylcholine me-

tabolism have already been discussed under Hydrolytic Reactions.

Species Differences

Species differences in drug metabolism are most commonly manifested either as differences in rates of metabolism (Table 4-8) or as differences in the metabolic products formed. In those instances in which multiple metabolic products can be formed, the ratios of the products may differ considerably among different animal species. For instance, the rabbit deaminates amphetamine to a biologically inactive ketone, while the rat produces the active vasopressor substance 4-hydroxyamphetamine (Fig. 4-8).

Species differences in drug metabolism may greatly complicate the extrapolation of data obtained in animals to humans. This is true from both the toxicological and therapeutic point of view. In the early 1940s, sulfanilamide was the only active antibacterial drug available. The drug was tested extensively in dogs and found to be safe and quite nontoxic, but administration to humans produced an alarming incidence of hematuria, anuria, renal failure, and death. The reason this problem was not picked up in the early toxicology studies was that, by a phylogenetic quirk, the dog, in contrast to most mammalian species, is almost totally incapable of acetylating foreign compounds and was excreting sulfanilamide in a chemically unchanged form; since the toxicity was due to the acetylated species, none was seen in the dog.

Disease

Hepatic drug metabolism is impaired in patients with malaria and schistosomiasis. Neoplastic disease, even in the absence of hepatic involvement, inhibits drug metabolism in liver, possibly by humoral factors. Biotransfor-

Figure 4-7. The bimodal distribution of patients into those who rapidly inactivate isoniazid and those who slowly metabolize it.

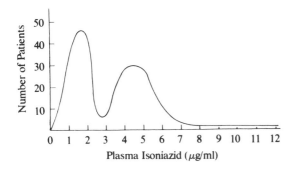

Table 4-8. Species Differences in the Duration of Action and Metabolism of Hexobarbital

Species	Duration of action (sleeping time, min)	Relative enzyme activity (μg hexobarbital metabolized/gm liver/hr)
Mouse	12 ± 8	598 ± 184
Rabbit	49 ± 12	196 ± 28
Rat	90 ± 15	134 ± 51
Dog	315 ± 105	36 ± 30

Source: G. P. Quinn et al., Species, strain, and sex differences in the metabolism of hexobarbitone, amidopyrine, antipyrine and aniline. *Biochem. Pharmacol.* 1:152, 1958.

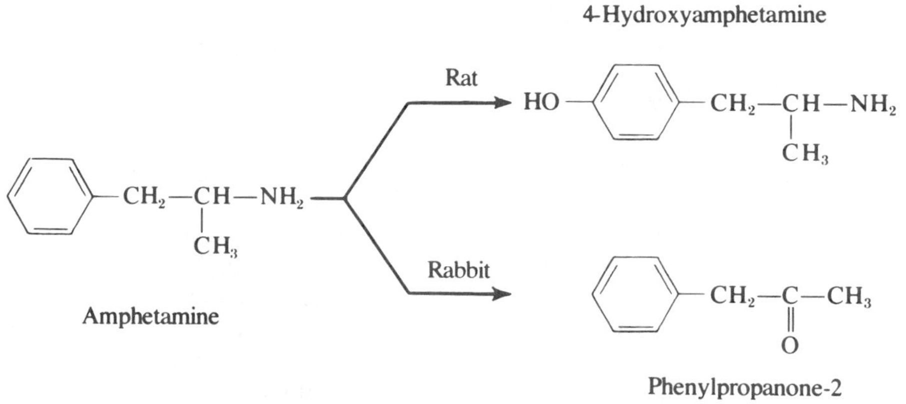

Figure 4-8. An example of species difference in the metabolism of drugs.

mation is also impaired by the presence of such pathological conditions as hepatitis, obstructive jaundice, or advanced cirrhosis. However, in the last-named conditions, whole-body clearance and duration of drug action are prolonged only in very severe cases.

Radiation

Hepatic drug metabolism is impaired by sublethal doses of whole-body x-irradiation or by radiation of the head region alone; the latter effect is presumably related to impaired secretion of adrenocorticotropic hormone (ACTH) by the pituitary.

Sex Differences

There are marked differences in the rates of biotransformation of many, but not all, drug substrates in male and female animals. In rats, the sex-related differences in rates of drug metabolism are clearly the result of a stimulatory effect of androgens, and they can be abolished by castration. The administration of testosterone to females will increase, and estradiol-17β to males will decrease, the rate of drug metabolism. Sex differences do not exist among newborn or very young rats ($<$3–4 weeks), but become prominent at sexual maturation.

Such a sex difference in rates of drug metabolism and duration of drug effect has only been reported in rats and some strains of mice. No sex differences in drug metabolism have been reported for humans.

Coadministration of Drugs

Kinetic studies reveal that one drug capable of being metabolized by the monooxygenase drug-metabolizing system can *competitively inhibit* the metabolism of a second coadministered drug. For example, the anticonvulsant phenytoin and the anticoagulant dicumarol are both metabolized by monooxygenase enzymes. Patients receiving a constant maintenance dose of phenytoin who later have dicumarol added to their regimen may experience severe central nervous system symptoms of phenytoin toxicity as a result of a dicumarol-associated inhibition of phenytoin metabolism. Similarly, diabetics being maintained with the hypoglycemic agent tolbutamide may experience a severe hypoglycemic crisis when phenylbutazone or dicumarol is added to their drug regimens.

The inhibitory effects of acute alcoholism on the metabolism of many drugs have been discussed above. The combined ingestion of a benzodiazepine and alcohol has a dual effect. Since both drugs are metabolized by the monooxygenase system, they inhibit each other's metabolism and therefore the duration of their pharmacological effects is prolonged. The central nervous system depressant effects of the two agents also are additive.

Hormonal Factors

Corticosteroids

In some species adrenalectomy impairs the metabolism of several drug substrates; this effect can be reversed by injection of cortisone, cortisol, or prednisolone. In many laboratory animals a diurnal variation (*circadian rhythm*) in hepatic drug metabolism may exist; this can be abolished by adrenalectomy. Hepatic drug-metabolizing activity appears to correlate inversely with plasma glucocorticoid levels.

Thyroxine

Thyroidectomy reduces the metabolism of a number of drug substrates. For example, barbiturate sleeping time and drug half-lives are significantly prolonged in thyroidectomized animals. Clinically, hypothyroid patients show reduced rates of plasma drug clearance.

Insulin

Animals made grossly diabetic by injection of alloxan or streptozotocin, agents that cause necrosis of pancreatic β cells, have prolonged barbiturate sleeping times and impaired drug metabolism. These alterations are reversed by insulin administration.

Estrogens and Progesterone

Studies in humans suggest impaired drug metabolism in the mother during pregnancy. For example, the administration of either meperidine (*Demerol*) or promazine (*Sparine*) to pregnant women shortly before term resulted in the excretion of more parent drug and markedly less metabolites than occurred in nonpregnant patients.

Intestinal Microflora

Therapeutic agents present in the gastrointestinal lumen come into intimate contact with the intestinal microflora. The anaerobic microflora, particularly those present in the distal ileum and colon, are rich in reductases and may be responsible for a significant proportion of the azoreductase and nitroreductase activity observed in humans. The role of the enzyme β-glucuronidase, present both in the intestinal contents and in the intestinal epithelium, in hydrolyzing a glucuronide conjugate has been discussed earlier in this chapter.

The side effects associated with the artificial sweetener cyclamate largely result from its conversion to the toxic metabolite cyclohexylamine, a biotransformation carried out by various microorganisms present in the intestinal lumen.

Formation of Reactive Intermediates

For many years it was believed that biotransformation resulted only in drug inactivation, that is, in the formation of biologically less active metabolites. Although this view is generally valid, it is not so invariably. There are notable instances in which xenobiotics are transformed into highly reactive metabolic products that can react with vital biological macromolecules. Chemically reactive metabolites generated in vivo may bind covalently to nucleic acids or proteins and thereby initiate such serious toxicity as cellular and tissue necrosis, anemias and blood dyscrasias, carcinogenesis, mutagenesis, teratogenesis, and fetal death.

It is now well established that many carcinogens are active only after their biotransformation to chemically re-

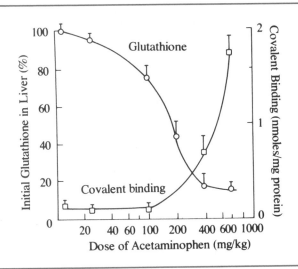

Figure 4-9. Relationship between hepatic glutathione levels and covalent binding of acetaminophen ^{3}H in the liver after the administration of increasing doses of acetaminophen to mice. O—O = glutathione concentration; □—□ = covalent binding of acetaminophen [3]H. (From J.R. Mitchell et al., *J. Pharmacol. Exp. Ther.* 187:211, 1973. Copyright 1973, The Williams & Wilkins Co., Baltimore.)

active metabolites. For example, the hydrocarbons 3-methylcholanthrene and benzo[*a*]pyrene are not themselves believed to be carcinogenic, but after their metabolism to highly reactive epoxide intermediates, they may bind covalently with DNA to initiate malignant transformation or mutation.

Acetaminophen, a relatively safe analgesic when taken in normal therapeutic doses, is bioactivated by a cytochrome P450-dependent monooxygenase to an active intermediate, possibly a semiquinone imine. Once formed, this active intermediate is usually rapidly conjugated with tissue glutathione (in the presence of a glutathione transferase), with the formation of a nontoxic product. However, as the dose of acetaminophen is increased, depletion of hepatic glutathione occurs. Once hepatic glutathione concentrations reach a critically low level, covalent binding of the reactive intermediate to hepatic macromolecules begins (Fig. 4-9). Apparently, it is this irreversible inactivation of vital tissue components that is the cause of an acetaminophen-associated, fatal hepatic necrosis after massive overdose. Similar bioactivation steps are required to initiate hepatic necrosis following large doses of the diuretic furosemide (*Lasix*) and to initiate bone marrow aplasia following the administration of chloramphenicol.

Supplemental Reading

Anders, M.W. (ed.). *Bioactivation of Foreign Compounds.* New York: Academic, 1985.

Benford, D., Gibson, G.G., and Bridges, J.W. (eds.). *Drug Metabolism from Molecules to Man.* Philadelphia: Taylor & Francis, 1987.

Gorrod, J.W., Oelschlager, H., and Caldwell, J. (eds.). *Metabolism of Xenobiotics.* Philadelphia: Taylor & Francis, 1988.

Gram, T.E. (ed.) *Extrahepatic Metabolism of Drugs and Foreign Compounds.* Jamaica, N.Y.: Spectrum, 1980.

Guengerich, F.P. (ed.). *Mammalian Cytochrome P-450.* Boca Raton, Fla.: CRC, 1987. Vols. 1 and 2.

Horai, Y., and Ishizchi, T. Pharmacogenetics and its clinical implications: *N*-Acetylation polymorphism. *Ration. Drug Ther.* 21:2, 1987.

Kalow, W., Goedde, H.W., and Agarwal, D.P. Ethnic Differences in Reactions to Drugs and Xenobiotics. New York: Liss, 1986.

Loi, C.M., and Vestal, R.E. Drug metabolism in the elderly. *Pharmacol. Ther.* 36:131, 1988.

Nebert, D.W., Nelson, D.R., and Feyereisen, R. Evolution of the cytochrome P450 genes. *Xenobiotica* 19:1149–1160, 1989.

Schmuckler, D.L. Aging and drug disposition: An update. *Pharmacol. Rev.* 37:133, 1985.

Sherlock, S. Hepatotoxicity caused by drugs. *Ration. Drug. Ther.* 22:1, 1988.

Turner, N., Scarpace, P.J., and Lowenthal, D.T. Geriatric pharmacology: Basic and clinical considerations. *Annu. Rev. Pharmacol. Toxicol.* 32:271, 1992.

Woods, W.G., and Strong, R. (eds.). *Geriatric Clinical Pharmacology.* New York: Raven, 1987.

Excretion of Drugs

William O. Berndt and Robert E. Stitzel

Despite the reduction in activity that occurs as a drug leaves its site of action, it may still remain in the body for a considerable period of time, especially if it is strongly bound to tissue components. Thus, reduction in pharmacological activity and drug elimination are to be seen as related, but separable, phenomena.

Excretion, as well as metabolism and tissue redistribution, is important in determining both the duration of drug action and the rate of drug elimination. Excretion is a process whereby drugs are transferred from the internal to the external environment, and the principal organs involved in this activity are the kidneys, lungs, biliary system, and intestines.

It is important to remember that the physicochemical considerations discussed previously (see Chap. 3) that govern the passage of drugs across biological barriers are applicable to both excretory and absorptive phenomena.

Renal Excretion

Although some drugs are excreted through extrarenal pathways, the kidney serves as the primary organ of removal for most drugs, and especially for those that are water soluble and nonvolatile. *The three principal processes that determine the urinary excretion of a drug are glomerular filtration, tubular secretion, and tubular reabsorption (mostly passive back-diffusion).* Active tubular reabsorption also may have some influence on the rate of excretion for a limited number of compounds.

Glomerular Filtration

The ultrastructure of the glomerular capillary wall is such that it permits a high degree of fluid filtration while concomitantly restricting the passage of compounds having relatively large molecular weights.

Several factors influence the glomerular filtration of large molecules, including molecular size, charge, and shape. The restricted passage of macromolecules can be thought of as a consequence of the presence of a glomerular capillary wall "barrier" with uniform pores each possessing a radius of approximately 50 Å. Since approximately 130 ml plasma water is filtered across the porous glomerular capillary membranes each minute (190 liters/day), the kidney is admirably suited for its role in drug excretion. As the ultrafiltrate is formed, any drug that is free in the plasma water, that is, not bound to plasma proteins or the formed elements in the blood (e.g., red blood cells), will be filtered as a result of the driving force provided by the cardiac action.

All unbound drugs will be filtered as long as their molecular size, charge, and shape are not excessively large. Compounds with an effective radius of greater than 20 Å may have their rate of glomerular filtration restricted; hindrance to passage increases progressively as molecular radius increases and will approach zero passage when the compound radius becomes greater than about 42 Å.

Charged substances (e.g., sulfated dextrans) are usually filtered at slower rates than neutral compounds (e.g., neutral dextrans), even when their molecular sizes are comparable. The greater restriction to filtration of charged molecules, particularly anions, is probably due to an electrostatic interaction between the filtered molecule and the presence of fixed negative charges within the glomerular capillary wall. These highly anionic structural components of the wall contribute to the existence of an electrostatic barrier and are most likely located in the endothelial or glomerular basement membrane regions.

Molecular configuration also may influence the rate of glomerular filtration of drugs. Differences in the three-dimensional shape of macromolecules result in a restriction of glomerular passage of globular molecules (e.g., proteins) to a greater extent than of random coil or extended molecules (e.g., dextrans). Thus, the very efficient retention of proteins within the circulation is attributed to a combination of factors, including their globular structure, their large molecular size, and the magnitude of their negative charge.

Factors that affect the glomerular filtration rate (GFR) of drugs also can influence the rate of drug clearance. For instance, inflammation of the glomerular capillaries may result in an increased GFR and hence a greater extent of drug filtration. Most drugs are at least partially bound to plasma proteins, and therefore their actual filtration rates are less than the theoretical GFR. Anything that alters drug-protein binding, however, will change the drug filtration rate. The usual range of half-lives seen for most drugs that are cleared solely by glomerular filtration is 1 to 4 hr. However, considerably longer half-lives will be seen if extensive protein binding occurs.

Additionally, since water constitutes a larger percentage of the total body weight of the newborn than of individuals in other age groups, the apparent volume of distribution of water-soluble drugs is greater in neonates. This results in a lower concentration of drug in the blood coming to the kidneys per unit time and hence a decreased rate of drug clearance. The lower renal plasma flow in the newborn also could result in a decreased glomerular filtration of drugs.

Passive Diffusion

An important determinant in the urinary excretion of drugs (i.e., weak electrolytes) is the extent to which substances diffuse back across the tubular membranes and reenter the circulation. In general, the movement of drugs is favored from the tubular lumen to blood rather than from blood to lumen. This is due, in part, to the reabsorption of water that occurs throughout most portions of the nephron, and this may result in an increased concentration of drug and other solutes in the luminal fluid. The concentration gradient thus established will facilitate movement of the drug out of the tubular lumen, given that the lipid solubility and ionization of the drug are appropriate.

The pH of the urine (usually between 4.5 and 8.0) can markedly affect the rate of passive diffusion and hence of drug excretion. The back-diffusion occurs primarily in the distal tubules and collecting ducts, where most of the urine acidification takes place. Since it is the nonionized form of the drug that diffuses from the tubular fluid across the tubular cells into the blood, it follows that acidification increases reabsorption (or decreases elimination) of weak acids such as salicylates and promotes elimination (decreases reabsorption) of weak bases such as alkaloids. However, should the nonionized form of the drug not have sufficient lipid solubility, urinary pH changes will have little influence on urinary drug excretion.

Effects of pH on urinary drug elimination may have important applications in medical practice, especially in cases of drug overdose or poisoning. For example, one can reduce the half-life of a barbiturate (a weak acid) by administering bicarbonate to the patient. This procedure alkalinizes the urine and thus promotes the excretion of the now more completely ionized drug. The excretion of bases can be increased by making the urine more acidic through the use of an acidifying salt such as ammonium chloride. The passive transfer of compounds across biological membranes is discussed extensively in Chap. 3.

Active Tubular Secretion

A number of drugs, for example, organic anions (Fig. 5-1) and organic cations, can serve as substrates for the two active secretory systems located in the proximal tubule cells. These transport systems, which actively transfer drugs from blood to luminal fluid, are independent of each other; one secretes organic anions, the other secretes organic cations. It should be noted that one anion can compete for transport with a simultaneously administered or endogenously present anion; this competition will result in a decrease in the overall rate of excretion of each compound. The secretory capacity of both the organic anion and organic cation secretory systems can be saturated at high drug concentrations. Each drug will have its own characteristic maximum rate of secretion (*transport maximum,* T_m).

Some drugs that are not candidates for active tubular secretion may be metabolized to compounds that are. This is true for some drug metabolites that are formed as a result of conjugative reactions. Because the conjugates are

Figure 5-1. Active renal elimination of an organic anion. Note that the transport mechanism is located in the peritubular portion of the membrane of the proximal tubular cell.

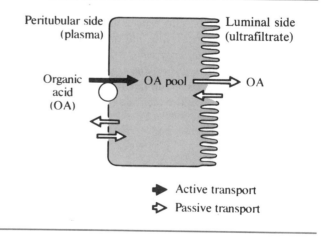

generally not pharmacologically active, increases in their rate of elimination through active secretion usually have little effect on the drug's duration of action, that is, duration of action is determined by metabolism.

These active secretory systems are important in drug excretion because *charged anions and cations are often strongly bound to plasma proteins* and therefore are not readily available for excretion by filtration. However, since the protein binding is usually reversible, the active secretory systems can rapidly and efficiently remove many protein-bound drugs from the blood and transport them into tubular fluid.

Any drug known to be largely excreted by the kidney that has a body half-life of less than 2 hr is probably eliminated, at least in part, by tubular secretion. Some drugs can be secreted *and* have long half-lives, however, because of extensive passive reabsorption in distal segments of the nephron (see Passive Diffusion).

Pharmacologically active drugs known to be secreted by the organic anion secretory system include penicillins, salicylates, ethacrynic acid, acetazolamide, and a number of the thiazide diuretics. Cations that are actively secreted include mecamylamine, tolazoline, hexamethonium, morphine, and the endogenous compounds—catecholamines, histamine, choline, and thiamine.

It is important to appreciate that these tubular transport mechanisms are not as well developed in the neonate as in the adult animal. In addition, their functional capacity may be diminished in the elderly. Thus, *compounds normally eliminated by tubular secretion will be excreted more slowly in the very young and in the older adult.* This age dependence of the rate of renal drug secretion may have important therapeutic implications and must be considered by the physician who prescribes drugs for these age groups.

In summary, the renal proximal tubule cell can actively transport certain anions and cations from blood to urine. At least with the anions, the movement of these substances involves a mediated transport step across the basolateral membrane, accumulation in the proximal tubular cell, and finally efflux across the brush border into the tubular fluid (Fig. 5-1). There still exists some uncertainty as to whether or not the mediated step for cation transport is on the basolateral or brush border side of the cell. In any event, these transport processes are against the electrochemical gradient for the compound (i.e., "uphill" transport) and require energy. Because discrete transporters are involved in the processes, coadministration of drugs that utilize the transporters can result in a reduced rate of renal secretion for each of the compounds, that is, competition occurs. Finally, it should be appreciated that compounds that undergo active tubular secretion also are filtered at the glomerulus (assuming protein binding is minimal). Hence, a reduction in secretory activity does not reduce

the excretory process to zero, but rather to a level that approximates the glomerular filtration rate.

Active Tubular Reabsorption

Some substances filtered at the glomerulus are subsequently reabsorbed by active transport systems found primarily in the proximal tubules. Active reabsorption is particularly important for endogenous substances that the body needs to conserve, such as ions, glucose, and amino acids (Fig. 5-2), although a small number of drugs also may be actively reabsorbed. The probable location of the active transport system is on the luminal side of the proximal cell membrane. *Bidirectional* active transport across the proximal tubule also occurs for some compounds; that is, a drug may be both actively reabsorbed and secreted. The occurrence of such bidirectional active transport mechanisms across the proximal tubule has been described for several organic anions, including the naturally occurring uric acid (see Chap. 44). The major portion of *filtered* urate is probably reabsorbed, whereas that eventually found in the urine is mostly derived from active tubular secretion.

In general, most drugs act by reducing active transport, rather than by enhancing it. Thus, drugs that promote uric acid loss (uricosuric agents, such as probenecid and sulfinpyrazone) probably inhibit active urate reabsorption, while pyrazinamide, which reduces urate excretion, may block the active tubular secretion of uric acid. A complicating observation is that a drug may primarily inhibit active reabsorption at one dose, and active secretion at another, frequently lower, dose. For example, small amounts of salicylate will decrease total urate excretion, while high doses have a uricosuric effect. This is offered

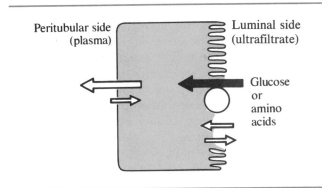

Figure 5-2. Active reabsorption of important substances that have been filtered at the glomerular membranes. Note that the transport mechanism is located in the luminal portion of the membrane of the proximal tubular cell. Solid arrow indicates active transport.

Peritubular side (plasma)

Luminal side (ultrafiltrate)

Glucose or amino acids

as an explanation of the apparently paradoxical effects of low and high doses of drugs on the total excretory pattern of compounds that are handled by renal active transport.

Summary of Renal Excretion

The rate of urinary drug excretion will depend on the drug's volume of distribution, its degree of protein binding, and the following renal factors:

1. Glomerular filtration rate
2. Tubular fluid pH
3. Extent of back-diffusion of the un-ionized form
4. Extent of active tubular secretion of the compound
5. Possibly, extent of active tubular reabsorption

Changes in any of these factors may result in clinically important alterations in drug action. In the final analysis, the amount of drug that finally appears in the urine will represent a balance between filtered, reabsorbed (passively and actively), and secreted drug. For many drugs, the duration and intensity of pharmacological effect will be influenced by the status of renal function because of the major role played by this organ in drug and metabolite elimination. Ultimately, whether or not dosage adjustment (e.g., prolongation of dosing interval, reduction in the maintenance dose, or some combination of these two) becomes necessary will depend on an assessment of the degree of renal dysfunction, the percentage of drug cleared by the kidney, and the potential for drug toxicity, especially under conditions of reduced renal function.

Biliary Excretion

The liver secretes about 1 liter of bile daily. Bile flow and composition depend on the secretory activity of the hepatic cells that line the biliary canaliculi. As the bile flows through the biliary system of ducts, its composition can be modified in the ductules and ducts by the processes of reabsorption and secretion, especially of electrolytes and water. In the gallbladder the composition of the bile is modified further through reabsorptive processes.

Osmotically active compounds, including bile acids, transported into the bile promote the passive movement of fluid into the duct lumen. After reaching the intestine, most of the bile acids are removed by an active intestinal epithelial transport system.

The passage of most foreign compounds from the blood into the liver normally is not restricted because the endothelium of the hepatic blood sinusoids behaves as a very porous membrane. Hence, drugs with molecular weights lower than those of most protein molecules readily reach the hepatic extracellular fluid from the plasma. A number of compounds are taken up into the liver by carrier-mediated systems, while other more lipophilic drugs pass through the hepatocyte membrane by diffusion. The subsequent passage of substances into the bile, however, is much more selective.

At least three groups of compounds enter the bile as determined by their concentrations in the bile compared to their concentrations in the blood. Compounds of group A are those whose concentration in bile and plasma are almost identical (bile-plasma ratio of 1). These include glucose, and ions such as Na^+, K^+, and Cl^-. Group B contains the bile salts, bilirubin glucuronide, sulfobromophthalein, procainamide ethobromide, and others, whose bile-blood ratio is much greater than 1, usually from 10 to 1,000. Group C is reserved for compounds for which the bile-blood ratio is less than 1, for example, insulin, sucrose, and proteins. Drugs can belong to any of these three categories. Only small amounts of most drugs reach the bile by diffusion. However, biliary excretion plays a major role (5–95% of the administered dose) in drug removal for three kinds of compounds: (1) anions, (2) cations, and (3) certain nonionized molecules, such as cardiac glycosides. In addition, biliary elimination also may be important for the excretion of some heavy metals.

Cardiac glycosides, anions, and cations are transported from the liver into the bile by three distinct and independent carrier-mediated active transport systems, the last two closely resembling those that secrete anions and cations into tubular urine. As is true for renal tubular secretion, protein-bound drug is completely available for biliary active transport. In contrast to the bile acids, the *actively secreted drugs* generally do not recycle, because they are not substrates for the intestinal bile acid transport system, and they are generally too highly charged to back-diffuse across the intestinal epithelium. Thus, the ability of certain compounds to be actively secreted into bile, without active or passive reabsorption from the intestinal tract, accounts for the large quantity of these drugs removed from the body by way of the feces.

On the other hand, most drugs that are secreted by the liver into the bile and then into the small intestine are not eliminated through the feces. The physicochemical properties of most drugs are sufficiently favorable for passive intestinal absorption to occur so that the compound will reenter the blood that perfuses the intestine and again be carried to the liver. Such recycling may continue (*enterohepatic cycle* or *circulation*) until the drug either undergoes metabolic changes in the liver or is excreted by the kidneys, or both. This process permits the conservation of such important endogenous substances as the bile acids, vitamins D_3 and B_{12}, folic acid, and estrogens (Table 5-1).

Table 5-1. Drugs that Undergo Enterohepatic Recirculation

Adriamycin	Methadone
Amphetamine	Metronidazole
Chlordecone	Morphine
1,25-Dihydoxyvitamin D$_3$	Phenytoin
Estradiol	Polar glucuronic acid conjugates
Indomethacin	Polar sulfate conjugates
Mestranol	Sulindac

Drugs known to undergo extensive enterohepatic cycling include cardiac glycosides, chlorpromazine, antibiotics, and indomethacin. An extensive amount of enterohepatic cycling may, in part, be responsible for a drug's long persistence in the body. Orally administered activated charcoal and anion-exchange resins have been used clinically to interrupt enterohepatic cycling and trap drugs in the gastrointestinal tract.

When foreign compounds enter the liver, many of them are either partially or extensively metabolized. The conjugation of a compound or its metabolites is an especially important factor in determining whether the drug will undergo biliary excretion. Frequently, when a compound is secreted into the intestine through the bile, it is in the form of a conjugate. *Conjugation generally enhances biliary excretion* since it both introduces a strong polar (i.e., anionic) center into the molecule and increases its molecular weight. Molecular weight may, however, be of less importance in the biliary excretion of organic cations. Conjugated drugs will not be reabsorbed readily from the gastrointestinal tract unless the conjugate is hydrolyzed by gut enzymes such as β-glucuronidase. Chloramphenicol glucuronide, for example, is secreted into the bile, where it is hydrolyzed by gastrointestinal flora and largely reabsorbed. Such a continuous recirculation may lead to the appearance of drug-induced toxicity.

The kidney and liver are, in general, capable of actively transporting the same organic anion substrates. However, there are certain quantitative differences in drug affinity for the transporters present in each of the two organs. It has been suggested that several subsystems of organic anion transport may exist and that the binding specificities of the transporters involved are not absolute, but overlapping.

Liver disease or injury may impair bile secretion and thereby lead to the accumulation of some drugs, for example, probenecid, digoxin, glutethimide, ouabain, and diethylstilbestrol. Impairment of liver function can lead both to decreased rates of drug metabolism and to decreased rates of secretion of drugs into bile. These two processes, of course, are frequently interrelated since many drugs are candidates for biliary secretion only after appropriate metabolism has occurred.

Decreases in biliary excretion have been demonstrated at both ends of the age continuum. For example, ouabain, a nonmetabolized cardiac glycoside that is secreted into the bile, is considerably more toxic in the newborn. This is largely due to a reduced ability of biliary secretion to remove ouabain from the plasma.

Increases in hepatic excretory function also may take place. After the chronic administration of either phenobarbital or the potassium-sparing diuretic spironolactone, the rate of bile flow is augmented. Such an increase in bile secretion can reduce blood levels of drugs that depend on biliary elimination.

Finally, the administration of one drug may influence the rate of biliary excretion of a second coadministered compound. These effects may be brought about through an alteration in one or more of the following factors: hepatic blood flow, uptake into hepatocytes, rate of biotransformation, transport into bile, or rate of bile formation. In addition, antibiotics may alter the intestinal flora in such a manner as to diminish the presence of sulfatase and glucuronidase-containing bacteria. This would result in a persistence of the conjugated form of the drug and hence a decrease in its enterohepatic recirculation.

Pulmonary Excretion

Any volatile material, irrespective of its route of administration, has the potential for pulmonary excretion. Certainly, gases and other volatile substances that enter the body primarily through the respiratory tract can be expected to be excreted by this route. *There are no specialized transport systems involved in the loss of substances in expired air; simple diffusion across cell membranes is predominant.* The rate of loss of gases is not constant, but depends on the rate of respiration and pulmonary blood flow.

The degree of solubility of a gas in blood also will affect the rate of gas loss. Gases such as nitrous oxide, which are not very soluble in blood, will be excreted rapidly, that is, almost at the rate at which the blood delivers the drug to the lungs. *Increasing cardiac output would have the greatest effect on the removal of poorly soluble gases;* for example, doubling the cardiac output nearly doubles the rates of loss. Agents with high blood and tissue solubility, on the other hand, are only slowly transferred from pulmonary capillary blood to the alveoli. Ethanol, which has a relatively high blood-gas solubility, is excreted very slowly by the lungs. *The arterial concentration of a highly soluble gas falls much more slowly, and its rate of loss is more dependent on respiratory rate than on cardiac output.* The importance of these and other physical and chemical factors is discussed in Chap. 29 for various anesthetic agents.

Most of the drugs undergoing removal by the pulmonary route are not metabolites but are usually the intact parent drug. A rise in cardiac output and, therefore, an increase in pulmonary blood flow, may substantially increase the rate of gas loss from the lung by presenting the alveoli with a greater amount of gas-containing blood per unit time. Since gas in the pulmonary capillaries equilibrates almost instantaneously with that in the alveoli, exercise or excitement may increase the rate of gas loss dramatically. However, if cardiac output is reduced, as occurs in shock, the reverse may be true. *When given anesthetic gases, patients in shock may require considerably more time before their blood levels fall to nonanesthetic concentrations.*

A more detailed discussion of the uptake, distribution, and elimination of inhalationally administered compounds can be found in Chap. 29.

Excretion in Other Body Fluids

Sweat and Saliva

Excretion of drugs into these two fluids occurs but is of only minor importance for most drugs. The mechanisms involved in drug excretion are similar for sweat and saliva. Excretion is primarily dependent on the diffusion of the nonionized, lipid-soluble form of the drug across the epithelial cells of the glands. Thus, the pK_a of the drug and the pH of the individual secretion formed in the glands are important determinants of the total quantity of drug appearing in the particular body fluid. It is not definitely established whether active drug transport occurs across the ducts of the glands.

Lipid-insoluble compounds, such as urea and glycerol, enter saliva and sweat at rates proportional to their molecular weight. This presumably occurs owing to filtration through the aqueous channels in the secretory cell membrane. Drugs or their metabolites that are excreted into sweat may be at least partially responsible for the dermatitis and other skin reactions observed as side effects of some therapeutic agents. Substances excreted into saliva are usually swallowed and therefore their fate is the same as that of orally administered drugs (unless expectoration is a major characteristic of a person's habits). The excretion of a drug into saliva accounts for the "drug taste" patients sometimes report after certain compounds are given intravenously.

Milk

Many drugs present in a nursing mother's blood will be detectable in her milk (Table 5-2). The ultimate concentration of the individual compound in milk will depend on many factors, including the amount of drug in the maternal

Table 5-2. Examples of Drugs that Appear in Breast Milk

Acetylsalicylic acid
Antithyroid uracil compounds
Barbiturates
Caffeine
Ethanol
Glutethimide
Morphine
Nicotine

blood, its lipid solubility, its degree of ionization, and the extent of its active excretion. Thus, the same physicochemical properties that govern the excretion of drugs into saliva and sweat also apply to the passage of drugs into milk.

Since milk is more acidic (pH 6.5) than plasma, basic compounds (e.g., alkaloids such as morphine, codeine, etc.) may be somewhat more concentrated in this fluid. In contrast, the levels of weak organic acids will probably be lower than those in plasma. In general, a high maternal plasma protein binding of drug will be associated with a low milk concentration. A highly lipid-soluble drug should tend to accumulate in milk fat. Low-molecular-weight un-ionized, water-soluble drugs will diffuse passively across the mammary epithelium and transfer into milk. There they may reside in association with one or more milk components, for example, bound to protein such as lactalbumin, dissolved within fat globules, or free in the aqueous compartment. Nonelectrolytes such as ethanol, urea, and antipyrene readily enter milk and reach approximately the same concentration as in plasma. Compounds used in agriculture also may be passed from cows to humans by this route. Finally, antibiotics such as the tetracyclines, which can function as chelating agents and bind calcium, will be found to have a higher milk than plasma concentration.

Both maternal and infant factors determine the final amount of drug present in the nursing child's body at any particular time. Variations in the daily amount of milk formed within the breast (e.g., changes in blood flow to the breast) as well as alterations in breast milk pH will affect the total amount of drug found in milk. In addition, the composition of the milk will be affected by the maternal diet; for example, a high-carbohydrate diet will increase the content of saturated fatty acids in milk.

The greatest drug exposure would occur when feeding has been initiated shortly after maternal drug dosing. Additional factors determining infant exposure would include milk volume consumed (~ 150 ml/kg/day) and milk composition at the time of feeding. Fat content is highest in the morning and then gradually decreases until about 10 P.M. A longer feed usually results in exposure of the infant to more of a fat-soluble drug since milk fat content increases somewhat during a given nursing period.

Whether or not a drug accumulates in a nursing child will, in part, be affected by the infant's ability to eliminate (via metabolism and excretion) the ingested compound. In general, the ability to carry out drug oxidation and conjugation reactions is low in the neonate and does not approach full adult rates until approximately age 6. It follows, therefore, that drug accumulation should be less in an older infant who breast-feeds than it is in a suckling neonate.

Although abnormalities in fetal organ structure and function can result from the presence of certain drugs in breast milk, it would be quite inappropriate to deny the breast-feeding woman appropriate and necessary drug therapy. A pragmatic approach on the part of both the physician and patient is necessary. *Breast-feeding should be discouraged when inherent drug toxicity is known or when adverse pharmacological actions of the drug on the infant are likely.* Infant drug exposure can be minimized, however, through short intermittent maternal drug use and by drug dosing immediately after breast-feeding.

Supplemental Reading

Bennett, P.N. (ed.). *Drugs and Human Lactation.* Amsterdam: Elsevier, 1988.

Cutler, R.E., et al. Extracorporeal removal of drugs and poisons by hemodialysis and hemoperfusion. *Annu. Rev. Pharmacol. Toxicol.* 27:169, 1987.

Klaassen, C.D., and Watkins, J.B. Mechanisms of bile formation, hepatic uptake, and biliary excretion. *Pharmacol. Rev.* 36:1, 1984.

Moller, J.V., and Sheikh, M.I. Renal organic anion transport system: Pharmacological, physiological and biochemical aspects. *Pharmacol. Rev.* 34:315, 1982.

Roberts, R.J. *Drug Therapy in Infants.* Philadelphia: Saunders, 1984.

Ross, C.R., and Holohan, P.D. Transport of organic anions and cations in isolated renal plasma membranes. *Annu. Rev. Pharmacol. Toxicol.* 23:65, 1983.

Walker, R.J., and Duggin, G.G. Drug nephrotoxicity. *Annu. Rev. Pharmacol. Toxicol.* 28:331, 1988.

Wilson, J.T. Determinants and consequences of drug excretion in breast milk. *Drug Metab. Rev.* 14:619, 1983.

6

Pharmacokinetics

Peter R. Gwilt

Pharmacokinetics is the mathematical description of the rate and extent of uptake, distribution, and elimination of drugs in the body. This area of study has developed primarily to clarify the relationship between the size and frequency of drug dose administration and the intensity and duration of the pharmacological effect. There has been increasing application of pharmacokinetics to clinical medicine, particularly with a view to individualization of dosing. For example, a patient develops a *Staphylococcus aureus* infection following surgery. Intravenous vancomycin, 750 mg every 8 hours, is prescribed. On the third dose, blood is drawn just before and shortly after dose administration. Vancomycin concentrations measured in these blood samples indicate that the drug levels are outside the therapeutic range. The same levels are then entered into a pharmacokinetic equation and a new dose of vancomycin is calculated that exactly matches the patient's needs. The use of such approaches to drug therapy clearly requires an understanding of the basics of pharmacokinetics, which are presented below. Clinical applications of the concepts and formulas discussed in this chapter are presented in the chapter appendix.

Basic Concepts

In order to employ relatively simple equations to describe drug uptake and disposition, the body is viewed as a single fluid-filled compartment (Fig. 6-1). An intravenous bolus injection of a drug is modeled by the instantaneous introduction of an amount of drug (D) into the compartment. It is further assumed that the drug is instantaneously distributed throughout the fluid in the compartment. The volume of the compartment is known as the volume of distribution of the drug. Simultaneous with distribution, the drug undergoes elimination from the body. This process might involve chemical conversion of the drug in the liver to a metabolite or physical removal

through the kidney. Collectively, this process is called *elimination* and is usually *a first-order process; that is, the rate of elimination of the drug from the body is proportional to the concentration of drug in the blood.* This is analogous to the common observation that the rate of drainage of water from a tank is proportional to the height of the water level. In mathematical terms, the rate of elimination proportional to C, the concentrations of drug in the blood, is expressed by

$$\frac{dC}{dt} \propto C \tag{1}$$

where dC/dt is the rate of decline of the drug concentration in the blood. The equation can be refined to include a proportionality term, K, to yield

$$\frac{dC}{dt} = -KC \tag{2}$$

The proportionality term is called the elimination rate constant. The negative sign is included, indicating that the drug concentration is decreasing with time.

Since the drug concentration, rather than its differential, is the focus of interest, equation (2) is solved to give

$$c = c_o e^{-Kt} \tag{3}$$

K is now incorporated into an exponential term and C_o is the concentration of drug in the blood immediately after dose administration. A plot of the concentration of drug in the blood after intravenous bolus administration is shown in Fig. 6-2. A comparison of this figure with innumerable examples in the literature of plots of drug concentration–time data following intravenous administration confirms the validity of this simple approach.

Returning to the fluid-filled compartment model, when the drug dose is placed in the compartment, it immediately distributes throughout the fluid-filled volume.

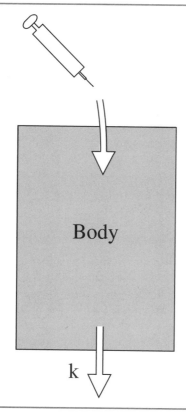

Figure 6-1. Configuration of the one-compartment pharmacokinetic model.

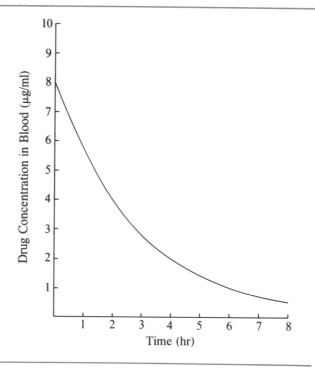

Figure 6-2. Decline in drug concentrations in the blood with time for a drug with one-compartment pharmacokinetics.

In mathematical terms, the volume of distribution of a drug in the body, V, can be expressed by

$$V = \frac{X}{C} \qquad (4)$$

where X is the amount of drug in the body and C is the concentration of drug in the blood. Since the only time that the amount of intact drug in the body is known with certainty is immediately after dose administration the volume of distribution is estimated by dividing the dose by the initial drug concentration in the blood C_o,

$$V = \frac{D}{C_o} \qquad (5)$$

To characterize the pharmacokinetics of a drug in a patient, it is necessary to determine the elimination rate constant as well as the volume of distribution. This is difficult to do from Fig. 6-2. A convenient way of estimating the elimination rate constant is to replot the data in Fig. 6-2 as the natural logarithm of the concentration against time

(ln C vs. t). Taking the natural logarithm of equation (3) gives

$$\ln C = \ln C_o - Kt \qquad (6)$$

This is the equation of a straight line. Therefore, a plot of the logarithm of drug concentration against time (Fig. 6-3) would yield a line, the slope of which is K, the elimination rate constant, and the intercept is equal to ln C_o.

In most cases in the literature, the half-life ($t_{1/2}$) rather than the elimination rate constant is recorded. *The half-life is defined as the time taken for the drug concentration in the blood to decline to one half of the current value.* Thus, if the concentration of drug in the blood is 10 mg per liter at 2 hr and 5 mg/L at 6 hr, the half-life of the drug is 4 hr. Half-life is related to the elimination rate constant by the following equation

$$t_{1/2} = \frac{0.693}{K} \qquad (7)$$

where 0.693 is the natural logarithm of 2.

One additional parameter required to describe the pharmacokinetics of a drug is clearance. This term has been used for many years in clinical medicine to characterize elimination or excretion. *Clearance is defined as the*

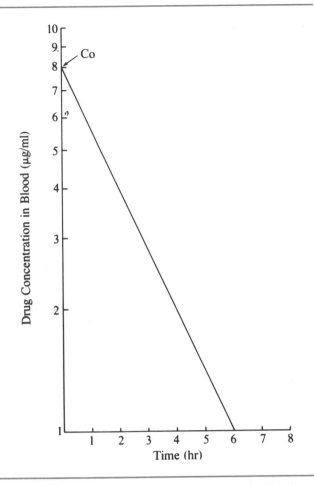

Figure 6-3. Decline in drug concentrations in the blood with time for a drug with one-compartment pharmacokinetics (semilogarithmic plot). Co = initial drug concentration.

theoretical volume of fluid from which drug is completely removed over a period of time. A well-known example is the use of creatinine clearance to estimate renal function. Creatinine clearance is determined by the following formula:

$$Cl_{cr} = U_{cr} \times \frac{V}{C_{cr}} \qquad (8)$$

where Cl_{cr} is creatinine clearance, C_{cr} is the serum creatinine concentration, V is the volume flow of urine, and U_{cr} is the concentration of creatinine in the urine. The product of U_{cr} and V is the excretion rate of creatinine. Rearranging equation (8) and expressing the creatinine excretion rate as dX_{cr}/dt, we get

$$\frac{dX_{cr}}{dt} = Cl_{cr}C_{cr} \qquad (9)$$

Since creatinine is almost exclusively removed from the body by the kidneys, dX_{cr}/dt is also the elimination rate. Using equation (4), equation (9) can be further modified to

$$\frac{d(VC_{cr})}{dt} = Cl_{cr}C_{cr} \qquad (10)$$

where V is the volume of distribution of creatinine. Rearranging equation (10) gives

$$\frac{dC_{cr}}{dt} = \frac{Cl_{cr}}{V} C_{cr} \qquad (11)$$

In general terms for a drug, the decline in drug concentrations in the blood can be described by

$$\frac{dC}{dt} = -\frac{Cl}{V} C \qquad (12)$$

Comparing this equation with equation (2), it follows that

$$K = \frac{Cl}{V} \qquad (13)$$

and from equation (7)

$$t_{1/2} = 0.693 \frac{V}{Cl} \qquad (14)$$

This is a very important relationship because it demonstrates that *the half-life of a drug is dependent on both the volume of distribution and the clearance.* Thus, a long half-life need not necessarily reflect slow elimination. A drug could have very efficient metabolism, but because it exhibits a large volume of distribution it may have a very long half-life.

Oral or First-Order Absorption

Most drugs are administered by mouth and most frequently in tablet form. Unlike intravenous bolus administration, in which the input to the circulation is instantaneous, oral administration delivers drug over a period of time. This input process can usually best be described by a first-order process similar to that characterizing elimination. Figure 6-4 shows the concentration-time curve of a drug following oral administration.

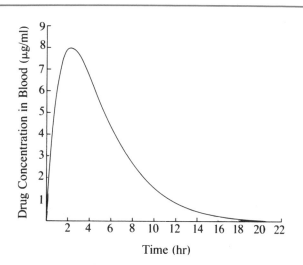

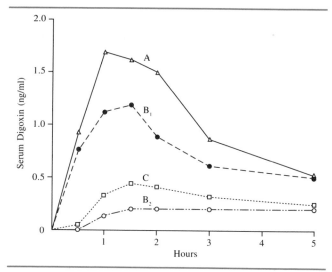

Figure 6-4. Drug concentration–time curve in the blood following oral administration.

Figure 6-5. Mean serum digoxin levels over a 5-hour period after oral administration of four digoxin products (0.5 mg digoxin as two 0.25-mg tablets) to four volunteers. Each line represents the mean of four curves. (From J. Lindenbaum et al., Variation in biologic availability of digoxin from four preparations *N. Engl. J. Med.* 285:1344, 1971.

The following equation describes the drug concentrations in the blood following oral administration:

$$C = \frac{Ka\ F\ D}{V(Ka - K)}\ (e^{-Kt} - e^{-Kat}) \qquad (15)$$

All of the parameters in equation (15), except for F and Ka, are the same as in equations (2) through (6). F is the fraction of the oral dose that is delivered to the systemic circulation and Ka is the first-order absorption rate constant.

Examination of Fig. 6-4 reveals certain parameters that characterize an oral absorption curve. These are (1) *the time to the peak concentration,* (2) *the peak concentration,* and (3) *the area under the drug concentration–time curve.* The time to the peak concentration depends on the relationship between the absorption rate constant and the elimination rate constant. The greater the absorption rate constant (or the smaller the elimination rate constant) the earlier the peak. Increasing the dose does not influence the time of the peak but will increase the peak concentration itself. The area under the drug concentration–time curve (AUC) is the ratio of the amount of drug that reaches the systemic circulation and the clearance of the drug. The greater the fraction of the dose that reaches the circulation the greater the AUC. Conversely, the higher the clearance the lower the AUC.

The AUC affords a method for estimating the fraction of an oral dose that is absorbed. The AUC following oral administration is compared to the AUC following intravenous administration. Since a dose given by the latter route is completely available to the systemic circulation, and the clearance of the drug is the same regardless of the route of administration, the ratio of the oral and intravenous AUCs gives F, that is,

$$F = \frac{AUC_{oral}}{AUC_{intravenous}} \qquad (16)$$

Similarly, one can compare the relative absorption (F_{rel}) of two formulations of the same drug, whether made by the same manufacturer or another pharmaceutical company, by comparing the AUCs following administration of both formulations to a panel of subjects.

$$F_{rel} = \frac{AUC_{oral}(1)}{AUC_{oral}(2)} \qquad (17)$$

The assessment of relative absorption or bioequivalence has become particularly important in evaluating the therapeutic equivalence of multisource (generic) drugs. The Food and Drug Administration (FDA) requires that two such formulations must not differ significantly with respect to the time to peak concentration, the peak concentration, and the AUC. Figure 6-5 illustrates differences in drug concentration–time curves following administration of different brands of digoxin.

Chronic Administration

Most drugs need repeated administration to be of therapeutic benefit. This may require continuous intravenous

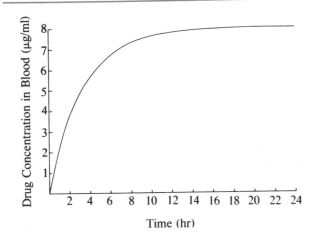

Figure 6-6. Drug concentrations in the blood resulting from a constant infusion.

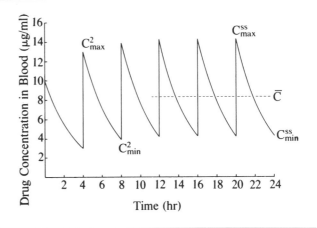

Figure 6-7. Drug concentration–time profile in the blood obtained following multiple intravenous administrations.

infusion or repeated oral or parenteral administration. Both methods of drug delivery are adequately described by pharmacokinetic equations.

Figure 6-6 shows the drug concentration–time profile obtained during continuous intravenous infusion. It can be seen that the drug concentration in the blood increases until it becomes constant. This steady-state concentration is achieved for the following reason: Drug is delivered at a constant rate, generally by an infusion pump. The drug elimination rate, however, is proportional to the drug concentration in the blood. As the drug concentration in the blood rises, the elimination rate also increases until the rate of elimination equals the rate of input. This steady-state level is given by

$$C_{ss} = \frac{K_0}{Cl} \qquad (18)$$

where C_{ss} is the steady-state drug concentration in the blood and K_o is the infusion rate.

This relationship is particularly useful in determining the optimal rate at which to infuse a drug. The desired therapeutic level for many drugs is known. Furthermore, the average clearance of a great number of drugs is established in the literature. This information allows an estimate of the appropriate infusion rate to achieve a desired therapeutic drug concentration in the blood. Furthermore, by taking a steady-state drug concentration in the blood during the infusion, immediate dose adjustment is possible when the clearance of the individual differs significantly from the population mean clearance value.

From Fig. 6-6 it can be seen that a significant period of time may elapse before the target drug concentration is attained. In fact, pharmacokinetic theory predicts that *four half-lives must elapse before steady state is achieved*. Thus, a pa-

tient may remain at subtherapeutic concentrations for a considerable period of time if the drug has a long half-life. To avoid this, a *loading dose* can be given at the start of the infusion, which will result in immediate attainment of steady-state drug concentrations. Theory indicates that the appropriate loading dose (D*) would be

$$D^* = C_{ss}V \qquad (19)$$

In addition to continuous intravenous infusion, drugs can be administered chronically by repeated administration of intravenous bolus, oral, or other doses. The equations for drug concentrations in the blood following single-dose administration previously developed in this chapter can be modified to include the dose interval, τ, and the number of doses administered, n. An equation describing the concentration of drug in the blood at any time during administration of multiple intravenous bolus doses is

$$C_n = \frac{D}{V}\left[\frac{1 - e^{-nKt}}{1 - e^{-Kt}}\right]e^{-Kt} \qquad (20)$$

where t is the time after the nth dose has been given and D is the dose given every τ hours. It can be seen that this equation is in fact equal to the equation of a single dose multiplied by the "multiple dose" function in brackets. The concentrations obtained during multiple IV bolus administration are depicted in Fig. 6-7.

As with chronic administration via continuous intravenous infusion, the concentrations increase until they achieve a steady-state level. The average steady-state drug level attained during chronic intravenous bolus administration is given by

$$C_{ss} = \frac{D/\tau}{Cl} \qquad (21)$$

There is an obvious similarity between this equation and equation (18). This is true because of the similarity between K_o and D/τ, the second term signifying the average rate of drug administration during repeated intravenous bolus administration.

Multicompartment Models

The time course of a drug in the blood cannot always be described by equation (3). This equation requires that the body be represented by a single compartment and that distribution of the drugs to the tissues is extremely rapid relative to the overall time course of the drug in the body.

Many drugs, because of their physicochemical characteristics, are not rapidly taken up by tissues in the body. Figure 6-8 represents the concentration profile of such a drug. Comparing this plot with Fig. 6-3, it is seen that at early time points the plot of log concentration against time is curvilinear and only at later times is the linear relation between log concentration and time attained.

Figure 6-8. Drug concentrations in the blood of a drug with two-compartment pharmacokinetics following an intravenous bolus dose. $\gamma_1 = 50\ \mu g/ml$; $\gamma_2 = 10\ \mu g/ml$.

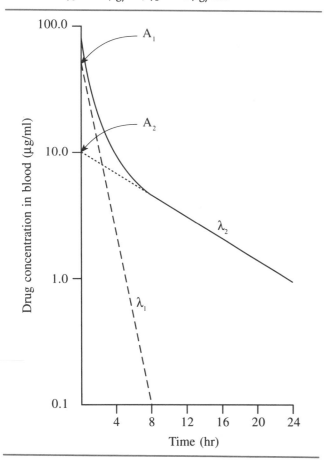

Upon administration, drug rapidly distributes to highly perfused tissues such as the lungs and liver. The curvilinear section of Fig. 6-8 represents redistribution of drug from these highly perfused regions to less accessible, poorly perfused tissues such as muscle and fat. Such drugs are therefore modeled by considering the body as two connected compartments; one compartment, the *central* compartment, consisting of blood and highly perfused tissues and a second compartment (the peripheral compartment) consisting of the less accessible, poorly perfused tissues (see Fig. 6-8). Since the eliminating organs are highly perfused, elimination is considered to occur exclusively from the central compartment.

Just as the single-compartment model requires a single exponent to describe the relationship between drug concentration and time [equation (3)], so the two-compartment model is expressed by two exponential terms or

$$C = C_1 e^{-\lambda_1 t} + C_2 e^{-\lambda_2 t} \tag{22}$$

This equation is best explained by examining Fig. 6-8.

The portion of the curve at later times is described by $C_2 e^{-\lambda_2 t}$ where λ_2 is similar to the elimination rate constant in equation (3). The half-life of the drug is given by $0.693/\lambda_2$. Early time points are largely dependent on $C_1 e^{-\lambda_1 t}$. Thus, the correct expression for each drug concentration time point is the sum of both exponential terms given in equation (22).

Physiological Determinants of Pharmacokinetic Parameters

Up to this point, pharmacokinetic terms have been introduced solely as mathematical parameters, whereas in fact they are intimately related to anatomical and physiological functions. An understanding of the effects of altered physiological states and disease on pharmacokinetics is not possible without an appreciation of this connection. The relationship between anatomy and physiology and the two primary determinants of drug disposition, volume of distribution and clearance, are now discussed.

Volume of Distribution

The volume of distribution of a drug relates the concentration of drug in the blood to the amount of drug in the body [equation (4)]. Any factor that increases the fraction of drug in the tissues relative to that in the blood will increase the volume of distribution. Thus, lipophilic drugs, which are able to penetrate the intracellular space, are more likely to have a larger volume of distribution than compounds that are restricted to the extracellular fluid. Also, if a drug exhibits greater affinity for tissue macromolecules than for those in the blood, the volume of distribution will tend toward higher values. *The volume of distribution* of a drug is therefore determined by the *physiological space into which it penetrates and the relative affinity of the drug for the tissues compared to the blood.* These relationships have been expressed by the equation

$$V = V_B + \frac{fu}{fu_T} V_T \qquad (23)$$

where V_B and V_T are the physiological spaces occupied by the blood and tissues and fu and fu_T are the fractions of unbound drug in the blood and tissues, respectively. Thus, it is clear that when there is no binding (fu = fu_T = 1) the volume of distribution equals total body water, or V_B + V_T. When binding in the tissue is much greater than that in the blood (fu_T < fu), the volume of distribution can greatly exceed total body water.

Hepatic Clearance

The rate at which the liver eliminates a drug depends on three primary physiological parameters—liver blood flow (Q); intrinsic clearance, that is, intrinsic enzyme activity (Clint); and the fraction of unbound drug in the blood (fu). These variables have been related to hepatic clearance by the following equation

$$Cl_H = \frac{Q \, fu \, Clint}{Q + fu \, Clint} \qquad (24)$$

This equation predicts that when intrinsic enzyme activity is large compared to blood flow, the latter term controls hepatic clearance and Cl_H = Q. Drugs for which this is true are designated highly extracted drugs. Conversely, when enzyme activity is low compared to blood flow, the product of the fraction of drug unbound in the blood and intrinsic clearance predominates, or Cl_H = fu Clint. Such drugs are described as poorly extracted drugs. If a poorly extracted drug also has high binding in the blood (fu < 0.1), it is further classified as binding sensitive. This term is used because slight changes in the binding of a highly bound drug can result in sizable changes in fu and therefore in hepatic clearance. For example, changing the binding of a drug from 99 to 98 percent binding doubles the fraction unbound (fu changes from 0.01 to 0.02) and consequently the clearance will double. Poorly extracted drugs, with low binding, are classified as binding insensitive, since changes in binding result in only slight changes in fu. Changes in the hepatic clearance of poorly extracted, binding-insensitive drugs directly reflect changes in enzyme activity or intrinsic clearance.

Pharmacokinetics in Disease States

Pharmacokinetic parameters are now available for most drugs. These parameters are obtained initially in studies using healthy, young volunteers. Other patient populations, such as the elderly, the very young, and pregnant women, may have very different kinetics. Furthermore, it should be remembered that many disease states can profoundly alter the kinetics of a drug.

Hepatic Disease

Hepatic disease can affect each of the three physiological parameters that determine hepatic clearance [equation (24)]. Hepatic blood flow, although highly variable, appears to be reduced during chronic liver failure, and the hepatic clearance of highly extracted drugs such as propranolol and lidocaine is correspondingly lower.

Poorly extracted, binding-sensitive drugs are affected by both changes in binding and intrinsic clearance. Chronic liver disease brings about an impaired synthesis of both albumin and many of the drug-metabolizing enzymes. The reduction in circulating albumin often results in decreased binding, particularly for acid drugs, which may offset any decrease in intrinsic clearance. In fact, for tolbutamide, the decrease in protein binding is greater than the reduction in intrinsic clearance, so that the clearance of this drug in patients with liver failure is greater than in those with normal hepatic function.

Drugs that are poorly extracted and have low binding in the blood are dependent only on changes in intrinsic clearance. It would be expected that all drugs of this class would exhibit a decreased clearance in liver failure. However, not all routes of metabolism are equally affected by liver disease. While phase I, oxidative metabolism, is reduced in chronic hepatic disease, glucuronidation (phase II) apparently is not.

Renal Disease

Although the major effect of renal disease on drug kinetics is a reduction in excretion, for many drugs absorption, distribution, and metabolism are also affected. The potential for altered drug absorption in patients with renal failure is substantial. Gastrointestinal problems such as gastroenteritis accompanied by anorexia, nausea, and vomiting are not uncommon. Furthermore, patients typically ingest copious amounts of aluminum-containing antacids, which are known to interfere with the absorption of many compounds. Unfortunately, very few carefully designed studies investigating the influence of renal failure on drug absorption have been reported.

The distribution of drugs in patients with renal disease, on the other hand, has been widely studied. Acidic drugs, such as phenytoin and warfarin, that are extensively bound to plasma albumin have larger volumes of distribution, increased clearances, and, consequently, lower drug concentrations in the blood. The binding of these drugs is generally reduced in renal failure. This is due either to a reduction in circulating plasma albumin levels, as in the nephrotic syndrome, or to the presence of endogenous inhibitors. These inhibitors, thought to be low-molecular-weight peptides, normally are efficiently cleared by the kidney. In renal failure they accumulate in the plasma and compete with acidic drugs for albumin-binding sites.

The binding of basic drugs for the most part does not appear to be affected by renal disease, although the acute-phase reactant, α_1-acid glycoprotein, has been observed to increase in uremia, and increased binding of some basic drugs has been reported.

Finally, nonrenal elimination also can be affected by renal disease. While the hepatic clearance of most drugs remains unchanged by kidney disease, several drugs commonly used in renal failure exhibit altered hepatic elimination. The extraction ratio of certain highly extracted drugs, including propranolol and propoxyphene, is reduced in renal failure.

Poorly extracted drugs that are binding sensitive, such as phenytoin, may have an increased hepatic clearance, largely due to decreased binding in the blood. The hepatic clearance of poorly extracted, binding-insensitive drugs directly reflects the intrinsic clearance of the drug by the liver and the activity of the various routes of metabolism. Most poorly extracted binding-insensitive drugs undergoing oxidation or conjugation appear to be unaffected by renal disease, although again there are exceptions, for example, the oxidation of antipyrine, which exhibits an increased clearance in subjects with renal failure. Other mechanisms of biotransformation such as reduction and hydrolysis are apparently depressed, as exemplified by the decreased reduction of cortisol and the diminished hydrolysis of procaine.

Cardiac Disease

Cardiac failure results in a blood flow that is insufficient to meet the needs of the tissues. This reduced blood flow and its compensatory sequelae can have profound effects on the absorption and disposition of drugs.

With regard to drug absorption, both a delay and a reduction in the amount of drug absorbed from extravascular sites may be expected. Sympathetically mediated vasoconstriction reduces blood flow to intramuscular

absorption sites. A similar reduction in mesenteric blood flow coupled with mucosal edema may account for the reduced oral absorption of drugs such as metolazone, hydrochlorothiazide, and prazosin in patients with cardiac failure. The apparent delay in the absorption of quinidine and procainamide may correspond to reduced gastrointestinal motility as a result of increased sympathetic and decreased parasympathetic activity.

The volume of distribution of several drugs, including lidocaine, disopyramide, procainamide, and quinidine, is significantly reduced in cardiac failure. It is thought that reduced blood flow to the muscles, a large storage site for lipid-soluble drugs, contributes to the smaller volume of distribution of these drugs. Increased binding of basic drugs to an α_1-acid glycoprotein that is elevated following myocardial infarction may also bring about reduced volumes of distribution.

With a reduction in the cardiac index of patients with cardiac failure, hepatic blood flow is reduced proportionally. It is not surprising, then, that drugs that are highly extracted by the liver, such as lidocaine, demonstrate reduced hepatic clearance in patients with congestive heart failure. Hepatocellular damage may also occur subsequent to hepatic congestion, hypoperfusion, and hypoxemia arising from heart failure. The intrinsic clearance of poorly extracted drugs may therefore be decreased in cardiac failure, and a reduced hepatic clearance of such drugs as aminopyrine and furosemide has been reported. Elevated α_1-acid glycoprotein may also contribute to the reduced clearance of basic drugs that are poorly extracted and binding sensitive.

Finally, blood flow to the kidneys is also diminished in patients with heart failure. This results in a decrease in glomerular filtration, and thus renal clearance. In addition, blood flow is redistributed within the kidney, with blood diverted from the cortical to the juxtamedullary region. Since the sites for tubular secretion are located in this area, this mechanism of excretion may feature more prominently in the overall renal clearance of drugs in patients with heart failure.

Supplemental Reading

Benet, L.Z., Massoud, N., and Gambertoglio, J.F. Pharmacokinetic basis for drug treatment. New York: Raven, 1984.

Evans, W.E., Schentag, J.J., and Jusko, W.J. (eds.). *Applied Pharmacokinetics* (3rd ed.). San Francisco: Applied Therapeutics, 1992.

Gibaldi, M. *Biopharmaceutics and Clinical Pharmacokinetics*. Philadelphia: Lea & Febiger, 1991.

Gibaldi, M., and Prescott, L. (eds.). *Handbook of Clinical Pharmacokinetics*. Balgowlah, New Zealand: ADIS Health Science, 1983.

Rowland, M., and Tozer, T.N. *Clinical Pharmacokinetics: Concepts and Applications* (2nd ed.). Philadelphia: Lea & Febiger, 1989.

Appendix

Example 1

An individual receives an intravenous bolus dose of 100 mg of a drug. Blood samples are drawn and analyzed for drug content. The following drug concentrations were found:

TIME (HR)	CONCENTRATION (μg/L)
0	500
2	250
4	125
6	62.5

Determine the volume of distribution, the elimination rate constant, the half-life, and the clearance of the drug.

Solution

The first step would be to plot ln C versus time. The parameters would then be estimated as follows:

1. Volume of distribution
   From equation (5),

$$V = \frac{D}{C_0} = \frac{100 \text{ mg}}{500 \text{ } \mu g/L}$$

$$= \frac{1,000 \times 100 \text{ } \mu g}{500 \text{ } \mu g/L} = 200 \text{ L}$$

2. Elimination rate constant
   Slope $= -K$

$$\text{Slope} = \frac{\ln C_1 - \ln C_2}{t_1 - t_2} = \frac{\ln 250 - \ln 125}{2 - 4}$$

$$\text{Slope} = \frac{5.521 - 4.838}{-2} = \frac{0.693}{-2} = -0.346 \text{ hr}^{-1}$$

   Therefore, $K = 0.346 \text{ hr}^{-1}$.
3. Half-life
   From equation (7)

$$t_{1/2} = \frac{0.693}{K} = \frac{0.693}{0.346} = 2 \text{ hr}$$

4. Clearance
   From equation (13)

$$K = \frac{Cl}{V}$$

Therefore,

$$Cl = KV = 0.346 \text{ hr}^{-1} \times 200 \text{ L} = 69 \text{ L/hr}$$

Example 2

A patient requires intravenous infusion of a drug. The average clearance of the drug is 27 L/hr, the steady-state target concentration is 10 mg/L, and the volume of distribution is 40 L. Calculate a suitable infusion rate to achieve the target concentration and a loading dose.

Solution

Rearranging equation (18), $C_{ss} = \frac{K_0}{Cl}$,

$$K_0 = C_{ss}Cl = 10 \text{ mg/L} \times 27 \text{ L/hr} = 270 \text{ mg/hr}$$

The loading dose is estimated from equation (19),

$$D^* = C_{ss}V = 10 \text{ mg/L} \times 40 \text{ L} = 400 \text{ mg}$$

Twelve hours later, the patient is experiencing nausea and agitation, both toxic effects of this drug. A blood sample is drawn and a drug level of 30 mg/L is returned. Estimate a new infusion rate suitable for this patient.

Evidently, this patient has a clearance that is lower than normal. The clearance can be calculated by rearranging equation (18)

$$Cl = \frac{K_0}{C_{ss}} = \frac{270 \text{ mg/hr}}{30 \text{ mg/L}} = 9 \text{ L/hr}$$

The new K_0 can now be calculated:

$$K_0 = ClC_{ss} = 9 \text{ L/hr} \times 10 \text{ mg/L} = 90 \text{ mg/hr}$$

Example 3

A drug has a clearance of 3 L/hr and a half-life of 6 hr. The therapeutic range of the drug in the blood is 10 to 20 mg/L. At what rate would you administer the drug?

Solution

Let the target concentration be midway between the upper and lower limits of the therapeutic range, that is, 15 mg/L. Rearranging equation (21), $C_{ss} = \dfrac{D/\tau}{Cl}$,

$$\frac{D}{\tau} = C_{ss}Cl = 15 \text{ mg/L} \times 3 \text{ L/hr} = 45 \text{ mg/hr}$$

The dose could be administered in a number of ways. For example, it could be given as 1080 mg every 24 hr, 540 mg q12h, or 270 mg q6h. Each combination would result in the same C_{ss} but different peak and trough concentrations. A rule of thumb for determining the dosing interval that would keep the peak and trough concentrations within the therapeutic range is that the maximum dosing interval possible (τ_{max}) for the drug to stay in the therapeutic range at steady state is given by

$$\tau_{max} = 1.44 \, t_{1/2} \ln TI$$

where TI is the therapeutic index and is equal to the ratio of the upper to the lower limit of the therapeutic range. Since in this case TI is 2, and $t_{1/2}$ is 6 hr, τ_{max} is 6 hr. Therefore, a safe and effective dosage regimen for this drug would be 270 mg q6h. Equation (20) could now be used to generate the exact time course of the drug concentrations in the blood during the entire dosage regimen.

7

Drug Delivery Systems

Peter R. Gwilt

For many drugs there is a direct relationship between the pharmacological response and the drug concentration at the receptor site. The concentration depends not only on the disposition kinetics of the drug but also on the efficiency and the design of the drug delivery system. The *drug delivery system* is the sequence of events that culminates in the delivery of drug to the site of drug action. This process includes the administration of the drug product, the release of the active ingredient by the product, and the subsequent transport of the active ingredient across biological membranes to the site of action. Improving the efficiency of the system in increasing the rate and extent of drug delivery should result in increased rate of onset and an elevated intensity of drug response. With specially designed drug delivery systems, such as prolonged-release medication, the duration of drug action may be greater than that attained with conventional formulations.

Bioavailability and Bioequivalence

Different formulations of the same drug will not necessarily produce identical pharmacological responses. The availability of a drug may be affected by the dosage form in which it is contained. The term *bioavailability* refers to the rate and extent of drug absorption from a dosage form.

There is much evidence indicating that a drug's absorption, and therefore therapeutic performance, can be markedly affected by the materials and methods used in the manufacture of the dosage form. The physician must therefore realize that generically equivalent preparations (containing the same quantity of active drug) from different commercial sources cannot be assumed to have the same clinical effect or result in identical blood levels.

The most reliable and sensitive method of determining bioavailability involves an analysis of plasma or serum concentrations of the drug at various times after oral administration (Fig. 7-1). Several components of the curve that describes serum drug concentration as a function of time (see Fig. 7-1) provide important information on bioavailability. For example, *the peak drug concentration* (peak height) in blood is the highest concentration achievable with a particular formulation. The *rate* of drug absorption is reflected by the time required to achieve the maximum concentration following drug administration. Figure 7-2 illustrates how differences in bioavailability may affect the therapeutic performance of a formulation.

The area under the serum concentration–time curve (see Fig. 7-1) also provides pertinent information on drug bioavailability. The area is proportional to the total amount of drug absorbed. *For products to be considered bioequivalent, the areas under the curves derived after administration of different formulations of the same drug, the peak concentration, and time to reach peak concentration should not be significantly different.*

Differences in bioavailability will be significant depending on the potency and toxicity associated with the individual drug under evaluation. *The clinical importance of bioavailability and bioequivalence data is greatest for drugs with a low therapeutic index,* such as antiarrhythmics, anticonvulsants, and bronchodilators. Bioequivalence data for drugs with large therapeutic indices (e.g., antimicrobials), however, do not have the same clinical importance. Differences of less than 25 percent in absorption parameters among several formulations will usually have no significant effect on clinical outcome.

Oral Medication

Drug administration most frequently involves the gastrointestinal tract. Absorption may occur from buccal, sublingual, and rectal dosage forms as well as from the more common oral medication. Commonly encountered oral dosage forms are solutions, suspensions, capsules, tablets, or coated tablets; the rate of appearance of a drug in

65

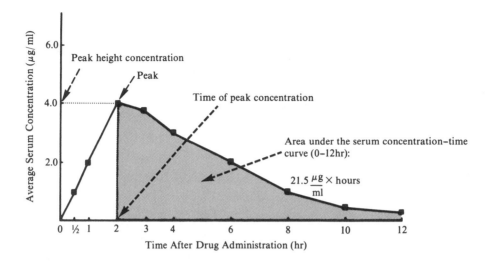

Figure 7-1. A model drug-blood level curve such as might be seen following oral administration of a drug. The parameters important in evaluating the bioavailability of this drug are (1) peak height concentration, (2) time of peak concentration, and (3) area under the serum concentration–time curve. (From D.J. Chodos and A.R. DiSanto, *Basics of Bioavailability*. Kalamazoo, Mich.: Upjohn, 1973.)

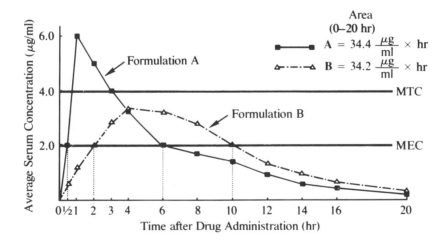

Figure 7-2. A comparison of the drug-blood level curves of two formulations of a hypnotic compound. MTC = minimum toxic concentration; MEC = minimum effective concentration. The areas under the serum concentration curves are identical for the two formulations; therefore, equal amounts of both are absorbed. Formulation A, however, would produce its effects sooner; it would produce toxic effects (i.e., levels exceed MTC); and its effects would be terminated earlier than those of formulation B (i.e., levels fall below MEC). Formulation B would induce sleep later (about 2 hr following administration); it would not be expected to produce any signs of toxicity; and its effects would persist much longer. (From D.J. Chodos and A.R. DiSanto, *Basics of Bioavailability*. Kalamazoo, Mich.: Upjohn, 1973.)

the systemic circulation following administration of these dosage forms is roughly in the order given above. Drug delivery is generally fastest by solution and slowest by coated tablet.

Solutions

Liquid dosage forms such as solutions and suspensions are particularly useful in the administration of drugs to children and other patients who are either unable or unwilling to ingest a tablet or capsule.

Drug delivery by the oral route is generally most rapid when the drug is administered in solution. The initial steps of drug release from the dosage form, that is, disintegration and dissolution, are not required. *Since drug absorption is usually most rapid in the proximal small intestine, the rate-limiting step in the overall absorption of a drug from solution is frequently gastric emptying.*

Not all drugs are inherently soluble in water, and they must, therefore, be solubilized either by converting the drug to a soluble form such as a salt or by adding a cosolvent (e.g., alcohol) to aid solution. The solution dosage form poses problems for drugs that are unpalatable and unstable in solution.

Suspensions

A suspension consists of a dispersion of relatively coarse particles, usually in an aqueous vehicle. Like solutions, suspensions are useful in patients who cannot tolerate a solid dosage form. An additional advantage of a suspension is that the dose can usually be contained in a smaller volume than that of a solution. Because the drug is in an insoluble form, unpalatable drugs are better tolerated and drugs that are unstable in solution exhibit a slower rate of degradation.

Water-insoluble drugs such as phenytoin can be suspended directly in an aqueous medium. Other drugs require formulation as an insoluble ester or salt. Suspensions of relatively large particles tend to settle and necessitate addition of a suspending agent. Suspending agents prevent settling, usually by increasing the viscosity of the medium or by reducing the attractive forces between the particles.

Drugs are normally readily available for absorption when administered as a suspension. Disintegration is not required for drug release, and the rate-limiting step in the absorption process is usually dissolution. Thus, factors that decrease the rate of dissolution—increase in particle size, increase in vehicle viscosity, coating of particles by wetting or suspending agents—will usually result in slowed absorption.

Capsules

Drugs are most commonly administered in solid dosage forms, such as capsules and tablets. The advantages of a drug in a solid dosage form include convenience of administration, accuracy and reproducibility of dosing, increased drug stability, and ease of mass production.

A capsule is a hard gelatin shell consisting of a base and a tightly fitting cap. Capsules rarely contain solid drug alone. To ensure physical stability, *diluents* or fillers such as lactose are added to fill the capsule. Diluents also aid in the rapid dispersal of drugs into the gastrointestinal fluids. *Lubricants* such as magnesium stearate are included during the manufacturing process to ensure the flow of powders. Unfortunately, some lubricants are very hydrophobic and can significantly slow drug dispersal into the gastrointestinal fluids. *Disintegrants* such as starch are necessary for prompt capsule disintegration. When a capsule comes into contact with the fluids of the gut, the gelatin starts to dissolve. As the aqueous fluids invade the capsule contents, disintegrants rapidly swell, causing the capsule to burst and discharge its contents into the gastrointestinal fluids.

Unlike the hard-shell gelatin capsule, soft-shell capsules can contain liquids. The absorption of a number of drugs with poor bioavailability may be improved by solubilizing the drug and administering it in a soft-shell gelatin capsule. The bioavailability of digoxin is greatly increased by the drug's formulation in a soft-shell capsule. Absorption appears to be equal to or greater than that obtained following administration of a solution of the drug.

Tablets

The tablet is the most frequently used means of administering a drug. High compression of the drug and excipients make for a convenient and, usually, therapeutically effective dosage form. The compression, however, also results in the major problem in drug delivery by tablets—that of redispersing the drug following ingestion.

As was described for capsules, ingredients other than the active therapeutic agent are contained within a tablet formulation to contribute to the ease of manufacturing and the in vivo performance of tablets. These substances include diluents, lubricants, and disintegrants.

Dissolution is usually the rate-limiting step in the delivery of drug from a tablet to the systemic circulation. The solubility of the drug is a major determinant of the dissolution rate. The rate may be increased by using a more soluble form of the drug, such as a salt, or by decreasing the particle size.

Coated Tablets

Tablets may be further modified by adding an extra coating to the tablet. This may be done to improve appearance, palatability, or the physicochemical stability of the product. In some cases, however, disruption of the coating is the rate-limiting step in the overall absorption process (Fig. 7-3).

A special type of coating, *enteric coating,* is designed to delay disintegration of the dosage form until it reaches the small intestine (see Fig. 7-3). This may be done to protect the drug from the acidic environment of the stomach or to protect the stomach from the drug. The tablet (or capsule) is coated with a polymer, such as cellulose acetate phthalate, that is insoluble between pH 1 to 3 but dissolves between pH 5 to 7. Absorption of drugs from enteric-coated formulations is typically quite variable. The variability is attributed to individual differences in gastric emptying rate. Efforts to overcome this problem have led to the coating of individual granules rather than the whole dosage form, resulting in a gradual but continual transfer of drug from the stomach to the small intestine.

Nonoral Medication

Buccal and Sublingual Administration

Drugs that are destroyed by the gastrointestinal fluids or are subject to substantial presystemic degradation may be formulated into tablets to be placed in the buccal pouch or under the tongue. *Buccal* tablets are usually small, flat, and oval in shape. They are generally designed to dissolve or erode slowly. Hormones such as progesterone have been formulated as buccal tablets. *Sublingual* tablets are relatively small and dissolve rapidly. Nitroglycerin and organic nitrates are commonly administered by this route.

Rectal Administration

Drugs are administered rectally either to treat local conditions such as hemorrhoids or to achieve systemic absorption. This route of administration is suitable for patients who cannot or will not tolerate oral medication and is an alternative to parenteral drug administration.

Drugs are normally administered rectally in the form of a suppository made with a variety of bases ranging from cocoa butter to polyethylene glycol derivatives. Soft gelatin capsules are also finding use in rectal drug delivery. The major factor determining the extent of absorption of a drug that is administered rectally is the time between insertion of the dosage form and defecation. Fecal matter can bind drugs, preventing absorption, but, more importantly, defecation removes the dosage form from the absorption site. Prior enema administration can substantially improve absorption.

Intravenous and Intraarterial Administration

Intravenous bolus administration of drugs is indicated when a rapid onset of action is required and when careful control of drug concentrations in the blood is necessary. *A slow intravenous administration of drug avoids excessively high transient concentrations and minimizes sudden precipitation of insoluble drugs* such as phenytoin, thereby reducing the formation of emboli. A constant intravenous infusion may be required for acute therapy when a drug has a narrow therapeutic range and sustained, controlled blood concentrations are necessary. This mode of drug delivery is particularly appropriate for drugs with short half-lives. There has been increasing interest in the intraarterial administration of antineoplastic agents. The site of injection is usually a small artery with relatively slow blood flow proximal to the tumor. High concentrations of drug can be achieved in the target organ while minimizing total body exposure.

Intramuscular Administration

A requirement for drug absorption after an intramuscular injection is some degree of water solubility. Lipophilic drugs usually gain rapid access to the capillaries. If, however, they precipitate in the interstitial fluid of the muscle on injection, slow and erratic absorption results. Drugs such as digoxin and diazepam are very poorly soluble in an aqueous medium, whereas others, such as chlordiazepoxide and phenytoin, are soluble only at a pH far from the physiological medium. Other factors that influence absorption rate are the volume and osmolarity of the solution injected and blood flow to the muscle tissue.

Subcutaneous Administration

A number of drugs and other therapeutic agents can be conveniently administered by injection into the loose tissue located immediately below the dermis. *The most important drug administered in this manner is insulin.* The clearance of low-molecular-weight compounds from the injection site is generally blood flow limited. The clearance of other drugs, generally those of high molecular

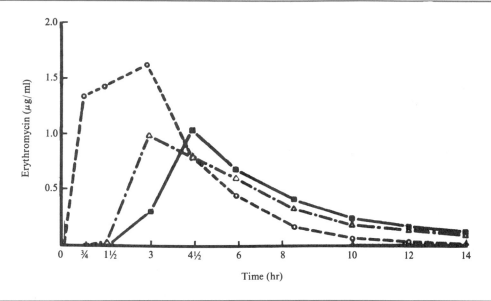

Figure 7-3. Mean serum concentrations obtained after administration of two 250-mg erythromycin tablets. Uncoated tablets, O; film-coated tablets, △; and enteric-coated tablets, ■. (From A.R. DiSanto, Chap. 76. Bioavailability and Bioequivalency Testing. In A. Osol et al. (eds.), *Remington's Pharmaceutical Sciences* [17th ed.]. Easton, Pa.: Mack Publishing Co., 1985.)

weight, is limited by the rate of diffusion through connective tissue from the injection site to the capillaries.

Percutaneous Absorption

Drugs are applied to the skin to treat or ameliorate dermatological disorders or to gain access to the systemic circulation (see Chap. 46). In recent years this latter aspect has received considerable attention and has resulted in the development of "patches" that release drug from a reservoir into the skin at a rate at least partially controlled by the device. By this means, controlled, sustained blood concentrations of scopolamine, nitroglycerin, nicotine, and other drugs have been achieved.

The two major potentially rate-limiting steps in drug delivery through the skin appear to be the release of drug from the formulation and passage across the stratum corneum. Ideally, the drug should be soluble in the vehicle. Poor solubility results in slow dissolution of suspended particles, resulting in a decrease in the rate of absorption. If the drug is extremely soluble in the vehicle, the drug will remain in the vehicle rather than diffusing into the skin.

The other major barrier to most drugs is the stratum corneum. Most of the epidermal mass is concentrated in this compact, dense, horny layer. Removal or disruption of the stratum corneum by mechanical or chemical injury or by disease leads to very rapid percutaneous transport of most drugs. Furthermore, in areas of the skin where this layer is very thin, for example, the scrotum, face, and

scalp, and where there is a high density of hair follicles, percutaneous transport is rapid.

Inhalation

Surprisingly, this route of administration is rarely used to deliver drugs systemically but is almost entirely restricted to drugs that act locally on the lungs. The reason for this lies principally in the extremely effective barriers that exist to prevent deep penetration of the lung by airborne particulate matter. Such particles must pass through a labyrinth of ever-narrowing passages starting with the oral and nasal cavities and leading successively to the trachea, bronchi, bronchioles, and finally the alveoli. The airway from the nasal cavity to the lower bronchi is lined with mucus and cilia that trap particles and move them to the pharynx to be swallowed or expectorated. Such barriers impede predictable drug delivery to the systemic circulation.

Most drugs intended for inhalation are administered by a pressurized aerosol or, less frequently, a powder inhaler. Drug is either dissolved or suspended in a fluorohydrocarbon propellant or mixed with a lactose diluent in the powder inhaler. Critical to the efficient delivery of drug to the lung is the penetration of the barriers just described. *The principal determinant is particle size distribution.* Large particles of diameter 10 μ or greater deposit in the upper airways by impaction and never reach the site of drug absorption. Equally ineffective are formulations consisting of particles 0.6μ or less in size. These particles will penetrate the lung but have too small a mass to settle on the lung surface by sedimentation and are removed with the next exhalation.

Patient education is another critical factor in assuring effective drug delivery from aerosols and powder inhalers. Patients should be instructed in the preliminary clearing of mucus, correct prior exhalation techniques, coordination between inhalation and product actuation, breath holding, and exhalation after administration. Failure to comply with these techniques invariably results in less than satisfactory drug response.

Finally, although the delivery of drugs by inhalation is usually indicated for patients with pulmonary disease, *disorders such as asthma will obstruct airflow and prevent optimal drug delivery.* Emphysema, however, results in a destruction of the integrity of the lung wall and increased permeation of drug may result.

Prolonged-Release Medication

Theoretical Background

Most disorders require chronic medication. The duration of therapy may last from a few days to a lifetime of dependence on a drug. In many instances optimal therapy is achieved only when plasma drug concentrations are maintained within a restricted range. This range is bounded by a maximum concentration above which unacceptable toxicity is experienced by the patient (C_{TOX}) and a lower concentration below which a pharmacological response is not evident (C_{MIN}).

The maximum allowable dosage interval depends on the half-life and the therapeutic index of the drug. The smaller the value of these parameters the more frequently the drug must be administered to maintain concentrations within the therapeutic range. For example, the half-life of procainamide is 3 hr; procainamide must, therefore, be given every 3 hr or less to maintain therapeutic concentrations. Strict compliance to such a dosage regimen is practically impossible, particularly when one realizes that such a schedule must be maintained throughout the night. A less than optimal therapy would have to be accepted as inevitable were it not for the existence of specialized dosage forms such as *prolonged-release medication.*

The time course of a drug in the body may be prolonged by decreasing the rate of absorption of the drug. This is usually achieved by administration of dosage forms with slower but sustained rates of drug release. Such dosage forms contain more drug than conventional doses but release the drug over a longer period of time and hence can be administered less frequently.

Prolonged-release medication, therefore, has the advantage of reducing dosing frequency while maintaining therapeutic drug concentrations. Compliance is increased and a reduction in plasma fluctuations is usually observed, resulting in a more uniform pharmacological response (Fig. 7-4).

Oral Medication

Several different techniques have been used to produce oral prolonged-release products. One of the earliest approaches was to prepare *coated release beads.* Small inert beads made of a combination of sugar and starch are coated with a drug. A capsule will typically contain from 50 to 500 such beads with diameters ranging from 1 to 2 mm. Before the capsule is filled, the beads undergo further coating with layers of material that is resistant to dissolution in the gastrointestinal fluids. The beads are divided into four groups. The first group receives no additional coating of resistant material and provides an initial bolus of drug. The other three groups receive enough layers to resist dissolution for 3, 6, and 9 hours, respectively. A more recent variant of this approach is *microencapsulation.* Solids and liquids can be encapsulated into microscopic-sized particles through formation of relatively insoluble materials around the substance. By varying the thickness of the wall, the dissolution of the particles can be varied. Needless to say, a large number of more sophisticated and more reliable products are now available.

Parenteral Medication

The earliest attempt to produce a parenteral prolonged-release formulation was the injection of slowly dissolving drug suspensions into muscle or subcutaneous tissue. For example, a single intramuscular injection of an aqueous suspension of the decanoate ester of fluphenazine, an antipsychotic, provides effective results in schizophrenics for 1 to 3 weeks. The oral dose, by contrast, must be administered one to four times per day.

The rate of drug absorption from injected suspensions is limited by the rate of dissolution. By choosing a relatively insoluble form of the drug, formulating with large particle size, and suspending in a viscous medium, slow drug release can be produced. A similar approach is to dissolve or suspend the drug in an oil such as sesame or peanut oil. Drug release into the body is controlled by the rate at which the drug partitions out of the oily vehicle into the aqueous interstitial fluid.

Sustained drug release can also be effected by injecting or surgically placing solid pellet *implants.* The drug is incorporated into a matrix that slowly erodes over time,

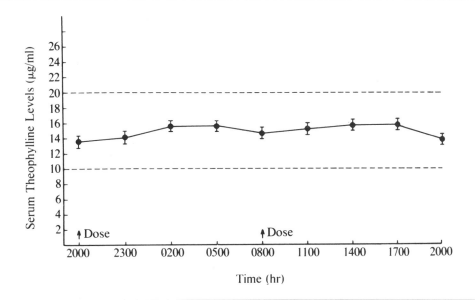

Figure 7-4. Mean steady-state serum theophylline concentrations in 20 asthmatic children receiving an oral prolonged-release formulation every 12 hr. (From H. W. Kelly and S. Murphy, Efficacy of a 12-hour sustained-release preparation in maintaining therapeutic serum theophylline levels in asthmatic children. *Pediatrics* 66:97, 1980.)

steadily releasing the drug. Better control has been achieved by placing the drug in a silicone rubber capsule. Lipophilic, low-molecular-weight substances, such as progesterone, ethinylestradiol, and testosterone, diffuse slowly and at an almost constant rate through the silicone wall.

In special situations *portable* or *implantable pumps* may be required to provide constant drug delivery. Portable insulin pumps are now available to diabetics for whom conventional subcutaneous administration fails to produce acceptable blood glucose control. The pump consists of a motor-driven syringe that empties into a catheter. The catheter is attached to a needle that is secured subcutaneously. The pump can be programmed to deliver insulin at a faster rate before than after meals.

An implantable heparin pump has been developed for patients with severe clotting problems. Both portable and implantable pumps have been used to deliver antineoplastic agents intraarterially to target organs such as the liver.

The most recent development in parenteral prolonged-release formulation is the *transdermal drug delivery system.* The prototype product provides controlled delivery of scopolamine to treat motion sickness. The drug is suspended in a liquid vehicle that is contained in a reservoir. The reservoir is separated from the skin by a microporous rate-limiting membrane. The system is designed for application to the postauricular area of the skin. At this location the skin is thin and relatively permeable to lipophilic drugs. Similar devices are now available to deliver nitroglycerin and other compounds.

Finally, special devices are available for local controlled, prolonged drug delivery. The first of these systems (*Ocusert*) delivers pilocarpine, used in the treatment of glaucoma. Traditional treatment requires administration of 2% pilocarpine eye drops every 6 hours. The *Ocusert* consists of a waferlike pilocarpine core held between two flexible ethylene-vinyl acetate copolymer membranes that control the rate of drug delivery to the eye. The unit is placed either under the eyelid or in the cul-de-sac of the eye. Pilocarpine levels in ocular tissue remain essentially constant over a period of 7 days. Advantages of this system are that the myopia and the miotic effects of pilocarpine are reduced and the total dose of pilocarpine is decreased by a factor of 8.

Working on a similar principle, *Progestasert* is a T-shaped intrauterine device that releases progesterone at a rate of 65 μg per day. It is a small, flexible, multicomponent unit consisting of a membrane-enclosed drug reservoir that delivers progesterone to the lining of the uterus. This device can provide contraception for up to 2 years.

Prodrugs as Delivery Systems

The systems described above improve drug delivery by controlling the rate and amount of drug released, the duration of its release, and, in some cases, limiting its sphere of influence by placing the device directly into the target area. Prodrugs accomplish some of these same objectives. In general, *prodrugs are made by synthesizing an inactive chem-*

ical derivative that after administration can be converted under the influence of biological fluids or enzymes to an active drug.

Prodrugs avoid disadvantages inherent in the physical properties of the parent drug by modifying drug transport, distribution, site localization, metabolism, or excretion. Bioavailability may be improved by increasing the drug's aqueous solubility or ability to penetrate membranes. In addition, patient acceptance may be enhanced by eliminating the drug's unpleasant taste, odor, or ability to irritate the gastrointestinal tract.

Supplemental Reading

Baker, R.W. *Controlled Release of Biologically Active Agents.* New York: Wiley, 1989.

Daemen, M.J.A.P., et al. Pharmacokinetic considerations in target organ-directed drug delivery. *Trends Pharmacol. Sci.* 9:138, 1988.

Ensminger, W.D., and Wollner, I.S. Implantable drug delivery devices (pumps, ports) in cancer therapy. *Ration. Drug Ther.* 22:1, 1988.

Fara, J.W., and Karim, A. Short and Long Term Transdermal Delivery Systems. In J. McClosky, (ed.), *Drug Delivery Systems; Proceedings of An International Conference.* Springfield, Ore.: Aster, 1983. P. 28.

Friend, D.R. *Oral Colon-Specific Drug Delivery.* Boca Raton, Fla.: CRC, 1992.

Hollenbeck, R.G., and Wiser, T.H. Inhalation Drug-Delivery Systems. In G.S. Banker and R.K. Chalmers (eds.). *Pharmaceutics and Pharmacy Practice.* Philadelphia: Lippincott, 1982. P. 391.

Langer, R. New methods of drug delivery. *Science* 249:1527, 1990.

Rosoff, M. (ed.). *Controlled Release of Drugs.* New York: VCH, 1989.

Shaw, J.M. (ed.). *Lipoproteins as Carriers of Pharmacologic Agents.* New York: Marcel Dekker, 1991.

Struyker-Boudier, H.A.J. (ed.). *Rate-Controlled Drug Administration and Action.* Boca Raton, Fla.: CRC, 1986.

Yacobi, A., and Halperin-Walega, E. (eds.). *Oral Sustained Release Formulations.* New York: Pergamon, 1987.

8

Principles of Toxicology

Mark J. Reasor and Mary E. Davis

As with therapeutic effects, the toxicity of drugs and other chemicals (*xenobiotics*) is a function of the concentration of the compound achieved at the site of action. For locally acting external irritants, this means that the magnitude of toxicity produced is proportional to the substance's concentration in the external medium (air or water); for systemically acting agents, the magnitude of the adverse effect produced is proportional to the dose of the toxicant. The analysis of toxicity dose-response relationships is quite similar to that already described for therapeutic dose-response relationships (see Chap. 2).

The target organ for the expression of xenobiotic toxicity is not necessarily that tissue or organ in which the drug produces its therapeutic effect, nor is it necessarily the tissue that has the highest concentration of the agent. For example, lead accumulates in bone but produces no toxicity there; certain chlorinated pesticides accumulate in adipose tissue but produce no local adverse effects.

Toxic metabolites can be produced during a variety of biotransformation reactions, including those catalyzed by monooxygenases, epoxide hydrolases, and enzymes involved in conjugation reactions. For those xenobiotics that form reactive intermediates, enzyme distribution may affect site specificity and toxicity. Drugs such as acetaminophen cause necrosis in the centrilobular portion of the liver at a site where the monooxygenase enzymes that bioactivate the analgesic are located.

It is necessary to distinguish between the intrinsic toxicity of a chemical and the hazard it poses. While a chemical may be of high intrinsic toxicity, it may pose little or no hazard if exposure is low. In contrast, a relatively nontoxic chemical may be quite hazardous if exposure is large.

Health professionals may be asked to provide an opinion on the cause and effect relationship between exposure to a xenobiotic and an adverse health effect ranging from symptoms of toxicity to a disease state. Certain principles should be considered in such an evaluation including an assessment of temporality. Do the symptoms or disease follow the exposure within a proper time frame? In addition, an evaluation of the toxicological properties of the substance should be included. Does the xenobiotic possess properties that can logically be expected to cause the damage or disease in question? For many chemicals, the qualitative consideration of the types of symptoms, injury, or disease that may occur after exposure can be predicted based on the available toxicological data or known biological activity of the chemicals. If the toxicity or disease does not fit into this known profile, a causal relationship between the chemical and the problem should be questioned further. If the xenobiotic has the appropriate toxicological properties, quantitative consideration of the total dose received must be carefully evaluated. Was the dose realistically high enough to produce health effects? Finally, the possibility of alternate causes for the health problems must be investigated carefully. Are there other, more logical, explanations for the symptoms? If appropriate, drug side effects should be considered as a possible cause of the adverse health effects. Lifestyle and avocations also must be evaluated. Alternate causation is ideally evaluated by a thorough, and frequently tedious, review of complete medical, occupational, and social records of the patient.

Manifestations of Toxicity

Organ Toxicity

Drugs or chemicals may cause cell death, which can lead to failure of the organ. The events that initiate cell death are not understood. The common final stages of cell death are disruption of normal metabolic processes, followed by an inability to maintain intracellular electrolyte homeostasis. If the insult is severe or prolonged enough, the cell will not regain normal function. Some drugs are metabolized to reactive products that bind to cellular macromolecules. If such binding impairs the function of crucial macromolecules, cell viability is lost. How severely organ function will be impaired depends on the reserve capacity of that organ. For example, more than 80 percent

Table 8-1. Xenobiotics that can Cause Pulmonary Toxicity

Drugs	Chemicals
Amiodarone	Asbestos
Bleomycin	Beryllium
Busulfan	Cadmium oxide
Cyclophosphamide	Chlorine gas
Methotrexate	Nitrogen dioxide
	Ozone
	Paraquat
	Phosgene
	Silica
	Sulfur dioxide

of renal function must be lost before impairment is suspected or detected on routine examination.

The ultimate outcome will depend on the affected organ's regenerative capacity and response to damage. A single, large dose of a hepatotoxin may cause liver necrosis and possibly failure, yet resolve with little or no tissue scarring. Continued exposure to the toxic agent, however, can result in hepatic cirrhosis and permanent scarring. During repair, damaged lung alveolar epithelium may be replaced by fibrous tissue that does not allow for gas exchange, thus intensifying the damage caused by the initial lesion. Since damaged neural tissue cannot easily replicate, glial and other nonconducting cells may proliferate and occupy the space of the dead neurons, and the damage will be expressed as deficits of sensory and motor functions and behavior. Alternatively, other neurons may take on the functions of the damaged neurons such that there is little or no perceptible damage.

Pulmonary Toxicity

The lungs are highly susceptible to a wide array of xenobiotics that enter the lungs by inhalation. Gases, solid particles, or liquid aerosols may deposit throughout the respiratory system, depending on their chemical and physical properties. The large surface area of the respiratory passages and alveolar region and the large volume of air delivered to that area (approximately 6–7 liters per minute in a young male adult) provide great opportunity for interaction between inhaled materials and lung tissue. Examples of inhaled xenobiotics that cause lung damage include silica, asbestos, ozone, nitrogen dioxide, sulfur dioxide, toluene diisocyanate, phosgene, and chlorine gas.

Xenobiotics also may reach the lungs through delivery by the bloodstream. Since the lungs receive the entire cardiac output of blood, the tissue may be exposed to xenobiotics that have entered the body by ingestion or injection. Bleomycin, amiodarone, cyclophosphamide, and paraquat are examples of xenobiotics that can injure the lungs through systemic exposure. Examples of chemicals

that can cause pulmonary toxicity are presented in Table 8-1. Exposure of the lungs to xenobiotics may result in bronchitis, emphysema, asthma, hypersensitivity pneumonitis, pneumoconiosis, and cancer. In most instances, the disorders result from chronic exposure to the causative agents.

Hepatotoxicity

Both hepatic anatomy and function contribute to the susceptibility of the liver to the toxic effects of xenobiotics. The liver has a high blood flow (receiving approximately 30% of cardiac output while it contributes approximately 5% of body mass). Moreover, the blood draining the stomach and small intestine is delivered directly to the liver via the hepatic portal vein, thus exposing the liver first to relatively large concentrations of ingested drugs or toxicants. Examples of xenobiotics that can cause hepatotoxicity are given in Table 8-2.

The liver has the highest activity of cytochrome P450–mixed function oxidase enzymes, and because of its large size, it carries out the bulk of xenobiotic biotransformation. Therefore, hepatic exposure to those agents that undergo bioactivation to toxic species can be significant.

Hepatic necrosis can be classified by the zone of the liver tissue affected. Xenobiotics such as acetaminophen or chloroform that undergo bioactivation to toxic intermediates particularly cause necrosis of the cells surrounding the central veins (*centrilobular*) because the components of the cytochrome P450 system are found in those cells in abundance. At higher doses or in the presence of agents that increase the synthesis of cytochrome P450 (inducers), the area of necrosis may incorporate the *midzonal* area (midway between the portal triad and central vein). Necrosis to cells around the portal triad (*periportal*), an area that is perfused first, occurs with other agents, such as endotoxin.

In contrast to chemically induced hepatotoxicity, allergic reactions to drugs produce foci of necrosis that are scattered diffusely throughout the liver. Other agents

Table 8.2 Xenobiotics that can Cause Hepatotoxicity

Drugs	Chemicals
Acetaminophen	Carbon tetrachloride
Nitrofurantoin	Chloroform
Chlorpromazine	Beryllium
Estrogens	Allyl formate
Ethanol	Vinylidene chloride
Halothane	
Urethane	
Isoniazid	
Phenylbutazone	
6-Mercaptopurine	

Table 8-3. Xenobiotics that can Cause Nephrotoxicity

Drugs	Chemicals
NSAIDs	Hexachlorobutadiene
Gentamicin	Mercuric chloride
Cephalothin	Chloroform
Cephalexin	Citrinin
Cyclosporine A	
Cisplatin	
Ifosfamide	
Streptozocin	

Key: NSAIDs = nonsteroidal antiinflammatory drugs.

Table 8-4. Xenobiotics that can Cause Neurotoxicity

Drugs	Chemicals
Cocaine	Acrylamide
Doxorubicin	Carbon disulfide
Isoniazid	Carbon monoxide
Quinine	Hexane
	Lead
	Mercury
	Methanol
	Organochlorine insecticides
	Organophosphate insecticides
	Trichloroethylene

cause severe (chlorpromazine) or mild (estrogens) cholestatic liver damage, including cholestasis and inflammation of the portal triad and hepatocellular necrosis.

Nephrotoxicity

Similar to the liver, the kidneys are susceptible to toxicity from xenobiotics because they too have a high blood flow (22% of cardiac output) relative to their mass (0.5% of body mass). Cells of the tubular nephron also face double-sided exposure, to agents in the blood on the basolateral side and in the filtered urine on the luminal side. Cells in the proximal tubule are generally the site of nephrotoxicity. These cells have the greatest abundance of cytochrome P450 in the nephron, and they have the ability to transport organic anions and cations from the blood into the cells, concentrating these chemicals manyfold. Examples of nephrotoxic xenobiotics are given in Table 8-3.

Chemically induced kidney damage is typically seen as acute tubular necrosis (ATN). The cells in the proximal tubule are affected. Reabsorption of water, electrolytes, glucose, and amino acids is impaired. The cells of the macula densa sense that the urine is dilute and cause a renin-angiotensin–mediated constriction of the afferent arterioles. This decreases glomerular filtration and thus prevents delivery of large volumes of water to nephron segments unable to reabsorb the load. Depending on the accuracy of the feedback, urine output will be increased, decreased, or unchanged. Markers of glomerular filtration, *blood urea nitrogen (BUN)* and *creatinine,* are increased. The urine may contain glucose and protein, including proteinaceous casts formed in the nephron of tubular debris.

Neurotoxicity

The central nervous system is protected from a number of xenobiotics by the blood-brain barrier. The barrier is not effective, however, against lipophilic compounds such as chlorinated solvents or insecticides. While the peripheral nervous system also is protected by a blood-neural barrier, it is less extensive than that for the central nervous system (CNS). The barriers are less well developed in the immature nervous system, rendering the fetus and neonate even more susceptible to neurotoxicants. Toxicity can occur in neural tissues following exposure to a wide range of xenobiotics including drugs, gases, metals, pesticides, solvents, and hydrocarbons. Examples of neurotoxicants are given in Table 8-4. The susceptibility of neural tissue is due in large part to its high metabolic rate, high lipid content, and, for the central nervous system, high rate of blood flow (14% of the cardiac output to about 2% of body mass).

Neurotoxicity to the central nervous system may manifest itself as structural-level damage, such as lead-induced encephalopathy; molecular-level damage, such as enzyme inhibition by cyanide; or functional-level damage, as exhibited by behavioral dysfunction.

Immunotoxicity

Chemical interaction with the immune system can result in two principal types of toxicity. If the immune system is functionally damaged, immunodeficiency may result, leading in severe cases to increased susceptibility to infection or decreased surveillance against precancerous or cancerous cells. The immune system can also be affected in such a way that it initiates or participates in tissue-damaging reactions. Allergic and autoimmune reactions are examples of this form of toxicity.

A number of drugs and environmentally and occupationally important chemicals can impair the activity of one or more components of the immune system (see Chap. 63). Table 8-5 contains examples of xenobiotics that are known to be immunosuppressive.

Immunological reactions that cause tissue damage can be initiated in a variety of ways. Table 8-6 presents a suggested classification of the different types of immune injury. Rarely does one mechanism operate independently from others, and the same chemical may elicit a different reaction in different persons. Other processes, such as nonspecific complement activation, may contribute to the toxicity. Host factors, such as genetic determinants responsible for hypersensitivity, may be of major importance.

Table 8-7 is a partial list of substances capable of inducing immunopathological reactions. The diversity of chemical structures is apparent. A multitude of materials—numerous plant and animal products, industrial chemicals—can induce immunologically mediated respiratory diseases, including occupational asthma and hypersensitivity pneumonitis. Allergic contact dermatitis may result from exposure to mercury, beryllium, platinum, nickel, chromium, epoxides, and ethylenediamine. Clinical expressions of cutaneous allergic reactions occur in a variety of ways. Eczematous, indurate-inflammatory, and urticarial eruptions are the most common reactions to

such allergens. Irritant responses causing direct damage to the skin may be confused with allergic responses involving immune mechanisms. An important difference is that allergic reactions require an initial exposure to sensitize the individual; dermatitis is then elicited by minimal subsequent exposure to the agent.

Toxic Effects on Genetic Material and Cell Replication

Mutagenesis, teratogenesis, and carcinogenesis are different manifestations of damage to genetic material (*genotoxicity*) or cell replication. Chemically induced genotoxicity occurs in several steps, and at each step there is opportunity for repair. Generally, xenobiotics are not themselves mutagenic, but rather they must be bioactivated to metabolites that are sufficiently reactive to bind to DNA and disrupt its coding. The reactive intermediates must be formed close enough to the DNA to interact with it before interacting with other, less important macromolecules or before being further metabolized to inactive forms.

Reproductive Toxicity

Since the placenta is readily permeated by molecules with a molecular weight smaller than 600, most drugs and chemicals pose a threat to the developing fetus (see Chap. 3). An estimated 4 to 5 percent of developmental defects

Table 8-5. Chemicals that Suppress the Immune System in Humans and Animals

Drugs	Chemicals
Azathioprine	Arsenic
Corticosteroids	Benzene
Cyclophosphamide	Dibenzodioxins (TCDD)
Cyclosporine A	Lead
Methotrexate	Organophosphate and organochlorine insecticides
	Ozone
	Polybrominated and polychlorinated biphenyls

Table 8-6. Classification of Immunopathological Reactions

Gell and Coombs type	Description	Mechanism(s)	Clinical examples
I	Anaphylactic hyper-sensitivity (reaginic allergy)	IgE-mediated noncytotoxic mediator release from basophilic leukocytes and tissue mast cells	Anaphylaxis Urticaria "Extrinsic" asthma Allergic rhinoconjunctivitis
II	Cytolysis or cyto-toxic damage	Complement-mediated injury involving antibodies (IgM and IgG) and any cell with isoantigen	Rh hemolytic disease of the newborn Interstitial nephritis Some drug-induced cytopenias Goodpasture's syndrome
III	Immune complex	Complement-mediated inflammatory response initiated by soluble antigen-antibody complexes (mainly IgG)	Serum sickness Lupus nephritis Drug fever Some glomerulonephritis
IV	"Delayed" or cellular hypersensitivity	Injury directly (cytolysis) and indirectly (lymphokines) from sensitized small lymphocytes and macrophages	Contact dermatitis Tuberculin hypersensitivity Allograft rejection Tumor immunity

Source: N. F. Adkinson, Jr., Environmental influences on the immune system and allergic reactions. *Environ. Health Perspect.* 20:97, 1977.

in humans result from prenatal exposure to drugs or environmental chemicals. This is particularly important since women with irregular menstrual cycles may be exposed to teratogens and enter the sensitive period of *organogenesis* before pregnancy is suspected.

Gestation is generally considered to consist of three periods of development, each with differing sensitivities to chemicals. During the *preimplantation* or predifferentia-

Table 8-7. Agents Capable of Inducing Immunopathological Reactions

"Natural" allergens
  Aeroallergens: pollens, animal danders, organic dusts, fungal
    spores, infectious agents
  Contactants: poison ivy (oleoresin), infectious agents
  Injectants: stinging insect venoms
  Ingestants: foods; infectious agents including parasites
Occupational agents
  Fungal spores
  Animal proteins (blood, urine, feces)
  Toluene diisocyanate (TDI)
Industrial chemical allergens
  Detergent enzymes
  Heavy metal salts
  Polyvinyl chloride (PVC) fumes
Drugs, food additives, cosmetics
  Penicillins
  Sulfonamides
  Photosensitizing chemicals
  Fragrance chemicals
  Sulfites

Source: Adapted from N. F. Adkinson, Jr., Environmental influences on the immune system and allergic reactions. *Environ. Health Perspect.* 20:97, 1977.

tion phase, expression of toxicity is an all-or-none phenomenon; damage to the embryo results either in death or no effect. *Organogenesis* occurs during the embryonic period (the first 3 months of pregnancy) and, therefore, susceptibility to teratogenesis is high; the embryo is particularly vulnerable to teratogens on days 25 through 40. The *fetal period* consists of the last 6 months of gestation and is a time of reduced susceptibility to teratogenic alterations. Certain organs, such as the genitals and the nervous system, however, are still undergoing differentiation during this period. Functional impairment in tissues, without marked structural damage, and growth retardation are the most common effects of chemical exposure during the fetal period.

The male is also susceptible to reproductive toxins. Spermatogenesis is the usual target for male reproductive toxins. Chemicals, such as 1,2-dibromo-3-chloropropane, can disrupt spermatogenesis leading to impaired reproductive function, including sterility. Men undergoing cancer chemotherapy with alkylating drugs are at increased risk for sterility.

Treatment of Poisonings

Specific antidotes are available for only a few toxic agents (Table 8-8). Even these are not always effective, particularly if the poisoning is severe. The best treatment begins with supportive care. This includes resuscitation (if necessary) and maintenance of respiration and cardiovascular function. Imbalances in fluid and electrolytes may need to be corrected. An approach to the treatment of poisoned victims is presented in Table 8-9.

Table 8-8. Some Specific Antidotes for Toxic Drugs and Chemicals

Agent	Antidote	Mechanism of antidotal action
Drugs		
Heparin	Protamine	Ionically neutralizes heparin
Acetaminophen	N-acetylcysteine	Inactivates toxic metabolite
Narcotics and opioids	Naloxone	Displaces drugs from receptors
Insulin/oral hypoglycemics	Glucose	Reverses glucose depletion
Chemicals		
Methanol	Ethanol	Blocks metabolism to toxic metabolite
Ethylene glycol	Ethanol	Blocks metabolism to toxic metabolite
Botulinum toxin	Antiserum	Immunologically neutralizes toxin
Cyanide	Sodium nitrite	Forms methemoglobin, which binds cyanide, thus removing it from active pool
	Sodium thiosulfate	Provides a source of sulfur to detoxify cyanide
Organophosphates	Atropine	Displaces acetylcholine from its receptor
	Pralidoxime	Reactivates acetylcholinesterase
Carbon monoxide	Oxygen	Displaces toxin from hemoglobin
Nitrites	Methylene blue	Reduces methemoglobin to hemoglobin
Arsenic	Dimercaprol	Forms inactive complex with metal
Iron	Deferoxamine	Forms inactive complex with metal
Lead	Calcium disodium edetate	Forms inactive complex with metal
Warfarin	Vitamin K_1	Stimulates coagulation factor synthesis

Table 8-9. A General Approach to the Treatment of Acute Poisoning

Provide emergency management
  Perform cardiopulmonary resuscitation if necessary
  If victim is in a coma, administer naloxone hydrochloride (in narcotic or opioid overdose) and 50% glucose (in case of insulin shock)
Evaluation
  Identify the toxic agent and dose if possible
  Assess vital signs and level of consciousness
  Conduct laboratory tests
Reduce absorption and enhance removal of poison
  Irrigate eyes and skin if involved
  Induce emesis with syrup of ipecac if victim is conscious and has not ingested acids, alkali, or hydrocarbons/petroleum distillates
  Perform gastric lavage if victim is unconscious or in some instances when conscious
  Administer activated charcoal to bind poison
  Administer milk or water if alkali, acid, or hydrocarbon/petroleum distillates have been ingested
  Administer antidote, if one exists, that is specific for the poison
  Consider forced diuresis, urine acidification, or alkalinization if specific antidotes are not available
  Hemodialysis or charcoal hemoperfusion may be appropriate for rapid elimination if antidotes are not available

Exposure to Nontherapeutic Toxicants

Worldwide production of chemicals has increased dramatically in the last four decades, resulting in increased human exposure. This applies not only to workers who manufacture the chemicals and final products but also to those who use the products (such as painters, printers, secretaries, and hobbyists) as well as to the general population through contamination of surface and ground water and air.

The chemical industry is regulated by the Environmental Protection Agency (EPA). Worker safety is overseen by the Occupational Safety and Health Administration (OSHA) of the Department of Labor. States may have their own regulatory agencies and reporting requirements. The EPA regulates the production and use of pesticides and chemicals, disposal of hazardous wastes, control of air and water pollution, and availability of chemical inventory information to emergency personnel and the community. OSHA sets limits for human exposure to hazardous chemicals in the workplace.

Chemicals used in industrial settings often are not pure, and after exposure, damage may be due to contaminants rather than to the primary components. The health concern over exposure to Agent Orange is not with the herbicide, but with the contaminant, dioxin. Furthermore, the toxic chemical may be generated during use.

For example, phosgene is formed when certain halogenated solvents used in metal degreasing come in contact with hot metal during welding.

Air Pollution

Industrialization has resulted in pollution of the outdoor air with a number of chemicals known to be hazardous to human health. These include a variety of gases, such as carbon monoxide, ozone, and the oxides of sulfur and nitrogen. Unacceptable levels of air pollutants can occur in the indoor environment as well. While some of these pollutants may be the same as for the outdoor air, most appear limited to the indoor environment, and include biological agents (fungal spores, viruses, bacteria, actinomycetes, etc.), volatile organic compounds, carbon dioxide, and formaldehyde. Sources of indoor pollutants include household cleaning products, personal care products, and off-gassing from construction materials or furnishings. Pollutants may either build up from inadequate ventilation or be introduced by poor maintenance of ventilation systems.

Individuals with compromised respiratory or cardiovascular function are at greatest risk when exposed to excessive air pollution. Such individuals should minimize their activity and remain indoors during pollution conditions. Vigorous manual labor or exercise should be curtailed, since it increases pulmonary exposure to pollutants in air.

Gases

Carbon monoxide arises from the incomplete combustion of organic material. Of principal concern is its generation by the internal combustion engine and by home heating units, particularly in poorly ventilated areas. Carbon monoxide emission by automobiles in closed garages and by unvented space heaters results in numerous deaths each year. Following inhalation, carbon monoxide binds to hemoglobin, displacing oxygen and forming carboxyhemoglobin. This decreases the oxygen-carrying capacity of the blood and impairs the blood cells' ability to release bound oxygen. The resulting hypoxia is the principal mechanism involved in carbon monoxide toxicity. Carbon monoxide can be formed endogenously during the metabolism of solvents such as methylene chloride.

Nitrogen oxides (principally nitrogen dioxide) and ozone are classified as oxidizing pollutants. The major source of nitrogen dioxide is the internal combustion engine. Photolysis of nitrogen dioxide by ultraviolet radiation liberates oxygen atoms, which can then combine with molecular oxygen to form ozone. Both gases cause irritation of the deep lung and can result in increased susceptibility to respiratory infection, pulmonary edema, and impaired lung function.

Oxides of sulfur (principally sulfur dioxide) are generated during the burning of fossil fuels, most notably coal, and are classified as reducing pollutants because of the types of reactions they undergo. The presence of particulate matter associated with most emissions promotes the conversion of sulfur dioxide to the more toxic sulfuric acid and facilitates deposition in the deep lungs. The acid can cause bronchospasm and lung damage, including alveolitis. Asthmatic episodes can be exacerbated by sulfur dioxide and sulfuric acid.

Particulates

Industrial processes, such as milling and mining, construction work, and the burning of wood or fossil fuel, generate particulates that can have adverse effects on health. They can be directly toxic themselves or serve as a vector for the transfer of bound material such as sulfuric acid, metals, and hydrocarbons into the lungs. Natural products such as pollen and animal dander can elicit toxic reactions on inhalation or skin contact. The inhalation of asbestos, silica, or coal dust can cause pneumoconiosis, which may develop into serious lung disease. The size of the particle, ventilatory rate, and depth of breathing determine the extent of pulmonary deposition.

Food Additives and Contaminants

Virtually thousands of substances are added to foods to enhance their marketability (appearance, taste, texture, etc.), storage properties, or nutritive value. The Delaney Clause of the 1958 Food Additives Amendment to the Food, Drug and Cosmetics Act prohibits the use of any additive found to induce cancer in animals or humans. Chemicals in use at the time were listed as Generally Recognized as Safe (*GRAS*), subject to future testing; this testing resulted in the banning of certain food colors and the artificial sweetener cyclamate. Microbial or fungal contamination of food can result in the introduction of powerful toxins into food. Contamination with microorganisms or their toxins occurs on the raw produce as well as during processing and storage. Some examples are given in Table 8-10.

Metals

When present in high enough concentrations, virtually all metals can produce some toxicity in humans. Exposure to most metals, however, is quantitatively and qualitatively minor. Several do pose important hazards to humans. Characteristics of toxicity for a number of metals are presented in Table 8-11. While the exact tissue and molecular site of the toxic action of each metal is different, toxicity generally results from the interaction of the metal with specific functional groups on macromolecules in the cell. These groups include sulfhydryl, carboxyl, amino, phosphoryl, and phenolic moieties. Interactions of such groups with metals can lead to disruption of enzyme activities and transport processes, and eventually to loss of such cellular functions as energy production and ion regulation.

In general, toxicity is related to the form of the metal (inorganic, organic, or elemental), the route of exposure, and the route of excretion. An exception to this principle is lead, which concentrates in bone but has no toxicity in that tissue. The carcinogenic activity of metals is now recognized. There is evidence that arsenic, chromium, and nickel can cause cancer in humans; cadmium and beryllium are probable carcinogens.

Solvents

Solvents are generally classified as aliphatic or aromatic, and either type may be halogenated, most commonly with chlorine; bromine, fluorine, and iodine sub-

Table 8-10. Examples of Food Additives and Contaminants

Agent	Type	Source and effects
Nitrate/nitrite	Preservative	Present in vegetables; form carcinogenic nitrosamines
Botulinum toxin	Contaminant	Produced by *Clostridium botulinum* in improperly canned vegetables; nausea, vomiting, diarrhea, paralysis
Salmonella	Contaminant	Improper processing of food allows *Salmonella* from intestinal tract to survive; the most common cause of gastroenteritis
Aflatoxins	Contaminant (mycotoxin)	Produced by *Aspergillus flavus,* especially grains, corn, and peanuts; carcinogenic and hepatotoxic
Ochratoxin, citrinin	Contaminant (mycotoxin)	Produced by *Penicillium* strains; nephropathy (endemic Balkan nephropathy)
Polybrominated biphenyls (PBBs)	Contaminant	Fire retardant inadvertently substituted for feed supplement in Michigan; livestock loss, undetermined effect on human health

stituents are also found. Exposure to solvents is generally through inhalation of vapors, although direct skin contact also occurs. The concentration of solvent in air is determined by the vapor pressure of the solvent, the ambient temperature, and the effectiveness of ventilation systems. These factors and the rate of pulmonary air exchange will affect the extent of exposure. Because exposure is usually through the air, the ability to detect the presence of hazardous concentrations is important. For some chemicals, odor can be used as a warning signal. Other solvents, however, produce damage at concentrations below the odor threshold.

Solvents are generally lipid soluble, and therefore they are readily absorbed across the skin. Once absorbed, they tend to concentrate in the brain, and CNS dysfunction is common at high exposures. Symptoms can range from confusion to unconsciousness. The toxicity of representative solvents is summarized in Table 8-12.

Aliphatic Solvents

Chloroform, a halomethane solvent, was widely used as an anesthetic agent between 1847 and 1894 until the association between postsurgical jaundice and chloroform was made. Trichloroethylene, until recently, was widely used as a degreasing agent. Adverse effects of trichloroethylene are quite rare. Workers chronically exposed to trichloroethylene (from inadequate ventilation) report increased sensitivity to alcohol because trichloroethylene metabolites effectively compete with ethanol for metabolism by alcohol dehydrogenase. Trichloroethylene also increases the sensitivity of the myocardium to the arrhythmogenic effects of epinephrine. Fatal arrhythmias have occurred after exertion. The use of trichloroethylene has decreased markedly since it was found to be carcinogenic in a National Cancer Institute screening test.

Aromatic Solvents

Benzene is the typical example of this class of compounds, which also includes toluene, xylene, and crude petroleum distillates. Acute overexposure causes giddiness and euphoria. Headache, nausea, unconsciousness, and death follow with increasing doses. Chronic exposure to low doses of benzene results in a decreased synthesis of formed elements of the blood, aplastic anemia, or leukemia.

Benzene is used in the synthesis of other cyclic compounds, in printing chemicals, adhesives, and paint removers, and occurs as a contaminant of toluene, xylene,

Table 8-11. Characteristics of Toxicity of Selected Metals*

Metal	Selected features of toxicity
Arsenic	
Inorganic	Diarrhea, hyperkeratosis, garlic breath, Mees' lines on fingernails
Arsine gas	Hemolysis
Beryllium	Pneumonitis, chronic granulomatous disease, contact dermatitis
Cadmium	Pneumonitis, emphysema, kidney damage
Iron	Gastric irritation, liver damage
Lead	Peripheral and central neurotoxicity, kidney damage, anemia
Mercury	Pneumonitis, neuropsychiatric toxicity
Elemental	(excitability, emotional instability, depression, insomnia), motor dysfunction (tremors)
Organic	Sensory neuropathy (dysarthia, paresthesia, constriction of visual field, loss of taste, hearing, smell), motor dysfunction (tremors)
Inorganic	Kidney damage, irritation of oral cavity and gastrointestinal tract

*Representative toxicities are presented; for most metals, other symptoms of toxicity may be demonstrated. Nature of the toxicities is dependent on level of exposure, whether the exposure is acute or chronic, and the route of exposure.

Table 8-12. Toxicity of Selected Solvents

Solvent	Uses	Effect and mechanism
Aliphatic solvents		
Chloroform	Drug purification	Hepatic centrilobular necrosis, likely from reactive metabolites
Trichloroethylene	Degreasing, dry cleaning	Sensitizes the myocardium to epinephrine, interferes with alcohol metabolism
Methylene chloride	Degreasing, paint stripping, aerosol propellant	Metabolized to CO, resulting in formation of carboxyhemoglobin
Hexane, methyl n-butyl ketone	Wood glue, plastics manufacturing	Polyneuropathy from their metabolite, 2,5-hexanedione
Aromatic solvents		
Benzene	Petroleum product, adhesives and coatings	Leukemia, aplastic anemia, likely from reactive intermediates
Toluene	Adhesives	Cerebellar degeneration with repeated high-dose exposure (glue sniffing)

Table 8-13. Toxicity of Selected Pesticides

Class and examples	Effect and mechanism

Organochlorine insecticides
    DDT, chlordane, aldrin,
        heptachlor
	Neuronal hyperactivity; convulsions; impaired vision, concentration, and memory
	Altered membrane permeability to Na^+, K^+
	Block repolarization by inhibiting Na^+, K^+-ATPase
	Block GABA-stimulated chloride uptake

Organophosphate insecticides
    Bromophos, chlorpyrifos, para-
        thion, malathion, diazinon
	Bronchoconstriction and secretion, muscular weakness or paralysis, CNS depression, including respiratory centers
	Inhibition of acetylcholinesterase (reversible or irreversible)

Carbamate insecticides Carbaryl	Same as organophosphate insecticides Inhibition of acetylcholinesterase (reversible)

Pyrethrin and pyrethroid insecticides
    Pyrethrin I, II; fenvalerate,
        permethrin
	Neuronal hyperactivity, incoordination, tremors with hyperthermia, seizures
	Delayed inactivation of channels in excitable tissues, causing repetitive firing and, at high doses, depolarization
	Block GABA-stimulated chloride uptake

Chlorophenoxy herbicides 2,4-D; 2,4,5-T	Muscle weakness, aching, and tenderness; hypotonia
Bipyridyl herbicides Paraquat, diquat	Delayed respiratory distress, fibrosis, and atelectasis Gastrointestinal, liver, and kidney toxicity Formation of reactive oxygen species

Rodenticides
    Compound 1080, warfarin,
        strychnine
	Block tricarboxylic acid cycle (fluoroacetates)
	Prevent blood clotting
	Induce seizures

Key: ATP = adenosine triphosphatase; GABA = gamma-aminobutyric acid; 2,4-D = 2,4-dichlorophenoxyacetic acid; 2,4,5-T = 2,4,5-tetrachlorodibenzodioxin.

and other petroleum products. The extent of benzene contamination varies from batch to batch. Benzene is a by-product of the coking process, during which exposure is most difficult to control and reduce.

Pesticides

Pesticides are chemicals used to eliminate unwanted or undesirable organisms. Common targets for pesticides include insects, weeds (herbicides), fungi, and rodents. Commercial use and sale of pesticides is controlled by the EPA through its pesticide registration program. Poisoning from pesticides often involves professional exterminators, agricultural workers, and consumers. Over half of the poisonings due to agricultural pesticides involve children. Some states require physicians to report pesticide poisonings of agricultural workers to the state labor department. The toxicity of representative pesticides is summarized in Table 8-13.

Insecticides

Most insecticides are lipid soluble, so that the insecticide can be absorbed through the chitinous exoskeleton of the insect. Some insecticides require metabolic activation

before they can exert their toxic effects. Insects possess monooxygenase enzymes similar to those found in the mammalian liver and therefore are able to metabolize insecticides similarly to humans. Inhibitors of monooxygenase activity, especially the methylene-dioxybenzene derivative piperonyl butoxide, are incorporated into insecticide formulations to decrease the rate of inactivation of the insecticide by the insect. These compounds are referred to as *insecticide synergists*.

The prototypical *organochlorine insecticide* is DDT. It was first used in World War II for vector control of malaria. Other organochlorine insecticides include chlordane, heptachlor, lindane, mirex, chlordecone, aldrin, and dieldrin. The organochlorine insecticides are very stable in the environment. This persistence allows toxic concentrations to build up in nontarget organisms. Human adipose tissue samples taken between 1976 and 1980 had detectable amounts of DDT, and residues of aldrin/dieldrin were found in more than 90 percent of the adipose samples. Similarly, DDT and its metabolites are still found in samples of raw agricultural commodities grown in California. The organochlorine insecticides alter electrolyte movements across nerve cells.

Organophosphate insecticides take their name from the phosphate triester group that is essential for their action. Many organophosphates undergo metabolic activation through desulfuration and oxidation of the phosphate to yield a species that will react with the serine residue on the active site of acetylcholinesterase (AChE) (see Chap. 16). This reaction is irreversible if AChE undergoes aging (for instance, malathion, parathion, diazinon). Symptoms of poisoning, due to excessive stimulation of cholinergic receptors, include increased salivation, bronchoconstriction and secretion, bradycardia, muscular weakness and fatigue, and depression of central respiratory and circulatory centers. In cases of lethal poisoning, death is from respiratory failure. Distal neuropathy of the lower limbs, involving axonal degeneration followed by myelin degeneration, has been seen in pesticide workers who have had repeated exposure to some organophosphates. This toxicity is independent of AChE inhibition and occurs with other organophosphate compounds that do not inhibit AChE.

The *carbamate insecticides* also inhibit AChE. The mechanism of inhibition is similar, but the reaction is reversible. The enzyme is carbamylated, and the carbamyl group dissociates from the enzyme more readily so that a chemically induced reactivation of the enzyme is neither necessary nor desirable, as the reactivators are also substrates for AChE.

Herbicides and Rodenticides

The mechanisms of herbicidal activity generally involve interference with plant-specific biochemical reactions. Thus, toxicities in mammals are generally low and not predictable from the mechanism of herbicidal action. In contrast, for rodenticides target selectivity is not based on differences of biochemistry or physiology between humans and rodents, but rather on behavior, especially feeding behavior.

The *chlorophenoxy herbicides*, 2,4-dichlorophenoxyacetic acid (2,4-D) and 2,4,5-trichlorophenoxyacetic acid (2,4,5-T), act as growth hormones, stimulating plant growth beyond that which the plant can support. Both were used in defoliating operations in Vietnam and the adverse health effects of the contaminant 2,3,7,8-tetrachlorodibenzodioxin (dioxin) continues to be controversial. Although use of 2,4,5-T has been severely restricted, 2,4-D continues to be used, particularly for controlling plant growth on power line rights-of-way. The chlorophenoxyacetic herbicides are toxic to mammals only at high doses, as they are rapidly eliminated by renal secretion.

The *bipyridyl herbicides* paraquat and diquat are broadspectrum herbicides. Paraquat poisoning typically occurs following accidental ingestion of solution in beverage containers. As little as 10 ml paraquat concentrate is lethal in adults. Paraquat damages the lungs and may result in the appearance of a delayed respiratory distress syndrome;

symptoms often appear 1 or 2 weeks after poisoning. Therapy for paraquat poisoning includes eliminating as much of the compound as possible (by gastric lavage and hemoperfusion) and supportive care. Since paraquat toxicity is enhanced by oxygen, oxygen supplementation should be used only as necessary. Diquat has a very different spectrum. Lung damage is minimal, as diquat does not selectively accumulate in the lung. Acute renal failure, liver toxicity, and gastrointestinal damage are sequelae to diquat poisoning.

Warfarin, a coumarin anticoagulant, is incorporated into cornmeal for use as a rat poison. Repeated exposure results in sufficient inhibition of prothrombin synthesis to cause fatal internal hemorrhage.

Cyanide

Cyanide is found in a variety of commercial preparations, including rodenticides; cyanide gas may be liberated during certain industrial processes. It is sometimes used as a means of suicide.

Cyanide impairs tissue oxygen utilization by blocking the cellular electron transport chain through inhibition of the terminal enzyme cytochrome oxidase. While its delivery to the tissues is normal, oxygen cannot be utilized because of the enzymatic blockade. The victim suffers from hypoxia and will complain of headache, ataxia, and elevated respiratory effort, which can progress to coma and death.

Cyanide poisoning is treated by administering amyl nitrite by inhalation or sodium nitrite by injection. These agents convert a portion of blood hemoglobin to methemoglobin, which has a high affinity for cyanide. The methemoglobin liberates some of the cyanide from its complex with cytochrome oxidase. The subsequent intravenous administration of sodium thiosulfate then results in the dissociation of cyanide from methemoglobin with the formation of the nontoxic thiosulfate, which is readily excreted in the urine. Some evidence suggests that placing the victim in an oxygen-rich atmosphere may hasten recovery.

Drug Interactions

Perhaps the major toxicological problem in our society is drug interaction, owing to the frequent use of more than one therapeutic agent by patients, particularly the elderly. Drug interactions may increase toxicity by a number of mechanisms, including increases or decreases in drug metabolism, changes in renal or hepatic clearance, reduction in binding to plasma proteins, and augmented release or impaired neuronal uptake of neurotransmitters. The number of possible drug interactions is much too large to describe in this chapter. Numerous references exist on this subject, including:

- Hansten, P.D., and Horn, J.R. *Drug Interactions* (6th ed.). Philadelphia: Lea & Febiger, 1989.
- Stockley, I.H. *Drug Interactions* (2nd ed.). Oxford, England: Blackwell, 1991.
- Tatro, D.S. *Drug Interaction Facts* (3rd ed.). St. Louis: Facts and Comparisons, 1992.

The health professional should be aware of these sources and utilize them regularly.

Supplemental Reading

Amdur, M.O., Doull, J., and Klaassen, C.D. (eds.). *Casarett and Doull's Toxicology, the Basic Science of Poisons* (4th ed.). New York: Pergamon, 1991.

Ellenhorn, M.J., and Barceloux, D.G. *Medical Toxicology.* New York: Elsevier, 1988.

Gosselin, R.E., Smith, R.P., and Hodge, H.C. *Clinical Toxicology of Commercial Products* (5th ed.). Baltimore: Williams & Wilkins, 1984.

Haddad, L.M., and Winchester, J.F. *Clinical Management of Poisoning and Drug Overdose* (2nd ed.). Philadelphia: Saunders, 1990.

Hayes, A.W. (ed.). *Principles and Methods of Toxicology* (2nd ed.). New York: Raven, 1989.

Hayes, W.J., and Law, E.R. (eds). *Handbook of Pesticide Toxicology.* New York: Academic, 1991.

9

Drug Testing in Humans

Joseph J. McPhillips

Before the twentieth century, most government controls were concerned not with drugs but with impure and adulterated foods. Medicines were thought to pose problems similar to those presented by foods, but their control was believed to be the concern of the pharmacy profession. Safety considerations arose in relation to the therapeutic use of toxic substances—for example, the use of hydrocyanic acid in the treatment of pulmonary tuberculosis. Efficacy was questioned in two respects: adulteration of active medicines by addition of inert fillers and false claims made for the so-called patent (secret) medicines or nostrums. These early interests in safety and efficacy foreshadowed later and greater concerns about the same issues. Indeed, much of the development of the science of pharmacy in the nineteenth century involved standardizing and improving prescription drugs.

Drug Control and Development

The profession of pharmacy also played a key role in the earliest attempts at voluntary regulation and in instituting federal controls. The Philadelphia College of Pharmacy, the nation's first (founded in 1821), was, from its beginning, greatly concerned about "spurious and inert medicines." Interest in the control of drug quality was written into the college's constitution, whose writers viewed with alarm the varying methods for preparing the same drug, the availability of differing strengths of given drugs under the same names, and the difficulty of detecting adulterations, all of which, they declared, offered "great incitements to cupidity and . . . a wide door to abuses." The college's constitution provided for expulsion of any member "guilty of adulterating or sophisticating any articles of medicine or drugs, or of knowingly vending articles of that character." This supervision implied group self-discipline rather than government intervention. Voluntary self-regulation by the pharmaceutical

profession was one of the earliest control measures exerted over drugs.

Formularies (books containing lists of medicinal substances and formulas) played an important part in the specification of drug standards. They were spontaneous products of the medical and pharmacy professions. The first *United States Pharmacopeia* was the result of a national convention held in 1820 representing all the state medical societies, colleges of physicians and surgeons, and medical schools then existing in the United States. By the 1842 edition, colleges of pharmacy had formally joined the endeavor. Unlike the *Pharmacopeia,* the *National Formulary* was from the beginning prepared principally by pharmacists.

Early Drug Legislation

A landmark in the control of drugs was the 1906 Pure Food and Drug Act. Food abuses, however, were the primary target. Less than one quarter of the first thousand decisions dealt with drugs, and of these, the majority were concerned with patent medicines. Nostrums had for some time been considered the greatest menace in the field of drugs. Patent medicines joined catsup and whiskey as a theme for congressional debate.

The 1906 law defined *drug* broadly and governed the labeling, but not the advertising, of any substance used to affect disease. This law gave the *Pharmacopeia* and the *National Formulary* equal recognition as authorities for drug specifications. In the first contested criminal prosecution under the law, action was taken against the maker of a headache mixture bearing the beguiling name of Cuforhedake-Brane-Fude. In 1912, Congress passed an amendment to the Pure Food and Drug Act that banned false and fraudulent therapeutic claims for patent medicines. Shortly thereafter, this amendment was tested in the courts. A court ruling stated that a manufacturer who believed his product to be effective had no intent to defraud and, hence, could not be said to be acting fraudulently. Thus, the modest degree of control that had been gained through this amendment was quickly lost.

Prescription drugs were also subject to control under the 1906 law. In fact, until 1953 there was no fixed legal boundary drawn between prescription and nonprescription medications. Prescription medications received a lower priority since food and patent medicine abuses were judged to be the more urgent problems. Under the 1906 law, all prescription drugs had to meet the standards for composition of the *United States Pharmacopeia* or the *National Formulary*. The Federal Bureau of Chemistry assumed the task of examining drugs for compliance.

For the next 30 years, drug control was viewed primarily as a problem of prohibiting the sale of dangerous drugs and tightening regulations against misbranding. Until the 1930s, new drugs posed little problem because there were few of them.

Modern Drug Legislation

The modern history of United States drug regulation began with the Food, Drug and Cosmetic Act of 1938, which superseded the 1906 Pure Food and Drug Act. In the 1938 act, control over new drugs was viewed not as a way of equipping the government to cope with a rising tide of new and hazardous drugs, but rather as a means of preventing the marketing of untested, potentially harmful drugs. An obscure proviso of the 1938 act was destined to be the starting point for some of the most potent controls the Food and Drug Administration (FDA) now exercises in the drug field. This was the power of the agency to exempt drugs from the requirement that their labeling give adequate directions for use. This allowed the prescription drug to come under special control by requiring that it carry only the legend, "Caution—to be used only by or on the prescription of a physician."

A major defect of the generally strong 1938 law was its lack of adequate control over advertising. In 1944, regulations were enacted on how information on prescription drugs should be disseminated. Current regulations requiring that "labeling on or within the package from which the drug is to be dispensed" bear adequate information for its use explain the existence of the "package insert." If the pharmaceutical manufacturer makes claims for its product beyond those contained in an approved package insert, the FDA may institute legal action against the deviations in advertising.

The 1938 act required manufacturers to submit a New Drug Application (NDA) to the FDA for its approval before the company is permitted to market a new drug. The original requirement for NDA approval was satisfaction of safety criteria, which at that time largely meant animal

safety. *Efficacy* (proof of effectiveness) became a requirement in 1962 with the Kefauver-Harris Drug Amendments. These amendments established a requirement that drugs show "substantial evidence" of efficacy before receiving NDA approval. "Substantial evidence" was further defined in the amendments as

> . . . evidence consisting of adequate and well-controlled investigations, including clinical investigations, by experts qualified by scientific training and experience to evaluate the effectiveness of the drug involved, on the basis of which it could fairly and responsibly be concluded by such experts that the drug will have the effect it purports or is represented to have under the conditions of use prescribed, recommended, or suggested in the labeling or proposed labeling thereof.

In addition to establishing the requirement for efficacy, the 1962 amendments introduced the Investigational New Drug (IND) procedure, a measure that controls both the preclinical and clinical phases of new drug investigations. Federal regulations specify that only drugs approved by the FDA for marketing may be shipped across state lines. The IND is an exemption to the federal regulations that permit a pharmaceutical company to send unapproved or investigational drugs to investigators for the purpose of conducting studies in human subjects. To obtain the exemption, the company must provide evidence that it is reasonably safe to conduct such studies. The evidence consists of the results of toxicity studies conducted in animals as well as the results of any clinical studies that may have been conducted outside of the United States. The company must also provide data on the composition and stability of the formulation to be used in the studies. The FDA monitors the conduct of clinical studies by requiring immediate reporting of serious adverse events and annual progress reports with particular attention to safety data.

Drug regulation in the United States is continuing to evolve rapidly both in promulgation of specific regulations and in the way regulations are implemented. Recent developments include the establishment of the FDA's Biomonitoring Program, which is designed to enhance federal surveillance of both clinical and preclinical studies and to refine the concepts of safety and efficacy.

In some ways, Congress has been conspicuously successful in its legislation and regulation. The abolition of patent medicines is an outstanding example, as is control over the accuracy of claims made for drugs. Since the 1962 amendments, the advertising of prescription drugs in the United States has been increasingly controlled—to a greater extent than in most other countries. Untested new medicines are a thing of the past; all the new drugs introduced since 1962 have some proof of efficacy. The 1962

Table 9-1. Major Congressional Legislation Enacted to Regulate Drug Development in the United States

Act of Congress	Major goal
Pure Food and Drug Act, 1906	Set guidelines for drug labeling
Food, Drug and Cosmetic Act, 1938	Required establishment of safety and need for FDA approval for new drugs
Kefauver-Harris Drug Amendments, 1962	Required demonstration of efficacy in addition to safety; introduced IND procedure

amendments have ensured that the available drugs are, on the average, more effective than the totally ineffective ones, which have been eliminated. This is not to say that misleading drug advertisements no longer exist; manufacturers still occasionally make unsubstantiated claims. The FDA, however, has the power to force drug companies to publish, in the same journals in which the advertisement originally appeared, a statement disclosing that the FDA considered the previous advertisement to be misleading. A summary of major legislative events is provided in Table 9-1.

Clinical Testing of Drugs

Experiments conducted in animals are essential in the development of new chemicals for the management of disease. The safety and efficacy of new drugs, however, can be established only by adequate and well-controlled studies conducted in human subjects. Since findings in animals do not always accurately predict the human response to drugs, subjects* who participate in clinical trials are put at some degree of risk. The risk involved comes not only from the potential toxicity of the new drug, but also from a potential lack of efficacy, with the result that the condition under treatment becomes worse. Since risk is involved, the primary consideration in any clinical trial should be the welfare of the subject. As a consequence of unethical or questionably ethical practices committed in the past, most countries have established safeguards to protect the rights and welfare of persons who participate in clinical trials. Two of the safeguards that have been established are the *institutional review boards* and the use of the *informed consent form*.

---

*The term *subject* is used to indicate the participant in a clinical trial. The subject may be a normal healthy individual who participates in a bioavailability study or a patient who participates in a therapeutic study.

Institutional Review Boards

The institutional review board (IRB), also known as the ethics committee or human subjects committee, originally was established to protect people who are confined to hospitals, mental institutions, nursing homes, and prisons who may be used as subjects in clinical research. In the United States any institution conducting clinical studies supported by federal funds is required to have proposed studies reviewed and approved by an IRB. The regulations were amended subsequently to apply to outpatients and healthy subjects who volunteer to participate in clinical studies. The FDA also requires that studies involving investigational new drugs performed on human subjects be reviewed and approved by an IRB.

The duties of the IRB are to review proposed studies and decide if such studies are appropriate medically, scientifically, and ethically. The IRB is required to ensure that the risks involved are reasonable in relation to any benefits, that informed consent is adequate and obtained from all subjects, and that there is continuous monitoring of the progress of the study to ensure the safety of the subjects. The membership of the committee should consist of a physician, scientist, lawyer, ethicist, or member of the clergy, and at least two other members of the community in which the institution is located.

Informed Consent

People who volunteer to be a subject in a drug study have a right to know what can and will happen to them if they participate. The investigator is responsible for ensuring that each subject receives a full explanation, in easily understood terms, of the purpose of the study, the procedures to be employed, the nature of the substances being tested, and the potential risks, benefits, and discomforts. For example, if venipuncture or endoscopy is to be done, the risks and discomforts of such procedures should be explained. If a placebo is to be used, the subjects should be told the probability of receiving the placebo. In a therapeutic trial in which subjects are patients, they should be made aware of alternative therapy if available. For example, if a new antiulcer drug is being tested subjects should be told that established treatment for ulcers is available and that they have the option to choose it.

It should be clear that participation in the trial is voluntary and that refusal to participate will not affect a patient's medical treatment. Subjects also should be told that they are free to withdraw from the trial at any time without prejudice. If they risk injury, the subjects should know whether or not medical treatment is available and of what the treatment will consist. *The entire consent process involves giving the subject adequate information, providing adequate op-*

portunity for the subject to consider all options, and allowing the subject to ask questions. With rare exception, consent in the United States is obtained in writing.

Drug Development

New chemical entities intended for the treatment of disease emerge from the laboratories of government, academic institutions, private research foundations, and the chemical and pharmaceutical industry. Part of the development process involves clinical testing and, in the United States and most other countries, the provision by the drug manufacturer of "substantial evidence of safety and efficacy" before a new drug can be released for general use.

In most instances an adequate and well-controlled investigation is the *randomized controlled* clinical trial. Although widely used and generally accepted, it is not without pitfalls. Nevertheless, it is the technique most frequently employed in clinical trials of new drugs. The essence of such studies involves selecting subjects; assigning them to experimental groups, usually of equal size; administering the test drug and control substance to the appropriate experimental groups; and then evaluating the outcome to determine if there is an effect that is attributable to the test drug. The critical elements of the randomized controlled clinical trial are described as follows:

Randomization

The term *randomization* means that subjects are assigned to treatment or control groups by a scheme over which neither the investigator nor the subject has any control. The purpose of randomization is to ensure that bias of the investigator or subject does not influence the composition of the treatment groups and, therefore, the outcome of the experiment. Assignment of subjects is accomplished usually by employing a table of random numbers or a randomization scheme generated by a computer. In a biological experiment any number of variables can influence the outcome of the experiment and the investigator cannot identify all variables ahead of time. Randomization tends to ensure that possible confounding variables are equally distributed among the experimental groups.

Control Groups

A well-designed study contains a *control group* with whom the treatment or experimental group is compared. The conditions and procedures to which both groups are exposed should be identical except for administration of the test drug. In the absence of a control group, changes observed after administration of the experimental drug may be attributed erroneously to the drug when, in fact, the changes may be related to factors other than treatment. For example, resolution of a respiratory tract infection following administration of a new antibiotic cannot appropriately be attributed to treatment in the absence of a control group because the infection may be self-limiting and would have resolved without treatment.

The control groups can be treated with a *placebo* (from the Latin, "I will please"), which is a formulation identical in appearance and composition to the test material, but without the drug. Alternatively, individuals may be treated with a standard drug of established efficacy and similar pharmacological activity (positive control).

The ideal situation is to have two control groups, one a placebo and the other a positive control. Comparison with the placebo group would establish efficacy, and comparison with the positive control would provide an estimate of how the new drug compares with established treatment. While the use of a placebo is not always acceptable or practical, comparisons only with a positive control group pose special problems if at the conclusion of the study there is no difference between the experimental group and the positive control group. The absence of a difference between the experimental and positive control groups may indicate either that both drugs were effective or that neither was effective. Occasionally, even established therapeutic agents will fail to show superiority over a placebo. This is particularly true of drugs (e.g., analgesics) whose potential beneficial effects may be interpreted subjectively by the patient. In addition, statistical problems are associated with trials that fail to show a difference between the treatment group and the positive control group.

Single- and Double-Blind Techniques

Single- and double-blind techniques are employed to reduce or eliminate bias while the study is in progress. The possibility exists that the investigator or the subject will intentionally or unintentionally create circumstances that may favor one treatment or outcome over another. In a *single-blind* study only the subject is unaware of the identity of the treatment. In a *double-blind* study neither the investigator nor the subject knows the identity of the treatment. When the appearance and composition of the formulation for both the control and the experimental drug can be made indistinguishable, there is no difficulty in using single- or double-blind techniques in a clinical study. There are times, however, when these procedures cannot be used. In such cases a third party, presumably uninterested in the outcome, can administer the drugs and perform the clinical assessments.

The purpose of the randomized controlled clinical trials is to eliminate bias in the interpretation of results.

Phases of Clinical Investigation

The clinical development of new drugs usually takes place in steps or phases conventionally described as clinical pharmacology (*phase I*), clinical investigation (*phase II*), clinical trials (*phase III*), and postmarketing studies (*phase IV*).

Phase I

When a new drug is administered to humans for the first time, the studies usually are conducted in healthy men between 18 and 45 years of age. For certain types of drugs, such as antineoplastic agents, it is not appropriate to use normal subjects because the risk of injury is too high. Women of childbearing potential are normally excluded from phase I studies. *The purpose of phase I studies is to establish the dose level at which signs of toxicity first appear.* The initial studies consist of administering a single dose of the test drug and closely observing the subject in a hospital or clinical pharmacology unit equipped with emergency facilities. If no adverse reactions occur, the dose is increased progressively until a predetermined dose or serum level is reached or toxicity supervenes. Ideally, such studies should be placebo controlled and single- or double-blind techniques should be used because the conditions under which such studies are conducted and the unusually close supervision used may tend to elicit a high incidence of adverse effects in the placebo group. Phase I studies are usually confined to a group of 20 to 80 subjects. If no untoward effects result from single doses, short-term multiple-dose studies are initiated.

Phase II

If the results of phase I studies show that it is reasonably safe to continue, *the new drug is administered to patients for the first time.* Ideally, these individuals should have no medical problems other than the condition for which the new drug is intended. Efforts are concentrated on evaluating efficacy and on establishing an optimal dose range. Therefore, dose-response studies are a critical part of phase II studies. Monitoring subjects for adverse effects is also an integral part of phase II trials. The number of subjects in phase II studies is usually between 80 and 100.

Phase III

When an effective dose range has been established and serious adverse reactions have not occurred, large numbers of subjects can be exposed to the drug. In phase III studies the number of subjects may range from several hundred to several thousand, depending on the drug. *The purpose of phase III studies is to verify the efficacy of the drug* and to detect effects that may not have surfaced in the phase I and II trials, during which exposure to the drug was limited.

A New Drug Application is submitted at the end of phase III. However, for drugs intended to treat patients with life-threatening or severely debilitating illnesses, especially when satisfactory therapy does not presently exist, the FDA has established procedures designed to expedite development, evaluation, and marketing of new therapies. In the majority of cases, the procedure would apply to drugs being developed for the treatment of cancer and acquired immunodeficiency syndrome (AIDS). Under the procedure, drugs could be approved on the basis of phase II studies conducted in a limited number of patients. Examples of recent approvals under this procedure are interleukin-2 for the treatment of renal cell cancer and taxol for the treatment of recurrent or refractory ovarian cancer. Under these provisions, the FDA may ask for phase IV studies to obtain additional data on risks, benefits, and optimal use.

Phase IV

Controlled and uncontrolled studies often are conducted after a drug is approved and marketed. Such studies are intended to broaden the experience with the drug and compare it to other drugs. Table 9-2 summarizes the four phases of clinical evaluation.

Special Populations

One of the goals of drug development is to provide sufficient data to devise prescribing information that will allow safe and effective use of the drug. Therefore, the pa-

Table 9-2. Phases of Clinical Investigation

Phase	Purpose
I	Establish safety
II	Establish efficacy and dose
III	Verify efficacy and detect adverse effects
IV	Obtain additional data following approval

tient population that participates in clinical trials should be representative of the patient population that will receive the drug when it is marketed. However, to a varying extent, *women, children, and patients over 65 years of age have been underrepresented in clinical trials of new drugs.* The reasons for exclusion vary but the consequence is that prescribing information for these patient populations is often deficient. For example, in the 1990 edition of the *Physicians' Desk Reference* fewer than 10 percent of the drugs listed have prescribing information for children even though many of the drugs are commonly prescribed for this group. Adjustments in the adult dose based on age or body surface area are not always appropriate and may result in toxicity or treatment failure. The lack of pediatric labeling has been attributed to the difficulties, some real and some perceived, in conducting adequate and well-controlled studies in children. However, the FDA has recently proposed new regulations that would allow data from studies in adults to provide substantial evidence of effectiveness in children if there is evidence that the disease course is the same in adults and children. Clinical studies still will be necessary to establish the dose in children.

Patients over the age of 65 years are often systematically excluded from clinical studies of new drugs. Provided patients meet functional criteria, there is no reason to exclude them only on the basis of age. While individuals 65 years of age and older represent only 12 percent of the population, they are responsible for approximately 30 percent of prescription drug use and 40 percent of nonprescription drug use. In addition, the prevalence of multiple diseases and diminished organ function increases with increasing age, which makes it inappropriate to extrapolate conclusions drawn from studies on younger patients. In developing new drugs, therefore, it is important to include patients over the age of 65 years because data on pharmacokinetics and on drug-drug and drug-disease interactions obtained from such studies are important in devising dosing instructions. In 1989, the FDA published guidelines to encourage "routine and thorough evaluation of the effects of drugs in the elderly population so that physicians will have sufficient information to use drugs properly in their elderly patients."

A recent report of the US General Accounting Office states that, although women generally are included in clinical studies, the percentage of women in the trials is lower than the percentage of women who have the disease being studied. Women who are pregnant and women of childbearing potential, with few exceptions, are excluded from studies of investigational drugs. In some studies women may participate if they are using "adequate" birth control measures; in others women may participate only if they have been sterilized surgically or if they are postmenopausal. This in effect excludes a high percentage of women between 18 and 50 years of age. The primary reason for excluding women is the concern that a drug given during pregnancy will cause injury to the fetus, either directly or indirectly. Consequently, drug labeling frequently contains a statement that controlled trials have not been conducted in pregnant women and that the physician should use the drug only if the benefit outweighs the risk. In many instances, the information available to make that judgment is inadequate. Nevertheless, women will require drug therapy during pregnancy because they acquire the same illnesses acquired by the general population. One study indicates that more than 60 percent of women receive at least one drug during pregnancy. There is no easy solution to this problem because controlled clinical trials of investigational drugs during pregnancy are unacceptable.

Adverse Reaction Surveillance

Almost all drugs have adverse effects associated with their use that range in severity from mild inconvenience to severe morbidity and death. Some adverse effects are extensions of the drug's pharmacological effect and are predictable, for example, orthostatic hypotension with some antihypertensive agents, arrhythmias with certain cardioactive drugs, and electrolyte imbalance with diuretics. Other adverse effects are not predictable and may occur rarely or be delayed for months or years before the association is recognized. Examples of such adverse reactions are aplastic anemia associated with chloramphenicol and clear cell carcinoma of the uterus in offspring of women treated with diethylstilbestrol during pregnancy. Postmarketing surveillance programs and adverse reaction reporting systems may be effective in detecting such events only if the attending physician is sufficiently observant. The best defense against devastating adverse reactions is still the vigilance and suspicion of the physician.

For final evaluation, new drugs must be tested in humans. Therefore, a responsible attitude toward the use of drugs in clinical practice demands that the physician be aware of the legal, ethical, philosophical, and economic issues involved in the introduction, testing, and distribution of new drugs.

Supplemental Reading

Guarino, R.A. (ed.). *New Drug Approval Process.* New York: Marcel Dekker, 1992.

Guideline for the Study of Drugs Likely to be Used in the Elderly. Center for Drug Evaluation and Research, Food and Drug Administration, November 1989.

Lemberger, L. Of mice and men: The extension of animal models to the clinical evaluation of new drugs. *Clin. Pharmacol. Ther.* 40:599, 1986.

Melman, K., et al. (eds.). *Clinical Pharmacology—Basic Principles in Therapeutics.* New York: McGraw-Hill, 1992.

O'Graby, J., and Linet, D. (eds.). *Early Phase Drug Evaluation in Man.* Boca Raton, Fla.: CRC, 1990.

O'Shaughnessy, J.A., et al. Commentary concerning demonstration of safety and efficacy of investigational anticancer agents in clinical trials. *J. Clin. Oncol.* 9:2225, 1991.

Spilker, B. *Guide to Clinical Trials.* New York: Raven, 1991.

Temple, R. Government viewpoint of clinical trials of cardiovascular drugs. *Med. Clin. North Am.* 73:495, 1989.

10

Ethics in Pharmacology

Janet Fleetwood

The well-publicized cases of scientific misconduct, the violations of patients' rights under the rubric of "clinical research," and the sometimes troubling relationship between researchers and drug companies all raise complicated ethical questions for the field of pharmacology. Although at first glance pharmacology may seem to be devoid of moral issues, the discipline cannot remain isolated from the ethical complexities arising from the recent growth in scientific technology and medicine. Any serious analysis of pharmacology should examine how professionals conduct their work, report their discoveries, and manage the relationships between colleagues, the public, and the pharmaceutical industry. This chapter outlines a theoretical framework for applying biomedical ethics in pharmacology, describes some of the field's ethical problems, and delineates some areas for further ethical inquiry.

Applying Biomedical Ethics in Pharmacology

Biomedical ethics is the study of ethical issues associated with providing health care or pursuing biomedical research. Studying biomedical ethics can enable one to recognize ethical issues in their medical and scientific contexts; provide critical, reasoned analysis; and resolve complex ethical questions.

Biomedical ethics, a branch of the philosophical discipline of ethics, is an interdisciplinary area involving concepts from theology, law, medicine, and the basic sciences. Although biomedical ethics is closely intertwined with these areas, it is important to recognize its independent standing as an academic discipline. Bioethics uses ethical principles that are separate from religious premises and presuppose no particular theological perspective. Similarly, although the law is often a consideration in bioethical decision making, laws in themselves do not determine the morality of an action, as they are developed and modified on the basis of moral concerns. Thus, while religion and law provide guidelines for acceptable behavior, religious beliefs and knowledge of the law are frequently insufficient to guide moral action. Solving problems that arise in the scientific and clinical contexts requires a knowledge of ethical principles and the methodology for applying them.

Three moral principles play key roles in bioethical analysis. These principles were developed from a pluralistic framework that itself presupposes no particular theological perspective. Although not every problem will involve all three principles, an understanding of the principles of autonomy, beneficence, and justice will build a solid framework for critical analysis.

The *principle of autonomy* entails that persons be treated as inherently valuable individuals with the moral right to make decisions about their own lives. To the extent that one's actions and choices do not negatively affect others, individuals with the capacity to make their own decisions should be free to do as they wish, even if their choices are risky or harmful to themselves. Many moral obligations for professionals engaged in scientific research or health care are derived from the principle of autonomy, such as the physician/researcher's obligation to elicit informed consent from patients and research subjects, and the clinician's duty to uphold a patient's wishes about accepting or refusing treatment. Each obligation is founded on the principle that individuals are the appropriate decision makers for choices that do not harm others.

The *principle of beneficence* entails helping people to further their own interests and refraining from injuring others. As the primary moral principle quoted in medical codes and oaths, the principle of beneficence is fundamental to the practice of medicine and clinical research. Concerns about beneficence motivate pharmacologists, pharmacists, and clinical researchers, all of whom share the goal of protecting subjects from harm while conducting studies that will ultimately benefit society by producing or refining effective treatments. Moreover, drug approval procedures, such as those implemented by the Food and Drug Administration (FDA), are designed to protect patients from harm while facilitating the marketing of drugs that have maximal therapeutic benefits.

The *principle of justice* is the final foundational principle. It states that individuals should be given what they deserve, be that benefit or burden. Cases that are alike should be treated similarly, and relevant distinctions should be drawn consistently. The principle of justice does not specifically state what distinctions are fair or which criteria are reasonable; it simply requires that, once criteria are determined, they be applied fairly. The principle is important in many areas, such as recruitment of subjects for a clinical study. Researchers must guard against distributing the burden of participation disproportionately among populations that are poorly equipped to give informed consent, such as children or the mentally incompetent.

The principles of autonomy, beneficence, and justice form a foundation for analysis of ethical quandaries. The principles must be weighed and balanced in each moral decision to provide guidance for the researcher's moral choices.

Pharmacology and Scientific Misconduct

At times scientists may make choices that go against commonly held moral beliefs and fall into the realm of scientific misconduct. Scientific misconduct includes plagiarism, data fabrication or falsification, inappropriate authorship attribution, violation of the rights of study subjects, and other departures from standard scientific procedures. Misconduct can occur in proposing, conducting, or reporting research. Its broad scope includes deliberate fraud, such as "dry labbing," in which one invents laboratory data without performing any studies, to failing to fully inform subjects in a research study of the risks of participation.

Misconduct differs from inadvertent scientific error primarily in its intent, as the goal of misconduct is to promulgate information that is not substantiated by the evidence provided or is substantiated by evidence that was illegitimately obtained. The truth or falsity of the scientist's claim is not what determines misconduct; what matters is that the evidence mustered does not support the claim asserted or that moral principles were violated in the process of obtaining the supporting data. In contrast, scientific error or sloppiness is unintentional, although responsible scientists have the duty to guard against error by carefully following procedures.

Instances of misconduct invariably involve violation of at least one ethical principle. For example, if subjects are poorly informed about the risks of a study before agreeing to participate, their autonomy has been restricted. Similarly, if patients are randomized into a placebo control group yet are under the misimpression that the physician is serving primarily as their advocate and providing the best care possible for them, then the doctor may be violating the duty of beneficence. Likewise, if research data are fabricated by an unscrupulous scientist, the dishonest researcher takes an unfair advantage over his or her colleagues, violating the principle of justice.

While scientific misconduct has received considerable public attention in the last decade, it is not new, and can be traced at least as far back as the early twentieth century case of Dawson's Piltdown man, which involved a hoax that led scientists to believe erroneously that early man was British. Recently, public attention has focused on several egregious cases of misconduct, such as Dr. William Summerlin's famed "painted mice" at the Sloan-Kettering Institute for Cancer Research, in which an ink marker was used to darken mouse skin grafts, and Dr. John Darsee's research fabrication of results of animal studies in cardiology at Harvard University.

Unfortunately, the area of drug research has not escaped its share of scandal, with the most publicized case of misconduct occurring in Dr. Stephen Breuning's infamous submission of false data to obtain a National Institute of Mental Health grant to study the use of drugs to control hyperactivity in retarded children. Breuning's studies, based on his "evidence" from hundreds of human subjects, asserted that stimulant drugs were more effective than tranquilizers. His work, published while he was at the Coldwater Regional Center for Developmental Disabilities and at the University of Pittsburgh, was widely respected and cited in the literature. However, an investigation by the National Institute of Mental Health found that Breuning had engaged deliberately in misleading and deceptive practices, and that the studies of psychopharmacological treatment he cited had in fact never been carried out. Breuning, a respected senior researcher, had himself practiced "dry labbing," generating his research data without performing the actual studies. Breuning pleaded guilty to making false statements on federal grant applications, and was sentenced to 60 days in a halfway house, 250 hours of community service, and 5 years of probation.

Moreover, scientific misconduct in pharmacology may be more widespread than just a few isolated, highly publicized examples like the Breuning case. A study of the extent and nature of scientific misconduct in clinical trials of investigational new drugs, which reviewed the FDA's records of 964 routine data audits conducted between June 1977 and September 1983, was published in *The New England Journal of Medicine* on March 14, 1985. Routine audits, in contrast to for-cause audits, are conducted by the FDA as part of their practice of monitoring investigators conducting clinical drug trials. The review of these FDA audits showed that 11.5 percent of the drug trials audited by the Food and Drug Administration evidenced serious deficiencies, including problems with patients' consent, drug accountability, adherence to the protocol, and accuracy or availability of records. Those researchers who were eventually disciplined by the FDA for their misconduct were guilty of a range of unacceptable activities, most commonly failing to maintain adequate case histories for data verification, failure to adhere to the protocol, and falsification of data.

Conducting research responsibly entails a commitment to the scientific method, including the formulation and testing of hypotheses, controlled observations or experiments, and careful analysis, interpretation, and presentation of data. A thorough understanding of scientific integrity and misconduct requires an awareness of the distinctions among fraud, misconduct, and sloppiness; a recognition of what constitutes accurate and complete data management including data preservation and reporting; an understanding of the ethically appropriate treatment of research subjects; a familiarity with the guidelines for attributing authorship credit and responsibility in scientific publications; a knowledge of the standards of ethical behavior proposed by organizations such as the American Association for the Advancement of Science, the National Science Foundation, the National Academy of Sciences, and the United States Public Health Service; and an understanding of the appropriateness of whistle blowing and criteria of due process for suspected violators.

Ethics of Research Involving Human and Animal Subjects

The protection of human and animal research subjects has received considerable attention in the literature and is one of the primary areas of concern for pharmacological research. In 1948 the Nuremberg Code set forth guidelines for the acceptable conduct of scientific research involving humans in response to the atrocities perpetrated by Nazi experimentation, and in 1964 the World Medical Association adopted the Declaration of Helsinki, which specifically guided physicians in biomedical research.

These documents specify basic moral guidelines ultimately founded on concerns for autonomy, beneficence, and justice. The guidelines require that

- Subjects give voluntary consent before being entered into any study after being fully advised of the study's aims, methods, benefits, risks, and discomforts
- Proposed studies have sufficient scientific merit to warrant their risks

- Studies be designed to avoid all unnecessary physical and mental suffering
- There be a clear balance of benefits over risks to subjects
- The researcher ensure subjects' privacy and confidentiality
- Subjects have the right to withdraw from the study at any time
- The researcher be obligated to stop the study if continuation is likely to result in subjects' injury

The guidelines further require that research on human subjects be conducted by qualified individuals and be reviewed by an independent committee, which in practice is generally the Institutional Review Board.

In pharmacokinetic studies, specific ethical concerns focus on the need for investigators to use noninvasive and minimally painful means of determining drug disposition, on minimizing the frequency of bodily fluid sampling, and on choosing study subjects who are representative of the target population whenever possible rather than exposing healthy volunteer subjects. In addition, investigators need to consider the safety of laboratory personnel and ensure that they have adequate training and protective supplies.

Research involving animals is similarly scrutinized, and the National Institutes of Health requires Animal Care and Use Committees to review institutional studies. Although some question the general morality of using animals for research, *the scientific community is largely supportive of animal use provided that certain safeguards are implemented.* Scientists' ethical concerns focus on issues including the use of anesthetics and tranquilizers to prevent inflicting pain, compassionate procedures for euthanasia, adequate training of staff who provide animal care, and appropriate selection of animals.

Science, Industry, and Conflicts of Interest

A conflict of interest occurs when an individual's private goals are inconsistent with his/her official responsibilities. Pharmacology, unlike other basic science disciplines, has a unique status when it comes to potential conflicts because the pursuit of pharmacological research is frequently tied to the pharmaceutical industry. Company-sponsored research is often directly linked to product development and sales, as frequently the eventual goal of the pharmaceutical company is to obtain the patent for a new product. The pharmaceutical company is therefore willing to offer financial incentives to researchers and clinicians who would be helpful in product development and testing. This financial compensation may compromise a scientist's professional judgment in conducting, analyzing, or reporting research.

Although pharmacology, as a scientific discipline, and the pharmaceutical industry share the objective of development and distribution of clinically effective products, the science and the industry are marked by potentially conflicting goals. The pharmaceutical industry combines a profit motive with a desire for discovery, development, and marketing. Scientists, be they pharmacologists, pharmacists, or physician/researchers, share the desire for drug discovery and development; however, scientists are primarily motivated by the desire to contribute to scientific advancement and by beneficent interests in improving patient care rather than concern about corporate profits. Naturally, pharmaceutical companies are concerned about patient care and want their products rigorously tested, but the commercial pressures of product marketing cannot help but affect their perspective.

Researchers and drug companies are mutually interdependent. The pharmaceutical industry depends on scientists and clinicians for research, development, and marketing. Conversely, the medical profession depends on research that is largely financed by the pharmaceutical industry. While this interdependence often benefits industry, research, and patient care, conflicts of interest may arise in two main areas: (1) drug research and development and (2) clinical education and product marketing.

The broad area of drug research and development frequently raises ethical concerns. For example, often a pharmaceutical company will contract with a clinical researcher to conduct a drug study. While in itself this arrangement is relatively unproblematic and frequently offers patients access to treatment that might otherwise be unavailable, the potential conflict may ultimately result in lack of objectivity in study design, data interpretation, and dissemination of research results. For example, a 1986 study in the *Journal of General Internal Medicine* found a statistically significant relationship between drug company funding and outcomes favoring a new therapy.

One typical situation in which a conflict of interest may occur is when a drug company offers payment in the form of cash or other inducements to a clinician willing to recruit patients for a company-designed drug study. The inducements, provided as a capitation payment or lump sum, often exceed the expenses incurred by the researcher in conducting the study. This money can provide a temptation for a clinician to enter patients into a drug trial before other, clinically recognized, therapeutic options have been exhausted.

In cases in which the physician enters into an agreement with the pharmaceutical company to do sponsored research, the doctor assumes a position of responsibility to the company while simultaneously maintaining duties to protect and benefit his or her patients. *The usual relationship between doctor and patient places the physician in the position of patient advocate, a position that can easily be compromised by undue influence from pharmaceutical companies.* The physician is in a special relationship with the patient, who depends on the doctor to protect his/her interests and may be unaware of countervailing forces on the physician's motives. At minimum, the principle of autonomy requires that patients be fully informed about the financial arrangements between their physician and the pharmaceutical company. In addition, the principles of autonomy and beneficence require that patients be told the source of funding for sponsored studies, and be made aware of the potential conflict between the physician's research interests and treatment recommendations.

Research sponsored by a drug company should undergo the same scientific scrutiny as other research, and should not simply be a ruse to get patients started on a particular manufacturer's product. In addition, industry sponsorship needs to be noted in any publication reporting study results. Finally, researchers or clinicians who are invited to conduct studies supported by drug companies and present their data at company-sponsored educational events need to take special care to conduct the study meticulously, analyze the data rigorously, and present the data as objectively as possible.

The second area for ethical concern is that of clinical education and product marketing. The line between "education" and "marketing" is frequently a blurry one, and it is often difficult to separate a company's desire to educate physicians about products that may enhance patient care from the company's desire to simply increase profits. *As the "gatekeepers" for all prescription drugs, physicians have the power to determine which drugs will compete successfully in the marketplace, making doctors the logical targets for marketing efforts by pharmaceutical firms.* Many company-sponsored arrangements may conflict with the physician's responsibility to act in the best interest of the patient, and physicians must take extreme care to ensure that participation in industry-sponsored activities does not negatively affect their prescribing habits, thereby violating the principle of beneficence.

In addition to direct product advertising in medical journals, pharmaceutical company sales representatives frequently visit physicians. Although the salesperson's goal is clearly to promote sales, often these visits take the form of "education" for busy clinicians. Company representatives present "educational" information, offer samples, and may give gifts or incentives to the doctor. Although such visits may keep clinicians informed about current products, they may also present the opportunity for conflicts of interest to arise. *Gifts of more than token value, trips to resort areas for "educational" programs with little scientific merit, and cash incentives for prescribing a drug or having it added to a hospital formulary all are cause for concern.* The line between a "gift" and a "bribe" is not a sharp one, and clinicians and drug company employees need to strive to avoid any impropriety.

Physicians should not accept gifts from companies if

the gift might, or might appear to, compromise the physician's objectivity. A helpful criterion suggested by the American College of Physicians when considering the ethical appropriateness of a particular interaction between a physician and drug company is to ask whether one would be willing to have the arrangement generally known. If not, the action falls outside the realm of ethical acceptability and should be avoided.

Medical students and residents are not exempt from the influence of drug companies, and need to be as vigilant as their more senior colleagues. Many students and residents are offered gifts of educational books or equipment or are invited to attend company-sponsored events. Young professionals need to be extremely careful to avoid impropriety, and should receive specific instruction about the ethically appropriate scope and limits of interactions with drug company representatives.

The area of continuing medical education is similarly mired with controversy, as educational "meetings" may be simply soft sells at company expense to encourage physicians to prescribe one company's product over the competition's. While some industry-sponsored education provides a good opportunity for unbiased scientific exchange, such as when a drug company underwrites the cost of an educational program but places no restrictions on topics discussed or speakers chosen, too often "education" is just a euphemism for product marketing.

The FDA is currently working on guidelines for industry-sponsored events, and will soon have regulations for company-sponsored promotional activities. To determine whether an activity is educational or primarily promotional, the FDA will look at the criteria of independence, objectivity, balance, and scientific rigor. These criteria require that company sponsors may not control the scientific content of the program; should only underwrite activities in organizations known to be objective, such as professional societies; should include experts representing a range of qualified medical opinions; and should only support those activities that reflect research of sufficient scientific rigor.

Speakers at company-sponsored events need to subject their presentation to the same level of scientific rigor as those they would give to a presentation at a professional meeting, and refrain from allowing the drug company to influence the data they present, the means of presenting it, or the outcomes drawn. If a speaker wishes to mention a specific product, he or she should be sure to avoid any appearance of impropriety by comparing it fairly and completely with its competitors. Speakers should avoid accepting lecture invitations to events at which the audience is paid to attend by the drug company, and should object if the company's marketing representatives conduct sales activities, such as distributing samples or brochures about a specific product, at the time of the lecture. Finally, both attendees and speakers should demand that financial sponsorship be revealed before registration, and that financial relationships between speakers and the promoter be plainly stated.

Attendees at company-sponsored events have obligations as well. Researchers and clinicians who attend educational events are responsible for assessing the objectivity and rigor of the information presented and should object to educational offerings that appear to be unduly biased. Attendees should assure themselves that the time spent in an educational setting is more than commensurate with the time spent in recreational activities, and that attending the company-sponsored event is not simply an excuse for a vacation or meal at company expense. Moreover, a 1982 study in the *American Journal of Medicine* has shown that doctors who rely on industry-provided information for drug education are more likely to prescribe drugs for indications that are not supported by the scientific literature. This leads to the conclusion that *doctors should get their information primarily from professional, peer-reviewed journals and not rely solely on material provided by drug companies.*

Ultimately, prescribing practices are the main source of concern, as physicians may be induced to prescribe some products rather than others based on factors other than therapeutic effectiveness or cost. Specifically, clinicians should monitor their own practices for signs of undue influence. Free drug samples provided by drug companies should be used cautiously, and the choice of drugs should be made on the basis of medical indications and not sample availability. The patient, as a health care consumer, is not in an educated position to assess the need for a certain drug, decide whether it is prescribed appropriately, or determine whether it is successful. Thus, *the patient deserves to be protected by the physician, whose primary role is that of patient advocate.*

Supplemental Reading

Beauchamp, T. and Walters, L. *Contemporary Issues in Bioethics.* Belmont, Calif.: Wadsworth Publishing, 1989.

Guarding the guardians: Research on editorial peer review. *J.A.M.A.* 263:1317, 1990.

Kessler, D.A. Drug promotion and scientific exchanges: The role of the clinical investigator. *N. Engl. J. Med.* 325:201, 1991.

Shapiro, M., and Charrow, R. Scientific misconduct in investigational drug trials. *N. Engl. J. Med.* 312:731, 1985.

Shimm, D., and Spece, R. Industry reimbursement for entering patients into clinical trials: Legal and ethical issues. *Ann. Intern. Med.* 115:148, 1991.

Sigma Xi, The Scientific Research Society. *Honor in Science,* 1986. Available from the Publications Office, Sigma Xi, The Scientific Research Society, P.O. Box 13975, Research Triangle Park, NC 27709.

Svensson, C. Ethical considerations in the conduct of clinical pharmacokinetic studies. *Clin. Pharmacokinet.* 17:217, 1989.

Drugs Affecting the Autonomic Nervous System

11

Introduction to the Autonomic Nervous System

William W. Fleming

General Organization and Functions of the Nervous System

The nervous system is divided into two parts: the central nervous system (CNS) and the peripheral nervous system (PNS). The CNS consists of the brain and spinal cord. The peripheral nervous system consists of all *afferent* (sensory) neurons, which carry nerve impulses into the CNS from sensory end organs located in peripheral tissues, and all *efferent* (motor) neurons, which carry nerve impulses from the CNS to effector cells in peripheral tissues. The peripheral efferent system is further divided into the *somatic nervous system* and the *autonomic nervous system*. The effector cells innervated by the somatic nervous system are skeletal muscle cells. The autonomic nervous system innervates three different types of effector cells: (1) smooth muscle, (2) cardiac muscle, and (3) exocrine glands. While the somatic nervous system can function on a reflex basis, voluntary control of skeletal muscle is of primary importance. In contrast, in the autonomic nervous system voluntary control can be exerted, but reflex control is paramount.

Both somatic and autonomic effectors may be reflexly excited by nerve impulses arising from the same sensory end organs. For example, when the body is exposed to cold, heat loss is minimized by vasoconstriction of blood vessels in the skin and by the curling up of the body. At the same time, heat production is increased by an increase in skeletal muscle tone and shivering and by an increase in metabolism owing, in part, to secretion of epinephrine.

In general terms, the function of the autonomic nervous system is to maintain the constancy of the internal environment (*homeostasis*). This includes the regulation of the cardiovascular system, digestion, body temperature, metabolism, and the secretion of the exocrine glands.

Differences Between the Somatic and Autonomic Nervous Systems

There are anatomical differences between the peripheral somatic and autonomic nervous systems that have led to their classification as separate divisions of the nervous system. Besides the different effector cells innervated, the nature of the link between the CNS and the effector cells differs between the somatic and autonomic nervous systems. The axon of a somatic motor neuron leaves the CNS and travels without interruption to the innervated effector cell (i.e., a skeletal muscle cell, Fig. 11-1). In contrast, two neurons are required to connect the CNS and a visceral effector cell (i.e., smooth muscle, cardiac muscle, or exocrine gland cell) of the autonomic nervous system. The first of these two neurons, its cell body within the CNS, sends out an axon, which makes a synaptic connection with a second neuron located outside the CNS in a collection or mass of nerve cells known as a *ganglion*. The first neuron in this sequence is called the *preganglionic* neuron. The second neuron, whose cell body is located within the ganglion, travels to the visceral effector cell; it is called the *postganglionic* neuron (see Fig. 11-1).

Autonomic Nervous System

The cell bodies of the preganglionic neurons of the two divisions of the autonomic nervous system are found in different parts of the CNS. The preganglionic neurons of the *sympathetic* nervous system have their cell bodies in the thoracic and lumbar regions of the spinal cord. This division of the autonomic nervous system is frequently referred to as the thoracolumbar division. The sympathetic

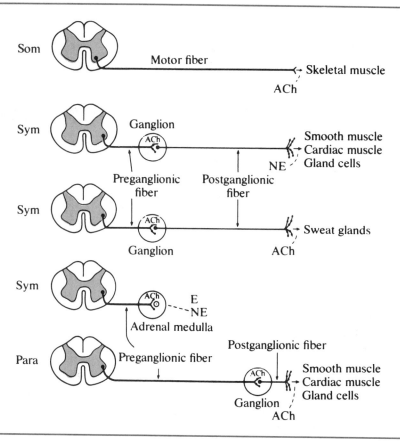

Figure 11-1. Anatomical characteristics and neurotransmitters of the somatic (Som), sympathetic (Sym), and parasympathetic (Para) divisions of the peripheral nervous systems. ACh = acetylcholine; E = epinephrine; NE = norepinephrine.

preganglionic cell bodies are found in all segments of the thoracic region of the spinal cord and in the upper two or three segments of the lumbar cord, largely in the intermediolateral cell column of the gray matter.

The preganglionic neurons of the *parasympathetic* division have their cell bodies in the brainstem and in the sacral region of the spinal cord. This division of the autonomic nervous system is frequently also called the craniosacral division. The cranial part of the parasympathetic nervous system innervates structures in the head, neck, thorax, and abdomen (e.g., the stomach, part of the intestines, and pancreas). The cranial parasympathetic fibers leave the CNS in the oculomotor, facial, glossopharyngeal, and vagal cranial nerves. The sacral division of the parasympathetic nervous system innervates the remainder of the intestines and the pelvic viscera.

Location of the Autonomic Ganglia

Characteristically, the sympathetic ganglia consist of two chains of 22 segmentally arranged ganglia located lat-

erally to the vertebral column. The preganglionic fibers leave the spinal cord in adjacent ventral roots and enter neighboring ganglia where they make synaptic connections with postganglionic neurons. Some preganglionic fibers pass through the vertebral ganglia without making synaptic connections and travel by way of splanchnic nerves to paired prevertebral ganglia situated in front of the vertebral column, where they make synaptic connections with postganglionic neurons. In addition, some sympathetic preganglionic fibers pass through the splanchnic nerves into the adrenal glands, and make synaptic connections on the chromaffin cells of the adrenal medulla. (The relationship of this endocrine gland to the sympathetic nervous system is discussed under The Adrenal Medulla in this chapter.)

Because sympathetic ganglia lie close to the vertebral column, sympathetic preganglionic fibers are generally short. Postganglionic fibers are generally long, since they arise in vertebral ganglia and must travel to the innervated effector cells, which may be located a considerable distance from the ganglion. An example of such effector cells is the vascular smooth muscle in the hands or feet. There are exceptions to this generalization. A few sympathetic ganglia lie near the organs innervated (e.g., urinary bladder and rectum); thus, these preganglionic fibers are long and the postganglionic fibers are short.

It is characteristic of the parasympathetic ganglia that they lie very close to, or actually within, the organs innervated by the parasympathetic postganglionic neurons. The ganglia of the cranial division of the parasympathetic division of the autonomic nervous system are located in the head near the organs innervated, with the exception of the ganglia associated with the vagus nerves, which contain the synapses for parasympathetic nerves to organs in the thorax (e.g., heart, bronchial tree) and abdomen (e.g., gastrointestinal tract). The vagal ganglia are located within these organs. The ganglia of the sacral division of the parasympathetic nervous system are also found within the organs innervated. Thus, the parasympathetic preganglionic fibers are generally longer than postganglionic fibers because the latter must travel only short distances to the cells innervated by them.

Ratio of Preganglionic to Postganglionic Neurons

A single sympathetic preganglionic fiber branches a number of times after entering a ganglion and makes synaptic connection with a number of postganglionic neurons. Furthermore, some branches of this preganglionic fiber may ascend or descend to adjacent vertebral ganglia and terminate on an additional number of postganglionic neurons in these ganglia as well. The number of postganglionic neurons with which a given preganglionic fiber of the sympathetic nervous system makes synaptic connection varies considerably in different species. In human superior cervical ganglia, a single preganglionic fiber may connect with 63 to 196 postganglionic neurons. Therefore, activity in a single sympathetic preganglionic neuron may result in the activation of a number of effector cells in widely separated regions of the body. Anatomically, *the sympathetic nervous system is designed to produce widespread physiological activity.*

By contrast, parasympathetic preganglionic neurons are extremely limited in their distribution. In general, a single parasympathetic preganglionic fiber makes a synaptic connection with only one or two postganglionic neurons. For this reason, along with the fact that the ganglia are near or embedded in the organs innervated, individual *parasympathetic preganglionic neurons influence only a small region of the body or affect only specific organs.*

Physiological Significance

The physiological importance of the morphological features discussed above is clear from a comparison of the physiological responses produced by activation of the sympathetic and parasympathetic systems. The sympathetic nervous system prepares the body for strenuous muscular activity, stress, and emergencies. The parasympathetic nervous system is involved with the accumulation, storage, and preservation of body resources.

When the sympathetic integrative centers in the brain are activated (by anger, stress, or emergency situations), the body's resources are mobilized for combat or for flight. Obviously, *widespread activation of the sympathetic nervous system is beneficial to the individual under appropriate circumstances.* Stimulation of the sympathetic nervous system results in an acceleration of the heart rate and an increase in the contractile force of the heart muscle. There is increased blood flow (*vasodilation*) through skeletal muscle and decreased blood flow (*vasoconstriction*) through the skin and visceral organs. Activity of the gastrointestinal tract, such as peristaltic and secretory activity, is decreased, and intestinal sphincters are contracted. The pupils are dilated. The increased breakdown of glycogen (*glycogenolysis*) in the liver produces an increase in blood sugar, while the breakdown of lipids (*lipolysis*) in adipose tissue produces an increase in blood fatty acids; these biochemical reactions make energy available for active tissues. In addition to a generalized activation of the sympathetic system in response to stress, there can also be more discrete homeostatic activation of the sympathetic system. For example, a selective reflex-associated alteration in the sympathetic outflow to the cardiovascular system can occur.

Stimulation of the parasympathetic nervous system decreases heart rate. The tone and peristaltic and secretory activities of the gastrointestinal tract increase at the same time that the sphincters of the intestine relax. The pupils of the eye are constricted, and accommodation for near vision occurs. The smooth muscle of the bronchial tree is constricted. Glandular cells, such as lacrimal, salivary, and mucous, are stimulated to secrete.

Widespread activation of the parasympathetic system would not serve a useful purpose. The parasympathetic system is designed to function more or less on an organ system basis, usually under conditions of minimal stress. For example, the activation of the gastrointestinal tract takes place during the digestion of a meal; constriction of the pupil and accommodation for near vision are essential for reading.

Autonomic Neurotransmitters

Two chemical substances have been established as neurotransmitters in the peripheral nervous system. These are acetylcholine and norepinephrine. Both transmitters are synthesized and stored primarily in the nerve terminals until released by a nerve impulse. It should be noted, to avoid confusion, that in the United States the transmitter in the sympathetic nervous system is referred to as *norepinephrine* and the major adrenal medullary hormone is referred to as *epinephrine*. In Europe and most of the world these two substances are called *noradrenaline* and *adrenaline*, respectively.

Neurotransmission in the peripheral nervous system occurs at four major sites. Acetylcholine is the transmitter released at a majority of these sites. These are (1) preganglionic synapses in both parasympathetic and sympathetic ganglia, (2) parasympathetic postganglionic neuroeffector junctions and a few sympathetic neuroeffector junctions, and (3) all somatic motor end-plates on skeletal muscle.

All neurons that release acetylcholine are called *cholinergic* (i.e., working like acetylcholine) neurons. Norepinephrine is the transmitter released at most sympathetic postganglionic neuroeffector junctions, and neurons that release this substance are called *adrenergic* or *noradrenergic* (working like noradrenaline) neurons.

Not all sympathetic postganglionic neurons are noradrenergic neurons. The sympathetic postganglionic neurons that innervate the sweat glands and some of the blood vessels in skeletal muscle are cholinergic neurons; that is, they release acetylcholine rather than norepinephrine, even though anatomically they are sympathetic neurons (see Fig. 11-1).

It is common practice in modern pharmacology to refer to drugs that mimic the actions of acetylcholine as *cholinomimetic* drugs and those that mimic epinephrine and/or norepinephrine as *adrenomimetic* drugs. The cholinomimetic drugs are also called cholinergic or parasympathomimetic drugs. The adrenomimetic drugs are often called adrenergic or sympathomimetic drugs.

The receptors with which acetylcholine or other cholinomimetic drugs interact are called *cholinoceptors*, while the receptors with which norepinephrine, epinephrine, or other adrenomimetic drugs combine are called *adrenoceptors*. It is common both in textbooks and the scientific literature to see these receptors referred to as cholinergic or adrenergic receptors. This is, however, improper usage of the terms cholinergic and adrenergic since it implies that the receptors function like acetylcholine or norepinephrine (or epinephrine).

Drugs that antagonize the actions of acetylcholine are known as *cholinoceptor antagonists;* those that antagonize norepinephrine are known as *adrenoceptor antagonists*.

A number of other substances are released by sympathetic and parasympathetic neurons, often the very same neurons that release norepinephrine or acetylcholine. These substances include adenosine triphosphate (ATP), neuropeptide Y, and substance P. In general, these modulate the release and/or the postsynaptic effects of the primary neurotransmitter. Each of these neuromodulators has its own selective receptors. At present, there are no therapeutically used drugs that mimic or antagonize the new modulators.

Innervation of Various Organs by the Sympathetic and Parasympathetic Nervous Systems

Many visceral organs are innervated by both divisions of the autonomic nervous system. In most instances, when an organ receives a dual innervation, the two systems work in opposition to one another. In some tissues or organs, the two innervations exert an opposing influence on the same effector cells (e.g., the sinoatrial node in the heart), while in other tissues opposing actions come about because different effector cells are activated (e.g., the circular and radial muscles in the iris). Some organs are innervated by only one division of the autonomic nervous system.

Many neurons of both divisions of the autonomic nervous system are tonically active; that is, they are continually carrying some impulse traffic. The moment-to-moment activity of an organ such as the heart, which receives a dual innervation by sympathetic (noradrenergic) and parasympathetic (cholinergic) neurons, is controlled by the level of tonic activity of the two systems. A change in the activity of the sympathetic and parasympathetic systems depends on information conveyed to the cardiac center of the brain from sensory end-organs such as the baroreceptors, or from higher brain centers. Acceleration of the heart rate (*tachycardia*) occurs when there is an increase in sympathetic and a decrease in parasympathetic activity. Slowing of the heart rate (*bradycardia*) occurs when there is an increase in parasympathetic and a decrease in sympathetic activity.

Blood Vessels

Most vascular smooth muscle is innervated solely by the sympathetic (noradrenergic) nervous system. Exceptions to this general rule exist, however. Some blood vessels in the face, tongue, and urogenital tract (especially the penis) are innervated by parasympathetic (cholinergic) as well as sympathetic (noradrenergic) neurons. The parasympathetic innervation of blood vessels has only regional importance, for example, in salivary glands, where increased parasympathetic activity causes vasodilation that supports salivation. The primary neural control of total peripheral resistance is through sympathetic nerves. The caliber (diameter) of blood vessels is controlled by the tonic activity of noradrenergic neurons. There is a continuous outflow of noradrenergic impulses to the vascular smooth muscle, and therefore some degree of constant vascular constriction is maintained. An increase in impulse outflow causes further contraction of the smooth muscle, resulting in greater vasoconstriction. A decrease in impulse outflow permits the smooth muscle to relax, leading to a vasodilation.

Heart

The heart is innervated by both sympathetic and parasympathetic neurons; however, their distribution in the heart is quite different. Postganglionic noradrenergic fibers from the stellate and inferior cervical ganglia innervate the sinoatrial (S-A) node and myocardial tissues of the atria and ventricles. Activation of the sympathetic outflow to the heart results in an increase in rate (*positive chronotropic effect*), in force of contraction (*positive inotropic effect*), and in conductivity of the atrioventricular (A-V) conduction tissue (*positive dromotropic effect*).

The postganglionic cholinergic fibers of the parasympathetic nervous system terminate in the S-A node, atria, and A-V conduction tissue. Cholinergic fibers do not innervate the ventricular muscle to any significant degree. Activation of the parasympathetic outflow to the heart results in a decrease in rate (*negative chronotropic effect*) and a prolongation in the A-V conduction time (*negative dromotropic effect*). There is a decrease in the contractile force of the atria, but little effect on ventricular contractile force.

The effect of a drug on the heart is dependent on the balance of sympathetic and parasympathetic activity at the time the drug is administered. An example is the effect of the ganglionic blocking agents (see Chap. 17), which nonselectively inhibit transmission in both sympathetic and parasympathetic ganglia. Normally, under conditions of rest or mild activity, the heart is predominantly under the influence of the vagal parasympathetic system. Blockade of the autonomic innervation of the heart by the administration of a ganglionic blocking agent accelerates the heart rate. Conversely, if sympathetic activity is dominant, as in exercise, ganglionic blockade will decrease the heart rate and also reduce ventricular contractility.

Cardiovascular Reflexes

Any sudden alteration in the mean arterial blood pressure tends to produce compensatory reflex changes in heart rate, contractility, and vascular tone, which will oppose the initial pressure change and restore the homeostatic balance. The primary sensory mechanisms to detect changes in the mean arterial blood pressure are stretch receptors (*baroreceptors*) located in the carotid sinus and aortic arch. These baroreceptor reflexes play an important role in modifying the cardiovascular responses to drugs that alter the blood pressure.

The injection of a vasoconstrictor, which causes an increase in mean arterial blood pressure, results in activation of the baroreceptors and increased neural input to the cardiovascular centers in the medulla oblongata. The reflex compensation for the drug-induced hypertension involves an increase in parasympathetic nerve activity and a decrease in sympathetic nerve activity. This combined alteration in neural firing results in a decrease in cardiac rate and force and a reduction in the tone of vascular smooth muscle. As a consequence of the altered neural control of both the heart and the blood vessels, the rise in blood pressure induced by the drug is opposed and blunted.

The injection of a drug that causes a fall in the mean arterial blood pressure triggers diametrically opposite reflex changes. There is decreased impulse traffic from the cardiac inhibitory center, stimulation of the cardiac accelerator center, and augmented vasomotor center activity. These changes in cardiac and vasomotor center activity accelerate the heart and increase sympathetic transmission to the vasculature; thus, the drug-induced fall in blood pressure is opposed and blunted.

The Eye

The smooth muscles that control the size of the pupil and the degree of visual accommodation are innervated by the autonomic nervous system. Two sets of smooth muscle in the iris control the diameter of the pupil. One set of muscles, which is arranged radially (dilator pupillae), is innervated by sympathetic (noradrenergic) fibers. These fibers arise from cells in the superior cervical ganglion, and their stimulation causes contraction of the radial smooth muscle cells, leading to dilation of the pupil (*mydriasis*). The other set of smooth muscle cells in the iris is arranged circularly (constrictor pupillae) and is innervated by parasympathetic neurons arising from cells in the ciliary ganglion. Stimulation of these cholinergic neurons causes contraction of the circular smooth muscle of the iris (working much like a sphincter), and this produces constriction of the pupil (*miosis*).

The lens, which aids in visual accommodation, is attached at its lateral edge to the ciliary body by suspensory ligaments. When the smooth muscles of the ciliary body are relaxed, the ciliary body exerts tension on the lens, causing it to flatten. Thus, the eye is accommodated for far vision. Stimulation of parasympathetic cholinergic neurons, which arise in the ciliary ganglion, causes contraction of the smooth muscle of the ciliary body; this decreases the lateral tension on the lens. Naturally elastic, the lens then thickens, and the eye accommodates for near vision. Drugs that block accommodation are called *cycloplegic* drugs. The parasympathetic system is dominant in the eye. Blockade of the parasympathetic system by atropine (see Chap. 15), or of both autonomic systems by a ganglionic blocking agent, will produce pupillary dilation and a loss of accommodative capacity.

Most dually innervated organ systems are dominated

by the parasympathetic division of the autonomic nervous system. Thus, ganglion blockade results in dilation of the bronchial tree, reduced tone and motility of the gastrointestinal tract, relaxation of the smooth muscle of the urinary bladder (detrusor muscle), and reduction in the secretion of the exocrine glands.

Pulmonary Smooth Muscle

The bronchial tree is innervated by both divisions of the autonomic nervous system. Postganglionic parasympathetic neurons innervate bronchial smooth muscle directly and produce bronchoconstriction when stimulated. Sympathetic noradrenergic neurons appear to innervate vascular smooth muscle and parasympathetic ganglion cells. The effect of noradrenergic fibers on ganglion cells is to inhibit their firing. There is some controversy concerning the role of noradrenergic fibers in the regulation of airway smooth muscle tone. There is no doubt, however, that adrenoceptors are present on bronchial smooth muscle and that epinephrine from the adrenal gland and drugs such as epinephrine and isoproterenol produce bronchodilation of the airway.

Gastrointestinal Tract

The innervation of the gastrointestinal tract is extremely complex (see Chap. 73). The myenteric and submucosal plexuses contain many interneurons. These possess a number of neurotransmitters and neuromodulators including several peptides, such as enkephalins, substance P, and vasoactive intestinal peptide (VIP). There is reflex activity within the plexuses that regulates peristalsis and secretion locally. The effects of sympathetic and parasympathetic nerve stimulation are superimposed on this local neural regulation.

The gastrointestinal tract receives a dual innervation. The cell bodies of postganglionic neurons, with which parasympathetic preganglionic neurons make synaptic connections, constitute a large proportion of the ganglion cells of the intramural or intrinsic nerves of the gut (the myenteric and submucosal plexuses). These ganglion cells give rise to excitatory cholinergic fibers that directly innervate the smooth muscle and gland cells of the gut. The sympathetic fibers that enter the gastrointestinal tract are postganglionic noradrenergic fibers, stimulation of which inhibits gut motility and gland secretion and contracts sphincters. Most of the noradrenergic fibers terminate either in blood vessels or on the cholinergic ganglionic cells of the intramural plexuses. These fibers alter gut motility by inhibiting acetylcholine release from the intramural

nerves. Direct noradrenergic innervation of smooth muscle of the nonsphincter portion of the gut is sparse.

Salivary Glands

One exception to the generalization that the two systems work in opposition to each other is secretion by the salivary glands; both sympathetic (noradrenergic) and parasympathetic (cholinergic) activation of these glands lead to an increase in the flow of saliva. However, the nature of the saliva produced by the two systems is qualitatively different. The saliva produced by activation of the sympathetic system is a sparse, thick, mucinous secretion, whereas that produced by parasympathetic activation is a profuse, watery secretion.

The Adrenal Medulla

The paired adrenal glands are composite endocrine glands that consist of an outer cortical and an inner medullary part. The adrenal cortex is considered in Chap. 66. The cells of the adrenal medulla, called *chromaffin* cells, are homologous with sympathetic postganglionic neurons. The adrenal medulla may, in fact, be considered to be a modified sympathetic ganglion. The similarity between the chromaffin cells and the sympathetic neurons is suggested by the following considerations: (1) Both the sympathetic postganglionic neurons and the chromaffin cells of the adrenal medulla have a common embryonic origin; that is, both arise from neural crest ectoderm. (2) Both are innervated by anatomically sympathetic preganglionic fibers that are cholinergic in nature (i.e., they release acetylcholine). (3) The adrenal medulla secretes two hormones. One is norepinephrine, which is also the primary neurotransmitter of sympathetic postganglionic neurons. The other medullary hormone is epinephrine (adrenaline). The term *sympathoadrenal system* is frequently used to indicate the close physiological relationship that exists between the sympathetic nervous system and the adrenal medulla.

Generalized activation of the sympathetic system occurs during stress, fear, or anxiety, and is accompanied by increased secretion of adrenal medullary hormones, which consist primarily of epinephrine in the human. In humans, the percentage ratio of epinephrine to norepinephrine in the adrenal medulla is approximately 80:20.

The secretory activity of the adrenal medulla is regulated by the CNS. Following denervation of the glands by sectioning of the splanchnic nerves, the hormone output is reduced and the glands become unresponsive to various

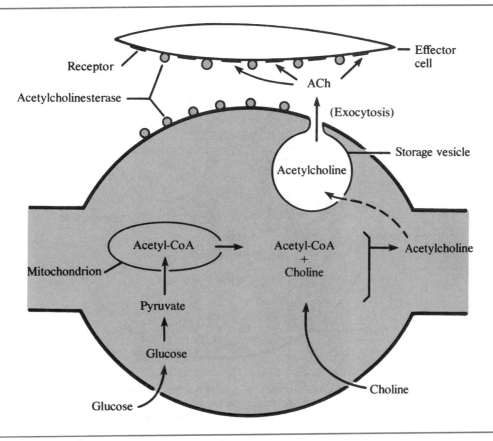

Figure 11-2. Varicosity, showing processes of synthesis and storage of acetylcholine within a cholinergic neuron. Also shown are the release of acetylcholine (exocytosis) and the location of acetylcholinesterase, which inactivates acetylcholine.

physiological stresses, such as hypoxia, hypoglycemia, hypotension, fear, and anxiety.

Some bloodborne substances of endogenous origin such as histamine, angiotensin, or bradykinin can directly stimulate the chromaffin cells to secrete epinephrine and norepinephrine. A variety of exogenously administered drugs such as cholinomimetic agents and caffeine can directly stimulate the secretion of adrenal medullary hormones. The neuronally induced secretion of medullary hormones is antagonized by ganglionic blocking agents.

Transmission of the Nerve Impulse

Microscopic studies of the structure of the terminal axons of the autonomic nerves have shown that the axons branch many times on entering the effector tissue, forming a plexus among the innervated cells. "Swollen" areas are found at intervals along the terminal axons, which

thus resemble strings of beads passing through the mass of effector cells. These swollen areas are referred to as *varicosities* (see Figs. 11-2 and 11-3). Within each varicosity are mitochondria and numerous small membrane-bound sacklike structures called *vesicles,* which contain neurotransmitters.

The vesicles are also intimately involved in the release of the transmitter into the *synaptic* or *neuroeffector cleft* in response to an action potential. Following release, the transmitter must then diffuse to the effector cells, where it interacts with receptors on these cells to produce a response. The distance between the varicosities and the effector cells varies considerably from tissue to tissue. Smooth muscle, cardiac muscle, and exocrine gland cells do not contain morphologically specialized regions comparable to the end-plate of skeletal muscle.

In the autonomic ganglia, the terminal branches of the preganglionic axons are varicose in nature, very much like the postganglionic terminals in autonomic effector tissues. There is an important difference, however, in that the varicosities of the preganglionic terminals come into

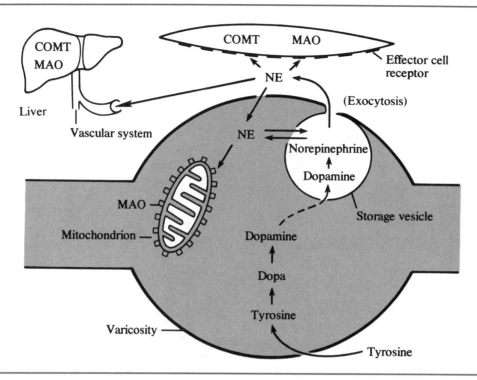

Figure 11-3. Varicosity of a noradrenergic neuron, showing processes of synthesis and storage of norepinephrine. Also shown is the release of norepinephrine (NE) and multiple routes for degradation. COMT = catechol-*O*-methyltransferase; MAO = monoamine oxidase.

close contact primarily with the dendrites of the ganglionic cells and make synaptic connection with them.

The transmission of nerve impulses across synapses that are located between neurons or at neuroeffector junctions described above is referred to as *neurochemical transmission.*

Steps in Neurochemical Transmission

Regardless of the type of neuron under consideration, the fundamental steps in chemical transmission are the same. Each of these steps is a potential site for pharmacological intervention in the normal transmission process. The steps are as follows:

1. Synthesis of the transmitter
2. Storage of the transmitter
3. Release of the transmitter by a nerve action potential
4. Interaction of the released transmitter with receptors on the effector cell membrane and the associated change in the effector cell

5. Rapid removal of the transmitter from the vicinity of the receptors
6. Recovery of the effector cell to the state that preceded transmitter action

Synthesis, Storage, Release, and Removal of Acetylcholine

The processes involved in neurochemical transmission in a cholinergic neuron are shown in Fig. 11-2.

The initial substrates for the synthesis of acetylcholine are *glucose* and *choline.* Glucose enters the neuron by means of facilitated transport. The molecules of choline, which are almost completely ionized at body pH, also enter by a transport system. There is some disagreement as to whether to call the transport of choline active or facilitated. Choline apparently enters the neuron in association with Na^+. The sodium gradient is dependent on the membrane Na^+-K^+ pump, which is an active transport system. Pyruvate derived from glucose is transported into mitochondria and converted to *acetylcoenzyme A (acetyl-CoA).* The acetyl-CoA is transported back into the cytosol. With the aid of the enzyme choline acetyltransferase, acetylcholine is synthesized from acetyl-CoA and choline. The acetylcholine is then transported to and stored within the storage vesicles. Thus far, experiments have failed to delineate the mechanism involved in the transport of acetylcholine into the vesicles.

Conduction of an action potential through the terminal branches of an axon causes depolarization of the varicosity membrane, resulting in the release of transmitter molecules by a process known as *exocytosis.* During exocytosis, vesicles come in contact with the varicosity membrane. At the point of contact, the membranes of the vesicles and the varicosity fuse together, and an opening develops through which the transmitter is extruded into the extracellular space. Once in the junctional extracellular space (biophase), acetylcholine interacts with cholinoceptors.

The interactions between transmitters and their receptors are readily reversible, and the number of transmitter-receptor complexes formed is a direct function of the amount of transmitter in the biophase. The length of time that intact molecules of acetylcholine remain in the biophase is short because *acetylcholinesterase,* an enzyme that rapidly hydrolyzes acetylcholine, is located in high concentrations on the outer surfaces of both the prejunctional (neuronal) and postjunctional (effector cell) membranes. A rapid hydrolysis of acetylcholine by the enzyme results in a lowering of the concentration of free transmitter, and a rapid dissociation of the transmitter from its receptors; little, if any, acetylcholine escapes into the circulation. If some acetylcholine does reach the circulation, it will be immediately inactivated by plasma esterases.

The rapid removal of transmitter is essential to the exquisite control of neurotransmission. As a consequence of rapid removal, the magnitude and duration of effect produced by acetylcholine are directly related to the frequency of transmitter release, that is, to the frequency of action potentials generated in the neuron.

Synthesis, Storage, Release, and Removal of Norepinephrine

The transmission process in noradrenergic neurons is somewhat more complex, particularly in regard to the mechanisms by which the transmitter is removed from the biophase subsequent to its release. Noradrenergic transmission is represented diagrammatically in Fig. 11-3.

Synthesis of norepinephrine begins with the amino acid *tyrosine,* which enters the neuron by active transport, perhaps facilitated by a permease. In the neuronal cytosol, tyrosine is converted by the enzyme *tyrosine hydroxylase* to *dihydroxyphenylalanine (dopa),* which is converted to *dopamine* by the enzyme *aromatic* L-*amino-acid decarboxylase,* sometimes termed dopa-decarboxylase. The dopamine is actively transported into storage vesicles. Within the ves-

icles, dopamine is converted to norepinephrine (the transmitter) by *dopamine β-hydroxylase,* an enzyme localized within the storage vesicle.

In noradrenergic neurons, the end product is norepinephrine. In the adrenal medulla, the synthesis is carried one step further. An enzyme found in that organ, *phenylethanolamine* N-*methyltransferase,* converts norepinephrine to epinephrine. The human adrenal medulla contains approximately four times as much epinephrine as norepinephrine. The absence of this enzyme in noradrenergic neurons accounts for the absence of significant amounts of epinephrine in noradrenergic neurons. The structures of these compounds are shown in Fig. 11-4.

Since the enzyme that converts dopamine to norepinephrine (dopamine β-hydroxylase) is located only within the vesicles, the transport of dopamine into the vesicle is an essential step in the synthesis of norepinephrine. This same transport system is essential for the storage of norepinephrine. There is a tendency for norepinephrine to leak from the vesicles into the cytosol. If norepinephrine remains in the cytosol, much of it will be destroyed by a mitochondrial enzyme, *monoamine oxidase (MAO).* However, most of the norepinephrine that leaks out of the vesicle is rapidly returned to the storage vesicles by the same transport system that carries dopamine into the storage vesicles. *It is important for a proper understanding*

Figure 11-4. Steps in the synthetic pathway of epinephrine and norepinephrine.

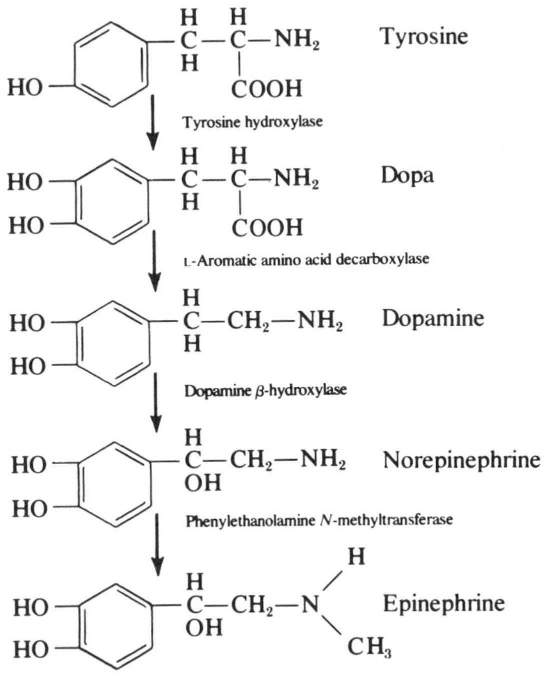

of drug action to remember that this single transport system, which will be referred to as vesicular transport, is an essential element of both synthesis and storage of norepinephrine.

Like the cholinergic transmitter, the noradrenergic transmitter is released by action potentials through exocytosis, the contents of entire vesicles being emptied into the biophase (synaptic or junctional region). Similarly, the formation of transmitter-receptor complexes is a direct function of the concentration of transmitter in the biophase and is readily reversible. In this instance, the receptors are adrenoceptors.

Three processes contribute to the removal of norepinephrine from the biophase.

1. Transport back into the noradrenergic neuron (*reuptake*), followed by either vesicular storage or by enzymatic inactivation by mitochondrial MAO. The transport of norepinephrine into the neurons is a sodium-facilitated process similar to that for choline transport.
2. Diffusion from the synapse into the circulation and ultimate enzymatic destruction in the liver.
3. Active transport of the released transmitter into effector cells (*extraneuronal uptake*), followed by enzymatic inactivation by catechol-*O*-methyltransferase.

The neuronal transport system is the most important mechanism for removing norepinephrine. This is true not only for neuronally released norepinephrine, but also for circulating norepinephrine and epinephrine. It is important to recognize that any norepinephrine or epinephrine in the circulation will equilibrate with the junctional extracellular fluid and thus become accessible to the receptors and to neuronal transport. Thus, neuronal transport is also an important mechanism for limiting the effect and duration of action of norepinephrine or epinephrine, whether these are released from the adrenal medulla or administered as drugs.

It is important to make a clear distinction between neuronal transport and vesicular transport. *Neuronal transport* occurs from the junctional extracellular fluid (biophase), across the cell membrane of the neuron, into the neuronal

cytosol. *Vesicular transport* (often referred to as granular uptake) is from the neuronal cytosol, across the membrane of the vesicle, into the vesicle. Although these two transport systems readily transport both norepinephrine and epinephrine, certain drugs will selectively inhibit one or the other transport system.

Neuronal uptake is primarily a mechanism for removing norepinephrine rather than conserving it. Under most circumstances, synthesis of new norepinephrine is quite capable of keeping up with the needs of transmission, even in the complete absence of neuronal reuptake.

The second most important mechanism for removing norepinephrine from the synapse is the escape of neuronally released norepinephrine into the general circulation and its subsequent metabolism in the liver. The liver has two enzymes that perform this function: *catechol-O-methyltransferase (COMT)* and *MAO.*

COMT is a very specific enzyme, accepting only catechols as substrates. A catechol is a substance with two adjacent hydroxyl groups on an unsaturated, six-member ring. S-Adenosyl methionine serves as the source of the methyl group; the end result of the action of COMT is the O-methylation of the *meta*-hydroxyl group on the catechol nucleus. Fig. 11-5 illustrates the action of COMT on norepinephrine. This reaction reduces the biological activity of norepinephrine or epinephrine at least 100-fold.

MAO is a much less discriminating enzyme, in that it will catalyze the removal of an amine group from a variety of substrates. The action of MAO on norepinephrine is indicated in Fig. 11-6. The list of its substrates is very large, including endogenous substances (norepinephrine, epinephrine, dopamine, tyramine, 5-hydroxytryptamine) as well as many drugs that are amines. At least in the brain, two separate forms of MAO have been described: MAO, type A and MAO, type B. The two types are differentiated on the basis of substrate and inhibitor specificity.

Metabolism of Catecholamines

Fig. 11-7 illustrates the possible pathways of metabolism of norepinephrine and epinephrine.

Although either COMT or MAO may act first on cir-

Figure 11-5. The O-methylation of norepinephrine by catechol-O-methyltransferase (COMT).

Norepinephrine   Normetanephrine

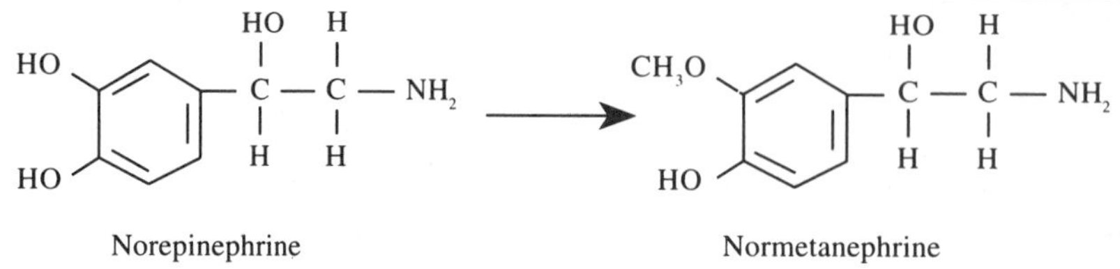

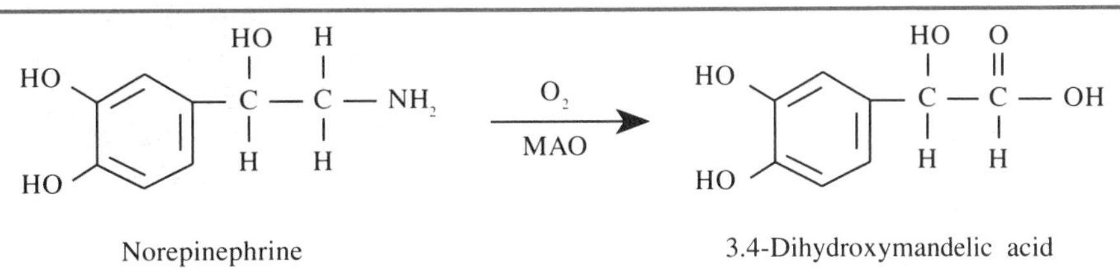

Figure 11-6. The deamination of norepinephrine by monoamine oxidase (MAO).

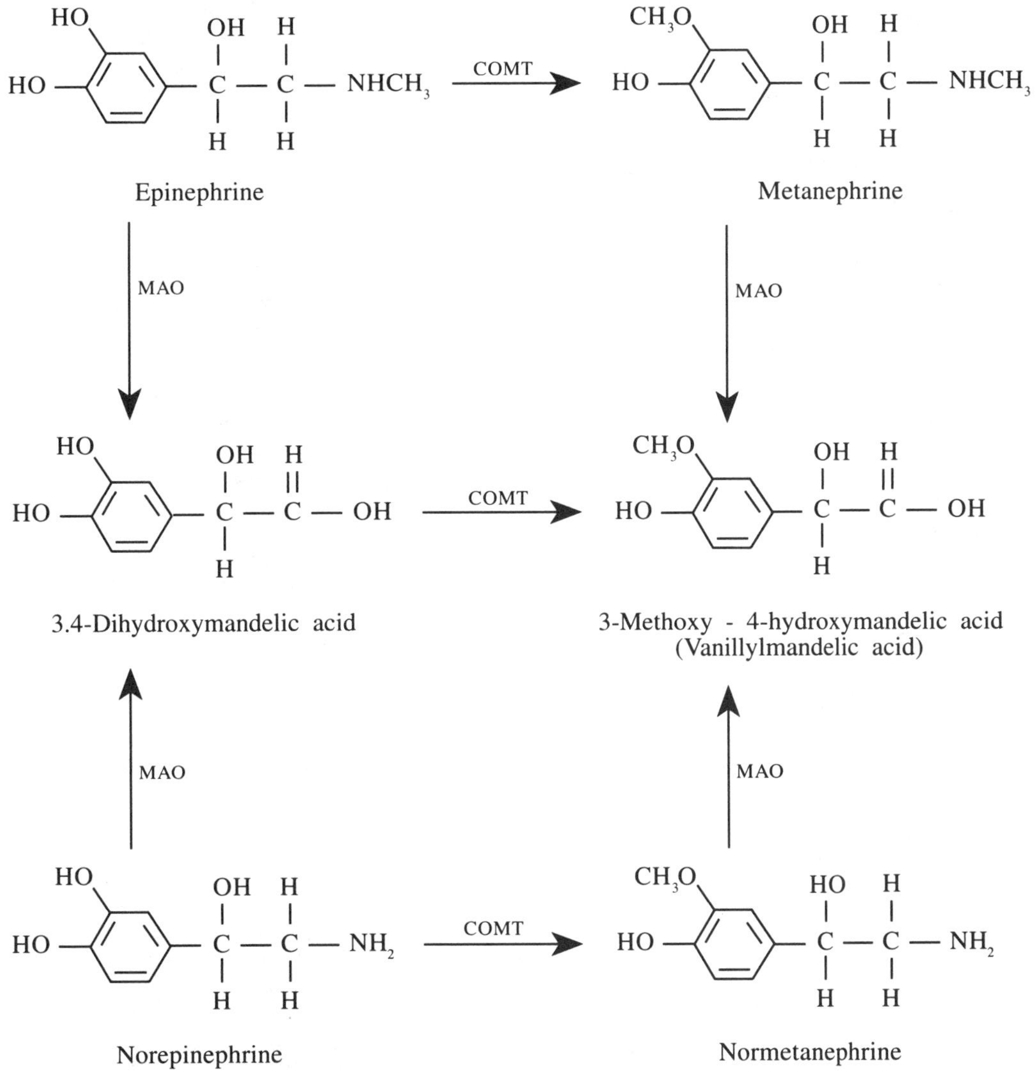

Figure 11-7. Primary route of metabolism of norepinephrine and epinephrine. COMT = catechol-O-methyltransferase; MAO = monoamine oxidase.

culating norepinephrine or epinephrine, COMT is the more rapidly acting enzyme, and therefore more molecules are O-methylated and then deaminated than the reverse. Some norepinephrine and epinephrine appear unchanged in the urine. The larger portion, however, is

metabolized and the products of metabolism are excreted in the urine, often as conjugates.

Measurements of norepinephrine, epinephrine, and their metabolites in the urine constitute valuable diagnostic aids, particularly in the detection of tumors that synthesize and secrete norepinephrine and epinephrine (e.g., pheochromocytoma).

Catecholamines can be transported into effector cells (*extraneuronal uptake*). These cells generally contain both COMT and MAO. The combined processes of extraneuronal uptake and *O*-methylation are believed to be a minor, but functionally significant, site of irreversible loss of catecholamines. The precise role of extraneuronal MAO in the inactivation of transmitter substrates remains to be elucidated.

Receptors on the Autonomic Effector Cells

The receptors for acetylcholine and related drugs (*cholinoceptors*) and for norepinephrine and related drugs (*adrenoceptors*) are different. Acetylcholine will not interact with receptors for norepinephrine, and norepinephrine will not interact with cholinoceptors. Not only are these receptors selective for their respective agonists, but they are also selective for their respective antagonist drugs; that is, drugs that antagonize or block acetylcholine at cholinoceptors will not antagonize norepinephrine at adrenoceptors and vice versa.

Cholinoceptors

Acetylcholine is the transmitter at several different sites: autonomic ganglia, all parasympathetic and some anatomically sympathetic postganglionic nerve terminals, and somatic motor nerve terminals. It was recognized by pharmacologists early in this century that the action of administered acetylcholine on effector systems innervated by parasympathetic postganglionic neurons (smooth muscle cells, cardiac muscle cells, and exocrine gland cells) resembled the actions produced by the naturally occurring plant alkaloid *muscarine*. The actions of both acetylcholine and muscarine on the visceral effectors were similar to those produced by parasympathetic nerve stimulation. Furthermore, the effects of acetylcholine, muscarine, and parasympathetic nerve stimulation on visceral effectors were antagonized by atropine, another plant alkaloid. It was also observed that the administration of acetylcholine mimicked the stimulatory effect of *nicotine,* the alkaloid from the tobacco plant, on autonomic ganglia and the adrenal medulla. It has become common practice for pharmacologists to refer to the effects of acetylcholine on visceral effectors as the *muscarinic* action of acetylcholine, and to its effects on the autonomic ganglia and adrenal medulla as the *nicotinic* action of acetylcholine. The respective receptors are called the muscarinic and nicotinic cholinoceptors or the muscarinic and nicotinic receptors of acetylcholine.

At the skeletal muscle motor end-plate, the action of acetylcholine resembles that produced by nicotine. Thus, the cholinoceptor on skeletal muscle is a nicotinic receptor. Based on antagonist selectivity, however, the autonomic and somatic nicotinic receptors are not pharmacologically identical (see Chap. 18).

Acetylcholine can stimulate a whole family of receptors. All of those receptors recognize acetylcholine and accept it as an agonist. However, these receptors are sufficiently chemically diverse (see Chaps. 14, 15, 17, and 18) that different exogenous agonists and antagonists can distinguish among them. Great therapeutic benefit has been obtained from this diversity because it allows the development of therapeutic agents that can selectively mimic or antagonize selected actions of acetylcholine. Fortunately, such a diversity of receptor subtypes exists for other neurotransmitters in addition to acetylcholine.

Adrenoceptors

Norepinephrine is the neurotransmitter released at noradrenergic nerve terminals. The adrenoceptors on the innervated tissues not only interact with norepinephrine but also with the adrenal medullary hormone epinephrine and a number of chemically related drugs. However, the responses produced by the drugs in different autonomic structures differ quantitatively or qualitatively from one another.

On the basis of the observed selectivity of action among agonists and antagonists, it was proposed that two types of adrenoceptors exist. These were designated as α(alpha)- and β(beta)-adrenoceptors. Subsequently, it has become necessary to further classify the adrenoceptors into α_1- and α_2- and β_1- and β_2-receptor subtypes. Table 11-1 indicates present knowledge of the distribution of the subtypes of adrenoceptors in various tissues.

The α_1-adrenoceptors are located at postjunctional (postsynaptic) sites on tissues innervated by adrenergic neurons. Originally, α_2-adrenoceptors were believed to have a presynaptic (i.e., neuronal) location exclusively, and to be involved in the feedback inhibition of norepinephrine release from nerve terminals. There is now evidence that α_2-receptors also can occur postjunctionally. The β_1-adrenoceptors are found chiefly in the heart and adipose tissue, while β_2-adrenoceptors are located in a number of sites including bronchial smooth muscle and skeletal muscle blood vessels.

Activation of α_1-adrenoceptors in smooth muscle of blood vessels leads to vasoconstriction while activation of β_2-adrenoceptors in blood vessels of skeletal muscle produces vasodilation. Activation of β_1-adrenoceptors on cardiac tissue produces an increase in the heart rate and contractile force.

Norepinephrine and epinephrine are potent α-adrenoceptor agonists, but isoproterenol, a synthetic adreno-

Table 11-1. Responses to Adrenergic and Cholinergic Nerve Stimulation

Organ or tissue function	Predominant adrenoceptor type	Adrenergic response	Cholinergic response[a]
Heart[b]			
Rate (chronotropic effect)	β_1	Increase	Decrease
Contractile force (inotropic effect)	β_1	Increase	None
Conduction velocity (dromotropic effect)	β_1	Increase	Decrease
Eye			
Pupil size	α_1	Constriction of radial muscle causing dilation (mydriasis)	Contraction of circular muscle (miosis)
Accommodation		No innervation	Contraction of ciliary muscle producing accommodation for near vision
Bronchial smooth muscle	β_2	Relaxation	Contraction
Blood vessels (arteries and arterioles)[c]			
Cutaneous	α_1	Constriction	No innervation[e]
Visceral	α_1	Constriction	No innervation[e]
Pulmonary	α_1	Constriction	No innervation[e]
Skeletal muscle	α_1, β_2	Constriction[d]	Dilation
Coronary	α_1, β	Constriction, dilation[f]	No innervation[e]
Cerebral	α_1	Constriction	
Veins	α_1	Constriction	No innervation
Gastrointestinal tract (tone, motility, and secretory activity)	α_2, β_2	Decrease[g]	Increase
Sphincters	α	Contraction	Relaxation
Splenic capsule	α_1	Contraction	No innervation
Urinary bladder			
Detrusor muscle	β	Relaxation	Contraction
Trigone-sphincter muscle	α_1	Contraction	Relaxation
Uterus	α_1, β_2	Contraction-relaxation[h]	Contraction-relaxation
Glycogenolysis			
Skeletal muscle	β_2	Increase	None
Liver	α_1, β_2	Increase	None
Lipolysis	β_1	Increase	None
Renin secretion	β_1	Increase	None
Insulin secretion	α_2	Decrease	Increase

[a]Muscarinic cholinoceptors.
[b]There are some β_2-receptors in the heart. The ratio of β_1/β_2 varies with the region and the species. In the human heart, the ratio of β_1/β_2 is about 3:2 in atria and 4:1 in ventricles.
[c]There are some α_2-receptors in some vascular smooth muscle.
[d]Low doses of epinephrine of endogenous or exogenous origin plus other β_2-receptor agonists dilate these blood vessels.
[e]Exogenously administered cholinergic drugs dilate these blood vessels.
[f]Dilation is the dominant in vivo response, owing to indirect effects.
[g]α_2-Adrenoceptors may be involved in hypersecretory responses.
[h]Responses depend on hormonal state.

mimetic that is selective for β_1- and β_2-adrenoreceptors, is not similarly active in therapeutic doses. Norepinephrine and epinephrine are thus potent vasoconstrictors of those vascular beds that contain predominantly α-adrenoceptors, while isoproterenol has little effect in these vessels.

Isoproterenol and epinephrine are potent β_2-adrenoceptor agonists; norepinephrine is a relatively weak β_2-adrenoceptor agonist. Isoproterenol and epinephrine produce vasodilation in skeletal muscle, but norepinephrine does not; rather it produces vasoconstriction through the α_1-adrenoreceptors.

Isoproterenol, epinephrine, and norepinephrine are potent β_1-adrenoceptor agonists; thus, all three can stimulate the heart. (See Table 11-1 and Chaps. 12 and 13 for further details.)

Presynaptic Receptors

It has long been recognized that in chemical neurotransmission, either from neuron to neuron or from neuron to effector cell, there are receptors on the postsynaptic membrane with which the transmitter (released by the presynaptic neuron) interacts. The activation of these

Table 11-2. Drugs that Interfere with Specific Steps in the Process of Chemical Transmission

Transmission step	Adrenergic nerves	Cholinergic nerves
Synthesis of transmitter	α-Methyldopa	Hemicholinium
Storage of transmitter	Reserpine	None known
Release of transmitter	Guanethidine	Botulinum toxin
Combination of transmitter with receptor	Phentolamine (α-receptors)	Atropine (muscarinic receptors)
	Propranolol (β-receptors)	d-Tubocurarine (nicotinic receptors)
Destruction or removal of transmitter from site of action	Pyrogallol (COMT inhibitor)	Physostigmine (cholinesterase inhibitor)
	Phenelzine (MAO inhibitor)	
	Tricyclic antidepressants (inhibit neuronal transport)	
Recovery of postsynaptic cell from the effects of the transmitter	None known	Succinylcholine

Key: COMT = catechol-O-methyltransferase; MAO = monoamine oxidase.

postsynaptic receptors determines the response of the postsynaptic element (neuron or effector cell).

A second population of receptors also plays a role in neurotransmission. These are called *presynaptic* or *prejunctional receptors;* they are located on the presynaptic nerve endings. Their function is to control the amount of transmitter released per nerve impulse, and in some instances to affect the rate of transmitter synthesis through some as yet undetermined feedback mechanism. For instance, during repetitive nerve stimulation, when the concentration of transmitter released into the synaptic or junctional cleft is relatively high, the released transmitter may activate presynaptic receptors and thereby reduce the further release of transmitter. Such an action could serve to prevent excessive and prolonged stimulation of the postsynaptic cell. In this case, the activation of the presynaptic receptor would be part of a *negative feedback mechanism.*

The presynaptic receptors are of potential pharmacological significance since several drugs may act, in part, either by preventing the transmitter from reaching the presynaptic receptor, thus causing excessive transmitter release, or by directly stimulating presynaptic receptors and thereby diminishing the amount of transmitter released per impulse.

The presynaptic α-adrenoceptors found on noradrenergic neurons are of the α_2 subtype. (As mentioned earlier in this chapter there is now evidence that α_2-adrenoceptors are not limited to a presynaptic location, but occur also on postjunctional effector cells.) Adrenoceptors of the β_2 subclass also occur presynaptically, and activation of these receptors leads to enhanced norepinephrine release. The physiological and pharmacological importance of these presynaptic β_2-receptors, however, is less certain than it is for presynaptic α_2-receptors.

Presynaptic receptors for nonadrenomimetic substances (e.g., acetylcholine, adenosine) also have been found on the sympathetic presynaptic nerve ending.

Their importance and role in the modulation of neurotransmission have not been definitively established.

Pharmacological Intervention in Neurotransmission

The drugs listed in Table 11-2 affect specific steps in cholinergic or adrenergic transmission. Many other drugs that alter transmission are considered in subsequent chapters.

Supplemental Reading

Appenzeller, O. *The Autonomic Nervous System* (4th ed.). Amsterdam: Elsevier, 1990.

Burnstock, G., and Griffith, S.G. *Noradrenergic Innervation of Blood Vessels.* Boca Raton, Fla.: CRC, 1988.

Ciriello, J., et al. *Organization of the Autonomic Nervous System: Central and Peripheral Mechanisms.* New York: Liss, 1987.

de Belleroche, J. *Presynaptic Receptors: Mechanisms and Functions.* New York: Wiley, 1982.

Furness, J.B., and Costa, M. *The Enteric Nervous System.* New York: Churchill Livingstone, 1987.

Goldberg, A.M., and Hanin, I. *Biology of Cholinergic Function.* New York: Raven, 1976.

Gootman, P.M. (ed.). *Developmental Neurobiology of the Autonomic Nervous System.* Clifton, N.J.: Humana, 1986.

Limbird, L.E. (ed.). *The Alpha-2 Adrenergic Receptors.* Clifton, N.J.: Humana, 1988.

Perkins, J.D. (ed.). *The Beta-Adrenergic Receptors.* Clifton, N.J.: Humana, 1991.

Rubanyi, G.M., and Vanhoutte, P.M. (eds.). *Endothelium-Derived Relaxing Factors.* Basel: Karger, 1990.

Ruffolo, R.R. (ed.). *The Alpha-1 Adrenergic Receptors.* Clifton, N.J.: Humana, 1987.

12

Adrenomimetic Drugs

Tony J.-F. Lee and *Robert E. Stitzel*

The *adrenomimetic drugs* mimic the effects of adrenergic sympathetic nerve stimulation on sympathetic effectors. Thus, these drugs are also referred to as *sympathomimetic agents.* The adrenergic transmitter norepinephrine and the adrenal medullary hormone epinephrine also are included under this broad heading. The adrenomimetic drugs are an important group of therapeutic agents that can be used to maintain blood pressure or to relieve a life-threatening attack of acute bronchial asthma. These drugs are also present in many over-the-counter preparations, in which advantage is taken of their ability to constrict mucosal blood vessels and thus relieve nasal congestion.

Chemistry

The adrenomimetic drugs can be divided into two major groups on the basis of their chemical structures: the catecholamines and the noncatecholamines. The catecholamines include norepinephrine, epinephrine, and dopamine, all of which are naturally occurring, and several synthetic substances, the most important of which is isoproterenol (isopropylnorepinephrine).

The skeletal structure of the catecholamines is shown in Fig. 12-1.

The term *catecholamine* is derived from the structure of the molecule, which consists of catechol (3,4-dihydroxybenzene) and a two-carbon side chain with a terminal amino group (ethylamine). The hydroxyl groups of the catechol moiety are meta (position 3) and para (position 4) to the ethylamine side chain. The carbon atoms of the side chain are designated as the α- and β-carbons starting from the amino group. The structures of the more important catecholamines are shown in Fig. 12-2.

The hydroxyl substituent on the β-carbon of the side chain makes possible the existence of stereoisomers of epinephrine, norepinephrine, and isoproterenol. The l isomers are the naturally occurring forms of epinephrine and norpinephrine. The l isomers of epinephrine, norepi-

nephrine, and isoproterenol also possess considerably greater pharmacological effects than do the d isomers. Throughout most of the rest of the world, epinephrine and norepinephrine are known as *adrenaline* and *noradrenaline,* respectively.

Noncatecholamine adrenomimetic drugs differ from the basic catecholamine structure by having substitutions on their benzene ring. While the majority of noncatecholamine adrenomimetic drugs retain the phenylethylamine skeleton, in some the benzene ring is replaced by a five- or six-member saturated ring, by naphthalene, or by an aliphatic chain.

Mechanism of Action

Many adrenomimetic drugs produce responses by interacting with the adrenoceptors on sympathetic effector cells. An examination of Table 11-1 in Chap. 11 reveals that sympathetic effectors have either α_1-, α_2-, β_1-, β_2-, or, in some cases, combinations of these adrenoceptors. Adrenomimetic drugs vary in their affinities for various subgroups of adrenoceptors. Some, like epinephrine, have a high affinity for all of the adrenoceptors. Others are relatively selective. For example, isoproterenol has a high affinity for β_1- and β_2-receptors but a very low affinity for α-receptors; isoproterenol is considered a nearly pure β-agonist. Norepinephrine has a high affinity for α- and β_1-adrenoceptors, but a relatively low affinity for β_2-receptors.

The effect of a given adrenomimetic drug on a particular type of effector cell depends on the receptor selectivity of the drug, the response characteristics of the effector cells, and the predominant type of adrenoceptor found on the cells. For example, the smooth muscle cells of many blood vessels have only or predominantly α-receptors. The interaction of compounds with these α-receptors initiates a chain of events in the vascular smooth muscle cells that leads to an activation of the contractile process. Thus,

115

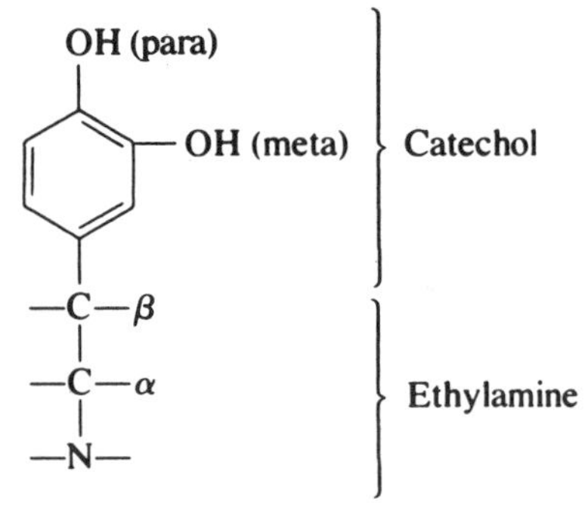

Figure 12-1. Skeletal structure of catecholamines.

norepinephrine and epinephrine, which have high affinities for α-receptors, cause the vascular muscle to contract and the blood vessels to constrict. Since bronchial smooth muscle contains β_2-receptors, the response in this tissue elicited by the action of β_2-receptor agonists is relaxation of smooth muscle cells. Epinephrine and isoproterenol, drugs that have high affinities for β_2-receptors, cause relaxation of bronchial smooth muscle. Norepinephrine, on the other hand, has a lower affinity for β_2-receptors and has relatively weak bronchiolar relaxing properties.

Adrenomimetic drugs can be divided into two major groups on the basis of their mechanism of action. Norepinephrine, epinephrine, and some closely related adrenomimetics produce responses in effector cells by directly interacting with α- or β-adrenoceptors and are referred to as *directly acting* adrenomimetic drugs.

Many adrenomimetic drugs, such as amphetamine, do not themselves interact with adrenoceptors, yet they are capable of producing sympathetic effects. They do so by releasing norepinephrine from neuronal storage sites (vesicles). The norepinephrine that is released by these compounds then interacts with the receptors present on the effector organ. These adrenomimetics are called *indirectly acting* adrenomimetic drugs. Their capacity to release norepinephrine depends on their ability to be taken up into the adrenergic neuron, and ultimately into the storage vesicles, by the same transport systems that normally take up norepinephrine. Once inside the vesicle, each molecule of an indirectly acting drug may displace a molecule of norepinephrine in the cytosol of the varicosity. Some of the norepinephrine released into the cytoplasm is metabolized by monoamine oxidase (MAO), but some escapes from the varicosity (nonexocytotically) and interacts with adrenoceptors to produce a biological response. *The effects elicited by indirectly acting drugs resemble those produced by norepinephrine.*

An important characteristic of indirectly acting adrenomimetic drugs is that repeated injections or prolonged infusion lead to *tachyphylaxis* (gradually diminishing responses to repeated administration). This occurs as a result of a gradually diminishing availability of releasable norepinephrine stores on repeated drug administration. If the indirectly acting drug is not metabolized by MAO, tachyphylaxis will develop more rapidly and a longer period is required for the return of activity than with drugs that are metabolized by MAO.

The actions of many indirectly acting adrenomimetic drugs are reduced or abolished by the prior administration of either cocaine or tricyclic antidepressant drugs (e.g., imipramine). These compounds can block the adrenergic neuronal transport system and thereby prevent the indirectly acting drug from reaching the norepinephrine storage vesicles. Lipophilic drugs (e.g., amphetamine), however, can enter nerves by diffusion and do not need membrane transport systems, and therefore, their indirect effects are not as readily blocked by cocaine or imipramine.

Destruction or surgical interruption of the adrenergic

Figure 12-2. Chemical structures of four important catecholamines.

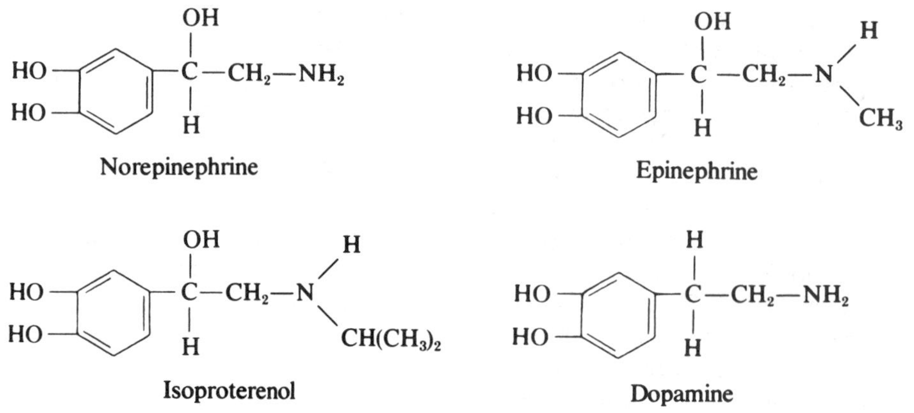

nerves leading to an effector tissue renders indirectly acting adrenomimetic drugs ineffective because neuronal norepinephrine is no longer available for release since the nerves have degenerated. Also, patients being treated for hypertension with reserpine or guanethidine, drugs that deplete the norepinephrine stores in adrenergic neurons (see Chap. 22), will respond poorly to administration of indirectly acting adrenomimetic drugs.

Some adrenomimetic drugs act both directly and indirectly; that is, they release some norepinephrine from storage sites and also activate tissue receptors directly. Such drugs are called *mixed-action* adrenomimetics. Most adrenomimetic drugs of therapeutic importance in humans, however, are usually either directly or indirectly acting.

Structure-Activity Relationships Among Adrenomimetic Drugs

The nature of the substitutions made on the basic phenylethylamine skeleton at the para and meta positions of the benzene ring or on the β-carbon of the side chain will determine whether an adrenomimetic drug will be either directly or indirectly acting. Direct action on adrenoceptors is the result of multiple (two or three) substitutions (usually hydroxyl groups) on the meta and para positions of the ring and the β-carbon of the side chain. Compounds with one or no such substitutions are primarily indirectly acting drugs.

Directly acting adrenomimetic drugs, which have two or more carbon atoms (e.g., isoproterenol) added to their amino group, are virtually pure β-receptor agonists. Directly acting drugs, which have only small substitutions on their amino groups (e.g., norepinephrine and epinephrine), are usually α-receptor agonists but may be β-receptor agonists as well. Norepinephrine has very weak actions on β2-adrenoceptors but strong β1-receptor actions. Epinephrine has a high affinity for both β1- and β2-receptors.

Adrenomimetic drugs with no substitutions on their benzene ring (e.g., amphetamine and ephedrine) are generally quite lipid-soluble compounds. Since they are lipid soluble, they cross the blood-brain barrier relatively easily and can cause CNS stimulation.

The structure of a particular adrenomimetic drug will influence its susceptibility to metabolism by catechol-O-methyltransferase (COMT) and MAO. The actions of COMT are specific for the catechol structure. If either the meta or para hydroxyl group is absent, the drug will not be metabolized by COMT. Such compounds will tend to have a prolonged duration of action since they are not metabolized by this enzyme. The presence of a substitution, such as a methyl group, on the α-carbon of the side chain reduces the affinity of the adrenomimetic drug for MAO.

Also, drugs with large substitution on the terminal nitrogen will not be degraded by MAO. A noncatecholamine that has a methyl group attached to its α-carbon will not be metabolized by either enzyme and will have a greatly prolonged duration of action (e.g., amphetamine).

The Role of Second Messengers in Receptor-Mediated Responses

The endogenous release or the exogenous administration of many chemicals, such as neurotransmitters, hormones, growth factors, and so forth, produces a biological response through an initial interaction with a specific receptor system. The adrenomimetic drugs, including the naturally occurring catecholamines, initiate their responses by combining with either α-, β-, or dopamine receptors. This interaction triggers a series of biochemical events starting within the effector cell membrane that eventually culminate in the production of a physiological response, for example, contraction, secretion, relaxation, altered metabolism, etc. The total process of converting the action of an external signal (e.g., norepinephrine released from a sympathetic neuron) to a physiological response (e.g., vascular smooth muscle contraction) is called *signal transduction.*

Following the binding of the agonist (the *first messenger*) to its appropriate receptor, located on the external surface of the effector cell, a *second messenger* is generated (or synthesized) and then participates in a particular series of biochemical reactions that ultimately results in the generation of a specific physiological response by that cell (Figs. 12-3 and 12-4). Some of the biochemical events involved in the coupling of neurotransmitter receptors to various effector functions have been discussed in Chap. 2. For both α- and β-adrenoceptors, the signal transduction process seems to involve the participation of G-proteins. These G-proteins may couple to ion channels in addition to or instead of involving specific second messengers.

The existence of specific second-messenger pathways constitutes a highly versatile signaling system that can modify (stimulate or inhibit) numerous cellular processes including secretion, contraction, metabolism, neuronal excitability, and cell growth. The second messengers that participate in signal transduction initiated by stimulation of the sympathetic nervous system (and by adrenomimetic drugs) are *cyclic adenosine monophosphate (cAMP), diacylglycerol,* and *inositol triphosphate.* Once liberated within the cell, second messengers will activate specific signal pathways. For example, inositol triphosphate functions by mobilizing calcium from intracellular stores or opening channels; the calcium can now be used to initiate vascular smooth muscle contraction, probably through a protein phosphorylation pathway (see Fig. 12-4). Diacylglycerol is known to stimulate an enzyme, protein kinase C, that

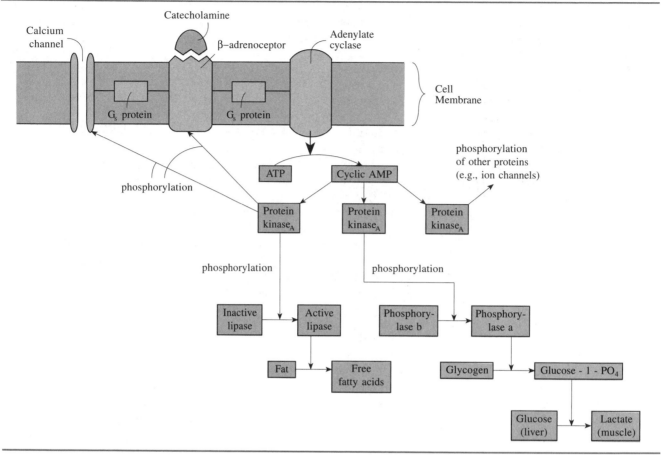

Figure 12-3. The role of cyclic 3′,5′–adenosine monophosphate (cAMP) as a second messenger in the actions of catecholamines acting on β-receptors. ATP = adenosine triphosphate.

phosphorylates specific intracellular proteins, some of which regulate ionic mechanisms such as the Na^+/H^+ exchanger and potassium channels.

The basic features of the signaling system found in different cells are remarkably similar, but what varies is the way in which a particular second-messenger pathway drives the different effector systems. It appears that protein phosphorylation represents a final common pathway in the molecular mechanisms through which neurotransmitters, hormones, and the nerve impulse produce many of their biological effects in target cells.

Pharmacodynamic Actions of Norepinephrine, Epinephrine, and Isoproterenol

Vascular Effects

The cardiovascular effects of these agents are shown in Table 12-1. Differences in the action of these three cate-

cholamines on various vascular beds are due both to the different affinities possessed by the catecholamines for α- and β-adrenoceptors and to differences in the relative distribution of the receptors in a particular vascular bed. The hemodynamic responses of the major vascular beds to these amines are shown in Table 12-2.

The blood vessels of the skin and mucous membranes predominantly contain α-adrenoceptors. Both epinephrine and norepinephrine produce a powerful constriction in these tissues, thus substantially reducing blood flow through them. Isoproterenol, which is almost a pure β-receptor agonist, has little effect on the vasculature of the skin and mucous membranes. The blood vessels in visceral organs, including the kidneys, contain predominantly α-receptors, although some $β_2$-receptors are also present. Consequently, epinephrine and norepinephrine cause vasoconstriction and a reduced blood flow though the kidneys and other visceral organs. Isoproterenol produces either no effect or a weak vasodilation.

The blood vessels in skeletal muscle contain both α- and $β_2$-adrenoceptors. Norepinephrine constricts these blood vessels and reduces blood flow through skeletal

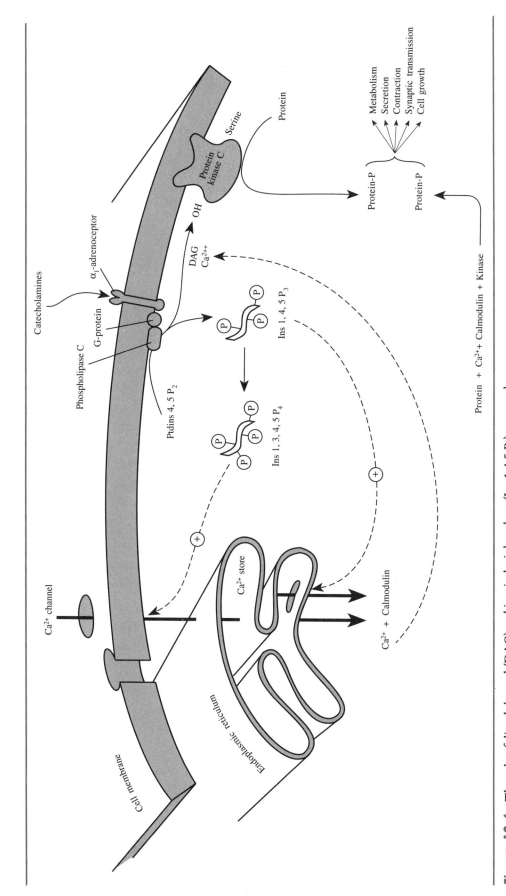

Figure 12-4. The role of diacylglycerol (DAG) and inositol triphosphate (Ins 1,4,5 P₃) as second messengers linked to agonist-receptor (α₁-adrenoceptor) interactions. Ptdins 4,5 P₂ is a phosphatidylinositol precursor found in cell membranes that is hydrolyzed following receptor activation to form the two second messengers, Ins 1,4,5 P₃ and DAG. Once liberated within the cell, these second messengers activate separate but interacting pathways. Ins 1,4,5 P₃ releases intracellularly stored Ca²⁺ and also can be phosphorylated to form a tetraphosphate (Ins 1,3,4,5 P₄), which can open Ca²⁺ channels in the membrane. DAG triggers protein phosphorylation through the activation of protein kinase C. A Ca²⁺-induced activation of the enzyme calmodulin also will result in protein phosphorylation. Note that adenylyl cyclase traverses the membrane. Cyclic AMP–dependent protein kinase can phosphorylate and inactivate the β-adrenoceptors. This kinase may have a role in homologous desensitization of Gₛ-protein–coupled β-adrenoceptors. It should be mentioned that β-receptor stimulation can (1) activate Ca²⁺ channels through an action of Gₛ proteins without the participation of cAMP, and (2) affect other ion channels through phosphorylation via kinases. (Modified from M. J. Berridge, Inositol triphosphate and diacylglycerol: Two interacting second messengers. *ISI Atlas of Science: Pharmacology,* 1:91, 1987.)

Table 12-1. Cardiovascular Effects of Catecholamines in Humans (in therapeutic doses of 0.1–0.4 μg/kg/min IV or 0.5–1.0 mg SC)

Cardiovascular function	Epinephrine	Norepinephrine	Isoproterenol
Systolic blood pressure	+ +	+ + +	0 +
Diastolic blood pressure	−	+ +	− −
Mean blood pressure	+ 0 −	+ +	− −
Total peripheral resistance	− −	+ + +	− − −
Heart rate (chronotropic effect	+	−	+ +
Stroke output (inotropic effect)	+ +	+	+ +
Cardiac output	+ + +	− 0	+ + +

Key: 0 = no effect; + = increased; − = decreased. The number of symbols indicates the approximate magnitude of the response.

Table 12-2. Response of the Major Vascular Beds to Usual Doses of the Catecholamines

Vascular bed	Receptor type*	Norepinephrine	Epinephrine	Isoproterenol
Cutaneous blood vessels	α	Constriction	Constriction	None
Visceral blood vessels	α	Constriction	Constriction	None (weak dilation)
Renal blood vessels	α	Constriction	Constriction	None (weak dilation)
Coronary blood vessels	α, β	Dilation	Dilation	Dilation
Skeletal muscle blood vessels	α, β_2	Constriction	Dilation	Dilation
Pial blood vessels	α, β_1	Constriction/dilation	Constriction/dilation	Dilation

*While virtually all blood vessels have α_1-receptors, some also have α_2-receptors. Stimulation of either subtype generally results in vasoconstriction.

muscle, an action that is initiated by the compound's interaction with α-receptors. Isoproterenol dilates the vessels in skeletal muscle and consequently increases blood flow through the tissue. This action of isoproterenol is mediated through its interaction with the β_2-receptors. Epinephrine has a more complex action on these blood vessels because of its high affinity for both α- and β_2-receptors. Whether epinephrine produces vasodilation or vasoconstriction in skeletal muscle depends on the dose administered. Low doses of epinephrine will dilate the blood vessels; larger doses will constrict them.

To explain the effects of epinephrine, it has been hypothesized that the threshold for activation of β_2-receptors is lower than that for α-receptors. Thus, low doses of epinephrine activate β_2-receptors, resulting in vasodilation. Increasingly large doses of epinephrine activate more and more α-receptors as well as β_2-receptors, until ultimately the balance between activation of β_2- and α-receptors favors the production of vasoconstriction. The secondary vasodilation that is seen following a vasoconstrictor response to epinephrine is due to the combined effects of (1) the decreasing activation of α-receptors as the concentration of epinephrine declines and (2) a reappearance of the β_2-receptor–mediated vasodilation as lower concentrations of epinephrine are again reached.

Although several factors can influence the flow of blood through the coronary vessels, the most important of these is the local production of vasodilator metabolites that occurs as a result of stimulation-induced increased work by the heart. Alpha- and β-adrenoceptors present in the coronary vascular beds do not play a major role in determining the vasodilator effects that result from the administration of epinephrine or norepinephrine. The increased coronary flow seen after administration of either of these two catecholamines results from the increased cardiac work that they bring about. Isoproterenol, which acts predominantly through β-receptors, produces an uncomplicated direct vasodilator effect on coronary blood vessels; it also increases the local production of vasodilator metabolites (see Chap. 22).

Effects on the Intact Cardiovascular System

An increase in sympathetic tone in nerves that innervate the cardiovascular system causes an increase in heart rate (positive chronotropic effect, or tachycardia) and an increase in the cardiac contractile force (positive inotropic effect) such that the stroke output is increased. Cardiac output, which is the result of rate and stroke output, is thus increased. It should be recalled that a physiological increase in sympathetic tone is almost always accompanied by a diminution of parasympathetic vagal tone; this allows full expression of the effects of increased sympathetic tone on the activity of the heart.

An increase in sympathetic tone causes a constriction of blood vessels in the major vascular beds and, therefore, a net increase in total peripheral resistance. Increased sympathetic tone results from an increased neural release of norepinephrine and its subsequent interaction both with β-adrenoceptors on cardiac cells and with α-receptors on vascular smooth muscle cells. As a consequence, the systolic and diastolic blood pressures are elevated. It follows that the mean arterial blood pressure must also be increased.

Norepinephrine

Norepinephrine, administered to a normotensive adult either subcutaneously or by slow intravenous injection, causes a constriction of blood vessels in all the major vascular beds in the body (see Table 12-2). Venules as well as arterioles are constricted. As a consequence, there is a net increase in the total peripheral resistance (see Table 12-1).

The effects of norepinephrine on cardiac function are complex because of the dynamic interaction of the direct effects of norepinephrine on the heart and the initiation of powerful cardiac reflexes. The baroreceptor reflexes, which are initiated by elevations in blood pressure such as those induced by vasoconstrictors like norepinephrine, are discussed in detail in Chap. 11.

Important considerations are: (1) *the direct effect of norepinephrine on the heart is stimulatory;* (2) *the reflex initiated is inhibitory,* that is, opposite to the direct effect; (3) the reflex varies with the level of sympathetic and parasympathetic activity existing just before the initiation of the reflex; and (4) the distribution of sympathetic and parasympathetic nerves is not uniform in the heart. The net result of the effect of norepinephrine on heart rate and ventricular contractile force, therefore, will vary depending on the dose of norepinephrine, the activity of the subject, existing cardiovascular and baroreceptor pathology, and the presence of other drugs that may alter reflexes.

In a normal, resting subject who is receiving no drugs, there is a moderate parasympathetic tone to the heart, and sympathetic activity is relatively low. The ventricular muscle receives little, if any, parasympathetic innervation. As the blood pressure rises in response to norepinephrine, the baroreceptor reflex is activated, parasympathetic impulses (which are inhibitory) to the heart are increased in frequency, and what little sympathetic outflow there is may be reduced. Heart rate is slowed so much that the direct effect of norepinephrine to increase the rate is masked and there is a *net* decrease in rate. Under the conditions described, however, the impact of the reflex on the ventricles is very slight because there is no parasympathetic innervation and the preexisting level of sympathetic activity is already low. A further decrease in sympathetic activity, therefore, would have little further effect on contractility in this subject. The direct effects of the norepinephrine, administered to increase contractility,

cannot be masked. Thus, a decrease in heart rate and an increase in stroke volume will occur. Cardiac output, the product of rate and stroke volume, will change very little (Table 12-1, Fig. 12-5).

The reflex nature of the bradycardia induced by parenterally administered norepinephrine can readily be demonstrated by administration of atropine, an equilibrium competitive antagonist of cholinoceptors. Atropine abolishes the compensatory vagal reflexes. Under conditions of vagal blockade, the direct cardiac stimulatory effects of norepinephrine are unmasked. There is a marked tachycardia, an increase in stroke volume, and, as a consequence, a marked increase in cardiac output. The systolic and mean blood pressures are more markedly elevated, primarily because of the greater increase in cardiac output.

Epinephrine

The qualitative nature of the blood pressure response to parenterally administered epinephrine is dose dependent. A small dose causes a fall in mean and diastolic pressure, with little or no effect on systolic pressure. The depressor action (fall in diastolic and mean blood pressure) produced by small doses of epinephrine is due to the net decrease in total peripheral resistance that results from the predominance of vasodilation in the skeletal muscle vascular bed. The intravenous infusion or subcutaneous administration of epinephrine in the range of doses used in humans generally increases the systolic pressure, but the diastolic pressure is decreased. Therefore, the mean pressure may either decrease, remain unchanged, or increase slightly, depending on the balance between the rise in systolic and fall in diastolic blood pressures (see Table 12-1, Fig. 12-5).

The cardiac effects of epinephrine are due to its action on β-receptors in the heart. The rate and contractile force of the heart are increased; consequently, cardiac output is markedly increased (see Table 12-1, Fig. 12-5). Because total peripheral resistance is decreased, the increase in cardiac output is largely responsible for the increase in systolic pressure. Since epinephrine causes little change in the mean arterial blood pressure, reflex slowing of the heart is usually not seen in humans.

Isoproterenol

Slow intravenous infusion of therapeutic doses of isoproterenol in humans produces a marked decrease in total peripheral resistance, owing to the predominance of vasodilation in skeletal muscle vascular beds. As a consequence, diastolic and mean blood pressures fall (see Fig. 12-5, Table 12-1). The depressor action of isoproterenol is more pronounced than that produced by epinephrine because isoproterenol causes no vasoconstriction whereas epinephrine does in some vascular beds. Systolic blood

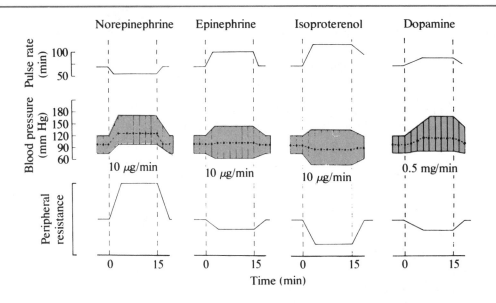

Figure 12-5. Cardiovascular effects of infusions of norepinephrine, epinephrine, isoproterenol, and dopamine in humans. Infusions were made intravenously during the time indicated by the broken lines. Heart rate is given in beats per minute, blood pressure in mm Hg, and peripheral resistance in arbitrary units. The dotted line in the blood pressure record is the calculated mean arterial blood pressure. (From M. J. Allwood, A. F. Cobbald, and J. Ginsburg, *Br. Med. Bull.* 19:132, 1963. Reproduced by permission of the Medical Department, The British Council.)

pressure may remain unchanged or may increase. When an increase in systolic blood pressure is seen, it is due to the marked increase in cardiac output produced by isoproterenol.

The effects of isoproterenol on the heart are similar to those produced by epinephrine. Isoproterenol usually increases the heart rate and stroke volume more than does epinephrine. This is partly due to the fact that it decreases mean blood pressure, which reflexly diminishes vagal activity, and partly because it is a more potent agonist in the heart.

Effects on Vascular Smooth Muscle

Our understanding of the types of adrenoceptors that participate in the control of vascular smooth muscle contractility has become increasingly complex in recent years. It is now known that both α_1- and α_2-receptor subtypes may exist at either the prejunctional or postjunctional site. However, the evidence demonstrating any functional role for the postjunctional α_2-adrenoceptors is poor, especially in the arterial system. Postjunctional α_1-adrenoceptors are always found in veins, arteries, and arterioles. Activation of postjunctional α_1-adrenoceptors results in the entry of extracellular calcium through receptor-operated channels

and in the release of intracellularly stored calcium; this is brought about through the participation of the inositol triphosphate second-messenger system. This system plays an important role in the regulation of blood pressure and vascular tone.

It is now recognized that the vascular endothelium also plays an important role in maintaining vascular tone. The endothelium appears to mediate or modulate both vasodilation and vasoconstriction through its ability to locally synthesize and release vasodilator and vasoconstrictor compounds, which in turn directly affect vascular smooth muscle activity. Stimulation of α_2-adrenoceptors located on the endothelial cells in certain vascular beds (such as the coronary artery) results in the release of endogenous vasodilator substances, *endothelium-derived relaxing factors* (EDRFs). Nitric oxide has been shown to be an EDRF. *Endothelium-derived constricting factors* (EDCFs) such as *endothelin* also have been demonstrated. Since nitrous oxide may inhibit the synthesis and release of endothelin, the role of endothelial α-adrenoceptors in the release of EDCF remains unknown.

In any blood vessel, the final integrated response to either neuronally released norepinephrine or to circulating epinephrine probably depends on the relative participation of at least four populations of α-adrenoceptors; postjunctional α_1- and α_2-adrenoceptors mediate constriction of vascular smooth muscle while prejunctional and endothelial α_2-adrenoceptors mediate vasodilation. In addition, it appears that an understanding of the total blood vessel response to adrenomimetic drugs must now also consider the effects of drugs on vascular endothelial cells and their production of either EDRF or EDCF.

Effects on Nonvascular Smooth Muscle

In general, the responses to administered catecholamines are similar to those seen after sympathetic nerve stimulation. The effects of norepinephrine, epinephrine, and isoproterenol on various types of nonvascular smooth muscle depend on the type of adrenoceptor present in the muscle (see Table 11-1).

Bronchial smooth muscle is relaxed by epinephrine and isoproterenol through their interaction with β_2-adrenoceptors. Epinephrine and isoproterenol are potent bronchodilators, while norepinephrine has a relatively weak action in this regard. The bronchodilator effects of these drugs are more readily observed when the airways are constricted, as in bronchial asthma, since it is difficult to observe relaxation in already relaxed smooth muscle.

Smooth muscle of the gastrointestinal tract is generally relaxed by catecholamines, but this may depend on the existing state of muscle tone. Usually motility of the gut is reduced by catecholamines while the gastrointestinal sphincters are contracted by these drugs. Catecholamines appear to produce relaxation of the gut through an action on α_2-adrenoceptors located on ganglionic cells. Activation of these receptors reduces acetylcholine release from cholinergic neurons. Catecholamines also may produce gastrointestinal relaxation through an action on β_2-adrenoceptors on smooth muscle cells. Contraction of the sphincters occurs through action on α_1-adrenoceptors. These effects are quite transient in humans and, therefore, are of no therapeutic value.

The radial (dilator) muscle of the iris contains α-adrenoceptors. Epinephrine—and to a somewhat lesser extent norepinephrine—causes dilation of the pupil (*mydriasis*) by contracting the radially arranged dilator muscle.

The *uterine muscle* contains both α- and β-adrenoceptors. The response of the human uterus to catecholamines is variable and depends on the endocrine balance of the individual at the time of amine administration. During the last stage of pregnancy and during parturition, epinephrine inhibits the uterine muscle, as does isoproterenol; norepinephrine contracts the uterus.

The *detrusor muscle* (which contains β-receptors), located in the body of the urinary bladder, is relaxed by epinephrine and isoproterenol. On the other hand, the trigone and sphincter (which contain α-receptors) are contracted by norepinephrine and epinephrine; this action inhibits the voiding of urine.

Central Nervous System Effects

Epinephrine, in therapeutic doses, mildly stimulates the central nervous system (CNS). The most noticeable features of this stimulation are apprehension, restlessness, and increased respiration. Both isoproterenol and norepinephrine, in therapeutic doses, also have minor CNS stimulant properties. Since these compounds do not easily cross the blood-brain barrier, the mechanism of their stimulatory effects is not clear. It is likely that the stimulating effects are primarily, if not entirely, due to actions in the periphery that alter the neural input to the CNS.

Metabolic Effects

The catecholamines, primarily epinephrine and isoproterenol, exert a number of important effects on metabolic processes. Most of these are mediated through an interaction with β-receptors. Norepinephrine is usually effective only in large doses. Epinephrine and isoproterenol in therapeutic doses increase oxygen consumption by 20 to 30 percent. Endogenous epinephrine secreted by the adrenal medulla, in response to stress such as exercise, increases blood levels of glucose, lactic acid, and free fatty acids.

Epinephrine is the most potent stimulant of hepatic glycogenolysis and gives rise to glucose 6-phosphate, which readily enters the circulation and increases the blood glucose level. Isoproterenol produces a relatively weak hyperglycemia. The identification of the adrenoceptor mediating liver glycogenolysis has presented problems. Administration of both α- and β-receptor blocking agents appears to be necessary to totally antagonize glycogenolysis in this tissue. In humans, the question of the relative importance of α- and β-receptors is not settled.

Isoproterenol is the most potent stimulant of skeletal muscle glycogenolysis, followed by epinephrine and norepinephrine. The adrenoceptor mediating muscle glycogenolysis is a β-receptor. Stimulation of skeletal muscle glycogenolysis will result in the elevation of blood lactic acid levels rather than blood glucose levels because skeletal muscle lacks the enzyme glucose 6-phosphatase, which catalyzes the conversion of glucose 6-phosphate to glucose.

The release of free fatty acids from adipose tissue (lipolysis) is mediated through β_1-adrenoceptors. Isoproterenol is the most potent agonist, followed by epinephrine and norepinephrine.

The β-receptor–mediated metabolic effects produced by catecholamines involve the activation of adenylate cyclase, an enzyme in the postjunctional cell membrane. This enzyme catalyzes the conversion of adenosine triphosphate (ATP) to cAMP. Increased levels of cAMP in the effector cell lead to the activation of a protein kinase that catalyzes the conversion of a previously inactive enzyme to an active enzyme; this enzyme then initiates the appropriate metabolic response. In the case of glycogenolysis, increased levels of cAMP lead to the conversion of inactive phosphorylase *b* to active phosphorylase *a*, which in turn catalyzes the breakdown of glycogen to glucose 1-phosphate (see Fig. 12-3).

Catecholamine-induced lipolysis in adipose tissue also occurs when increased cAMP levels activate a protein kinase. This kinase is different from the one involved in glycogen breakdown, because it catalyzes the breakdown of triglycerides in fatty tissue to free fatty acids (see Fig. 12-3).

It has been proposed that the ability of the second-messenger cAMP to alter a particular physiological process may depend on which specific protein kinase it activates, the nature of the protein that is phosphorylated, or both.

Potassium Homeostasis

The catecholamines can play an important role in the short-term regulation of plasma potassium levels. Stimulation of hepatic α-adrenoceptors will result in the release of potassium from the liver. In contrast, stimulation of β-adrenoceptors, particularly in skeletal muscle, will lead to the uptake of potassium into this tissue. The β-adrenoceptors appear to be of the β_2 subtype and are linked to the enzyme Na^+, K^+ adenosine triphosphatase (ATPase). Excessive stimulation of these β_2-adrenoceptors may produce a hypokalemia, which in turn can be a cause of cardiac arrhythmias.

Pharmacological Actions of Dopamine

Dopamine is a naturally occurring catecholamine; it is the immediate biochemical precursor of the norepinephrine found in adrenergic neurons and the adrenal medulla. It is also a neurotransmitter in the CNS, where it is released from dopaminergic neurons to act on specific dopamine receptors. These receptors may be either of the D_1 or D_2 subtype (see Chap. 38).

Dopamine is a unique adrenomimetic drug in that it exerts its cardiovascular actions by (1) releasing norepinephrine from adrenergic neurons, (2) interacting with α- and β_1-adrenoceptors, and (3) interacting with specific dopamine receptors.

The cardiovascular response to dopamine in humans is dependent on the concentration infused. Low rates of dopamine infusion can produce vasodilation in the renal, mesenteric, coronary, and intracerebral vascular beds with

little effect on other blood vessels or on the heart. The vasodilation produced by dopamine is not antagonized by the β-adrenoceptor blocking agent propranolol, but is antagonized by haloperidol and other dopamine-receptor blocking agents. Thus, the vasodilator action of dopamine on these vascular beds must be mediated by specific dopamine receptors.

Dopamine can exert pronounced cardiovascular and renal effects through the activation of both D_1- and D_2-receptor subtypes. Stimulation of the D_1 receptor, which is present on blood vessels and certain other peripheral sites, will result in vasodilation, natriuresis, and diuresis. D_2 receptors are found on ganglia, the adrenal cortex, and within the cardiovascular centers of the CNS; their activation produces hypotension, bradycardia, and regional vasodilation (e.g., renal vasodilation). The kidney appears to be a particularly rich source for endogenous dopamine in the periphery.

The infusion of moderately higher concentrations of dopamine increases the rate and contractile force of the heart and augments the cardiac output. This action is mediated by β_1-receptors and norepinephrine release, and it is antagonized by propranolol. In contrast to isoproterenol, which has a marked effect on both the rate and the contractile force of the heart, dopamine has a relatively greater effect on the force than on cardiac rate. The advantage of this relatively greater inotropic than chronotropic effect of dopamine is that it produces a smaller increase in oxygen demand by the heart than does isoproterenol. Systolic blood pressure is increased by dopamine, whereas diastolic pressure is usually not changed significantly. Total peripheral resistance is decreased owing to the vasodilator effect of dopamine.

At still higher concentrations, dopamine causes an α-receptor–mediated vasoconstriction in most vascular beds, as well as stimulation of the heart. Total peripheral resistance may be increased. If the concentration of dopamine reaching the tissue is high enough, vasoconstriction of the renal and mesenteric beds also occurs. The vasoconstrictive action of dopamine is antagonized by α-receptor blocking agents such as phentolamine.

Clinical Uses of Catecholamines

The clinical uses of catecholamines are based on their actions on bronchial smooth muscle, blood vessels, and the heart. Epinephrine is also useful for the treatment of allergic reactions that are due to liberation of histamine in the body, because it produces certain physiological effects opposite to those produced by histamine. It is the primary treatment for anaphylactic shock and is useful in the therapy of urticaria, angioneurotic edema, and serum sickness. Epinephrine and isoproterenol are useful in relieving the bronchoconstriction associated with acute and chronic bronchial asthma, pulmonary emphysema, and bronchitis.

Epinephrine also has been used to lower intraocular pressure in open-angle glaucoma. Its use promotes an increase in the outflow of aqueous humor. Because epinephrine administration will decrease the filtration angle formed by the cornea and the iris, its use is contraindicated in angle-closure glaucoma; under these conditions the outflow of aqueous humor via the filtration angle and into the venous system is hindered, and intraocular pressure may rise abruptly.

The vasoconstrictor actions of epinephrine and norepinephrine have been used to prolong the action of local anesthetics by reducing local blood flow in the region of the injection. Epinephrine has been used as a topical hemostatic agent for the control of localized hemorrhage. Norepinephrine is infused intravenously to combat systemic hypotension during spinal anesthesia or other hypotensive conditions in which peripheral resistance is low. It is not generally used to combat the hypotension due to most types of shock. In shock, marked sympathetic activity is already present, and perfusion of organs, such as the kidneys, may be jeopardized by norepinephrine administration.

Epinephrine and isoproterenol have been used to restore activity to the heart after cardiac arrest. Isoproterenol has been used to stimulate cardiac automaticity in cases of partial or complete heart block.

Dopamine is used in the treatment of shock owing to inadequate cardiac output (cardiogenic shock), which may be due to myocardial infarction or congestive heart failure. It is also used in the treatment of septic shock. An advantage of using dopamine in the treatment of shock is that it has an inotropic action that increases cardiac output while, at the same time, it dilates renal blood vessels and thereby increases renal blood flow. Renal circulation is frequently compromised during shock.

Adverse Reactions

Because they increase the force of the heartbeat, all three catecholamines may produce palpitations. Palpitations produced by epinephrine and isoproterenol are accompanied by tachycardia, whereas those produced by norepinephrine usually are accompanied by bradycardia owing to reflex slowing of the heart. Headache and tremor are also commonly experienced. Epinephrine is especially likely to produce feelings of anxiety, fear, and nervousness.

The greatest hazards of accidental overdosage with epinephrine and norepinephrine are cardiac arrhythmias, excessive hypertension, and acute pulmonary edema. Large doses of isoproterenol can produce such excessive cardiac

stimulation, combined with a decrease in diastolic blood pressure, that coronary insufficiency may result. It also may cause arrhythmias and ventricular fibrillation.

Tissue sloughing and necrosis due to severe local ischemia may occur following extravasation of norepinephrine at its injection site. The tissue damage can be minimized by infiltration of the affected area with a rapidly acting α-receptor blocking agent such as phentolamine.

Preparations and Dosage

Epinephrine

Epinephrine injection (*Adrenalin Chloride*) is epinephrine hydrochloride in a 1:1,000 sterile solution supplied in 1-ml ampules and 30-ml vials. When used with local anesthetics, epinephrine concentrations of 1:100,000 to 1:20,000 are generally employed.

Epinephrine for oral inhalation is available as epinephrine hydrochloride in a 1% nonsterile solution and as epinephrine bitartrate for oral inhalation as an aerosol. Solutions of epinephrine are unstable when exposed to light and are oxidized to adrenochrome. This pink solution should be discarded.

Norepinephrine

Norepinephrine (levarterenol) bitartrate injection is supplied in 4-ml ampules.

Isoproterenol

Isoproterenol hydrochloride injection (*Isuprel Hydrochloride*) is supplied in a 1:5,000 sterile solution in 1- and 5-ml ampules. The solution can be administered by the subcutaneous, intramuscular, intravenous, or intracardiac routes. Nebulizing units that deliver 0.075 mg for each oral inhalation are commercially available.

Dopamine

Dopamine hydrochloride (*Intropin*) is supplied in 5-ml ampules containing 40 mg/ml.

Other Adrenomimetic Agents

There are a number of adrenomimetic amines that are not catecholamines. Some of these are directly acting amines that must interact with adrenoceptors to produce a response in effector tissues. Some directly acting compounds, such as phenylephrine and methoxamine, activate α-receptors almost exclusively, whereas others, like albuterol and terbutaline, are nearly pure β-receptor agonists. Drugs that exert their pharmacological actions by releasing norepinephrine from its neuronal stores (indirectly acting) produce effects that are similar to those of norepinephrine. They tend to exert strong α-receptor activity, but β_1-receptor activity typical of norepinephrine, such as myocardial stimulation, also occurs (Table 12-3).

Some of the indirectly acting adrenomimetic amines are used primarily for their vasoconstrictive properties. They are applied locally to the nasal mucosa or to the eye. Other amines are used as bronchodilators, while still others are used exclusively for their ability to stimulate the CNS (Table 12-3). Many noncatecholamine adrenomimetic amines are resistant to enzymatic destruction, have prolonged actions, and are orally effective. The indirectly acting drugs are effective only when given in large doses, and they often produce tachyphylaxis.

Directly Acting Adrenomimetic Drugs

Phenylephrine, Metaraminol, and Methoxamine

These drugs are directly acting adrenomimetic amines that exert their effects primarily through an action on α-adrenoceptors, although phenylephrine has weak β-adrenoceptor activity as well. Consequently, these agents have little or no direct action on the heart. All three drugs increase both systolic and diastolic blood pressures through their vasoconstrictor action. The pressor response is accompanied by a reflex bradycardia, no change in the contractile force of the heart, and little change in cardiac output. They do not precipitate cardiac arrhythmias and do not stimulate the CNS.

Phenylephrine is not a substrate for COMT, while metaraminol and methoxamine are not metabolized by either COMT or MAO. Consequently, their durations of action are considerably prolonged compared to that of norepinephrine. Following intravenous injection, pressor responses to phenylephrine may persist for 20 min, while pressor responses to metaraminol and methoxamine may last for more than 60 min. Methoxamine generally produces the most persistent effects, probably because it is not taken up into adrenergic neurons. All three drugs are administered by intravenous, intramuscular, or subcutaneous injection. Phenylephrine is also frequently administered orally or by instillation to the eye or nose.

The clinical uses of these drugs are associated with their potent vasoconstrictor action. They are used to restore or maintain blood pressure during spinal anesthesia and certain other hypotensive states. The reflex bradycardia induced by their rapid intravenous injection has been used to terminate attacks of paroxysmal atrial tachycardia. Phenylephrine is commonly used as a nasal decongestant, although occasional nasal mucosal damage has occurred

Table 12-3. Adrenomimetic Drugs*

Generic name (proprietary name)	Therapeutic application
Phenylephrine (Neo-Synephrine)	Systemic vasoconstrictor; ophthalmic vasoconstrictor; nasal decongestant
Metaraminol (Aramine)	Systemic vasoconstrictor
Methoxamine (Vasoxyl)	Systemic vasoconstrictor; nasal decongestant
α-Methylnorepinephrine (Levonordefrin, Cobefrin)	Systemic vasoconstrictor (used as a vasoconstrictor in local anesthetics)
Dobutamine (Dobutrex)	Cardiogenic shock
Terbutaline (Bricanyl)	Bronchodilator (selective for β_2-adrenoceptors)
Albuterol (Ventolin, Proventil)	Bronchodilator (selective for β_2-adrenoceptors)
Ephedrine	Systemic vasoconstrictor; nasal decongestant; bronchodilator
Phenylpropanolamine (Propadrine)	Nasal decongestant; appetite suppressant (similar to ephedrine but less CNS stimulation)
dl-Amphetamine (Benzedrine) d-Amphetamine (Dexedrine)	CNS stimulant
Hydroxyamphetamine (Paredrine)	Ophthalmic vasoconstrictor (similar to ephedrine but with less CNS stimulation)
Cyclopentamine (Clopane)	Nasal decongestant
Tuaminoheptane (Tuamine)	Nasal decongestant
Tetrahydrozoline (Tyzine, Visine)	Nasal decongestant; ophthalmic vasoconstrictor
Oxymetazoline (Afrin)	Nasal decongestant

*This list of adrenomimetic drugs is by no means complete. Compounds are included primarily because of their therapeutic usefulness or because they represent a type of structure having adrenomimetic activity.

from injudicious use of the nasal spray. It is also employed in ophthalmology as a mydriatic agent. Phenylephrine, however, should not be given to patients with closed-angle glaucoma before iridectomy, since further increases in intraocular pressure may result. In dentistry, phenylephrine is used to prolong the effectiveness of a local anesthetic.

Phenylephrine hydrochloride (*Neo-Synephrine*) is supplied as an elixir, as a 10-mg/ml injectable solution, and in several concentrations for nasal and ophthalmic use.

Metaraminol bitartrate (*Aramine*) is supplied in 1- and 10-ml ampules (10 mg/ml).

Methoxamine hydrochloride (*Vasoxyl*) is supplied as aqueous solutions of 10 and 20 mg/ml for IM and IV injection.

Dobutamine

Dobutamine (*Dobutrex*), in contrast to dopamine, does not produce a significant proportion of its cardiac effects through the release of norepinephrine from adrenergic nerves; dobutamine acts directly on β_1-adrenoceptors in the heart. Dobutamine exerts a greater effect on the contractile force of the heart relative to its effect on the heart rate than does dopamine. Compared to dopamine, dobutamine increases the oxygen demands on the heart to a lesser extent. Like dopamine, it produces vasodilation of renal and mesenteric blood vessels. Dobutamine may be more useful than dopamine in the treatment of cardiogenic shock.

Dobutamine hydrochloride (*Dobutrex*) is supplied in 20-ml vials containing 250 mg of drug for injection.

Terbutaline and Albuterol

Terbutaline and albuterol are β-adrenoceptor agonists that have a relative selectivity for β_2-receptors. Both have a longer duration of action than isoproterenol because they are not metabolized by COMT. Like isoproterenol, they also are not metabolized by MAO and are not transported into adrenergic neurons. Terbutaline and albuterol are effective when administered either orally or subcutaneously. Because of their selectivity for β_2-adrenoceptors, they produce less cardiac stimulation than does isoproterenol but are not completely without effects on the heart.

Therapeutically, terbutaline and albuterol are used to treat bronchial asthma and bronchospasm associated with bronchitis and emphysema.

Side effects include nervousness, tremor, tachycardia, palpitations, headache, nausea, vomiting, and sweating. The frequency of appearance of these adverse effects is minimized, however, when the drugs are given by inhalation, a route that is available in the United States only for albuterol.

Terbutaline should not be used by individuals for whom adrenomimetic drugs in general are contraindicated, such as patients with hyperthyroidism or hypertension. It also should not be used in patients who are hypersensitive to adrenomimetics.

Terbutaline sulfate (*Bricanyl, Brethine*) is available as 2.5- and 5-mg tablets and as a 1:1,000 solution for injection.

Albuterol (*Ventolin, Proventil*) is available as 2- or 4-mg tablets and in canisters containing 17.0 gm for inhalation.

Indirectly Acting Adrenomimetic Drugs

Ephedrine

Ephedrine is a naturally occurring alkaloid obtained from plants of the genus *Ephedra*. It has been used in Chinese medicine for over 5,000 years. Ephedrine crosses the blood-brain barrier and thus exerts a strong CNS-stimulating effect in addition to its peripheral actions. The peripheral actions of ephedrine are primarily due to its indirect effects and depend largely on the release of norepinephrine. However, ephedrine may cause some direct receptor stimulation, particularly in its bronchodilating effects. Because it is resistant to metabolism by both COMT and MAO, its duration of action is more prolonged than is that of norepinephrine. As is the case with all indirectly acting adrenomimetic amines, ephedrine is much less potent than norepinephrine; in addition, tachyphylaxis develops to its peripheral actions. Unlike epinephrine or norepinephrine, however, ephedrine is effective when administered orally.

Pharmacological Actions
Ephedrine increases systolic and diastolic blood pressure; heart rate is generally not increased. Contractile force of the heart and cardiac output are both increased. Ephedrine produces bronchial smooth muscle relaxation of prolonged duration when administered orally. Aside from pupillary dilation, ephedrine has little effect on the eye.

Clinical Uses
Ephedrine is useful in relieving bronchoconstriction and mucosal congestion associated with bronchial asthma, asthmatic bronchitis, chronic bronchitis, and bronchial spasms. It is often used prophylactically to prevent asthmatic attacks and is used as a nasal decongestant, as a mydriatic, and in certain allergic disorders. Although its bronchodilator action is weaker than that of isoproterenol, its oral effectiveness and prolonged duration of action make it valuable in the treatment of these conditions. Because of their oral effectiveness and greater bronchiolar selectivity, however, terbutaline and albuterol are gradually replacing ephedrine for bronchodilation.

Adverse Effects
Symptoms of overdosage are related primarily to cardiac and CNS effects. Tachycardia, premature systoles, in-

somnia, nervousness, nausea, vomiting, and emotional disturbances may develop. Ephedrine should not be used in patients with cardiac disease, hypertension, or hyperthyroidism.

Preparation and Dosage
Ephedrine sulfate is available for oral use and as an injectable solution.

Amphetamine

Amphetamine exists as an *l* and a *d* isomer. The *l* isomer is slightly more potent in producing peripheral effects. On the other hand, the *d* isomer (dextroamphetamine) is three to four times more potent in producing CNS stimulation.

Pharmacological Actions
Amphetamine is an indirectly acting adrenomimetic amine that depends on the release of norepinephrine from noradrenergic nerves for its action. Its pharmacological effects are similar to those of ephedrine; however, its CNS stimulant activity is somewhat greater. Central nervous system stimulation is the dominant effect of this drug and is the basis for its therapeutic usefulness. Nevertheless, amphetamine has typical adrenomimetic properties that are commonly seen during its therapeutic use, especially when larger doses are employed. Both systolic and diastolic blood pressures are increased by oral dosage with amphetamine. The heart rate is frequently slowed reflexly. Cardiac output may remain unchanged in the low and moderate dose range.

Clinical Uses
The therapeutic uses of amphetamine are based on its ability to stimulate the CNS. It has been used in the treatment of obesity because of its anorexic effect, although tolerance to this effect develops rapidly. It prevents or overcomes fatigue and has been used as an analeptic. *Amphetamine is no longer recommended for these uses because of its potential for abuse,* and its use is restricted by law in some states. Amphetamine is useful in certain cases of narcolepsy or minimal brain dysfunction.

Amphetamine sulfate (*Dexedrine*) is available as tablets and as slow-release capsules.

Further discussion of amphetamine can be found in the chapters, Central Nervous System Stimulants (Chap. 34) and Contemporary Drug Abuse (Chap. 41).

Supplemental Reading

Burnstock, G., and Griffith, S.G. *Noradrenergic Innervation of Blood Vessels.* Boca Raton, Fla.: CRC, 1988.

Exton, J.H. Mechanisms involved in effects of catecholamines on liver carbohydrate metabolism. *Biochem. Pharmacol.* 28:2237, 1979.

Farah, A.E., Alousi, A.A., and Schwarz, R.A., Jr. Positive inotropic agents. *Annu. Rev. Pharmacol. Toxicol.* 24:275, 1984.

Gootman, P.M. (ed.). *Developmental Neurobiology of the Autonomic Nervous System.* Clifton, N.J.: Humana, 1986.

Limbird, L.E. (ed.). *The Alpha-2 Adrenergic Receptors.* Clifton, N.J.:Humana, 1988.

Moncada, S.R., Palmer, M.J., and Higgs, E.A. Nitric oxide: Physiology, pathophysiology, and pharmacology. *Pharmacol. Rev.* 43:109, 1991.

Moreland, R.S., and Bohr, D.F. Adrenergic control of coronary arteries. *Fed. Proc.* 43:2857, 1984.

Reinhart, P.H., Taylor, W.M., and Bygrave, F.L. The mechanism of α-adrenergic agonists action in liver. *Biol. Rev.* 59:511, 1984.

Rubanyi, G.M., and Botelho, L.H. Parker endothelins. *FASEB J.* 5:2713, 1991.

Wang, J.Y., and Lee, T.J.-F. Beta-receptor–mediated vasodilation in cerebral arteries of the pig. *Acta Physiol. Scand.* 127 (Suppl. 552):41, 1986.

13

Adrenoceptor Antagonists

David P. Westfall

Adrenoceptors

The notion that there exist in tissues specific elements with which drugs interact and that this interaction results in some characteristic tissue response is well entrenched in modern pharmacology (see Chap. 2). The "specific elements" are called *receptors*. Evidence favoring the existence of *adrenoceptors* (receptors with which adrenomimetic agents interact) is extensive and derives from both functional pharmacological and molecular biological studies. Drugs that produce responses by interacting with adrenoceptors are referred to as *adrenoceptor agonists* or *adrenergic agonists*. Norepinephrine and isoproterenol are examples of such compounds. Agents that inhibit responses mediated by adrenoceptor activation are known as *adrenoceptor antagonists, adrenergic antagonists,* or *adrenergic blocking agents*. Phentolamine and propranolol are examples of receptor-blocking drugs. The pharmacology of the adrenoceptor antagonists is described in this chapter.

Norepinephrine is released from the varicosities of the postganglionic sympathetic nerves during neural activity. Norepinephrine then interacts with the adrenoceptors of the effector organ, producing the characteristic response of the effector. This occurs because norepinephrine has an *affinity* for the receptors and possesses *intrinsic activity;* that is, it has the capacity to activate the receptors. Circulating catecholamines and other directly acting adrenomimetic drugs also interact with these receptors. Receptor activation initiates a series of events in the effector; these may include alterations in membrane conductance or formation of cyclic 3′, 5′-adenosine monophosphate (cAMP), or both; these initial events ultimately result in such responses as muscle contraction or glycogenolysis.

The adrenergic blocking agents also have an affinity for the adrenoceptors. The antagonists, however, have only limited or no capacity to activate the receptors; that is, they have little or negligible intrinsic activity. The blocking drugs compete with the adrenomimetic substances for access to the receptors. Thus, *these agents reduce the effects produced by both sympathetic nerve stimulation and by exogenously administered adrenomimetics*. This action forms the basis for their therapeutic and investigational use.

Competition for receptors, and hence receptor antagonism, is governed by the *law of mass action;* that is, the interaction between drug and receptor is dependent on the concentration of drug in the vicinity of the receptor and the number of receptors present. Because both agonist and antagonist have an affinity for the same receptors, the two substances compete for binding to the receptors.

For most adrenoceptor antagonists (and agonists), the attachment of the blocking agent to the adrenoceptor is by relatively weak forces, such as hydrophobic, hydrogen, or van der Waal's bonding. Because the drug easily dissociates from the receptor, the antagonism exhibited by these compounds is readily reversible on removal of the antagonists from the biophase. This type of antagonism is referred to as *reversible-competitive* or *equilibrium-competitive* (see Chap. 2). However, one group of antagonists, the haloalkylamines, is highly chemically reactive. These compounds are capable of forming covalent bonds with various chemical groupings on receptors. Removal of these antagonists from the biophase is not sufficient to restore the responsiveness of the effector to agonists. Full tissue responsiveness may not occur for several days. Because of the apparently irreversible nature of this drug antagonism, it is termed *irreversible-competitive* or *nonequilibrium-competitive* (see Chap. 2).

Adrenoceptor blocking agents have the ability to reduce the effectiveness of sympathetic nerve activity. They do not prevent the release of transmitters from adrenergic nerves as do the neuron-blocking agents such as guanethidine, and they are not catecholamine-depleting agents such as reserpine (see Chap. 22). They prevent the agonist from interacting with its receptor.

Classification of Blocking Drugs

The notion that more than one class of adrenoceptors may exist had its origin in Sir Henry Dale's studies of ergot alkaloids in the early 1900s. Dale noted that certain extracts of the fungus ergot not only inhibited the usual hypertensive response to epinephrine, but actually converted it to a hypotensive response. It was some 40 years before a conceptual framework was proposed to provide a basis for this ergot effect. By comparing a series of adrenomimetic amines in a variety of effector systems, Raymond Ahlquist demonstrated that there are two distinct orders of potency. This led him to suggest that there are two distinct types of receptors in sympathetically innervated tissue. He proposed the designations *alpha* and *beta* to distinguish between these two receptor populations. The adrenergic blocking agents that existed at the time were shown to antagonize responses mediated by the α-receptor, but not the β-receptor. The concept of multiple types of adrenergic receptors was solidified when agents such as dichloroisoproterenol were developed which antagonized those responses that had been classified by Ahlquist as β-adrenergic.

Classically, adrenoceptors are defined both on the basis of the order of potency of a series of adrenomimetics and by the drugs that antagonize sympathetic responses. An α-receptor is one that mediates responses for which the adrenomimetic order of potency is epinephrine $\geq$ norepinephrine $>$ isoproterenol, and that is susceptible to blockade by phentolamine and phenoxybenzamine. It follows from this definition that phentolamine and phenoxybenzamine are called α-adrenoceptor antagonists or α-blocking agents. A β-receptor mediates responses for which the adrenomimetic order of potency is isoproterenol $>$ epinephrine $\geq$ norepinephrine, and is susceptible to blockade by propranolol. Propranolol is, therefore, called a β-adrenoceptor antagonist or β-blocking agent.

Recent studies suggest that the division of adrenergic receptors solely into α and β types is too simplistic. Evidence has accumulated pointing to the existence of subclasses of both α- and β-receptors (see also Chap. 11).

β-Receptor Subtypes

On the basis of the study of relative potencies of a large series of agonists, it was shown that there are at least two types of β-receptors. The two types were given the designations β_1 and β_2. Among the responses mediated by β_1-receptors are cardiac stimulation and inhibition of intes-

tinal motility, whereas β_2-receptor stimulation mediates bronchodilation and relaxation of vascular and uterine smooth muscle (see Chap. 11). These findings are significant, since a number of both agonists and antagonists have been developed that have some degree of selectivity for either β_1- or β_2-receptors.

A comparison of the effects produced by propranolol, a nonselective β-receptor blocking agent, with those of metoprolol, a relatively selective β_1-receptor blocker, illustrates the clinical utility of such drugs. For example, a patient who is a candidate for β-blocker therapy (angina, hypertension) but who also has obstructive airway disease probably should not receive a nonselective β-blocking agent such as propranolol because of the possibility of aggravating bronchospasm. In this instance, metoprolol would be advantageous since β-receptors of the respiratory system are β_2 and would be less affected by metoprolol than by propranolol. It is important to recognize, however, that metoprolol's selectivity is only relative, and at high concentrations the drug will also antagonize β_2 responses.

It is likely that an absolute selectivity of drug action does not exist. Any given effector tissue probably contains more than one receptor subtype, and it is likely that the proportion of receptor subtypes varies within that effector. Nevertheless, the designation of a drug as either a β_1-receptor or β_2-receptor selective agent seems both useful and justified if one keeps in mind that the designation represents a shorthand notation for what is only a predominance of activities.

Molecular genetic techniques have confirmed the notion of multiple subtypes of β-adrenoceptors. β_1- and β_2-receptors have been cloned and important information about their structure has been learned. In addition, recent molecular biological evidence indicates the existence of at least one additional β-receptor subtype, called the β_3-receptor. Neither the physiological relevance nor the effector distribution of the β_3-receptor has been established. There is the suggestion that the β_3-receptor may mediate some of the metabolic effects of catecholamines. Although some experimental drugs exhibit selectivity for the β_3-receptor, none of the currently available β-blockers have been shown to rely on β_3-receptor antagonism for their therapeutic effectiveness. It should be borne in mind, however, that further characterization of the β_3-receptor, and perhaps other subtypes, may eventually lead to the development of additional selective and useful therapeutic agents.

α-Receptor Subtypes

Subclasses of α-receptors also exist. This knowledge evolved from the realization that α-receptors play a role in the regulation of norepinephrine release. When norepinephrine, which has been released by sympathetic nerve stimulation, achieves a certain concentration in the synaptic cleft, it will stimulate α-receptors located on the nerve terminals (i.e., *presynaptic receptors*) and cause a reduction in the further release of norepinephrine. This feedback regulation of transmitter release occurs at physiological rates of nerve stimulation. The administration of certain α-receptor blocking agents will antagonize the decreased transmitter release caused by norepinephrine (or any α-agonist) such that, in the presence of an α-receptor blocking agent, the neural release of norepinephrine actually is enhanced.

Once the existence of presynaptic α-receptors was recognized, a number of studies were undertaken to characterize them. The results indicate that there are differences between the α-receptors located on nerves (*presynaptic α-receptors*) and those found on effector cells (*postsynaptic α-receptors*). Furthermore, some α-agonists and antagonists exhibit selectivity for one of these α-receptor types.

A terminology has emerged that classifies α-receptors as either α_1 or α_2. α_1-Receptors are those whose stimulation has traditionally been associated with the postsynaptic α-receptors of smooth muscle while α_2-receptors are those originally associated with the presynaptic α-receptors of peripheral nerves. However, the classification of α-receptors is now based primarily on the characteristics of drugs that react specifically with each receptor type. It should be noted that the designation of receptors as either α_1 or α_2 cannot be categorized strictly by anatomical location (i.e., presynaptic or postsynaptic). The evidence now indicates that α_2-receptors, in addition to being on peripheral nerves, are located at a variety of sites, including smooth muscle, adrenal medullary cells, the brain, and melanocytes.

The existence of α-receptor subclasses and the receptor selectivity exhibited by certain α-blocking agents have therapeutic implications. Phentolamine is a disappointing antihypertensive drug because its administration results in a reflex increase in both heart rate and contractile force; these effects tend to negate the reduction in blood pressure that it produces. In contrast, prazosin, a more recently introduced α-blocker, is an effective antihypertensive drug because the reflex cardiac stimulation it induces is much less. The differing hemodynamic effects produced by phentolamine and prazosin appear to be related to their relative degree of selectivity for α_1- and α_2-receptors. Phentolamine is a relatively nonselective α-receptor blocking agent since, in addition to blocking postsynaptic α_1-receptors, it will block presynaptic α_2-receptors; the latter action results in an enhanced release of norepinephrine and, hence, an augmented cardiac rate and contractile force. Blockade of α_2-receptors may actually potentiate the cardiac effects of sympathetic nerve stimulation. Prazosin, in contrast to phentolamine, is relatively selective for α_1-receptors; that is, it preferentially blocks responses mediated by the postsynaptic α_1-receptors in the blood vessels without having a substantial effect on presynaptic

α_2-receptors. Thus, prazosin administration causes less stimulation of the heart than does phentolamine.

It is important to recognize that absolute selectivity of action for α_1- or α_2-receptors does not exist for the currently available α-agonists and antagonists. Furthermore, as is the case with β-receptors, a given effector tissue may contain more than one α-receptor subtype. Recent evidence suggests that in addition to α_1-receptors, vascular smooth muscle may possess α_2-receptors. Although the functional importance of α_2-receptors in blood vessels seems to be less than that of α_1-receptors, this can account for certain clinical observations, as, for example, the pressor response that occurs upon initiation of treatment with the α_2-agonist clonidine.

It is becoming increasingly clear that neither α_1- nor α_2-receptors are homogeneous. There seem to be at least three subtypes of both α_1- and α_2-receptors, for example, α_{1A}, α_{1B}, α_{1C}, α_{2A}, α_{2B}, and α_{2C}. The existence of these subtypes had been surmised from functional pharmacological studies and radioligand binding experiments and more recently confirmed by the cloning of the receptors. At this point, the pharmacology and therapeutic usefulness of the available α-antagonists can be reasonably well explained by considering their relative selectivity for the two main classes of α-receptors, α_1 and α_2, without considering their action at the subtypes. This is likely to change, however, and further characterization of these subtypes holds the promise of a clearer understanding of drug action and the development of additional therapeutically useful drugs.

α-Receptor Blocking Agents

A large number of compounds possess some α-receptor blocking activity. However, most of these drugs also have other actions that cannot be attributed directly to α-receptor antagonism, and these effects limit their usefulness as α-blockers. The benzodioxane derivatives piperoxan and dibozane and the antipsychotic agents chlorpromazine and haloperidol are examples of such drugs.

There are a few drugs whose therapeutic applications are the specific result of their α-blocking activity. The clinically important drugs fall into three chemical groups: the *haloalkylamines* (e.g., phenoxybenzamine), the *imidazolines* (e.g., phentolamine), and the *quinazoline derivatives* (e.g., prazosin). The structures of these compounds are shown in Fig. 13-1.

Haloalkylamines

Practically all members of the haloalkylamine series possess α-blocking activity, and their pharmacological actions are quite similar. The haloalkylamines are chemi-

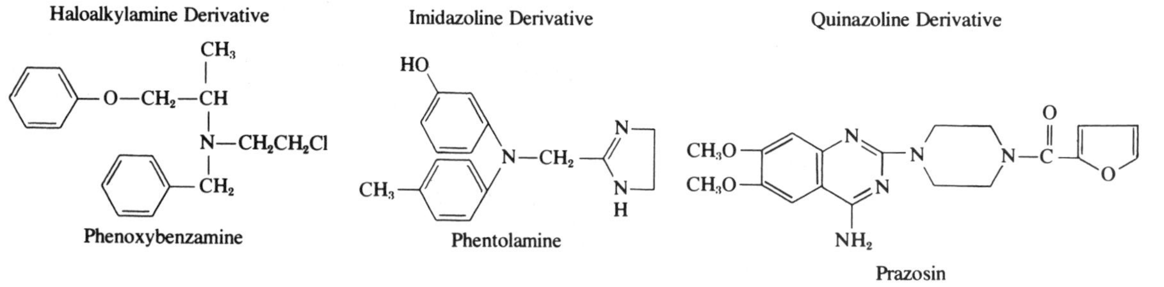

Figure 13-1. Structures of the principal α-blockers.

cally related to the highly reactive nitrogen mustards. Clinically, the most important drug is phenoxybenzamine.

Mechanism of Action

The haloalkylamines produce an *irreversible (nonequilibrium)-competitive antagonism* of responses mediated by α-adrenoceptors. Because of the irreversible nature of this antagonism, the duration of their action is much longer than that of other classes of α-blocking agents. In neutral or alkaline solution, this blocking effect is directly related to the loss of their β-halogen, with the subsequent cyclization of the tertiary amine to form reactive ethylenimino intermediates. These intermediates alkylate various groups on or near the α-receptors. *The long duration of their antagonism is due to the firm binding of the haloalkylamine to the receptor.* In essence, the haloalkylamines can be viewed as "removing" a portion of the α-receptors from the total pool available to interact with α-agonists.

Phenoxybenzamine has a somewhat greater affinity for α₁- than for α₂-receptors. Nevertheless, α₂-receptors can be blocked by the drug; therefore, in addition to blocking vascular smooth muscle contraction, phenoxybenzamine potentiates the release of norepinephrine from adrenergic nerves.

Phenoxybenzamine and the other haloalkylamines are not only capable of blocking α-receptors, but also of inhibiting responses mediated by several other receptor types. The antagonism of these other receptor-mediated responses is also of the nonequilibrium-competitive type and probably occurs as a result of *receptor alkylation.* For example, responses to acetylcholine, 5-hydroxytryptamine (serotonin; 5-HT), and histamine can be antagonized by phenoxybenzamine, although higher concentrations of phenoxybenzamine generally are required to antagonize responses to acetylcholine and 5-HT. Phenoxybenzamine is, however, a potent antagonist of histamine at usual doses.

Pharmacological Actions

Phenoxybenzamine will effectively antagonize those α-receptor-mediated effects produced either by sympathetic nerve stimulation or by adrenomimetic drugs. Although phenoxybenzamine will inhibit the contractions of smooth muscles contained in the spleen, ureter, and radial muscle of the iris, the most important effect therapeutically is its ability to antagonize the contraction of vascular smooth muscle. Phenoxybenzamine and the other α-blockers will produce vasodilation whenever blood vessels are constricted as a result of sympathetic (or adrenomimetic) stimulation.

The hemodynamic effects produced by phenoxybenzamine are similar in many respects to those produced by directly acting vasodilators (Chap. 22). The drug reduces blood pressure by diminishing systemic and pulmonary resistance; this effect is more prominent under conditions of high sympathetic activity, that is, as occurs in a standing rather than a recumbent individual. Since both venodilation and arteriodilation occur, postural hypotension is a conspicuous feature of phenoxybenzamine-induced α-blockade.

Phenoxybenzamine administration frequently results in increases in heart rate and myocardial contractile force that enhance cardiac output. Several factors contribute to this effect. First, a reflex increase in sympathetic stimulation of the heart is a normal consequence of decreased peripheral vascular resistance. Because the adrenoceptors that mediate the heart's response to neurally released norepinephrine are β-receptors, phenoxybenzamine does not antagonize the increased sympathetic stimulation. Second, the release of norepinephrine from the cardiac sympathetic nerves actually may be enhanced as a result of the α₂-blocking effects of phenoxybenzamine.

In general, if sympathetic tone is large, α-blockade will decrease resistance and will increase blood flow in most vascular beds. Cerebral blood flow, however, is little affected unless the blood pressure is greatly reduced.

Phenoxybenzamine modifies the blood pressure responses produced by most adrenomimetic amines. In some instances, it reduces the magnitude of the blood pressure rise caused by an agonist, while in other cases it may actually convert the response to the agonist from one of constriction to one of vasodilation. This latter effect will occur if epinephrine is the agonist, since epinephrine has the ability to activate β- as well as α-receptors in the vasculature. Thus, with α-receptors blocked by phenoxybenzamine, the β activity (vasodilating) of epinephrine will predominate. The pressure increase to norepinephrine is antagonized, but not reversed, by phenoxybenzamine; this is due to norepinephrine's low intrinsic activity for vascular β-receptors (β_2). Responses to isoproterenol are not antagonized by phenoxybenzamine, because isoproterenol produces responses that are mediated almost entirely by β-receptors.

Absorption, Metabolism, and Excretion

The haloalkylamines are effective by all routes of administration, but because of potential damage to muscle, intravenous injection is the preferred parenteral route. The absorption of phenoxybenzamine from the gastrointestinal tract, while sufficient to produce a pharmacological response, is incomplete and somewhat erratic. At best, only 20 to 30 percent of an orally administered dose will be absorbed in active form.

The onset of action of phenoxybenzamine occurs after a delay of about 1 hr. This lag presumably is due to the time required to form the reactive intermediates that bind to receptors. The duration of action after a single intravenous injection is quite long, generally ranging from 1.5 to 5 days. Although the haloalkylamines are quite lipid soluble and are stored in body fat, this probably does not account for their long duration of action. The prolonged action is more likely the result of their binding irreversibly to receptors. Unchanged, dealkylated, and conjugated forms of phenoxybenzamine all occur in the urine.

Adverse Reactions

Most side effects associated with the use of phenoxybenzamine and the other α-blockers are directly attributable to their α-receptor blocking ability. These effects include postural hypotension, tachycardia, miosis, nasal stuffiness, and failure of ejaculation. The most serious of these are hypotension and reflex-mediated tachycardia. These two effects are exaggerated by hypovolemia. If a patient exhibits signs of hypovolemia, phenoxybenzamine must be administered cautiously, and only after blood volume corrections have been made. Rapid intravenous injection may cause a precipitous fall in blood pressure, and, therefore, intravenous administration should be slow. Pa-

tients receiving phenoxybenzamine should be cautioned that any activity that increases sympathetic nerve activity (e.g., exercise, a large meal) may precipitate a fall in blood pressure. Similarly, because reflex sympathetic control of blood pressure is interfered with, phenoxybenzamine and the other α-blockers potentiate responses to drugs that cause vasodilation, such as the directly acting vasodilators, narcotics, and alcohol.

Phenoxybenzamine also may produce side effects that are not directly related to its α-receptor blocking action. These include local tissue irritation after parenteral administration and nausea after oral administration.

Preparations and Dosage

Phenoxybenzamine hydrochloride (*Dibenzyline*) is available in 10-mg tablets or in ampules (100 mg/2 ml) for intravenous use.

Imidazoline Derivatives

Phentolamine and tolazoline are the most important drugs of this class. They exhibit pronounced α-blocking activity but possess other actions as well. For example, tolazoline has considerable histaminelike and cholinomimetic activity. Of the two drugs, phentolamine is the more potent α-receptor blocking agent.

Mechanism of Action

In contrast to the haloalkylamines, imidazolines produce an *equilbrium-competitive antagonism* of the actions of the catecholamines. Responses mediated by receptors other than α-receptors are, in general, not as susceptible to blockade by imidazolines as they are by phenoxybenzamine. However, large doses of phentolamine can antagonize the action of several endogenous substances, including 5-HT.

The imidazolines do not show selectivity toward either α_1- or α_2-receptors. The amount of norepinephrine released per nerve impulse is enhanced by these agents; this effect probably contributes considerably to the adrenomimetic actions that accompany imidazoline administration. Tachycardia is prominent after administration of phentolamine or tolazoline.

Pharmacological Actions

The α-blocking activity of the imidazolines results in effects that are quite similar to those of phenoxybenzamine, with the exception that their onset of action is quicker and their duration of action is shorter. The degree of α-blockade that can be produced in humans by phentolamine and tolazoline is far from complete. This is not due to a lack of α-blocking effectiveness, but rather to the appearance of side effects that limit the amount of drug that can be administered. These side effects include stimulation of gastrointestinal motility (owing to cholinomimetic actions and parasympathetic predominance) and enhanced gastric secretory activity (owing to histaminelike activity).

Except for their duration, the hemodynamic effects resulting from phentolamine administration are quite similar to those caused by phenoxybenzamine. Phentolamine produces vasodilation by inhibiting the influence of sympathetic nerve stimulation on vascular smooth muscle. Both arterial and venous smooth muscle are affected, and postural hypotension is prominent. Reflex-initiated increases in cardiac rate and contractile force occur in response to the peripheral vasodilation. Cardiac stimulation is enhanced by the α_2-blocking activity of phentolamine. Imidazolines modify blood pressure responses to circulating catecholamines in a manner similar to that of phenoxybenzamine. The hemodynamic responses resulting from tolazoline administration are more variable, however, because this compound has more prominent adrenomimetic and histaminelike activities.

Absorption, Metabolism, and Excretion

Phentolamine and tolazoline can be administered either orally or parenterally, although an orally administered dose is only 20 percent as effective as an equivalent intravenous dose. Because the absorption of tolazoline from the gastrointestinal tract is slow, and because renal excretion through the tubular organic base secretory system is high, plasma levels of tolazoline are usually low. The plasma half-life of tolazoline is approximately 2 hr.

Adverse Reactions

Postural hypotension and cardiac stimulation are important adverse effects associated with phentolamine and tolazoline administration. Tachycardia can be considerable and, if uncontrolled, may lead to arrhythmias, myocardial ischemia, or both. The drugs should be used with great caution in patients with coronary artery disease. As with phenoxybenzamine, vasodilation produced by other drugs is potentiated by phentolamine and tolazoline.

Gastrointestinal disturbances resulting from both the cholinomimetic and histaminelike activities of these drugs can be quite prominent. Contractions are stimulated and may cause diarrhea; gastric secretion also is enhanced. Patients who suffer from gastritis or peptic ulcer should be treated cautiously, if at all, with imidazoline α-blocking

agents. In addition to the gastric glands, a number of other exocrine glands (e.g., lacrimal and salivary) also are stimulated by the imidazolines.

Curiously, the radial muscle of the iris seems to be resistant to the actions of tolazoline. Mydriasis, rather than the miosis typical of α-blockade, is sometimes observed following administration of tolazoline.

Preparations and Dosage

Phentolamine is available for both parenteral (phentolamine mesylate, *Regitine Mesylate*) and oral (phentolamine hydrochloride, *Regitine Hydrochloride*) administration. Tolazoline hydrochloride (*Priscoline Hydrochloride*) is available in 25-mg tablets and in 10-ml vials; it is rarely used parenterally, however.

Clinical Uses of the Haloalkylamines and Imidazolines

Although these drugs have limited usefulness in the treatment of primary hypertension, they are useful for the treatment of hypertension caused by catecholamine-secreting tumors (*pheochromocytoma*). The drugs are used for both the preoperative management and the prevention of paroxysmal hypertension caused by surgical manipulation of the tumor. Drug treatment is usually instituted several weeks before surgery. The drugs are used on a prolonged basis in the rare case of an inoperable tumor.

In the past, the blood pressure responses to phentolamine were used as a diagnostic test for pheochromocytoma (the *Regitine* test). Because these tumors usually secrete large amounts of epinephrine, phentolamine administration will produce a rapid reduction in blood pressure. However, in recent years the use of the Regitine test has declined, largely owing to the availability of sensitive techniques for the quantification of urinary catecholamines and their metabolites.

The α-blocking drugs have been widely employed for the treatment of various forms of peripheral vascular disease. However, since the term *peripheral vascular disease* actually encompasses a variety of conditions of diverse etiology, it is not surprising that the benefit achieved from the use of these agents has been somewhat variable. Success is more likely if the drugs are employed for conditions associated with a high degree of sympathetically induced vasoconstriction, as occurs in Raynaud's syndrome, acrocyanosis, and ulceration of the extremities caused by chronic peripheral vasospasm and the sequelae of frostbite.

Phenoxybenzamine finds some use in the management of benign prostatic obstruction, especially in patients who are not candidates for surgery. Blockade of α-adrenoceptors in the base of the bladder and the prostate apparently reduces the symptoms of obstruction and the urinary urgency that occurs at night.

Although use of a α-receptor blocking agents (particularly phenoxybenzamine) has been advocated in the treatment of shock, the drugs are used primarily as adjuncts to other forms of therapy, for example, blood volume replacement.

Quinazoline Derivatives

Drugs of this class exhibit selectivity for α_1-adrenoceptors and, therefore, are more useful than phenoxybenzamine and phentolamine for the treatment of primary hypertension. Their chief use is in the management of primary hypertension. Examples of quinazoline α-blockers include prazosin, trimazosin, terazosin, and doxazosin.

Mechanism of Action

The α-antagonism produced by prazosin and the other quinazoline derivatives is of the *equilibrium-competitive* type. The drugs are selective for α_1-adrenoceptors so that at usual therapeutic concentrations there is little or negligible antagonism of α_2-adrenoceptors. As with most adrenoceptor antagonists, however, selectivity is only relative and can be lost with high drug concentrations. While the majority of the pharmacological effects of prazosin are directly attributable to α_1-antagonism, at high doses the drug can cause vasodilation by a direct effect on smooth muscle independent of α-receptors. This action appears to be related to an inhibition of phosphodiesterases that results in an enhancement of intracellular levels of cyclic nucleotides.

Pharmacological Actions

As with other α-adrenoceptor antagonists, the most important pharmacological effect of prazosin is its ability to antagonize vascular smooth muscle contraction that is caused by either sympathetic nervous activity or the action of adrenomimetics. Hemodynamically, the effects of prazosin differ from those of phenoxybenzamine and phentalomine in that venous smooth muscle is not as much affected by prazosin. Postural hypotension during chronic treatment is also less of a problem than with classic α-blockers. Additionally, increases in heart rate and contractile force and plasma renin activity, which normally occur after the use of vasodilators and α-blockers, are much less prominent following chronic treatment with prazosin.

Prazosin exerts its antihypertensive effect through a relaxation of vascular smooth muscle. Although a direct relaxation of smooth muscle may occur, particularly at high doses, the vasodilation is primarily due to the drug's α-blocking activity.

The differences in the effects produced by prazosin and the classic α-blockers are related to differences in the proportion and characteristics among α-receptors present in various effector tissues. Phenoxybenzamine and phentolamine, in addition to blocking postsynaptic α-receptors, also block α_2-receptors on nerves and, therefore, can enhance the release of norepinephrine. In a situation in which norepinephrine exerts a postsynaptic action by means of β-adrenoceptors (e.g., cardiac stimulation, renin release), blockade of presynaptic α_2-receptors by phenoxybenzamine and phentolamine may actually potentiate the responses. Prazosin blocks responses mediated by postsynaptic α_1-receptors, but has no effect on the presynaptic α_2-receptors. Thus, stimulation of the heart and renin release are less prominent with this drug.

Absorption, Metabolism, and Excretion

Prazosin is readily absorbed after oral administration, and peak serum levels occur approximately 2 hr after a single oral dose. The antihypertensive effect of prazosin persists for up to 10 hr after an oral dose. Its half-life in plasma ranges from 2.5 to 4 hr, and elimination from plasma appears to follow first-order kinetics. The drug is extensively (perhaps as high as 97%) bound to plasma proteins; this partially explains the lack of correlation between plasma drug levels and persistence of antihypertensive effect.

The metabolic fate of prazosin in humans has not been completely established, but the drug is believed to be extensively metabolized in the liver, where O-dealkylation and glucuronide formation appear to be major pathways of biotransformation. Four metabolites are formed, all of which possess less than 25 percent of the parent compound's antihypertensive activity.

Only about 10 percent of orally administered prazosin is excreted in the urine. Curiously, however, plasma levels of prazosin are increased in patients with renal failure; the nature of this interaction is unknown. Clinically, therefore, it probably is advisable to reduce the dose of prazosin in such patients.

Adverse Reactions

Although less a problem than with phenoxybenzamine or phentolamine, symptoms of postural hypotension, such as dizziness and light-headedness, are the most commonly reported side effects associated with prazosin therapy. These effects occur most frequently during initial treatment and when the dosage is sharply increased. The appearance of postural hypotension seems to be more pronounced during Na^+ deficiency, as may occur in patients

Table 13-1. Comparative Information About the Three Classes of α-Adrenoceptor Antagonists

	Haloalkylamines	Imidazolines	Quinazolines
Prototype	Phenoxybenzamine *(Dibenzyline)*	Phentolamine *(Regitine)*	Prazosin *(Minipress)*
Others		Tolazoline *(Priscoline)*	Terazosin *(Hytrin)* Doxazosin *(Cardura)* Trimazosin *(Cardovar)*
Antagonism	Irreversible (nonequilibrium)-competitive	Equilibrium-competitive	Equilibrium-competitive
Selectivity	Somewhat selective for α_1	Nonselective	Selective for α_1
Hemodynamic effects	Decrease peripheral vascular resistance and blood pressure Venodilation is prominent Cardiac stimulation occurs because of cardiovascular reflexes and enhanced release of norepinephrine	Similar to phenoxybenzamine	Decrease peripheral vascular resistance and blood pressure Veins seem to be less susceptible to antagonism than arteries; thus, postural hypotension is less of a problem Cardiac stimulation is less because release of norepinephrine is not enhanced
Actions other than α-blockade	Some antagonism of responses to ACh, 5-HT, and histamine Blockade of neuronal and extraneuronal uptake	Cholinomimetic, adrenomimetic, and histaminelike actions Antagonism of responses to 5-HT	At high doses some direct vasodilator action, probably due to phosphodiesterase inhibition
Routes	Intravenous and oral Oral absorption incomplete and erratic	Similar to phenoxybenzamine	Oral
Adverse reactions	Postural hypotension, tachycardia, miosis, nasal stuffiness, failure of ejaculation	Same as phenoxybenzamine and in addition gastrointestinal disturbances	Some postural hypotension, especially with the first dose; less of a problem overall than with phenoxybenzamine or phentolamine
Therapeutic uses	Conditions of catecholamine excess such as pheochromocytoma Peripheral vascular disease	Same as phenoxybenzamine	Primary hypertension

Key: ACh = acetylcholine; 5-HT = 5-hydroxytryptamine.

on a low-salt diet, or in patients being treated with diuretics, β-blockers, or both.

Preparations and Dosage

Prazosin hydrochloride *(Minipress)* is available as 1-, 2-, and 5-mg capsules. Because the incidence of side effects is greatest when prazosin treatment is first instituted, the recommendation is to start with low doses.

Trimazosin hydrochloride *(Cardovar)*, terazosin hydrochloride *(Hytrin)*, and doxazosin mesylate *(Cardura)* are other quinazoline derivatives available for clinical use.

Clinical Uses

Prazosin is effective in reducing all grades of hypertension. The drug can be administered alone in mild and (in some instances) moderate hypertension. When hypertension is moderate or severe, it generally is given in combination with a thiazide diuretic and a β-blocker. The antihypertensive actions of prazosin are considerably potentiated by coadministration of thiazides or other types of antihypertensive drugs.

Prazosin may be particularly useful when patients cannot tolerate other classes of antihypertensive drugs or when blood pressure is not well controlled by other drugs. Since prazosin does not significantly influence blood uric acid or glucose levels, it can be used in hypertensive patients whose condition is complicated by diabetes mellitus or gout.

Comparative information concerning the three principal classes of α-blockers is presented in Table 13-1.

β-Adrenoceptor Blocking Agents

There are approximately a dozen β-blockers on the market in the United States. Of these, propranolol, a nonselective β-antagonist, was the first to be introduced and is the prototypical drug to which the others are compared. Metoprolol was the first β_1-selective drug and timolol the first β-blocker approved for ophthalmic use. The names of several of the other β-blockers are listed in Table 13-2. The structures of representative β-blockers are shown in Fig. 13-2.

As a class, β-blocking agents have greater structural similarity to their corresponding agonists than do the α-blockers. This structural similarity also accounts for the greater specificity of action exhibited by the β-receptor blocking drugs as compared to the α-blockers, which antagonize responses mediated by several receptor systems (histamine, 5-HT, acetylcholine).

Figure 13-2. Structures of isoproterenol and some β-blockers.

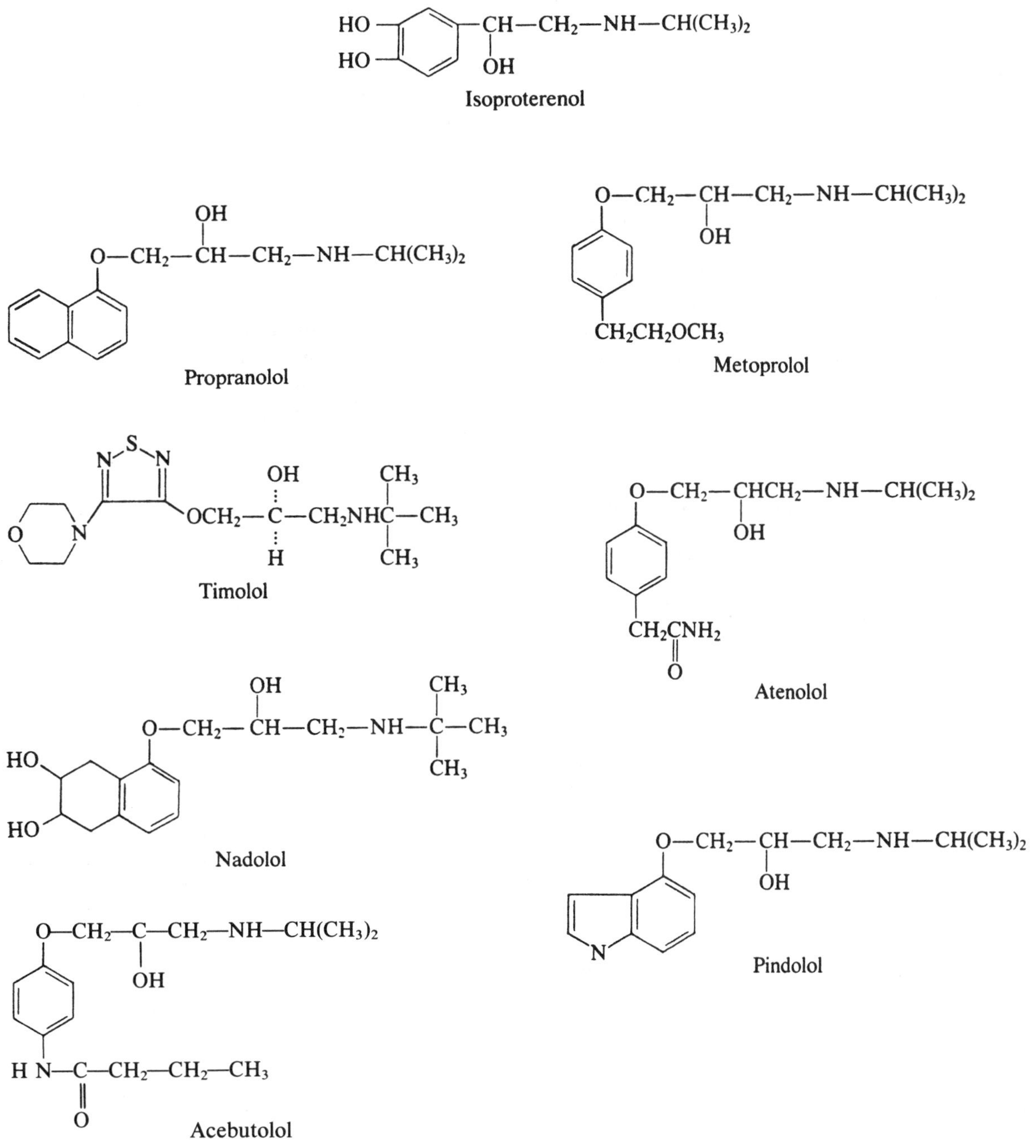

The similarity in structure to β-agonists is most certainly responsible for the finding that some β-blockers activate β-receptors; that is, they have some intrinsic agonistic activity. The intrinsic activity of these compounds is generally modest in comparison to an agonist such as isoproterenol, and they are generally referred to as *partial agonists* (see Chap. 2). The clinically important β-blockers are either devoid of or have only slight intrinsic activity.

Mechanism of Action

All the β-blockers exert an equilibrium-competitive antagonism of the actions of catecholamines and other adrenomimetics at β-receptors. β-blockers are more selective than α-blockers in terms of blocking nonadrenergic receptors. This does not mean that β-blockers are devoid of other effects, however. Probably the best recognized non-β-receptor-mediated action of these compounds is a depression of cellular membrane excitability. This effect has been described as a membrane-stabilizing action, a quinidinelike effect, or a local anesthetic effect. This action is not too surprising in view of the structural similarities that exist between β-blockers and local anesthetics.

While several β-receptor blocking agents do depress membrane excitability, the importance of this effect to the overall pharmacological actions of this class of compounds has been over-emphasized. With the usual thera-

peutic doses, the actions of the β-receptor blocking agents appear to be almost entirely accounted for by their β-receptor antagonism. This is particularly true of the antiarrhythmic properties of these compounds. Several observations support this notion. First, propranolol has antiarrhythmic activity at concentrations considerably lower than those necessary to depress membrane excitability. And, second, the d isomer of propranolol, which has membrane-stabilizing activity, but virtually no β-blocking activity, is not an effective antiarrhythmic. It is possible that some β-blockers, such as sotalol, have a component of their action, in addition to β-antagonism and membrane stabilizing activity, that contributes to their overall antiarrhythmic effectiveness.

Because the β-receptors of the heart are β_1 and those in the pulmonary and vascular smooth muscle are β_2, β_1-selective antagonists are frequently referred to as *cardioselective blockers*. The intrinsic activity, cardioselectivity, and membrane-stabilizing actions of a number of β-blockers are summarized in Table 13-2.

Pharmacological Actions

A number of physiological responses to sympathetic nerve stimulation and to adrenomimetic drugs are mediated by β-receptors (see Chap. 12). A knowledge of these β-mediated responses is essential to the appreciation of the

Table 13-2. Characteristics and Preparations of β-Blockers

β-Blocker	Cardioselective	Partial agonist activity	Membrane stabilizing activity	Trade name(s)	Preparations available
Propranolol	No	None	Yes	Inderal	Oral: 10-, 20-, 40-, 60-, 80-, 90-mg tablets; 80-, 120-, 160-mg time release capsules Intravenous: 1-mg/ml vials
Acebutolol	Yes	Slight	None	Sectral	Oral: 200-, 400-mg capsules
Atenolol	Yes	None	None	Tenormin	Oral: 50-, 100-mg tablets
Betaxolol	Yes	None	Slight	Betoptic Kerlone	Oral: 10-, 20-mg tablets Ophthalmic: 0.25% drops
Carteolol	No	Slight	None	Cartrol	Oral: 2.5-, 5.0-mg tablets
Esmolol	Yes	None	None	Brevibloc	Intravenous: 10 mg/ml for injection; 2.5-g ampules for dilution to 10 mg/ml for IV infusion
Levobunolol	No	None	None	Betagan Liquifilm	Ophthalmic: 0.5% drops
Metoprolol	Yes	None	Slight	Betaloc Lopressor	Oral: 50-, 100-mg tablets Intravenous: 1-mg/ml vials
Nadolol	No	None	None	Corgard	Oral: 20-, 40-, 80-, 120-, 160-mg tablets
Penbutolol	No	Slight	None	Levatol	Oral: 20-mg tablets
Pindolol	No	Yes	Slight	Visken	Oral: 5-, 10-mg, tablets
Timolol	No	Slight	None	Timoptic Blocadren	Oral: 5-, 10-, 20-mg tablets Ophthalmic: 0.25, 0.5% drops

pharmacology of the β-receptor blocking agents. Probably the most important actions of the β-blocking drugs are on the cardiovascular system. *β-Blockers decrease heart rate, myocardial contractility, cardiac output, and conduction velocity within the heart.* These effects are most pronounced when sympathetic activity is high or when the heart is stimulated by circulating agonists.

The actions of β-blockers on blood pressure are complex. After acute administration, blood pressure is only slightly altered. This occurs because of the compensatory reflex increase in peripheral vascular resistance that results from a β-blocker–induced decrease in cardiac output. It should be remembered that vasoconstriction is mediated by α-receptors, and α-receptors are not antagonized by β-receptor blocking agents. Chronic administration of β-blockers, however, results in a reduction of blood pressure, and this is the reason for their use in primary hypertension (see Chap. 22). The mechanism of this effect is not well understood, but may include such actions as a reduction in renin release, an antagonism of β-receptors in the central nervous system, or an antagonism of presynaptic facilitory β-receptors on sympathetic nerves.

Plasma volume and venous return to the heart tend to be reduced during treatment with β-blockers. This is presumably due to the unopposed stimulatory effects of catecholamines on vascular α-receptors. Postural hypotension is not a prominent feature of β-blockade.

Total coronary blood flow is reduced by the β-blockers. This effect may be due in part to the unopposed α-receptor–mediated vasoconstriction that follows β-receptor blockade in the coronary arteries. Additional contributing factors to the decrease in coronary blood flow are the negative chronotropic and inotropic effects produced by the β-blockers; this results in a decrease in the amount of blood available for the coronary system. The decrease in mean blood pressure may also contribute to the reduced coronary blood flow.

In view of the effects the β-receptor blocking agents have on coronary blood flow, it seems somewhat paradoxical that these drugs are useful for the prophylactic treatment of *angina pectoris,* a condition characterized by inadequate myocardial perfusion. The chief benefit of the β-blockers in this condition derives from their ability to decrease cardiac work and oxygen demands. The use of the β-blockers in angina is considered in Chap. 25.

The release of renin from the juxtaglomerular cells of the kidney is believed to be regulated in part by β-receptors; most β-blockers decrease renin release. While the drug-induced decrease in renin release may contribute to their hypotensive actions, it is probably not the only factor (see Chap. 22). Nevertheless, β-blockers are useful and logical agents to use when treating hypertension that is accompanied by high plasma renin activity.

The glycogenolytic and lipolytic actions of endogenous catecholamines are mediated by β-receptors and are subject to blockade by β-blockers. This metabolic antagonism exerted by the β-blockers is particularly pronounced if the levels of circulating catecholamines have been increased reflexly in response to hypoglycemia. Additionally, other physiological changes induced by hypoglycemia, such as tachycardia, may be blunted by β-blockers. These agents, therefore, must be used with caution in patients susceptible to hypoglycemia (e.g., diabetics treated with insulin). Because the metabolic responses to catecholamines are mediated by β_2-receptors, and possibly by β_3-receptors, β_1-selective antagonists such as metoprolol and atenolol may be better choices whenever β-blocker therapy is indicated for a patient who has hypoglycemia.

Propranolol increases airway resistance by antagonizing β_2-receptor–mediated bronchodilation. Although the resulting bronchoconstriction is not of great concern in patients with normal lung function, it can be quite serious in the asthmatic. *The cardioselective β-blockers produce less bronchoconstriction than do the nonselective antagonists.*

A recently discovered action of the β-blockers is their ability to reduce intraocular pressure in open-angle glaucoma and ocular hypertension. The mechanism by which these drugs decrease intraocular pressure is not fully understood, but it is believed to be related to a decreased production of aqueous humor. Timolol was the first β-blocker to be approved for the treatment of glaucoma. Other β-blockers that are used include levobunolol and betaxolol.

Absorption, Metabolism, and Excretion

Propranolol

Propranolol is suitable for both parenteral and oral administration. Absorption from the gastrointestinal tract is extensive. The peak therapeutic effect after oral administration occurs in 1 to 1.5 hr. The plasma half-life of propranolol is approximately 3 hr. The drug is concentrated in the lungs and, to a lesser extent, in the liver, brain, kidneys, and heart. Binding to plasma proteins is extensive.

The liver is the chief organ involved in the metabolism of propranolol, and the drug is subject to a significant degree of first-pass metabolism. Although the metabolic fate of propranolol has not been completely elucidated, at least eight metabolites have been recovered from the urine, the major excretory route, and one of these, 4-hydroxypropranolol, also exhibits a considerable degree of β-blocking activity.

Metoprolol

The pharmacokinetic profile of metoprolol is similar to that of propranolol. Metoprolol is readily and rapidly absorbed after oral administration and is subject to a significant amount of first-pass metabolism by the liver. Curiously, the duration of metoprolol's action is longer than one would predict from its plasma half-life, which ranges from 0.5 to 2.5 hr.

The degree of binding of metoprolol to plasma proteins is modest (10%) in comparison to that of propranolol (90%). The extensive distribution of metoprolol to the lungs and kidney is typical of a moderately lipophilic drug. Metoprolol undergoes considerable metabolism; only 3 to 10 percent of an administered dose is recovered as unchanged drug. The metabolites are essentially inactive as β-receptor blocking agents and are eliminated primarily by renal excretion. Small amounts of the drug are present in the feces.

Timolol

Timolol is almost completely absorbed from the gastrointestinal tract. Peak plasma levels occur 2 to 4 hr after oral administration; the plasma half-life of timolol is around 5.5 hr. The extensive tissue distribution of timolol into lung, liver, and kidney is similar to that of other β-blockers. Approximately 70 percent of the drug is excreted in the urine within 24 hr, mostly as highly polar, unconjugated metabolites. Only 6 percent of an administered dose is recovered in the feces.

Although timolol is approved for the *topical* treatment of elevated intraocular pressure, there is limited information about its pharmacokinetics following administration by this route. The drug apparently can reach the systemic circulation after intraocular instillation, but plasma levels are only about 7 percent of those achieved in the aqueous humor.

Acebutolol

About one half of an orally administered dose of acebutolol is absorbed. Approximately 25 percent of the drug is bound to plasma proteins, and the plasma half-life of acebutolol is about 4 hr. Metabolism of acebutolol produces a metabolite with β-blocking activity whose half-life is 10 hr.

Atenolol

Roughly one half of an orally administered dose of atenolol is absorbed. The drug is eliminated primarily by the kidney and, unlike propranolol, undergoes little hepatic metabolism. Its plasma half-life is approximately 6 hr, although if administered to a patient with impaired renal function, its half-life can be considerably prolonged.

Betaxolol

Absorption of an oral dose of betaxolol is almost complete. The drug is subject to a slight first-pass effect so that the absolute bioavailability of the drug is about 90 percent. As with many β-blockers, betaxolol binds to plasma proteins to the extent of about 50 percent. The plasma half-life of betaxolol is fairly long, approaching about 20 hr, and the drug is suitable for dosing once per day. The primary route of metabolism is by the liver, with only 15 percent of unchanged drug being excreted.

Carteolol

Carteolol is a long-acting β-blocker that is suitable for once-per-day dosing. It is almost completely absorbed and exhibits about 30 percent binding to plasma proteins. Unlike many β-blockers, carteolol is not extensively metabolized. Up to 70 percent of an administered dose is excreted unchanged.

Esmolol

This β-blocker is unusual in that it is very rapidly metabolized; its plasma half-life is only 9 min. This compound has an ester linkage in the alkyl side chain and is subject to hydrolysis by cytosolic esterases in red blood cells, which yields methanol and an acid metabolite, the latter having an elimination half-life of about 4 hr. Only 2 percent of the administered esmolol is excreted unchanged. Because of its rapid onset and short duration of action, esmolol is used by the intravenous route for the control of ventricular arrhythmias in emergency situations.

Nadolol

Nadolol is rather slowly and incompletely absorbed from the gastrointestinal tract. It is estimated that only 30 percent of an orally administered dose is absorbed. Appreciable metabolism does not seem to occur; the drug is excreted primarily unchanged in the urine and feces. The plasma half-life is quite long, approaching 24 hr, thus permitting dosing once per day.

Pindolol

Like propranolol, pindolol is extensively absorbed from the gastrointestinal tract. First-pass metabolism is estimated at about 15 percent. The plasma half-life of pindolol is also similar to that of propranolol, being on the order of 3 to 4 hr. The binding of pindolol to plasma proteins is approximately 50 percent. The metabolic fate of pindolol is not completely understood, although 50 percent of an administered dose is recovered primarily in the urine, as unchanged drug.

Clinical Uses of β-Blockers

The β-receptor blocking agents have widespread and important uses in the management of cardiac arrhythmias, angina pectoris, and hypertension. Their uses in these conditions are reviewed in Chaps. 26, 25, and 22, respectively. Other therapeutic applications of the β-blockers are discussed below.

Hyperthyroidism

The β-blockers have been shown to reduce significantly the peripheral manifestations of hyperthyroidism, particularly the elevated heart rate, increased cardiac output, and muscle tremors. Although the β-blockers can improve the clinical status of the hyperthyroid patient, it must be remembered that the patient remains "biochemically" hyperthyroid. The β-blockers should not be used as the sole form of therapy in hyperthyroidism. They are most logically employed in the management of hyperthyroid crisis, in the preoperative preparation for thyroidectomy, and during the initial period of administration of specific antithyroid drugs (also see Chap. 69).

Glaucoma

β-Blockers can be used topically to reduce intraocular pressure in patients with chronic open-angle glaucoma and ocular hypertension. The mechanism by which ocular pressure is reduced appears to depend on a decreased production of aqueous humor. Timolol was the first β-blocker approved for this use. Timolol has a somewhat greater ocular hypotensive effect than do the currently available cholinomimetic or adrenomimetic drugs. The effectiveness and safety of the β-blockers for the treatment of acute angle-closure glaucoma have not been established.

Anxiety States

Patients with anxiety experience a variety of psychic and somatic symptoms. The peripheral manifestations of anxiety may include a number of symptoms (e.g., palpitations) that are due in part to overactivity of the sympathetic nervous system. The β-blocking agents may be of some benefit in the treatment of anxiety because they reduce the intensity of these sympathetically induced symptoms and also provide relief of such somatic symptoms of anxiety as tremor and diarrhea.

Migraine

The value of the β-blockers in the treatment of migraine headache was discovered serendipitously when it was observed that patients being treated with β-blockers for various cardiovascular diseases experienced relief from migraine headaches. The mechanism of this antimigraine effect is not completely understood, but is thought to involve a blockade of craniovascular β-receptors that results in reduced vasodilation. The painful phase of a migraine attack is believed to be produced by vasodilation. The β-blockers are currently being employed in the prophylactic treatment of migraine, particularly when control of these attacks is difficult to achieve by other measures.

Adverse Reactions

The most prominent side effects associated with the administration of the β-blockers are those directly attributable to their ability to block β-receptors. Although the decreased heart rate and decreased cardiac output induced by these drugs may not be troublesome in patients with adequate cardiac reserve, they can be life threatening for a patient suffering from congestive heart failure. *Patients exhibiting frank signs of cardiac failure should not be treated with β-blockers.* Additionally, because conduction of impulses in the heart may be slowed by β-blockers, patients with conduction disturbances, particularly through the atrioventricular (A-V) node, should not be treated with β-blockers.

Caution must be exercised in the use of β-blockers in obstructive airway disease since these drugs promote further bronchoconstriction. Cardioselective β-blockers have less propensity to aggravate bronchoconstriction than do nonselective β-blockers.

β-Blockers have been shown to potentiate hypoglycemia by antagonizing catecholamine-induced mobilization of glycogen. The use of β-blockers in hypoglycemic patients is, therefore, dangerous and must be undertaken with caution. If β-blocker therapy is required, a cardioselective β-blocker is preferred.

Whenever β-blocker therapy is employed, the period of greatest danger for asthmatics or insulin-dependent diabetics is during the initial period of drug administration, since the greatest disruption of the existing autonomic balance will occur at this time. If marked toxicity does not occur during this period, further doses are less likely to cause problems.

The β-blockers produce a number of central effects, although it is not clear whether these effects are due to blockade of central β-receptors. After high doses, patients may experience hallucinations, nightmares, insomnia, and depression.

The topical application of timolol to the eye is also well tolerated. The incidence of side effects, which consist of burning or dryness of the eyes, is reported to be 5 to 10 percent.

In spite of the potential seriousness of some of their side effects, β-blockers as a class are well tolerated and patient compliance is good.

Preparations and Dosage

Information about preparations and dosage for the prototype nonselective β-blocker, propranolol; the β_1-selective agent, metoprolol; and the ophthalmic drug, timolol, is given below. Information about these and other available preparations of β-blockers is summarized in Table 13-2.

Propranolol hydrochloride (*Inderal*) is available as tablets and in 1-ml ampules (1 mg/ml) for IV use. A sustained-release formulation of propranolol has been introduced (*Inderal LA*). The pharmacokinetics of this long-acting preparation obviously differ from those of conventional tablets; therefore, patients may need to be retitrated when preparations are switched to the long-acting formulation.

Metoprolol tartrate (*Betaloc, Lopressor*) is commercially available in tablets containing 50 or 100 mg.

Timolol maleate (*Timoptic*) is available as an ophthalmic solution (0.25% or 0.5%) for topical application to the eye.

Drugs with Combined β- and α-Blocking Activity

Labetalol

Labetalol possesses both β-blocking and α-blocking activity, and is approximately one-third as potent as propranolol as a β-blocker and one-tenth as potent as phentolamine as an α-blocker. The ratio of β/α activity is about 3:1 when labetalol is administered orally and about 7:1 when it is administered intravenously. Thus, the drug can be most conveniently thought of as a β-blocker with some α-blocking properties.

Mechanism of Action

Labetalol produces an *equilibrium-competitive antagonism* at β-receptors. The drug does not exhibit selectivity for β_1- or β_2-receptors. Like certain other β-blockers (e.g., pindolol and timolol), labetalol possesses some degree of intrinsic activity. This intrinsic activity, or partial agon-

ism, especially at β_2-receptors in the vasculature, has been suggested to contribute to the vasodilator effect of the drug. The membrane-stabilizing effect, or local anesthetic action, possessed by propranolol and several other β-blockers is also possessed by labetalol and, in fact, the drug is a reasonably potent local anesthetic.

The α-blockade produced by labetalol is also of the equilibrium-competitive type. In a manner similar to prazosin, labetalol exhibits selectivity for α_1-receptors. Presynaptic α-receptors, which are of the α_2 subclass, are not antagonized by labetalol. The drug also has some intrinsic activity at α-receptors, although this action is less than its intrinsic β-receptor–stimulating effects.

Labetalol appears to produce relaxation of vascular smooth muscle not only by α-blockade but also by a partial agonist effect at β_2-receptors. In addition, labetalol may produce relaxation by a direct, nonreceptor-mediated effect.

In addition to receptor blockade and a possible direct effect on vascular smooth muscle, labetalol has been shown to block the neuronal uptake of norepinephrine and other catecholamines. This, plus its slight intrinsic activity at α-receptors, may account for the seemingly paradoxical, although infrequent, increase in blood pressure seen on initial administration of labetalol.

Pharmacological Actions

Although capable of antagonizing a variety of responses in a number of effectors that are mediated by both β- and α-receptors, *the most important actions of labetalol are on the cardiovascular system.* These effects may vary from individual to individual and will depend on the existing sympathetic and parasympathetic tone at the time of drug administration.

The usually observed hemodynamic effect of acutely administered labetalol in humans is a *decrease in peripheral vascular resistance and blood pressure without an appreciable alteration in heart rate or cardiac output.* This pattern differs from that seen with either a conventional β- or α-blocker. Acute administration of a β-blocker produces a decrease in heart rate and cardiac output with little effect on blood pressure, while acute administration of an α-blocker leads to a decrease in peripheral vascular resistance and a reflexly initiated increase in cardiac rate and output. Thus, the pattern of cardiovascular responses observed after labetalol administration combines the features of β- and α-blockade, that is, a decrease in peripheral vascular resistance (due to α-blockade and direct vascular effects) without an increase in cardiac rate and output (due to β-blockade).

Prolonged oral therapy with labetalol results in cardiovascular responses similar to those obtained following conventional β-blocker administration, that is, decreases in peripheral vascular resistance, blood pressure, and heart rate. Generally, however, the decrease in heart rate is less pronounced than that seen after administration of propranolol or other β-blockers.

Absorption, Metabolism, and Excretion

Labetalol is almost completely absorbed from the gastrointestinal tract. However, the drug is subject to considerable first-pass metabolism, which occurs in both the gastrointestinal tract and the liver, so that only about 25 percent of an administered dose reaches the systemic circulation. While traces of unchanged labetalol are recovered in the urine, most of the drug is metabolized to inactive glucuronide conjugates. The plasma half-life of labetalol is 6 to 8 hr, and the elimination kinetics are essentially unchanged in patients with impaired renal failure.

Clinical Uses

Labetalol is useful for the chronic treatment of primary hypertension. It can be used alone but is more often employed in combination with other antihypertensive agents. Labetalol also has been used intravenously for the treatment of hypertensive emergencies. Like conventional β-blockers, labetalol may be useful for patients with coexisting hypertension and anginal pain due to ischemia. The drug is also being investigated as a possible therapeutic modality for ischemic heart disease, even in the absence of hypertension. The benefit derives from its β-blocking activity, which serves to decrease cardiac work, as well as from its ability to decrease afterload by virtue of its α-blocking activity.

Labetalol, because it possesses both α- and β-blocking activity, is useful for the preoperative management of patients with a pheochromocytoma.

Adverse Reactions

There have been reports of excessive hypotension as well as paradoxical pressor effects following intravenous administration of labetalol. These latter effects may be due to a labetalol-induced blockade of neuronal amine uptake, thereby increasing concentrations of norepinephrine at receptors.

Approximately 5 percent of the patients who receive labetalol complain of side effects typical of noradrenergic nervous system suppression. These include postural hypotension, gastrointestinal distress, tiredness, sexual dysfunction, and "tingling" of the scalp. The majority of these effects are related to α-blockade, although the tingling of the scalp may be due to intrinsic activity at α-receptors. Side effects associated with β-blockade, such as induction of bronchospasm and congestive heart failure, may also occur, but generally at a lower frequency than α-receptor–associated effects.

Skin rashes have been reported, as has an increase in the titer of antinuclear antibodies. Despite the latter observation, the appearance of a systemic lupus syndrome is rare. Labetalol also has been reported to interfere with chemical measurements of catecholamines and metabolites.

Preparations and Dosage

Labetalol is marketed under several brand names, including *Trandate, Vescal,* and *Normodyne.* The usual starting dose for oral use is 100 mg twice per day. Maintenance therapy may require up to 800 mg per day.

Supplemental Reading

Benfield, P., and Sorkin, E.M. Esmolol: A preliminary review of its pharmacodynamic and pharmacokinetic properties, and therapeutic efficacy. *Drugs* 33:392, 1987.

Benfield, P., et al. Metoprolol. *Drugs* 31:376, 1986.

Brodde, O.-E. β₁- and β₂-adrenoceptors in the human heart: Properties, function, and alterations in chronic heart failure. *Pharmacol. Rev.* 43:203, 1991.

Harrison, J.K., et al. Molecular characterization of α₁- and α₂-adrenoceptors. *Tr. Pharmacol. Sci.* 12:62, 1991.

Limbird, L.E. *The Alpha₂ Adrenergic Receptors.* Clifton, N.J.: Humana, 1988.

Minneman, K.P. α₁-Adrenergic receptor subtypes, inositol phosphates, and sources of cell Ca²⁺. *Pharmacol. Rev.* 40:87, 1988.

Ruffolo, R.R., Jr. *The Alpha₁ Adrenergic Receptors.* Clifton, N.J.: Humana, 1987.

Ruffolo, R.R., Jr., et al. Structure and function of α-adrenoceptors. *Pharmacol. Rev.* 43:475, 1991.

van Zwieten, P.A. Antihypertensive drugs interacting with alpha- and beta-adrenoceptors: A review of basic pharmacology. *Drugs* 35:6, 1988.

14

Directly Acting Cholinomimetics

Brenda K. Colasanti

Drugs that produce end-organ responses similar to those produced by parasympathetic nerve stimulation are called *parasympathomimetics*. These agents also belong to the group of drugs known as *cholinomimetics*. They act directly at cholinergic receptor sites to produce their responses.

The cholinomimetic group of drugs (Fig. 14-1) contains additional agents that mimic the actions of acetylcholine at all cholinergic transmission sites, including some postganglionic sympathetic synapses. Thus, the cholinesterase inhibitors (see Chap. 16), which enhance the actions of endogenous acetylcholine by preserving it from enzymatic destruction, are also members of the cholinomimetic group of drugs. These agents act *indirectly* in producing their responses.

Receptor sites for acetylcholine released by nerve stimulation are discussed in detail in Chap. 11. It will be recalled that, since the receptors receiving input from postganglionic parasympathetic fibers are *muscarinic,* the actions of acetylcholine at these receptor sites (localized in smooth muscle, cardiac muscle, and most exocrine glands) are blocked by atropine. Muscarinic receptors are also present in the sweat glands, in the blood vessels of the major vascular beds, and at cortical and subcortical sites within the central nervous system. On the other hand, because the receptors with cholinergic input from preganglionic fibers and from somatic motor nerves are *nicotinic,* the actions of acetylcholine at these target organs (postganglionic sympathetic and parasympathetic neurons, the adrenal medulla, and skeletal muscle) are not blocked by atropine.

While the individual directly acting cholinomimetics that are used clinically possess varying degrees of muscarinic and nicotinic activity, the effects of all these agents, when they are administered in the usual therapeutic doses, are exclusively muscarinic. The pharmacological actions of the individual drugs differ primarily in the relative selectivity of each for a particular organ system. The directly acting cholinomimetics have traditionally been di-

vided into two main groups: the *choline esters* and the naturally occurring and synthetic *alkaloids*.

Choline Esters

Slight modifications of the structure of the acetylcholine molecule have led to the development of three clinically utilized choline esters: acetyl-β-methylcholine (methacholine), carbamylcholine (carbachol), and bethanechol (Fig. 14-2). These three compounds combine with cholinergic receptors in the same manner as does acetylcholine. Each has a cationic quaternary ammonium group for attachment at one site on the receptor. This structural feature is essential for the manifestation of both muscarinic and nicotinic activity of choline esters. Similarly, each agent has a two-carbon chain between the cationic head and the ester oxygen, allowing attachment of the latter at a second site on the receptor. Addition of a methyl group to the carbon adjacent to the ester oxygen, as in the case of methacholine and bethanechol, markedly reduces the susceptibility of the compound to enzymatic actions of cholinesterases. This structural change also markedly reduces nicotinic activity. Substitution of an amine group for the terminal methyl group of acetylcholine, as in the case of carbachol and bethanechol, renders the compound completely *resistant to hydrolysis* by any of the cholinesterases.

A primary therapeutic advantage afforded by the above structural modifications of the acetylcholine molecule resides in the resistance of these modified compounds to enzymatic destruction by cholinesterase. This property endows the analogues of acetylcholine with a much *longer duration of action* than that of the parent compound. The structural changes also confer greater selectivity for muscarinic sites.

The primary pharmacological actions of the choline esters are summarized in Table 14-1. Additional musca-

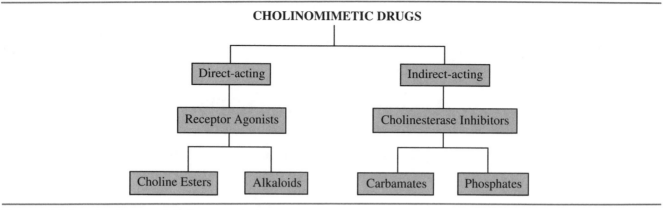

Figure 14-1. Classification of cholinomimetic drugs.

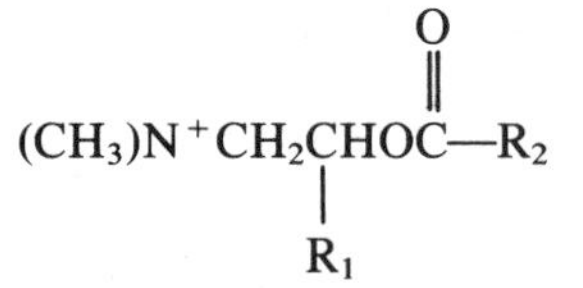

$$(CH_3)N^+CH_2CHOC\overset{\overset{\displaystyle O}{\parallel}}{—}R_2$$
$$\underset{R_1}{|}$$

	R_1	R_2
Acetylcholine	H	CH_3
Carbachol	H	NH_2
Bethanechol	CH_3	NH_2
Methacholine	CH_3	CH_3

Figure 14-2. Chemical structures of the choline esters currently in clinical use.

rinic effects of these agents in other organ systems are summarized in Table 14-2.

Acetylcholine

Pharmacological Actions

In order to obtain any systemic pharmacological effects from exogenously administered acetylcholine, it must be injected intravenously. Even after administration by this route, the effects are short lived because of the rapid destruction of acetylcholine by cholinesterases.

After intravenous administration, the muscarinic effects of acetylcholine predominate. The most prominent effects are exerted on the cardiovascular system. Low doses of acetylcholine produce vasodilation within the major vascular beds and thus a fall in peripheral resistance. Both systolic and diastolic blood pressure are subsequently lowered. Reflex activation of sympathetic activity by pressor-receptor mechanisms results in tachycardia.

In *higher doses,* acetylcholine additionally exerts a direct depressant effect on the heart, and this overrides the reflex effect. Heart rate is decreased by a reduction in the rate of diastolic depolarization at the sinoatrial (S-A) node, and the rate of conduction of action potentials through the atrial fibers to the atrioventricular (A-V) node is reduced. A-V conductivity is decreased, and there is also a decrease in the force of contraction of both atrial and ventricular muscle. Acetylcholine released by nerve stimulation has no effect on the ventricle only because this region has no cholinergic innervation.

The remaining muscarinic actions of injected acetylcholine on autonomic effector organs resemble those produced by postganglionic parasympathetic stimulation. At *moderate doses,* acetylcholine causes bronchial constriction and an increase in secretion. Thus, asthmalike attacks may be precipitated. Acetylcholine also stimulates the lacrimal, salivary, and sweat glands. Diaphoresis is profuse because acetylcholine's direct effect on the sweat gland is augmented by cutaneous vasodilation. Other prominent muscarinic effects seen after injection of moderate doses of this choline ester include urinary bladder contraction and decreased bladder capacity.

At *higher doses,* injected acetylcholine exerts stimulatory effects on the gastrointestinal tract. The resting tone of gastrointestinal smooth muscle and the force of contractions are both increased. The enhancement of contractile activity and gastric secretion may be accompanied by nausea and vomiting.

Acetylcholine administered intravenously has no effect on the iris, because this quaternary ammonium ion does not pass the blood–aqueous humor barrier. After direct local application within the eye, however, acetylcholine causes a transient miosis by acting at muscarinic receptors of the iris sphincter.

The nicotinic effects of acetylcholine cannot ordinarily be seen. Because acetylcholine is a quaternary ammonium

Table 14-1. Pharmacological Actions of Choline Esters

Pharmacological activity	Acetylcholine	Methacholine	Carbachol	Bethanechol
Muscarinic				
Cardiovascular (bradycardia, vasodilation)	+ +	+ +	+	+
Gastrointestinal (increased motility)	+ +	+ +	+ + +	+ + +
Urinary (contraction)	+ +	+ +	+ + +	+ + +
Nicotinic	+ +	−	+ + +	−

Key: − = no effect; + = activity. The number of symbols indicates the relative magnitude of the response.

Table 14-2. Miscellaneous Muscarinic Effects of Choline Esters

Organ	Effect
Eye	
Iris sphincter	Miosis
Ciliary muscle	Accommodation
Lung	
Bronchial muscle	Bronchoconstriction
Bronchial glands	Secretion
Glands	
Lacrimal	Secretion
Salivary	Secretion
Sweat	Secretion

ion, it is distributed primarily in extracellular spaces and does not readily penetrate the layers of fat surrounding skeletal muscle and autonomic ganglia. Doses of acetylcholine sufficient to ensure reaching most of the nicotinic receptors would probably result in death from excessive muscarinic stimulation.

If the muscarinic effects of acetylcholine are blocked by prior administration of atropine, the nicotinic effects of large doses can be seen. Following atropine pretreatment, acetylcholine can stimulate nicotinic receptors both in sympathetic and in parasympathetic ganglia. However, stimulation of the parasympathetic ganglia produces no end-organ response, even though acetylcholine release from the postganglionic parasympathetic nerves does occur, because the muscarinic receptors are blocked by atropine.

In contrast, stimulation of the nicotinic receptors in most *sympathetic* ganglia will result in a change in effector organ activity, since atropine cannot block the effects of the norepinephrine that is released from most postganglionic sympathetic nerve fibers. Actions of acetylcholine at nicotinic sites in the adrenal medulla result in the release of catecholamines from this organ.

Thus, the net effect of nicotinic stimulation in the presence of muscarinic blockade is massive sympathetic activity. The blood vessels become constricted, and blood pressure rapidly increases. Heart rate and force of contraction are increased. Norepinephrine, acting in the gastrointestinal tract, causes a decrease in gastrointestinal motility. Bronchodilation and pupillary dilation are also seen. An additional nicotinic action of high doses of acetylcholine is stimulation of skeletal muscle.

Clinical Uses

Because of its extremely short duration of action, acetylcholine has only one therapeutic application. Acetylcholine chloride (*Miochol*) is used during ophthalmic surgery, most frequently to obtain rapid and complete miosis during cataract removal. This agent is also occasionally employed during other surgical procedures within the anterior portion of the eye when immediate miosis is required.

Methacholine

Pharmacological Actions

With regard to muscarinic effects, the pharmacological spectrum of activity of methacholine is essentially identical to that of acetylcholine; however, because methacholine is highly *resistant* to enzymatic destruction by cholinesterases, cardiac arrest after intravenous administration of this agent will last longer and is therefore more likely to be lethal. In contrast to acetylcholine, methacholine exerts essentially no nicotinic activity.

Absorption of methacholine from the gastrointestinal tract is quite poor and irregular. Subcutaneous administration, the preferred route, offers two advantages. Absorption is slow, and therefore the drug's duration of action is prolonged. In addition, if toxicity develops, absorption can be stopped by application of a tourniquet.

Clinical Uses

Methacholine retains usefulness as a *diagnostic tool*. In cases of suspected poisoning due to belladonna alkaloids, the diagnosis is confirmed by failure of 10 to 30 mg methacholine, given SC, to elicit characteristic signs of flush, sweating, salivation, lacrimation, and enhanced gastrointestinal motility. In the diagnosis of familial dysautonomia, a disease characterized by degeneration of the autonomic nerves, a dose of methacholine that produces no change in pupil size in normal individuals will result in a significant degree of miosis in patients with dysautonomia.

Carbachol

Pharmacological Actions

The *nicotinic effects* of carbachol are greater than those of acetylcholine. At doses within the therapeutic range, this agent stimulates autonomic ganglia, the adrenal medulla, and skeletal muscle.

In contrast to methacholine, the *muscarinic effects* of carbachol differ quantitatively from those of acetylcholine. Carbachol produces more prominent actions on the gastrointestinal tract, the urinary bladder, and the iris than does acetylcholine. On the other hand, this choline ester affects the cardiovascular system less conspicuously than does acetylcholine or methacholine, although excessive doses of carbachol can lead to cardiac arrest. The muscarinic effects of carbachol are more resistant to blockade by atropine than are those of acetylcholine. Higher doses of atropine are thus required to counteract these actions.

It is now recognized that there are several subtypes of muscarinic cholinergic receptors, and that the relative proportion of each receptor subtype in a given tissue may vary (see Chap. 15). This finding may, in part, explain the quantitative differences seen in the actions of the individual choline esters since each ester may activate slightly different subgroups of muscarinic receptors.

Clinical Uses

Carbachol ophthalmic solution (*Isopto Carbachol*) is used to lower intraocular pressure in the treatment of glaucoma. The drug is applied locally to the eye. Carbachol is also used to produce miosis on intraocular application to the iris during eye surgery.

Bethanechol

Combining the structural changes in the acetylcholine molecule that gave rise to methacholine (i.e., a methyl substitution) and carbachol (i.e., an amine substitution) has resulted in the synthesis of bethanechol (see Fig. 14-1). The pharmacological spectrum of activity of this choline ester thus embraces properties unique to each of the above two analogues of acetylcholine.

Pharmacological Actions

The muscarinic effects of bethanechol resemble those of carbachol. Thus, bethanechol acts more selectively on the gastrointestinal tract and the urinary bladder than does acetylcholine. The cardiovascular effects of this agent are very slight at moderate doses. Like methacholine, bethanechol is virtually devoid of nicotinic activity.

Absorption and Metabolism

Bethanechol is completely resistant to breakdown by cholinesterases and is readily absorbed after oral administration. Absorption from the subcutaneous route is also quite good. The drug should not be administered by other parenteral routes.

Clinical Uses

The primary therapeutic indication for bethanechol (*Urecholine, Myotonachol*) is in the treatment of urinary retention, both that occurring postoperatively and that of neurogenic origin.

Adverse Reactions

Adverse effects occurring during therapy with bethanechol are direct extensions of its pharmacological actions. Flushing, sweating, epigastric distress, abdominal cramps, and salivation may be observed after therapeutic doses. While untoward cardiovascular effects are rarely seen at such doses, overdose with this agent may produce symptoms culminating in cardiac arrest.

Contraindications

Bethanechol is contraindicated in peptic ulcer and in cases in which the strength or integrity of the gastrointestinal wall is in question. Patients with asthma or coronary insufficiency should not be treated with bethanechol because of the obvious potential for aggravation of these conditions. In addition, bethanechol is contraindicated in patients with hyperthyroidism, because of the potential for precipitation of atrial fibrillation.

Caution should be exercised when bethanechol is administered concomitantly with several other drugs. Quinidine and procainamide may antagonize the effects of bethanechol. In patients being treated with ganglionic blocking agents (see Chap. 17), bethanechol may initially cause severe abdominal symptoms and may subsequently precipitate a critical fall in blood pressure. Use of bethanechol in patients maintained on drugs that deplete brain serotonin should be avoided because such a drug combination can result in a profound hypothermia.

Naturally Occurring Alkaloids and Synthetic Analogues

Several naturally occurring alkaloids and their synthetic analogues can produce parasympathomimetic activity of clinical importance. Although these compounds, which include muscarine, pilocarpine, and oxotremorine, are structurally more complex than the choline esters, nevertheless the distance between the presumed active portions of the molecule of each of these agents is similar to that in acetylcholine. This allows similar attachment to the cholinergic receptor. Muscarine is a quaternary ammonium compound. Pilocarpine and oxotremorine, on the other hand, are both tertiary amines.

The alkaloids produce muscarinic activity qualitatively similar to that of the choline esters (see Tables 14-1 and 14-2). In addition, they produce muscarinic effects within the central nervous system.

Muscarine

The naturally occurring substance that historically provided the basis for classification of muscarinic receptors is the alkaloid *muscarine.* This compound is essentially devoid of nicotinic activity. It has considerable clinical significance because it is the agent responsible for poisoning after ingestion of several species of mushrooms. Although the mushroom *Amanita muscaria,* the original source of muscarine, has a low content of the alkaloid, various species of *Inocybe* contain much higher concentrations.

Muscarine is well absorbed from the gastrointestinal tract and is approximately 100 times more potent than acetylcholine. Because it is not an ester, muscarine is not enzymatically destroyed by cholinesterases, and its duration of action is thus prolonged. Poisoning by muscarine is treated effectively by administration of atropine.

Unlike the highly water-soluble choline esters, muscarine crosses the blood-brain barrier and produces cortical arousal. This is a muscarinic response, as it is blocked by atropine.

Pilocarpine

Pharmacological Actions

The leaves of a species of South American shrub (*Pilocarpus jaborandi*) are the natural source of pilocarpine. This alkaloid exerts predominantly muscarinic effects, which are qualitatively similar to those of acetylcholine. The effects of pilocarpine on the sweat glands and salivary glands are prominent. Action within the eye produces miosis. Pilocarpine also has a marked ability to increase gastric secretion, and these secretions contain a high concentration of pepsin. Its effects on the cardiovascular system are less prominent than those of acetylcholine.

Like muscarine, pilocarpine also produces a cortical activation response.

Clinical Uses

The sole therapeutic use of pilocarpine (*Isopto carpine, Pilocar*) is in lowering intraocular pressure in the treatment of glaucoma.

Oxotremorine

Oxotremorine is a synthetic alkaloid that is of interest primarily because of its effects on the central nervous system. This agent exerts classic muscarinic effects in the periphery and is quite potent in this regard. Like other cholinomimetics that pass the blood-brain barrier, oxotremorine produces a cortical arousal response. In addition, it produces tremor, ataxia, and spasticity, symptoms similar to those seen in cases of parkinsonism. Oxotremorine has become very useful as a research tool in experimental studies aimed at the development of more effective antiparkinsonian drugs.

Supplemental Reading

Aquilonius, S.-M., and Gillberg, P.-G. (eds.). Cholinergic neurotransmission: Functional and clinical aspects. Proceedings of Nebel Symposium 76. *Progr. Brain Res.* 84, 1990.

Kumar, V., and Calache, M. Treatment of Alzheimer's disease with cholinergic drugs. *Int. J. Clin. Pharmacol. Ther. Toxicol.* 29:23, 1991.

McKinney, M., and Coyle, J.T. The potential for muscarinic receptor subtype-specific pharmacotherapy for Alzheimer's disease. *Mayo Clin. Proc.* 66:1225, 1991.

Palacios, J.M., Boddeke, H.W., and Pombo-Villar, E. Cholinergic neuropharmacology: An update. *Acta Psychiatr. Scand.* 366(Suppl.):27, 1991.

Ruoff, H.-J., et al. Gastrointestinal receptors and drugs in motility disorders. *Digestion* 48:1, 1991.

15

Muscarinic Blocking Drugs

Donald B. Hoover

Muscarinic blocking drugs are compounds that selectively antagonize the muscarinic receptor–mediated responses to acetylcholine (ACh) and other parasympathomimetics. These agents are also referred to as *muscarinic antagonists, antimuscarinic drugs, and anticholinergics.* The belladonna alkaloids, such as atropine, are the oldest known muscarinic blocking compounds, and their medicinal use preceded the concept of neurochemical transmission. Today, we have a vast number of natural and synthetic muscarinic blocking agents, most of which have actions very similar to those of atropine.

Muscarinic receptors are found at many sites in the peripheral and central nervous systems. They mediate the response to ACh at tissues receiving a postganglionic parasympathetic innervation (e.g., heart and bronchi) and at tissues innervated by postganglionic cholinergic fibers of the sympathetic nervous system (e.g., sweat glands). Muscarinic receptors in the brain are associated with cholinergic synapses in the cerebral cortex, limbic system (e.g., hippocampus and amygdala), striatum, and several other locations.

Although cholinergic nerves are absent in much of the vascular system, muscarinic receptors are present on the vascular endothelium. Binding of muscarinic agonists to these receptors causes the release of *endothelium-derived relaxing factor* (EDRF). The latter substance mediates the vasodilation that is produced by muscarinic agonists.

Pharmacological and molecular studies have established the existence of multiple subtypes of the muscarinic ACh receptor. Major evidence for muscarinic receptor subtypes resulted from pharmacological experiments with the muscarinic antagonist, pirenzepine. This drug is structurally distinct from atropine and, unlike atropine, has a higher affinity for muscarinic receptors in neuronal tissue than those in heart and smooth muscle. Pharmacological experiments with pirenzepine and other new muscarinic antagonists have led to the classification of muscarinic receptors as M_1, M_2, and M_3 (Fig. 15-1). It is anticipated that five subtypes will eventually be defined since molecular cloning studies have identified this number of muscarinic receptor genes. The obvious advantage of a selective antagonist is that it would more discretely affect cholinergic neurotransmission and thereby produce less adverse effects. However, the muscarinic antagonists currently marketed in the United States are not subtype selective and often differ in their pharmacokinetic properties and potency.

Chemistry

The best known of the muscarinic blocking drugs are the belladonna alkaloids, atropine and scopolamine (Fig. 15-2). They are both tertiary amines and contain an ester linkage. Atropine is the name applied to the racemic mixture *dl*-tropyl-tropate (*dl*-hyoscyamine). Scopolamine is the *l* isomer of tropyl-scopate (*l*-hyoscine). In both cases, the pharmacologically active isomer is levorotatory.

Numerous compounds with antimuscarinic activity have been synthesized and are currently on the market. Some are structurally related to the belladonna alkaloids, possessing the tropine or scopine moiety (e.g., ipratropium, Fig. 15-2), while others have chemically distinct structures (e.g., propantheline, Fig. 15-2). All of these antimuscarinic compounds have a tertiary or quaternary amine group and one or more large functional groups.

Mechanism of Action

Antimuscarinic drugs exert their effects through competitive antagonism of ACh binding to muscarinic receptors. These receptors appear to possess three separate regions capable of binding ACh. Two of these receptor sites interact with

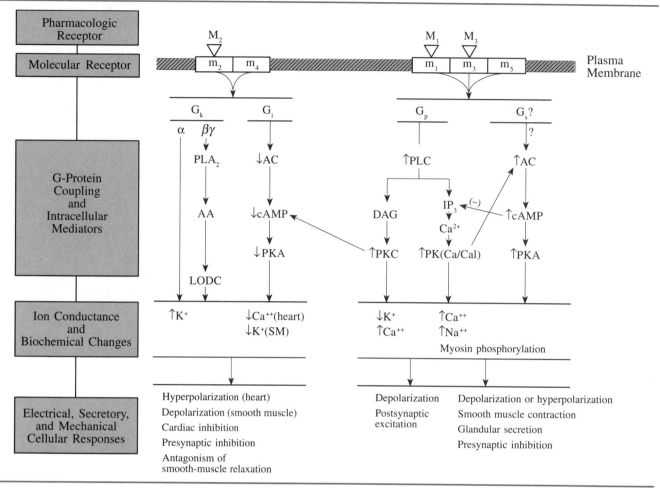

Figure 15-1. Subtypes of muscarinic receptors, intracellular mediators, and cellular responses. The pharmacologically defined subtypes correspond to the respective molecular subtypes. M_2/m_2 and m_4 are mainly coupled with G_k and G_i, whereas M_1/m_1, M_3/m_3, and m_5 are coupled with G_p and possibly with G_s, although the latter is doubtful. G_k is so named because it is coupled with potassium (K^+) channels; G_i and G_s are coupled with adenylate cyclase (AC), which they inhibit and stimulate, respectively. G_p is a family of putative G-proteins that are coupled with phospholipase C (PLC). The intracellular mediators involved depend on the type of G-protein activated. The changes in the mediators lead to ion conductance and biochemical changes, and subsequently to electrical, secretory, and mechanical cellular responses. There is interaction between the products of PLC stimulation and those of AC stimulation. α and $\beta\gamma$ = subunits of G_k; PLA_2 = phospholipase A_2; AA = arachidonic acid; LODC = lipooxygenase-derived compounds; PKA = protein kinase A; DAG = diacylglycerol; PKC = protein kinase C; IP_3 = inositol triphosphate; PK (Ca/Cal) = protein kinase that is sensitive to calcium and calmodulin; Sm = smooth muscle. (From R.K. Goyal, Muscarinic receptor subtypes. Physiology and clinical implications. *N. Engl. J. Med.* 321:1022, 1989.)

separate points in the acetyl group of ACh, whereas the third binds the quaternary nitrogen. The nitrogen site is anionic in nature and is apparently important for agonistic activity. Antimuscarinic drugs contain tertiary or quaternary amine groups that also are capable of binding to the anionic site, but these drugs do not activate the receptors. It has been suggested that the large groups present in antimuscarinic drugs play a major role in their receptor-blocking activity. These groups increase drug affinity for the receptor but decrease the fit of the blocking drug's amine group at the anionic site.

Pharmacological Actions

Muscarinic antagonists have no intrinsic activity and only produce effects through blockade of receptor stimu-

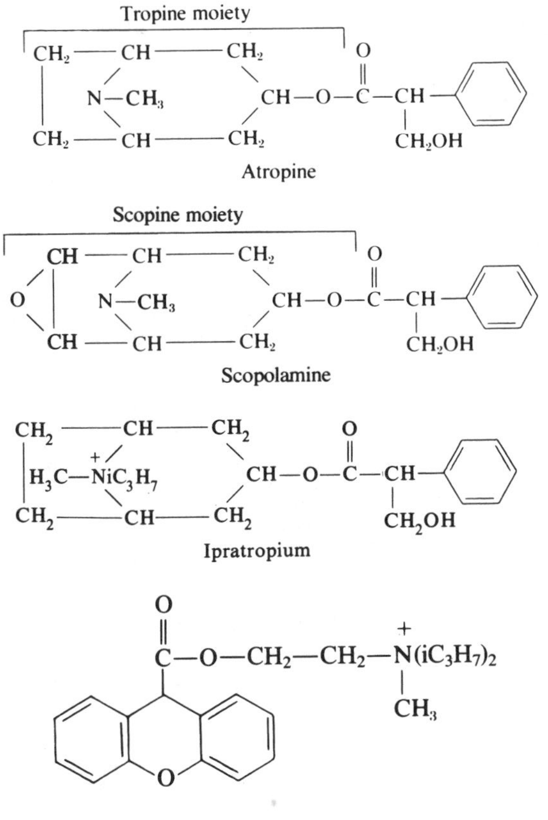

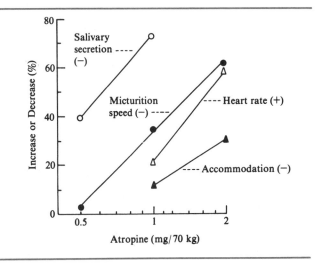

Figure 15-2. Structures of selected muscarinic blocking drugs.

Table 15-1. Effects of Muscarinic Blocking Drugs in Humans

Tissue or system	Effects
Skin	Inhibition of sweating (hyperpyrexia may result); flushing
Visual	Cycloplegia (relaxation of ciliary muscle); mydriasis (relaxation of sphincter pupillae muscle); increase in aqueous outflow resistance (increases intraocular pressure in many cases of glaucoma)
Digestive	Decreased salivation; reduced tone and motility in the gastrointestinal tract; decrease in vagus-stimulated gastric, pancreatic, intestinal, and biliary secretions
Urinary	Urinary retention (relaxation of the detrusor muscle); relaxation of ureter
Respiratory	Bronchial dilation and decreased secretions
Cardiovascular	Bradycardia at low doses (may be a CNS effect) and tachycardia at higher doses (peripheral effect); increased cardiac output if patient is recumbent
Central nervous system	Decreased concentration and memory; drowsiness; sedation; excitation; ataxia; asynergia; decrease in alpha EEG and increase in low-voltage slow waves (as in drowsy state); hallucinations; coma

lation by muscarinic agonists or by neuronally released ACh. Thus, the ability of these drugs to elicit a response depends on the ambient level of cholinergic nerve activity or the presence of muscarinic receptor stimulants. The nature of the response to muscarinic blockers can also depend on the innervation characteristics of the effector unit. Several tissues contain adrenergic and cholinergic nerves that produce opposing actions when stimulated (e.g., sinoatrial node). At these locations, adrenergic responses would be expected to predominate in the presence of muscarinic receptor blockade.

The effects of muscarinic blocking drugs on various human organ systems are summarized in Table 15-1. The tissues or systems affected by antimuscarinic drugs depend on the dose administered. This is demonstrated in Fig. 15-3, which shows the responses caused by the subcutaneous injection of different doses of atropine sulfate. At a low dose (0.5 mg/70 kg), atropine has a prominent inhibitory effect on salivary secretion but causes no change in micturition or accommodation. This dose is also without effect on gastric acid secretion. The unfortunate consequence of this type of relationship is that the use of *effective* doses of atropine in patients with peptic ulcers is accom-

Figure 15-3. Some effects in humans of varying doses of atropine sulfate given subcutaneously. The (+) and (−) signs signify increase or decrease, respectively. (From A. Herxheimer, A comparison of some atropine-like drugs in man, with particular reference to their end-organ specificity. *Br. J. Pharmacol.* 13:184, 1958.)

panied by side effects on systems that are equally or more sensitive to the drug.

Heart

Atropine and scopolamine administration can produce either increases or decreases in heart rate. A slight bradycardia is often seen following the intravenous administration of low doses, whereas higher doses, through their ability to block the parasympathetic input to the sinoatrial (S-A) node, produce tachycardia. Although it has been suggested that the bradycardia results from an effect of the drugs on the central nervous system (CNS), this appears unlikely, since methylatropine (a quaternary ammonium compound) produces similar responses. One plausible explanation for the *paradoxical bradycardia* produced by low doses of muscarinic blockers relates to presynaptic muscarinic receptors that mediate feedback inhibition of ACh release. Neuronal release of ACh is increased when presynaptic muscarinic receptors are blocked, and this effect may be dominant over postsynaptic muscarinic receptor blockade following low doses of antagonist. Antimuscarinic agents also can block parasympathetic effects on the cardiac conduction system.

Blood Vessels

The effects of atropine and other muscarinic blocking drugs on the circulation are minimal. This reflects the relatively minor role of cholinergic fibers in determining vascular smooth muscle tone. Atropine can produce a flushing in the blush area, owing to vasodilation. It is not known whether this is a direct effect or a response to the hyperpyrexia induced by the drug's ability to inhibit sweating.

Gastrointestinal Tract

Muscarinic blocking drugs have numerous effects on the digestive system. The inhibition of salivation by low doses of atropine results in a dry mouth and difficulty in swallowing. Antimuscarinic drugs also impair gastric secretion and gastrointestinal motility, because both processes are partly under the control of the vagus nerve. Since relatively large doses of atropine are required to inhibit acid secretion, side effects such as dry mouth, tachycardia, ocular disturbances, and urinary retention often accompany its use in the treatment of peptic ulcers.

Bladder

The antimuscarinic agents can cause urinary retention by blocking the excitatory effect of ACh on the detrusor muscle of the bladder. During urination, cholinergic input to this smooth muscle is activated by a stretch reflex.

Central Nervous System

Commonly employed doses of atropine (0.2–2.0 mg) have minimal central effects, while larger amounts may produce a constellation of responses collectively termed the *central anticholinergic syndrome*. At intermediate doses (2–10 mg), memory and concentration may be impaired, and the patient may become drowsy; the electroencephalogram is typical of drowsiness, showing a decrease in frequency and amplitude of alpha activity and a shift to slow activity. If doses of 10 mg or higher are used, the patient may exhibit confusion, excitement, hallucinations, ataxia, asynergia, and possibly coma.

Even low doses of scopolamine have central effects. Sedation, amnesia, and drowsiness are commonly observed during the clinical use of this drug. Large doses of scopolamine can produce all the responses seen with atropine. Other tertiary amine compounds with muscarinic receptor blocking activity have similar central effects.

Eye

Antimuscarinic drugs block the effects of ACh on the iris sphincter and ciliary muscles of the eye. This results in mydriasis and paralysis of accommodation (*cycloplegia*), responses that cause photophobia and blurred vision. Ocular effects are produced only after higher parenteral doses. Atropine and scopolamine produce prolonged responses (i.e., lasting several days) when applied directly to the eyes.

Lung

Both the secretions and smooth muscle activity in the respiratory system are affected by muscarinic blocking drugs. The parasympathetic innervation of respiratory smooth muscle is most abundant in larger airways and exerts a dominant constrictor action. In agreement with this innervation pattern, muscarinic blockers produce their major bronchodilator effect at large-caliber airways. In addition, these drugs are potent inhibitors of secretions throughout the respiratory system from the nose to the bronchioles. By this mechanism they can block reflex laryngospasm during surgery.

Nicotinic Receptors

Although the antimuscarinic drugs are normally selective for muscarinic cholinergic receptors, high concentrations of agents with a quaternary ammonium group (e.g., propantheline) may cause some blockade of nicotinic receptors on autonomic ganglia and skeletal muscles. However, these effects are generally not of clinical importance at usual therapeutic doses.

Absorption, Metabolism, and Excretion

Both atropine and scopolamine are tertiary amines that cross biological membranes readily. They are well absorbed from the gastrointestinal tract and conjunctiva and can cross the blood-brain barrier.

Only limited information is available concerning the metabolism of these alkaloids. After the intravenous injection of atropine (i.e., *dl*-hyoscyamine), the biologically inactive isomer, *d*-hyoscyamine, is excreted unchanged in the urine. The active isomer, however, can undergo dealkylation, oxidation, and hydrolysis. Corresponding metabolites found in the urine are *l*-norhyoscyamine, *l*-

hyoscyamine-*N*-oxide, and *l*-tropic acid plus tropine, respectively. The metabolism of atropine, therefore, appears to be stereoselective.

The quaternary amine derivatives of the belladonna alkaloids, as well as the synthetic quaternary amines, are incompletely absorbed from the gastrointestinal tract. Consequently, greater amounts of these compounds are eliminated in the feces following oral administration. The blood-brain barrier prevents quaternary amine muscarinic blockers from gaining significant access to the CNS.

Table 15-2 lists the names of selected muscarinic blocking drugs and some information on their clinical use.

Clinical Uses

Cardiovascular

Atropine can be of some value in patients with *carotid sinus syncope*. This condition results from excessive activity of afferent neurons whose stretch receptors are located

Table 15-2. Selected Muscarinic Blocking Drugs and Their Uses

Drug	Primary use(s) and corresponding route(s)	$t_{1/2\beta}$ (hr)	Other information
Tertiary amines			
Atropine	Preoperative medication (IM)	2.5	
	Intraoperative medication to correct bradyarrhythmia (IV)		
	Block muscarinic responses during reversal of neuromuscular blockade with anticholinesterase (IV)		
	Treatment of anticholinesterase poisoning (IV)		
Scopolamine	Preoperative medication (IM)	8	Transdermal, 72-hr duration
	Intraoperative medication (IV)		
	Prevention of motion sickness (transdermal)		
	Inhibit involuntary bladder contractions (transdermal, investigational use)		
Cyclopentolate	Produce mydriasis and cycloplegia (topical)		6- to 24-hr duration
Tropicamide	Produce mydriasis and cycloplegia (topical)		2- to 6-hr duration
Dicyclomine	Adjunct in treatment of irritable bowel syndrome (po, IM)	9–10	Also has direct relaxant effect on smooth muscle
	Inhibit involuntary bladder contractions (po, IM)		
Oxybutynin	Inhibit involuntary bladder contractions (po)		Also has direct relaxant effect and local anesthetic action
Quaternary amines			
Glycopyrrolate	Preoperative medication (IM)	1.7	
	Intraoperative medication (IV)		
	Block muscarinic responses during reversal of neuromuscular blockade with anticholinesterase (IV)		
Ipratropium	Bronchodilation in chronic obstructive lung disease (topical; metered-dose inhaler)	2	4 to 6-hr duration
	Adjunct to other bronchodilator therapy in asthma (topical; metered-dose inhaler)		
	Reduce rhinorrhea in patient with rhinitis (intranasal, investigational use)		
Propantheline	Adjunct in treatment of irritable bowel syndrome (po)	1.6	Taken before meals, to reduce postprandial pain, and before bedtime
	Inhibit involuntary bladder contractions (po)		

in the carotid sinus. By reflex mechanisms, this excessive afferent input to the medulla oblongata causes a pronounced bradycardia, which is reversible by atropine.

Under certain conditions, atropine may be of value in the treatment of acute myocardial infarction. A bradycardia frequently occurs after acute myocardial infarction, especially in the first few hours; this is probably due to excessive vagal tone. The increased tone may facilitate the development of ventricular ectopy. Atropine sulfate has proved beneficial in those patients whose bradycardia is accompanied by hypotension or ventricular ectopy. *However, atropine is generally not recommended in this condition unless hypotension or ventricular ectopy is present.* Use of atropine is not without hazard, since cardiac work can be increased without improved perfusion, and ventricular arrhythmias may occur.

Uses in Anesthesiology

At one time, atropine or scopolamine was routinely administered before the induction of general anesthesia, in order to block excessive salivary and respiratory secretions induced by certain inhalation anesthetics (e.g., diethyl ether). With the newer, less irritating anesthetics, anticholinergic premedication may not be routinely required as an *antisialagogue* (i.e., to counteract formation of saliva). Although such premedication may afford some protection from reflex vagal effects, the doses generally used do not produce complete vagal block. If bradycardia and hypotension are anticipated due to reflex activation of vagal efferents during surgery or administration of succinylcholine, atropine can be given as a prophylactic measure. Sedation can occur following scopolamine administration, and preanesthetic or postoperative agitation has been observed in some patients. High serum levels of drugs with antimuscarinic activity may produce postoperative delirium. Glycopyrrolate bromide has also been given intramuscularly as a preanesthetic medication, with satisfactory results. This agent is a quaternary amine and, therefore, produces no central effects. During reversal of competitive neuromuscular blockade with neostigmine or another anticholinesterase agent, atropine or another anticholinergic drug is given to prevent excessive stimulation of muscarinic receptors.

Uses in Ophthalmology

Anticholinergic drugs are widely used in ophthalmology to produce mydriasis and cycloplegia. These actions permit an accurate determination of the refractive state of the eye and are also useful in treating specific ocular diseases and for the postsurgical treatment of patients following iridectomy.

Atropine, scopolamine, cyclopentolate, and tropicamide are among the anticholinergic drugs used in ophthalmology. All of these agents are tertiary amines and penetrate well to the iris and ciliary body after topical application to the eye. Systemic absorption of these drugs from the conjunctival sac is minimal, but significant absorption and toxicity can occur if the anticholinergic drugs come into contact with the nasal and pharyngeal mucosa by route of the nasolacrimal duct. To minimize this possibility, pressure should be applied to the lacrimal sac for a few minutes after topical application of muscarinic blockers.

The mydriatic and cycloplegic actions of atropine and scopolamine may remain for over one week after topical application to the eye. Cyclopentolate and tropicamide have substantially shorter durations of action and are quite useful when prolonged effects are not required. Complete recovery of accommodation occurs within 6 to 24 hr for cyclopentolate and 2 to 6 hr for tropicamide.

Uses in Disorders of the Digestive System

Nonselective antimuscarinic drugs have been employed in the therapy of peptic ulcers because they can reduce gastric acid secretion. This is accomplished directly by blockade of cholinergic input to parietal cells and indirectly by blockade of the vagal stimulation of gastrin release. Effective doses of the muscarinic blockers generally produce a significant degree of anticholinergic side effects.

Antacids, H_2-receptor blockers, and sucralfate are currently the agents of choice for the initial therapy of peptic ulcers (see Chap. 73). Single-drug therapy with one of these agents is usually very effective. Anticholinergic drugs may be useful adjuncts to therapy in resistant cases.

Pirenzepine is an anticholinergic agent with a dose-dependent selectivity for M_1 muscarinic receptors that has been marketed outside the US for the treatment of peptic ulcers. Although the exact site of action for this drug has not been demonstrated, decreased acid secretion may result from blockade of ganglionic M_1 receptors on cholinergic neurons that innervate parietal cells. Pirenzepine produces fewer side effects than the nonselective muscarinic blockers, but is probably somewhat less effective than H_2-receptor antagonists and causes dry mouth in some patients.

Muscarinic blocking drugs are sometimes used as adjuncts in the treatment of irritable bowel syndrome. This is a fairly common disorder of gastrointestinal motility that results in symptoms such as constipation, diarrhea, and abdominal pain. Emotional factors may be involved and response to placebo is high. Anticholinergic drugs can decrease the pain associated with postprandial spasm of intestinal smooth muscle by blocking contractile responses to ACh. Some of the agents used for this disorder have only anticholinergic activity (e.g., propantheline), while other drugs have additional properties that contribute to their antispasmodic action. Dicyclomine has antimuscarinic activity and a direct smooth muscle relaxant effect, while oxybutynin has both of the latter properties plus local anesthetic activity.

Uses in Urology

Beneficial effects of anticholinergic drugs have been reported in uninhibited bladder syndrome, bladder spasm, enuresis, and urge incontinence. Propantheline, oxybutynin, dicyclomine, and several other agents have been used for these purposes. However, total prevention of involuntary bladder contractions is difficult to achieve. The participation of noncholinergic, nonadrenergic nerves in bladder contraction may explain this apparent resistance to muscarinic blocking agents.

Uses in Respiratory Disorders

The muscarinic receptor-blocking alkaloids of the *Solanaceae* family were used in the therapy of respiratory disorders at least as early as three centuries ago. Various methods of alkaloid inhalation were employed, including smoking of cigarettes prepared with leaves from *Datura stramonium*. Bronchodilation resulted from blockade of the cholinergic input to the respiratory smooth muscle. For a long time these alkaloids occupied a major place in the therapy of asthma, but they have now been largely displaced by the adrenergic drugs (see Chap. 45). The problems associated with the use of antimuscarinic alkaloids in respiratory disorders are low therapeutic index and impaired expectoration. The latter is a consequence of the effect of the alkaloids in reducing mucous secretion, ciliary activity, and mucous transport.

Ipratropium bromide is a synthetic muscarinic blocking drug that has gained widespread use in recent years for the treatment of respiratory disorders. The drug is a quaternary amine and is applied topically to the airways through the use of a metered-dose inhaler. A substantial portion of the dose is swallowed, but absorption from the airways and gastrointestinal tract is negligible and most of the drug is eliminated in the feces. Consequently, systemic anticholinergic effects are not observed with ipratropium. Dryness of the mouth, development of a cough, and a bad taste have been reported to occur in some patients, but the drug appears to have no other significant adverse effects. Furthermore, ipratropium does not affect mucociliary transport or the volume and viscosity of sputum. The reason for this clinically important distinction between ipratropium and atropine is currently unexplained.

Clinical studies have demonstrated the effectiveness of ipratropium in chronic obstructive lung disease, for which it is equal or better in effectiveness than β_2-adrenergic agonists. Half-maximal response occurs within several minutes of inhaling a dose of ipratropium, but the maximum bronchodilator response takes 1.5 to 2.0 hr to develop. Consequently, it would be less suitable than a rapidly acting β-adrenergic agonist in emergencies. Ipratropium is less effective than the β_2-receptor agonists in asthma, but may be useful when combined with other bronchodilators.

Uses in Parkinsonism

Antimuscarinic agents can have beneficial effects in the treatment of parkinsonism since there is an apparent excess of cholinergic activity in the striatum of patients suffering from this disorder due to the loss of inhibitory dopaminergic input. Primary therapy of Parkinson's disease is currently directed toward replacement of the dopaminergic deficiency rather than blocking the cholinergic excess. However, anticholinergics are sometimes employed for mild cases and in combination with other agents (e.g., levodopa) for treatment of more advanced cases. Side effects due to peripheral muscarinic blockade are common, and CNS side effects (e.g., confusion and hallucinations) may occasionally limit their use (see Chap. 38 for a more detailed discussion of the use of anticholinergic drugs in extrapyramidal disorders).

Uses in Motion Sickness

Scopolamine is useful for the prevention of motion sickness when the motion is very stressful and of short duration. A transdermal preparation, with a 72-hr duration of action, has been marketed for this purpose. Blockade of cholinergic sites in the vestibular nuclei and reticular formation may account for the effectiveness of this agent. When the motion is less stressful and of a longer duration, the antihistamines (H_1 antagonists) are probably preferable to the anticholinergic drugs, especially for the prophylactic treatment of motion sickness.

Uses as Antidotes for Poisoning

Atropine is used as an antidote in poisoning from an overdose of a cholinesterase inhibitor (see Chap. 16). It also is used in cases of poisoning from species of mushroom (e.g., *Clitocybe dealbata*) that contain high concentrations of muscarine and related alkaloids. Atropine should not be used indiscriminately, since the drug can aggravate symptoms caused by some mushrooms.

Adverse Reactions

As already noted, the antimuscarinic drugs rarely affect only the system toward which their use is directed. At a given dose, they may cause some blockade of cholinergic transmission in a number of tissues containing muscarinic receptors. The desired effect for one specific use may well be an adverse effect associated with another application. Depending on the dose of drug employed, a patient may have a dry mouth, visual disturbances (e.g., photophobia and blurred vision), constipation, difficulty in urinating, tachycardia, and CNS effects.

Cardiac arrhythmias, in addition to sinus tachycardia, can also occur following administration of muscarinic blocking agents. Atrioventricular (A-V) dissociation, A-V block, and ventricular extrasystoles have been seen in some patients after administration of atropine. Serious arrhythmias may occur when atropine is given to anesthetized patients. The incidence of these depends on the anesthetic employed; it is highest with cyclopropane. The likelihood of occurrence of arrhythmias is reduced if the dose of atropine is administered over a prolonged period of time.

Contact dermatitis of the eyelids and conjunctiva is occasionally seen after the ocular use of atropine. In older patients, it is especially important to determine that the anterior chamber angle is not narrow, since anticholinergic drugs may produce angle closure in such patients and increase intraocular pressure (narrow-angle glaucoma). Systemic effects can be observed after topical ophthalmic application of anticholinergics. For example, topically applied cyclopentolate has been reported to elicit such signs of CNS toxicity as convulsions and psychotic episodes.

Anticholinergic Poisoning

Anticholinergic poisoning can result from the intake of excessive doses of belladonna alkaloids, synthetic anticholinergic drugs, and drugs from other pharmacological groups that have significant antimuscarinic activity (Table 15-3). In addition, poisonings have occurred following intentional, as well as unintentional, ingestion of belladonna alkaloids derived from plants of the *Solanaceae* family (e.g., *Atropa belladonna,* the deadly nightshade, and *D. stramonium,* jimsonweed or stinkweed).

Signs of peripheral muscarinic blockade (e.g., speech disturbances, swallowing difficulties, cardioacceleration, and pupillary dilatation) are most common at lower doses, whereas CNS effects (e.g., headache, restlessness, ataxia, and hallucinations) are more apparent after large doses. Although a lack of responsiveness to methacholine injection is convincing evidence of anticholinergic poisoning,

Table 15-3. Sources of Anticholinergic Poisoning

Group	Examples
Antihistamines (H$_1$-receptor antagonists)	Diphenhydramine
	Chlorpheniramine
	Dimenhydrinate
Antiparkinsonian drugs	Benztropine
	Trihexyphenidyl
Antipsychotics	Chlorpromazine
	Thioridazine
	Loxapine
Antispasmodics	Dicyclomine
	Propantheline
Belladonna alkaloids and related drugs	Atropine
	Scopolamine
Belladonna alkaloid–containing plants	Deadly nightshade
	Angel's trumpet
	Jimsonweed
Cyclic antidepressants	Amitriptyline
	Doxepin
	Fluoxetine
Cycloplegics and mydriatics	Cyclopentolate
	Tropicamide
Muscle relaxants	Orphenadrine
	Cyclobenzaprine

Source: Modified from L. Goldfrank, *Goldfrank's Toxicologic Emergencies.* East Norwalk, CT: Appleton & Lange, 1990.

an evaluation of the symptom complex is usually sufficient to establish the diagnosis. Many cases of anticholinergic poisoning can be managed by removing unabsorbed drug and providing supportive therapy. However, the presence of serious toxic effects (i.e., seizures, severe hypertension, hallucinations, or life-threatening arrhythmias) would justify the use of specific antidotal therapy with the cholinesterase-inhibiting compound physostigmine. Special caution should be employed if disorders are present that might be aggravated by the cholinergic stimulation resulting from the use of physostigmine. Benzodiazepines can be used to sedate delirious patients.

Contraindications and Cautions

Muscarinic blocking agents are contraindicated in angle-closure glaucoma. Caution also should be used in individuals with open-angle glaucoma, cardiac disease, and prostatic hypertrophy. Muscarinic blockers can aggravate reflux esophagitis because they decrease the tone of the lower esophageal sphincter. Infants and children are especially sensitive to the hyperthermic action of muscarinic blockers. Phenothiazines and tricyclic antidepressants have anticholinergic activity and can produce effects that are additive to those of the muscarinic blocking drugs.

Supplemental Reading

Ali, H.H. Reversal—anticholinesterases and anticholinergics. *Curr. Opinion Anaesth.* 3:630, 1990.

Amitai, Y., et al. Atropine poisoning in children during the Persian Gulf crisis. A national survey in Israel. *J.A.M.A.* 268:630, 1992.

Doods, H.N. Selective muscarinic antagonists as bronchodilators. *Agents Actions* 34(Suppl.):117, 1991.

Freston, J.W. Overview of medical therapy of peptic ulcer disease. *Gastroenterol. Clin. North Am.* 19:121, 1990.

Friedman, G. Treatment of the irritable bowel syndrome. *Gastroenterol. Clin. North Am.* 20:325, 1991.

Goyal, R.J. Muscarinic receptor subtypes. Physiology and clinical implications. *N. Engl. J. Med.* 321:1022, 1989.

Gross, N.J. Ipratropium bromide. *N. Engl. J. Med.* 319:486, 1988.

Hulme, E.C., Birdsall, N.J.M., and Buckley, N.J. Muscarinic receptor subtypes. *Annu. Rev. Pharmacol. Toxicol.* 30:633, 1990.

Mei, L., Roeske, W.R., and Yamamura, H.I. Molecular pharmacology of muscarinic receptor heterogeneity. *Life Sci.* 45:1831, 1989.

Mirakhur, R.K. Anticholinergic drugs in anesthesia. *Br. J. Hosp. Med.* 46:409, 1991.

Ruckenstein, M.J., and Harrison, R.V. Motion sickness. Helping patients tolerate the ups and downs. *Postgrad. Med.* 89:139, 1991.

Smilkstein, M.J. As the pendulum swings: The saga of physostigmine (editorial). *J. Emerg. Med.* 9:275, 1991.

Tattersfield, A.E. Bronchodilators: New developments. *Br. Med. Bull.* 48:190, 1992.

Vanderhoff, B.T., and Mosser, K.H. Jimson weed toxicity: Management of anticholinergic plant ingestion. *Am. Fam. Physician* 46:526, 1992.

Wein, A.J. Practical uropharmacology. *Urol. Clin. North Am.* 18:269, 1991.

16

Cholinesterases and Cholinesterase Inhibitors

Donald B. Hoover

The drugs described in this chapter interact with cholinesterase enzymes and inhibit their catalytic activity. The major consequence of this inhibition is *enhanced* neurotransmission at cholinergic synapses. Since the predominant action of these drugs is mediated by the acetylcholine (ACh) that accumulates in their presence, cholinesterase inhibitors are also classified as *indirectly acting cholinomimetics.*

In addition to their clinical use, inhibitors of the cholinesterases have been employed as insecticides in the agriculture industry and as weapons of chemical warfare. Since an appreciation of the actions of the cholinesterases is important for a full understanding of the mechanisms by which these inhibitors exert their effects, a brief description of the properties of the cholinesterases precedes that of the drugs.

Characteristics of Cholinesterases

Cholinesterases are enzymes that, under optimum conditions, catalyze the hydrolysis of choline esters to a greater extent than other esters. These enzymes have been further classified on the basis of substrate specificity and sensitivity to various inhibitors. The cholinesterase of primary neuropharmacological importance is *acetylcholinesterase* (AChE), also called *true, specific,* or *erythrocyte cholinesterase.* This enzyme is the main factor responsible for terminating the action of ACh released from nerve terminals. The other major class of cholinesterase enzymes is that of the so-called *nonspecific* or *pseudocholinesterases.* Pseudocholinesterase (pseudo-ChE) has other names, including *serum cholinesterase,* as well as names based on substrate preference—for example, butyryl- and propionylcholinesterase. The function of pseudo-ChE is largely unknown.

Although ACh is generally the preferred substrate of AChE, the enzyme will also hydrolyze acetyl-β-methylcholine and acetylcarnitylcholine. AChE is a poor catalyst of butyrylcholine and benzoylcholine hydrolysis, while pseudo-ChE shows high activity toward both of these substrates and toward ACh. Acetyl-β-methylcholine is a poor substrate for pseudo-ChE.

The cholinesterases show different susceptibilities to inhibitors. Both AChE and pseudo-ChE are inhibited by physostigmine and isoflurophate (diisopropylphosphofluoridate, DFP), while pseudo-ChE is somewhat more sensitive to DFP. Pseudo-ChE can be selectively inhibited by proper concentrations of iso-OMPA (isooctamethylpyrophosphoramide) or ethopropazine.

By the judicious use of substrates and inhibitors, one can selectively measure the activity of either AChE or pseudo-ChE in any given tissue.

Distribution and Function

The only known function of AChE is in neurotransmission, and its distribution is well suited to this purpose. Histochemical methods have made it possible to visualize locations of AChE at both the light and electron microscopic level. Using such techniques, it has been clearly demonstrated that AChE is located on both the presynaptic and postsynaptic membranes of cholinergic synapses. AChE is also found at the basement membrane of cholinergic synapses. The action of the AChE found at cholinergic synapses is the primary means by which the action of ACh is terminated; there is no specific uptake system for this neurotransmitter such as that occurring in sympathetic nerves for norepinephrine. AChE is also found in the cisternae of the endoplasmic reticulum and on the plasma membranes of cholinergic neurons. Within the central nervous system, AChE is largely associated with cholinergic neurons. Although some noncholinergic neurons also contain this enzyme, many of these are cholinoceptive cells. The function of the AChE present in erythrocytes and placenta is not as yet understood.

Pseudo-ChE has a widespread distribution, with enzyme especially abundant in liver, where it is synthesized, and serum. Although pseudo-ChE in the brain is mainly associated with glial cells and capillaries, some neurons also possess the enzyme. In the periphery, Schwann cells contain pseudo-ChE, as do some neurons, muscles, and other tissues. In spite of its presence in these and other regions, its function has not been established. It does, however, have a clinically important function in drug metabolism. Succinylcholine, procaine, and numerous other esters are metabolized by pseudo-ChE.

Acetylcholinesterase Structure and Mechanism of Catalysis

Acetylcholinesterase is a macromolecule that appears to consist of several subunits. Each molecule has a number of active centers where the hydrolysis of ACh takes place (Fig. 16-1). These active centers have two areas that interact with ACh: the *anionic site* and the *esteratic site*. The anionic site contains a negatively charged amino acid that binds the positively charged quaternary amine group of ACh through coulombic forces. This probably serves to bring the ester group of ACh in apposition to the esteratic site of AChE.

The esteratic site of the enzyme contains a serine molecule, which is made more reactive by hydrogen bonding to a nearby histidine molecule. The nucleophilic oxygen of serine can react with the carbonyl carbon of ACh, thereby breaking the ester linkage. During this reaction, choline is liberated and an *acetylated* AChE is formed. The latter intermediate is rapidly hydrolyzed to regenerate free enzyme and produce acetic acid. The entire process takes about 100 microseconds.

Cholinesterase Inhibitors

Chemistry

The cholinesterase inhibitors can be grouped into three broad classes, based on their structure. These are the mono-quaternary and bis-quaternary amines, the carbamates, and the organophosphates. These structures are important determinants of the mechanisms by which the drugs inhibit AChE.

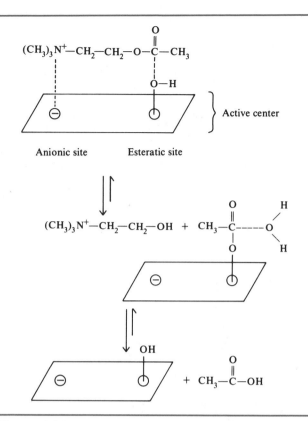

Figure 16-1. Simplified scheme of acetylcholine hydrolysis at the active center of acetylcholinesterase. Rectangular area represents the active center of the enzyme with its anionic and esteratic sites. At the top the initial bonding of acetylcholine at the active center is depicted. Coulombic forces are represented by the dashed line at the left. The dashed line at right represents the beginning interaction between the serine oxygen of the enzyme and the carbonyl carbon of acetylcholine. The ester linkage is broken, choline is liberated, and an acetylated enzyme intermediate is formed (middle). Finally, the acetylated intermediate undergoes hydrolysis to free the enzyme and generate acetic acid (bottom).

The mono-quaternary amine compounds have only one nitrogen atom with four carbons linked to it (e.g., edrophonium), while the bis-quaternary amines have two such nitrogens (e.g., ambenonium). Mono-quaternary amines and bis-quaternary amines remain charged over the entire physiological pH range and are, therefore, very water soluble.

Carbamates have the general structure:

$$R_2-\underset{\underset{\displaystyle R}{|}}{N}-\underset{\underset{\displaystyle O}{\|}}{C}-O-R_3$$

The R_1 and R_2 groups either may be organic radicals or may consist simply of a hydrogen atom. R_3 is frequently an aromatic ring structure containing a tertiary or quaternary amine. As would be expected from their structures, the carbamates are water soluble.

The organophosphate compounds have the general structure:

$$\begin{matrix} R_1 & O \\ \diagdown & \| \\ & P \\ \diagup & \diagdown \\ R_2 & X \end{matrix}$$

R_1 and R_2 are alkoxy groups in all clinically useful organophosphates. Examples of X groups are fluorine in isoflurophate and thiocholine in echothiophate. Parathion and malathion are thionophosphates

$$\begin{matrix} & S \\ \diagdown & \| \\ \diagup & P- \end{matrix}$$

that must be converted to oxyanalogues to be active. The organophosphates, as a group, are very lipid soluble. Echothiophate contains a quaternary amine group and is an exception to this generalization.

Mechanisms of Action

The compounds that inhibit AChE bind at the active center of this enzyme and prevent ACh from gaining access to it. *Blockade at either the anionic or esteratic site will prevent the hydrolysis of ACh.*

Quaternary Ammonium Compounds

Several mono-quaternary and bis-quaternary amines inhibit AChE by forming a noncovalent bond at the active center of the enzyme. Edrophonium is a clinically useful quaternary amine that competes with ACh for binding at the anionic site of the active center. Although edrophoniumlike compounds are effective for only a few minutes, the bis-quaternary amines may inhibit cholinesterases for several hours. Little is known concerning the reasons for the increase in duration of cholinesterase inhibition produced by the bis-compounds, but the distance between the quaternary nitrogens appears important in establishing a very tight binding of the drug to AChE.

Carbamates

Carbamate anticholinesterase agents interact with the esteratic site of AChE in a fashion similar to that of ACh. The clinically useful carbamates generally contain a tertiary or quaternary amine group that can bind noncova-

lently to the anionic site of the enzyme. The inhibition of AChE by neostigmine illustrates the general mechanism. The quaternary amine group of this molecule forms a noncovalent bond with the anionic site of the enzyme. The serine oxygen at the esteratic site of the enzyme reacts with the carbonyl carbon of neostigmine just as it would with that of ACh. A *carbamylated* intermediate is formed instead of an acetylated one. This carbamylated enzyme, however, undergoes hydrolysis much more slowly than does the acetylated one; the acetylated enzyme is hydrolyzed instantaneously, while the half-time for hydrolysis of this particular carbamylated intermediate is about 1 hr.

The key features of the inhibition caused by the carbamate inhibitors are covalent bonding to the esteratic site of AChE and their destruction during the interaction with the enzyme. *Physostigmine* (also called *eserine*) and *pyridostigmine* are two other agents in this class.

Organophosphates

The organophosphate inhibitory compounds also react at the esteratic site of AChE. In general, however, they are much less selective than are the carbamates, inhibiting many enzymes that contain a serine molecule at the active center. *Isoflurophate* is one agent in this group. In the interaction of isoflurophate with AChE, a phosphorylated intermediate is formed and fluoride is released. An important characteristic of the organophosphate-induced inhibition is that the bond between the phosphate and the enzyme is very stable. While the regeneration of most carbamylated enzymes occurs with a half-time of minutes or hours, the recovery of a phosphorylated enzyme is generally measured in days. These agents are referred to, therefore, as *irreversible inhibitors.*

Although the spontaneous hydrolysis of a phosphorylated enzyme is generally very slow, compounds called *oximes* can cause dephosphorylation. Oximes have the general structure R-CH = N-O-H and contain an oxygen that is much more nucleophilic than that of water. Pralidoxime chloride (2-PAM) (*Protopam Chloride*) is an oxime used in therapeutics to reactivate phosphorylated AChE. It has the additional feature that its quaternary amine group binds to the anionic site of the enzyme and thereby promotes dephosphorylation. If the oxime is not administered soon enough (minutes to hours) after AChE has been inhibited, an alkoxy group may be lost from the phosphorylated enzyme. This latter reaction is called *aging.* Once aging has occurred, oximes can no longer regenerate free enzymes. The rate of aging appears to depend both on the nature of the enzyme (AChE or pseudoChE) and on the particular inhibitor employed. Since pralidoxime is a quaternary amine, significant amounts of this drug will not cross the blood-brain barrier. Pralidoxime, therefore, is not considered useful for reactivating cholinesterases in the central nervous system.

A   No Drug   **B AChE Inhibitor ($-\!\!/\!\!\!\to$)**

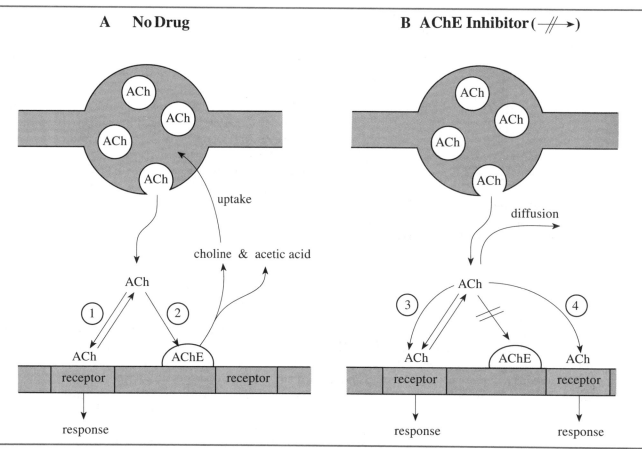

Figure 16-2. Action of AChE at a cholinergic neuroeffector junction and effects of AChE inhibition. Panel A shows key features of cholinergic neurotransmission in the absence of drugs. After release from a cholinergic varicosity, ACh can (1) bind reversibly to cholinergic receptors in the postsynaptic membrane and elicit a response or (2) bind to AChE and undergo hydrolysis to choline and acetic acid (inactive metabolites). The survival time of released ACh is quite brief due to the abundance and effectiveness of AChE. Panel B depicts the consequences of AChE inhibition. Since ACh no longer has access to the active site of AChE, the concentration of ACh in the synaptic cleft increases. This can result in enhanced transmission due to (3) repeated activation of receptors and (4) activation of more cholinergic receptors.

Pharmacological Actions

Inhibition of AChE potentiates and prolongs the effects of cholinergic neuronal stimulation (Fig. 16-2, Table 16-1). The sites at which anticholinesterase agents act include the neuromuscular junction, adrenal medulla, autonomic ganglia, cholinergic synapses at effector tissues of the autonomic nervous system, and cholinergic synapses in the central nervous system. The degree and range of effects observed depend on the inhibitor chosen, the dose employed, and the route of exposure or administration.

Cholinesterase inhibitors produce miosis by enhancing cholinergic input to the iris sphincter, and they blur vision through an action on the ciliary muscle. Other effects of cholinesterase inhibition on the eye are discussed under Glaucoma.

The activity of various glands is increased owing to enhanced cholinergic transmission. This results in lacrimation, salivation, increased secretion of gastric acid and pancreatic enzymes, and a generalized augmentation of intestinal secretions. Bronchial secretion is also enhanced by the action of cholinesterase inhibitors.

Neuromuscular transmission at skeletal muscle is enhanced by low concentrations of anticholinesterase agents, whereas high concentrations result in cholinergic blockade. This blockade is initially due to a persistent membrane depolarization, but if ACh levels remain high, the cholinergic receptors can become desensitized. Although anticholinesterase agents will facilitate cholinergic transmission at autonomic ganglia, their action at these sites is less marked than at the neuromuscular junction.

Table 16-1. Effects of Anticholinesterase Agents in Humans

Tissue or system	Effects
Skin	Sweating
Visual	Lacrimation, miosis, blurred vision, accommodative spasm
Digestive	Salivation; increased gastric, pancreatic, and intestinal secretions; increased tone and motility in gut (abdominal cramps, vomiting, diarrhea, and defecation)
Urinary	Urinary frequency and incontinence
Respiratory	Increased bronchial secretions, bronchoconstriction, weakness or paralysis of respiratory muscles
Skeletal muscle	Fasciculations, weakness, paralysis (depolarizing block)
Cardiovascular	Bradycardia (due to muscarinic predominance), decreased cardiac output, hypotension; effects due to ganglionic actions and activation of adrenal medulla also possible
Central nervous system	Tremor, anxiety, restlessness, disrupted concentration and memory, confusion, sleep disturbances, desynchronization of EEG, convulsions, coma, circulatory and respiratory depression

In addition to these indirect effects of cholinesterase inhibitors, the quaternary amine compounds also can cause direct stimulation of nicotinic receptors on skeletal muscle. The dose required to demonstrate a direct action in vitro is higher than that required to increase the amplitude and duration of end-plate potentials (i.e., effects attributed to AChE inhibition). Nevertheless, it has been suggested that a direct action on skeletal nicotinic receptors might contribute to the clinical effectiveness of quaternary amine cholinesterase inhibitors at the neuromuscular junction. Direct effects on autonomic effector organs are not observed.

Anticholinesterase agents of all classes have been shown to initiate *antidromic* firing of action potentials in motor neurons. It has been proposed that this is due to an activation of prejunctional ACh receptors. The inhibition of AChE permits ACh to reach these receptors. Quaternary amine inhibitors also may be agonists at these sites. The initiation of antidromic firing may be a mechanism by which cholinesterase inhibitors produce muscle fasciculation.

Actions of the cholinesterase inhibitors on smooth muscle and parasympathetic ganglionic cells in the gut result in increased intestinal tone and motility. In the urinary system, the cholinesterase inhibitors increase peristaltic activity in the ureters and contract the detrusor

muscle of the bladder. Inhibition of AChE likewise results in contraction of tracheal and bronchial smooth muscle.

The effects of anticholinesterase agents on the cardiovascular system are complex. The primary effect produced by these drugs is a bradycardia, with a consequent decrease in cardiac output and blood pressure. In addition to these effects, actions at the autonomic ganglia and adrenal medulla may further alter cardiovascular status. Activation of reflexes also may complicate the total cardiovascular response to cholinesterase inhibitors.

Absorption, Metabolism, and Excretion

Physostigmine, a tertiary amine, is rapidly absorbed from the gastrointestinal tract and distributed throughout the body. Quaternary amines, on the other hand, are poorly absorbed after oral administration, and therefore relatively large amounts of drug are often eliminated in the feces. Nevertheless, quaternary ammonium compounds like neostigmine and pyridostigmine are orally active if larger doses are employed.

Physostigmine and most organophosphates readily enter the central nervous system, whereas the quaternary amines are charged compounds and do not easily penetrate the blood-brain barrier. Because of their high lipid solubility, most of the organophosphates are absorbed by all routes of administration; even percutaneous exposure can result in the absorption of sufficient drug to permit the accumulation of toxic levels of these compounds.

A portion of an administered dose of edrophonium is metabolized to a glucuronide conjugate in the liver. Some of this metabolite is excreted in bile. Carbamates undergo both nonenzymatic and enzymatic hydrolysis in the body, with enzymatic hydrolysis generally resulting from an interaction of the drug with cholinesterase enzymes. The pseudo-ChE in plasma and liver is particularly important in this respect. Organophosphates are metabolized to inactive products by hydrolytic enzymes in the plasma, kidney, liver, and lungs. In contrast, the organophosphate insecticide parathion requires metabolism to become an effective insecticide. It is oxidatively desulfurated in insects and humans to form the active compound paraoxon.

Metabolites of the cholinesterase inhibitors and, in some instances, significant amounts of the parent compound are eliminated in the urine. Renal excretion is very important in the clearance of agents such as neostigmine, pyridostigmine, and edrophonium. This is demonstrated by a two- to threefold increase in elimination half-lives for these drugs in anephric patients. Renal elimination is largely the result of glomerular filtration, but probably also involves, at least in the case of quaternary amines, transport via the renal cationic transport system.

Table 16-2 lists the names of selected cholinesterase inhibitors and some information on their clinical use.

Table 16-2. Selected Cholinesterase Inhibitors and Their Uses

Drug	Primary use(s) and corresponding route(s)	$t^{1/2}_\beta$ (min)	Other information
Reversible inhibitors			
Mono- and bis-quaternary amines			
Ambenonium (Mytelase)	Treatment of myasthenia gravis (po)		Duration 3–8 hr
Demecarium (Humorsol) (also a carbamate)	Treatment of open-angle glaucoma (topical) Diagnosis and treatment of accommodative esotropia (topical)		Long duration
Edrophonium (Tensilon)	Reversal of nondepolarizing neuromuscular blocking agents (IV) Diagnosis of myasthenia gravis (IM or IV)	108	IV duration about 10 min
Carbamates			
Neostigmine (Prostigmin)	Treatment of myasthenia gravis (po) Reversal of nondepolarizing neuromuscular blocking agents (IV) Treatment of postoperative nonobstructive urinary retention and postoperative gastrointestinal ileus (SC or IM)	54	po duration 3–6 hr Parenteral duration 2–4 hr
Physostigmine (Antilirium)	Antidote to muscarinic blocking drugs (IV)	22	1- to 2-hr duration Can enter the CNS
Pyridostigmine (Mestinon)	Treatment of myasthenia gravis (po) Reversal of nondepolarizing neuromuscular blocking agents (IV)	84	po duration 3–6 hr (6–12 hr for extended-release tablets) Parenteral duration 2–4 hr
Irreversible inhibitors			
Organophosphates			
Isoflurophate (Floropryl)	Treatment of open-angle glaucoma (topical) Diagnosis and treatment of accommodative esotropia (topical)		Irreversible inhibitor
Echothiophate (Phospholine)	Treatment of open-angle glaucoma (topical) Diagnosis and treatment of accommodative esotropia (topical)		Irreversible inhibitor

Clinical Uses

Reversal of Neuromuscular Blockade

Anticholinesterase agents are widely used in anesthesiology to reverse the neuromuscular blockade caused by nondepolarizing muscle relaxants (see Chap. 18) like curare. The blockade produced by curare is competitive and can, therefore, be overcome by increasing the concentration of ACh at the cholinergic receptors located in the neuromuscular junction. Neostigmine, pyridostigmine, and edrophonium are anticholinesterase agents that are used for this purpose. Atropine or glycopyrrolate is administered in conjunction with the anticholinesterase agents to prevent the bradycardia and other side effects that result from excessive stimulation of muscarinic receptors.

Myasthenia Gravis

Myasthenia gravis is an autoimmune disease in which neuromuscular transmission at skeletal muscles is im-paired. Muscle weakness and rapid fatigue of muscles during use are characteristics of the disease. The primary immune response is toward ACh receptors on skeletal muscles. This leads to a decrease in the number of receptors and, consequently, a decreased sensitivity of the muscle to ACh. Anticholinesterase agents help to compensate for the sensitivity problem by elevating the concentration of ACh in the synaptic cleft. By contrast, thymectomy, plasmapheresis, and corticosteroid administration are treatments that are directed at the immune system.

Anticholinesterase agents play a key role in the diagnosis and therapy of myasthenia gravis, because they increase muscle strength. During diagnosis, the patient's muscle strength is examined before and immediately after the intravenous injection of edrophonium chloride. In myasthenics, an increase in muscle strength is obtained for a few minutes.

The pronounced weakness that may result from inadequate therapy of myasthenia gravis (*myasthenic crisis*) can be distinguished from that due to anticholinesterase overdose (*cholinergic crisis*) by the use of edrophonium. In cholinergic crisis, edrophonium will briefly cause a further weakening of muscles, whereas improvement in muscle strength is seen in the myasthenic patient whose anticholinesterase therapy is inadequate. Means for artificial respiration should be available when patients are being tested for the presence of cholinergic crisis.

Pyridostigmine and neostigmine are the major anticholinesterase agents used in the therapy of myasthenia gravis, but, ambenomium can, on rare occasions, be used if the others are found inadequate. When it is feasible, these agents are given orally. Pyridostigmine has a slightly longer duration of action than neostigmine and causes fewer muscarinic side effects. Ambenonium may act for a somewhat longer time than pyridostigmine, but it produces more side effects and tends to accumulate.

In general, patient-drug requirements must be individualized, since responsiveness will vary with external conditions, including physical activity, stress, and presence of infection.

Glaucoma

Glaucoma is a disease characterized by increased intraocular pressure, which, if untreated, will ultimately result in damage to the optic nerve. Two major categories of primary glaucoma are *angle-closure* and *open-angle*. Treatment of angle-closure glaucoma is surgical, but drugs, usually pilocarpine, are used to normalize intraocular pressure before surgery. The primary therapy of open-angle glaucoma is pharmacological.

Miotics are useful in open-angle glaucoma because they improve outflow facility. The most probable mechanism involved in the drug-associated improvement in aqueous humor outflow is an increased opening of lamina of the trabecular meshwork due to the stretching produced by contraction of the ciliary muscle.

Although anticholinesterase agents were commonly used in the therapy of open-angle glaucoma, they have been largely replaced by less toxic drugs. Either pilocarpine, a directly acting miotic (see Chap. 14), or timolol, a nonselective β-adrenergic blocker (see Chap. 13), is the agent of choice for initial therapy. If a single drug fails to control intraocular pressure, it may be necessary to combine two or more drugs from different classes. Epinephrine and a carbonic anhydrase inhibitor are additional agents used to treat open-angle glaucoma. If intraocular pressure is still not reduced on a multidrug regimen including a carbonic anhydrase inhibitor, some physicians would try one of the long-acting cholinesterase inhibitors (e.g., echothiophate, isoflurophate, or demecarium) while others would opt for surgical treatment.

Topical application of long-acting cholinesterase inhibitors to the eye can cause the development of cataracts, and this is a primary reason for reluctance to use these drugs even in resistant cases of glaucoma. The mechanism for this toxicity is currently unknown. Other side effects

of these drugs are related to accumulation of ACh. Accommodative spasm, dimness of vision, eyelid twitch, and headache are common. Blood vessels of the iris and conjunctiva become dilated and more permeable, and there is some breakdown of the blood–aqueous humor barrier. These actions result in congestion of the eye. Cholinesterase inhibitors may also cause a pupillary block by increasing the area of contact between the lens and iris. Finally, the potential exists for systemic effects after topical application of long-acting cholinesterase inhibitors to the eye.

Strabismus

Drug treatment of *strabismus* (turning of one or both eyes from the normal positions) is largely limited to certain cases of accommodative *esotropia* (inward deviation). Long-acting anticholinesterase agents, such as isoflurophate, echothiophate, or demecarium, are employed to potentiate accommodation by blocking ACh hydrolysis at the ciliary body. This results in reduced accommodative convergence. The same side effects and precautions mentioned for the use of these drugs in glaucoma apply to the therapy of strabismus.

Smooth Muscle Atony

Anticholinesterase agents can be employed in the treatment of adynamic ileus and atony of the urinary bladder, both of which may result from surgery. Neostigmine can be administered subcutaneously or intramuscularly in these conditions. Cholinesterase inhibitors are, of course, contraindicated if any mechanical obstruction of the intestine or urinary tract is known to be present.

Antimuscarinic Toxicity

A number of drugs in addition to atropine and scopolamine have antimuscarinic properties. These include tricyclic antidepressants, phenothiazines, and antihistamines. Physostigmine has been used in the treatment of acute toxicity produced by these compounds. However, physostigmine can produce cardiac arrhythmias and other serious toxic effects of its own. The drug should, therefore, be considered as an antidote only in life-threatening cases of anticholinergic drug overdose.

Adverse Reactions

Cholinesterase inhibitors are widely used as agricultural and household insecticides, and accidental poisoning sometimes occurs during their manufacture and use. Overdose can also occur during the therapeutic use of the anticholinesterase compounds. In addition, a number of cholinesterase inhibitors have been used in chemical warfare. These are the so-called nerve gases such as *sarin* and *soman.* The acute toxicity of all of the above-mentioned chemicals is entirely due to the buildup of ACh at cholinergic synapses. Maintaining adequate ventilation is of primary importance in cholinesterase poisoning. If enough enzyme is inhibited, there will be bronchoconstriction, accumulation of respiratory secretions, weakened or paralyzed respiratory muscles, and central respiratory paralysis.

In addition to the acute toxic effects that result from inhibition of AChE, certain of the organophosphorus compounds can produce delayed neurotoxicity, which is unrelated to inhibition of any cholinesterase. Recent work has prompted the hypothesis that phosphorylation of Ca^{2+}/calmodulin kinase II by the neurotoxic organophosphates is the initial step that triggers a series of biochemical effects leading to axonal degeneration. Clinically, this syndrome is characterized by muscle weakness that begins a few weeks after acute poisoning. This may progress to a flaccid paralysis, and eventually a spastic paralysis. The latter effect is a consequence of spinal cord damage. There is no specific therapy for organophosphate-induced neuropathy and clinical recovery only occurs in the mildest cases.

Treatment of Anticholinesterase Poisoning

In treating anticholinesterase poisoning, one should take steps to prevent or reduce any further absorption of the inhibitor. Contaminated clothing should be removed, and exposed skin washed with soap and water. Gastric lavage with water can be used if the inhibitor has been orally ingested; some form of respiratory assistance may also be required. Pharmacological measures include the use of atropine and, possibly, reactivating agents.

If the poisoning is due to an organophosphate, prompt administration of pralidoxime chloride will result in dephosphorylation of cholinesterases in the periphery. The primary importance of this measure is that it will decrease the degree of the blockade existing at the neuromuscular junction. Since pralidoxime is a quaternary amine, it will not enter the central nervous system and therefore cannot reactivate centrally located cholinesterases. In addition, pralidoxime is effective only if there has been no aging of the phosphorylated enzyme. Pralidoxime is administered IV over a 30-min interval in a dose of 1 to 2 gm. Since its half-life in the blood is only about 1 hr, a second injection may be necessary.

Atropine sulfate should be administered to block effects that stem from the accumulation of ACh at muscarinic receptor sites. Atropine administration will antagonize salivation, bronchial secretion, and bronchoconstriction, but will not influence skeletal and respiratory muscle paralysis. A dose of 2 to 4 mg is given IM or IV, depending on the severity of symptoms. Further doses of atropine should be given until muscarinic effects have been eliminated and a slight muscarinic blockade exists, but, in general, heart rate should not be allowed to exceed 100. In cases of organophosphate poisoning, this mild atropinization should be continued for 1 or more days.

Contraindications and Cautions

Although the anticholinesterase agents are employed in the treatment of atony of the bladder and adynamic ileus, they are contraindicated in cases of mechanical obstruction of the intestine or urinary tract. Caution should be used in giving these drugs to a patient with bronchial asthma or other respiratory disorders since they will further constrict the smooth muscle of the bronchioles and stimulate respiratory secretions.

Because anticholinesterase agents also inhibit plasma pseudo-ChE, they will potentiate the effects of succinylcholine by inhibiting its breakdown. This is important, for example, when succinylcholine is to be employed in patients who have previously received cholinesterase inhibitors for the treatment of myasthenia gravis or glaucoma.

Supplemental Reading

Abou-Donia, M., and Lapadula, D.M. Mechanisms of organophosphorus ester-induced delayed neurotoxicity: Type I and type II. *Annu. Rev. Pharmacol. Toxicol.* 30:405, 1990.

Ali, H.H. Reversal—anticholinesterases and anticholinergics. *Curr. Opinion Anaesth.* 3:630, 1990.

Ames, R.G., et al. Protecting agricultural applicators from overexposure to cholinesterase-inhibiting pesticides: Perspectives from the California programme. *J. Soc. Occup. Med.* 39:85, 1989.

Arena, J.M. (ed.). Insecticides. In *Poisoning: Toxicology, Symptoms, Treatments* (5th ed.). Springfield, Ill.: Thomas, 1986. P. 174.

Drugs Used for Glaucoma. In D.R. Bennett (ed.), *AMA Drug Evaluations Annual.* Chicago: American Medical Association, 1992. P. 1963.

Hartvig, P., et al. Clinical pharmacokinetics of acetylcholinesterase inhibitors. *Prog. Brain Res.* 84:139, 1990.

Marrs, T.C. Toxicology of oximes used in treatment of organophosphate poisoning *Adverse Drug React. Toxicol. Rev.* 10:61, 1991.

Osterman, P.O. Current treatment of myasthenia gravis. *Prog. Brain Res.* 84:151, 1990.

Smilkstein, M.J. As the pendulum swings: The saga of physostigmine (editorial). *J. Emerg. Med.* 9:275, 1991.

Trundle, D., and Marcial, G. Detection of cholinesterase inhibition. The significance of cholinesterase measurements. *Ann. Clin. Lab. Sci.* 18:345, 1988.

17

Ganglionic Blocking Agents

Thomas C. Westfall

Ganglionic Transmission

A brief review of ganglionic anatomy and physiology seems warranted to better understand the actions of drugs that stimulate or antagonize transmission through autonomic ganglia. Transmission through autonomic ganglia is more complex than neurotransmission at the neuromuscular and postganglionic neuroeffector junctions (see Chaps. 11 and 18) and is subject to numerous pharmacological and physiological influences. In some ganglionic synapses, especially at parasympathetic ganglia, there is a simple presynaptic to postsynaptic cell relationship; in others, the presynaptic to postsynaptic cell relationship can be quite complicated, and may involve neurons interposed between the pre- and postsynaptic elements (*interneurons*).

In a variety of sympathetic and certain parasympathetic ganglion cells (e.g., vagal ganglia in the sinoatrial node), cells exhibiting the characteristic catecholamine fluorescence spectrum have been found. These cells are referred to as *small intensely fluorescent* (SIF) cells. At some autonomic ganglia, the SIF cell is a true interneuron, receiving afferent innervation from preganglionic cholinergic neurons and forming efferent synapses with postganglionic neurons. At other autonomic ganglia, the function of the SIF cell is not completely understood, but is believed to play a role in modulation of ganglionic transmission. *Many of the SIF cells are thought to contain dopamine as their neurotransmitter.*

Unlike the receptors at postganglionic neuroeffector junctions or at skeletal neuromuscular junctions, *both types of cholinergic receptors, that is, nicotinic and muscarinic, are present on the cell bodies of the postganglionic neurons.* Stimulation of the preganglionic neuron results in the release of acetylcholine (ACh) from the preganglionic nerve terminal, which in turn activates postganglionic cholinergic receptors and leads ultimately to the formation of a propagated action potential down the postganglionic axon. At the more complicated synapses, the release of ACh from preganglionic neurons results in the appearance of complex postsynaptic potential changes consisting of several temporally arranged components. There is an initial fast excitatory postsynaptic potential (fast EPSP) followed by a succession of much slower postsynaptic potential changes, including a slow EPSP that lasts for 2 to 5 sec, a slow inhibitory postsynaptic potential (slow IPSP) lasting about 10 sec, and a late slow EPSP lasting for 1 to 2 min.

It is known that cholinergic-nicotinic receptors in skeletal muscle are different from those in autonomic ganglia and the central nervous system. Such receptors at the skeletal muscle consist of four subunits (α, β, γ, and δ), while in the autonomic ganglion there are only α and β subunits, which are not the same as those in skeletal muscle. There are now known to be α_2, α_3, α_4, and α_5 subunits as well as β_2, β_3, and β_4 subunits. Functional receptors appear to be produced when any combination of α_2, α_3, or α_4 with either β_2 or β_4 is produced. Like the receptor in muscle, the subunits are thought to form a pentamer surrounding an inner core or ion channel. It is still unclear what the correct nature of the subunits is that forms the physiologically relevant receptor.

Excitatory and Inhibitory Potentials

The interaction of ACh with the postsynaptic nicotinic receptor results in a depolarization of the membrane, an influx of Na^+ and Ca^{2+}, and the generation of the fast EPSP. This change in postsynaptic potential is principally responsible for the generation of the propagated action potential in the postganglionic neuron. Generally, several presynaptic terminals innervate a single ganglion cell, and several preganglionic axon terminals must fire simultaneously for transmission to take place. *Ganglionic blocking agents prevent transmission by interfering with the postsynaptic action of ACh.* The drugs either interact with the nicotinic-cholinergic receptor itself or with the associated ionic channel complex. It is still not clear what combinations of subunits are responsible for the fast EPSP. The most likely candidates are the α_3/β_4 and α_4/β_2 combinations.

Interaction of ACh with the postsynaptic ganglionic cell muscarinic receptor is responsible for a slowly developing depolarization, the slow EPSP, which lasts for 2 to 5 sec. The signaling mechanisms leading to the slow EPSP are complicated. The S-EPSP is due to inhibition of a voltage-dependent K^+ current called the M current, and inhibition of the M current involves activation of G-proteins. In addition, there is stimulation of phospholipase C with subsequent production of the second messengers inositol 1,4,5-triphosphate (IP_3) and diacylglycerol (DAG). There are now known to be at least four types of muscarinic receptors (M_1, M_2, M_3, and M_4) that have been

Figure 17-1. Composite schematic drawing of ganglionic neurotransmission. For simplicity, it has been divided into a type A synapse containing interneurons or small intensely fluorescent (SIF) cells and a type B synapse, lacking interneurons. In the type A synapse, ACh is released from the preganglionic neuron and activates nicotinic and muscarinic receptors on the SIF cells (when present), leading to the release of a catecholamine, presumably dopamine. Dopamine subsequently activates a receptor on the postganglionic nerve. The insert depicts the temporal postganglionic action potential, consisting of a fast excitatory postsynaptic potential (EPSP) due to activation of nicotinic receptors by ACh, a slow inhibitory postsynaptic potential (IPSP) due to dopamine or another catecholamine activating the appropriate receptor, and a slow EPSP due to activation by ACh of an M_1 muscarinic cholinergic receptor located on the postganglionic nerve cell body. The muscarinic receptor on the SIF cell is either an M_1 or M_2 muscarinic cholinergic receptor. The postganglionic nerve cell body also contains autacoid receptors that generate a late slow EPSP. The dashed line and X represent the appropriate receptor antagonists. ACh = acetylcholine; DA = dopamine. The type B synapse is similar to the type A synapse but lacks interneurons or SIF cells. In this case, ACh activates nicotinic receptors leading to the fast EPSP as well as activating muscarinic receptors leading to both the slow IPSP and slow EPSP. The receptor type leading to the slow IPSP is either an M_1 or M_2 receptor while that leading to the slow EPSP is an M_1 receptor.

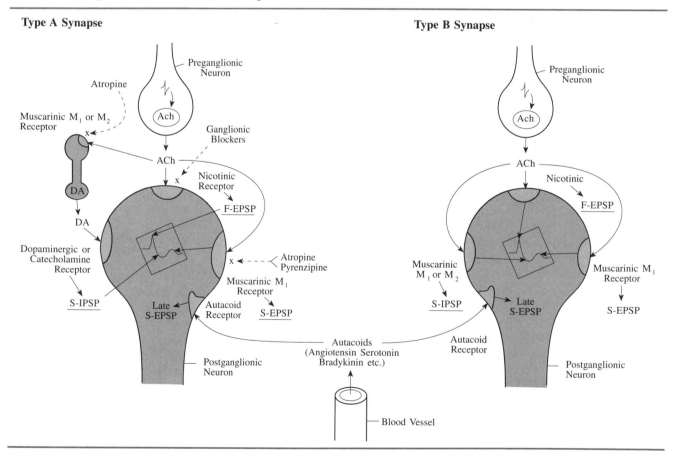

identified using functional studies, and at least five subtypes (m_1, m_2, m_3, m_4, and m_5) identified by molecular cloning techniques. The receptor generating the slow EPSP has a high affinity for the m_1 selective agent, pirenzepine, and, therefore, the m_1 receptor appears responsible for inhibiting the M current. The phosphoinositol response could be mediated by the m_1 or m_3 receptor.

The slow IPSP consists of hyperpolarization of the membrane lasting about 10 sec. The receptor mediating the slow IPSP has a low affinity for pirenzepine and therefore does not appear to be an M_1 receptor. Current evidence suggests that M_2 receptors mediate the hyperpolarization although a role for M_4 receptors has not been ruled out. The mechanism for the slow hyperpolarization may involve an increase in potassium conductance or a reduction in chloride conductance.

In some species and at some ganglionic synapses, an additional neurotransmitter may also be involved in mediating the slow IPSP. Release of acetylcholine may activate SIF cells located between preganglionic and postganglionic neurons. In this case activation of a muscarinic receptor located on SIF cells results in the release of a catecholamine; this in turn activates a receptor on the postganglionic cell, leading to the slow IPSP.

The catecholamine most frequently released from SIF cells appears to be dopamine, although norepinephrine, epinephrine, adenosine, or adenosine triphosphate (ATP) also may serve as the neurotransmitter at some synapses. It should be noted that the role of a catecholamine in mediating the slow IPSP following stimulation of the preganglionic neuron is not universally accepted. It is also possible that ACh acts directly on the principal ganglion cell to produce the slow IPSP.

Finally, a late slow EPSP, lasting for 1 to 2 min, can be seen at some ganglionic synapses. The mediator is unclear, but most likely involves peptides such as substance P or α-luteinizing hormone releasing hormone (LHRH)–like peptide. Both the slow EPSP and the slow IPSP seem to modulate ganglionic transmission by altering membrane potential during subsequent depolarizations. Pharmacological blockade of muscarinic and catecholamine recep-

tors will alter ganglionic potentials, but not greatly influence the fast EPSP or excitation of postganglionic cells.

There are suggestions that the fast EPSP, the slow EPSP, and the slow IPSP are elicited by different stimulation parameters. Therefore, the regulation and modulation of ganglionic transmission may be quite complex.

In addition to the cholinergic and adrenergic receptors on autonomic ganglion cells, there also appear to be receptors for a variety of excitatory and inhibitory substances, including angiotensin, bradykinin, histamine, 5-hydroxytryptamine, and substance P. Although receptors for these substances exist, the role of these receptors in ganglionic neurotransmission is far from clear; however, they provide an opportunity for a wide variety of options to modulate ganglionic transmission. Agonists for these receptors most likely reach the ganglia through the circulation. A composite picture of the current status of ganglionic transmission is represented diagrammatically in Fig. 17-1. For simplicity, the figure has been divided into a type A synapse, which includes SIF cells, and a type B synapse, which lacks SIF cells. Table 17-1 summarizes the type of ganglionic action potential generated at various ganglion synapses, the type of receptor mediating the response, and the primary transmitter or mediator that activates the receptor.

Ganglionic Stimulants

A variety of agents, including nicotine, lobeline, and dimethylphenyl piperazinium (DMPP), can stimulate ganglionic nicotinic receptors. Nicotine and lobeline are naturally occurring substances found in the leaves of tobacco and lobelia plants, respectively. Although drugs capable of stimulating ganglionic nicotinic receptors have little or no therapeutic use, they remain of considerable interest for several reasons. First, drugs such as nicotine that have the ability both to stimulate and to block ganglionic receptors have proved valuable as an aid in identifying and localizing postganglionic fibers. Second,

Table 17-1. Type of Ganglionic Action Potential per Synapse Type

Neurotransmitter/neuromodulator	Ganglionic receptor	Ganglionic action potential
Acetylcholine (from preganglionic neuron)	Nicotinic cholinergic	Fast EPSP
Acetylcholine (from preganglionic neuron)	Muscarinic cholinergic	Slow EPSP
Acetylcholine (from preganglionic neuron)	Muscarinic cholinergic or interneuron	Slow IPSP
Norepinephrine, epinephrine, dopamine (from interneuron)	Adrenergic/dopaminergic	Slow IPSP
Autacoid (angiotensin, etc.) or peptide (LHRH, etc.)	Autacoid or peptide receptor	Late slow EPSP

nicotine's use as a potent insecticide and rodenticide has endowed it with considerable toxicological interest. Finally, there are clear indications that tobacco smoking, especially cigarette smoking, is injurious to health. Smokers experience a higher incidence of such cardiovascular diseases as coronary heart disease, cerebrovascular disorders, and hypertension.

Mechanism of Ganglionic Stimulation

Nicotine and such related drugs as lobeline, trimethylammonium, and dimethyl-4-phenylpiperazine stimulate *all* autonomic ganglia by simple combination with ganglionic nicotinic receptors on the postsynaptic membrane. This leads to a membrane depolarization, an influx of sodium and calcium ions, and the generation of a fast EPSP. These agents produce a generalized stimulation of autonomic ganglia and a complex pattern of mixed sympathetic and parasympathetic responses.

In addition to autonomic ganglia, nicotinic receptors are also found in a variety of organs, and their stimulation will produce quite different results in these different tissues. Activation of nicotinic receptors on the plasma membrane of the cells of the adrenal medulla leads to the exocytotic release of epinephrine and norepinephrine; stimulation of nicotinic receptors at the neuromuscular junction results in the contraction of skeletal muscle (see Chap. 18); stimulation of nicotinic receptors in adrenergic nerve terminals leads to the release of norepinephrine; activation of nicotinic chemoreceptors in the aortic arch and carotid bodies causes nausea and vomiting. Finally, nicotinic receptors present in the central nervous system are capable of mediating a complex range of excitatory and inhibitory effects.

Mechanism of Ganglionic Blockade

Doses of nicotine greatly in excess of those inhaled from tobacco smoke produce a prolonged blockade of ganglionic nicotinic receptors. Unlike the blockade of ganglionic transmission produced by most ganglion-blocking agents, which is a nondepolarizing competitive antagonism, the blockade produced by nicotine consists of two phases.

The *initial phase (phase 1)* can be described as a persistent depolarization of the ganglion cell. The initial application of nicotine to the ganglion cells produces depolarization of the cell, which results in the initiation of an action potential. After a few seconds, however, this discharge stops and transmission is blocked. At this time, antidromic stimuli will fail to induce an action potential. In fact, during this phase, the ganglia will fail to respond to the administration of any ganglionic stimulant, regardless of the type of receptor it activates. The main reason for the loss

of electrical or receptor-mediated excitability during a period of maintained depolarization is that the voltage-sensitive sodium channel becomes inactivated and is no longer able to open in response to a brief depolarizing stimulus. During the latter part of phase 1, all nonnicotinic ganglionic stimulants, such as histamine, angiotensin, bradykinin, and serotonin, become effective.

Phase 1 is followed by a *postdepolarization phase (phase 2)* during which only the actions of nicotinic receptor agonists are blocked. This phase takes place after nicotine has acted for several minutes. At this time, the cell partially repolarizes and its electrical excitability returns. The main factor responsible for phase 2 block appears to be receptor *desensitization*. Desensitization results in the receptor becoming desensitized to ACh, thereby resulting in transmission failure.

Pharmacological Actions of Nicotine

Nicotine is present in varying amounts in all forms of tobacco smoke, and neither use of protective filters nor attempted denicotinization of the tobacco has eliminated the pharmacological responses attributable to nicotine inhalation. Following its absorption from the lungs, the blood nicotine levels achieved are sufficient to cause stimulation, not blockade, of nicotinic receptors. In addition to stimulating receptors on autonomic ganglia, all the other nicotinic receptors mentioned above also can be activated. Thus, *tobacco smoking has stimulatory effects on the cardiovascular, respiratory, and nervous systems.*

Cardiovascular System

The effects of nicotine on the cardiovascular system mimic those seen after activation of the sympathoadrenal system, and they are principally the result of release of epinephrine and norepinephrine from the adrenal medulla and adrenergic nerve terminals. These include a positive inotropic and chronotropic effect on the myocardium as well as an increase in cardiac output. In addition, both systolic and diastolic blood pressures are increased secondarily to stimulation of the sympathoadrenal system. These effects are the end result of a summation of adrenergic and cholinergic stimulation.

Respiratory System

Low doses of nicotine stimulate respiration through an activation of chemoreceptors located in the aortic arch and carotid bodies. High doses directly stimulate the respiratory centers. In toxic doses, nicotine depresses respiration, owing to inhibition of the respiratory centers in the brainstem as well as to a complex action at the receptors at the neuromuscular junction of the respiratory muscles. At these neuromuscular receptors, nicotine appears to occupy the receptors, and the end-plate is depolarized. After this, the muscle accommodates and relaxes in a fashion similar to that seen after administration of succinylcholine. As a result of these central and peripheral effects, there is paralysis of the respiratory muscles.

Central Nervous System

The actions of nicotine on the central nervous system are the result of a composite of stimulatory and depressant effects. These can include tremors, convulsions, respiratory stimulation or depression, and release of antidiuretic hormone from the pituitary. Nausea and emesis are frequently observed after the initial use of nicotine in the form of tobacco smoke. However, tolerance to these effects rapidly develops. This is in contrast to the effects of nicotine on the cardiovascular system, where tolerance develops much more slowly.

Other Systems

Additional effects of nicotine include an increase in gastric acid secretion and an increase in the tone and motility of the gastrointestinal tract. These effects are produced because of the predominance of cholinergic input to these effector systems.

Absorption, Distribution, and Excretion of Nicotine

Nicotine is well absorbed from the mucous membranes located in the oral cavity, gastrointestinal tract, and respiratory system. If tobacco smoke is held in the mouth for two seconds, 66 to 77 percent of the nicotine present in the smoke will be absorbed across the oral mucosa. If tobacco smoke is inhaled, approximately 90 to 98 percent of the nicotine will be absorbed. Nicotine is distributed throughout the body, readily crossing the blood-brain and placental barriers. Approximately 80 to 90 percent of the alkaloid is metabolized by the liver, kidney, and lung. Nicotine and its metabolites are rapidly eliminated by the kidney.

Ganglionic Nicotinic Blocking Drugs

Although a number of drugs possessing ganglionic blocking properties have been developed, only a few are currently available for clinical use. The prototypical ganglionic blocking agent was the bis-quaternary ammonium compound *hexamethonium.* There are currently no bis-quaternary ammonium compounds available in the

United States. *Trimethaphan* is a triethylsulfonium derivative; *mecamylamine* is a secondary amine. The ganglionic blocking agents vary in their ability to act as competitive antagonists at the nicotinic cholinergic receptor or to act directly on the associated ionic channel complex. They also may vary in potency, in duration of action, or in their primary route of administration. In addition, there are other drugs, such as curare, that are not employed as ganglionic blocking agents, although they have the ability to block ganglionic nicotinic receptors, especially at high doses.

Mechanism of Action

Drugs can block autonomic ganglia by any one of several mechanisms. They may act *presynaptically* by affecting nerve conduction or neurotransmitter synthesis, release, or reuptake. Acting *postjunctionally,* drugs may affect the interaction between ACh and its receptor; or they may affect depolarization of the ganglion cell or initiation of a propagated action potential. Ganglionic nicotinic blockers can be divided into two groups. The first group, characterized by nicotine and related drugs (e.g., lobeline, tetramethylammonium), initially stimulates the ganglia and then blocks them (see above). These agents are not therapeutically useful. The second group of drugs, which have some therapeutic usefulness, act to inhibit the postsynaptic action of ACh and do not themselves produce depolarization, thereby blocking transmission without causing initial stimulation. In the past, it was largely held that drugs such as hexamethonium acted as competitive antagonists at the receptor site. Recently, however, *the site of action of many blocking drugs has been shown to be at the associated ionic channel rather than at the receptor.* This second group of drugs neither directly modifies impulse conduction in either preganglionic or postganglionic neurons nor alters the release of acetylcholine from cholinergic terminals. Furthermore, these drugs do not antagonize ganglionic muscarinic receptors or receptors on the SIF cells.

Prolonged administration of ganglionic blocking drugs leads to the development of tolerance to their pharmacological effects. An interesting possible explanation for this tolerance is that the ganglionic muscarinic receptor responsible for the slow EPSP may take over the functional role of ganglionic neurotransmission normally carried out by the nicotinic receptor.

Pharmacological Actions

The effects of inhibition of ganglionic neurotransmission are widespread and include virtually all the tissues and organs innervated by the autonomic nervous system.

The physiological effects brought about by ganglionic blocking agents can best be understood through a knowledge of which division of the autonomic nervous system is dominant when a given tissue is innervated by both sympathetic and parasympathetic nerves. An overview of this topic is presented in Table 17-2, which also lists the effects resulting from ganglionic blockade. The magnitude of the response produced by ganglionic blocking drugs depends largely on the quantity and relative proportion of the total autonomic input coming from sympathetic and parasympathetic nerves at the time of drug administration. For example, if cardiac vagal tone is high at the time ganglion blockade is induced, tachycardia results. On the other hand, if heart rate is high, a decrease in rate may be seen.

The extent of the hypotension (especially postural hypotension) produced by a ganglionic blocking agent also depends on the degree of sympathetic tone existing at the time of drug administration. For instance, patients with normal cardiac function may have their cardiac output diminished after ganglionic blockade, while patients in cardiac failure often respond to ganglionic blockade with an increase in cardiac output.

To date, *it has not been possible to develop ganglionic blocking drugs that have a high degree of selectivity for either sympathetic or parasympathetic ganglia.* However, since these drugs do not affect all of the various ganglia equally, and since the time at which their peak effect occurs will vary among the various types of ganglia, some degree of selectivity of action does, in fact, exist.

Table 17-2. Predominant Autonomic Tone at Various Neuroeffector Junctions and the Effect Produced by Ganglionic Blockade

Site	Effect of ganglionic blockade
Tissues predominantly under parasympathetic (cholinergic) tone	
Myocardium	
Atrium; S-A node	Tachycardia
Eye	
Iris	Mydriasis
Ciliary muscle	Cycloplegia
GI tract	Decrease in tone and motility; constipation
Urinary bladder	Urinary retention
Salivary gland	Dry mouth
Tissues predominantly under sympathetic (adrenergic) tone	
Myocardium	
Ventricles	Decrease in contractile force
Blood vessels	
Arterioles	Vasodilation; increase in peripheral blood flow; hypotension
Veins	Vasodilation; pooling of blood; decrease in venous return; decrease in cardiac output
Sweat glands*	Decrease in secretion

*Anatomically sympathetic; transmitter is ACh.

Clinical Uses

Hypertensive Cardiovascular Disease

Ganglionic blockers were once widely used in the management of essential hypertension and represented an important advance in the treatment of that disease. Unfortunately, the development of tolerance to these drugs and their numerous undesirable side effects, resulting from their nonselective ganglion-blocking properties, have led to a decline in their use in essential hypertension (see Chap. 22); they have now been completely replaced by more effective and less toxic drugs. They do retain some usefulness, however, in the emergency treatment of hypertensive crisis.

Controlled Hypotension

Ganglionic blocking agents have been used to achieve controlled hypotension in plastic, neurological, and ophthalmological surgery. They are most commonly used in surgical procedures involving extensive skin dissection.

Autonomic Hyperreflexia (Autonomic Neurovegetative Syndrome)

This condition is a clinical syndrome that develops in up to 85 percent of patients with spinal cord injury, particularly if such injury results in quadriplegia or high-level (T5 or above) paraplegia. The syndrome consists of the paroxysmal onset of sweating, flushing, piloerection, and severe headache. Clinical signs may include marked increases in systemic arterial pressure, bradycardia, alterations in the level of consciousness, convulsions, or cessation of respiration. The increase in arterial pressure can be precipitous and may result in retinal hemorrhage, myocardial infarction, or a cerebrovascular accident.

Both ganglionic blocking agents, such as pentolinium and mecamylamine, and α-adrenoceptor antagonists have been used successfully in treating autonomic hyperreflexia. Generally, bradycardia and bladder spasticity are more readily controlled than is hypertension. This suggests that the cholinergic innervation is more sensitive to blockade than is the adrenergic input.

Adverse Reactions

All the responses summarized in Table 17-2 can be produced by administration of ganglionic blocking agents. Many of these responses represent undesirable effects, which can limit, and have seriously limited, the therapeutic usefulness of these agents. Mild untoward responses include mydriasis, difficulty in vision accommodation, dry mouth, urinary hesitancy, constipation, diarrhea, abdom-

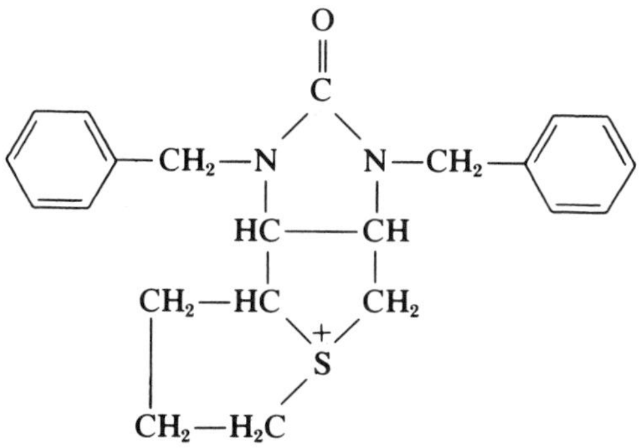

Figure 17-2. Trimethaphan.

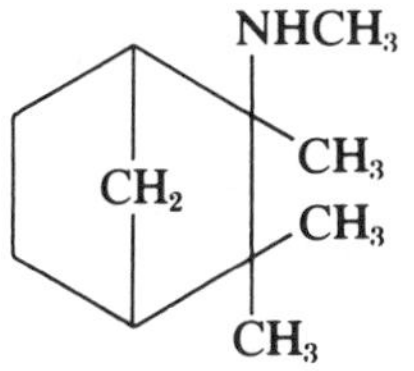

Figure 17-3. Mecamylamine.

inal discomfort, anorexia, and syncope. More serious, but less frequent, disturbances can include marked hypotension, constipation, paralytic ileus, urinary retention, and anginal pain. In addition, the nonquaternary ammonium-blocking agent mecamylamine (see below) can produce such central nervous system effects as mania, depression, and seizures.

Preparations and Dosage

Trimethaphan camsylate (*Arfonad*) possesses ganglionic blocking properties (Fig. 17-2). It is an extremely short-acting agent and is available only in parenteral form (50 mg/ml). Its major therapeutic use is in the production of controlled hypotension in certain surgical procedures or in the emergency treatment of hypertensive crisis. Continuous infusion may be employed to maintain its antihypertensive effect, especially in patients with acute dissecting aortic aneurysm. In addition to the effects that result from the drug's ganglionic blocking properties, high doses of trimethaphan release histamine and cause a direct vasodilation. Much of the decrease in blood pressure seen following trimethaphan administration is thought to be due to its direct vasodilating properties. In vitro, trimethaphan is an inhibitor of pseudocholinesterase, and it may be metabolized by this enzyme. In some patients, trimethaphan has produced a prolonged neuromuscular blockade and, therefore, it should be used with caution as a hypotensive agent during surgery. It has been reported to potentiate the neuromuscular blocking action of tubocurarine. Because of its histamine-releasing properties,

trimethaphan also should be used with caution in patients with allergies.

Mecamylamine hydrochloride (*Inversine*) is a secondary amine and can more easily penetrate cell membranes. It is more complete and less erratic in its absorption from the gastrointestinal tract than are quaternary ammonium compounds. Mecamylamine (Fig. 17-3) is well absorbed orally and crosses both the blood-brain and placental barriers; its distribution is not confined to the extracellular space. High concentrations of the drug accumulate in the liver and kidney, and it is excreted unchanged by the kidney. In contrast to most of the highly ionized ganglionic blocking agents, mecamylamine can produce central nervous system effects, including tremors, mental confusion, seizures, mania, and depression. The mechanisms by which these central effects are produced are unclear. Mecamylamine is very rarely used today as an antihypertensive drug because it blocks both parasympathetic and sympathetic ganglia.

Supplemental Reading

The Biology of Nicotine Dependence. CIBA Foundation Symposium No. 152. New York: Wiley, 1990.

Buckley, N., and Caufield, M. In G. Brunstock and C.H.V. Hoyle (eds.), *Transmission: Acetylcholine in Autonomic Neuroeffector Mechanisms* Chur, Switzerland: Harwood Academic Publishers, 1992. Pp. 257–322.

Dun, N.J. Ganglionic transmission: Electrophysiology and pharmacology. *Fed. Proc.* 39:2982, 1980.

Elfvin, L.G. *Autonomic Ganglia.* New York: Wiley, 1983.

Lippiello, P.M., Colins, A.C., and Gray, J.A. (eds.). *The Biology of Nicotine.* New York: Raven, 1992.

Martin, W.R., et al. (eds.). *Tobacco Smoking and Nicotine.* New York: Plenum, 1987.

Nordberg, A., et al. (eds.). Nicotinic receptors in the brain: Their role in synaptic transmission. *Prog. Brain Res.* 79:3, 1989.

18

Drugs Affecting Neuromuscular Transmission

Robert L. Volle and Michael D. Miyamoto

Acetylcholine (ACh) release from the motor nerve terminal and the generation of end-plate currents (EPCs) are pivotal events in neuromuscular transmission. When EPCs attain adequate intensity, excitation of the skeletal muscle membrane occurs and leads, ultimately, to muscle contraction. EPCs are local, graded currents that result from the conversion of the receptor complex from a closed to an open, ion-conducting configuration (Fig. 18-1). The binding of two ACh molecules to the receptor protein is required to initiate the opening of an ion channel.

The amplitude and time course of the EPCs are determined by the junctional concentration of both ACh and receptors. An effective ACh concentration is determined by the amount of ACh released, by the rate at which enzymatic (acetylcholinesterase, AChE) inactivation of ACh occurs, and by the rate of diffusion of ACh from the synaptic cleft. *Drugs modify transmission by affecting transmitter release or by altering the interaction between ACh and its receptor.*

Junctional morphology (Fig. 18-2) shows an orderly array of the axonal and end-plate entities that participate directly in transmission. Active zones in the terminal are surrounded by attachment and release sites for the ACh-containing vesicles. The ACh receptors are located on the surface of junctional folds at sites in juxtaposition to the active zones, sites favorable for an optimal response to junctional ACh. AChE is present in high concentrations predominantly in the junctional folds (Fig. 18-2).

Spontaneous release of ACh is manifest by the random occurrence of low-amplitude (miniature) EPCs. It is thought that transmitter release takes place in a *quantal* fashion and that the miniature EPC represents the response of many ACh receptor channels to a quantum (the ACh contained in a *single* vesicle) of transmitter. When the motor nerve is stimulated, many quanta are released simultaneously to produce a large-amplitude EPC.

Drugs that alter electrogenic events in the motor nerve terminal affect ACh release. Substances that prevent action potential generation will impair transmitter release. Similarly, drugs that induce repetitive firing in the motor nerve or prolong action potential duration will enhance release. Because Ca^{2+} is essential to the transmitter release process, drugs that affect Ca^{2+} conductance in the nerve terminal have marked effects on release.

In general, drugs that modify the *frequency* of miniature EPCs do so by altering transmitter release. For example, elevated extracellular concentrations of K^+ increase miniature EPC frequency by a Ca^{2+}-dependent process; Mg^{2+} depresses release and reduces miniature EPC frequency by interfering with Ca^{2+} availability.

Drugs that change the *amplitude* of miniature EPCs do so either by preventing the destruction of ACh or by reducing the number of functional ACh receptors. AChE inhibition results in larger and more prolonged miniature EPCs; ACh receptor blockade results in reduced miniature EPC amplitude. Some drugs enter the open channel of the ACh receptor to block current flow; in this case, miniature EPC duration is reduced. Thus, *changes in miniature EPC frequency, amplitude, and duration can be used to locate the site of drug action.*

Enhancement of Acetylcholine Release

Aminopyridines

The aminopyridines, of which 4-aminopyridine (4-AP) is a prototype, increase the number of quanta released by an action potential and cause bursts of miniature EPCs. 4-Aminopyridine enhances transmitter release in autonomic ganglia and in postganglionic sympathetic and parasympathetic nerve endings. There are marked increases in vesicle fusion with nerve terminal membranes

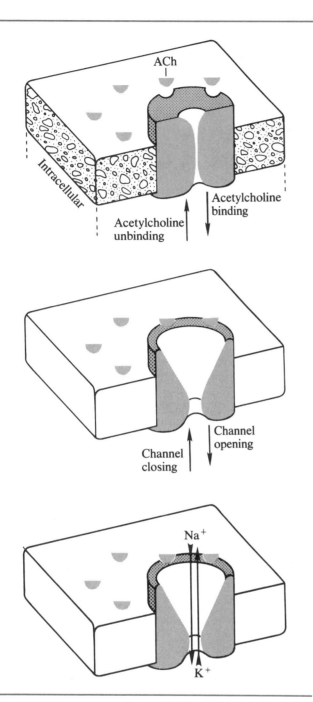

Figure 18-1. Schema of acetylcholine (ACh) receptor showing the two ACh-binding sites on the protein- and the ion-conducting component of the receptor. Sequence: (1) reversible ACh binding to protein, and (2) opening and closing of the channel for NA^+ and K^+ current flow.

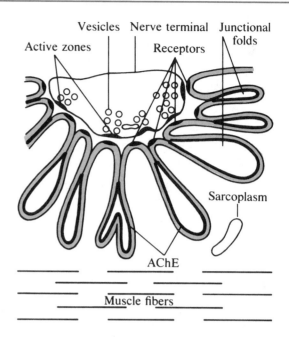

Figure 18-2. Schema of neuromuscular junction. Axonal terminal contains vesicles, mitochondria, and active zones. End-plate folds contain ACh receptors and acetylcholinesterase (AChE).

and an acceleration of exocytosis at central and peripheral synapses treated with 4-AP.

At concentrations higher than those required to alter nerve terminal excitation, 4-AP depresses K^+ conductance and prolongs action potential duration in peripheral nerves, skeletal muscle fibers, and cardiac cells. Thus, enhanced transmitter release probably results from the abil-

ity of 4-AP to prolong action potential duration and increase Ca^{2+} conductance in the terminals.

In patients with the myasthenic syndrome and in others poisoned with the botulinum type E toxin, muscle strength has been improved by 4-AP (however, the beneficial effects of 4-AP in botulinum poisoning are transient). Side effects that limit clinical utility include convulsions, restlessness, insomnia, and elevated blood pressure.

Guanidine

Guanidine hydrochloride is the drug of choice in the management of patients with myasthenic syndrome (see below) and may be of utility in the treatment of botulinum intoxication. The enhancement of transmitter release by guanidine may involve a blockade of K^+ channels and prolongation of the nerve terminal action potential.

Depression of Acetylcholine Release

Botulinum Toxin

Neuromuscular paralysis caused by the neurotoxin component of the botulinum toxin protein occurs 12 to

36 hr after ingestion of the toxin. Early signs are related to the paralysis of the bulbar muscle group and include diplopia, ptosis, dysphagia, and dysarthria. Paralysis may descend to include proximal and limb muscles and result in dyspnea and respiratory depression. Pupil size may or may not be normal, but, importantly, mental and sensory functions are unimpaired. This potent neurotoxin causes paralysis by depressing the release of ACh from the motor nerve terminal. Recovery from paralysis, when it occurs, requires days to weeks.

The toxins produced by *Clostridium botulinum* are classified into eight antigenically distinct types. Ingestion of improperly canned food is the most common mode of intoxication. However, botulinum poisoning may occur after wound contamination with the *Clostridium* organism. The toxins do not cross the placental barrier but do enter the central nervous system.

The neurotoxins *block ACh release at all cholinergic junctions,* including central and peripheral synapses. Choline uptake, ACh synthesis, and excitability at the nerve terminal are not impaired. Moreover, nicotinic and muscarinic receptors are not affected by the toxin. Rapid, repetitive nerve stimulation accelerates the onset of paralysis. The neurotoxin reduces the number of quanta released by the action potential, decreases the frequency of miniature EPCs, and prevents the release of ACh induced by K^+.

The botulinum neurotoxins consist of a single polypeptide chain of about 150,000 daltons. All but one are nicked by trypsin-type enzymes to give a dichain molecule, that is, a light (50,000 daltons) and a heavy (100,000 daltons) chain linked by a disulfide bridge. One end of the heavy chain mediates binding to the nerve membrane and the other end initiates internalization of the toxin. The light chain produces the actual inhibition of ACh release at the intracellular site. This may involve enzymatic inhibition of a substrate critical for exocytosis.

Reliable antidotes for botulinum toxin poisoning are not available. In some cases, anticholinesterase drugs improve muscle strength and restore function, albeit temporarily. Guanidine and 4-AP have been useful. Management depends primarily on supportive measures, such as those needed to maintain respiration and airways and, when possible, to promote elimination of the toxin.

Myasthenic (Lambert-Eaton) Syndrome

Muscle weakness in this autoimmune disorder results from diminished ACh release. At the end-plates of affected muscles the amplitude of miniature EPCs is normal, indicating that the postjunctional receptors are normal. The motor nerve terminal contains the usual number of vesicles and appears to have a normal morphology. The frequency of miniature EPCs and the number of quanta in an EPC are low, suggesting a defect in ACh release.

The *myasthenic syndrome* is often associated with bronchogenic carcinoma of the small cell type. It is possible that immunoglobulin G antibodies, elaborated in patients with this syndrome, are able to block calcium channels at the motor nerve and depress the release of ACh.

Drugs available to treat the myasthenic syndrome are limited to those that promote transmitter release, for example, guanidine. Clinical improvement, increased muscle strength, and decreased fatigability are seen 3 to 4 days after initial treatment using guanidine. Common side effects of treatment include paresthesia of the lips, face, hands, and feet; gastrointestinal distress; skin eruptions; bone marrow depression; renal tubular necrosis; hyperirritability; tremor; ataxia; and seizures. The aminopyridines have been used in clinical studies, with some positive results. The anticholinesterase agents are marginally effective.

Drugs That Act on End-Plate Acetylcholine Receptors

Langley wrote in 1905 that "both nicotine and curare abolish the effect of nerve stimulation, but do not prevent contraction from being obtained by direct stimulation of the muscle. . . . It may be inferred that neither the poison nor the nerve impulse acts directly on the contractile substance of the muscle but on some accessory substance. . . . We may speak of it as the receptive substance of the muscle."

The nicotinic ACh receptor is a glycoprotein with a molecular weight of about 290,000 daltons. It consists of five polypeptide subunits (denoted as α_1, β, α_2, γ, and δ), each about 55,000 daltons, and carbohydrate constituents of about 20,000 daltons. The binding sites for ACh are found on the two α subunits. The complex appears as a cylindrical unit, with a diameter of about 8 nm and a central, ion-conducting pore (see Fig. 18-1). The unit spans the plasma membrane, in keeping with its function as a cation-selective channel. Receptor densities at mammalian and amphibian end-plates are on the order of $10^4/\mu m^2$.

Toxins that selectively bind, in an irreversible manner, to the ACh receptor reveal much about receptor morphology, chemistry, and function. α-Bungarotoxin (α-BTX), isolated from the venom of the snake *Bungarus multicinctus,* is a protein that binds to the same sites on the receptor as does ACh. *Because α-BTX is selective for end-plate nicotinic receptors, distribution of α-BTX binding reflects receptor distribution.* Because α-BTX binding is irreversible, recovery from receptor blockade reflects shedding, synthesis, and insertion into the end-plate membrane of a newly synthesized ACh receptor.

Another toxin, histrionicotoxin (HTX), obtained from a Panamanian frog, has been used to study the conducting component of the ACh receptor. HTX has no effect on α-

BTX binding, but blocks the ACh receptor when the channel is in the open or conducting configuration. Nicotinic agonists increase HTX binding, presumably by increasing the frequency of channel openings.

ACh causes end-plate currents that result from increased inward Na^+ and outward K^+ conductances (see Fig. 18-1). Micropipettes filled with low concentrations of agonists can be used to initiate channel openings and to record single-channel conductances. The single-channel current activated by ACh persists for 1 msec; for carbachol, a stable choline ester, single-channel current flow persists for 0.4 msec. Thus, channel lifetime depends on intrinsic properties of the agonist-receptor binding. After AChE inhibition, end-plate currents caused by released ACh are prolonged, but single-channel lifetime measured with exogenous ACh is unaffected. This means that *enzyme inhibition prolongs ACh survival and permits repetitive ACh binding to the receptor, resulting in repeated ion channel openings.*

Channel Blockade

Ion channels opened by ACh can be blocked by a variety of drugs, including local anesthetics, atropine, barbiturates, and some psychoactive drugs. *These drugs do not prevent ACh or α-BTX binding to the receptor but block transmission by shortening the duration of current flow.* Phencyclidine and ketamine are good examples of drugs with this action. Single-channel lifetime is reduced because these drugs move into open channels to reduce ion flow; these drugs interfere with HTX binding.

Depolarization Blockade and Desensitization

Succinylcholine (SCh) (Fig. 18-3) binds to the ACh receptor, opens ion channels, causes current flow, and depolarizes the end-plate. For this reason, it is known as a *depolarizing* neuromuscular blocking drug. When used to produce neuromuscular block, SCh may cause muscle contraction that precedes the block. Denervated muscle is especially sensitive to depolarizing drugs because of the increased numbers of ACh receptors present on the sarcolemma of denervated skeletal muscle.

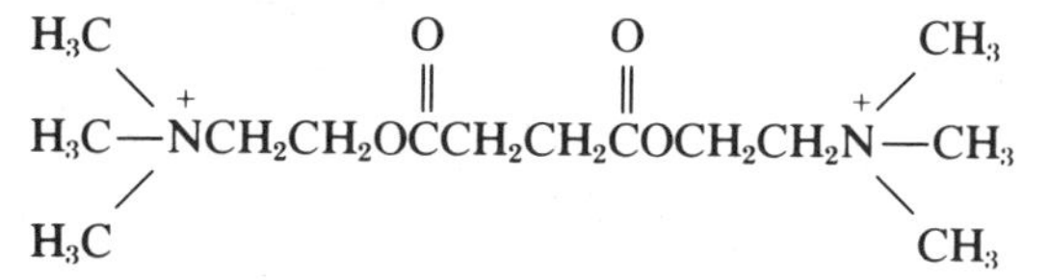

Neuromuscular blockade during end-plate depolarization results from inactivation of voltage-sensitive Na^+ channels in the muscle membrane. Muscle membrane action potentials in response to both direct and neural stimulation are suppressed. Blockade during depolarization is called *phase I block*. In the continued presence of the drug,

Figure 18-3. Succinylcholine.

depolarization may subside so that Na^+ channel inactivation is reduced or reversed and muscle membrane excitability is restored. Nonetheless, the neuromuscular block persists, a condition described as *phase II block.*

Although the mechanism for phase II block is not understood, a model of receptor desensitization has been proposed. An SCh · R_C complex is formed causing associated channels to open (SCh · R_O). Most complexes dissociate, restoring R_O to a natural state (R_C); however, *some complexes convert to a nonconducting state (SCh · R_D) that leads to a desensitized receptor state, R_D.* The continued presence of SCh favors the formation of R_D. With time, in the absence of SCh, R_D is transformed spontaneously to R_C, the natural state of the receptor. There is some evidence that phosphorylation of the ACh receptor by cyclic adenosine monophosphate–dependent protein kinases regulates receptor desensitization.

Succinylcholine

Pharmacological Actions

Succinylcholine, a drug that produces a depolarizing neuromuscular blockade, is a dicholine ester that is rapidly hydrolyzed by plasma pseudocholinesterase. Under normal circumstances, its actions are brief (5–10 min), but anticholinesterase drugs or abnormal plasma cholinesterase activity may prolong its action. *Succinylcholine has little effect on autonomic ganglia or postganglionic cholinergic junctions.* Actions at these sites attributed to succinylcholine may arise from the effects of choline. Succinylcholine does not enter the central nervous system (CNS).

Metabolism

The liver is the site of synthesis of pseudocholinesterase, the enzyme largely responsible for the rapid metabolism of succinylcholine. Neuromuscular blockade by succinylcholine may be prolonged in patients with liver disease. Within the general population is a group of individuals whose response to succinylcholine is prolonged due to diminished or abnormal pseudocholinesterase activity. Diminished *levels* of the enzyme have been associated with a heterozygous state while an *abnormal variant* of the enzyme has been associated with a homozygous state. The incidence of the abnormal variant alone may be 1/2,500.

Adverse Reactions

Postoperative muscle pain after the use of succinylcholine may be related to the level of general body fitness. Myoglobinuria associated with succinylcholine use suggests that the pain results from muscle fasciculations. Because succinylcholine causes contractions of extraocular muscles, the danger of transient elevated intraocular pressure exists. Hyperkalemia may occur in patients with large masses of denervated skeletal muscle. Succinylcholine may induce cardiac arrhythmia or arrest when plasma K^+ (normally 4 mM) is increased to 7 or 10 mM, respectively. Malignant hyperthermia may be precipitated by succinylcholine, and contracture is an early sign of succinylcholine-induced malignant hyperthermia (not to be confused with the neuroleptic malignant or parkinsonism hyperpyrexia syndrome, which involves dopamine systems in the CNS). Prolonged contraction of the affected muscles is caused by succinylcholine in patients with myotonia and amyotrophic lateral sclerosis.

Preparations

Succinylcholine chloride (*Anectine, Sucostrin Chloride, Quelicin*) is available as a sterile solution (20 mg/ml) and in individual packages with 500 mg powder per package.

Acetylcholine Receptor Blockade

Compounds in this group block neuromuscular transmission by reversibly occluding ACh-binding sites on the ACh receptor. These drugs do not induce changes in end-plate currents, but prevent ACh and related agonists from doing so. Neuromuscular block by these agents is reversed by administration of anticholinesterase agents and other procedures that preserve or increase the concentration of junctional ACh. The drugs listed below are *nondepolarizing, competitive* neuromuscular junction–blocking drugs.

d-Tubocurarine

The curares are alkaloids found in plants of the family Menispermaceae and genus *Strychnos*. Crude preparations of these drugs were named after the containers in which they were stored, for example, *tubo*-curare, in bamboo tubes; *pot*-curare, in earthenware pots; *calabash*-curare, in gourds made from calabashes.

Mechanism of Action

d-Tubocurarine (Fig. 18-4), the most important of the curare alkaloids, blocks nicotinic ACh receptors in muscle end-plates, autonomic ganglia, and adrenergic neurons, but has no effect on muscarinic ACh receptors. *d*-Tubocurarine has no effect on the excitability of muscle or nerve and does not alter the conduction of action potentials. It penetrates cells poorly and does not enter the central nervous system. However, if applied directly to brain and spinal cord, *d*-tubocurarine will block nicotinic receptors present in those tissues.

Pharmacological Actions

d-Tubocurarine given intravenously causes progressive flaccid paralysis, affecting head and neck muscles initially and, ultimately, the muscles of respiration. In humans, *d*-tubocurarine has a very rapid onset of action (3–5 min) causing ptosis, strabismus, and diplopia, with dysarthria and dysphagia (i.e., muscle paralysis in the head and neck). Limb muscles are affected next and respiration then becomes largely diaphragmatic. After cessation of drug administration recovery follows in reverse order.

At doses (0.2–0.5 mg/kg) used to block neuromuscular transmission, *d*-tubocurarine causes incomplete block of ganglionic transmission. Blockade of sympathetic ganglia and the adrenal medulla contributes to the fall in blood pressure caused by *d*-tubocurarine. In addition, *d*-tubocurarine provokes histamine release, an occurrence that also contributes to the hypotensive response.

Drugs or procedures enhancing ACh concentration in the junction antagonize neuromuscular blockade by *d*-tubocurarine and related muscle relaxants. Tetanic motor nerve stimulation or drugs that promote transmitter release (e.g., 4-AP) restore transmission. Similarly, the inactivation of end-plate AChE by edrophonium or neostigmine antagonizes the block by prolonging the survival of ACh. As would be expected, the antagonism of blockade

Figure 18-4. *d*-Tubocurarine.

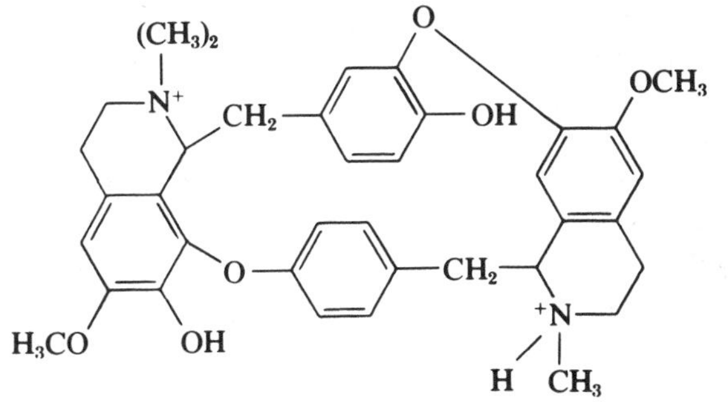

by edrophonium is transient; that caused by neostigmine, prolonged.

Clinical Uses

Neuromuscular block is used to relax skeletal muscle for surgical procedures, to prevent dislocations and fractures associated with electroconvulsive therapy, and to control muscle spasms in tetanus. These drugs do *not* produce anesthesia or analgesia.

The degree of blockade can be influenced by the status of body pH and electrolyte balance. Low extracellular K^+ such as that which occurs with diarrhea, renal disease, or the use of diuretics potentiates the effect of nondepolarizing drugs. In contrast, increased extracellular K^+ may enhance the end-plate response to succinylcholine and oppose the actions of *d*-tubocurarine.

The effect of pH changes on the activity of neuromuscular blocking agents is not understood. There are reports that alkalosis reduces the effectiveness of *d*-tubocurarine.

The inhalation anesthetics potentiate the action of nondepolarizing agents, either through a modification of the end-plate or by an alteration in local blood flow. The extent of potentiation depends on the anesthetic used and the depth of anesthesia. The following anesthetics potentiate neuromuscular blockade: isoflurane, enflurane, halothane, and nitrous oxide. Some antibiotics (e.g., aminoglycosides, macrolides, polymyxins, and lincomycin) enhance nondepolarizing blockade, either by decreasing ACh release or by a curarelike action. Procainamide and phenytoin also increase the effects of *d*-tubocurarinelike drugs.

Newborn children are extremely sensitive to the nondepolarizing muscle relaxants and, by contrast, may require three times as much depolarizing agent, on an mg/kg basis, as an adult for an equivalent degree of block. Like newborn children, patients with myasthenia gravis are very sensitive to paralysis by *d*-tubocurarine but resistant to succinylcholine. It is likely that this altered responsiveness is due to a reduced number of end-plate ACh receptors.

Preparations and Dosage

Tubocurarine chloride (*d*-tubocurarine chloride, *Tubarine*) is available in two concentrations: 15 mg/ml and 3 mg/ml. The usual dose is dependent on the other anesthetic agents or drugs being administered, the weight of the patient, and the distribution volume for the drug. Blood flow, pH, and body temperature will also affect its action. A reasonable dose range is 0.2 to 0.7 mg/kg body weight for an adult. It should be recalled that since neonates are very sensitive to this agent, the dosage must be reduced and the degree of neuromuscular blockade closely monitored. *d*-Tubocurarine is usually administered intra-

venously, but can be given intramuscularly as well. In the latter case, the drug will produce a prolonged weak paralysis. Full paralysis generally occurs within 3 to 4 min after adequate intravenous dosage.

Curarelike Drugs

Metocurine iodide (dimethyl tubocurarine; *Metubine Iodide*) is a semisynthetic derivative that has twice the potency and a slightly longer duration of action than *d*-tubocurarine. Otherwise, metocurine is similar to *d*-tubocurarine.

Pancuronium (*Pavulon*) is a synthetic bis-quaternary neuromuscular blocking agent that is five times more potent than *d*-tubocurarine. Like *d*-tubocurarine, it is a competitive antagonist of ACh at the cholinergic receptor but, unlike *d*-tubocurarine, it does not cause histamine release or block ganglionic transmission.

Vecuronium bromide (*Norcuron*) is a mono-quaternary analogue of pancuronium and is a moderately short-acting, nondepolarizing, competitive neuromuscular junction–blocking drug. The drug does not block ganglia or vagal neuroeffector junctions and does not release histamine.

Atracurium besylate (*Tracrium*) is a moderately short-acting bis-quaternary ester with actions similar to those of *d*-tubocurarine. Atracurium is rapidly destroyed in the plasma by hydrolysis of the ester group or by elimination of the bridging chain from the quaternary nitrogen. The drug has a half-life of about 20 min and can be used in patients with impaired renal and hepatic disease.

Gallamine triethiodide (*Flaxedil*) differs structurally from the others in that it contains three quaternary nitrogen groups. In addition to neuromuscular paralysis, gallamine blocks muscarinic receptors under cardiac vagal influence. As a result, gallamine may cause sinus tachycardia and occasional arrhythmias. It is available in a sterile solution.

Pharmacology of Antispasticity Agents

Muscle relaxants are of some value for the relief of spastic muscle disorders, that is, a state of increased muscle tone that results from an imbalance between central and spinal control of muscle tone. *Spasticity* is the result of a general release from supraspinal control and is characterized by heightened excitability of alpha and gamma motor systems and the appearance of primitive spinal cord reflexes. Treatment presents a difficult therapeutic problem, since often relief can be achieved only at the price of increased muscle weakness.

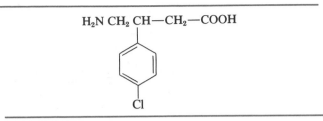

Figure 18-5. Baclofen.

Baclofen

Baclofen (Fig. 18-5) is the parachlorophenyl analogue of the naturally occurring neurotransmitter γ-aminobutyric acid (GABA).

Mechanism of Action

The mechanism by which baclofen affects the neuromuscular axis has not been established. However, it appears to act directly on sensory efferents, gamma motor neurons, and collateral neurons in the spinal cord to inhibit both mono- and polysynaptic reflexes. At primary sensory afferents, inhibition of the release of excitatory neurotransmitters (by activation of presynaptic $GABA_B$ receptors) may be involved.

Absorption, Metabolism, and Excretion

Baclofen is rapidly and effectively absorbed after oral administration. It is lipophilic and able to penetrate the blood-brain barrier. Approximately 35 percent of the drug is excreted unchanged in the urine and feces.

Clinical Uses

Baclofen is an agent of choice for treating spinal spasticity and spasticity associated with multiple sclerosis. It is not useful for treating spasticity of central origin. Doses should be increased gradually to a maximum of 100 to 150 mg per day, divided into four doses. Elderly patients and patients with multiple sclerosis may require lower doses and may display increased sensitivity to the central side effects. The drug has also been noted to increase the frequency of seizures in epileptics.

Adverse Reactions

Side effects are not a major problem and can be minimized by graduated dosage increases. They include tiredness, lassitude, slight nausea, and mental disturbances (including confusion, euphoria, and depression). The drowsiness is less pronounced than that produced by diazepam—an important therapeutic advantage. Hypotension has been noted, particularly following overdose.

Preparation

Baclofen (*Lioresal*) is available in 10-mg tablets.

Benzodiazepines

Benzodiazepines also possess muscle relaxant activity. Their pharmacology is discussed in Chap. 33. Diazepam and clonazepam have been used for control of flexor and extensor spasms, spinal spasticity, and multiple sclerosis. The muscle relaxant effect of the benzodiazepines may be mediated by an action on the primary afferents in the spinal cord, resulting in an increased level of presynaptic inhibition of muscle tone. Polysynaptic reflexes are inhibited. The most troublesome side effect is drowsiness, which is dose dependent. Tolerance develops to both the therapeutic effects and the side effects. Patients are treated with 15 to 60 mg diazepam per day.

Dantrolene Sodium

Dantrolene sodium acts directly on the skeletal muscle contractile mechanism. It blocks Ca^{2+} release from the sarcoplasmic reticulum and uncouples muscle excitation and contraction. Fast muscle fibers are more sensitive to this drug than are slow muscle fibers. It is used in the treatment of spasticity due to stroke, spinal injury, multiple sclerosis, or cerebral palsy. Another major use is in the prophylaxis or treatment of malignant hyperthermia (see above).

The most prominent, and often limiting, feature of dantrolene administration is a dose-dependent muscle weakness. Other side effects are drowsiness, dizziness, malaise, fatigue, and diarrhea. Evidence of minor liver dysfunction with transient elevations of serum glutamic-oxaloacetic transaminase (SGOT) is a disturbing side effect. Symptomatic hepatitis is reported in 0.5 percent of patients receiving the drug, and fatal hepatitis in up to 0.2 percent. Contraindications include respiratory muscle weakness or liver disease. It is suggested that patients on dantrolene therapy be given regular liver function tests.

Dantrolene (*Dantrium*) is active orally, although its absorption is slow and incomplete. Its biological half-life ($t_{1/2}$) is 8.7 hr in adults. The drug is metabolized by liver microsomal enzymes and is eliminated in the urine and bile.

Central Skeletal Muscle Relaxants

These are a chemically diverse series of compounds that have limited utility in relieving the signs and symp-

Table 18-1. Some Central Skeletal Muscle Relaxants

Official name	Trade name(s)
Carisoprodol	Rela, Soma
Chlorzoxazone	Paraflex
Cyclobenzaprine hydrochloride	Flexeril
Methocarbamol	Robaxin, Delaxin
Orphenadrine citrate	Norflex
Meprobamate	Miltown, Equanil

toms of localized muscle spasm. None has been shown to be superior to analgesic-antiinflammatory agents for the relief of acute or chronic muscle spasm, although all are superior to placebo. Most of these drugs have mild sedative properties and their muscle relaxant activity may be a direct result of sedation. One, meprobamate, has been widely used for the treatment of anxiety.

Experimentally, all centrally active skeletal muscle relaxants preferentially depress spinal polysynaptic reflexes over monosynaptic reflexes.

Most of the agents have similar actions and therefore the same adverse reactions are seen. These consist most commonly of drowsiness, dizziness, and light-headedness. One agent, cyclobenzaprine, has a prominent anticholinergic component and frequently causes dryness of the mouth, along with sedation and dizziness.

In addition to being employed alone, many of these compounds are available in combination with a nonnarcotic analgesic, or caffeine, or both. Because of their limited utility, the drugs will not be considered individually. The currently approved agents are given in Table 18-1.

Miscellaneous Agents

Chlorpromazine provides muscle relaxation but generally produces too much sedation. Fonazine mesylate is claimed to be a nonsoporific antihistaminic phenothiazine. Side effects include photosensitivity, weight gain, and increased flexor spasms. Sclerosant agents, including phenol and alcohol, have also been employed to destroy sensory or motor nerves in severe, disabling spasticity. The agents are injected into motor points or peripheral nerves, or intrathecally.

Supplemental Reading

Augustine, G.J., Charlton, M.P., and Smith, S.J. Calcium action in synaptic transmitter release. *Ann. Rev. Neurosci.* 10:633, 1987.

Engel, A.G. Myasthenia gravis and myasthenic syndromes. *Ann. Neurol.* 16:519, 1984.

Evered, D., and Whelan, J. (eds.). *Plasticity of the Neuromuscular System. CIBA Foundation Symposium No. 138.* New York: Wiley, 1988.

Heiman-Patterson, T.D. Malignant hyperthermia. *Semin. Neurol.* 11:220, 1991.

Jones, R.M. Neuromuscular transmission and its blockade. Pharmacology, monitoring and physiology updated. *Anaesthesia* 40:964, 1985.

Kharkevich, D.A. (ed.). *New Neuromuscular Blocking Agents.* Vol. 79: *Handbook of Experimental Pharmacology.* New York: Springer-Verlag, 1986.

Kim, Y.I., and Neher, E. IgG from patients with Lambert-Eaton syndrome blocks voltage-dependent calcium channels. *Science* 239:405, 1988.

Kunath, W., Giersig, M., and Hucho, F. The electron microscopy of the nicotinic acetylcholine receptor. *Electron Microsc. Rev.* 2:349, 1989.

Sakmann, B. Nobel Lecture. Elementary steps in synaptic transmission revealed by currents through single ion channels. *Neuron* 8:613, 1992.

Thesleff, S. Transmitter release at the neuromuscular junction. *P.R. Health Sci. J.* 7:67, 1988.

Ward, A., Chaffman, M.O., and Sorkin, E.M. Dantrolene. A review of its pharmacodynamic and pharmacokinetic properties and therapeutic use in malignant hyperthermia, the neuroleptic malignant syndrome and an update of its use in muscle spasticity. *Drugs* 32:130, 1986.

Drugs Affecting the Cardiovascular System

19

Vasoactive Substances: Renin, Angiotensin, and Kinins

Lisa A. Cassis and *Michael J. Peach*

A variety of naturally occurring substances of diverse chemical structure possess biological and, in larger doses, potential pharmacological activity. In this chapter, we focus on some of those substances, other than hormones and well-established neurotransmitters, that are present in humans. Most of these chemicals exert their effects through as yet ill-defined physiological and biochemical mechanisms.

For the forseeable future, it is likely that individual endogenous substances will play a lesser role in clinical medicine than will their antagonists. The actions of many other substances, such as polypeptides (e.g., endothelin, endothelium-derived relaxing factor, kallidin, bradykinin, and atriopeptin), lipids (e.g., leukotrienes, prostaglandins, and platelet activating factor), and nucleotides (e.g., adenosine triphosphate [ATP] and adenosine) are beginning to be appreciated, and their possible roles in cardiovascular, pulmonary, gastrointestinal, and neural physiology are beginning to be clarified.

Although the physiological and clinical significance of these endogenous substances is not entirely recognized, the presence of such potent substances points to their importance in normal mammalian systems and, possibly, in disease states, since they may act either directly or as important causative agents in the expression of pathological symptoms.

Renin

In 1827, Richard Bright suggested that a relationship existed among kidney disease, left ventricular hypertrophy, and elevated arterial blood pressure. By the 1880s, investigators had begun to search for an endogenous material of renal origin that could affect blood pressure. The name *renin* was first used to describe a saline-extractable pressor substance obtained from kidney homogenates. This observation received little attention until 1934, when it was demonstrated that experimentally induced renal arterial stenosis would result in arterial hypertension. Subsequent experiments revealed that renin is an enzyme that is synthesized and stored in the renal juxtaglomerular apparatus and catalyzes the formation of a decapeptide, *angiotensin I,* from a plasma protein substrate. Renin is considered to control the rate-limiting step in the ultimate production of angiotensin II. It thus has a narrow substrate specificity that is limited to a single peptide bond in angiotensinogen, a precursor of angiotensin I. Angiotensin I is recognized now as the first in a series of peptides generated by a cascade of enzymes working in concert (Fig. 19-1).

Chemistry

The structures of human kidney renin and its precursor forms have been deduced from the complementary DNA sequence. The product of messenger RNA (mRNA) translation has a molecular weight of 45,000 and is referred to as *preprorenin.* Rapid intracellular proteolysis of preprorenin results in the removal of a 20-amino acid presequence and the formation of *prorenin* (mol wt 42,500). Further posttranslational modification occurs (proteolysis and glycosylation) and prorenin is processed to mature renin, which has a molecular weight of 37,235. The half-life of renin in the circulation is from 10 to 30 min, with inactivation occurring primarily in the liver. Small amounts of renin are eliminated by the kidneys.

Pure human renin has been used to develop specific inhibitors of the enzyme. Low-molecular-weight, orally effective renin inhibitors are in clinical trials.

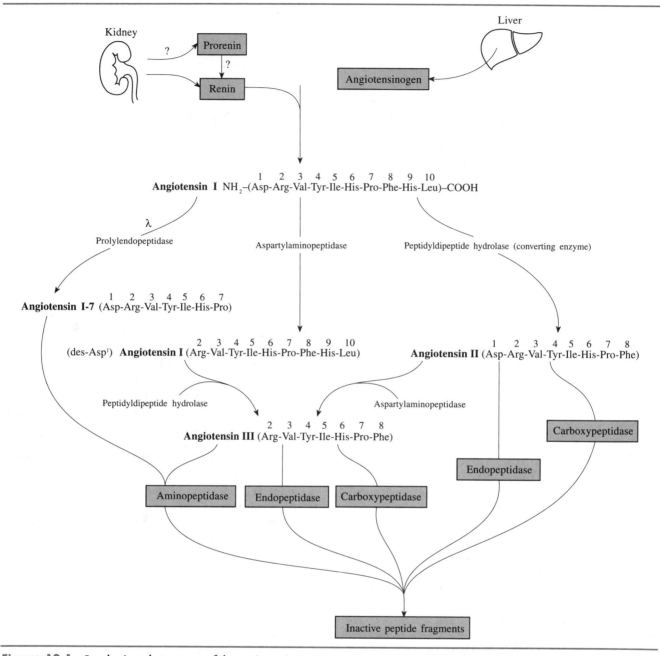

Figure 19-1. Synthesis and structures of the angiotensins.

Renin Release

Three generally accepted mechanisms are involved in the regulation of renin secretion by the renal juxtaglomerular apparatus (Fig. 19-2). The first mechanism depends on renal afferent arterioles that act as stretch or baroreceptors. Increased intravascular pressure and increased volume in the afferent arterioles inhibit the release of renin, whereas a diminished pressure and decreased volume induce the release of the enzyme. The second controlling mechanism is based on the modulation of renin secretion as a result of changes in the amount of filtered sodium that reaches the macula densa. *Plasma renin activity correlates inversely with dietary sodium intake.* The third control for renin release is neurogenic and involves the dense sympathetic innervation of the juxtaglomerular cells in the afferent arteriole; renin release is increased following activation of β-adrenoceptors.

Vasopressor agents, such as angiotensin II, act on the juxtaglomerular cells to inhibit the release of renin; this process is therefore a negative feedback mechanism. The prostaglandin synthesis inhibitor, indomethacin, reduces

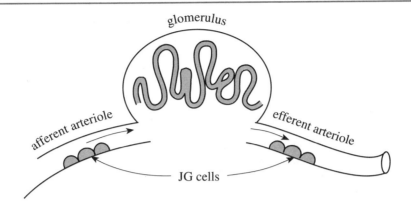

MECHANISMS

1.	2.	3.
Increased pressure in afferent arteriole leads to decreased renin release by JG cells.	Increased NaCl at macula densa in distal tubule leads to decreased renin release by JG cells.	Decreased sympathetic nerve activity in afferent arteriole leads to decreased renin release.

Figure 19-2. Mechanisms involved in regulation of renin secretion. JG = juxtaglomerular.

plasma renin activity, suggesting that prostacyclin (PGI_2), a product of cyclooxygenase-mediated arachidonic acid metabolism, is most likely the endogenous renal eicosanoid messenger between the macula densa and the juxtaglomerular cells.

Angiotensinogen

Human plasma contains a glycoprotein with a molecular weight of 56,000 called *angiotensinogen,* which serves as the substrate for renin. Angiotensinogen is synthesized in the liver, brain, kidney, and fat. Its gene transcription and plasma concentration increase following treatment with adrenocorticotropic hormone (ACTH), glucocorticoids, thyroid hormone, and estrogens, as well as during pregnancy and inflammation, and after nephrectomy. Angiotensinogen also has been found in large quantities in cerebrospinal and amniotic fluid.

Converting Enzyme (Peptidyldipeptide Hydrolase)

Angiotensinogen must undergo proteolysis before active portions of the protein are sufficiently unmasked to exert biological effects. Angiotensinogen is the only known substrate for the kidney enzyme renin, which cat-

alyzes its metabolism to the decapeptide *angiotensin I.* This relatively inactive peptide is then acted on by a dipeptidase "converting enzyme" to produce the very active octapeptide *angiotensin II.* In addition to converting enzyme, angiotensin I can also be acted on by prolylendopeptidase, which removes the first amino acid to produce angiotensin 1-7, a peptide primarily active in the brain.

Converting enzyme has been identified in vascular endothelial cells, epithelial cells of the proximal tubule and small intestine, male germinal cells, and the central nervous system. This enzyme has been purified to homogeneity, and the gene has been cloned. A single gene for converting enzyme gives rise to two isozymes, one produced by endothelial and epithelial cells (somatic) and the other produced by developing male germinal cells (testis). While the precise function of converting enzyme in the testis is unknown, it is thought to play a role in sperm development. Somatic converting enzyme is a zinc-containing glycoprotein with a molecular weight of about 130,000. Although converting enzyme was originally thought to be specific for the conversion of angiotensin I to II, this enzyme is now known to be a rather nonspecific peptidyldipeptide hydrolase that cleaves dipeptides from the carboxy terminus of a number of endogenous peptides. Peptides with penultimate prolyl residues are not cleaved by converting enzyme; this accounts for both the biological stability of angiotensin II and the relatively long half-life of some peptide inhibitors of the hydrolysis of angiotensin I. Inhibition of converting enzyme results in an elevated pool of angiotensin I.

The Angiotensins

Chemistry

The amino acid composition of the peptides and the enzymes involved in the synthesis and metabolism of the angiotensins is shown in Fig. 19-1. Angiotensin I is believed to have little direct biological activity and must be converted to angiotensin II or angiotensin 1-7 before characteristic responses of the renin-angiotensin system are manifested. Angiotensin I and II are degraded at their amino terminus by *aspartylaminopeptidase,* an enzyme present in plasma and numerous tissues. Angiotensin II is inactivated rapidly by aspartylamino-, endo-, and carboxy-peptidases, while angiotensin III is hydrolyzed by amino-, endo-, and carboxypeptidases (see Fig. 19-1). The biological activity of angiotensin III is one-fourth to equipotent with angiotensin II, depending on the response being monitored.

Once the structure of angiotensin II was known, several analogues were synthesized in an attempt to identify structural features necessary for biological activity. The side chains of tyrosine and histidine as the fourth and sixth residues, respectively, are vital for receptor affinity. A secondary contribution is made to binding by the first and second amino acids, asparagine and arginine. The aromatic rings of phenylalanine (at the COOH terminus) and tyrosine are important for intrinsic activity. The NH_2-terminal residue is a determinant of duration of action (i.e., susceptibility to aminopeptidase). The neutral side chains of valine, isoleucine, and proline are major determinants of the conformation of the peptide in solution.

Pharmacological Actions

The following discussion addresses the pharmacology of angiotensin II, but most of these responses also occur following administration of angiotensin III. Generally, angiotensin III is less potent than angiotensin II. Angiotensin 1-7 is similar to angiotensin II in its actions in the central nervous system, but devoid of peripheral vasoconstrictor activity.

Cardiovascular System

Arterial Blood Pressure

The intravenous injection of angiotensin results in a sharp rise in systolic and diastolic pressures. The response is consistently reproducible when small doses of angioten-

sin II are injected; however, larger amounts of the peptide produce *tachyphylaxis* (loss of response on repeated administration). The mechanism underlying tachyphylaxis to angiotensin II is unknown. Subcutaneous and intramuscular injections are much less potent and have a longer duration of action than do comparable doses given intravenously. Infusions that cause an immediate pressor response tend to result in tachyphylaxis over a period of several hours. On a molar basis, angiotensin II is about 40 times more potent than norepinephrine. The pressor response to angiotensin II is caused by its direct receptor-mediated effect on vascular smooth muscle. The peptide stimulates the formation of the second messenger inositol 1,4,5-triphosphate, to release intracellular Ca^{2+}, which results in smooth muscle contraction.

Heart Rate

The administration of angiotensin II to an animal with intact baroreceptor reflexes results in a reflex bradycardia. When baroreceptor reflexes are depressed (barbiturate anesthesia) or if vagal tone is inhibited (atropine or vagotomy), angiotensin induces cardiac acceleration.

Contractile Force

Angiotensin stimulates the influx of Ca^{2+} into cardiac cells and its direct inotropic actions are blocked by Ca^{2+} channel blockers. Additionally, interactions of angiotensin with the sympathoadrenal system also may contribute to the increase in myocardial contractility.

Cardiac Output

In spite of the positive chronotropic and inotropic effects produced by angiotensin II, cardiac output rarely is increased. In fact, angiotensin II may decrease cardiac output through a reflex bradycardia induced by the rise in peripheral resistance that it causes. In contrast, centrally administered angiotensin II increases both blood pressure and cardiac output.

Vascular Permeability

Angiotensin II can cause a net fluid accumulation in tissues and has been shown to increase the permeability of the endothelium in large arteries and to induce a widening of the interendothelial spaces in the aorta, coronary, mesenteric, and peripheral arteries. This response to angiotensin probably reflects the effect of elevated pressure on the endothelial permeability barrier. The peptide also stimulates the release of PGI_2 from arterial endothelial cells.

Central Nervous System

Pressor Response

The peripheral administration of angiotensin II increases arterial blood pressure. The central administration of angiotensin II into the vertebral circulation increases peripheral blood pressure. This hypertensive action, mediated by the central nervous system, is primarily the result of an increase in central efferent sympathetic activity to the periphery. The area postrema of the caudal medulla appears to be the structure responsible for the central cardiovascular actions of angiotensin II.

Dipsogenic Response

Angiotensin II produces changes in body hydration and thirst by a direct action in the central nervous system. The administration of angiotensin II into the septal, anterior hypothalamic, and medial preoptic areas stimulates drinking behavior in several species. Part of the volume response also may be caused by antinatriuretic and antidiuretic effects of angiotensin.

Endocrine Response

Angiotensin II, administered into the central nervous system, increases the release of luteinizing hormone, adrenocortical hormone, thyroid-releasing hormone, β-endorphin, vasopressin, and oxytocin from the anterior pituitary. In contrast, centrally administered angiotensin II inhibits the release of anterior pituitary growth hormone and prolactin.

Sympathetic Nervous System

Angiotensin, acting at presynaptic receptors of the nerve terminal, potentiates the release of norepinephrine during low-frequency sympathetic nerve stimulation. Aside from its action on nerve terminals of postganglionic sympathetic neurons, angiotensin also directly stimulates sympathetic ganglia and the adrenal medulla.

Adrenal Cortex and Aldosterone Secretion

Angiotensin II stimulates aldosterone synthesis. The aldosterone secretion induced by angiotensin II in humans is not accompanied by an increase in glucocorticoid plasma levels. Chronic administration of angiotensin will maintain elevated aldosterone secretion for several days to weeks unless hypokalemia ensues.

Inhibitors of the lipooxygenase pathway of amino acid metabolism prevent angiotensin II–induced aldosterone synthesis, suggesting that a lipooxygenase product is the primary mediator of this angiotensin II effect. The adrenal gland possesses all of the necessary components for synthesis of angiotensin II, suggesting that part of the angiotensin II–induced aldosterone production in the adrenal may be independent of circulating angiotensin II. Angiotensin II–induced adrenal aldosterone production is increased when plasma sodium is low or plasma potassium is high.

Clinical Uses

Angiotensin II is a potent pressor agent that will sustain an increase in arterial pressure during prolonged infusion. It has been used to increase blood pressure in hypotension; however, the use of pressor agents in shock is controversial. Although an enhanced pressor sensitivity to angiotensin II by pregnant women has been suggested as a test for the identification of subjects in whom preeclampsia and eclampsia may develop, the potential risk of precipitating a severe hypertensive response must be considered carefully.

Antagonists of the Renin-Angiotensin System

A summary of the agents that inhibit the renin-angiotensin system and their sites of action is provided in Fig. 19-3.

Renin Inhibitors

The acid protease inhibitor *pepstatin* and some transition-state peptide analogues of the amino terminal tetradecapeptide of angiotensinogen can inhibit competitively the formation of angiotensin I by human renin. Two of these compounds, enalkiren and CGP38560A, have been shown to block renin activity when given as an intravenous infusion to human subjects. Highly specific renin inhibitors may prove beneficial as antihypertensive agents or in the treatment of congestive heart failure.

Several agents that impair the effects of sympathetic nervous system stimulation (methyldopa, clonidine, and propranolol) attenuate the release of renin. Inhibitors of prostaglandin synthesis (indomethacin) inhibit renin release, especially renin release that is induced by diuretics and vasodilators.

Peptidyldipeptide Hydrolase (Converting Enzyme) Inhibitors

Several peptides isolated from the venom of the snake *Bothrops jararaca* block the effects of the renin-angiotensin system by inhibiting the conversion of angiotensin I to angiotensin II. The nonapeptide teprotide (Glu-Trp-Pro-Arg-Pro-Gln-Ile-Pro-Pro) is a potent competitive inhibitor of peptidyldipeptide hydrolase. Teprotide is an experimental agent that has an immediate onset of action after intravenous administration; it has a biological half-life of 60 to 90 min.

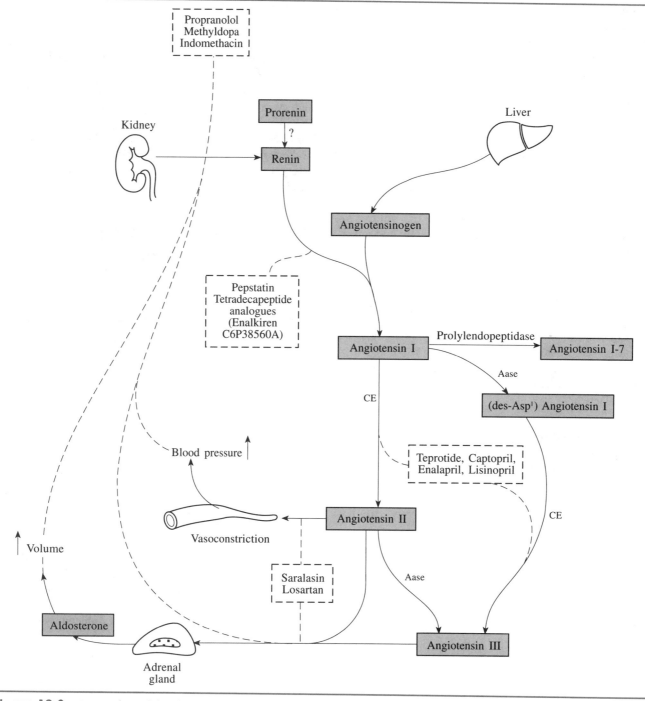

Figure 19-3. Agents that inhibit the renin-angiotensin system and points at which they act. CE = converting enzymes; Aase = aspartylaminopeptidase.

Teprotide reduces blood pressure in "renin-dependent" hypertension and is of benefit in models of congestive heart failure. The only side effect or toxicity reported for teprotide to date is a severe hypotensive response.

The orally active peptidyldipeptide hydrolase inhibitors currently prescribed differ in the form in which the drug is administered (prodrug: pentopril, quinapril, benzapril, ramipril, enalapril), and the presence of sulfhydryl groups (captopril, lisinopril) that are involved in the binding of the drug to the active site of the enzyme. The properties of the various agents are shown in Table 19-1.

Captopril

This compound (Fig. 19-4) is an orally effective inhibitor of peptidyldipeptide hydrolase. Captopril blocks the

Table 19-1. Properties of Angiotensin Converting Enzyme Inhibitors

Inhibitor (trade name)	Contains sulfhydryl groups	Form	
		Prodrug	Nonprodrug
Captopril (*Capoten*)	X		X
Quinapril (*Accupril*)		X	
Ramipril (*Altace*)		X	
Fosinopril (*Monopril*)	X		X
Benzapril (*Lotensin*)		X	
Enalapril maleate (*Vasotec*)		X	
Lisinopril (*Prinivil, Zestril*)			X

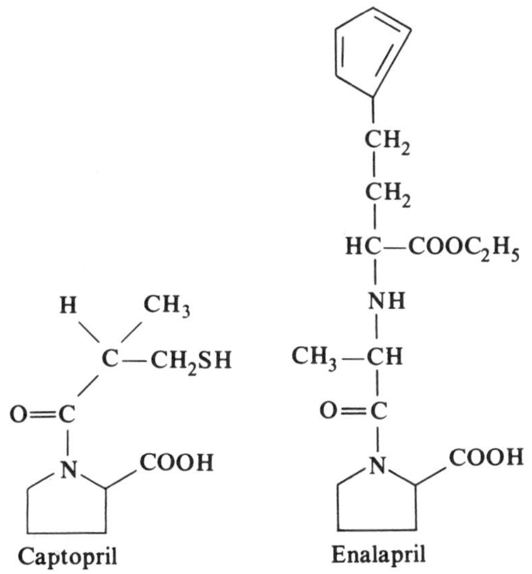

Figure 19-4. Captopril and enalapril.

blood pressure responses caused by the administration of angiotensin I. The onset of its action following oral administration is about 15 min, with peak blood levels achieved in 30 to 60 min. Its apparent biological half-life is approximately 2 hr, with the duration of its antihypertensive effects observed for 6 to 10 hr. The kidneys appear to play a major role in the inactivation of captopril.

Treatment with captopril reduces blood pressure in patients with renovascular disease and in patients with essential hypertension. The decrease in arterial pressure is related to a reduction in total peripheral resistance.

The hypotensive response to captopril is accompanied by a fall in plasma aldosterone and angiotensin II levels and an increase in plasma renin activity. There is no effect on serum potassium levels unless potassium supplements or potassium-sparing diuretics are used concomitantly; this can result in severe hyperkalemia. In response to the decrease in pressure, there is no baroreflex-associated increase in heart rate, cardiac output, or myocardial contractility, presumably because captopril decreases the sensitivity of the baroreceptor reflex. Captopril enhances cardiac output in patients with congestive heart failure by inducing a reduction in ventricular afterload and preload. Converting enzyme inhibitors have been shown to decrease the mass and wall thickness of the left ventricle in both normal and hypertrophied myocardium. These agents lack metabolic side effects and do not alter serum lipids.

Although peptidyldipeptide hydrolase is a relatively nonspecific enzyme that may have multiple endogenous substrates in addition to angiotensin I, most studies demonstrate a good correlation between the hypotensive effect of inhibitors and the blockade of the renin-angiotensin system.

Approximately 10 percent of the patients treated with captopril report the occurrence of a maculopapular rash. The appearance of the rash is dose related and often disappears when the dosage of captopril is reduced. Other common adverse effects are fever, a persistent cough, and a loss of taste that may result in anorexia. These effects are reversed when drug therapy is discontinued. More serious toxicities include a 1 percent incidence of proteinurea and glomerulonephritis; less common are leukopenia and agranulocytosis. All converting enzyme inhibitors are contraindicated in patients with bilateral renal artery disease or with unilateral renal artery disease and one kidney. Use under these circumstances may result in renal failure or a paradoxical malignant hypertension.

Captopril (*Capoten*) is available in tablets containing 25, 50, or 100 mg.

Lisinopril

Lisinopril (*Prinivil*) is an orally active inhibitor of peptidyldipeptide hydrolase. The molecule contains sulfhydryl groups that are important in binding the drug to the active site of the enzyme. Except for the decrease in cardiac output it produces, the pharmacologic effects and clinical indications for lisinopril are quite similar to those of captopril and enalapril.

Enalapril, Pentopril, Quinapril, Benzapril, and Ramipril

These orally effective inhibitors of peptidyldipeptide hydrolase are prodrug ester compounds that must be hydrolyzed in plasma to the active moiety (Table 19-1). The ester function promotes absorption of the compound from the gastrointestinal tract. In contrast to captopril, the recommended dosing interval for these prodrug compounds is once to twice daily. Otherwise, these compounds are generally similar to captopril in their mechanisms of action, side effects, and contraindications.

Angiotensin Receptor Blocking Agents

Saralasin

Sar-Arg-Val-Tyr-Val-His-Pro-Ala

The NH_2-terminal sarcosyl substitution in this analogue of angiotensin II imparts resistance to enzymatic hydrolysis by aminopeptidase and retards the rate of saralasin's dissociation from angiotensin receptors. The aliphatic amino acid alanine replaces the aromatic residue phenylalanine at the COOH terminal of the peptide. This modification has little or no effect on receptor affinity, but it markedly decreases intrinsic activity of the compound. Saralasin has been shown to be a competitive inhibitor of angiotensin receptors in a variety of tissues and species.

Due to its peptide nature, saralasin acetate (*Sarenin*) must be administered by intravenous bolus injection or by infusion. In hypertensive patients with high plasma renin activity, saralasin has a plasma half-life of 3.2 min and a pharmacological half-life of 8.2 min. As a charged peptide, saralasin does not cross the blood-brain barrier. It is distributed in the vascular space and extracellular fluid and is not selectively taken up by any tissue.

Saralasin may cause an initial increase in blood pressure followed by a decrease. The pressor response generally can be minimized by pretreatment with a diuretic, except in low-renin forms of hypertension. The pressor effects of saralasin may be mediated by an action (partial agonist properties) on vascular angiotensin receptors. Rarely, a sustained or rebound pressor response is observed following termination of the saralasin infusion. This effect is thought to result from the increase in plasma renin activity induced by saralasin and from the fact that renin has a longer plasma half-life than does saralasin.

Major side effects include severe hypotension, rebound hypertension (most often in patients with accelerated or malignant hypertension), and acute hypertension (most pronounced in patients with low-renin forms of hypertension).

Saralasin has been proposed as a diagnostic aid in the identification of angiotensin-dependent hypertension. It may have significant value in identifying surgical candidates with renovascular hypertension. Finally, this angiotensin receptor blocking agent may be useful in the hospital management of malignant hypertension and hypertensive crisis.

Recently discovered orally active nonpeptide angiotensin II receptor antagonists are a new class of potentially therapeutic drugs for the treatment of hypertension and congestive heart failure. These antagonists are imidazole compounds that are potent and selective for the angiotensin II receptor. One of these compounds, losartan, is currently in clinical trials.

Plasma Kinins (The Kallikrein-Kinin System)

History

In the 1920s and 1930s, a depressor substance was identified in several body fluids and tissues. The pancreas was a particularly rich source of this material, which was eventually given the name *kallikrein*. By the late 1930s, it was established that kallikrein had no direct agonist activity, but was an enzyme whose substrate was an inactive precursor in plasma. The product of the kallikrein reaction with plasma was identified as a polypeptide and was given the name *kallidin*. Certain venoms react with a plasma globulin to produce a second vasodilating polypeptide that has smooth muscle contractile properties when applied to the intestine in vitro. Because the contraction induced in the gut was very slow to develop, the name *bradykinin* was given to this substance. Subsequent studies led to the isolation, determination of the amino acid sequence, and synthesis of kallidin and bradykinin. These two polypeptides are known collectively as the *plasma kinins*.

Chemistry

Plasma kallikrein is an enzyme that has a molecular weight of about 100,000; it is formed from prekallikrein by an activator. The activator is stimulated by kallikrein as well as Hageman factor and plasmin. Plasma kallikrein hydrolyzes a plasma glycoprotein, known as high-molecular-weight kininogen, to yield a number of peptides. High-molecular-weight kininogen is an essential factor in the contact-mediated activation of factor XII of the intrinsic pathway for blood coagulation (see Chap. 27).

The peptides kallidin (lysyl-bradykinin) and bradykinin refer to a decapeptide and nonapeptide, respectively. These are two of probably several peptides that have been split from plasma glycoprotein substrates by a group of enzymes given the collective name kininogenases, the most prominent member of which is the alkaline esterase enzyme kallikrein. Bradykinin can be formed either directly by the action of plasma kallikrein on high-molecular-weight kininogen or by plasma and tissue aminopeptidases that can convert kallidin (decapeptide) to bradykinin (nonapeptide). The structures of these two peptides are shown below:

Kallidin
  Lys-Arg-Pro-Pro-Gly-Phe-Ser-Pro-Phe-Arg
Bradykinin
  Arg-Pro-Pro-Gly-Phe-Ser-Pro-Phe-Arg

Kallikrein also can hydrolyze proteins that are not related to kininogens. These substrates include big-renin, high-molecular-weight atriopeptin, and high-molecular-weight adrenal medullary peptide. It is not clear whether these actions of kallikrein are important functions for the enzyme.

The usual circulating levels of these two peptide kinins are quite low because the kallikrein enzymes are present largely in inactive forms, that is, prekallikreins. An additional factor in the low levels of free kinins observed in blood is their very short half-life, about 15 sec.

Two separate kallikrein molecules exist: tissue (or glandular) kallikrein and plasma kallikrein. Tissue kallikrein differs from plasma kallikrein in that it has a molecular weight of 24,000 to 44,000 and hydrolyzes both a low- and a high-molecular-weight plasma kininogen. This enzyme is activated from tissue prekallikrein by an activator. Glandular kallikrein cleaves kallidin from low-molecular-weight kininogen. Kallidin is converted to bradykinin in tissues by removal of the NH_2-terminal lysine residue by a tissue and plasma aminopeptidase. Both kallidin and bradykinin are inactivated by COOH-terminal degradation through the catalytic action of both plasma and tissue kininase I, a carboxypeptidase, and peptidyldipeptide hydrolase (angiotensin converting enzyme or kininase II). The routes for synthesis and subsequent inactivation for the plasma kinins are shown in Fig. 19-5. Numerous analogues of the plasma kinins have been synthesized and evaluated for biological activity. Several peptide analogues have been synthesized that are specific, competitive antagonists of bradykinin.

Pharmacological Actions

Kinins are potent peptides that stimulate the endothelium to release PGI_2 and endothelium-derived relaxing factor(s) that induce relaxation of arterial smooth muscle.

Figure 19-5. Two routes of synthesis and inactivation of bradykinin (see text for description).

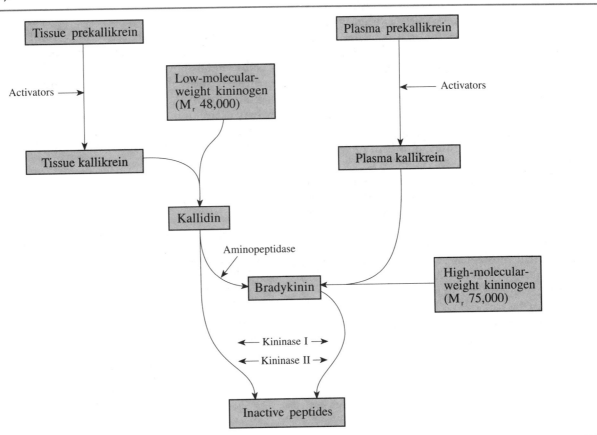

They increase blood flow to the brain, heart, viscera, skeletal muscle, and glands. The plasma kinins increase vascular permeability by increasing the size of intraendothelial junctions in small venules, thereby producing edema. In most nonvascular smooth muscle (intestine, uterus, airways), bradykinin induces a contractile response.

Kinins cause intense pain when applied to the base of a blister or superficial cut; pain also occurs when they are administered either into an artery or intraperitoneally. High doses directly stimulate autonomic ganglia and the adrenal medulla. Kinins also are considered to play a primary role in inflammation due to their release of cytokines (interleukin-1, tumor necrosis factor), as well as their ability to alter vascular permeability with subsequent production of edema.

The kallikrein-kinin system also has been shown to impinge importantly on the blood clotting system. Furthermore, in the kidney and other tissues, the kinins can activate the prostaglandin synthesizing system. The apparent coupling of the kallikrein-kinin and prostaglandin systems within the kidney is particularly intriguing, suggesting that the prostaglandins may mediate some of the actions of the kinins and modulate others. It also suggests that, at least in the kidney, the intrarenal generation of kinins may determine the local concentration and biological effects of prostaglandins, including perhaps their effects on peripheral vasculature.

The physiological significance of the tissue kallikrein-kinin system is uncertain. A role has been proposed in blood pressure homeostasis and the regulation of organ blood flow. Recent studies also have focused on the renal kallikrein-kinin system. Plasma bradykinin and angiotensin II concentrations respond in a parallel fashion to changes in posture, dietary sodium depletion, and saline loading. Urinary kallikrein is increased in conditions characterized by elevated mineralocorticoid levels; patients with Bartter's syndrome, or primary hyperaldosteronism, have high urinary kallikrein excretion.

The increased urinary kallikrein excretion in response to mineralocorticoid treatment does not occur for several days, suggesting that some other factor(s) controls renal kallikrein excretion. Urinary kallikrein levels are reduced by treatment with indomethacin, and this suggests regulation by renal prostaglandin synthesis. At present, any role of the renal or plasma kallikrein-kinin systems in salt and water excretion remains obscure.

Defects in the kallikrein-kinin system may be involved in human hypertension. Evidence comes from the observation that kallikrein excretion is low in essential hypertension and often high in patients with primary hyperaldosteronism and pheochromocytoma.

Bradykinin is a potent dilator of arterioles, but it may induce venous constriction. Intravenous administration generally causes a decreased peripheral resistance and blood pressure, an increased heart rate, and an increased cardiac output. The force of myocardial contraction also is increased. At least part of the cardiac actions of bradykinin may be secondary to a reflex activation of the sympathetic nervous system.

Involvement of kinins in inflammation, anaphylactic reactions, and shock also has been proposed. Additionally, it has been suggested that bradykinin plays a role in the adaptation of fetal circulation to extrauterine life, for example, through constriction of the umbilical artery, veins, and ductus arteriosus, and through dilation of the pulmonary artery. The neonate has been shown to be capable of synthesizing bradykinin.

Clinical Uses

At present there is no use for bradykinin or kallidin in clinical medicine. Although there is a commercially produced pancreatic kallikrein (*Padutin*), no clinical benefit has ever been demonstrated convincingly.

Inhibitors of the Kallikrein-Kinin System

Aprotinin (*Trasylol*) is an inhibitor of kallikrein that is prepared from bovine lung. It inhibits the hydrolysis of substrates by both plasma and tissue kallikreins. It has not proved to be useful in the in vivo control of the kallikrein-kinin system. Aprotinin and other protease inhibitors are very useful in in vitro studies of kallikrein.

While specific kinin receptor blocking agents do exist, there are no specific clinical indications for their use.

Supplemental Reading

Bhoola, K., et al. Bioregulation of kinins: Kallikreins, kininogens, and kininases. *Pharmacol. Rev.* 44:1, 1992.

Delabays, A., et al. Hemodynamic and humoral effects of the new renin inhibitor enalkiren in normal humans. *Hypertension* 13:941, 1989.

Fisher, J.W. *Kidney Hormones*. New York: Academic Press, 1986. Vol. 3.

Mulinari, R., et al. Bradykinin antagonism and prostaglandins in blood pressure regulation. *Hypertension* 13:960, 1989.

Peach, M.J. Renin-angiotensin system: Biochemistry and mechanisms of action. *Physiol. Rev.* 57:313, 1977.

Wong, P., et al. Angiotensin II receptor antagonists and receptor subtypes. *Trends in Medicine* 3:211, 1992.

20

Cholesterol and Hypocholesterolemic Drugs

Richard J. Cenedella

People with hyperlipidemias (especially those with high concentrations of plasma cholesterol) have more severe atherosclerosis and more frequent heart attacks than do people with normal or low plasma lipid levels (Fig. 20-1). Lowering elevated plasma cholesterol levels, specifically *low-density lipoprotein (LDL) cholesterol,* with drug treatment and diet decrease the incidence of coronary heart disease (CHD). Increasing high-density lipoprotein cholesterol by drug treatment also decreases heart attacks. Furthermore, lowering of high blood cholesterol by dietary modification and drugs may promote regression of coronary atherosclerosis.

This chapter reviews the rationale for the use of drugs in the control of plasma lipid levels and describes the drugs available for this purpose.

Lipoproteins

Hyperlipidemias (actually, hyperlipoproteinemias) can be classified into six types (Table 20-1). Each type carries a different risk factor for coronary heart disease, the etiology of each differs, and different therapeutic measures are used to treat each one.

Lipids are insoluble in aqueous systems; they must be solubilized by association with proteins to be transported in blood. The resulting complexes, *lipoproteins,* are *spherical or ellipsoid particles composed of a core of nonpolar lipid surrounded by protein and polar lipids.* Lipoproteins differ from one another in size, shape, and in the type and amount of protein and lipid they contain. Blood plasma lipoproteins are classified as chylomicrons, β-lipoproteins, pre–β-lipoproteins, or α-lipoproteins (Fig. 20-2). Chylomicrons and pre–β-lipoproteins play important roles in the transport of cholesterol and triglyceride. Alpha, or high-density, lipoproteins (HDLs), contain lower concentrations of cholesterol and triglyceride than the other lipoproteins but are very important for lipid transport.

Chylomicrons, the least dense of the lipoproteins, are composed almost entirely of triglyceride derived from the diet (Table 20-2). Chylomicrons are produced in the intestines and gain access to the systemic circulation through the lymphatics; their triglycerides are hydrolyzed through the action of lipoprotein lipase, an enzyme located at the endothelial surface of capillary blood vessels (Fig. 20-3). A chylomicron remnant is the end product of chylomicron degradation in the circulation. This particle possesses specific surface proteins, apoproteins B-48 and E; apoprotein E is recognized by receptors on liver plasma membranes. The remnant particles, rich in cholesterol of dietary origin, are bound and internalized and then degraded by lysosomal enzymes. By this process, cholesterol of dietary origin is delivered to the liver.

Very low density lipoproteins (VLDLs) are the second lowest density class of lipoproteins and are synonymous with pre–β-lipoproteins. VLDLs are derived mainly from the liver and function to transport triglyceride manufactured in this tissue. VLDLs also transport significant amounts of cholesterol derived from synthesis de novo and, indirectly, from the diet. Triglycerides of VLDLs, like those of chylomicrons, are degraded by lipoprotein lipase (see Fig. 20-3). A VLDL remnant or IDL (*intermediate-density lipoprotein*) remains after removal of much of the triglyceride. This particle is enriched with specific proteins (apoproteins B-100 and E). IDL is either directly removed from the circulation by interaction with the hepatic apoprotein B/E receptor or is converted to LDL. The conversion of IDL to LDL involves removal of triglyceride and apoprotein E, and apparently occurs at the surface of hepatocytes through the action of the enzyme hepatic lipase. A defect in the E apoproteins of human

VLDLs results in the accumulation of an atherogenic VLDL remnant (β-VLDL), type III hyperlipoproteinemia (see Table 20-1).

Low-density lipoprotein retains most of the cholesterol and apoprotein B-100 originally present in VLDLs, and thus it is enriched with both cholesterol and apoprotein B-100. LDL is removed from the circulation through binding with plasma membrane B-100/E receptor (the LDL receptor) in the liver and extrahepatic tissues (see Fig. 20-3). Most appears to be removed by the liver. The cholesterol in LDL is delivered to these tissues, where it suppresses the cellular synthesis of new cholesterol molecules. A deficiency of LDL receptor activity results in type IIa hypercholesterolemia (also termed *familial hypercholesterolemia*). This is perhaps the most common serious genetic disorder in humans.

The precursors of HDLs (nascent HDL) are produced by the liver and converted to mature HDL in the circulation as a consequence of acquiring cholesterol ester and apoproteins from other lipoproteins. HDL plays a role in the metabolism of chylomicrons and VLDL, and also could be important for transport of cholesterol out of peripheral tissues (including arteries) to the liver for disposal (Fig. 20-4). In fact, this *reverse cholesterol transport could be the basis of the inverse correlation between coronary heart disease and plasma HDL levels.* Having very high levels of HDL (upper 95th percentile) is positively correlated with longevity. A plasma HDL cholesterol level below 35 mg/dl is considered low.

In the postabsorptive state, essentially all of the triglyceride and cholesterol in the circulation have entered the blood plasma from the liver as part of a VLDL particle. The triglyceride of a typical VLDL particle is removed from the circulation by the extrahepatic tissues in an average time of 2 to 3 hr or less. In the normal state, most of the circulating triglyceride is present in VLDLs and, be-

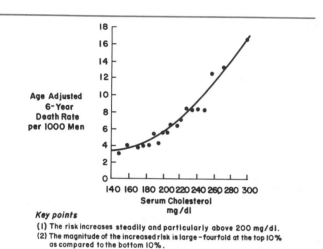

Figure 20-1. Relationship of serum cholesterol to deaths from coronary heart disease in 361,662 men aged 35-37 years during an average follow-up period of 6 years. Each point represents the median value for 5 percent of the population. (From *Report of the Expert Panel on Detection, Evaluation and Treatment of High Blood Cholesterol in Adults.* NIH Publication No. 88-2925, 1988.)

Table 20-1. Classification of Hyperlipoproteinemias

Type	Lipoprotein increased	Main plasma lipids increased	Classification	Incidence	Relationship to increased CHD[a]
I	Chylomicrons	Triglyceride	Familial (exogenous) hypertriglyceridemia (lipoprotein lipase deficiency)	1:10	None
IIa	LDL	Cholesterol	Familial hypercholesterolemia (LDL receptor defects)	1:500	Positive
			Multifactorial hypercholesterolemia	1:4[a]	
IIb	LDL + VLDL	Cholesterol and triglyceride	Familial multiple-type or combined hyperlipoproteinemia	1:300	Positive
III	VLDL (IDL)	Cholesterol and triglyceride	Familial dysbetalipoproteinemia	?	Positive
IV	VLDL	Triglyceride	Familial (endogenous) hypertriglyceridemia	1:500	Questionable[b]
V	VLDL and chylomicrons	Triglyceride	Mixed hypertriglyceride	?	Questionable

Key: CHD = coronary heart disease; LDL = low-density lipoprotein; VLDL = very low density lipoprotein; IDL = intermediate-density lipoprotein.
[a]Over one fourth of middle-aged Americans are estimated to have plasma cholesterol levels above 240 mg/dl.
[b]High triglyceride when coupled with low plasma concentration of high-density lipoprotein is associated with premature coronary heart disease.

cause of the much slower plasma clearance of LDL (days), most of the cholesterol is found in LDL.

Hyperlipoproteinemias

Hyperlipoproteinemia means an abnormally high concentration of lipoproteins in the plasma. *Hyperlipidemia* is a more general term designating high levels of plasma lipids. Elevated concentrations of plasma cholesterol or cholesterol plus triglycerides can be associated with enhanced development of atherosclerosis and increased risk of heart disease. A plasma cholesterol level between 200 and 239 mg/dl is considered to be borderline-high and above 240 mg/dl is high.

In selecting a dietary or drug therapy for a patient with high plasma cholesterol or triglyceride levels, it is essential to know the identity of the lipoprotein fraction transporting the lipid. For example, a hypertriglyceridemia due to high levels of chylomicrons is treated very differently from that due to high concentrations of VLDL. Six different hyperlipoproteinemias are recognized (see Table 20-1).

An individual's tendency toward development of a given hyperlipoproteinemia depends in part on his or her genetic background and nutritional status. For example, type IV hyperlipoproteinemia may be a genetically linked condition that could be brought into clinical expression by excessive caloric intake, often to the point of obesity, or excessive alcohol consumption. Type IIa hypercholesterolemia is usually familial, and when the disorder is genetically determined, the clinical manifestations appear early in life, with a tremendous increase in risk of myocardial infarction before age 50. In fact, type IIa homozygous individuals rarely survive beyond the second decade.

Although six well-characterized classes of hyperlipoproteinemias are identified, the great majority of patients treated with drugs for hyperlipidemia are, paradoxically, not well described by one of these specific classes. Over one fourth of all middle-aged Americans are estimated to possess a plasma total cholesterol level above 240 mg/dl. This elevation of cholesterol, pervasive in western society, is due to many factors (dietary, lifestyle, and genetic) and can be identified as multifactorial hypercholesterolemia. *The typical American diet, which is high in animal fats and calories, can aggravate a genetic predisposition to any one of the hyperlipoproteinemias.*

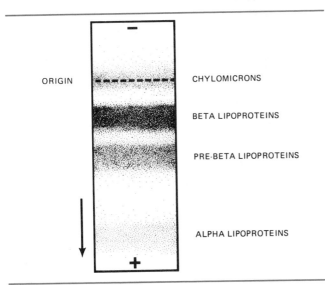

Figure 20-2. Electrophoretic separation of plasma lipoproteins. When a sample of blood plasma is placed at the origin and the preparation is developed in the direction of the arrow, the various lipoproteins will migrate at different rates, owing mainly to differences in net charge on their protein moieties. Chylomicrons, if present, remain at the origin; α-lipoproteins (HDLs, high-density lipoproteins) migrate most rapidly; β- and pre–B-lipoproteins (LDLs, low-density lipoproteins; and VLDLs, very low density lipoproteins) migrate at rates that are intermediate between those of chylomicrons and α-lipoproteins.

Table 20-2. Description of Plasma Lipoproteins

| Lipoprotein identity* | | | Lipid content (% by wt) | | |
By electrophoresis	By ultracentrifugation	Approx. size (diameter Å)	Total cholesterol	Total triglyceride	Site of origin
Chylomicrons	Chylomicrons	800–2,000	3	90	Small intestines
Pre-β	Very low density (VLDL)	300–900	16	55	Liver
β	Low density (LDL)	200	60	9	Membrane surface of liver cells (?)
α	High density (HDL)	70–100	17	8	Liver

*Intermediate-density lipoproteins (IDLs) are formed during the conversion of VLDLs to LDLs but normally do not accumulate in plasma. They possess electrophoretic mobility, density, and chemical composition intermediate between those of VLDLs and LDLs.

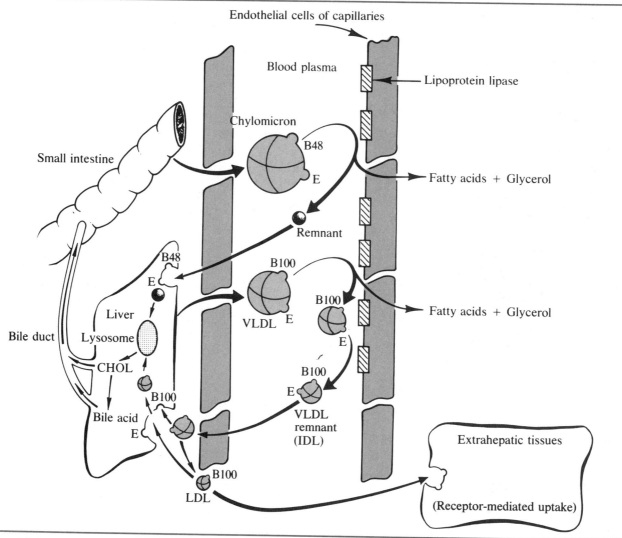

Figure 20-3. Partial summary of lipoprotein metabolism in humans. CHOL = cholesterol; IDL = intermediate-density lipoprotein.

Regulation of Plasma Lipid Levels: Basic Concepts

The concentration of a lipid present in blood plasma at any moment depends on both the transporting lipoprotein's rate of entry into the circulation and its rate of removal or clearance from the circulation. Thus, *any treatment that lowers the plasma concentration of a lipid must do so either by decreasing the input of the lipoprotein into plasma or by increasing its rate of removal from the plasma.*

The rate at which cholesterol and triglyceride enter the circulation from the liver and small intestines depends on the supply of the lipids and proteins necessary to form the lipoprotein complexes. Although the proteins must be synthesized, the lipids can be derived either from the diet or from biosynthesis de novo in these tissues. Obviously, then, *dietary manipulation can decrease the availability of lipids,* and drugs that decrease the biosynthesis of lipids or the protein components of lipoproteins (apoproteins) can decrease the input of lipoproteins into the circulation (Fig. 20-5).

Secretion of lipoproteins by the liver and small intestines also can be influenced by factors that interfere with the actual assembly of lipid and protein into a lipoprotein particle. Stimulation of the activity of lipoprotein lipase could result in an increased rate of removal both of chylomicrons and VLDL-triglycerides from the circulation. *Factors that promote catabolism and excretion of cholesterol from the body or enhance clearance of the LDL particles from the cir-*

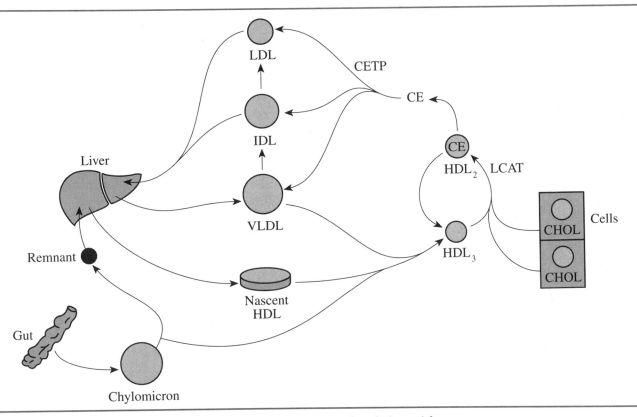

Figure 20-4. HDL metabolism. HDL_3 = HDL fraction that accepts free cholesterol from cell plasma membranes; HDL_2 = the larger HDL particle, which donates cholesterol ester to other lipoproteins; LCAT = lecithin-cholesterol acyltransferase. This enzyme esterifies the free cholesterol in HDL_3. CE = cholesterol ester; CETP = cholesterol ester transfer protein, which transfers cholesterol from HDL_2 to other lipoproteins for eventual removal by the liver.

culation could contribute to a reduction in plasma cholesterol. In particular, factors that decrease the hepatic content of cholesterol can cause increased formation of LDL receptors by the liver, and this will result in increased removal of LDL from blood.

Diet Versus Drugs

The control of plasma lipid levels is indeed complex, and the ways by which dietary modification and drug therapy result in lowered lipid concentrations are incompletely understood. Most hyperlipoproteinemias can be reduced by strict control of diet; however, the extent of reduction will depend on the specific condition being treated. A period of at least 6 months is usually reserved for evaluating the effect of diet, and *drug therapy should begin only if the dietary approach is found inadequate.* Continuation of dietary therapy along with the drug is essential, since the combined effects of both forms of therapy are additive. The use of drugs to treat hyperlipoproteinemias should always be approached and conducted with caution,

since this therapy can involve lifelong administration of drugs whose long-term effects are poorly understood.

Reduction of body weight in most individuals is accompanied by a lowering of the concentration of plasma lipids. Caloric restriction is probably the single most important aspect of dietary therapy. As a general rule, a *weight-controlling diet that is low in cholesterol and fats should decrease lipid levels to nearly normal values in most cases of moderate hyperlipoproteinemia.* The importance of dietary cholesterol intake in controlling plasma cholesterol levels can vary greatly among individuals.

Diets that are high in saturated fats increase plasma cholesterol levels, whereas polyunsaturated fatty acids have the opposite effect. Polyunsaturated fatty acids could increase conversion of free cholesterol in liver cells to inert cholesterol ester. A decrease in hepatic free cholesterol (the metabolically active form of cholesterol) leads to increased LDL receptor synthesis and, therefore, to decreased plasma LDL levels.

There is recent interest in the ability of dietary polyunsaturated fatty acids (PUFA) of fish oil (the omega-3 PUFA) to decrease the incidence of heart attacks by inhibiting platelet functions. Consuming fish oil also mark-

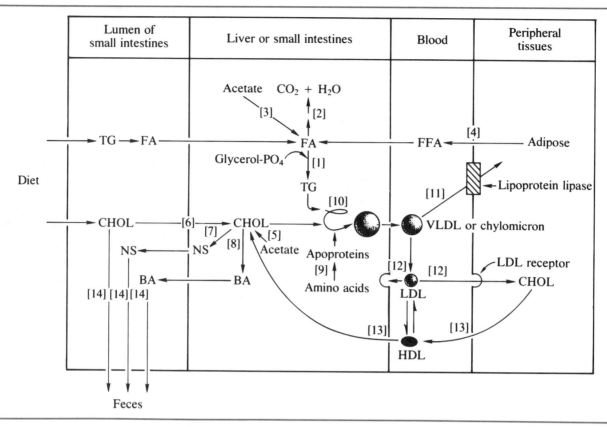

Figure 20-5. Some potential sites of action of hypolipidemic drugs. TG = triglyceride; CHOL = cholesterol; FA = fatty acid; FFA = free fatty acid; NS = neutral sterol; BA = bile acid. Hypolipidemic drugs have been suggested to reduce plasma lipoprotein concentrations by (1) direct inhibition of triglyceride synthesis; (2) reducing the supply of fatty acids for triglyceride synthesis by stimulating fatty acid catabolism; (3) reducing the supply of fatty acids for triglyceride synthesis by inhibiting synthesis de novo of fatty acids; (4) reducing the supply of fatty acids for triglyceride synthesis by decreasing the release of free fatty acids from adipose tissue; (5) direct inhibition of cholesterol synthesis de novo; (6) inhibition of intestinal absorption of cholesterol; (7) stimulation of cholesterol catabolism to neutral sterols; (8) stimulation of cholesterol catabolism to bile acids; (9) direct inhibition of the synthesis of apoproteins; (10) inhibition of assembly of the lipoprotein particles; (11) stimulation of lipoprotein lipase activity, which increases the rate of clearance from plasma of triglyceride-rich lipoproteins; (12) stimulation of receptor-mediated uptake of LDL particles by the liver and peripheral tissues; (13) increasing circulating HDL levels, which can result in increased removal of cholesterol from peripheral tissues and the blood; and (14) stimulation of the excretion of cholesterol, neutral sterols, or bile acids in the feces.

edly lowers plasma triglyceride levels in type IV hyperlipoproteinemia.

Special attention is given to restricting alcohol and carbohydrate intake in individuals with type IV disorder since excessive consumption of these substances can lead to increased VLDL-triglyceride production.

Treatment of an individual with type I disease demands dietary modification, since drugs are ineffective in this condition. Type I hyperlipoproteinemia is characterized by the presence of high concentrations of chylomicrons in the postabsorptive state. Triglyceride levels exceed 1,000 mg/dl plasma. Clearance of chylomicrons is impaired in this condition, apparently owing to a genetic abnormality of lipoprotein lipase.

Hypolipidemic Drugs

The individual drugs available to reduce the concentrations of plasma lipids generally decrease either the level of cholesterol or of triglycerides, but not both; that is, they affect either the circulating levels of LDL or VLDL. Niacin (nicotinic acid) is an exception in that it reliably reduces both classes of lipoproteins. Drugs can be recommended for treatment of patients when the plasma LDL cholesterol rises above 160 mg/dl (equivalent to 240 mg/dl total cholesterol). The goal is to reduce LDL cholesterol to below 130 mg/dl. Guidelines for initiating drug therapy are outlined in Table 20-3, and an overview of the drugs and their use is presented in Table 20-4.

Before initiation of drug treatment for a hyperlipidemia, one must be certain that the elevation of plasma lipid is directly due to a problem in lipid metabolism and not the consequence of other pathology, such as diabetes mellitus, hypothyroidism, or alcoholism. Therapy should be initiated with the minimum effective dosage to limit side effects.

Table 20-3. Treatment Guidelines for Patients with Hypercholesterolemia

Treatment guidelines	LDL cholesterol[a]	
	Initiation level (mg/dl)	Minimal goal (mg/dl)
Dietary treatment		
Without CHD or two other risk factors[b]	≥160	<160[c]
With CHD or two other risk factors[b]	≥130	<130[d]
Drug treatment		
Without CHD or two other risk factors[b]	≥190	<160
With CHD or two other risk factors[b]	≥160	<130

Key: LDL = low-density lipoproteins; CHD-coronary heart disease.
[a]Classification: <130 mg/dl = desirable LDL cholesterol level; 130–159 mg/dl = borderline-high–risk LDL cholesterol; >160 mg/dl = high-risk LDL cholesterol.
[b]Patients have a lower initiation level and goal if they are at high risk because they already have definite CHD, or because they have any two of the following factors: male sex, family history of premature CHD, cigarette smoking, hypertension, low high-density lipoprotein (HDL) cholesterol, diabetes mellitus, definite cerebrovascular or peripheral vascular disease, or severe obesity.
[c]Roughly equivalent to total cholesterol level of <240 mg/dl.
[d]Roughly equivalent to total cholesterol level of <200 mg/dl.
Source: Adapted from *Arch. Intern. Med.* 148:36, 1988, with permission.

Drugs for Reduction of Plasma Cholesterol

Cholestyramine, lovastatin, colestipol, niacin, and probucol are the principal drugs now available.

Cholestyramine

Cholestyramine is a quaternary ammonium exchange resin that, in the chloride form, exchanges chloride for other anions. One gram of the drug can bind about 100 mg bile salts. Long-term use of cholestyramine has been shown to reduce fatal heart attacks by about 20 percent.

Mechanism of Action

After oral ingestion, cholestyramine remains in the gastrointestinal tract, where it readily exchanges chloride ions for bile salts in the small intestine and markedly increases excretion of the salts in the feces. The decreased

Table 20-4. Summary of Major Hypolipidemic Drugs

Drug	Reduced CHD risk	Principal use	Hyperlipidemia type treated	Special precautions
Bile acid Sequestrants	Yes	Reduction of LDL	IIa	Can alter absorption of other drugs; can increase triglyceride levels and should not be used in patients with hypertriglyceridemia
Gemfibrozil	Yes	Reduction of VLDL and IDL (raises HDL)	IV, V, and III	May increase LDL cholesterol in hypertriglyceridemic patients; should not be used by patients with gallbladder disease
Nicotinic acid	Yes	Reduction of VLDL and LDL	IIb, IIa, IV, and V	Test for hyperuricemia, hyperglycemia, and liver function abnormalities
Probucol	Unknown	Reduction of LDL	IIa	Lowers HDL cholesterol, although the significance of this has not been established; prolongs QT interval
Vastatins	Unknown	Reduction of LDL	IIa	Monitor for liver function abnormalities, and possible lens capacities

Source adapted from *Arch. Intern. Med.* 148:36, 1988, with permission.

concentration of bile acids returning to the liver lowers the feedback inhibition of 7-α-hydroxylase, the rate-limiting enzyme in the conversion of cholesterol to bile acids, and results in increased breakdown of hepatic cholesterol. This increased catabolism of cholesterol leads to increased activity of hepatic 3-hydroxy-3-methylglutaryl CoA (HMG CoA) reductase, the rate-limiting enzyme in cholesterol biosynthesis. In most individuals, the increased synthesis of cholesterol is presumably insufficient to compensate for the increased catabolism, and cellular cholesterol levels decrease. The decrease in cholesterol leads to increased removal of LDL particles from the circulation. Thus, *cholestyramine ultimately lowers plasma levels of LDLs by stimulating their receptor-mediated catabolism.*

Absorption, Metabolism, and Excretion

Because cholestyramine is insoluble in water and has a molecular weight of over 1 million, it is neither absorbed from the intestines following an oral dose nor metabolically altered in its passage through the intestines. Thus, its effects on tissue biochemistry must be secondary to its ability to promote bile acid loss from the body. For this reason and because of its low toxicity, cholestyramine is often combined with other hypocholesterolemic drugs to treat severe hypercholesterolemias.

Clinical Uses

Cholestyramine is effective and safe for the treatment of type IIa hypercholesterolemia. Plasma cholesterol levels are routinely decreased by 20 to 25 percent, and skin xanthomas may disappear if they are present. Enhanced response of type IIa individuals to cholestyramine has been obtained by combining this therapy with niacin. Unfortunately, cholestyramine has little effect on plasma cholesterol levels of the homozygous form of familial type IIa hypercholesterolemia, a condition that is often fatal in childhood. These individuals totally lack functional LDL receptors on cell membranes. Because of the propensity to elevate VLDLs, cholestyramine is not recommended for treatment of hypercholesterolemias associated with elevated concentrations of VLDLs (types IV and V). If a patient's plasma triglyceride level is above 250 mg/dl, bile acid sequestrants should not be given.

Adverse Reactions

Cholestyramine is generally well tolerated, and most side effects are minor. The most frequent complaint is constipation. In older patients, and particularly those with heart disease, routine use of a laxative, such as psyllium, is often recommended. No significant increase in gallstones or cholecystectomy has been identified with its use.

Because cholestyramine can bind many anions, a mild steatorrhea can develop as a result of increased fecal excretion of long-chain fatty acids. Also, impaired intestinal absorption of fat-soluble vitamins (particularly A, D, and K) can occur with use of larger doses.

Drug Interactions

Cholestyramine can decrease or delay the intestinal absorption of digitoxin, phenobarbital, chlorothiazide, phenylbutazone, warfarin, flufenamic acid, mefenamic acid, and the tetracyclines. Other drugs should always be taken at least 1 hr before, or 4 to 6 hr after, cholestyramine.

Preparations and Dosage

Cholestyramine resin (*Questran*) is given orally in two or four divided doses before meals. The drug must be mixed in a fruit juice or other beverage before use. A "candy bar" formulation (*Cholybar*) may increase patient compliance.

Colestipol

Colestipol hydrochloride (*Colestid*) is a high-molecular-weight anion exchange resin that is very similar to cholestyramine in efficacy, mechanism of action, and toxicity. Colestipol decreases plasma cholesterol (but not triglyceride) levels through its ability to bind intestinal bile acids and increase their excretion in the feces. This anion exchange resin is given orally in the form of water-insoluble beads at a dose of 12 to 25 gm per day in three or four divided doses. Colestipol is not absorbed from the gastrointestinal tract. Side effects are mainly gastrointestinal distress. Colestipol, like cholestyramine, should not be ingested simultaneously with other drugs.

Niacin

Niacin, or nicotinic acid (Fig. 20-6), lowers both plasma cholesterol and triglyceride levels. The hypolipidemic properties of niacin are separate from its vitamin activity and are seen only at doses much higher than those used for vitamin supplementation.

Mechanism of Action

The hypolipidemic effects of niacin are due to the decreased hepatic secretion of VLDLs that results from a reduction of triglyceride synthesis. Since LDL, the choles-

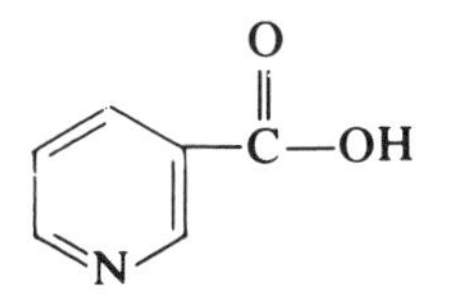

Figure 20-6. Niacin (nicotinic acid).

terol-rich lipoprotein, is derived from VLDLs, a reduction of plasma VLDL concentration can lead to a decrease in circulating levels of LDL and thus of cholesterol. In fact, *plasma triglyceride levels decrease within a few hours after a patient is given niacin, whereas reduction of cholesterol levels is seen only after several days of therapy.*

The ability of niacin to decrease formation of triglycerides in the liver could be due to a lowering of the plasma concentration of free fatty acid. Circulating free fatty acid is derived almost totally from adipose tissue, and niacin is a potent inhibitor of lipolysis in adipose tissue. Circulating free fatty acids are a main source of the fatty acid used for synthesis of triglycerides in the liver; thus, a reduction of free fatty acid levels in plasma can decrease triglyceride synthesis.

Absorption, Metabolism, and Excretion

Niacin is readily absorbed from all parts of the intestinal tract. Peak blood levels of about 30 μg/ml are reached within about a half-hour of receiving 1 gm. Niacin is metabolized to *N*-methylniacinamide, which is further metabolized to other products, all of which are excreted in the urine. At low doses, little free niacin is excreted in the urine, but significant amounts appear at high doses.

Clinical Use

Niacin (*Nicolar*) is used effectively for the treatment of both hypercholesterolemias and hypertriglyceridemias. Therefore, it has value in the treatment of type IIb hyperlipoproteinemia, in which both VLDL and LDL are increased. Decreases of plasma cholesterol of 15 to 30 percent, and of triglyceride of up to 60 percent, are seen. A reported ability to increase HDL levels could be an added benefit of niacin, since high HDL levels are inversely correlated with coronary heart disease. Although it is most effective against hypertriglyceridemias, niacin is used to treat severe hypercholesterolemias that do not respond to cholestyramine. Also, some clinicians recommend use of niacin in combination with either clofibrate or a bile acid sequestrant. In fact, combining nicotinic acid and colestipol can promote the regression of atherosclerotic lesions.

Adverse Reactions

The most common and annoying adverse reaction is the production of an intense cutaneous flush and pruritus. This reaction develops within 1 to 2 hr after drug administration. Because of the cutaneous symptoms, patient acceptance of niacin can be poor. However, with continued use, these symptoms will disappear in most patients. The cutaneous flush may be caused by prostaglandins and can be decreased by aspirin. Gastrointestinal distress is often encountered with drug therapy, but can be decreased by taking the medication with meals and by use of antacids. More severe, but less frequent, side effects of niacin include abnormal liver function tests, decreased glucose tolerance, glycosuria, hyperuricemia, and jaundice. Niacin is contraindicated in patients with hepatic dysfunction, active peptic ulcer, or hyperuricemia. It should be used with caution in individuals with diabetes mellitus, since it can result in deterioration of blood glucose control in non–insulin-dependent patients.

Lovastatin

Lovastatin (Fig. 20-7) is a potent competitive inhibitor of the rate-controlling enzyme in cholesterol biosynthesis, *HMG CoA reductase*. It is one of several HMG CoA reductase inhibitors, broadly called vastatins, currently available. Because of similarities in action and effectiveness, the newer vastatins (pravastatin and simvastatin) are not discussed separately.

Mechanism of Action

By inhibiting cholesterol synthesis in the liver, lovastatin decreases the cellular concentration of cholesterol, which leads to an increased synthesis of hepatic LDL receptors through derepression of the LDL receptor gene. This results in increased removal of LDL particles from the circulation.

Figure 20-7. Lovastatin.

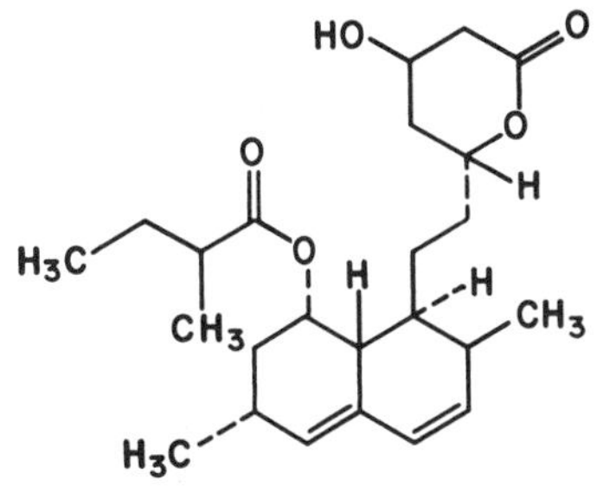

Absorption, Metabolism, and Excretion

Lovastatin is given as a lactone that is hydrolyzed in vivo to active β-hydroxyacid derivatives. About 30 percent of an oral dose is absorbed, with most of the drug cleared from blood by the liver in a single pass. Thus, lovastatin appears to concentrate in its target organ, the liver. Peak plasma levels are achieved within 2 to 4 hr of its administration, and with continued use the steady-state plasma concentration of drug reaches about 1.5 times the single dosage level. Lovastatin is metabolized by hydroxylation and excreted through the bile, with about 80 percent of an oral dose appearing in the feces; this represents drug excreted in bile as well as unabsorbed drug.

Clinical Uses

Lovastatin (*Mevacor*) is useful for treating hypercholesterolemia due to elevated LDL, particularly heterozygous familial hypercholesterolemia (type IIa). Thirty to 40 percent reductions of LDL cholesterol can be obtained. When lovastatin is used in combination with a bile acid sequestrant, LDL cholesterol levels have been decreased by 50 to 60 percent and regression of coronary atherosclerosis can occur. Lovastatin is currently the most prescribed hypolipidemic drug in the United States. Over 90 percent of patients have experienced a greater than 20 percent reduction of plasma LDL cholesterol at a dose of 40 mg twice a day.

Adverse Reactions

Lovastatin appears to produce a low incidence of acute adverse effects. Liver dysfunction has been seen in about 2 percent of patients. Myositis, inflammation of skeletal muscle marked by elevated creatine phosphokinase, can be a serious concern in about 0.5 percent of patients. The risk increases when lovastatin is used in combination with gemfibrozil.

The possibility of ocular damage with long-term use of lovastatin is a concern. The ocular lens and the cornea, unlike other tissues, must synthesize most of the cholesterol they require. Inhibition of lens cholesterol synthesis has been associated with the development of cataracts in animals. However, an increased incidence of human cataracts has not been observed to date. Because inhibition of cholesterol synthesis could be damaging during fetal and early postnatal development, lovastatin is contraindicated in pregnancy and lactation.

Probucol

Probucol (*Lorelco*) (Fig. 20-8), a bis-phenol, is lipid soluble and poorly absorbed after oral dosage. When two

Figure 20-8. Probucol.

500-mg tablets are given daily, moderate reductions in plasma cholesterol levels can be expected; however, the reductions in LDL cholesterol (15–20%) are smaller than those achieved with the bile acid-binding resins or nicotinic acid. Probucol lowers LDL levels by a unique mechanism: Treatment with probucol results in the production of a structurally altered LDL, which is more rapidly removed from the circulation than normal LDL. In spite of only a moderate effect on LDL cholesterol, probucol can produce a regression in cholesterol xanthomas. Probucol may lower HDL levels, an undesirable effect, but does not alter plasma triglycerides.

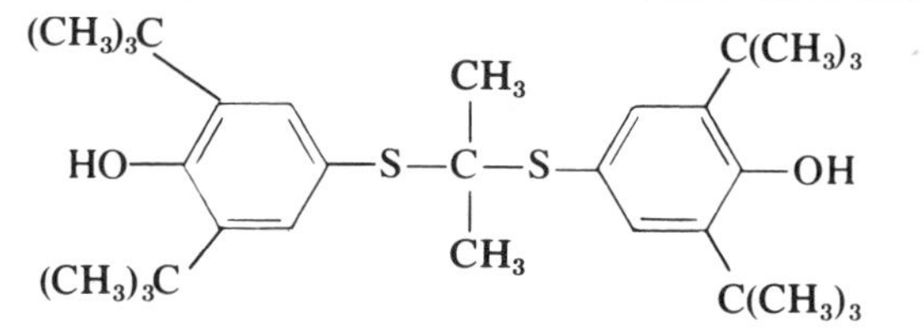

Probucol can reduce the development of aortic atherosclerotic lesions in experimental animals and appears to antagonize the oxidative modification of LDL particles that is thought to be important in the atherogenic process. Because of its high lipid solubility, several weeks are required to eliminate the drug from body fat stores after discontinuation of therapy. Probucol should be considered a second-line drug for lowering plasma cholesterol.

Probucol produces few side effects other than diarrhea, which occurs in about 10 percent of patients taking the drug.

Drugs for Reduction of Plasma Triglycerides

Niacin, described previously as a hypocholesterolemic agent, is also one of the most effective agents for lowering elevated plasma triglyceride levels due to its ability to decrease VLDL secretion by the liver. It is, therefore, particularly valuable in treating hypertriglyceridemias caused by hepatic overproduction of VLDLs.

Mild hypertriglyceridemia (<500 mg/dl), without concurrent depression of HDL cholesterol, is not a proven risk factor for coronary heart disease, and, therefore, drug therapy is not justified in this condition. Severe hypertriglyceridemia (500–1,500 mg/dl) is probably caused by an overproduction of VLDLs coupled with a defective clearance of VLDL triglyceride. If dietary therapy alone fails to adequately lower extreme levels of plasma triglycerides, drug therapy is recommended, since a high risk of pancreatitis accompanies this condition. Dietary fish oil (omega-3 PUFA) also is effective in lowering plasma triglycerides.

Moderately elevated triglyceride levels, when accompanied by low HDL cholesterol levels (<35 mg/dl), should be treated, since this blood lipid pattern appears to be associated with premature coronary heart disease. Both niacin and gemfibrozil are effective agents for reversing this pattern.

Gemfibrozil

While gemfibrozil (Fig. 20-9) has little effect on plasma LDL levels, it does appear to raise blood concentrations of HDL. This finding may account for the observation (Helsinki Heart Study) that use of gemfibrozil for 5 years decreased the incidence of heart attack by 34 percent.

Mechanism of Action

Gemfibrozil reduces blood levels of VLDL triglycerides by 35 percent or more by inhibiting VLDL production by the liver, and by enhancing the clearance of VLDLs from the circulation. The mechanism of its modest effect on plasma LDL levels is unexplained. Gemfibrozil's ability to raise HDL may be related to its stimulation of lipoprotein lipase and VLDL catabolism, since components of VLDL appear to contribute to HDL formation.

Absorption, Metabolism, and Excretion

More than 90 percent of orally administered gemfibrozil is absorbed and most of the absorbed drug is excreted unchanged in the urine. Its plasma half-life is about 1.5 hr, and peak blood levels are reached 1 to 2 hr after ingestion.

Clinical Uses

Until recently, gemfibrozil was largely used to treat hyperlipoproteinemias involving marked elevation of VLDLs, that is, in the treatment of severe hypertriglyceridemia. Because it both inhibits production of VLDL triglycerides and stimulates VLDL clearance from plasma, gemfibrozil should be of value in the treatment of type III, IV, and V hyperlipoproteinemias. It can be effective in preventing acute pancreatitis in patients with severe hypertriglyceridemia. Gemfibrozil does not have value in the treatment of type I hyperlipoproteinemia. Although gemfibrozil raises LDL levels in patients with hypertriglyceridemias, it slightly lowers LDL cholesterol (5–10%) in many patients with predominant hypercholesterolemia. *The ability of gemfibrozil to significantly reduce the incidence of heart attacks (Helsinki Heart Study) in patients with hypercholesterolemia correlated better with an increase in plasma HDL than with a decrease in LDL.*

Adverse Reactions

Gastrointestinal distress is the most frequently reported adverse reaction to the drug. Because gemfibrozil is structurally similar to drugs that increase the incidence of gallbladder disease, there has been concern over its long-term safety. However, increased gallbladder disease was not seen in the Helsinki Heart Study. The carcinogenicity of gemfibrozil is unclear.

Drug Interactions

Gemfibrozil, like clofibrate, potentiates the activity of anticoagulants. Care must be taken to reduce the dose of simultaneously administered anticoagulants, and plasma prothrombin should be measured frequently until the level is seen to stabilize.

Preparations

Gemfibrozil (*Lopid*) is available as 300-mg capsules.

Clofibrate

Chemistry

Clofibrate (Fig. 20-9) is a clear, water-insoluble liquid.

Figure 20-9. Gemfibrozil and clofibrate.

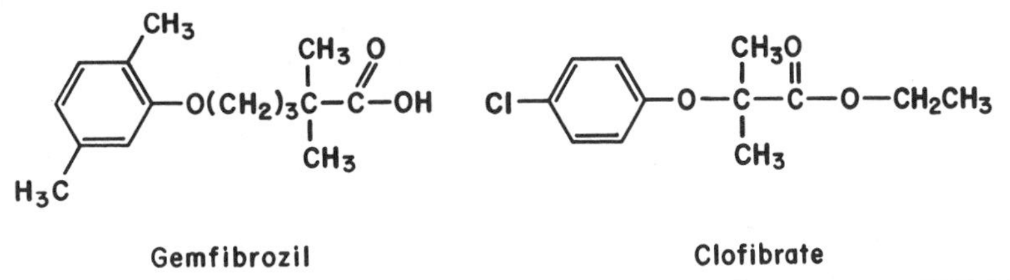

Mechanism of Action

Clofibrate can lower the plasma concentrations of both cholesterol and triglyceride. However, the effects on triglycerides are much greater and more consistently obtained. The hypotriglyceridemic effect is due to enhanced removal of VLDL triglycerides from the circulation secondary to the drug's ability to stimulate lipoprotein lipase.

Absorption, Metabolism, and Excretion

Clofibrate is well absorbed after oral dosage and is completely hydrolyzed to clofibric acid by intestinal and serum esterases. Clofibric acid binds to plasma proteins, chiefly albumin, and becomes widely distributed in body tissues. After a single oral dose of clofibrate (two 500-mg capsules), peak concentrations of 50 to 60 μg/ml plasma are reached in about 6 hr. The plasma half-life of the drug in humans is 15 to 20 hr.

Almost 100 percent of an oral dose is excreted in the urine as clofibric acid and its glucuronide conjugate. Trace amounts of clofibric acid are excreted in the bile.

Clinical Use

Clofibrate (*Atromid-S*) is useful in the treatment of hypertriglyceridemias, producing 30 to 40 percent reductions of plasma triglycerides. It is especially useful in the treatment of type III hyperlipoproteinemia, because it stimulates degradation of the β-VLDL particles that accumulate in this condition. Since these particles are also rich in cholesterol, clofibrate can significantly reduce total cholesterol levels in this hyperlipoproteinemia. However, the effects of clofibrate on the concentration of plasma cholesterol are more variable, and its usefulness in treating familial hypercholesterolemias has been limited. Paradoxically, clofibrate can increase plasma LDL cholesterol levels in some hyperlipidemias, for example, type IV. This effect apparently results from an accelerated degradation of VLDL triglyceride with a concomitant increase in LDL formation.

Adverse Reactions

The incidence of *acute* side effects from clofibrate is low and those produced are relatively mild (e.g., nausea, diarrhea, and weight gain); *chronic* toxicities may limit its usefulness. Of special concern, however, is that patients taking clofibrate have a two- or threefold increase in the incidence of gallbladder disease, possibly owing to the drug's ability to increase the concentration of cholesterol in bile. Concern over long-term use of clofibrate also comes from a large clinical trial that found a higher overall mortality in the clofibrate-treated groups. Clofibrate is reported to induce hepatic tumors in rodents and its use

may increase the risk of cancer in humans. For these reasons, clofibrate should only be used in type III hyperlipoproteinemia and in those patients with markedly elevated triglyceride levels; its use should be discontinued if a significant lowering of lipids is not obtained.

Drug Interactions

Clofibrate, like gemfibrozil, potentiates the anticoagulant activity of the coumarin anticoagulants by displacing them from their binding sites on plasma proteins. When administered with clofibrate, the dose of anticoagulant must be reduced by one-third to one-half and prothrombin should be measured frequently.

Combination Therapy

Although therapy of a hyperlipoproteinemia is usually begun with one drug, combinations of two drugs are often necessary to achieve a significant reduction in plasma lipids (15% or more reduction of LDL cholesterol and 30% or greater reduction of triglyceride levels). Drug combinations are routinely required for the treatment of heterozygous familial hypercholesterolemia (type IIa).

The objective of therapy is to decrease the production of LDL and to simultaneously increase removal of LDL from plasma. Niacin combined with cholestyramine or colestipol is an effective drug treatment of familial hypercholesterolemia. Niacin decreases VLDLs (and, therefore, eventually LDL production) while the bile acid-binding drug increases LDL receptors (and thus plasma clearance). LDL levels can be decreased by 55 percent with this combination.

For patients who are intolerant to nicotinic acid, the combination of lovastatin with a bile acid-sequestering agent has also produced a 50 percent or greater reduction in plasma LDL cholesterol. For patients who are intolerant to bile acid sequestrants and require multiple drug therapy, lovastatin and nicotinic acid can be combined. Triple therapy with colestipol, lovastatin, and nicotinic acid has produced 60 percent decreases of LDL cholesterol in heterozygous familial hypercholesterolemia.

Familial combined hyperlipidemia (type IIb), which involves elevation of both VLDLs and LDLs, can also be treated effectively with a combination of niacin with a bile acid-binding resin or lovastatin. Hypertriglyceridemias due to elevation of VLDLs (types IV and V) could be treated by the combined use of drugs that decrease the formation of VLDLs (niacin) and enhance removal of VLDLs from the circulation (clofibrate or gemfibrozil). Of course, use of drugs to control hypertriglyceridemia is warranted only if the plasma triglyceride levels are extremely high, that is, over 500 or perhaps even 1,000 mg/dl plasma.

Dysbetalipoproteinemia arises from a problem in the metabolism of VLDLs to LDLs and involves the accumulation of atherogenic β-VLDL particles. Drug therapy of this condition usually involves use of a single agent, either gemfibrozil or clofibrate, to increase lipoprotein lipase activity and thereby stimulate conversion of VLDLs to LDLs.

Summary

Lowering elevated plasma levels of LDL cholesterol and raising HDL cholesterol significantly reduce the incidence of heart attacks and decrease the progression of coronary atherosclerosis. Even partial reversal of atherosclerosis has been reported. Although diet alone is often effective in controlling moderately elevated plasma cholesterol, reduction of very high levels requires use of drugs.

Hypocholesterolemia drugs, singly or in combination, can usually reduce very high LDL cholesterol levels to the normal range in most patients. However, drug therapy is generally ineffective in homozygous familial hypercholesterolemia. *Normalization of high blood cholesterol, particularly when recognized at earlier ages, should retard the progression of atherosclerosis and decrease the incidence of premature heart disease.*

Pharmacological approaches to the prevention of atherosclerotic heart disease could soon expand beyond only controlling plasma LDL cholesterol levels to also include use of drugs to directly antagonize the atherosclerotic processes (probucol) and to raise plasma levels of HDL (gemfibrozil).

Supplemental Reading

Brown, G., et al. Regression of coronary artery disease as a result of intensive lipid-lowering therapy in men with high levels of apolipoprotein B. *N. Engl. J. Med.* 323:1289, 1990.

Grundy, S.M. Cholesterol and coronary heart disease, future directions. *J.A.M.A.* 264:3053, 1990.

Illingworth, D.R., and Bacon, S. Treatment of heterozygous familial hypercholesterolemia with lipid lowering drugs. *Atherosclerosis* 9 (Suppl.):121, 1989.

Kane, J.P., et al. Regression of coronary atherosclerosis during treatment of familial hypercholesterolemia with combined drug regimens. *J.A.M.A.* 264:3007, 1990.

Kichura, G.M., and Cohen, J.D. Guidelines for the use of cholesterol-lowering drugs. *Drug Ther.* 21:17, 1991.

Manninen, V., et al. Lipid alteration and decline in the incidence of coronary heart disease in the Helsinki Heart Study. *J.A.M.A.* 260:641, 1988.

Report of the Expert Panel on Detection, Evaluation and Treatment of High Blood Cholesterol in Adults. NIH Publication No. 88-2925, 1988.

Pravastatin, simvastatin and lovastatin for lowering serum cholesterol concentrations. *Med. Lett. Drugs Ther.* 34:57, 1992.

21

Water, Electrolyte Metabolism, and Diuretic Drugs

William O. Berndt and *Robert E. Stitzel*

The kidneys have the vital task of preserving, within relatively narrow limits, the concentrations of ions, amino acids, glucose, and other substances present in the plasma and lymph. Most of the 180 liters (L) of water filtered daily—along with essential anions, cations, and nutrients—are reabsorbed along the nephron. Filtered wastes and substances that are actively secreted, primarily by cells of the proximal tubule, remain in a relatively small volume of water and are eliminated as urine. *It is through the development of this rapidly functioning filtration-reabsorption-secretion system that the kidney has become almost entirely responsible for the maintenance of the composition of the internal environment.* Thus, the kidney excretes wastes not because it evolved for this purpose but because it accomplishes this as part of the overall process of regulation of the internal environment. In addition, the kidneys produce erythropoietin, renin, and prostaglandins and are involved in the synthesis of 1,25-dihydroxyvitamin D.

Quantitatively, the reabsorptive function of the kidney is the most important. More than 50 percent of renal oxygen consumption is in support of sodium chloride reabsorption. Because reabsorption of the glomerular filtrate is quantitatively so important, disorders of renal function are most easily detected as abnormalities of salt and water balance.

Diuretic drugs are most commonly thought of as agents that increase the volume of urine excreted. It is important, however, to realize that these drugs do more than just increase the amount of water that is eliminated. In fact, *the therapeutic action of most clinically important diuretics is intimately involved with a change in renal electrolyte reabsorptive or secretory capacity.* Thus, diuretics, by altering the total solute content of the extracellular fluid compartment, indirectly affect water balance.

Body Water and Electrolyte Metabolism

The electrolyte concentrations of intracellular and extracellular fluids are quite dissimilar (see Table 21-1). Intracellular fluid contains about 28 times the K^+ concentration and 24 times the Mg^{2+} concentration of extracellular fluid, whereas the latter has an Na^+ concentration that is 14 times greater than the intracellular fluid. The main anions of the extracellular compartment are bicarbonate (HCO_3^-) and chloride (Cl^-), whereas the intracellular fluid is richer in phosphates and negatively charged protein molecules.

The kidneys play a major role in the maintenance of these ion distributions. The functioning unit of the kidney that performs this homeostatic function is the *nephron*. The nephron is a complex tubular structure made up of distinct structural regions and a variety of distinct cell types.

For the kidney to accomplish its homeostatic function, it must receive a large blood supply. Under resting conditions, about one fifth of the blood ejected from the left ventricle perfuses the kidneys. This means that about 650 ml of plasma flows through the kidneys each minute. Of this plasma volume, approximately 125 ml/min is filtered through the glomeruli. The remainder of the plasma circulates through the efferent arterioles to bathe the peritubular surface of the nephron tubules. Of the 125 ml of ultrafiltrate formed, an average of only 1 ml/min is excreted as urine. This volume can be increased to about 16 ml/min after ingestion of excessive amounts of fluids, or it can be reduced to about 0.3 ml/min in cases of severe and prolonged fluid deprivation. At average rates of urine

Table 21-1. Approximate Electrolyte Content of Body Fluids

Ions	Extracellular fluid (mEq/L)	Intracellular fluid (mEq/L)	Extracellular-intracellular ratio
Cations			
Sodium	140	10	14
Potassium	4.5	125	0.04
Magnesium	1.7	40	0.04
Anions			
Bicarbonate	25	10	2.5
Chloride	100	25	4.00
Phosphate	3	150	0.02
Protein	15	40	0.38

flow in humans, more than 99 percent of the liquid filtered at the glomeruli is reabsorbed by the renal tubules.

Glomerular Filtration

The filtering force in the glomerulus is the hydrostatic pressure of the blood, which depends, in turn, on the work done by the heart. All the plasma constituents, with the exception of the blood cells, large proteins, and lipids, gain access to the tubular system; that is, a virtually protein-free *ultrafiltrate* of plasma is formed. The concentration of the readily filterable substances is practically the same in the glomerular filtrate as it is in the plasma.

The endothelial cells of the glomerular capillaries are arranged in such a way that large pores, or fenestrations (up to 100 nm in diameter), exist between the cells. These pores present little barrier to the passage of low-molecular-weight substances from the plasma.

In studying glomerular permeability to macromolecular substances, a number of factors are important. The shape of the molecule as well as its size and charge must be considered. The globular hemoglobin molecule (mol wt 64,500) readily filters through the glomerular capillary wall, whereas serum albumin (mol wt 68,000), which is an elongated molecule, filters much less readily. Molecular charge on the macromolecules also seems to be important. Hence, the glomerulus discriminates with respect to both size and charge while filtering large molecules.

Tubular Reabsorption

The primary work of the kidney is to reabsorb a large variety of the plasma constituents filtered at the glomerulus. Nearly 99 percent of the filtered water and salt is reabsorbed. In addition, nearly all the filtered bicarbonate, glucose, and amino acids are returned to the plasma. Although energy is required for many of these processes, passive reabsorption also occurs. For example, much of the reabsorption of sodium is active, while much of the

chloride and all of the water are reabsorbed passively. For those substances for which reabsorption is the predominant activity, renal clearances will be less than glomerular filtration. Similarly, the fractional excretion (i.e., urinary excretory rate divided by the filtered load) of such substances will be low.

Tubular Secretion

Secretion occurs when the amount of substance in the urine is larger than can be accounted for by filtration. Hence, if the filtered load of a substance is 5 mg/min [plasma concentration (0.05 mg/ml) × glomerular filtration rate (100 ml/min)], and its urinary excretion rate is 15 mg/min, secretion has occurred. Active tubular secretion of various organic anions and cations is well established. However, it should not be concluded that because secretion has occurred, active transport was involved. Potassium, for example, is secreted, at least in part, by purely passive means; that is, potassium moves down its electrochemical gradient.

Blood Supply

The blood perfusing the kidney represents 20 percent of the cardiac output. Anatomically, the blood reaches the kidney through the renal artery, which branches from the descending aorta. After entering the kidney, the renal artery branches in such a way that each nephron becomes supplied by a single *afferent arteriole* (Fig. 21-1). The afferent arteriole, in turn, further subdivides into the numerous porous capillary loops of the *glomerulus.*

The blood vessel that leaves the glomerulus is not a vein but an arteriole, the *efferent arteriole.* It traverses to the tubule portion of the nephron, where it divides again into a capillary system that surrounds the tubules and forms their blood supply. Renal blood becomes venous blood only after passing through this second renal capillary system. *The afferent and efferent arterioles function as though they aid in the rapid transfer of material from blood into the tubular system.*

Proximal Tubule

This section of the mammalian nephron extends from the glomerulus to the descending limb of Henle's loop and can be divided into a convoluted portion and a *pars recta* or straight portion. The proximal tubule, which consists of a single layer of cuboidal cells, has, on its luminal side, a plasma membrane formed into a brush border arrangement. The peritubular side of the cells has large numbers of mitochondria near the basement membrane and a peritubular capillary in close contact. Mammalian proximal tubules have the ability, both actively and passively, to reabsorb large amounts of substances that appear in the ultrafiltrate, including amino acids, glucose, NaCl, and H_2O. The proximal tubules also secrete substances into the tubular fluid, including many organic anions and cations including drugs (e.g., penicillin and furosemide). At least three types of epithelial cells can be found lining the proximal tubule, and these different types of cells may well be related to specific characteristics and perhaps sites of drug action. The three cell types have been designated SI (nearest the glomerulus), SII, and SIII (*para recta*).

Perhaps the most striking functional characteristic of the convoluted part of the proximal tubule is isosmotic fluid reabsorption. This relatively leaky epithelium transports solute and water in the same proportions that exist in the plasma. That is, *the total solute concentration of the fluid in the proximal convoluted tubule does not change as the fluid moves toward the descending loop of Henle,* and this fluid concentration remains approximately the same as that in the plasma. This is an important consideration for an understanding of the actions of osmotic diuretics.

Loop of Henle

An abrupt disappearance of the brush border from the luminal side of the cells marks the transition from the proximal tubule to the thin descending limb of the loop of Henle. The ascending portion follows the hairpin turn of this tubule segment in the inner medullary region. The two different types of junctions found between cells of the descending loop (relatively loose junction) and the ascending loop (tight junction) probably form the ultrastructural basis for the renal countercurrent mechanism (Fig. 21-2).

The proximal tubule delivers an *isotonic* fluid to the descending limb. This limb is quite permeable to water and solutes, and the fluid in the lumen equilibrates with the interstitium by the movement of water out of the lumen and the addition of NaCl from the interstitium to the lumen. The luminal fluid becomes *hypertonic* as a result of this water loss and NaCl gain. The ascending limb is com-

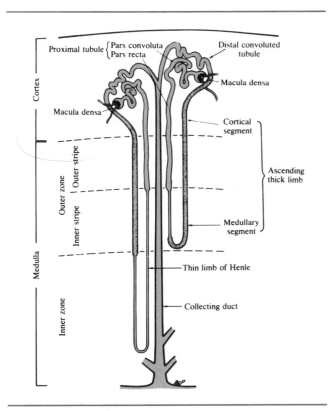

Figure 21-1. The structural organization of the mammalian kidney. (From C.C. Tisher, Anatomy of the Kidney. In B.M. Brenner and F.C. Rector, Jr. [eds.], *The Kidney* (2nd ed.) Philadelphia: Saunders, 1981.)

were variable resistors and aid in keeping glomerular filtration pressure relatively constant.

Role Of Nephron Segments In Salt and Water Balance

The tubular portion of the nephron is long and unbranched (Fig. 21-1) and consists of a single layer of epithelial cells lining the lumen. It extends from Bowman's capsule, which surrounds the glomerular capillaries in the cortical region of the kidney, through four distinct tubular segments: proximal tubule, loop of Henle, distal tubule, and collecting duct.

Bowman's Capsule

Bowman's capsule is in intimate contact with the capillary network that makes up each individual glomerulus. The walls of the capsule are continuous with the lumen of the proximal tubule. *The combination of hydrostatic pressure, the numerous pores of the glomerular endothelium, and the narrow separation between glomerulus and Bowman's capsule all*

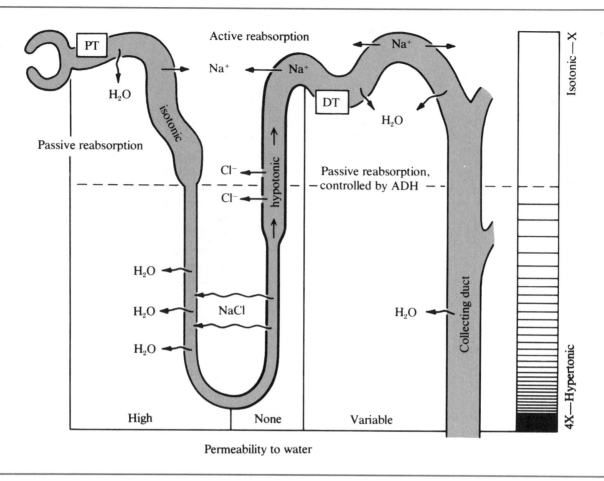

Figure 21-2. Renal countercurrent system. The increasing osmolarity observed when intratubular fluid travels from cortical to medullary regions is largely the result of the countercurrent system formed by the loop of Henle. Straight arrows represent active transport; wavy arrows represent passive transport. PT = proximal tubule; DT = distal tubule; ADH = antidiuretic hormone.

posed of a thin segment that begins near the corticomedullary junction. *Both segments of the ascending limb are relatively impermeable to water.* The thin ascending limb permits the passive equilibration of NaCl. The thick ascending limb is involved in the active transport of Cl^- out of the lumen through the mediation of the Na^+-K^+-$2Cl^-$ transporter; this ultimately results in a hypertonic fluid in the interstitium and a hypotonic fluid in the lumen.

The major portions of the proximal and distal tubules are in contact with interstitial fluid that is essentially isotonic with plasma. However, in the deeper regions of the medulla, the concentration of total solutes (mainly NaCl and urea) in the interstitial fluid rises, until a hypertonicity of approximately 1,200 mOsm is reached (3–4 times that of plasma). The active transport of Cl^- and its attendant Na^+ from lumen to interstitial fluid by the ascending loop of Henle, along with a relatively sluggish blood flow in the medullary region of the kidney (which prevents a

rapid removal of interstitial NaCl and urea), is responsible for the increasing hypertonicity of the interstitium, which occurs from the corticomedullary junction to the papilla tip.

Distal Tubule and Collecting Duct

The last 5 percent of ultrafiltrate that is going to be reabsorbed will be reabsorbed in the distal tubule and collecting duct. The tubular fluid that enters the distal tubule is *hypotonic.* In contrast to those of the previously discussed tubular segments of the nephron, the aqueous permeability characteristics of the distal and collecting duct epithelia are not constant but are hormone dependent. In the presence of the posterior pituitary hormone, antidiuretic hormone (ADH, vasopressin), the permeability of the luminal membrane increases, and water will enter both the cells and the intercellular spaces and be reabsorbed into the blood. The action of ADH is permissive; that is, it permits water to flow from the more dilute tubular fluid to the more concentrated interstitium. In the absence of ADH, these cells remain relatively impermeable to water, and there will be a marked increase in the volume of urine, of reduced osmolarity, that is voided.

At normal ADH levels, water diffuses out of the lumen of the collecting ducts as they pass through the hypertonic medullary interstitium. This water reabsorption results in the final elimination of a hypertonic urine, which is equivalent in volume to only 1 percent of the amount that was originally filtered at the glomerulus. It is important to understand that ADH levels can significantly modify the total urine volume as well as the osmolar character of that urine.

Urinary acidification and potassium secretion also occur in the late distal tubule or collecting duct, or both. The secretion of potassium is at least in part a passive event in response to the generation of an appropriate electrochemical gradient that permits K^+ to move from within the cells to the tubular fluid. The generation of the electrochemical gradient is related to sodium reabsorption, which helps explain how many natriuretic drugs also promote potassium loss.

Sodium Conservation

The volume of extracellular fluid is largely determined through the maintenance of a balance between the intake and excretion of Na^+. In the healthy individual, excessive Na^+ intake quickly initiates a complex interplay of factors, including decreased angiotensin and aldosterone formation (which promotes Na^+ loss) and increased ADH release (which promotes water retention). Excessive Na^+ loss, on the other hand, results in a reversal of the above processes.

Since Na^+ is the ion present in the highest concentration in the extracellular fluid and is, therefore, readily available for glomerular filtration, it is vital to prevent excessive urinary loss of this important ion. The cellular mechanisms responsible for sodium conservation are discussed below (Fig. 21-3).

1. *Proximal reabsorption.* Approximately two thirds of the Na^+, Cl^-, and water that is filtered is reabsorbed isosmotically by the proximal tubule cells, with reabsorption of water and Cl^- being passive physicochemical processes. Water is reabsorbed by the osmotic gradients produced by ion transport, while Cl^- reabsorption is accomplished by the electrochemical potential generated by the active transport of Na^+. In addition, Na^+ also is reabsorbed through its coupled transport with organic compounds and by a H^+-Na^+ antiport system. Further-

more, about one third of the Na^+ reabsorbed from the proximal tubule may result from passive reabsorption.

2. *NaCl and the loop of Henle.* The tubular fluid reaching the loop of Henle is still isosmotic with plasma, but it is reduced in total volume by two-thirds compared to that volume that was filtered across the glomerulus. The fluid in the descending limb of the loop of Henle passively equilibrates with the surrounding interstitium through a net water loss and net addition of solutes. The end result of water loss and *passive* Na^+ entry in this limb is that the fluid that enters the ascending limb is relatively *hypertonic* and has a high NaCl content. As mentioned previously, active transport of Cl^- out of the ascending limb occurs by an Na^+-K^+-$2Cl^-$ transporter. Exactly how this transporter functions is still debated, but electrophysiological data suggest that Cl^- movement is the primary event. The lack of concomitant water reabsorption in the ascending limb results in a *hypotonic* solution reaching the distal tubule. Although the total volume and salt content of the tubular fluid leaving the loop of Henle are not much diminished compared to that which entered, *Henle's loop has accomplished the vital function of establishing the cortex-medulla osmolar gradient that is essential for fluid reabsorption and the excretion of a concentrated urine.*

3. *Na^+-H^+ exchange.* In the proximal and distal tubules and collecting ducts, another mechanism exists for the conservation of Na^+: a coupled reabsorption of Na^+ in exchange for the secretion of H^+, that is, the Na^+-H^+ antiport system. This transfer involves no net change in electrical potential, since two positively charged ions are simply being exchanged across a membrane. No accompanying anion is necessary to maintain electrical neutrality. In addition to accomplishing Na^+ conservation, this ion exchange serves two other important homeostatic functions: (1) distal tubule urine acidification and (2) HCO_3^- reabsorption. The Na^+-H^+ exchange system appears to be located, at least in the proximal tubule, in the microvillus portion of the luminal membrane.

4. *Na^+-K^+ exchange.* A second coupled exchange system located in the distal tubule and collecting duct also exists (Fig. 21-4). This system exchanges Na^+ from the tubular fluid for K^+ found within the distal nephron cells. Since most of the filtered K^+ had been reabsorbed from the ultrafiltrate before it reached the loop of Henle, *the distal secretion of K^+, in exchange for the conservation of Na^+, is responsible for almost all the K^+ that is finally excreted.* As indicated above, it is quite likely that the K^+ secretion that occurs in this segment is, at least in part, a secondary,

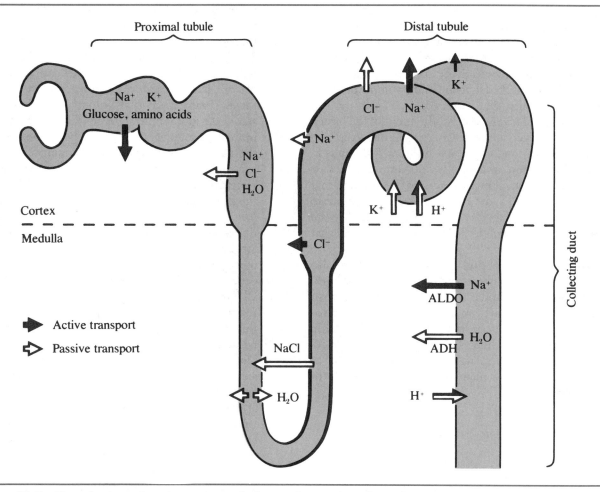

Figure 21-3. Sites of active and passive transport of solutes and water along the nephron.
ALDO = aldosterone; ADH = antidiuretic hormone.

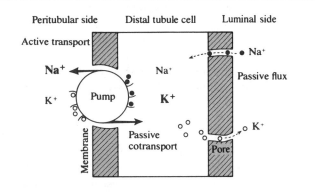

Figure 21-4. Coupled Na^+-K^+ exchange in the distal tubule cell. The dark and light circles represent Na^+ and K^+ ions, respectively. Na^+ is actively transported across the peritubular membrane of the tubular cell, whereas K^+ is passively cotransported in the opposite direction. Luminal side Na^+ can be either actively or passively transported into the distal tubule cell.

passive phenomenon, due to the transepithelial potential that is generated during the primary process, that is, active Na^+ reabsorption. Na^+ reabsorption from the lumen produces an electrical potential gradient across the tubular epithelium (lumen-negative) that permits passive K^+ movement from the cells into tubular urine. The mineralocorticoid *aldosterone* can stimulate this distal tubular reabsorption of Na^+. This exchange mechanism can be contrasted to Na^+-H^+ exchange, in which H^+ must be actively secreted into the tubular urine, often against its concentration gradient.

Potassium Regulation

Potassium is the major *intracellular* ion. It is under homeostatic control by both renal and extrarenal mechanisms. Although long-term control of K^+ balance is regulated largely by the kidneys, the response to an acute (4–6 hr) K^+ overload is largely determined in extrarenal tissues. Potassium uptake by liver and muscle cells as well as gastrointestinal secretion of K^+ are the most important of the extrarenal mechanisms involved in K^+ balance.

The renal regulation of K^+ is unusual, in that this ion undergoes *both* tubular reabsorption (proximal tubule) and secretion (distal tubule). Since the major portion (90%) of filtered K^+ is reabsorbed, the amount of K^+ excreted will ultimately depend on the following three factors: (1) serum K^+ concentration, which affects the amount filtered; (2) body Na^+ balance, which affects the amount of Na^+ reaching the distal exchange site; and (3) level of circulating aldosterone, which also influences Na^+ reabsorption and K^+ secretion.

Excessive urinary K^+ loss is an especially important clinical problem that often follows the use of several classes of diuretic drugs. Since disturbances in serum K^+ are fairly frequently observed in clinical practice, it is useful to review some of the basic processes that facilitate potassium loss.

1. The extent of Na^+ reabsorption occurring at the distal K^+ secretory site will influence K^+ secretion; this secretion rate will be *enhanced by the presence of increased amounts of Na^+* appearing in the distal tubule. Conversely, an individual placed on a low-Na^+ diet will have a reduced Na^+ delivery to the distal areas. Even though a low-Na^+ diet will stimulate aldosterone secretion, a diminution of Na^+ entering the distal tubule will reduce the exchange taking place, and thus K^+ may actually be retained under these conditions.
2. K^+ loss is increased if the Na^+ in the distal tubular fluid is accompanied by a nondiffusible anion rather than by the easily permeable Cl^- ion. The inability of a nonpermeable anion (e.g., SO_4^{2-}) to cross membranes in company with the actively transported, positively charged Na^+ ion results in the development of an electrochemical potential difference that eventually will inhibit further Na^+ transfer. Thus, if Na^+ is to be conserved under these conditions, this can only be done by stimulating cation exchange, since this type of exchange is independent of electrochemical potential differences. For example, if large amounts of the poorly diffusible anion HCO_3^- accompany Na^+ in the tubular fluid, K^+ loss will be increased. This occurs after the administration of carbonic anhydrase inhibitor diuretics.
3. Primary (e.g., adrenal tumor) or secondary (e.g., congestive heart failure, cirrhosis) hyperaldosteronism will cause a specific enhancement in distal K^+ loss. This occurrence involves a stimulation of distal Na^+ reabsorption in exchange for K^+ secretion.
4. A relatively constant 8 to 15 mEq per day of K^+

is lost through the feces. If diarrhea is present, however, considerably greater amounts of K^+ can be lost by this route. Some of the conditions that may result in hypokalemia are ulcerative colitis, pyloric obstruction, chronic laxative ingestion, tropical sprue, and severe diarrhea of any cause.

Hypokalemia

The chronic use of some diuretics may require the oral administration of potassium supplements. This is especially true for patients with congestive heart failure and cirrhosis, who are particularly sensitive to K^+ loss. The presence or absence of clinical symptoms is quite closely related to serum K^+ concentrations, and even small changes in extracellular K^+ can have marked effects. Most patients will begin to show symptoms when serum K^+ levels fall below 2.5 mEq/L (from a normal value of approximately 5 mEq/L).

Neurological symptoms include drowsiness, irritability, confusion, loss of sensation, dizziness, and coma. Other important symptoms of hypokalemia are muscular weakness, cardiac arrhythmias, tetany, respiratory arrest, and increased sensitivity of the myocardium to digitalis-like drugs.

Treatment

Treatment of hypokalemia can be accomplished by supplying exogenous K^+ through the diet, drug treatment, or both. Replacement should be gradual, with frequent evaluation of both serum K^+ concentrations and cardiac activity (ECG monitoring). K^+ supplements can be administered in several forms. Since KCl solutions have a rather bitter and unpleasant taste, this salt was formerly given as an enteric-coated tablet. However, the rapid release of KCl from the tablet after it entered the small intestine was responsible for a severe local ulceration, hemorrhage, and stenosis, especially when there was a delay in gut transit time; therefore, the enteric-coated tablet has been withdrawn.

Sugar-coated products have been marketed that contain KCl in a wax matrix (*Slow-K* and *Kaon-Cl*) and are purportedly slow- and controlled-release preparations. Available evidence indicates that these slow-release forms of KCl are occasionally capable of causing local tissue damage and, therefore, probably should be used with caution for K^+ supplementation. Solutions of potassium gluconate, like the tablets, also have been associated with intestinal ulceration. A microencapsulated KCl preparation is available (*Micro-K*) and appears to be superior to the wax-matrix formulation.

Potassium-rich foods are the easiest and most generally advised means of counteracting a K^+ deficit. Table 21-2 provides a list of foods that are suitable for K^+ supplementation.

Table 21-2. Foods Rich in Potassium (approximately 0.5-gm portion)

Prune juice (1 cup)
Orange juice (1 cup)
Grapefuit juice (1 cup)
Prunes (7)
Banana (1)
Dates (7)
Figs (4)
Raisins (½ cup)
Apricots (6)
Sweet potato (1)
White potato (1)

Table 21-3. Potassium Supplementation

Product	Manufacturer	Dosage form
Kaochlor	Adria	Liquid
Kay Ciel elixir	Berlex	Liquid
Potassium Triplex	Lilly	Liquid
KCl 10%	Purepac	Liquid
KCl 20%	Stanlabs	Liquid
K-Lor	Abbott	Powder*
K-Lyte	Mead Johnson	Tablets*

*This product, although supplied as a solid dose, is dissolved in water before ingestion.

In general, a normal diet plus about 40 mEq per day of K^+ are frequently adequate to prevent hypokalemia. If K^+-rich foods prove inadequate in replacing large quantities of the electrolyte or if the increased caloric intake that is part of the dietary supplementation is not desirable, oral *liquid* therapy is the formulation of choice. A listing of these solutions is given in Table 21-3. Although patients may find many of these products unpalatable, their further dilution with water or fruit juice can be helpful. Finally, the addition of a K^+-sparing diuretic (see below) to the therapeutic regimen may prove useful.

Hyperkalemia

Increased serum K^+ may result from excessive intake, diminished excretion, or increased cellular breakdown (necrosis or hemolysis), but most often it is due to a decrease in the renal excretion of K^+, which is caused by reduced renal perfusion. Disturbances in the functioning of the cardiovascular system (e.g., altered rhythm and excitability and depression of conductivity) and skeletal muscle system (e.g., depolarization of neuromuscular junction and decreased membrane potential) are particularly evident. Immediate, but short-term, correction of hyperkalemia may be accomplished by the infusion of sodium bicarbonate. This results in both elevated extracellular pH and Na^+, and both these conditions favor a shift of K^+

from extracellular to intracellular compartments. In the nondigitalized patient, Ca^{2+} salts can be given to antagonize the cardiac toxicity of hyperkalemia. Longer-lasting therapy may include the addition of oral sodium polystyrene sulfonate, a cation exchange resin (*Kayexalate*), to the therapeutic management. Each gram of this resin can remove approximately 30 mEq of K^+ from the body. Sodium polystyrene sulfonate is constipating, however, and should be given with a stool softener.

Uses Of Diuretics In Fluid Abnormalities

The ability of certain drugs to increase both fluid and electrolyte loss has led to their use in the clinical management of fluid and electrolyte disorders, for example, edema. Regardless of the cause of the syndrome associated with edema, the common factor is almost invariably an increased retention of Na^+. The aim of diuretic therapy is to enhance Na^+ excretion, thereby promoting a negative Na^+ balance. This net Na^+ (and fluid) loss leads to a contraction of the overexpanded extracellular fluid compartment.

Congestive Heart Failure

Diuretics may have considerable value in reducing the edema associated with congestive heart failure (CHF); however, each patient must be evaluated individually, since diuresis is not considered mandatory in all patients. Digitalis and salt restriction may be sufficient to decrease the associated symptoms of pulmonary congestion and peripheral edema. In patients who require a diuretic as adjunctive therapy, the usual drug choice should be a *benzothiadiazide* rather than one of the *loop diuretics* (e.g., bumetanide or furosemide). This is especially true in mild forms of CHF. The more efficacious compounds probably should be reserved for those who fail to respond to one of the thiazides. A K^+-sparing diuretic also can be given with the thiazide to maintain serum K^+ levels, which might otherwise be depleted. Hypokalemia predisposes patients to digitalis intoxication.

Hypertension

The use of diuretic drugs, either alone or in combination with other agents, in the management of mild to moderate hypertension is a frequently used form of therapy. Diuresis and restriction of salt intake are often sufficient therapeutic measures for all hypertensive patients except those with severe, malignant, or complicated hypertension. The mechanisms by which the diuretics lower arterial pressure are not precisely known, although it is thought that the initial response is caused by a reduction in plasma volume, with a consequently diminished cardiac output. However, after a few weeks, the initial degree of extracellular volume reduction is not maintained, probably owing to a gradual increase in aldosterone production (i.e., increased Na^+ retention and K^+ loss). Nonetheless, the antihypertensive effect remains.

Although the arterial pressure in hypertensive patients is related to intravascular volume, the changes in plasma volume are primarily caused by alterations in total body Na^+. *Strict dietary Na^+ restriction can lower arterial pressure in hypertensive patients, whereas a large Na^+ intake will reverse the hypotensive effects of the thiazide diuretics.* It appears quite plausible that all of the hypotensive effects of the diuretics can be attributed to some aspect of Na^+ depletion, that is, either directly on extracellular fluid volume or perhaps indirectly through the effects that Na^+ loss has on autonomic nervous function (e.g., diminished norepinephrine storage capacity in sympathetic nerves) or vascular smooth muscle reactivity.

Diuretics are frequently used in combination with other antihypertensive agents. The appropriateness of this combination becomes even more apparent when it is realized that nondiuretic antihypertensives (e.g., hydralazine or diazoxide) produce some increase in plasma volume, which, if not corrected, would lead to an eventual decrease in their activity.

Hepatic Ascites

Cirrhosis and other liver diseases may result in the formation of excessive amounts of fluid in the abdomen (*ascites*). The primary causes of ascites are usually an elevation of pressure in the portal vein and a decreased amount of hepatic plasma protein production. Both factors tend to reduce the ability of the vascular compartment to retain fluid. The resultant ascites may contribute to decreased appetite and respiratory difficulties, among other symptoms. When these difficulties are present, careful reduction in the fluid volume through the use of diuretics is desirable.

Since patients with cirrhosis vary widely in their responsiveness to diuretics, conservative initial diuretic therapy is called for. The mainstay of treatment, however, remains a restriction of dietary Na^+. A common finding in patients with cirrhosis is decreased glomerular filtration, despite the increase in total blood volume caused by the extensive pooling of blood in the splanchnic vessels. Diminished renal perfusion leads to increased aldosterone secretion, which, in turn, increases Na^+ retention and K^+ loss. Thus, in addition to diuretics, most patients will re-

quire K^+ supplementation. The *thiazides* remain the drugs of first choice. The use of a high-ceiling drug, such as furosemide, leads more frequently to such complications as hypokalemia, hyponatremia, and azotemia. K^+-sparing diuretics may be useful adjunctive (but not sole) agents if extensive hypokalemia is present.

Pulmonary Edema

The usual cause of pulmonary edema is acute left ventricular failure. The sequelae of events after left heart failure roughly follow the pattern of reduced stroke volume, leading to increased end-systolic and diastolic volume, which elevate left ventricular end-diastolic pressure. Pressure then increases in the left atrium, pulmonary vein, and finally, in the pulmonary capillaries. Elevated pressure in the last-named vascular bed results in the passing of more fluid into the pulmonary interstitial space, and this causes a compromised gas exchange, diminished total lung gas volume, and increased airway resistance. With acute pulmonary edema of cardiac origin, the traditional treatment has included administration of the efficacious, rapidly acting, loop diuretics. These agents, given parenterally, can reduce total blood volume rapidly and thus may help to prevent recurrence of pulmonary congestion. The value of immediate and vigorous use of the loop diuretics has been questioned. The problems of excessive fluid and K^+ loss indicate a conservative approach to diuresis even in this medical emergency situation.

Increased Intracranial Pressure

A rise in intracranial pressure results in the appearance of a number of symptoms, including headache, vomiting, edema of the optic discs, changes in vital signs, and possibly death. Dehydrating measures, including the use of diuretics, can help lower the pressure, particularly if the elevated intracranial pressure is of a nontraumatic origin. The parenteral administration of a hypertonic solution of the *osmotic diuretics,* urea or mannitol, can relieve the pressure through its osmotic effects. The oral administration of glycerol also has been used in neurosurgical procedures when increases in intracranial pressure are anticipated.

Renal Edema

Nephrotic Syndrome

This condition is characterized by proteinuria and edema due to some form of glomerulonephritis. The resulting fall in plasma protein concentration decreases vascular volume, which leads to diminished renal blood flow.

This, in turn, causes a secondary aldosteronism characterized by Na^+ and water retention and K^+ depletion. Rigid control of dietary Na^+ is of prime importance. Therapy of the nephrotic syndrome using a thiazide (possibly with a K^+-sparing diuretic) to control the secondary aldosteronism, is a useful initial approach to treatment. Since nephrotic edema is frequently more difficult to control than edema of cardiac origin, it may be necessary to switch to a loop diuretic (and spironolactone) to obtain adequate diuresis.

Chronic Renal Failure

The loop diuretics are usually required in treating this disorder, since drugs with lesser intrinsic activity are not sufficiently effective when tubular function has been compromised greatly. Larger than normal amounts of furosemide are frequently employed, and thus it is especially important to monitor the patient for excessive volume depletion. Intermittent therapy may be the best approach.

Acute Renal Failure

The principal rationale for the use of diuretics in acute renal failure is the prevention of complete renal shutdown. Whether renal failure is caused by some underlying disease or by a drug-induced renal toxicity, the continued production of even a small amount of urine is probably important in reducing further kidney tubular damage. Most commonly employed are the osmotic diuretics, with intravenous mannitol generally being the agent of choice. Osmotic diuresis is only possible if glomerular damage, tubular damage, or both have not progressed too far.

Premenstrual Edema and Edema of Pregnancy

Many women show signs of fluid retention during pregnancy and during the last days of the menstrual cycle. Breast fullness and subcutaneous swelling or puffiness are the most commonly observed symptoms; they are largely the result of elevated circulating hormone levels in the blood. Estrogens possess some mineralocorticoid activity and, thus, when present in relatively high concentrations, may produce some expansion of the extracellular fluid compartment. Excessive premenstrual edema frequently responds well to thiazide therapy. *Recent experience has diminished enthusiasm for use of any diuretics in pregnant women.* Since the edema of pregnancy is frequently well tolerated by the patient, worries of compromises in uteroplacental perfusion, possible ineffectiveness of diuretics in preeclampsia, and the potential risk of adverse effects of diuretics on the newborn (e.g., thiazides can both cross the placental barrier and appear in breast milk, producing electrolyte disturbances and thrombocytopenia in newborns) have led to lessened routine use of these agents in pregnancy.

Drugs Affecting Renal Function

Many drugs can enhance urine flow. For example, by increasing cardiac output in the patient with CHF, digitalis administration will cause a mobilization of edema fluid and diuresis. The term *diuretic,* however, is generally restricted to those agents that have a direct action on the kidney. From a therapeutic point of view, diuretics are considered to be those substances that aid in removing excess extracellular fluid and electrolytes. In the main, they accomplish this by decreasing salt and water reabsorption in the tubules.

Resistance To Diuretic Administration

Since the effectiveness of many diuretics ultimately depends on establishing a negative Na^+ balance in order to mobilize edema fluid, *restriction of dietary Na^+ intake is generally an essential part of diuretic therapy.* Therefore, one cause of therapeutic failure or apparent patient refractoriness to diuretics could be the patient's continued ingestion of large quantities of NaCl.

Some of the older diuretic drugs were self-limiting; that is, their prolonged use resulted in gradual diminution in their effectiveness. This problem was corrected through the use of intermittent diuretic therapy. Such a program of several days of diuresis followed by several days of drug withdrawal delayed refractoriness to the drug by preventing excessive disturbances in body electrolyte composition.

Many diuretics (e.g., thiazides and loop diuretics) must reach the tubular lumen before they begin to be effective. Because these compounds are organic acids and are bound to plasma proteins, they are not readily filtered at the glomerulus. However, they reach the luminal fluid by secretion. Any disease condition or drug that impairs *secretion* will affect the access of the diuretics to the luminal fluid and hence to their ultimate site of action (e.g., distal tubule or ascending loop). For example, renal dysfunction may lead to a buildup of *endogenous* organic acids that decrease drug secretion and thereby alter the patient's expected response to the diuretic. Patients with azotemia frequently require larger doses of organic acid diuretics to achieve a satisfactory response. The concomitant administration of other drugs that are substrates for the organic acid secretory system (e.g., probenecid or penicillin) may result in an apparent resistance to diuretic action. It should now be ob-

Table 21-4. Solutions Resembling Extracellular Fluid*

Solution	Manufacturer
Normosol-R	Abbott
Plasma-Lyte	Baxter
Inosol D-CM	Abbott
Polysal	Cutter
Lactated Ringer's	(Several)

*Most of these solutions contain electrolytes in the following mEq range: sodium (130–150), potassium (4–12), chloride (98–109), bicarbonate (50–55), calcium (3–5), and magnesium (0–3).

vious that, *in addition to disease and electrolyte imbalances, the pharmacodynamic handling of the diuretics themselves may be a factor in diuretic resistance.*

Excessive Diuresis

Excessively vigorous diuresis may lead to intravascular dehydration before removal of edema fluid from the rest of the extracellular compartment. This is an especially dangerous situation if the patient is suffering from significant liver or kidney disease. *Once the initial correction of fluid and electrolyte derangement has been achieved, the effect sought is maintenance of homeostasis, not dehydration.* Drug dosage, frequency of administration, and Na^+ intake now should be adjusted to achieve homeostasis.

If diuresis has been too vigorous, as may occur after injudicious use of loop diuretics, or if extensive fluid and electrolyte loss has occurred following severe diarrhea or vomiting, replacement therapy may be required. A number of solutions are available that resemble extracellular fluid and are useful for the repair of water and electrolyte deficits (Table 21-4).

Since the 1950s, diuretic therapy has changed dramatically. Earlier, the major diuretics were acid-forming salts, xanthines, organomercurial compounds, and carbonic anhydrase inhibitors. Either because of toxicity or lack of efficacy, these agents are rarely, if ever, used.

Osmotic Diuretics

Ideally, these would be water-soluble compounds, well absorbed after oral administration, freely filtered at the glomerulus, poorly reabsorbed by the tubule, and devoid of pharmacological effects. Since these osmotic agents act, in part, to retard tubule fluid reabsorption, *the amount of diuresis produced is proportional to the quantity of osmotic diuretic administered.* Therefore, unless large quantities of a particular osmotic diuretic are given, the increase in urinary volume will not be marked.

Ideally, distribution of osmotic diuretics should be largely confined to the vascular system, although this can lead to excessive expansion of the vascular compartment. Such an overexpansion could precipitate pulmonary edema or increase the cardiac work, or both. This is largely the result of a rapid transfer of fluid from the interstitial to the vascular compartment. These agents, therefore, should be given cautiously to patients with compromised cardiac function.

Mechanism of Action

The renal response to osmotic diuretics is probably due to the interplay of several factors. The primary effect involves an *increased fluid loss* caused by the osmotically active diuretic molecules; this results in reduced Na^+ and water reabsorption from the proximal tubule.

An additional contributing factor to the diuresis induced by osmotic diuretics is the *increase in renal medullary blood flow* that occurs following their administration. This medullary hyperemia reduces the cortex-medullary osmolar gradient by carrying away interstitial Na^+ and urea. This partial reduction of the osmolar gradient impairs normal reabsorption of tubular water, which occurs from the descending limb of Henle and the collecting duct.

Finally, there is an additional *increase in electrolyte excretion* due to impairment of ascending limb and distal tubule Na^+ reabsorption; this occurs as a result of a lowered tubular Na^+ concentration and the increased tubular fluid flow rate.

Individual Agents

Mannitol

Mannitol (*Osmitrol*) is a six-carbon sugar that does not undergo appreciable metabolic degradation. It is not absorbed from the gastrointestinal tract and therefore must be given intravenously. Mannitol is somewhat more osmotically active than urea, since in humans it is not reabsorbed in the proximal tubules.

Mannitol is particularly useful in those clinical conditions characterized by hypotension and decreased glomerular filtration. These symptoms are usually the result of some physical trauma or surgical procedure. Mannitol is useful in maintaining kidney function under these conditions since, even at reduced rates of filtration, a sufficient amount of the sugar may enter the tubular fluid to exert an osmotic effect and thus continue urine formation. However, if circulatory failure is profound and glomerular filtration is severely compromised or absent, not enough mannitol may reach the tubules to be effective. The ability to maintain a urine flow under conditions in which renal shutdown might otherwise be expected aids in preventing kidney tubular damage. In addition, mannitol has been used to reduce cerebral edema during neurosurgery, to reduce intraocular pressure before eye surgery for glaucoma, and to promote the elimination of ingested toxic substances.

The major characteristics of the renal response to mannitol diuresis include a fall in urine osmolality and a decrease in the osmolality of the interstitial fluid of the renal medulla. *The quantity of urine formation and Na^+ excretion is generally in proportion to the amount of mannitol excreted.* Although there is a significant inhibition of proximal water reabsorption, the effects of mannitol on proximal Na^+ reabsorption are not marked.

The major adverse reactions associated with mannitol administration are headache, nausea, vomiting, chest pain, and hyponatremia. Too rapid administration of large amounts may cause an excessive shift of fluid from the intracellular to the extracellular compartment and result in congestive heart failure.

Glycerin

The primary use of anhydrous glycerin (*Ophthalgan*) is as an osmotic agent that is applied topically to reduce corneal edema. Orally administered glycerin (*Glycerol, Osmoglyn*) is used to reduce intraocular pressure and vitreous volume before ocular surgical procedures.

Urea

The use of urea has declined in recent years owing both to its disagreeable taste and to the increasing use of mannitol for the same purposes. When used to reduce cerebrospinal fluid pressure, urea is generally given by IV drip as a 30% solution (*Ureaphil, Urevert*). Because of its potential effects on expansion of the extracellular fluid volume, urea is contraindicated in patients with severe impairment of renal, hepatic, or cardiac function or active intracranial bleeding.

Isosorbide

Isosorbide (*Ismotic*) is an orally effective, osmotically active drug that is most commonly used for the emergency treatment of acute angle-closure glaucoma. It is supplied as a 45% solution. This drug should not be confused with isosorbide dinitrate, an antianginal drug.

Aquaretics

These drugs promote the excretion of water in excess of electrolytes. By one mechanism or another aquaretics interfere with the action of ADH. For example, demeclocycline blocks cyclic adenosine monophosphate (cAMP) formation, which occurs as a result of ADH-receptor binding. Other drugs still in development block ADH-receptor interaction. This class of drugs has only limited clinical usefulness at present, but has proved useful in treating hyponatremia.

Carbonic Anhydrase Inhibitors

In the late 1930s, it was reported that sulfanilamide and other *N*-unsubstituted sulfonamides could induce a diuresis characterized by the excretion of an alkaline urine that is high in sodium bicarbonate. It was soon realized that these compounds inhibited *carbonic anhydrase,* an enzyme highly concentrated in renal tissue, and that this enzyme was important in the tubular reabsorption of bicarbonate. These findings led to the synthesis of a series of compounds capable of inhibiting carbonic anhydrase, the most useful of which was *acetazolamide.* This compound was the first orally active, nonmercurial diuretic drug developed. Although the clinical use of carbonic anhydrase inhibitors has greatly diminished since the 1960s, they have been vitally important in helping to delineate our understanding of the physiological role that carbonic anhydrase plays in electrolyte conservation and acid-base balance.

Inhibition of proximal tubule brush border carbonic anhydrase decreases bicarbonate reabsorption, and this accounts for the diuretic effect. In addition, carbonic anhydrase inhibitors affect both distal tubule and collecting duct H^+ secretion through inhibition of intracellular carbonic anhydrase.

Renal excretion of Na^+, K^+, and HCO_3^- are considerably increased by carbonic anhydrase inhibition. The major effect of the inhibitors on electrolyte and water excretion can be explained by an increased delivery of nonreabsorbable sodium bicarbonate to the ascending limb, distal tubule, and collecting ducts. *Potassium loss is particularly marked following carbonic anhydrase inhibition* both because of the presence of a nonreabsorbable ion (HCO_3^-) accompanying Na^+ and the inhibition of the Na^+-H^+ exchange mechanism, two effects that combine to stimulate greatly Na^+ reabsorption and K^+ secretion. Elevated urinary HCO_3^- loss leads to the formation of an alkaline urine and to metabolic acidosis as a result of both HCO_3^- loss and impairment of H^+ secretion.

The main therapeutic use of carbonic anhydrase inhibitors is not for the production of diuresis, but in the *treatment of glaucoma.* Because the formation of aqueous humor in the eye is highly dependent on carbonic anhydrase, acetazolamide has proved to be a useful adjunct to the usual therapy for lowering intraocular pressure. Although acetazolamide has been used in the treatment of epilepsy (particularly absence), it is not known whether the beneficial results are due to carbonic anhydrase inhibition or to the resulting acidosis that it produces.

Adverse reactions are minor; they include loss of appetite, drowsiness, confusion, and tingling in the extremities. Animal studies have shown some teratogenic potential and therefore the use of carbonic anhydrase inhibitors is not recommended during the first trimester of pregnancy.

Acetazolamide (*Diamox, Diamox Parenteral*) is marketed as tablets and as a powder for dissolution.

Benzothiadiazides—The Thiazide Diuretics

Chlorothiazide (Fig. 21-5) was synthesized during the search for new compounds possessing carbonic anhydrase inhibiting activity. It was soon recognized that this compound had properties different from those of classic carbonic anhydrase inhibitors. Although chlorothiazide and its subsequently developed congeners retain the sulfamyl group (SO_2NH_2), which is necessary for carbonic anhydrase inhibition, their primary effect did not rely on carbonic anhydrase inhibition.

In addition to the structurally related derivatives of chlorothiazide, several nonthiazide compounds (e.g., chlorthalidone, quinethazone, metolazone) that have similar mechanisms of action are available. All these agents exhibit pharmacological activities that are essentially identical with those of chlorothiazide, but they differ in their duration of action, the degree of carbonic anhydrase inhibition produced, and the dosage required for maximum natriuretic activity.

Mechanism Of Action

Evidence strongly suggests that *the major site of action of this group of drugs is the distal portion of the ascending limb or the distal tubule.* The thiazides must reach the luminal fluid before they can exert any diuretic effect. This is accomplished by the proximal tubule organic acid secretory system, since the thiazides are largely bound to plasma proteins and therefore are not readily filtered across the glomeruli. Although a proximal site cannot be ruled out, at usual therapeutic doses the major portion of the diuresis is due to an inhibition of reabsorption in the more distal parts of the nephron. The specific mechanism(s) of action is unknown. However, an inhibition of Na^+, K^+-adenosine triphosphatase (ATPase) or glycolysis (or both), actions that would limit the energy supply available for active transport, have been suggested. A thiazide-caused inhibition of phosphodiesterase, the enzyme involved in cAMP breakdown, also has been put forth as being involved in thiazide-induced diuresis. The last-named phe-

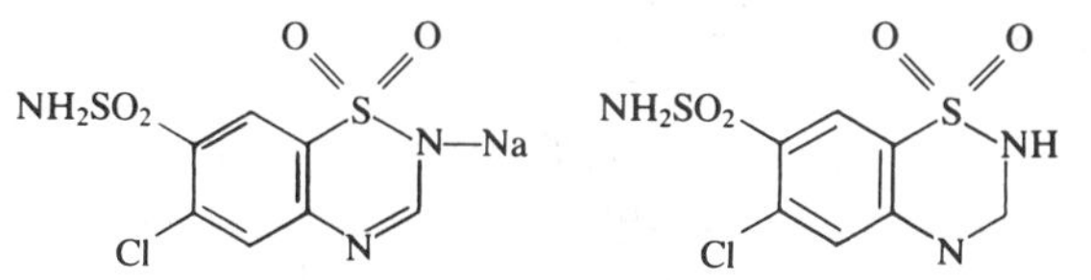

Figure 21-5. Two thiazide diuretics.

nomenon is interesting in light of the known ability of cAMP to inhibit tubular fluid reabsorption.

Especially at higher doses, administration of some of the thiazides results in some degree of carbonic anhydrase inhibition. However, *at usual doses only chlorothiazide shows any significant carbonic anhydrase inhibitory activity.*

Renal Response

When administered in maximal doses, chlorothiazide will markedly increase excretion of H_2O, Na^+, K^+, Cl^-, and HCO_3^-. Maximal diuresis may approach values as high as 10 percent of the filtered load. At usual clinical doses, however, the thiazide diuretics generally produce Na^+, K^+, and Cl^- loss.

The urinary loss of K^+ induced by the thiazides is primarily a consequence of the increased Na^+ delivered to the distal tubule.

There are two renal responses that appear to be unique for the thiazide diuretics. Most diuretics that cause an increase in Na^+ excretion similarly increase Ca^{2+} excretion. With the thiazides, Ca^{2+} excretion is decreased (probably because of increased distal Ca^{2+} reabsorption), making this class of diuretics useful in treating hypercalciuria. This effect is particularly beneficial in individuals who are potential calcium stone formers.

A second unusual response is the utility of these agents to treat nephrogenic diabetes insipidus. Patients who have an adequate supply of ADH, but whose kidneys fail to respond to ADH, excrete large volumes of very dilute urine, not unlike those individuals who have an ADH deficiency. The thiazides reduce glomerular filtration modestly and decrease positive free water formation. These actions combine to cause patients with nephrogenic diabetes insipidus to excrete a somewhat reduced urine volume with an increased osmolality.

Absorption and Elimination

Orally administered thiazides are rapidly absorbed from the gastrointestinal tract and begin to produce a diuresis in about 1 hr. Approximately 50 percent of an oral dose is excreted in the urine within 6 hr. These compounds are organic acids and are secreted. There also appears to be an extrarenal pathway for their elimination. This pathway involves the hepatic-biliary acid secretory system; this system becomes particularly important for thiazide elimination when renal function is impaired.

The thiazides have a variable effect on uric acid elimination, a substance that also is secreted by the renal acid secretory system. Especially at low doses, administration of thiazide diuretics may elevate serum uric acid levels and cause goutlike symptoms. In addition to its active proximal secretion, uric acid is unusual in that much of the uric acid present in the tubular fluid also is actively reabsorbed from the proximal tubule (see Chap. 44). Following large doses, thiazides may compete with uric acid for active reabsorption. Thus, under those conditions, the thiazides may promote uric acid elimination rather than impair it.

Clinical Uses

These agents are useful adjunctive therapy in controlling the edema associated with CHF, cirrhosis, premenstrual tension, and hormone therapy. They are widely used in the treatment of hypertension with or without edema (see Chap. 22). They can be used in patients with renal disease; however, their activity is proportional to the remaining tubular functional capacity of the kidney. The thiazides do not prevent the development, nor are they useful in the treatment, of toxemia in pregnancy.

Adverse Reactions

Thiazides should be used cautiously in the presence of severe renal and hepatic disease, since azotemia and coma may result. *The most important toxic effect associated with this class of diuretics is hypokalemia,* which may result in muscular and central nervous system (CNS) symptoms, as well as cardiac sensitization (see Hypokalemia). Periodic examination of serum electrolytes for the presence of possible imbalances is strongly recommended. Appropriate dietary and therapeutic measures for controlling hypokalemia have been described earlier in this chapter. The thiazides also possess some diabetogenic potential, and although pancreatitis during thiazide therapy has been reported in a few cases, the major mechanism contributing to this diabetogenic potential is not known.

Preparations

A large number of thiazides are available for use. A list of thiazides on the market in the United States is given in Table 21-5.

Table 21-5. Some Commonly Prescribed Thiazide and Thiazidelike Diuretics

Generic name	Trade names
Bendroflumethiazide	Naturetin
Benzthiazide	Aquatag, Exna
Chlorothiazide	Diuril
Hydrochlorothiazide	Esidrix, HydroDIURIL
Hydroflumethiazide	Saluron, Diucardin
Methyclothiazide	Enduron, Aquatensen
Polythiazide	Renese
Trichlormethiazide	Naqua, Metahydrin
Chlorthalidone	Hygroton
Indapamide	Lozol
Metolazone	Zaroxolyn
Quinethazone	Hydromox

Potassium-Sparing Diuretics

The three principal members of the potassium-sparing subgroup of diuretic agents (Fig. 21-6) produce similar effects on urinary electrolyte composition. Through actions in the distal segment of the nephron, they cause a mild natriuresis and a decrease in K^+ and H^+ excretion. Despite their similarities, these agents actually constitute two groups with respect to their mechanisms of action.

Aldosterone Antagonists— Spironolactone

The mechanism by which Na^+ is reabsorbed in coupled exchange with H^+ and K^+ in the distal tubule has been discussed previously; that is, Na^+-driven K^+ secretion is partially under mineralocorticoid control. Aldosterone and other compounds that possess mineralocorticoid activity bind to a specific receptor protein (*aldosterone-binding protein*) in the cytoplasm of distal tubule cells. This hormone-receptor complex is transported to the cell nucleus, where it induces protein synthesis through stimulation of a DNA-directed RNA synthesis. In some as yet unexplained manner the receptor-hormone complex regulates distal Na^+ reabsorption by supplying the energy for active extrusion of Na^+ across the peritubular membrane of distal tubule cells.

Mechanism of Action

Spironolactone is structurally related to aldosterone and acts as a competitive inhibitor to prevent binding of aldosterone to the specific cellular binding protein. Spironolactone thus blocks the hormone-induced stimulation of protein synthesis necessary for Na^+ reabsorption and K^+ secretion. *Spironolactone, in the presence of circulating*

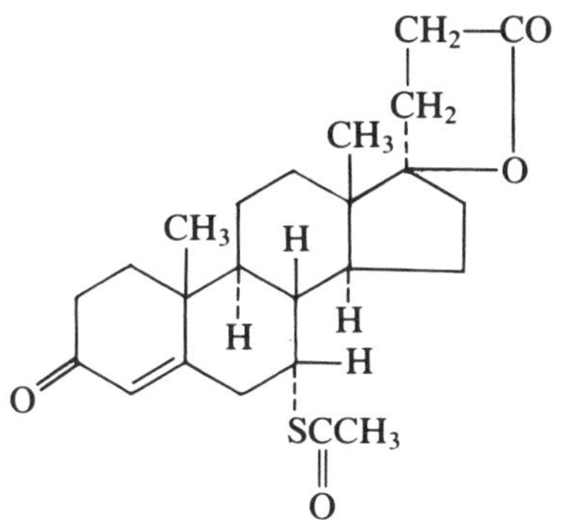

Figure 21-6. Potassium-sparing diuretics.

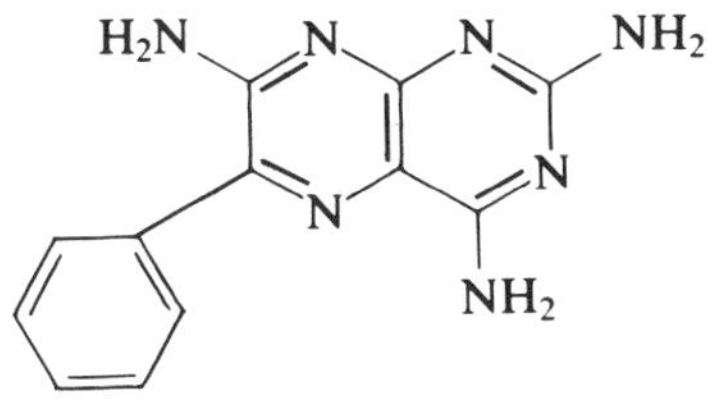

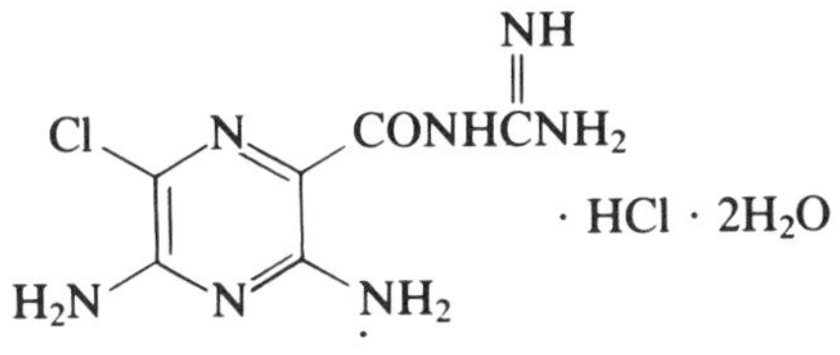

aldosterone, promotes a modest increase in Na$^+$ excretion associated with a decrease in K$^+$ elimination. The observations that spironolactone is ineffective in adrenalectomized patients and that the actions of spironolactone can be reversed by raising circulating aldosterone blood levels (surmountable antagonism) support the conclusion that spironolactone acts by competitive inhibition of the binding of aldosterone with receptor sites in the target tissue. *Spironolactone acts only when mineralocorticoids are present.*

Pharmacokinetic Properties

Spironolactone is poorly absorbed after oral administration and has a delayed onset of action; it may take several days until a peak effect is produced. It has a somewhat slower onset of action when compared to triamterene and

amiloride, but its natriuretic effect is a bit more pronounced, especially during long-term therapy. Spironolactone is rapidly and extensively metabolized, largely to the active metabolite *canrenone*. This metabolite has a half-life of approximately 10 to 35 hr. The metabolites of spironolactone are excreted in both the urine and feces.

Clinical Uses

Spironolactone has been used clinically in the following conditions:

1. *Primary hyperaldosteronism.* Used as an aid in preparing patients with adrenal cortical tumors for surgery.
2. *Hypokalemia.* Potassium-sparing diuretics have been used in patients with low serum K$^+$ resulting from diuretic therapy with other agents. Their use, however, should be restricted to patients who are unable to supplement their dietary K$^+$ intake or adequately restrict their salt intake, or who cannot tolerate the unpalatability of the orally available KCl preparations.
3. *Hypertension and congestive heart failure.* Although spironolactone may be useful in combination with thiazides, the latter remain the drugs of first choice. Fixed-dose combinations of spironolactone and a particular thiazide (e.g., *Aldactazide*) generally offer no therapeutic advantage over either component given separately and tend to restrict the ability of the clinician to determine the optimal dosage of each drug for a particular patient. This is particularly true because spironolactone acts as an aldosterone antagonist.
4. *Cirrhosis and nephrotic syndrome.* Spironolactone is a mild diuretic and may be useful in edema resulting from these two clinical conditions when excessive K$^+$ loss is to be avoided.

Adverse Reactions

Serum electrolyte balance should be monitored periodically, since *hyperkalemia* may occur, especially in patients with impaired renal function or excessive K$^+$ intake (including the K$^+$ salts of coadministered drugs, e.g., potassium penicillin). Hyponatremia, gastrointestinal upset, elevated blood urea nitrogen, drowsiness, and menstrual irregularity can occur. Painful *gynecomastia* (directly related to dosage level and duration of therapy), which is generally reversible, may necessitate termination of therapy. Recent animal studies demonstrating tumorigenic potential support the clinical judgment that spironolactone alone or in combination should not be used for most patients who require diuretic therapy and that its unnecessary use should be avoided.

Nonsteroidal Potassium-Sparing Drugs

Triamterene or *amiloride* administration results in changes in urinary electrolyte patterns that are qualitatively similar to those produced by spironolactone. The mechanism by which these agents bring about the alterations in electrolyte loss, however, is quite different. *Triamterene and amiloride can produce their effects whether or not aldosterone or any other mineralocorticoid is present.* The action of these two drugs is clearly unrelated to endogenous mineralocorticoid activity, and *these drugs are effective in adrenalectomized patients.*

Mechanism of Action

Although recent evidence suggests some differences in the site of action between triamterene and amiloride, both agents appear to affect Na^+ reabsorption in the mineralocorticoid-independent portion of the distal tubule. A site in the collecting duct also may be involved. *These two diuretics apparently can interact with a component in the luminal cell membrane to decrease permeability to Na^+.* The reduced rate of Na^+ reabsorption reduces the gradient that facilitates K^+ secretion. It should be remembered that K^+ secretion at this site is a passive phenomenon that is dependent on, and secondary to, the active reabsorption of Na^+.

In addition to their effects on distal Na^+ and K^+ transport, all of the K^+-sparing diuretics are capable of inhibiting urinary H^+ secretion in the distal tubule and cortical collecting duct. The mechanism involved in this inhibitory action is not totally clear, but inhibition of the Na^+-H^+ antiporter is a likely explanation.

Pharmacokinetic Properties

Both triamterene and amiloride are effective after oral administration. Diuresis ensues within 2 to 4 hr after administration, although a maximum therapeutic effect may not be seen for several days. Both drugs cause a modest (2–3%) increase in Na^+ and HCO_3^- excretion, a reduction in K^+ and H^+ loss, and a variable effect on Cl^- elimination. Approximately 80 percent of an administered dose of triamterene is excreted in the urine as metabolites; amiloride is excreted unchanged.

Clinical Uses

Triamterene can be used in the treatment of CHF, cirrhosis, and the edema caused by secondary hyperaldosteronism. It is frequently used in combination with other diuretics, except spironolactone. Amiloride, but not triamterene, possesses antihypertensive effects that can add to those of the thiazides.

Adverse Reactions

Because the actions of triamterene and amiloride are independent of plasma aldosterone levels, their prolonged administration is more likely to result in hyperkalemia. Triamterene should not be given to patients with impaired renal function. Potassium intake also must be reduced, especially in nonhospitalized patients. A folic acid deficiency has been reported to occur occasionally following the use of triamterene.

Preparations

These K^+-sparing diuretics are of low efficacy when used alone, since only a small amount of total Na^+ reabsorption occurs at more distal sites of the nephron. These compounds are used *primarily in combination* with other diuretics, such as the thiazides and loop diuretics, to prevent or correct hypokalemia. The availability of fixed-dose mixtures of thiazides with nonsteroidal K^+-sparing compounds has proved a rational form of drug therapy.

Triamterene (*Dyrenium*) is available alone or in combination with hydrochlorothiazide (*Dyazide, Maxzide*). Amiloride hydrochloride (*Midamor*) is marketed alone and in combination with hydrochlorothiazide (*Moduretic*).

High-Ceiling, or Loop, Diuretics

The compounds known as *high-ceiling* or *loop diuretics* are the most efficacious agents available for inducing marked water and electrolyte excretion. They can increase diuresis even in patients who are already responding maximally to other diuretics. The drugs in this group include furosemide, bumetanide, and ethacrynic acid (Fig. 21-7). Although differences exist among these agents, they share a common primary site of action, which underlies their effectiveness.

Mechanism of Action

The major site of action of loop diuretics is the thick ascending limb of the loop of Henle, and diuresis is brought about through an inhibition of the Na^+-K^+-$2Cl^-$ transporter. This segment of the nephron is critical in determining the final magnitude of natriuresis. As much as 20 percent of the filtered Na^+ may be reabsorbed in the loop of Henle. The importance of the loop is further emphasized by the realization that drugs that primarily inhibit proximal Na^+ and fluid reabsorption have their natriuretic response reduced due to the ability of the ascending limb to increase its rate of Na^+ reabsorption in the presence of an increased tubular Na^+ load. Thus, any agent that greatly impairs active re-

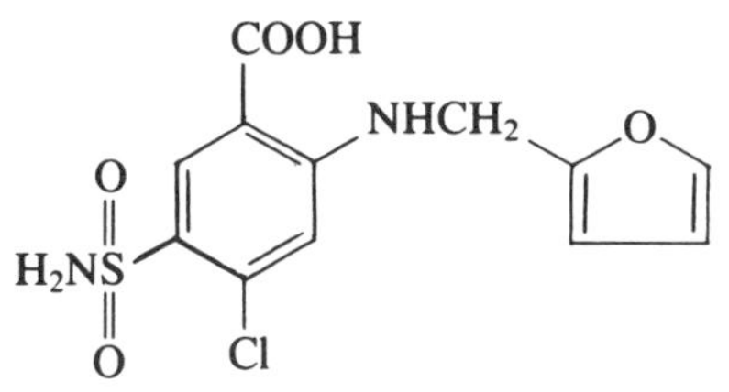

Figure 21-7. High-ceiling, or loop, diuretics.

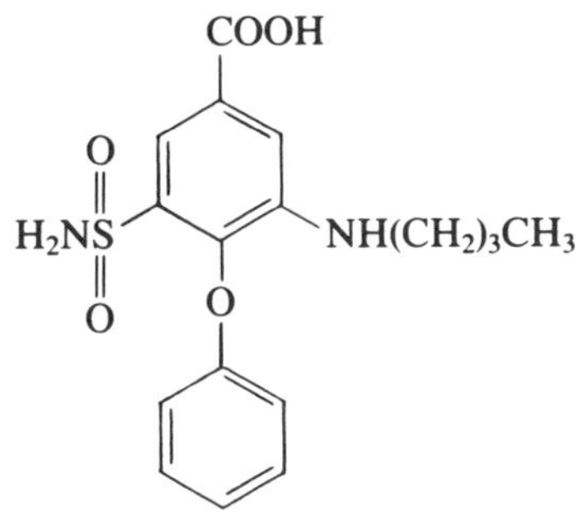

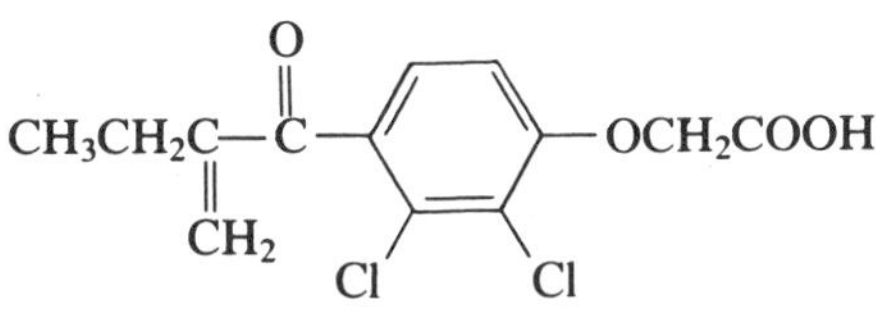

absorption in the thick ascending limb may induce a very large Na^+ and water loss. Furthermore, the relatively limited capacity of the distal tubule and collecting duct for Na^+ reabsorption makes it impossible to recapture much of the suddenly increased tubular Na^+ reaching them.

Since the thick ascending limb is responsible for initiating events that lead to the hyperosmolar medullary interstitium (and therefore providing the driving force for water reabsorption under the influence of ADH), it is this nephron segment that underlies urinary concentration. Thus, drugs that interfere with this concentrating function will have marked effects on urinary output.

Diuretic Response

During the peak effect of the loop diuretics, urine flow is greatly augmented, as is the excretion of Na^+ and Cl^-, corresponding to as much as 20 to 30 percent of their filtered load. K^+ loss also occurs (probably an indirect effect due to the large Na^+ load reaching the distal tubules) and is 2 to 5 times above normal levels of K^+ loss. With low or moderately effective doses, these drugs do not appreciably affect HCO_3^- or H^+ excretion.

Furosemide and bumetanide do possess some carbonic anhydrase–inhibiting activity (about one-tenth that of chlorothiazide). This property may account for the increased bicarbonate and phosphate excretion seen after large doses of these diuretics. The elevated HCO_3^- loss probably indicates some proximal tubular effects for furosemide and bumetanide.

Pharmacokinetic Properties

All of the loop diuretics are available for both oral and parenteral administration. Their onset of action is rapid, usually within 30 min after oral, and 5 min after intravenous, administration. They produce a peak diuresis in about 2 hr, with a total duration of diuretic action of approximately 6 to 8 hr. Loop diuretics are bound to plasma proteins and are eliminated in the urine by both glomerular filtration and tubular secretion. Approximately one third of an administered dose is excreted by the liver into the bile, from where it may be eliminated into the feces. Only small amounts of these compounds appear to be metabolized in the liver.

The loop diuretics must be present in the fluid in the tubular lumen before they can become effective. Because of their extensive binding to plasma proteins, filtration across the glomerular capillaries is restricted. Like the thiazides, however, these organic acids are substrates for the organic acid secretory system in the proximal tubule. A consequence of this active secretion is that the presence of other organic acids or certain forms of renal disease may impair the therapeutic usefulness of the loop diuretics. Studies with isolated perfused nephrons indicate that furosemide and bumetanide act as the parent compound; ethacrynic acid is metabolized extensively and probably acts as a cysteine conjugate.

Clinical Use

Because diuresis may be extensive, small doses should be administered initially, and multiple doses, if needed, should be given in early morning and early afternoon. During the remainder of the day, when the drug is not acting, the body can begin to compensate for any derangements in fluid and electrolyte balance that may have occurred as a result of drug therapy. These drugs should be restricted to patients who require greater diuretic potential than can be achieved by other diuretic drugs. In addition to being used in the usual edematous states associated with CHF, cirrhosis, and renal disease, the loop diuretics can be used in emergency situations, such as acute pulmonary edema, where rapid onset of action is essential. They are not recommended for use during pregnancy.

Adverse Reactions

Frequent serum electrolyte analysis is essential during therapy with the high-ceiling diuretics. Overdose may result in a rapid reduction of blood volume, dizziness, headache, orthostatic hypotension, hyponatremia, and hypokalemia. Gastrointestinal symptoms of nausea, vomiting, diarrhea, and loss of appetite are especially common with ethacrynic acid.

Ototoxicity has been reported to occur during therapy with all three loop diuretics. This effect seems to be dose related and is more common in patients with renal insufficiency. Deafness is usually reversed when these drugs are discontinued, but irreversible hearing loss has been reported after administration of ethacrynic acid, and this has led to a marked decrease in its use.

Furosemide and bumetanide are sulfonamide derivatives and, therefore, are chemically related to the thiazides. They share the thiazides' adverse effects of serum uric acid elevation and diabetogenic potential. Ethacrynic acid is chemically unrelated to other diuretics and does not appear to have diabetogenic potential.

Preparations

Furosemide (*Lasix*) is available as tablets and as an injectable solution. Bumetanide (*Bumex*) is supplied as tablets and as a sterile solution for IV or IM administration. Ethacrynic acid (*Edecrin*) is marketed both as oral tablets and as a powder for injection.

Supplemental Reading

Brater, D.C. Resistance to loop diuretics: Why it happens and what to do about it. *Drugs* 30:427,1985.

Brenner, B.M., and Rector, F.C. (eds.) *The Kidney* (4th ed.). New York: Saunders, 1990.

Dirks, J.H., and Sutton, R.A.L. (eds.). *Diuretics: Physiology. Pharmacology and Clinical Use.* Philadelphia: Saunders, 1986.

Eknoyan, G., and Martinez-Maldonado, M. (eds.). *The Physiological Basis of Diuretic Therapy in Clinical Medicine.* New York: Grune & Stratton, 1986.

Hyams, D.E., The elderly patient: A special case for diuretic therapy. *Drugs* 31:138,1986.

Puschett, J.B., and Greenberg, A. (eds.). *Diuretics II: Chemistry, Pharmacology, and Clinical Applications.* New York: Elsevier, 1987.

Rose, B.D. Diuretics. *Kidney Int.* 39:336,1991.

Ward, A., and Heel, R.C. Bumetanide: A review of its pharmacodynamic and pharmacokinetic properties and therapeutic use. *Drugs* 28:426,1984.

22

Antihypertensive Drugs

David P. Westfall

Hypertension is one of the most serious concerns of modern medical practice. It is estimated that, in the United States, about 60 million people are hypertensive or are being treated with antihypertensive drugs. Among the growing population of elderly Americans, some 13 million have high blood pressure. The level of blood pressure in itself is not a chief concern, since individuals with high blood pressure may be asymptomatic for many years. What is of prime significance is that *hypertension has been shown convincingly to be the single most important contributing factor to cardiovascular disease,* the leading cause of morbidity and untimely death in the United States.

The actual level of pressure that can be considered hypertensive is somewhat difficult to define; it depends on a number of factors, including the patient's age, sex, race, and lifestyle. As a working definition, many cardiovascular treatment centers consider that a diastolic pressure of 90 mm Hg or higher or a systolic pressure of 140 mm Hg or higher represents hypertension. In this chapter, reference is made to *mild, moderate,* or *severe hypertension,* particularly in relation to the indications for use of specific drugs.

Hypertension is considered to be mild if the diastolic pressure is 90 to 104 mm Hg, moderate if 105 to 114 mm Hg, and severe if it exceeds 115 mm Hg. These values should not be considered as absolute ranges but rather as indicators for facilitating discussion. Since, in general terms, *hypertension* can be defined as that level of blood pressure at which there is risk, the ultimate judgment concerning the severity of hypertension in any given individual must also include a consideration of factors other than diastolic or systolic pressure.

In view of the large number of hypertensive people in the general population and the serious consequences when hypertension remains untreated, the unequivocal evidence that antihypertensive drug therapy is effective in preventing complications and prolonging life is quite important. Hypertension, with its attendant cardiovascular disorders, is one of the few chronic abnormalities for which effective therapy exists.

The aim of therapy is straightforward—*a lowering of blood pressure to within the normal range.* In cases in which hypertension is secondary to a known organic disease, such as renovascular disease or pheochromocytoma, therapy is directed toward correction of the underlying malady. Unfortunately, about 90 percent of all hypertensive cases are of unknown etiology. The therapy of *primary,* or *essential hypertension,* as these cases are generally called, is often empirical.

There are three general approaches to the pharmacological treatment of primary hypertension. The first involves the use of diuretics to reduce blood volume. The second employs drugs that interfere with the renin-angiotensin system, and the third is aimed at a drug-induced reduction in peripheral vascular resistance, cardiac output, or both. A reduction in peripheral vascular resistance can be achieved directly by relaxing vascular smooth muscle with drugs known as vasodilators. The vasodilators are a heterogeneous group of compounds that possess a variety of mechanisms of action, including calcium channel antagonism, membrane hyperpolarization, and elevation of intracellular levels of cyclic guanosine $3',5'$-monophosphate (cGMP). These drugs have in common the vascular smooth muscle cell as a site of action. A reduction in peripheral vascular resistance can also be achieved indirectly by modifying the activity of the sympathetic nervous system. Table 22-1 summarizes these various pharmacological approaches to the treatment of hypertension.

The directly acting vasodilators, with the exception of calcium channel antagonists, and sympathetic nervous system depressants receive the bulk of attention in this chapter. The reader is referred to other chapters for addi-

Table 22-1. Pharmacological Approaches to the Treatment of Hypertension

Categories	Examples
I. Diuretics to reduce blood volume	Chlorothiazide (*Diuril*)
II. Drugs that interfere with the renin-angiotensin system	
A. Converting enzyme inhibitors	Captopril (*Capoten*)
B. Angiotensin-receptor antagonists	Saralasin (*Sarenin*)
III. Decrease peripheral vascular resistance and/or cardiac output	
A. Directly acting vasodilators	
1. Calcium channel blockers	Nifedipine (*Procardia*)
2. Potassium channel activators	Minoxidil (*Loniten*)
3. Elevation of cGMP	Nitroprusside (*Nipride*)
4. Others	Hydralazine (*Apresoline*)
B. Sympathetic nervous system depressants	
1. α-Blockers	Prazosin (*Minipress*)
2. β-Blockers	Propranolol (*Inderal*)
3. Norepinephrine synthesis inhibitors	Metyrosine (*Demser*)
4. Norepinephrine storage inhibitors	Reserpine (*Serpasil*)
5. Transmitter release inhibitors	Guanethidine (*Ismelin*)
6. Centrally acting: decrease sympathetic outflow	Clonidine (*Catapres*)

tional information on diuretics (Chap. 21), the renin-angiotensin system (Chap. 19), and the calcium channel antagonists (Chap. 23).

Diuretics

Diuretics have a vital role in the management of hypertension. They can be used alone, in the case of mild hypertension, or in combination with other classes of antihypertensive drugs.

The exact mechanism by which diuretics lower blood pressure is not entirely understood. Initially, diuretics produce a mild degree of Na$^+$ depletion, which leads to a decrease in extracellular fluid volume and cardiac output. However, it is unlikely that a decrease in cardiac output per se is responsible for the initial decrease in blood pressure. Even though cardiac output is one determinant of blood pressure (blood pressure = cardiac output × peripheral vascular resistance), the efficient cardiovascular reflexes should be able to compensate for a modest decrease in cardiac output. The effectiveness of diuretic therapy in mild hypertension may involve either an interference with, or a blunting of, cardiovascular reflexes.

As therapy with diuretics continues, there is a decrease in peripheral vascular resistance and a readjustment of fluid volume such that cardiac output may return to predrug levels. While Na$^+$ depletion and fluid volume reduction may wane during chronic treatment, these alterations do persist and are believed to contribute substantially to the antihypertensive effect of the diuretics. Regardless of the details, there is general agreement

that the blood pressure-lowering effects of diuretics do ultimately depend on the production of diuresis. High salt intake or low rates of glomerular filtration will eliminate the antihypertensive effects of the drugs. Furthermore, diuretics are not effective antihypertensive agents in anephric patients.

Diuretics are commonly used in combination with other classes of antihypertensive drugs. Their value lies in their ability to reverse the Na$^+$ retention commonly associated with many antihypertensive drugs that probably induce Na$^+$ retention and fluid volume expansion as a compensatory response to blood pressure reduction.

When diuretic therapy is indicated for the treatment of primary hypertension, the thiazide-type compounds (e.g., chlorothiazide, hydrochlorothiazide) are generally the drugs of choice. They can be used alone or in combination with other antihypertensive agents. Approximately 30 percent of patients with mild hypertension (diastolic pressures between 90 and 104 mm Hg) may be treated effectively with thiazide therapy alone.

The combined use of the thiazides and other types of antihypertensive drugs is common and beneficial. The effectiveness of these other agents, however, depends on the prevention of the salt and water retention that commonly results from chronically lowering the blood pressure. Antihypertensive drugs known to produce salt and water retention are the directly acting vasodilators and drugs that depress the functioning of the sympathetic nervous system.

Thiazide diuretics are not the drugs of choice in patients who suffer from renal insufficiency (generally defined as a creatinine clearance of less than 30 ml/min). In this situation, the loop diuretics, furosemide and bumetanide, are recommended; they have greater intrinsic natriuretic potency than do thiazides and do not depress renal blood flow.

About 15 percent of patients with primary hypertension have high plasma levels of *renin*. Renin, through its ability to increase the formation of the potent vasoconstrictor angiotensin and to stimulate aldosterone secretion (see Chap. 19), may contribute to hypertension. Since many diuretics, including the thiazides, elevate plasma renin levels, some clinical investigators believe that diuretics should not be used in high-renin hypertensives. Whether the elevated renin levels in primary hypertension constitute a contraindication to the use of diuretics is not clear, however. In situations of known renin-angiotensin-aldosterone involvement, such as in hypertension secondary to renal pathology (i.e., renovascular hypertension), agents that further elevate renin probably should not be used.

The percentage of tubular reabsorption of Na^+ subject to regulation in the distal tubule is small. It is not unexpected, therefore, that the magnitude of diuresis produced by compounds such as *triamterene, amiloride,* and *spironolactone* is modest in comparison to that of the thiazides and loop diuretics. The important feature of the action of these drugs is that the loss of Na^+ is not accompanied by loss of K^+. Thus, these compounds are referred to as *potassium-sparing diuretics.*

The K^+-sparing action of spironolactone, triamterene, and amiloride serves as the basis for their occasional use in the therapy of primary hypertension. The drugs can be employed in conjunction with other types of diuretics to help alleviate the K^+ loss caused by them. Under these conditions, K^+ balance is improved while natriuresis is maintained. Additional information concerning details of mechanism of action, metabolism, preparations, and dosage of diuretics is found in Chap. 21.

Vasodilators

Included for discussion in this section are drugs that produce a direct relaxation of vascular smooth muscle and thereby result in vasodilation. This effect is called *direct* because it is not dependent on the innervation of vascular smooth muscle and is not mediated by receptors for the classical transmitters and mediators, such as adrenoceptors, cholinoceptors, or receptors for histamine. The use of these agents represents a logical approach to the management of primary hypertension.

Primary hypertension is characterized by an increase in total peripheral vascular resistance. The vasodilators decrease resistance and thus correct the hemodynamic abnormality that is responsible for the elevated blood pressure. In addition to their effectiveness in primary hypertension, the vasodilators, because they act directly on vascular smooth muscle, are *effective in lowering blood pressure, regardless of the etiology of the hypertension.* Unlike many other antihypertensive agents, the vasodilators do not inhibit the activity of the sympathetic nervous system; therefore, orthostatic hypotension and impotence are not problems. Additionally, most vasodilators relax arterial smooth muscle to a greater extent than venous smooth muscle, thereby further minimizing postural hypotension.

Although vasodilators would appear to be ideal drugs for the treatment of hypertension, their effectiveness, particularly when they are used chronically, is severely limited by neuroendocrine and autonomic reflexes that tend to counteract the fall in blood pressure. How these reflexes compromise the fall in blood pressure produced by the vasodilators is shown in Fig. 22-1. The diagram does not show all the possible interrelationships but, rather, is meant to draw attention to the most prominent reflex changes that occur. These reflexes include an augmentation of sympathetic nervous activity that leads to an increase in heart rate and cardiac output. Large increases in cardiac output, occurring as a result of vasodilator therapy, will substantially counter the drug-induced reduction of blood pressure. Increased reflex sympathetic input to the heart also augments myocardial oxygen demand; this is especially serious in patients with coronary insufficiency and little cardiac reserve.

Plasma renin activity is elevated after treatment with vasodilators. The hyperreninemia appears to be due, in part, to enhanced sympathetic nervous activity. Elevated renin levels lead to an increase in the concentration of circulating angiotensin, a potent vasoconstrictor, and thus an increase in peripheral vascular resistance.

Thus, it seems that the lack of sympathetic nervous system inhibition by the vasodilators, which is advantageous in some ways, can also be a disadvantage in that reflex increases in sympathetic nerve activity will lead to hemodynamic changes that reduce the effectiveness of the drugs. *As the sole therapy for hypertension, therefore, the vasodilators are generally inadequate.* However, many of the factors that limit the usefulness of the vasodilators can be obviated when they are administered in combination with a β-adrenoceptor antagonist, such as propranolol, and a *diuretic.* Propranolol reduces the cardiac stimulation that occurs in response to increases in sympathetic nervous activity, and the large increase in cardiac output caused by the vasodilators will be reduced. Propranolol also reduces plasma renin levels, and that is an additional benefit. The reduction in Na^+ excretion and the increase in plasma volume that occurs with vasodilator therapy can be reduced by concomitant treatment with a diuretic. These relationships are shown in Fig. 22-1.

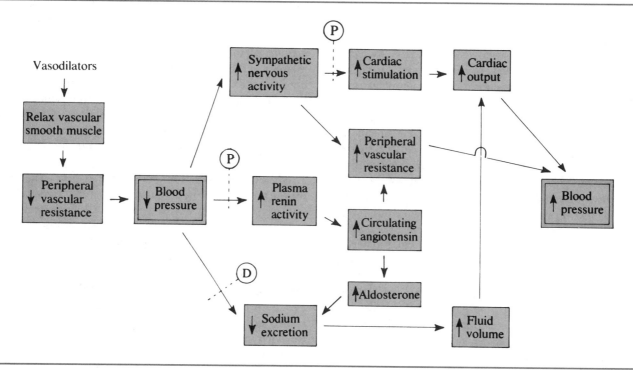

Figure 22-1. Neuroendocrine pathways that are activated when vasodilators decrease blood pressure. These pathways lead ultimately to an increase in blood pressure and thus compromise the effectiveness of the vasodilators. The effectiveness can be preserved by coadministration of propranolol (P) and a diuretic (D).

Mechanism of Action

Available evidence suggests that a single unifying mechanism does not exist but, rather, that various vasodilators may act at different places in the series of processes that couple excitation of vascular smooth muscle cells with contraction. For example, the vasodilators known as calcium channel antagonists block or limit the entry of calcium through voltage-dependent channels in the membrane of vascular smooth muscle cells. In this way the calcium channel blockers limit the amount of free intracellular calcium available to interact with smooth muscle contractile proteins.

Other vasodilators, such as diazoxide and minoxidil, cause dilation of blood vessels by activating potassium channels in vascular smooth muscle. An increase in potassium conductance results in a hyperpolarization of the cell membrane, which will cause relaxation of vascular smooth muscle.

Another group of drugs, the so-called nitrovasodilators, of which nitroprusside is an example, activate a soluble guanylate cyclase in vascular smooth muscle, which brings about an increase in the intracellular levels of cGMP. Increases in cGMP are associated with vascular smooth muscle relaxation. The action of the nitrovasodilators appears to be quite similar to that of the endogenous vasodilator released by a variety of stimuli from endothelial cells of blood vessels. This substance, originally named endothelial-derived relaxing factor, or EDRF, is nitric oxide, or a closely related nitrosothiol compound. The knowledge that the nitrovasodilators generate nitric oxide in vivo suggests that this substance may be the final common mediator of a number of vascular smooth muscle relaxants.

In this chapter, four vasodilators are described in detail (Fig. 22-2). Two of these agents, *hydralazine* and *minoxidil*, are effective orally and are used for chronic treatment of primary hypertension. The other two drugs, *diazoxide* and *sodium nitroprusside*, are not effective orally, but only intravenously. They are generally used in the treatment of hypertensive emergencies or during surgery.

Hydralazine

Hydralazine is a phthalazine derivative whose mechanism of action is not completely understood. There is some evidence that the vasodilation produced by hydralazine depends in part on the presence of an intact endothelium in blood vessels. This implies that hydralazine causes the release of EDRF, which then acts on the vascular smooth muscle to cause relaxation.

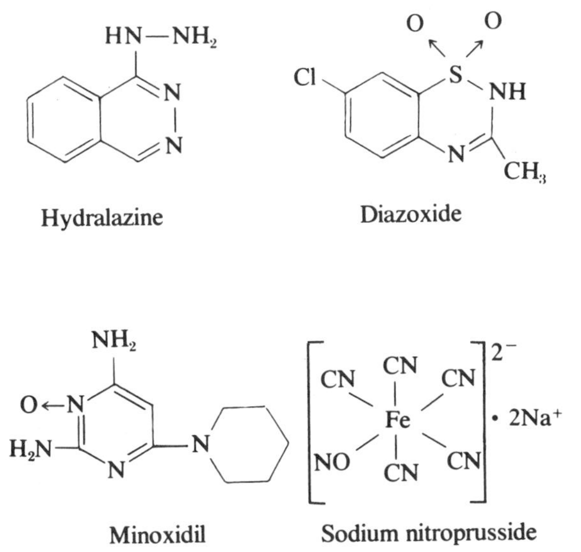

Figure 22-2. Chemical structures of some vasodilators.

Pharmacological Actions

Hydralazine produces a widespread, but apparently nonuniform, vasodilation; that is, vascular resistance is decreased more in cerebral, coronary, renal, and splanchnic beds than in skeletal muscle and skin. Renal blood flow and, ultimately, glomerular filtration rate may be slightly increased after acute treatment with hydralazine. However, after several days of therapy, the renal blood flow is usually no different from before drug use.

In therapeutic doses, hydralazine produces little effect on nonvascular smooth muscle or on the heart. Its pharmacological actions are largely confined to vascular smooth muscle and occur predominantly on the arterial side of the circulation; venous capacitance is much less affected. Because cardiovascular reflexes and venous capacitance are not affected by hydralazine, postural hypotension is not of clinical concern. Hydralazine treatment does, however, result in an increase in cardiac output. This action is brought about by the combined effects of a reflex increase in sympathetic stimulation of the heart, an increase in plasma renin, and salt and water retention. These effects limit the hypotensive usefulness of hydralazine to such an extent that *it is rarely used alone.*

Absorption, Metabolism, and Excretion

Hydralazine is well absorbed after oral administration (65–90%). Its peak antihypertensive effect occurs in about 1 hr, and its duration of action is about 6 hr.

The major pathways for its metabolism include ring hydroxylation, with subsequent glucuronide conjugation

and *N*-acetylation. Although some renal metabolism occurs, approximately 90 percent of hydralazine biotransformation is carried out in the liver. Hydralazine exhibits a first-pass effect in that part of an orally administered dose is metabolized before the drug reaches the systemic circulation. The first-pass metabolism occurs in the intestinal mucosa (mostly *N*-acetylation) and the liver. The primary excretory route is through renal elimination, and about 80 percent of an oral dose appears in the urine within 48 hr. About 10 percent is excreted unchanged in the feces.

Approximately 85 percent of the hydralazine in plasma is bound to plasma proteins. Although this does not appear to be a major therapeutic concern, the potential for interactions with other drugs that also bind to plasma proteins exists. The plasma half-life of hydralazine in patients with normal renal function is 1.5 to 3 hr. Interestingly, the half-life of the antihypertensive effect is somewhat longer than the plasma half-life. This may occur because hydralazine is accumulated specifically in artery walls, where it may continue to exert a vasodilator action even though plasma concentrations are low.

Because of their therapeutic implications, two aspects of the metabolism and excretion of hydralazine are particularly noteworthy. First, in patients with renal failure, the plasma half-life of hydralazine may be increased four- or fivefold. If renal failure is present, therefore, both the antihypertensive and toxic effects of hydralazine may be enhanced, and difficulties in maintaining a desired hypotensive effect can be encountered. Second, *N*-acetylation of hydralazine is an important metabolic pathway that is dependent on the activity of the enzyme *N*-acetyltransferase. Since genetically determined differences in the activity of this enzyme are known to occur (in some regions or ethnic groups, perhaps as high as 50% of the population), these individuals (known as "slow acetylators") will have higher plasma levels of hydralazine; therefore, the drug's therapeutic or toxic effects may be increased.

Clinical Uses

The chief use of hydralazine (*Apresoline*) is in the treatment of ambulatory patients with primary hypertension of moderate severity. Hydralazine is generally reserved for those moderately hypertensive patients who are not well controlled either by diuretics or by drugs that interfere with the sympathetic nervous system. It is almost always administered in combination with a diuretic (to prevent Na$^+$ retention) and a β-blocker, such as propranolol (to attenuate the effects of reflex cardiac stimulation and hyperreninemia). *The triple combination of a diuretic, β-blocker, and hydralazine constitutes a unique hemodynamic approach in the treatment of hypertension,* since three of the chief determinants of blood pressure are affected: cardiac output (β-blocker), plasma volume (diuretic), and peripheral vascular resistance (hydralazine).

Although hydralazine is available for intravenous administration and has been used in the past for hypertensive emergencies, it is not now generally employed for hypertensive emergencies. The onset of action after intravenous injection is relatively slow, and its actions are somewhat unpredictable in comparison to several other vasodilators.

Adverse Reactions

Most side effects associated with hydralazine administration are due to vasodilation and the reflex hemodynamic changes that occur in response to vasodilation. These side effects include headache, flushing, nasal congestion, tachycardia, and palpitations. More serious manifestations include myocardial ischemia and heart failure. These untoward effects of hydralazine are greatly attenuated when the drug is administered in conjunction with a β-blocker.

When administered chronically in high doses, hydralazine may produce a rheumatoidlike state, which, when fully developed, resembles disseminated lupus erythematosus. In patients receiving 400 mg per day or more, the incidence of lupus erythematosus is quite high (10–20%). This hydralazine syndrome is clearly dose related, since doses of 200 mg per day or less rarely result in the appearance of the rheumatoidlike condition.

Minoxidil

Minoxidil is an orally effective vasodilator. It is more potent and longer acting than hydralazine and does not accumulate significantly in patients with renal insufficiency. The drug is a piperidinopyrimidine derivative that depends on in vivo metabolism by hepatic enzymes to produce an active metabolite, minoxidil sulfate. Minoxidil sulfate activates potassium channels, resulting in hyperpolarization of vascular smooth muscle and relaxation of the blood vessel.

Pharmacological Actions

The hemodynamic effects of minoxidil are generally similar to those of hydralazine, with the noteworthy exception that a greater decrease in peripheral vascular resistance and, consequently, a larger reduction in blood pressure can be achieved with minoxidil. Well-tolerated doses of minoxidil can reduce mean blood pressure by 35 mm Hg, compared to only 10 to 20 mm Hg with hydralazine. Minoxidil produces no important changes in either renal blood flow or glomerular filtration rate. The drug has little or no effect on venous capacitance and does not inhibit the reflex activation of the sympathetic nervous system. Orthostasis and other side effects of sympathetic blockade are, therefore, not a problem. As with hydral-

azine, there is a significant increase in cardiac output that is secondary to reflex increases in sympathetic activity, hyperreninemia, and salt and water retention. These effects can reduce substantially the effectiveness of minoxidil when it is used alone. The addition of a β-blocker and a diuretic to the therapeutic regimen will preserve minoxidil's antihypertensive action while attenuating some of the undesirable side effects.

Absorption, Metabolism, and Excretion

Peak concentrations of minoxidil in the blood occur 1 hr after oral administration, although the therapeutic effect may take up to 2 or more hr to be manifest. This is probably related to the time it takes to metabolically convert minoxidil to minoxidil sulfate. The antihypertensive action after an oral dose of minoxidil lasts from 12 to 24 hr. The long duration of action allows the drug to be administered only once or twice a day, a regimen that may be beneficial to patient compliance. Interestingly, the therapeutic half-life is considerably longer than the plasma half-life. This may occur, as has been suggested for hydralazine, as a result of accumulation of the drug and its active metabolite in arterial walls or a longer plasma half-life of the sulfated metabolite, or both.

Minoxidil is extensively metabolized by the liver, with minoxidil sulfate, one of several metabolites, being the active species. The major inactive metabolite is a glucuronide conjugate. The ultimate disposition of minoxidil depends primarily on hepatic metabolism and only slightly on renal excretion of unchanged drug. Because of this, pharmacological activity is not cumulative in patients with renal failure.

Clinical Uses

The major indications for the use of minoxidil (*Loniten*) are (1) severe hypertension that may be life threatening or (2) hypertension that is resistant to milder forms of therapy. Compromises in renal function do not prolong either the plasma or therapeutic half-life of minoxidil and, therefore, the drug seems to be of particular importance for hypertensive patients with chronic renal failure.

Adverse Reactions

Signs of toxicity common to vasodilator therapy in general also occur with minoxidil and are attributable to vasodilation and reflex increases in sympathetic nerve activity. These include headache, nasal congestion, tachycardia, and palpitations. These effects do not have great clinical importance, since minoxidil is almost always administered in combination with a β-blocker, which antagonizes the indirect cardiac effects. A more troublesome side effect, particularly in women, is the growth of body hair. The original notion was that minoxidil promoted hair growth because of increased blood flow to hair follicles. More recent evidence suggests that minoxidil may also directly stimulate the growth and maturation of cells that form hair shafts. Apparently, minoxidil activates a specific gene that regulates hair shaft protein. In any case this particular side effect has been capitalized upon and minoxidil is now marketed for the treatment of male pattern baldness. For promoting hair growth minoxidil is marketed as a cream for topical application (*Rogaine*).

Diazoxide

Diazoxide is a benzothiadiazine derivative and is, therefore, chemically similar to the thiazide diuretics. It is devoid of diuretic activity, however, and, in fact, causes Na^+ and water retention. Diazoxide is a very potent vasodilator when administered intravenously. When given by mouth, it produces only a slight decrease in blood pressure. It is available only for intravenous use in the treatment of hypertensive emergencies.

The mechanism by which diazoxide relaxes vascular smooth muscle is related to its ability to activate potassium channels and produce a hyperpolarization of the cell membrane.

Pharmacological Actions

The hemodynamic effects of diazoxide are similar to those of hydralazine and minoxidil. It produces a direct relaxation of arteriolar smooth muscle, with no substantial effect on capacitance beds. Since the drug does not impair cardiovascular reflexes, orthostasis (standing upright) is not a problem. Its administration is, however, associated with a reflex increase in cardiac output that partially counters its antihypertensive effects. Propranolol and other β-blockers potentiate the vasodilating properties of the drug. Diazoxide has no direct action on the heart. Although renal blood flow and glomerular filtration may fall transiently, they generally return to predrug levels within 1 hr.

Absorption, Metabolism, and Excretion

The effect of diazoxide on the lowering of blood pressure occurs within 3 to 5 min after a rapid intravenous injection, and its duration may be from 4 to 12 hr. Interestingly, if diazoxide is either injected slowly or infused, its hypotensive action is quite modest. This is believed to be due to a rapid and extensive binding of the drug to plasma proteins. Both the liver and kidney contribute to the metabolism and excretion of diazoxide. The plasma half-life is, therefore, prolonged in patients with chronic renal failure.

Clinical Uses

Diazoxide (*Hyperstat*) is administered intravenously for the treatment of *hypertensive emergencies,* particularly malignant hypertension, hypertensive encephalopathy, and eclampsia. It is effective in 75 to 85 percent of the patients to whom it is administered and rarely reduces blood pressure below the normotensive range.

In patients with coronary insufficiency, a β-blocker can be given in conjunction with diazoxide to decrease the cardiac work associated with reflex increases in sympathetic stimulation of the heart. It should be noted, however, that β-blockers potentiate the hypotensive effect of diazoxide, and therefore the dose of the vasodilator should be lowered. The dose of diazoxide should also be lowered if the patient has recently been treated with guanethidine or another drug that depresses the action of the sympathetic nervous system. Such drugs enable a greater hypotensive effect to occur because they reduce the increase in cardiac output that normally partially counteracts the fall in pressure.

Diazoxide appears to have a direct antinatriuretic action. This direct action, coupled with the neuroendocrine reflexes that are activated by a decrease in peripheral vascular resistance, leads to a severe retention of Na^+ and water. Since tolerance to diazoxide can develop rapidly, it is frequently administered in conjunction with a diuretic.

Adverse Reactions

Since diazoxide is not often used for long-term treatment, toxicities associated with chronic use are rare. Of chief concern are the side effects associated with the increased workload on the heart, which may precipitate myocardial ischemia, and Na^+ and water retention. These undesirable effects can be controlled by concurrent therapy with a β-blocker and a diuretic.

Diazoxide may cause hyperglycemia, especially in diabetics, so if the drug is used for several days, blood glucose levels should be measured. Tolbutamide, an orally effective antidiabetic agent, may be given if necessary.

When used in the treatment of toxemia, diazoxide may cause labor to stop, because it relaxes uterine smooth muscle. Oxytocic drugs can be used to overcome this difficulty.

Sodium Nitroprusside

Sodium nitroprusside is chemically unusual in that it consists of an iron coordination complex. It is a hydrated nitrosylpentacyanoferrate compound that has a net negative charge and is prepared in association with two sodium ions. Sodium nitroprusside is a potent, directly acting vasodilator capable of reducing blood pressure in all patients, regardless of the cause of hypertension. It is used only by the intravenous route for the treatment of *hypertensive emergencies*. The pharmacological activity is caused by the nitroso moiety. The actions of the drug are similar to, although not identical with, those of the nitrites and nitrates that are used as antianginal agents (see Chap. 25). The action of the nitrovasodilators is dependent on the intracellular production of cGMP.

Pharmacological Actions

In contrast to hydralazine, minoxidil, and diazoxide, sodium nitroprusside produces relaxation of venules as well as arterioles. Thus, in addition to a decrease in peripheral vascular resistance, venous return to the heart is reduced. This action limits the increase in cardiac output that normally follows vasodilator therapy. Sodium nitroprusside does not inhibit sympathetic reflexes, so heart rate may increase following its administration even though cardiac output is not increased. Renal blood flow remains largely unaffected by sodium nitroprusside, because the decrease in renal vascular resistance is proportional to the decrease in mean arterial pressure. As with all vasodilators, plasma renin activity increases.

Absorption, Metabolism, and Excretion

The onset of the hypotensive action of sodium nitroprusside is very rapid, occurring within 30 sec after intravenous administration. If a single dose were given, the action would last for only a couple of minutes. The drug, therefore, must be administered by continuous intravenous infusion. After the infusion is stopped, the blood pressure returns to predrug levels within 2 to 3 min.

Nitroprusside is metabolically degraded by the liver, yielding thiocyanate. Because thiocyanate is excreted by the kidney, toxicities due to this compound will be more likely in patients with impaired renal function.

Clinical Uses

Sodium nitroprusside (*Nipride*) is used in the management of hypertensive crisis. Although it is effective in every form of hypertension, owing to its relatively favorable effect on cardiac performance sodium nitroprusside has special importance in the treatment of severe hypertension with acute myocardial infarction or left ventricular failure. Because the drug reduces preload (due to venodilation) and afterload (due to arteriolar dilation), it improves ventricular performance and, in fact, is sometimes used in patients with refractory heart failure, even in the absence of hypertension.

Adverse Reactions

The most commonly encountered side effects with sodium nitroprusside are those associated with extensive vasodilation and hypotension. These side effects include nausea, vomiting, and headache; they quickly dissipate when the infusion is terminated. When sodium nitroprusside treatment extends for several days, some danger of toxicity exists owing to the accumulation of thiocyanate, a metabolite of nitroprusside. Thiocyanate intoxication includes signs of delirium and psychosis; hypothyroidism also may occur. If nitroprusside is administered for several days, thiocyanate levels should be monitored. The drug is administered by continuous IV infusion.

Close supervision is required when nitroprusside is used because of the drug's potency and short duration of action.

Drugs That Impair Sympathetic Nervous System Functioning

The drugs discussed in the sections that follow reduce blood pressure by depressing the activity of the sympathetic nervous system. This is accomplished in four ways: (1) by reducing the number of impulses traveling in the sympathetic nerves, (2) by inhibiting neurotransmitter release, (3) by depleting the stores of norepinephrine, and (4) by antagonizing the actions of norepinephrine on the effector cells. The sites of action of these drugs are diverse and may best be appreciated by considering the sympathetic arc concerned with blood pressure regulation (Fig. 22-3).

Afferent fibers arising from baroreceptors and chemoreceptors in the carotid body and aortic arch regions are carried, mainly by the vagus nerve, to the medulla oblongata. These afferent fibers can modify the number of adrenergic impulses that come from a number of brain centers in the complex integrative and vasomotor areas of the brainstem. The adrenergic impulses descend in bulbospinal tracts, terminating in the gray matter of the cord, particularly in the intermediolateral cell columns between the first thoracic and second lumbar segments. Efferent fibers emerge from the spinal cord, forming synapses in the paravertebral ganglia. Acetylcholine (ACh) is the principal neurotransmitter at these ganglionic synapses. Acetylcholine interacts primarily with nicotinic receptors, and this stimulates the postganglionic neurons. These postganglionic fibers course to the heart and the vasculature. The transmitters at these sites include norepinephrine as well as several cotransmitters. One such cotransmitter is adenosine triphosphate (ATP). Recent evidence indicates that both norepinephrine and ATP contribute to transmission at the vascular neuroeffector junction. The cotransmitters are released from the nerve varicosities, with norepinephrine interacting with α- or β-receptors and ATP with purinoceptors of the P_2 class. Together these cotransmitters initiate the characteristic response of the effector (see Chap. 11 for additional discussion).

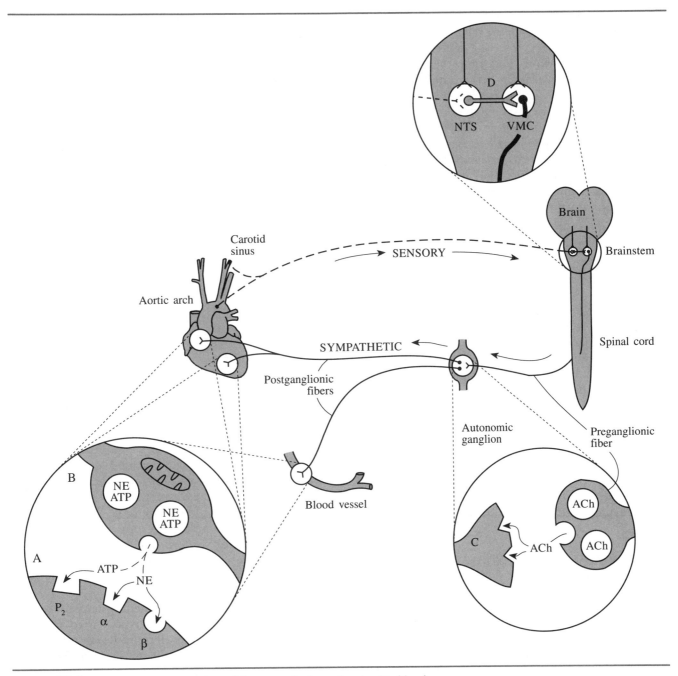

Figure 22-3. Schematic representation of the sympathetic arc involved in blood pressure regulation and sites where drugs may act to influence the system. (1) Receptors on effector cell; (B) adrenergic varicosity; (C) nicotinic receptors (postganglionic fibers); (D) brainstem nuclei. NTS = nucleus of the tractus solitarii; VMC = vasomotor center; ACh = acetylcholine; NE = norepinephrine; α = α-adrenoceptors; β = β-adrenoceptors; P_2 = P_2-purinoceptors; ATP = adenosine triphosphate.

The sympathetic nervous system plays an important role in the regulation of the cardiovascular system. Sympathetic stimulation of the heart results in increases both in cardiac rate and force of contraction, thus augmenting cardiac output; a reduction in sympathetic stimulation decreases cardiac output. The smooth muscle cells of the blood vessels receive sympathetic adrenergic innervation, and the tone of most blood vessels is directly related to the level of sympathetic activity. Impulses pass over the adrenergic fibers, keeping the vessels in a constant state of moderate constriction. An increase in the number of impulses reaching the muscle raises the tone of the vasculature and increases blood pressure, whereas a reduction in the number of impulses leads to a relaxation of the smooth muscle (vasodilation) and lowering of blood pressure.

It is important to realize that, while there may be some involvement of the adrenergic nervous system in primary hypertension, there is no clear evidence that a malfunction of this system is causally involved in the etiology of primary hypertension. Therefore, *even though drugs may depress the sympathetic system and thus lower blood pressure, it should not be assumed that this therapeutic approach "corrects" the cause of the elevated pressure.* Only in a few specific cases, such as pheochromocytoma, can hypertension be directly related to abnormalities in the functioning of the sympathetic system.

Adrenoceptor Antagonists

The adrenoceptor-blocking agents are described in detail in Chap. 13. The use of these agents in the treatment of hypertension is briefly described here. Drugs of this group are subdivided into α-adrenoceptor antagonists (α-blockers) and β-adrenoceptor antagonists (β-blockers). Both α- and β-blockers have uses as antihypertensive agents.

α-Blocking Drugs

There are three principal classes of α-blockers: the haloalkylamines (e.g., phenoxybenzamine), the imidazolines (e.g., phentolamine), and the quinazolines (e.g., prazosin).

Pharmacological Actions

The effects of the α-blocking drugs on the circulation are similar in many respects to those produced by the directly acting vasodilators. The α-blockers reduce systemic and pulmonary resistance and thus lower blood pressure. Their effects on regional blood flow depend on the degree of existing sympathetic tone in the vascular smooth muscles. In general, if sympathetic tone is high, the α-blockers will decrease resistance and increase blood flow in most vascular beds. Cerebral blood flow is little affected by α-blocking agents unless blood pressure is greatly reduced.

Unlike the vasodilators, which have a more prominent effect on arterial beds than on venous beds, the α-blockers prevent vasoconstriction in both vascular beds. Because of the venous dilation, postural hypotension is a prominent feature of α-blockade. This is especially true for the classic α-blockers such as phenoxybenzamine and phentolamine, but less so for the prazosinlike α-blockers. Venous smooth muscle is not as much affected by prazosin, and postural hypotension, while it occurs with prazosin, is not as severe as with the other types of α-blockers.

Administration of α-blockers will result in reflex increases in heart rate, contractile force, and plasma renin activity. This occurs with all α-blockers but less so with prazosin and other agents in its class. This is because prazosin and the other quinazoline α-blockers are selective for α_1-adrenoceptors, whereas the classic α-blockers, such as phenoxybenzamine and phentolamine, antagonize responses mediated by both α_1- and α_2-receptors. The significance of this is that the presynaptic α-receptors, whose activation limits the amount of transmitter release upon nerve stimulation, are of the α_2 type; antagonism of these presynaptic α_2-receptors results in enhanced transmitter release. In a situation in which norepinephrine exerts a postsynaptic action by means of β-receptors (e.g., cardiac stimulation, renin release), blockade of presynaptic α_2-receptors actually potentiates the response to sympathetic stimulation. Prazosin, being selective for α_1-receptors, will not potentiate the release of norepinephrine and, thus, the stimulation of the heart and renin release are less with this drug.

Clinical Uses

Postural hypotension and a somewhat erratic oral absorption limit the usefulness of phenoxybenzamine and phentolamine in the treatment of primary hypertension. They are of some use in the management of patients with a pheochromocytoma (see Chap. 13). Prazosin and the other quinazoline derivatives that are selective for α_1-adrenoceptors are quite useful for the management of primary hypertension. The α_1-receptor selective antagonists can be used alone in mild hypertension. When hypertension is moderate or severe, prazosin is generally administered in combination with a thiazide and a β-blocker. The antihypertensive actions of prazosin are considerably potentiated by coadministration of thiazides or other types of antihypertensive drugs.

Prazosin may be particularly useful when patients cannot tolerate other types of antihypertensive agents or when blood pressure is not well controlled by other drugs. Since prazosin does not significantly influence blood uric acid or glucose levels, it can be used in hypertensive patients whose condition is complicated by gout or diabetes mellitus. Prazosin treatment is associated with favorable effects on plasma lipids. Thus, this drug may be of particular importance in managing patients with hyperlipidemia.

Further information about the pharmacokinetics, adverse reactions, and preparations of α-blockers is given in Chap. 13.

β-Blocking Drugs

β-Blockers are drugs that competitively antagonize the responses to catecholamines that are mediated by β-receptors (see Chap. 13). These drugs have a number of clinical uses, including treatment of cardiac arrhythmias (Chap. 26) and angina pectoris (Chap. 25). Their use in these conditions is rational in that the therapeutic benefit is directly related to the blockade of β-receptors in the myocardium.

β-Blockers are also used in the treatment of hypertension, although this seems to be somewhat paradoxical in that blockade of vascular smooth muscle β-receptors might be expected to unmask, or leave unopposed, responses to catecholamines that occur through vascular α-receptors. Unopposed α-mediated responses would be expected to increase rather than decrease blood pressure. Nevertheless, *β-blockers have proved to be quite effective antihypertensive agents,* and they have an important place in the treatment of primary hypertension.

Quite a number of β-blockers are on the market or in the last phases of clinical testing. In the United States, *propranolol,* the prototype β-blocker, was the first approved for the treatment of hypertension. Other β-blockers are listed in Chap. 13. While there may be some differences among individual β-blockers in their relative selectivity for β_1- or β_2-receptors, their partial agonistic activity, or their ability to stabilize membranes (see Chap. 13), these factors have little bearing on their antihypertensive effectiveness. The common denominator for their antihypertensive actions is antagonism of β-receptors. Thus, a patient who fails to respond to one β-blocker will almost certainly fail to respond to another.

Pharmacological Actions

Decreases in heart rate and cardiac output are the most obvious results of administration of β-blockers. Initially, blood pressure is not much affected since peripheral vascular resistance will be reflexly elevated as a result of the drug-induced decrease in cardiac output. The reduction of blood pressure that occurs in chronic treatment correlates best with changes in peripheral vascular resistance rather than with drug-induced variation in heart rate or cardiac output.

Plasma volume and venous return tend to be reduced during treatment with propranolol. The reduction in plasma volume produced by β-blockers contrasts with the increased volume seen with other types of antihypertensives. Tolerance to the antihypertensive actions of β-blockers, therefore, is not as great a problem as occurs with the vasodilating drugs. An additional difference from the vasodilators is that *plasma renin activity is reduced,* rather than increased, by propranolol.

Both standing and recumbent blood pressures and coronary blood flow are reduced by the β-blockers; orthostatic hypotension does not occur. The reduction in coronary blood flow that follows β-blocker administration is either the result of β-blockade in the coronary vasculature or is related to the drugs' negative chronotropic and inotropic actions on the heart. More important, cardiac oxygen consumption is reduced because of the direct myocardial effects of the drugs.

Mechanism of Antihypertensive Action

It is not well understood how β-blockers produce a *persistent* reduction of blood pressure. Because blood pressure is reduced only with chronic treatment, some investigators believe that there is an adaptation of peripheral resistance as a consequence of reduced blood flow. This would result in a persistently reduced peripheral vascular resistance, regardless of the level of cardiac output.

Another suggestion to explain the antihypertensive effects of β-blockers is that they reduce plasma renin activity, thereby counteracting the effects of that substance, which may be a contributor to primary hypertension. The release of renin from the juxtaglomerular cells of the kidney is believed to be regulated in part by sympathetic nerves; the transmitter norepinephrine interacts with β-receptors. Propranolol, by antagonizing norepinephrine's effects, would reduce renin release. While this effect is beneficial in hypertensive patients with high plasma renin activity, it is uncertain whether such an activity can account for the hypotensive actions of propranolol.

There is evidence to suggest that noradrenergic nerves possess presynaptic β-receptors that, when activated, facilitate neurotransmitter release. If these presynaptic β-receptors play a functional role in the regulation of norepinephrine release, then antagonizing this facilitative effect could limit transmitter release and thereby limit sympathetically induced vasoconstriction.

Central, rather than peripheral, actions also have been proposed to account for the antihypertensive effects of the β-blockers. One such mechanism is that β-blockers somehow may reset the sensitivity of central baroreceptors to a lower level. Another hypothesis suggests that the drugs have a direct antagonistic action at central β-receptors.

Clinical Uses

The β-blockers are quite popular antihypertensive drugs. The drugs are well tolerated, and serious side effects are seldom observed. When used alone over a period of several weeks, β-blockers produce a significant reduction in blood pressure in approximately 30 percent of patients with mild to moderate hypertension. Thus, β-blockers can be employed as a first step in the management of high blood pressure. However, the drugs are often used in conjunction with a diuretic when therapy with a single agent is not satisfactory. Clinical evidence indicates that the combination of a β-blocker, thiazide diuretic, and vasodilator provides significant control of moderate to severe hypertension in approximately 80 percent of patients.

From a hemodynamic viewpoint, there are several obvious advantages to using a β-blocker in combination with a vasodilator. Reflex-mediated cardiac stimulation is a common feature of vasodilator treatment, and it can severely limit the antihypertensive effectiveness of the vasodilator. A β-blocker will reduce the cardiac stimulation and thus preserve the effectiveness of the vasodilator. Conversely, the increase in peripheral vascular resistance that occurs on initiation of treatment with a β-blocker will be prevented by the vasodilator. Furthermore, vasodilator treatment initiates reflexes that lead to an increase in plasma renin activity. Thus, β-blockers such as propranolol that reduce plasma renin activity are of obvious value.

Contraindications

Patients who exhibit signs of cardiac failure should not be treated with β-blockers. By reducing the effects of sympathetic stimulation on the heart, β-blockers will obtund an important compensatory mechanism and the failure will be worsened.

Their use is also contraindicated in patients with severe bradycardia or atrioventricular (A-V) conduction disturbances. A similar warning applies in the case of a patient suffering from asthma or obstructive airway disease. Sympathetic stimulation of bronchial smooth muscle leads to a relaxation that is mediated by β-receptors. β-Blocking agents may promote further bronchoconstriction. In this regard, cardioselective β-blockers (i.e., β_1), such as metoprolol, may have a slight advantage over a nonselective blocker, such as propranolol. The adrenoceptors of the respiratory system are classified as β_2 and those of the heart as β_1.

The β-blockers not only can interfere with some physiological symptoms produced by acute hypoglycemia, but they may exacerbate the hypoglycemia by antagonizing catecholamine-induced mobilization of glycogen. Extreme caution must be exercised when using the drugs in patients with diabetes mellitus.

In spite of the potential seriousness of the effects noted, the β-blockers have proved to be well-tolerated drugs, and patient compliance is good. The most frequently reported side effects are those associated with altered CNS function, such as hallucinations, nightmares, insomnia, and depression (see also Chap. 13).

Adrenergic Neuron-Blocking Drugs

These drugs are antihypertensive because they prevent the release of transmitters from peripheral postganglionic sympathetic nerves. The contraction of vascular smooth muscle due to sympathetic nerve stimulation is thereby re-

duced, and blood pressure decreases. Guanethidine is the prototypical member of this class and it, along with guanadrel, are approved for treatment of hypertension.

The maximum antihypertensive effectiveness of guanethidine and related drugs is greater than that produced by the adrenoceptor antagonists. This is likely due to the fact that guanethidine, by preventing exocytotic release, interferes with the postsynaptic action of the cotransmitters, such as ATP, as well as norepinephrine. The adrenoceptor antagonists reduce the postsynaptic action of only norepinephrine, not ATP.

Guanethidine

Guanethidine (Fig. 22-4) is a powerful antihypertensive agent that is quite effective in the treatment of moderate to severe hypertension. It is most frequently used in the treatment of severe hypertension that is resistant to other agents.

Pharmacological Actions

Guanethidine reduces blood pressure by its ability to diminish vascular tone; both the arterial and venous sides of the circulatory system are involved. The resulting venous pooling contributes to orthostatic hypotension, a prominent feature of guanethidine treatment. The reduction in blood pressure is more prominent when the patient is in the standing position rather than in the recumbent position.

A reduction in cardiac output, attributable to a decreased venous return, and the inability of sympathetic nerve impulses to release enough transmitter to stimulate the heart, occur during the early stages of guanethidine therapy. Accompanying the reduction in cardiac output is a proportional decrease in renal, splanchnic, and cerebral blood flow. With prolonged therapy, cardiac output, but not peripheral resistance, tends to return to pretreatment levels as a result of circulatory readjustments. There are no significant changes in renal function.

Mechanism of Action

Guanethidine exerts its effects at peripheral sympathetic nerve endings after its active transport into the nerve varicosities by the neuronal amine transport system. This is the same uptake system that transports norepinephrine into the varicosity (see Chap. 11). The accumulation of guanethidine in adrenergic neurons leads, through an as yet unexplained mechanism, to a disruption of the process by which action potentials trigger the release of stored norepinephrine and other cotransmitters from nerve terminals. It is this action of guanethidine that

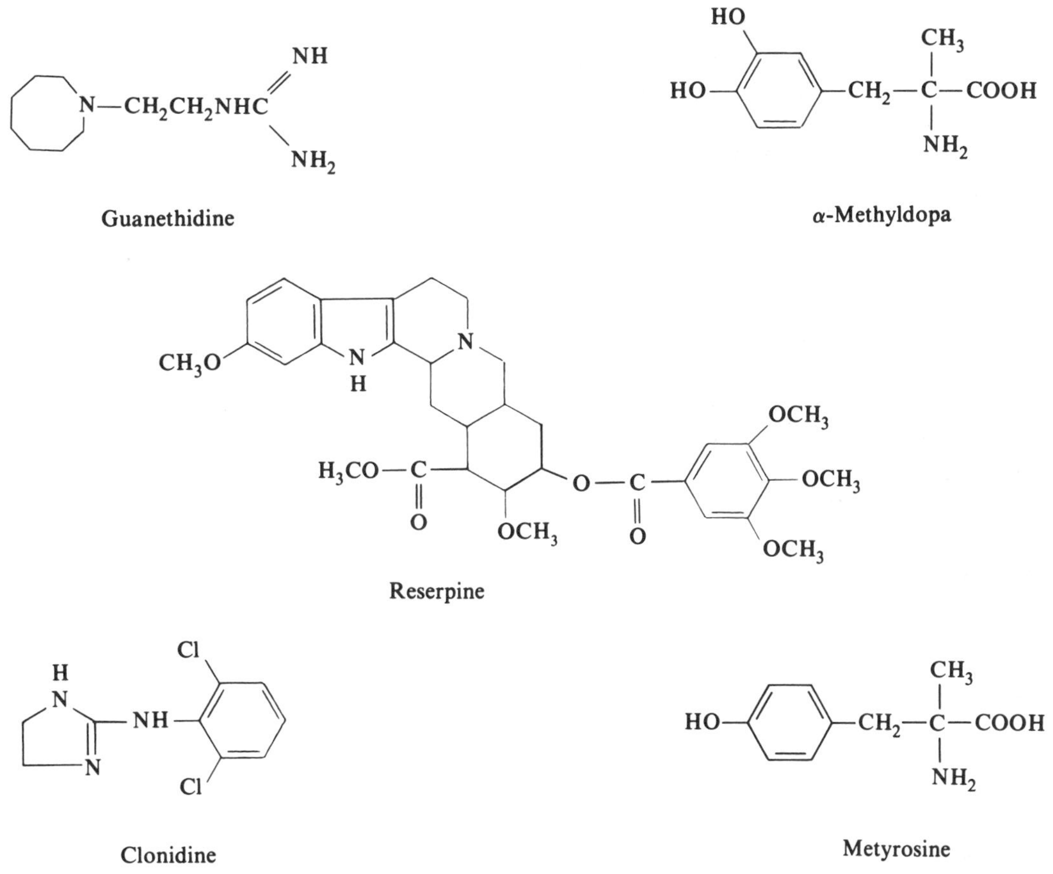

Figure 22-4. Structures of various sympathetic depressant drugs.

is primarily responsible for its antihypertensive properties. Parasympathetic function is not altered, a fact that distinguishes guanethidine from the ganglionic blocking agents.

A second consequence of the accumulation of guanethidine in noradrenergic varicosities is that the drug initially displaces norepinephrine from storage vesicles and thus releases this transmitter. This action accounts for the observation that an acute intravenous injection of guanethidine causes a transient pressor response. With chronic therapy, the displacement of norepinephrine by guanethidine leads to a reduction in transmitter concentration. Once sufficient amounts of norepinephrine are lost, guanethidine will no longer produce a pressor response. While the depletion of norepinephrine may contribute to the reduction in blood pressure that occurs as a result of long-term guanethidine therapy, depletion is not an absolute requirement of the drug's antihypertensive action.

Guanethidine neither releases nor depletes catechol-

amines from the adrenal medulla. However, it may provoke the release of catecholamines from a pheochromocytoma, resulting in a hypertensive crisis. Therefore, the drug is contraindicated in patients with pheochromocytoma.

Absorption, Metabolism, and Excretion

Guanethidine is suitable for oral use, and this is its usual route of administration. However, absorption from the gastrointestinal tract is rather variable and inefficient; 3 to 30 percent of the total oral dose is absorbed. Despite this variability among patients, absorption in an individual is reasonably constant.

The half-life of guanethidine is 5 days, with about one seventh of the total administered dose eliminated per day. The slow elimination contributes to the cumulative and prolonged effects of the drug.

Approximately half of an administered dose of guanethidine is excreted unchanged in the urine. Guanethidine is a strongly basic molecule and is eliminated in part by active tubular secretion. The remainder of the dose can be accounted for by hepatic metabolism. The two major metabolites produced are more polar than guanethidine and possess little antihypertensive activity.

In cases of liver disease or impaired kidney function, careful titration with guanethidine is necessary. Generally, these situations require a reduction in dose.

Clinical Uses

With the possible exception of minoxidil, guanethidine is the most potent orally effective antihypertensive drug. Guanethidine (*Ismelin, Hylorel*) effectively reduces blood pressure in three fourths of patients with severe primary hypertension. When combined with a thiazide diuretic, its effectiveness is reported to be as high as 85 percent.

Because guanethidine produces a number of side effects, which are due primarily to the imbalance between sympathetic and parasympathetic function it produces, the drug is generally reserved for the treatment of severe hypertension. Some clinicians, however, believe guanethidine occasionally could be considered for the treatment of moderate hypertension, since it produces minimal central nervous system (CNS) depression (a finding commonly associated with a number of other sympathetic depressants) and its long half-life permits administration once a day.

Chronic treatment with guanethidine, like treatment with other sympathetic depressants and vasodilators, leads to an intravascular volume expansion and a tolerance to the drug's antihypertensive effects. For this reason, guanethidine is almost always administered in conjunction with a diuretic. A vasodilator is sometimes added to this regimen to aid in the management of blood pressure when the patient is in the supine position.

Adverse Reactions

Up to 15 percent of the patients receiving guanethidine discontinue its use because they cannot tolerate the side effects, most of which are attributable to excessive impairment of sympathetic function and unopposed parasympathetic activity. Orthostatic hypotension associated with dizziness when the patient is standing is reported to occur in 35 to 40 percent of guanethidine-treated patients. This postural hypotension is most prominent in the morning and tends to wane during the day. Exercise-induced hypotension may also occur. Sexual impotence does occur and male patients may experience difficulty in ejaculation. Symptoms of unopposed parasympathetic activity include such gastrointestinal disturbances as diarrhea and increased gastric secretion.

Guanethidine may aggravate congestive heart failure or actually precipitate failure in patients with marginal cardiac reserve, owing to its ability to produce vascular volume expansion, edema, and a reduced effectiveness of sympathetic cardiac stimulation.

Contraindications

Guanethidine is contraindicated in patients with frank signs of congestive heart failure unrelated to hypertension and in patients with pheochromocytoma. The concomitant use of monoamine oxidase (MAO) inhibitors and guanethidine is also to be avoided, since this combined drug treatment eliminates two of the principal mechanisms for terminating the actions of the catecholamines and certain other adrenomimetic drugs, that is, biotransformation and neuronal uptake. Dangerously high concentrations of catecholamines at receptor sites could then occur.

Drug Interactions

The tricyclic antidepressants (e.g., desipramine and amitriptyline) and some phenothiazines block the sympathetic neuronal amine uptake system; they thereby would also block the uptake of guanethidine and thus reduce its hypotensive effectiveness. Conversely, guanethidine competitively inhibits the uptake of drugs that are substrates for neuronal uptake, such as the indirectly acting adrenomimetics (sympathomimetics; see Chap. 12).

Drugs That Interfere With Norepinephrine Storage

Reserpine

Rauwolfia serpentina (snakeroot), which is indigenous to India, Sri Lanka, Burma, and Java, contains at least 20 antihypertensive alkaloids. A number of *Rauwolfia* extracts and preparations are currently available for the treatment of hypertension; these include those derived from the whole root (*Raudixin*) and several purified or semisynthetic alkaloids, such as syrosingopine, rescinnamine, deserpidine, and reserpine. *Reserpine* (see Fig. 22-4) is the best-studied compound and is the alkaloid most frequently employed clinically. The actions and indications for use of other *Rauwolfia* alkaloids are essentially identical to those of reserpine.

Pharmacological Actions

The result of reserpine administration is diminished noradrenergic function. Vascular smooth muscle tone is reduced and therefore vascular resistance is decreased. Venous as well as arterial tone is reduced. The combination of reduction in venous tone and reduction in effective sympathetic stimulation of the heart leads to postural hypotension. This hypotension is generally less severe than that produced by guanethidine, possibly because reserpine affects transmission due to norepinephrine and not that due to ATP. Guanethidine affects both.

During long-term therapy with reserpine, the percentage decrease in blood pressure may be greater than the percentage decrease in cardiac output. The reduction in blood pressure produced by reserpine develops slowly over a period of weeks. A slight reduction in renal blood flow also may be a consequence of reserpine administration.

Mechanism of Action

The mechanism by which reserpine lowers blood pressure is reasonably well understood. The drug reduces norepinephrine concentrations in the noradrenergic nerves in such a way that less norepinephrine is released during neuron activation. Reserpine does not interfere with the release process per se as guanethidine does.

Under normal circumstances, when an action potential invades the sympathetic nerve terminal, a portion of the released norepinephrine is recycled. This event requires two successive steps: (1) Norepinephrine is transferred across the neuronal membrane into the cytosol by an energy-dependent, carrier-mediated active process, and (2) the recaptured amine is then transported from the cytosol into the noradrenergic storage vesicles, where it is stored until needed. *Reserpine inhibits only the second uptake process.* As a consequence of this inhibition of vesicular uptake, norepinephrine cannot be stored intraneuronally, and much of the cytosolic amine is metabolized by MAO.

In addition to impairing norepinephrine storage and thereby enhancing its catabolism, reserpine also impairs the vesicular uptake of dopamine, the immediate precursor of norepinephrine. Since dopamine must be taken up into the adrenergic vesicles in order to undergo hydroxylation to form norepinephrine, reserpine administration impairs norepinephrine synthesis. *The combined effects of the blockade of dopamine and norepinephrine vesicular uptake lead to transmitter depletion.*

Depletion of norepinephrine requires some time to occur, so that the onset of the antihypertensive action of reserpine is slow. A week or more may be necessary for the therapeutic effect to be fully manifest. Similarly, normal adrenergic function may require several weeks to be fully restored on cessation of treatment.

Reserpine-induced amine depletion is not restricted to peripheral noradrenergic nerves. Reserpine also will cause a reduction in adrenal medullary catecholamine concentrations, although the medulla is somewhat more resistant than are sympathetic nerves to the depleting action of the drug. Reserpine also interferes with the neuronal storage of a variety of central transmitter amines such that significant depletion of norepinephrine, dopamine, and 5-hydroxytryptamine (serotonin) occurs. This central transmitter depletion is responsible for the sedation and other CNS side effects associated with reserpine therapy.

The depletion of brain amines also may contribute to the antihypertensive effects of reserpine, but this action by itself is not believed to be essential; the peripheral effects are considered to be more important in producing hypotension. Reserpine has no direct effect on parasympathetic nerves.

Absorption, Metabolism, and Excretion

Orally administered reserpine is readily absorbed from the gastrointestinal tract and thereby gains rapid access to most body compartments. However, blood levels of the drug decline rapidly owing both to the lipophilic character of the molecule (which favors drug redistribution from blood to more highly lipid tissues) and to rapid drug biotransformation. It is now apparent that small amounts of reserpine remain selectively and tightly bound to the membranes of the monoamine storage vesicles. This binding, although representing only a small fraction of the administered dose, apparently is sufficient to impair the vesicular membrane uptake system.

Reserpine is extensively metabolized, and only a small amount of the administered drug is eliminated unchanged, with much of this being found in the feces. The principal urinary metabolites are trimethoxybenzoic acid and methyl reserpate. They are the products of ester hydrolysis, reactions that occur in the plasma, liver, and, to a small degree, in the intestinal mucosa. Hepatic oxidative and conjugative enzymes also may contribute to the metabolism of reserpine.

Clinical Uses

The chief use of reserpine (*Rau-Sed, Serpasil,* and others) is in the treatment of mild to moderate hypertension. As with other sympathetic depressant drugs, tolerance to the antihypertensive effects of reserpine can occur, owing to a compensatory increase in blood volume that frequently accompanies decreased peripheral vascular resistance. Reserpine, therefore, should be used in conjunction with a diuretic.

Because of its sedative properties, reserpine is of special benefit to hypertensive patients who exhibit symptoms of agitated psychotic states and who may be unable to tolerate therapy with phenothiazine derivatives.

Adverse Reactions

It is estimated that about 5 percent of all patients treated with *Rauwolfia* drugs discontinue therapy because of side effects. The most troublesome untoward effects involve the CNS: sedation and depression are the most common, although nightmares and thoughts of suicide also occur. Reserpine treatment, therefore, is contraindicated in patients with a history of severe depression. The occasional report of reserpine-induced extrapyramidal symptoms, which are similar to those seen in patients with Parkinson's disease (see Chap. 38), is believed to be a result of dopamine depletion from neurons in the CNS.

Peripheral nervous system side effects also occur. These are the result of a reserpine-induced reduction of sympathetic function and an unopposed parasympathetic activity; symptoms include nasal congestion, postural hypotension, diarrhea, bradycardia, increased gastric secretion, and occasional impotence. Because of the increased gastric secretion, reserpine is contraindicated for patients with peptic ulcer. In patients with little cardiac reserve, reserpine must be administered with caution because of its ability to interfere with sympathetic stimulation of the heart.

In 1974, several reports appeared that suggested an association between the use of *Rauwolfia* drugs and breast cancer. Subsequent studies have failed to substantiate such an association.

Drugs That Interfere With Norepinephrine Synthesis

Metyrosine

Chemically, metyrosine (Fig. 22-4) is α-methyl tyrosine. The drug blocks the action of tyrosine hydroxylase, the rate-limiting enzyme in the synthesis of catecholamines (see Chap. 11). Unlike α-methyldopa, metyrosine is not itself incorporated into the catecholamine synthetic pathway. The ultimate action of the drug is to decrease the production of catecholamines.

Metyrosine is well absorbed from the gastrointestinal tract. The drug-induced reduction in norepinephrine concentration requires several days to fully develop and thus there is a delay in the onset of the antihypertensive effect. Metyrosine is excreted in the urine largely as unchanged drug.

Metyrosine (*Demser*) is not employed for the treatment of essential hypertension but rather is used for the management of pheochromocytoma. It is useful for preoperative treatment and for long-term therapy when surgery is not feasible.

Sedation is the most common adverse effect of metyrosine. Other CNS disturbances, such as anxiety, confusion, and disorientation have also been reported. Symptoms of sympathetic nervous system depression in general, such as nasal congestion and dryness of mouth, can also occur with metyrosine.

Ganglionic Blocking Agents

The basis for the antihypertensive activity of these compounds lies in their ability to block transmission through autonomic ganglia (see Fig. 22-3, site C). This action, which results in a decrease in the number of impulses passing down the postganglionic sympathetic (and parasympathetic) nerves, decreases vascular tone, cardiac output, and blood pressure. These drugs prevent the interaction of acetylcholine (the transmitter of the preganglionic autonomic nerves) with the nicotinic receptors on postsynaptic neuronal membranes of both the sympathetic and parasympathetic nervous systems.

The ganglionic blocking agents are extremely potent antihypertensive agents and can reduce blood pressure, regardless of the extent of hypertension. Limiting the release of both norepinephrine and ATP, by virtue of reducing impulses traveling down vascular postganglionic sympathetic nerves, probably contributes to the extreme antihypertensive potency of the ganglion blocking agents.

Unfortunately, blockade of transmission in both the sympathetic and parasympathetic systems produces numerous untoward responses, including marked postural hypotension, blurred vision, dryness of mouth, constipation, paralytic ileus, urinary retention, and impotence. Owing both to the frequency and severity of these side effects and also to the development of other powerful antihypertensive agents, most notably the directly acting vasodilators, the ganglionic blocking agents are rarely used. The orally effective ganglionic blocking agents are, in fact, not recommended for the treatment of primary hypertension. However, certain intravenous preparations, such as the short-acting agent trimethaphan camsylate (*Arfonad*), are used occasionally for hypertensive emergencies or in surgical procedures in which hypotension is desirable in order to reduce the possibility of hemorrhage. A more complete description of trimethaphan and other ganglionic blocking agents can be found in Chap. 17.

Centrally Acting Hypotensive Drugs

Using drugs that interfere with the *peripheral* component of the sympathetic nervous system obviously represents an important approach to the treatment of hypertension. In recent years, however, a second approach has been demonstrated. At present, there are two important antihypertensive agents, α-methyldopa and clonidine, that act predominantly in the *brain* (see Fig. 22-3, site D). Although the details of their actions may differ in some respects, *their antihypertensive activity is ultimately due to their ability to decrease the sympathetic outflow from the brain to the cardiovascular system.*

α-Methyldopa

The spectrum of activity of α-methyldopa lies between the more potent agents, such as guanethidine, and the milder antihypertensives, such as reserpine. α-Methyldopa (see Fig. 22-4) is a structural analogue of dihydroxyphenylalanine (dopa) and differs from dopa only by the presence of a methyl group on the α-carbon of the side chain.

Pharmacological Actions

The primary hemodynamic alteration responsible for the hypotensive effects of α-methyldopa remains in dispute. Some investigators believe that blood pressure falls as a result of a reduction in peripheral vascular resistance with no change in cardiac output. Others believe, however, that such an action may account for hypotension during short-term treatment, but that long-term drug therapy leads to a decreased cardiac output with little or no alteration in vascular resistance. Part of the controversy may be related to the conditions under which the cardiovascular parameters are measured. When the patient is in the supine position, the reduction in blood pressure produced by α-methyldopa correlates best with a decrease in peripheral vascular resistance, cardiac output being only slightly reduced. When the patient is in the upright position, the fall in blood pressure corresponds more closely with a reduced cardiac output.

An important aspect of α-methyldopa's hemodynamic effects is that renal blood flow and glomerular filtration rate are not reduced. Because blood flow to the kidney is maintained with its use, α-methyldopa is especially valuable in treating hypertensive patients with renal insufficiency. As occurs with most sympathetic depressant drugs and vasodilators, long-term therapy with α-methyldopa leads to fluid retention, edema formation, and plasma volume expansion. While there are some conflicting data, it is generally thought that α-methyldopa suppresses plasma renin activity.

Mechanism of Action

A number of theories have been put forward to account for the hypotensive action of α-methyldopa. An early hypothesis suggested that since α-methyldopa is an inhibitor of the enzyme 1-aromatic amino acid decarboxylase (dopa decarboxylase), it may impair the conversion of dopa to dopamine in sympathetic neurons, a reaction catalyzed by this enzyme. Unfortunately, the drug's hypotensive ef-

fects do not correlate well with the extent of inhibition of dopa decarboxylase produced and therefore other explanations have been sought.

A second theory is based on the observation that α-methyldopa is itself a substrate for dopa decarboxylase. Thus, α-methyldopa rather than dopa is acted upon by dopa decarboxylase, and this results in the conversion of α-methyldopa to α-methyldopamine. A further enzymatically catalyzed reaction (dopamine hydroxylase, DBH) leads to formation of α-methylnorepinephrine, a compound that may be both retained in sympathetic nerve storage vesicles and displace some norepinephrine from these vesicles.

If α-methylnorepinephrine were to be released in conjunction with norepinephrine after sympathetic nerve stimulation, and if α-methylnorepinephrine were less potent than norepinephrine, effects of nerve stimulation would be reduced. By such a hypothesis, α-methylnorepinephrine would function as a *false transmitter*. Although there is no question that α-methylnorepinephrine is formed in noradrenergic tissues, it is now recognized that under most circumstances peripheral adrenergic effectors are just as sensitive to the actions of α-methylnorepinephrine as they are to norepinephrine. Thus, the false-transmitter hypothesis is no longer considered a workable explanation for the antihypertensive effects of α-methyldopa.

Current evidence agrees that in order for α-methyldopa to be an antihypertensive agent, it does need to be converted to α-methylnorepinephrine; however, *its site of action appears to be in the brain rather than in the periphery.* Systemically administered α-methyldopa rapidly enters the brain, where it accumulates in noradrenergic nerves, is converted to α-methylnorepinephrine, and is then released. Released α-methylnorepinephrine activates CNS α-adrenoceptors whose function is to decrease sympathetic outflow. Why α-methylnorepinephrine decreases sympathetic outflow more effectively than does the naturally occurring transmitter is not entirely clear. One explanation may be that α-methylnorepinephrine is longer acting than norepinephrine because it is less quickly metabolized. Additionally, activation of central α$_2$-receptors may lead to a decrease in sympathetic outflow; α-methylnorepinephrine also has a greater affinity for α$_2$-receptors than does norepinephrine.

The specific sites in the brain where α-methyldopa exerts its effects are not fully elucidated, although many investigators believe that the nucleus of the tractus solitarius (NTS) in the medulla oblongata is intimately involved.

Absorption, Metabolism, and Excretion

Approximately 50 percent of an orally administered dose of α-methyldopa is absorbed from the gastrointestinal tract. Both peak plasma drug levels and maximal blood pressure-lowering effects are observed 2 to 6 hr after oral administration. A considerable amount of unchanged α-methyldopa as well as several conjugated and decarboxylated metabolites can be found in the urine. In the presence of azotemia, however, urinary excretion of α-methyldopa is generally decreased and the drug's plasma half-life will be increased. The dose of α-methyldopa may need to be reduced in those circumstances.

Clinical Uses

When α-methyldopa is used alone for short-term treatment of hypertension, approximately two thirds of patients with mild to moderate primary hypertension respond with a significant decrease in blood pressure. Because plasma volume increases as the duration of α-methyldopa therapy is extended, the drug should be used in conjunction with a diuretic to produce a significantly greater fall in blood pressure than would occur with either drug used alone. Because α-methyldopa lowers blood pressure without compromising either renal blood flow or the glomerular filtration rate, it is particularly valuable in hypertension complicated by renal disease. However, if a condition of end-stage renal failure exists along with severe hypertension, α-methyldopa may not be effective.

The presence of α-methyldopa and its metabolites in the urine reduces the diagnostic value of urinary catecholamine measurements as an indicator of pheochromocytoma. These substances interfere with the fluorescence assay for catecholamines, since they have fluorescence spectra that are quite similar to those of the endogenous amines.

Adverse Reactions

α-Methyldopa is relatively well tolerated by most patients; the most commonly encountered side effects are sedation and drowsiness. The degree of sedation tends to decrease with continued therapy, whereas drowsiness may be a more persistent problem. These CNS effects are probably the result of reductions in brain catecholamine levels. Other side effects, also typical of sympathetic depression, are dry mouth, nasal congestion, orthostatic hypotension, and impotence. The orthostasis and impotence occur less frequently than with guanethidine therapy.

Side effects unrelated to sympathetic depression have also been reported. A relatively large number of patients exhibit a positive direct antiglobulin (Coombs') test. Fortunately, this is only rarely associated with hemolytic anemia. Other autoimmune reactions associated with α-methyldopa treatment include thrombocytopenia and leukopenia. Even though the incidence of the effects is quite low, occasional blood tests should be performed. A few cases of an α-methyldopa–induced hepatitis also have occurred. α-Methyldopa, therefore, is contraindicated in

patients with active hepatic disease. Flulike symptoms, treatable with salicylates, also are known to occur. Methyldopa (*Aldomet*) is also available as methyldopate hydrochloride (*Aldomet Ester Hydrochloride*).

Clonidine and Related Drugs

Clonidine is effective orally and is used primarily for the treatment of moderate hypertension. It is an imidazoline derivative (see Fig. 22-4) that is structurally related to the α-adrenoceptor antagonists phentolamine and tolazoline. *Clonidine, however, is not an α-blocker, but is actually an α-agonist.* Its antihypertensive effectiveness appeared paradoxical until it was recognized that clonidine activated central α_2-receptors, thus reducing sympathetic outflow to the periphery.

Guanabenz and *guanfacine* are two drugs with considerable structural similarity to clonidine. These agents also are central α_2-agonists and exhibit an antihypertensive profile similar to that of clonidine.

Pharmacological Actions

An acute intravenous injection of clonidine may produce a transient pressor response that apparently is due to stimulation of peripheral vascular α-receptors. The pressor response does not occur after oral administration, because the drug's centrally mediated depressor action overrides it.

The decrease in blood pressure produced by clonidine correlates better with a decreased cardiac output than with a reduction in peripheral vascular resistance. The reduction in cardiac output is the result of both a decreased heart rate and reduced stroke work; the latter effect is probably caused by a diminished venous return. Although orthostatic and exercise-induced hypotension may occur in some patients, it generally is not a problem. Clonidine apparently does not inhibit baroreceptor reflexes and may, in fact, enhance them.

Renal blood flow and glomerular filtration are not decreased, although renal resistance is diminished. Clonidine's effects on renal hemodynamics, therefore, are similar to those produced by α-methyldopa. Thus, it also is a useful agent for hypertension complicated by renal disease. Plasma renin activity is reduced by clonidine, presumably as a result of a centrally mediated decrease in sympathetic stimulation of the juxtaglomerular cells of the kidney.

Mechanism of Action

Although clonidine can produce effects on peripheral tissues, these effects do not account for its hypotensive activity. It does not produce catecholamine depletion or α- or β-receptor blockade, and does not inhibit ganglionic transmission.

The antihypertensive activity of clonidine can be ascribed solely to a decrease in the sympathetic activity transmitted from the brain to the peripheral vasculature. After clonidine administration, direct measurements of sympathetic nerve activity show that electrical discharge is reduced in a number of sympathetic nerves, including the cardiac, splanchnic, and cervical nerves.

It is generally agreed that clonidine acts in the same general area in the brain as does α-methyldopa, that is, somewhere in the medulla oblongata. The principal difference between clonidine and α-methyldopa would be that clonidine acts directly on α_2-receptors, whereas α-methyldopa first must be converted by synthetic enzymes to α-methylnorepinephrine.

Recent evidence indicates that another receptor type in the brainstem, similar to the α_2-receptor, may play a role in modulating sympathetic outflow to the peripheral vasculature. This receptor, referred to as an imidazoline-preferring receptor, although exhibiting some similarity to α_2-receptors, appears to be distinct. Clonidine, being an imidazoline derivative, has affinity for the imidazoline receptor as well as for α_2-receptors. The possibility exists that the antihypertensive effect of clonidine may be due in part to activation of both receptor types.

Absorption, Metabolism, and Excretion

Clonidine is well absorbed after oral administration. Peak plasma levels occur between 2 and 4 hr and correlate well with pharmacological activity. The plasma half-life in patients with normal renal function is 12 hr. Urinary excretion of clonidine and its metabolites accounts for almost 90 percent of the administered dose, and fecal excretion accounts for the rest. Approximately 50 percent of an administered dose is excreted unchanged; the remainder is oxidatively metabolized in the liver.

Reports vary somewhat concerning the influence of renal insufficiency on the biological fate of clonidine. The plasma half-life, and thus the drug's hypotensive action, is not much affected by mild azotemia, presumably because of a compensatory increase in hepatic metabolism. If azotemia is severe, however, it may be necessary to reduce the dose, because plasma half-life will be lengthened.

Clinical Uses

The primary indication for clonidine (*Catapres*) use is in mild and moderate hypertension that has not responded adequately to treatment with a diuretic alone. Since clonidine causes sodium and water retention and plasma volume expansion, it generally is administered in combination with a diuretic. A vasodilator can be added to the clonidine-diuretic regimen in the treatment of more resistant forms of hypertension. Such drug combinations can be quite effective, since the reflex increases in heart rate and cardiac output that result from vasodilator administration are reduced or negated by clonidine-induced decreases in heart rate and cardiac output.

For severely hypertensive patients, clonidine has been used in combination with a diuretic, a vasodilator, and a β-blocker. Some care must be taken, however, because the coadministration of clonidine and a β-blocker may cause excessive sedation. Clonidine is especially useful in patients with renal failure, since its duration of action is not appreciably altered by renal disease and it does not compromise renal blood flow.

Adverse Reactions

It is estimated that about 7 percent of all patients receiving clonidine discontinue the drug because of side effects. Although the symptoms are generally mild and tend to subside if therapy is continued for several weeks, as many as 50 percent of the patients complain of drowsiness and dryness of mouth. Other untoward effects include constipation, nausea or gastric upset, and impotence. These effects, characteristic of interference with the functioning of the sympathetic nervous system, are generally infrequent.

A potentially dangerous effect, and one that has received a lot of attention, is *rebound hypertension,* which occurs following abrupt withdrawal of clonidine therapy. This posttreatment hypertension appears to be the result of excessive sympathetic activity. The genesis of the syndrome is not well understood. A contributing factor could be the development of a supersensitivity in either the sympathetic nerves or the effector organs of the cardiovascular system due to the clonidine-caused chronic reduction in sympathetic activity. Thus, when the drug is abruptly withdrawn, an exaggerated response to "normal" levels of activity could occur. Other characteristics of the rebound syndrome, also suggestive of enhanced sympathetic activity, include insomnia, restlessness, and tremor. Either reinstitution of clonidine treatment followed by gradual drug withdrawal, or administration of α- and β-blocking agents, can effectively control the symptoms of this phenomenon. If treatment with clonidine is always terminated gradually, rebound hypertension is unlikely to occur. However, patients should be warned of the potential danger of abruptly discontinuing clonidine treatment.

Clonidine is also marketed as a transdermal patch (*Catapres-TTS*) that provides systemic delivery of the drug for 7 days.

Guanabenz acetate (*Wytensin*) is administered orally as tablets. The usual oral dose for starting treatment is 4 mg twice a day.

Guanfacine hydrochloride (*Tenex*) is also available in

tablets. The starting dose is 1 mg once a day usually at bed-time.

Supplemental Reading

Antonaccio, M.J. (ed.). *Cardiovascular Pharmacology* (3rd ed.). New York: Raven, 1990.

Cook, N.S. The pharmacology of potassium channels and their therapeutic potential. *Tr. Pharmacol. Sci.* 9:21, 1988.

Fregly, M.J., and Kare, M.R. (eds.). *The Role of Salt in Cardiovascular Hypertension.* New York: Academic, 1982.

Furchgott, R.F. Studies on endothelium-dependent vasodilation and the endothelium-derived relaxing factor. *Acta Physiol. Scand.* 139:257, 1990.

Ignarro, L.J., et al. Mechanism of vascular smooth muscle relaxation by organic nitrates, nitrites, nitroprusside and nitric oxide: Evidence for the involvement of S-nitrosothiols as active intermediates. *J. Pharmacol. Exp. Ther.* 218:739, 1981.

Ignarro, L.J., et al. Endothelium-derived relaxing factor produced and released from artery and vein is nitric oxide. *Proc. Natl. Acad. Sci.* 84:9265, 1987.

Joint National Committee on Detection, Evaluation, and Treatment of High Blood Pressure: The 1988 report. *Arch. Intern. Med.* 148:1023, 1988.

Laragh, J.H. (ed.). Imidazoline receptors: A new regulatory concept in blood pressure control. *Am. J. Hyperten.* 5:455, 1992.

Luther, R.R. New perspectives on selective alpha$_1$-blockade. *Am. J. Hyperten.* 2:729, 1989.

Meisheri, K.D., et al. Mechanism of action of minoxidil sulfate–induced vasodilation: A role for increased K^+ permeability. *J. Pharmacol. Exp. Ther.* 245:751, 1988.

Murad, F. Cyclic guanosine monophosphate as a mediator of vasodilation. *J. Clin. Invest.* 78:1, 1986.

Robertson, J.I.S. (ed.). *Clinical Aspects of Essential Hypertension.* New York: Elsevier, 1983.

Robertson, J.I.S. (ed.). *Clinical Aspects of Secondary Hypertension.* New York: Elsevier, 1983.

Stokes, G.S., and Marwood, J.F. Review of the use of alpha-adrenoceptor antagonists in hypertension. *Methods Find. Exp. Clin. Pharmacol.* 6:197, 1984.

Westfall, D.P., Dalziel, H.H., and Forsyth, K.M. ATP as a Neurotransmitter, Cotransmitter and Neuromodulator. In J.W. Phillis (ed.), *Adenosine and Adenine Nucleotides as Regulators of Cellular Function.* Boca Raton, Fla.: CRC Press, 1991, P. 295.

Wollam, G., and Hall, D.W. *Hypertension Management: Clinical Practice and Therapeutic Dilemmas.* Chicago: Year Book, 1988.

23

Calcium Channel Blockers

Vijay C. Swamy and *David J. Triggle*

The agents commonly referred to as the calcium channel blockers comprise an increasing number of agents, including the prototypical verapamil, nifedipine, and diltiazem. These agents are a chemically and pharmacologically heterogeneous group of synthetic drugs (Fig. 23-1), but they possess the common property of selectively antagonizing Ca^{2+} movements that underlie the process of excitation-contraction coupling in the cardiovascular system. *The primary use of these agents is in the treatment of angina, selected cardiac arrhythmias, and, increasingly, hypertension* (Table 23-1).

Although the Ca^{2+} channel blockers are potent vasodilating drugs, they lack the properties of other vasodilators of causing fluid accumulation and of persistent activation of the sympathetic and renin-angiotensin-aldosterone axes. Furthermore, the broad potential range of activities, both within and without the cardiovascular system, suggests that they may be clinically useful in disorders from achalasia to vertigo.

A number of second-generation analogues are known, particularly in the nifedipine (1,4-dihydropyridine) series, including nimodipine, nicardipine, felodipine, and amlodipine. These agents differ from nifedipine principally in their potency, pharmacokinetic characteristics, and selectivity of action. Nimodipine has selectivity for the cerebral vasculature, amlodipine exhibits very slow kinetics of onset and offset of blockade, and felodipine is a vascular-selective 1,4-dihydropyridine.

Calcium Antagonism: Pharmacological Principles

The concept of calcium antagonism as a specific mechanism of drug action was pioneered by Albrecht Fleckenstein and his colleagues, who observed that verapamil, and subsequently other drugs of this class, mimicked in reversible fashion the effects of Ca^{2+} withdrawal on cardiac excitability. These drugs inhibited the Ca^{2+} component of the ionic currents carried in the cardiac action potential. Because of this activity these drugs are also referred to as *slow channel blockers, calcium channel antagonists,* and *calcium entry blockers.*

The actions of these drugs must be viewed from the perspective of cellular Ca^{2+} regulation (Fig. 23-2). Ca^{2+} is fundamentally important in serving as a cellular messenger, linking cellular excitation and cellular response. This role is made possible by the high inwardly directed Ca^{2+} concentration and electrochemical gradients, by the existence of specific high-affinity Ca^{2+} binding proteins (e.g., calmodulin) that serve as intracellular Ca^{2+} receptors, and by the existence of Ca^{2+}-specific influx, efflux, and sequestration processes. Calcium, in excess, serves as a mediator of cell destruction and death during ischemia, neurodegeneration, cell toxicity, and so forth. The control of excess Ca^{2+} mobilization is thus an important contributor to cell and tissue protection.

The currently available Ca^{2+} channel blockers exert their effects primarily at voltage-gated Ca^{2+} channels of the plasma membrane. There are at least four types of channels—L, T, N, and P—distinguished by their electrophysiological and pharmacological characteristics. The blockers act at the L-type channel at three distinct receptor sites (Fig. 23-2). These different receptor interactions underlie, in part, the qualitative and quantitative differences exhibited by the three principal classes of channel blocker.

Cellular stimuli that involve Ca^{2+} mobilization by other processes, such as intracellular stores, will be insensitive or less sensitive to the channel blockers than is Ca^{2+} mobilization through the L-type voltage-gated channel. This differential sensitivity contributes to the variable sensitivity of vascular and nonvascular smooth muscle to these drugs, including regional vascular selectivity and the general lack of activity of these agents in respiratory smooth muscle disorders.

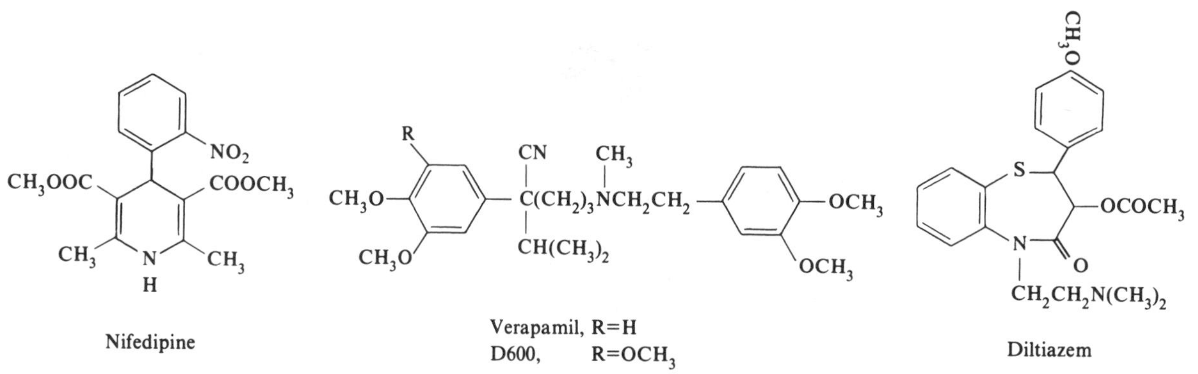

Figure 23-1. Chemical formulas of some Ca^{2+} antagonists.

Table 23-1. Therapeutic Uses of Calcium Channel Antagonists

Uses	Antagonist		
	Verapamil	Nifedipine	Diltiazem
Angina			
Exertional	+++	+++	+++
Prinzmetal's variant	+++	+++	+++
Paroxysmal supraventricular tachyarrhythmias	+++	−	+++
Atrial fibrillation and flutter	++	−	++
Hypertension	++	+++	+
Hypertrophic cardiomyopathy	+	−	−
Raynaud's phenomenon	++	++	++
Cardioplegia	+	+	+
Cerebral vasospasm (posthemorrhage)*	−	+	−

Key: +++ = used very commonly; − = not used.
*Use of nimodipine.

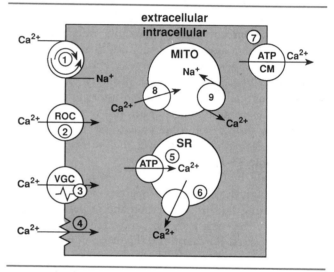

Figure 23-2. Schematic representation of cellular calcium regulation. Depicted are several sites that control calcium entry, efflux, and sequestration. 1: Na^+, Ca^{2+} exchange; 2: receptor-operated channels; 3: voltage-gated channels; 4: "leak" pathways; 5, 6: entry and efflux in sarcoplasmic reticulum; 7: plasma membrane pump; 8, 9: entry and efflux in mitochondria. ATP = adenosine triphosphate; CM = cell membrane.

The Selectivity of Action of Calcium Channel Blockers

Although the available Ca^{2+} channel blockers exert their effects through an interaction at one type of channel, they do so at different sites. Figure 23-3 shows the channel blockers acting at three discrete receptor sites to mediate channel blockade indirectly rather than by a direct or physical channel block or "plug." Support for this view is provided by the existence of analogues of nifedipine that serve to activate or open the channel and by the phenomenon of use-dependent blockade of the channel by verapamil, nifedipine, and diltiazem.

The existence of the different receptor sites is one basis for the different pharmacological profiles exhibited by these agents. Additionally, the activity of the Ca^{2+} blockers increases with increasing frequency of stimulation or intensity and duration of membrane depolarization. *This use-dependent activity is consistent with a preferred interaction of the antagonists with the open or inactivated states of the Ca^{2+} channel rather than with the resting state.* This activity is not shared equally by all Ca^{2+} blockers and, thus, may provide a further basis for the therapeutic differences between them. For example, verapamil and diltiazem are approximately equipotent in cardiac and vascular smooth muscle, whereas nifedipine and all other agents of the 1,4-dihy-

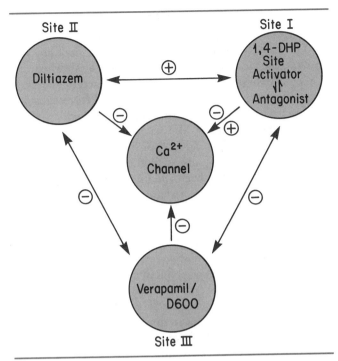

Figure 23-3. The principal receptors or drug binding sites at the calcium channel. These sites are linked to the opening and closing of the channel and to each other by activating [+] or inhibitory [−] allosteric mechanisms. The 1,4-DHP site is a receptor site for a number of 1,4-dihydropyridine compounds; D600 is the designation for a close chemical relative of verapamil.

dropyridine class are significantly more active in vascular smooth muscle. Furthermore, different members of the 1,4-dihydropyridine class have different degrees of vascular selectivity. These differences are broadly consistent with observation of verapamil and diltiazem acting preferentially through the open channel state, and nifedipine and its analogues acting through the inactivated state.

The Ca^{2+} channel blockers also differ in the extent to which they possess additional pharmacological properties. Verapamil and, to a lesser extent, diltiazem possess a number of receptor-blocking properties, together with Na^+ and K^+ channel-blocking activities, that may contribute to their pharmacological profile. Nifedipine and other 1,4-dihydropyridines are more selective for the voltage-gated Ca^{2+} channel, but they may also affect other pharmacological properties because their nonpolar properties may lead to cellular accumulation. Together with their channel-blocking properties, these additional pharmacological properties may contribute to the recently described antiatherogenic actions of the channel blockers in clinical states.

Pharmacological Effects on the Cardiovascular System

The effects of the prototypical calcium channel blockers are seen most prominently in the cardiovascular system (Table 23-2), although calcium channels are widely distributed among excitable cells.

Vascular Effects

Vascular tone and contraction are determined largely by the availability of calcium from extracellular sources (influx via calcium channels) or from the intracellular stores (see Fig. 23-2). Drug-induced inhibition of calcium influx via voltage-gated channels results in widespread dilatation and a decrease in contractile responses to stimulatory agents. In general, arteries and arterioles are more sensitive to their relaxant action than are the veins, and some arterial beds (e.g., coronary and cerebral vessels) show greater sensitivity than others. Peripheral vasodilatation, and the consequent fall in blood pressure, is commonly accompanied by reflex tachycardia when nifedipine and its analogues are used; this observation contrasts to verapamil and diltiazem, whose effects on peripheral vessels are accompanied by cardiodepressant effects.

Table 23-2. Cardiovascular Effects of Calcium Channel Blockers*

	Nifedipine	Diltiazem	Verapamil
Blood pressure	−	−	−
Vasodilation	+ + +	+ +	+ +
Heart rate	+ +	−	±
Contractility	0/+	0	0/−
Coronary vascular resistance	−	−	−
Blood flow	+ + +	+ + +	+ +

Key: + = increase; − = decrease; 0 = no significant effect.
*Changes are those seen commonly following oral doses used in therapy of hypertension or angina. The magnitude of response is indicated by number of symbols.

Cardiac Effects

Calcium currents in cardiac tissues serve the functions of inotropy, pacemaker activity (sinoatrial [S-A] node), and conduction at the atrioventricular (A-V) node. In principle, the blockade of calcium currents should result in decreased function at these sites. In clinical use, dose-dependent depression is seen only with verapamil and diltiazem and not with nifedipine, reflecting, in the main, differences in the kinetics of their interaction at calcium channels (see section on calcium antagonism). Characteristic cardiac effects include a variable slowing of the heart rate, strong depression of conduction at the A-V node, and inhibition of contractibility, especially in the presence of preexisting heart failure.

Therapeutic Applications

Hypertension

The calcium channel blocking drugs are effective antihypertensive agents and enjoy widespread use both as a single medication or in combination in a "stepped-care" regimen. Their effectiveness is related to a decrease in peripheral resistance accompanied by increases in cardiac index. The magnitude of their effects is determined partly by pretreatment blood pressure levels; maximum blood pressure lowering generally is seen 3 to 4 weeks after the start of treatment. These drugs possess some distinct advantages relative to other vasodilators, including:

1. Their relaxant effect on large arteries results in greater compliance, which is of benefit in older persons.
2. Tolerance associated with renal retention of fluid does not occur; an initial natriuretic effect is often observed, especially with the nifedipine group of blockers.
3. They do not have significant effects on the release of renin or cause long-term changes in lipid or glucose metabolism.
4. Postural hypotension, "first-dose" effect, or rebound phenomenon is not commonly seen.

Their antihypertensive efficacy is comparable to that of β-adrenergic blockers and angiotensin-converting enzyme (ACE) inhibitors. The choice of a calcium channel blocker, especially when used in combination therapy, is largely influenced by the effect of the drug on cardiac pacemakers and contractility. An additional benefit is that these drugs reduce left ventricular hypertrophy and the progression of atherosclerosis, thereby decreasing the risk associated with these developments.

Ischemic Heart Disease

The effectiveness and use of calcium channel blockers in the management of angina are well established (see Chap. 25); their benefit in postinfarction stages is less certain. Efficacy in angina is largely derived from their hemodynamic effects, which influence the supply and demand components of the ischemic balance by: (1) increasing blood flow directly or by increasing collateral blood flow and (2) by decreasing afterload and reducing oxygen demand. All three agents are useful in the management of stable, exertional angina, with their vasodilatory and cardiac effects making beneficial contributions. Given the differences in their relative effects (Table 23-2), the response of the patient can vary with the agent used and the preexisting cardiac status.

All agents are also very effective in the control of variant (Prinzmetal's) angina where spasm of the coronary arteries is the main factor. Their usefulness in the more complex unstable (preinfarction) angina is less definite and is dependent on the hemodynamic status and the susceptibility of the patient to infarction.

Cardiac Arrhythmias

The prominent depressant action of verapamil and diltiazem at the S-A node and the A-V node finds use in specific arrhythmias. They are of proven efficacy in acute control and long-term management of paroxysmal supraventricular tachycardia (see also Chap. 26), in which they are very effective in the conversion to sinus rhythm. Their ability to inhibit conduction at the A-V node is employed in protecting ventricles from atrial tachyarrhythmias, often in combination with digitalis or propranolol. Their potential for ventricular arrhythmias based on their ability to suppress slow calcium currents is under intensive investigation; their benefit in a clinical setting has not yet been established.

Miscellaneous and Potential Uses

The calcium channel blocking drugs have been investigated for an unusually wide number of clinical applications, which may be based, at least partly, on their actions unrelated to calcium antagonism. Verapamil-induced improvement of diastolic function has proved to be beneficial in the treatment of hypertrophic cardiomyopathy. Vasodilatory properties of these drugs are utilized in the treatment of peripheral vasoconstrictive disorders (Raynaud's disease) and in relieving vasospasm following subarachnoid hemorrhage. There is ongoing interest in investigating protective effects of the drugs on renal

Table 23-3. Pharmacokinetics of Calcium Channel Blockers

	Verapamil	Nifedipine	Diltiazem
Absorption, oral (%)	>90	>90	>90
Bioavailability (%)	20	60–80	~40
Onset of action: oral (min)	90–120	<20	<30
Peak effect	5 hr	1–2 hr	3–5 hr
Protein binding (%)	90	90	90
Plasma half-life	4–8 hr	5 hr*	5 hr
Metabolism	80% 1st-pass active metabolites	Inactive metabolites	60% of 1st dose; 10% steady state
Excretion			
Renal (%)	70	90	30
Fecal (%)	15	10	70

*Six to 11 hours after oral tablets; above value for capsules.

Table 23-4. Adverse Effects of Calcium Channel Blockers

	Verapamil	Diltiazem	Nifedipine
Tachycardia	0	0	+
Decreased heart rate*	+	+	0
Depressed A-V nodal conduction*	+ + +	+ +	0
Negative inotropy	+ +	+	0
Vasodilation (flushing, edema, hypotension, headaches)	+	+/0	+ + +
Constipation, nausea	+ +	+	+/0

Key: + = increase; 0 = no change.
*Marked effect in presence of sick sinus syndrome and A-V nodal disease.

function, and in their ability to reduce deleterious vascular changes in diabetes mellitus. Similarly, the potential benefit afforded by their selective vasodilatory action (especially the second-generation agents) in the management of heart failure is an area of current interest. These drugs are of some benefit in a variety of noncardiovascular conditions characterized by hyperactivity of smooth muscle (e.g., achalasia).

Pharmacokinetics

A comparison of the pharmacokinetic properties of these agents is listed in Table 23-3. All three drugs are well absorbed following oral administration. Verapamil and diltiazem undergo greater first-pass metabolism relative to nifedipine, resulting in lower bioavailability of the former two drugs. Hepatic metabolism of nifedipine is complete, yielding inactive metabolites; this is unlike verapamil and diltiazem, whose metabolites have pharmacological activity. Verapamil is metabolized stereoselectively in favor of the more active (−) enantiomer, thus requiring higher plasma concentrations after oral administration.

Toxicity

The common side effects seen in chronic therapy (Table 23-4) are mostly related to vasodilation—headaches, dizziness, facial flushing, hypotension, and so forth. High doses of verapamil in elderly patients are known to cause constipation. Serious side effects, especially following the intravenous use of verapamil, include marked negative inotropic effects and depression of preexisting sick sinus syndrome, A-V nodal disease, or enhancement of the action of other cardiodepressant drugs. Their use is generally contraindicated in obstructive conditions (e.g., aortic stenosis). No consistent or significant changes in lipid and glucose levels have been reported with chronic therapy.

Preparations and Dosage

Diltiazem hydrochloride (*Cardizem, Dilacor*) is available as tablets, sustained-release capsules, and injectable forms. Therapy is individualized and generally begins with 30 mg four times a day up to a maximum of 360 mg daily. Intravenous therapy usually begins with a dose of 0.2 mg/kg over 2 min, followed by an additional dose of 0.35 mg/kg. Infusions are usually given in doses of 10 mg per hour and can be maintained for up to 24 hr.

Nifedipine (*Procardia, Adalat*) is available in the form of capsules. Treatment is initiated with 10-mg doses three times a day and the usual range is 10 to 20 mg three times a day.

Nicardipine (*Cardene*) is marketed as tablets or as sustained-release capsules. The usual daily dose is 20 to 40 mg and adjustments in dosage are made at 3-day intervals.

Nimodipine (*Nimotop*) is available in the form of capsules. Treatment is initiated within 96 hours of subarachnoid hemorrhage and with doses of 60 mg every 4 hr for 21 days.

Verapamil (*Isoptin, Calan*) is supplied as tablets, extended-release tablets, and injectable forms. Oral administration usually is in the range of 8 to 120 mg three times a day up to a maximum of 480 mg. Intravenous use in supraventricular tachyarrhythmias usually requires 5 to 10 mg over at least 2 min, which can be repeated 30 min later.

Amlodipine (*Norvac*) is available as tablets. Treatment of hypertension or angina requires 5 mg per day, with adjustments in dosage made over 7 to 14 days.

Isradipine (*Dynacirc*) is supplied as 2.5- or 5-mg capsules. Dosage is individualized, with the usual dose being 2.5 two times a day.

Supplemental Reading

Billman, G.E. The antiarrhythmic and antifibrillatory effects of calcium antagonists. *J. Cardiovasc. Pharmacol.* 18 (Suppl. 10):5107, 1991.

Katz, A.M. Molecular basis of calcium channel blockade. *Am. J. Cardiol.* 69:17E, 1992.

Kern, M.J. Perspective: The cellular influences of calcium antagonists on systemic and coronary hemodynamics. *Am. J. Cardiol.* 69:3B, 1992.

Klaus, D. The role of calcium antagonists in the treatment of hypertension. *J. Cardiovasc. Pharmacol.* 20 (Suppl. 6):55, 1992.

Triggle, D.J. Calcium Antagonists. In M. Antonaccio (ed.), *Cardiovascular Pharmacology* (3rd ed.). New York: Raven, 1990.

24

Cardiac Glycosides and Other Drugs Used in Myocardial Insufficiency

Ernst Seifen

The first modern clinical use of digitalis glycosides was described by William Withering in his classical treatise, *An Account of the Foxglove and Some of its Medical Uses: Practical Remarks on Dropsy and Other Diseases,* published in 1785 in London. Glycosides from foxglove (*Digitalis purpurea* and *Digitalis lanata*) have been the mainstay drugs for the treatment of myocardial failure ever since. In the clinical jargon, therefore, the name "digitalis" became synonymous with steroidal drugs with positive iontropic properties. The following terms have been applied to cardioactive steroids of varying chemical nature: cardiac glycosides, cardioactive steroids, cardenolides, digitalis glycosides, and digitalis. If not specified otherwise, these terms generally denote cardioactive glycosides; in this chapter, the term *cardiac glycosides (CGs)* is used.

Physiology and Pathophysiology of Cardiac Muscle Function

An inability of the heart to generate adequate force, that is, myocardial insufficiency or dysfunction, leads in its final stage to congestive heart failure. This is a common pathophysiological disorder that affects from 6 to 10 percent of the United States population and is still associated with a mortality of 30 percent or higher in patients with congestive heart failure.

Myocardial insufficiency can be induced by very different means, including bacterial, viral, and chemical (drugs, toxicants) pathogens; elevated afterload due to outflow restrictions or increased systemic vascular resistance (valvular or vascular disease processes, hypertension); impaired coronary perfusion (hypoxia or ischemia); pathogenic mechanisms that lead to a persistent increase in circulating blood volume (e.g., volume overload in-

duced by endocrine disorders); and aberrations in cardiac rate or rhythm. A significant percentage of patients have no known cause for this disease, and it is classified as "idiopathic," "essential," or "genuine" cardiomyopathy.

Independently from the varying etiologies, the pathophysiology of untreated myocardial insufficiency progresses inevitably in the same way. Major systemic changes are summarized in Fig. 24-1. Reduced generation of force triggers compensatory mechanisms, which tend to restore cardiac output to ensure adequate tissue perfusion. Compensatory mechanisms are largely twofold (not including myocardial hypertrophy in this discussion). First, *sympathetic nervous system tone is increased* via reflex activation in response to the diminished rate of pressure rise of the pulse wave passing through baroreceptor areas in the carotid sinus, aorta, and so forth. This is a very effective means to activate baroreceptor reflexes under conditions in which a reduction in systemic arterial blood pressure is not significant. Since established myocardial insufficiency is generally irreparable, the associated sympathetic activation will persist and become chronic in nature. Without therapeutic intervention, chronic sympathetic activation leads to increased circulating catecholamine concentration; down-regulation of β_1-adrenoceptors, that is, a reduction in the available receptor pool; and depletion of the overall myocardial catecholamine content. In other words, this compensatory mechanism eventually will be exhausted and become ineffective. Recent studies in patients indicate that the reduction in cardiac β_1-adrenoceptors is accompanied by an increase in α_1-adrenoceptors; the latter have been implicated in the production of arrhythmias, especially in the ventricular myocardium.

If the sympathetic activation is unable to restore adequate cardiac function, the second compensatory safeguard, *the Frank-Starling mechanism,* will take over. This mechanism makes use of a basic principle of muscle phys-

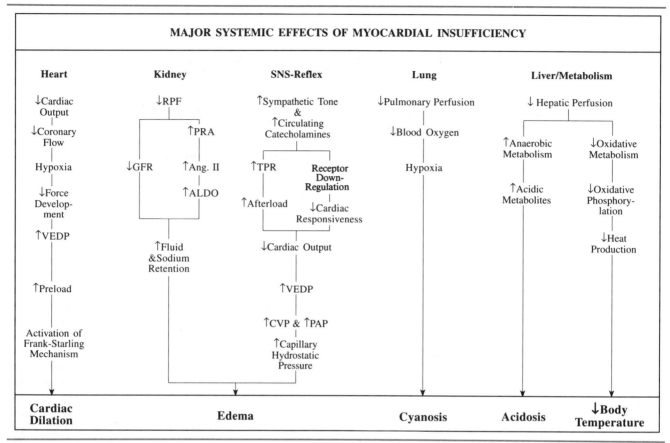

Figure 24-1. Major pathophysiological changes associated with myocardial insufficiency. *SNS* = sympathetic nervous system; *RPF* = renal plasma flow; *PRA* = plasma renin activity; *GFR* = glomerular filtration rate; *Ang. II* = angiotensin II; *TPR* = total peripheral resistance; *ALDO* = aldosterone; *VEDP* = ventricular end-diastolic pressure (this term is used instead of *LVEDP* to indicate that both left and right ventricles may be affected); *CVP* = central venous pressure; *PAP* = pulmonary artery pressure; Temp. = temperature; ↑ = increase; ↓ = decrease. Note: Edema stands for peripheral (ankle edema), abdominal (ascites), and pulmonary edema. (For further explanation see text.)

iology, namely, that lengthening of the muscle fiber increases its contractile force development. The reduction of cardiac output leads to a progressive engorgement of the chambers of the heart. This puts tension on the walls, which leads to increased stretch of the individual sarcomeres of the myocardium. Cardiac output then increases, as predicted by the Frank-Starling mechanism.

Unfortunately, there are limits to this compensatory mechanism. If lengthening of the muscle fiber surpasses "optimal" fiber length, force development will decline. Sarcomere length (proportional to fiber length) governs the overlap of actin and myosin filaments, which determines the number of cross-links that can be formed and, thus, the degree of force generation. Below 2.0 μ, an increase in sarcomere length augments cross-link formation. The greatest possible number of cross-links, that is, optimal cross-link formation, occurs at sarcomere lengths from 2.0 to 2.2 μ; at this point, the Frank-Starling curve

reaches its maximum. An increase in sarcomere length beyond 2.2 μ reduces cross-link formation and force development declines.

If the Frank-Starling mechanism is adequate to restore the ability of the heart to cope with venous return, cardiac output can be maintained within the normal range for some time. However, near-normal cardiac output will be maintained at the expense of increased ventricular end-diastolic pressure (preload) and reduced efficiency of the heart.

If compensatory mechanisms fail to restore and maintain adequate cardiac output, congestive heart failure develops, with the following classical triad of symptoms: (1) *edema* (usually starting in the lower extremities), (2) *cyanosis* (inadequate lung perfusion and blood oxygenation), and (3) *shortness of breath* (a result of [1] and [2]).

The pathophysiological sequelae of decompensated myocardial insufficiency are intricate and not completely understood. Myocardial insufficiency causes a reduction of the stroke volume and of the ejection fraction (the ratio of stroke volume over end-diastolic volume). The result is a rise in end-systolic resting volume and thus an augmented preload. Under this condition, cardiac output no longer matches venous return, and blood will be backed up into the capacitance vessels and into the capillary region, causing an increase in intracapillary hydrostatic pressure. The ensuing imbalance of the forces regulating the capillary fluid movement favors an increased net shift of fluid into the extravascular space, that is, edema formation. Edema may occur in the extremities (e.g., ankle edema), in the abdominal cavity (ascites), and in the lung (alveoli) under more severe conditions.

Reduced cardiac output results in diminished tissue perfusion and oxygenation. In the kidneys, reduced perfusion pressure may increase renin release. Renin release can be further raised by sympathetic stimulation of β_1-adrenoceptors of the juxtaglomerular apparatus and by a reduction in the sodium concentration in the distal convolution of the nephron, which is in close contact with the *macula densa*. All these mechanisms may be activated during myocardial insufficiency.

Increased renin release, that is, elevation of the plasma renin activity (PRA), results in the elevation of circulating angiotensin II (Ang.-II). Ang.-II may induce increased aldosterone release from the adrenal cortex, which, in turn, augments sodium retention and, therefore, supports fluid retention. Thus, fluid retention, i.e., edema formation, is not only the direct result of impaired hemodynamic parameters, but also is sustained by the renin-angiotensin-aldosterone system.

Other concomitant events need to be considered. Ang.-II does not only elevate aldosterone release from the adrenal medulla, but induces pituitary release of arginine vasopressin (AVP), which, like Ang.-II, increases peripheral resistance and promotes renal water retention.

Finally, it should be considered that enlargement of the heart, specifically stretch of atrial muscle fibers, induces release of atrial natriuretic factor (ANF, also known as atrial natriuretic peptide, ANP). This peptide promotes renal sodium excretion and peripheral vasodilatation, and reduces PRA. It appears, therefore, that ANF may counteract some of the actions of the renin-angiotensin-aldosterone system.

Among other events associated with myocardial insufficiency, a critical one is a reduction in blood oxygen content (hypoxemia, cyanosis). This may be the result of inadequate blood flow through the lungs, but may be aggravated by edema formation in the pulmonary interstitial tissue (impairing oxygen diffusion) or by fluid accumulation in the alveoli. Hypoxemia, and thus reduced oxygen delivery, further curtails the ability of the heart to maintain adequate cardiac output. Hypoxemia also tends to diminish oxidative, and increase anaerobic, metabolism; these actions reduce oxidative phosphorylation and heat production, and favor the accumulation of acidic metabolites, that is, acidosis.

Additional pathophysiological changes are associated with myocardial insufficiency or congestive heart failure, or both. Recent research suggests that the endothelium-derived relaxing factor (EDRF) has modulator functions on myocardial contractility. Many of those changes are not well defined or sufficiently understood to have significant impact on presently practiced therapeutic interventions. Therefore, they are not discussed in the confines of this textbook.

Therapy of Myocardial Insufficiency

Based on the major pathophysiological events evolving around myocardial insufficiency, three basic therapeutic goals need to be achieved: (1) improvement of myocardial contractility, (2) reduction of afterload, and (3) reduction of preload. Which of these goals will be pursued primarily is dictated by the severity of the disease state. Acute myocardial failure (e.g., myocardial infarction) requires a combination of all three therapeutic interventions, whereas a chronic, stable myocardial insufficiency may require only improvement of contractility, that is, administration of a positive inotropic drug.

Positive Inotropic Agents

Under physiological conditions the amount of Ca^{2+} made available during the electromechanical coupling process for contraction of cardiac muscle is never sufficient to form all possible cross-links that could be formed at any given overlap of actin and myosin filaments. Therefore, agents that interact with the electromechanical coupling to increase Ca^{2+} availability or sensitize the myofilaments to Ca^{2+} can increase contractile force development.

Intracellular Ca^{2+} can be increased pharmacologically by agents that: (1) inhibit the Na^+, K^+–adenosine triphosphatase (ATPase) or Na^+ pump, (2) increase intracellular cyclic adenosine monophosphate (cAMP), (3) promote calcium influx, and (4) promote sodium influx. Agents that can elicit effects such as these produce a positive inotropic action; however, not all of these agents can be safely used to treat myocardial insufficiency because of possible adverse reactions and severe side effects.

Sodium Pump Inhibitors: Cardiac Glycosides

Among the agents that inhibit Na^+, K^+-ATPase, only cardiac glycosides are in clinical use. They are the drugs

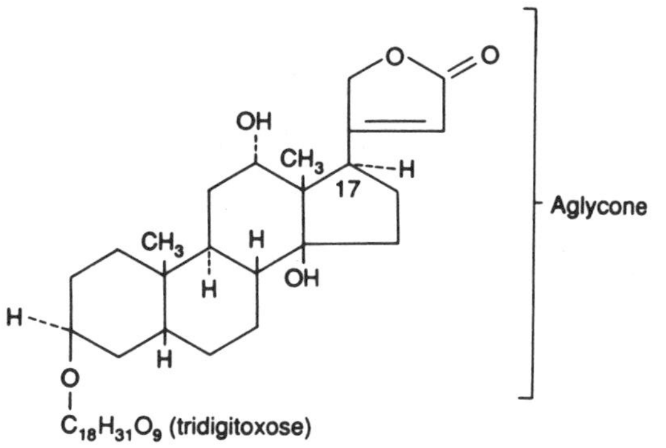

Figure 24-2. Structural formula of digoxin showing the sugar moiety, steroid nucleus, and lactone ring that compose the glycoside.

of choice in treating congestive heart failure, and judicious use of cardiac glycosides can reverse the self-supporting pathophysiological changes initiated by inadequate force development of the heart muscle.

Chemistry

The basic chemical structure of the cardiac glycosides consists of a steroid nucleus with two rings in "cis" and two in "trans" configuration (Fig. 24-2). Attached to the four-ring nucleus, at C-17, is either a five-membered or six-membered lactone ring (unsaturated). Opening of this lactone ring abolishes pharmacological activity.

Naturally occurring cardiac glycosides carry a chain of one to four sugar moieties (3 digitoxoses for digoxin and digitoxin) in 1–4 glycosidic connection—hence, the name "glycoside." Removal of the sugar moieties converts the glycoside into an "aglycone" or "genin." Genins have the same pharmacodynamic properties as the parent glycosides; however, they may differ greatly in pharmacokinetic properties, that is, bioavailability, protein binding, and elimination rates. Pharmacodynamic properties are also greatly influenced by the number of OH groups attached to the glycoside nucleus.

Pharmacokinetics

The pharmacokinetics for three cardioactive steroids, digoxin and digitoxin, which are widely used clinically, and the rarely used g-strophanthin (ouabain, which is a common research tool), are summarized in Table 24-1.

Both digitoxin and digoxin have a relatively high lipophilicity and are well absorbed when taken orally (high bioavailability). They can cross cellular barriers, including the blood-brain barrier and placenta, and will be found in breast milk. Digitoxin shows a significantly higher protein binding than does digoxin, which is in part responsible for its longer plasma half-life. Both these agents show a significant amount of enterohepatic recirculation (up to 30% or more); that is, they are excreted via the bile into the intestine, reabsorbed, and returned into the bloodstream. This "recycling" also contributes to their comparatively long plasma half-lives.

Digoxin is almost completely excreted unchanged via the kidney. Hence, in patients with renal insufficiency (increased blood urea nitrogen), a normal treatment schedule may result in higher than usual digoxin plasma levels and increased toxicity; therefore, a reduction in drug intake is required. Digitoxin, on the other hand, is converted (hydroxylated) by the liver into digoxin, which then is excreted by the kidney. Hepatic conversion occurs at such a slow rate that digoxin buildup rarely occurs even in the presence of significant renal insufficiency. However, under usual treatment schedules, digitoxin serum levels and toxicity may be elevated in patients with impaired liver function.

Renal clearance of digoxin is age dependent; in children, elimination rate may be 1.5 to 3 times faster than in adults, and in elderly or aged persons it may be reduced to one half or one third that of younger adults.

Digoxin and digitoxin levels in tissues are generally slightly higher (2- to 3-fold) than those in plasma; however, several tissues—especially kidney, gastrointestinal tract, and cardiac and skeletal muscle—may accumulate cardiac glycosides at a ratio of 30:1 or even higher. It is unlikely that this reflects a greater density of specific binding sites for cardiac glycosides on the membrane-bound Na^+, K^+-ATPase.

Table 24-1. Pharmacokinetic Properties of Digoxin, Digitoxin, and Ouabain

Drug (sugars)	No. of OH groups	Bioavailability (%)	Protein binding (%)	Vol of distrib. (L/kg)	Plasma half-life	Plasma clearance (ml/kg/min)	Elimination
Digitoxin (3)	1	>90	>95	0.4–0.6	7–11 days	0.04–0.07	Liver metabolism
Digoxin (3)	2	50–70	20–30	4–6	30–36 hr	0.7–1.5	Renal excretion
Ouabain (1)	5	<10	<10	1–1.5	14–20 hr	NA	Renal excretion

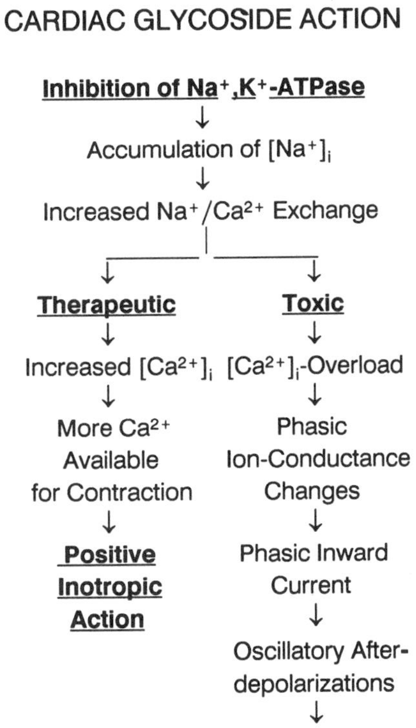

CARDIAC GLYCOSIDE ACTION

Inhibition of Na⁺,K⁺-ATPase
↓
Accumulation of $[Na^+]_i$
↓
Increased Na^+/Ca^{2+} Exchange
↓

Therapeutic	**Toxic**
↓	↓
Increased $[Ca^{2+}]_i$	$[Ca^{2+}]_i$-Overload
↓	↓
More Ca^{2+}	Phasic
Available	Ion-Conductance
for Contraction	Changes
↓	↓
Positive	Phasic Inward
Inotropic	Current
Action	↓
	Oscillatory After-
	depolarizations
	↓

Figure 24-3. Scheme of direct effects of cardiac glycosides induced by inhibition of Na⁺, K⁺-ATPase. (See text for detail.)

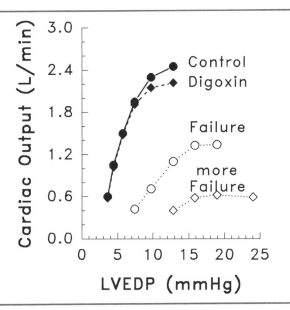

Figure 24-4. Effect of digoxin on cardiac output. Note the steep slope of the cardiac function curve under nonfailing conditions (control); during two stages of myocardial failure induced with a low and high concentration of a general anesthetic, the slope of the ventricular function curve flattens progressively, and maximal cardiac output is drastically reduced. Digoxin (1.7 ng/ml), given while continuing administration of the high concentration of the anesthetic (labeled "more failure"), returned the ventricular function curve back to its original position; that is, it restored normal cardiac function in the presence of the failure-inducing anesthetic. (Based on data obtained in the dog heart-lung preparation.) LVEDP = left ventricular end-diastolic pressure.

Mechanism of Action

As indicated earlier, individual cardiac glycosides do not differ significantly in their pharmacological actions. In order to understand the full range of their pharmacodynamics, therapeutic activity, and toxicity, it is important to understand their direct (inhibition of Na⁺, K⁺-ATPase activity) and indirect (vagal enhancement, interaction with adrenergic mechanisms) effects.

The *direct effects* of cardioactive steroids result from their ability to bind to specific sites on the membranal Na⁺, K⁺-ATPase (= transport ATPase or sodium pump)—and probably other ATPases—to inhibit the enzyme's transport function. Specifically, they interfere with the potassium-activated sodium release, causing a conformational change in the enzyme's steric configuration that prevents further cycling to the inactive and back to the active state. The degree of ATPase inhibition appears to determine not only therapeutic, but also toxic, actions. Reduction up to approximately 30 percent induces mainly therapeutic effects with little toxicity, while higher degrees of ATPase inhibition, especially when approaching or exceeding 60 to 80 percent, cause marked adverse effects and toxicity, as indicated in the accompanying scheme (Fig. 24-3).

Reduction of the Na⁺, K⁺-ATPase transport function causes intracellular accumulation of Na⁺. Elevated intra-cellular Na⁺ levels, in turn, cause increased export of Na⁺ by the electrogenic Na⁺/Ca²⁺ exchanger while importing Ca²⁺ (Na⁺:Ca²⁺ exchange ratio 3:1). This results in an elevation of the free cytosolic calcium concentration. Under physiological conditions, there is a "shortage" of Ca²⁺ in cardiac muscle; that is, the amount of Ca²⁺ mobilized during the excitation-contraction coupling process is not sufficient to initiate cross-link formation at all possible sites for a given actin-myosin overlap, i.e., sarcomere length. Making more free intracellular Ca²⁺ available, therefore, increases the number of cross-links formed and, thus, augments contractile force development (Fig. 24-4).

Cardiac glycosides increase contractile force development in the healthy heart as well as in the failing heart. Since the normal heart works under near optimal conditions, increased contractile force generation cannot be detected as a change in cardiac output (CO) or parameters derived from CO; in a healthy heart, CO is determined by venous return (VR), and since VR is not altered by the glycosides, CO remains unchanged. The insufficient heart, however, cannot cope with venous return; that is, CO is smaller than the potential VR; therefore, improve-

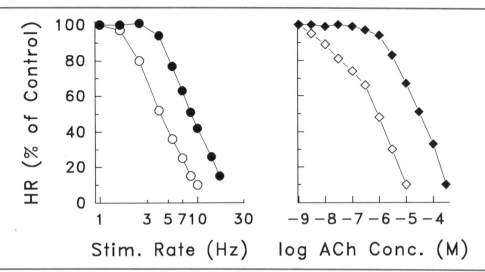

Figure 24-5. Effects of vagal stimulation *(left panel)* and acetylcholine (ACh; *right panel*) on S-A–nodal pacemaker activity in an isolated guinea pig heart. Responses without ouabain are denoted by filled symbols, and responses in the presence of a therapeutic concentration of ouabain (2×10^{-8} M) are indicated by open symbols. Note: Both response curves show a marked shift to the left, indicating the increased sensitivity to cholinergic stimulation in the presence of ouabain; the ouabain-induced sensitization can be completely abolished with atropine, a muscarinic antagonist, in therapeutic concentration of ouabain. (Based on data obtained in isolated guinea pig Langendorf preparations with intact vagal nerve supply.) HR = heart rate.

ment of contractile force development improves cardiac output. The positive inotropic effect of the cardiac glycosides can, however, be easily detected as a steeper rise in pressure during the isometric phase of ventricular contraction, and as an increase in the amplitude and steepness of the pressure rise during the ejection phase of an intraventricular pressure curve.

The direct effects of the glycosides also induce increased sinoatrial (S-A) pacemaker activity by increasing the slope of the pacemaker potential. This positive chronotropic effect is usually not observed in the intact organism, since it is outweighed by the glycoside-induced vagal enhancement; however, increased pacemaker activity occurring at high serum drug concentrations may be an expression of this effect.

If the cellular mechanisms that remove Ca^{2+} from the cytosol (sarcoplasmic reticular Ca^{2+}-ATPase, sarcolemmal Ca^{2+} transport, etc.) are able to lower cytosolic calcium levels quickly, then the major effect of the glycoside-induced transient elevation of intracellular Ca^{2+} concentration will be a positive inotropic action; that is, an increase in myocardial contractile force. If, however, the intracellular accumulation of Ca^{2+} exceeds the rate or capacity of diastolic calcium elimination, calcium overload ensues, which may be associated with a slowing of muscle relaxation, an increase in resting tension, and a reduction of maximal force development.

Intracellular Ca^{2+} overload also affects sarcolemmal

ion channel functions, and promotes uptake of Ca^{2+} into mitochondria and inhibition of mitochondrial enzyme activities. Extreme calcium overload in cardiac muscle presents as contracture, that is, an inability of the muscle to relax.

With respect to the electrophysiological properties of the heart, calcium overload may induce transient depolarizations following an action potential. The mechanism(s) involved are not fully understood, but may involve the sodium/calcium exchange current ($I_{Na/Ca}$) and the pacemaker current. If these glycoside-induced depolarizations reach threshold, they elicit premature, conducted action potentials, which initiate muscle contraction, such as premature atrial or ventricular contractions. They are a major cause of arrhythmias induced by cardiac glycosides.

Indirect effects of cardiac glycosides affect cholinergic and adrenergic autonomic nervous system functions; it is presently not clear to what extent these digitalis-induced alterations are central or peripheral in nature. The glycosides can increase baroreceptor sensitivity, leading to a reflexly increased efferent vagal tone that is further augmented by a direct stimulation of central vagal nuclei. The glycosides also have a direct effect on peripheral cholinergic receptors that enhances their sensitivity both to vagal stimulation or the agonist action of acetylcholine (Fig. 24-5).

The indirect cholinergic effects of the cardiac glycosides include slow S-A–nodal pacemaker activity (negative chronotropic effect), slow atrioventricular A-V conduction velocity (negative dromotropic effect), and promotion of ectopic atrial beat formation (positive bathmotropic action).

Ventricular effects of cholinergic enhancement are similar to those observed in the atria but normally are unnoticeable; they may become overt in the presence of agents that inhibit cholinesterase activity (organophosphates, cholinesterase inhibitors). Enhancement of cholinergic muscarinic action occurs also in other organ systems, for example, in the gastrointestinal and urogenital tract, and is responsible for some of the glycoside-associated side effects.

Interactions of cardiac glycosides with *adrenergic* mechanisms are less obvious at low therapeutic serum concentrations, but become more pronounced at higher and toxic serum levels. Therapeutic levels cause a reflex-induced reduction in sympathetic tone (enhanced baroreceptor sensitivity, mentioned above) and diminish the response of peripheral adrenoceptors to sympathetic stimulation. At higher and toxic drug levels, there appears to be a centrally induced increase in sympathetic tone and a release of catecholamines and probably other biogenic amines.

The diminished sympathetic activity induced by low levels of glycosides is synergistic with the enhancement of cholinergic activity. The increased sympathetic activity elicited by higher glycoside concentrations may induce or facilitate the occurrence of arrhythmias, especially premature ventricular contractions (PVCs), ventricular tachycardia, and tachyarrhythmia. There is some evidence suggesting that α_1-adrenoceptors may be involved in this arrhythmogenic effect. This is of interest because the down-regulation of β_1-adrenoceptors during myocardial failure is accompanied by an increase in α-adrenoceptors that may predispose the heart to arrhythmias.

The *combination* of the *direct* plus *indirect* cardiac effects induced by cardiac glycosides can be summarized as follows:

1. Initially, and at lower serum drug concentrations, predominantly vagal enhancement is observed, which causes
   a. *Bradycardia* (negative chronotropic effect)
   b. Prolonged P–R interval, i.e., *first-degree block* (negative dromotropic effect slowing A-V conduction velocity)
   c. Occasional *ectopic atrial beats* (positive bathmotropic effect)
2. As serum concentration increases, more obvious indirect effects will be observed; enhancement of vagal effects, reduction in sympathetic activity, and direct effects are becoming stronger, causing:
   a. More predominant slowing of A-V conduction, leading to *second-degree block*

(skipped beats, bigeminal, trigeminal pulse), and perhaps *third-degree block* (no A-V conduction)
   b. Increased probability of *ectopic atrial* and *ventricular* beat formation (atrial flutter or fibrillation, PVCs, ventricular arrhythmia)
3. At high glycoside concentrations the direct effects become more predominant and, in combination with a now increased sympathetic activity and still greater enhancement of vagal actions, will initiate or maintain *third-degree block*. A S-A–nodal tachycardia may occur, as well as a host of aberrations in cardiac rate and rhythm due to automaticity originating either from the atria, the conduction system, and/or the ventricles. Ventricular *tachycardia* or *tachyarrhythmia* can be life threatening because they are both apt to compromise cardiac output or convert into *ventricular fibrillation* with no cardiac output. At very high serum levels, automaticity may slow down or cease completely, most likely a result of calcium overload.

Clinical Uses

For the treatment of myocardial insufficiency and congestive heart failure, digoxin is the preferred drug. The goal of treatment is to restore normal or near-normal cardiac output. Adequate improvement of myocardial contractility can be achieved in more than 90 percent of patients treated properly with digoxin, and adequate treatment alleviates all sequelae of myocardial insufficiency. Treatment with digoxin is symptomatic; it does not eliminate the cause of the disease and, therefore, cannot be discontinued when cardiac function appears to return to normal. Thus, treatment must be continued for the remainder of the patient's life.

Supraventricular arrhythmias can be treated with cardiac glycosides. The term *supraventricular arrhythmia* applies to abnormal rates and rhythms originating in the atria or the A-V–nodal/His bundle region, or both. If abnormal supraventricular impulses are conducted to the ventricles and cause ventricular arrhythmias, especially tachycardia or tachyarrhythmia, associated with impaired cardiac output, treatment is indicated. The cardiac glycosides, by virtue of their indirect actions, can effectively inhibit conduction of high-frequency impulses to the ventricles, and thus protect the ventricles from supraventricular arrhythmias. This treatment, too, is symptomatic; that is, it does not eliminate the cause of the supraventricular arrhythmias. Digoxin can be used to treat this type of arrhythmia; digitoxin is, however, given preference, especially if recurrent attacks of arrhythmias require treatment for longer periods.

Since the *therapeutic index* of glycosides ranges from *1.6*

Table 24-2. Serum Concentrations for Digoxin and Digitoxin in Patients

Drug	Serum concentration	
	Therapeutic (ng/ml)	Toxic (ng/ml)
Digoxin	0.5–2.5	>2.5
Digitoxin	5–20	>20

to 2.5, it is recommended that oral therapy not be initiated with a single large loading dose, which would raise a patient's serum concentration, at least transiently, to toxic levels. Generally, oral administration is started with a "maintenance" dose that establishes desired steady-state serum levels within four to six half-lives. If it is necessary to establish adequate therapeutic levels within a shorter time period, it is recommended that oral therapy be started with subdivided "maintenance" doses administered at shorter time intervals. Intravenous bolus administration will raise serum concentration promptly. With digoxin, the onset of action will be observed within 5 to 15 min, and a maximal effect may be achieved within less than 1 hr; the danger of eliciting adverse or toxic effects with this regimen is, however, drastically increased.

When starting cardiac glycoside therapy, every patient should be "titrated" to a maintenance dose that is the optimal balance between a dose that produces the best possible improvement in cardiac function (output or rate) and a dose that induces the fewest side effects (or at least a level of side effect that can be tolerated). In order to establish an adequate therapeutic maintenance regimen, serum concentration can be determined. The values found in Table 24-2 can serve as a guide. Significant overlap exists, however, between concentrations that produce sufficient therapeutic benefit and concentrations that cause adverse or toxic effects (see Fig. 24-5).

Side Effects and Toxic Effects

Side effects and toxic effects of cardiac glycosides are frequently observed and may occur at any serum concentration (Fig. 24-6). Central nervous system (CNS) symptoms include weakness, fatigue, visual disturbances (green-yellow halos around bright objects), dizziness, nausea, headache, and anorexia. Other side effects reported are abdominal cramps, diarrhea, vomiting, peripheral vasoconstriction, gynecomastia, and hypokalemia. Cardiac toxicity may range from bradycardia to A-V block, atrial fibrillation, ventricular tachycardia, ventricular fibrillation, and cardiac arrest.

Treatment of Toxicity

Intolerable extracardiac side effects/toxicity can usually be alleviated by cessation of glycoside administration, followed by adjustment of the maintenance dose. Less se-

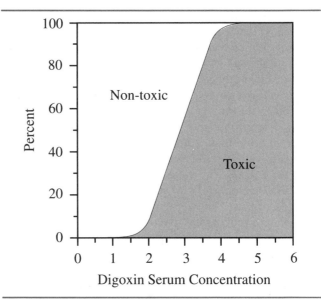

Figure 24-6. Schematic representation of the relationship between serum digoxin concentrations and approximate percentage of patients showing significant clinical toxicity under long-term digoxin treatment. Note: At 1.0 ng/ml digoxin, approximately 4 percent of the patients show signs of toxicity; above 1.5 ng/ml, toxicity rises steeply, and all patients show signs of toxicity at serum levels above 4 ng/ml.

vere cardiac disturbances can be treated with either oral or IV KCl. K^+ inhibits the binding of cardiac glycosides to their specific binding sites on Na^+, K^+-ATPase; however, the effectiveness of K^+ is limited by its own toxicity. Only a moderate elevation above physiological (3.5–5.2 mEq/L) serum K^+ level can be tolerated. Use of KCl is contraindicated in the presence of A-V conduction disturbances or hyperkalemia.

Lidocaine is used to treat ventricular arrhythmias, since it does not slow A-V conduction, which already may be impaired by the glycosides. Quinidine and procainamide may be especially helpful in treating rhythm disorders that are the result of glycoside-induced atrial and/or ventricular automaticity; however, caution is advised since the atropinelike properties of both these drugs may speed up A-V conduction and increase ventricular rate transiently. β-Blockers may be of special value in treating arrhythmias of sympathoadrenergic origin. Calcium channel blockers can be used for treatment of supraventricular rhythm disturbances, while atropine effectively counteracts the glycoside-induced enhancement of parasympathetic effects. Magnesium salts have recently gained renewed interest in the treatment of cardiac arrhythmias since magnesium ions are physiological antagonists to many calcium-induced systemic effects.

Severe toxicity induced by accidental or intentional poisoning with digitalis (serum digoxin levels well beyond 3.5 ng/ml) can be very effectively treated with digitalis-specific antibodies (*Digibind*). Purified Fab fragments are preferred because of their low antigenicity. Following IV administration, serum digitalis levels drop acutely and symptom reversal starts within minutes.

Preparations and Dosage

Digoxin (generic formulations, *Lanoxin*) is available for oral administration in tablet form, as an elixir for children, and for IV use. Digitoxin (generic formulations, *Crystodigin*) is also available in tablet form and for IV use.

Therapy with cardiac glycosides should be started with an oral maintenance dose. Rapid "digitalization" as well as use of a "loading dose" should be avoided to minimize the risk of severe toxicity. In certain clinical situations, faster than usual digitalization may require IV administration; such treatment should be done under strict supervision in a hospital environment. Determination of serum levels is widely practiced, but—as discussed earlier—is of limited usefulness for many patients. However, surveillance of the patient (response to drug, changes in cardiac performance, occurrence of side effects, or toxic effects) is imperative for good patient management.

Agents That Increase cAMP Levels

There are two major ways to increase intracellular cAMP—by increasing formation of cAMP (e.g., β-adrenergic agonists) or by inhibition of enzymatic degradation of cAMP by phosphodiesterase III (e.g., theophylline, caffeine).

Adrenergic Agonists

Isoproterenol, dopamine, and dobutamine are β_1-adrenergic agonists that can be used as positive inotropic agents. They increase cAMP formation by receptor-mediated stimulation of adenylate cyclase activity. Increased formation of cAMP leads to activation of cAMP-dependent protein kinase activity, which, in turn, promotes phosphorylation of voltage-dependent calcium channels. The resulting increase in calcium entering the cell during an action potential augments the force of contraction in heart muscle (for details on mechanism of action, see Chap. 12).

Isoproterenol (*Isuprel*) is a nonselective β-adrenoceptor agonist and is used to induce short-term positive inotropic or chronotropic effects, or both. It also diminishes peripheral resistance (β_2-adrenoceptors). Its use should be avoided in patients with myocardial infarction since its tendency to increase myocardial oxygen demand may increase infarct size. In the presence of cardiac glycosides, isoproterenol may precipitate ectopic impulse generation or increase the frequency of existing abnormal pacemaker activity. It should be avoided in the presence of atrial fibrillation (supraventricular arrhythmias), since it will increase A-V conduction and thus may increase the ventricular response rate.

Dobutamine (*Dobutrex*) can be used for short-term myocardial support in congestive heart failure and myocardial infarction. It is both an α_1- and β-adrenoceptor agonist. Action on β_1-adrenoceptors causes a mild to moderate positive inotropic effect, and speeds A-V–nodal and myocardial impulse conduction, but induces only a small positive chronotropic response. Peripheral resistance is usually not affected; most likely α_1-adrenoceptor–induced vasoconstriction is counteracted by dilation mediated by β_2-adrenoceptors. (See Chap. 12 for details.) Dobutamine has no effect on dopamine receptors.

In patients with impaired renal functions (oliguria, anuria), dopamine (*Intropin*) can be used instead of dobutamine. It has cardiac actions similar to those of dobutamine, but acts in addition on dopaminergic receptors to reduce norepinephrine release from sympathetic nerve terminals (D_2 receptors) and causes vasodilatation in the splanchnic region (D_1 receptors), which increases renal perfusion and thus may improve impaired kidney function.

Phosphodiesterase Inhibitors

Phosphodiesterase inhibitors increase cAMP by interfering with the degradation of cAMP to 5'-AMP by phosphodiesterase (PDE). Phosphodiesterase inhibitors may impede activity of any of the five isoforms I to V; however, it appears that only inhibition of PDE III activity is associated with positive inotropic action. Increase of cAMP in smooth muscle is associated with inactivation (phosphorylation) of myosin–light chain kinase, which leads to inhibition of smooth muscle contraction. Therefore, PDE inhibitors produce peripheral vasodilatation and reduce arterial blood pressure.

Amrinone (*Inocor*) and milrinone (*Corotrope*) are both PDE III inhibitors that produce mild to moderate positive inotropic effects without increasing heart rate markedly; however, their major systemic action appears to reside in peripheral vascular dilation. Long-term use of these drugs has not proved very effective in combating myocardial insufficiency. Amrinone has been approved for short-term treatment of congestive heart failure in patients who failed to respond to other treatment (digitalis, diuretics, and other vasodilators). Both agents induce a series of adverse and side effects (due to their PDE-inhibitory potential), including GI tract disturbances, hepatotoxicity, fever, and thrombocytopenia; more importantly, these drugs, especially milrinone, may increase the incidence of cardiac glycoside–induced arrhythmias. Even though a great deal of research is devoted to development of more adequate PDE inhibitors, it seems unlikely that congeners of PDE inhibitors with less potential for side effects will be introduced in the near future. The classical methylxanthine PDE inhibitors, such as theophylline, have a mild positive inotropic and chronotropic effect, but are rarely used for cardiac treatment.

A new agent, flosequinan (*Manoplax*), is now available

in the United States for treatment of congestive heart failure. It inhibits PDE and may have other mechanisms as well. Currently, it is approved only for patients who cannot tolerate or have not responded adequately to an angiotensin-converting enzyme (ACE) inhibitor.

Other Agents Used to Treat Congestive Heart Failure

ACE Inhibitors

Since the renin-angiotensin-aldosterone system appears to play an important role in the pathophysiology of myocardial insufficiency and the maintenance of sodium and volume retention, present therapeutic management of myocardial insufficiency and congestive heart failure also includes the use of ACE inhibitors, such as captopril or enalapril. ACE inhibitors not only interfere with the conversion of angiotensin I into the very potent vasoconstrictor octapeptide angiotensin II, but they also inhibit the enzymatic inactivation of bradykinin, which is a vasodilator peptide. Thus, ACE inhibitors counteract not only the vicious cycle of the renin-angiotensin-aldosterone system, but decrease cardiac workload by vasodilatation, that is, by reducing afterload. ACE inhibitors also can delay the development of myocardial hypertrophy. The agents commonly employed are either enalapril (*Vasotec*) or captopril (*Capoten*). For more detailed information about ACE inhibitors, see Chap. 19.

Vasodilators

A very effective approach to acutely reduce the workload of an insufficiently functioning heart is to lower the afterload, that is, to decrease both peripheral vascular resistance and venous return. Several classes of drugs, including nitrates and antihypertensives, possess such an action.

Among the nitrates, sodium nitroprusside, nitroglycerin, or sodium nitrate can be used. Their advantage is immediate onset of action when given IV and their short half-life (3–5 min). Thus, nitrate-induced effects can be easily controlled and adjusted. Side effects of nitrates are rare, but tolerance may develop. Different nitrates vary with respect to their preferential action on resistance or capacitance vessels (see Chap. 25). Adverse reactions to these agents may counteract their beneficial effects. For example, nitrate-induced hypotension may reflexly increase sympathetic nervous system tone to cause an increase in heart rate and contractility, thus increasing cardiac oxygen demand; it may also compromise coronary perfusion (which is dependent on aortic blood pressure) and reduce myocardial contractility.

Antihypertensive agents such as hydralazine (*Apreso-*

line), a directly acting smooth muscle relaxing agent, and prazosin (*Minipress*), an α_1-adrenoceptor antagonist, have been used to lower peripheral resistance for more extended periods than is feasible with nitrates. Both agents affect preferentially, but not solely, resistance vessels. Hydralazine is available for IV and oral use; prazosin is only used orally. For more detail see Chap. 22.

Diuretics

Reduction of the increased circulating volume resulting from myocardial insufficiency will be achieved by adequate improvement of cardiac functions with cardiac glycosides. However, the relatively slow onset of action and establishment of full action of the glycosides may not be sufficient to alleviate acute cardiac distress symptoms. If fast action is required, the circulating volume can be acutely and effectively reduced using IV administration of loop diuretics, for example, furosemide (*Lasix*). Reduction of circulating volume for extended periods can be achieved by oral administration of benzothiazide diuretics such as chlorothiazide (*Diuril*).

The predominant adverse effect associated with the use of diuretics in the treatment of myocardial insufficiency and congestive heart failure is their potential to induce or intensify existing hypokalemia as well as their potential to lower serum calcium levels (furosemide). More information concerning diuretics can be found in Chap. 21.

Supplemental Reading

Bryson, P.D. Cardiac Glycosides. In P.D. Bryson (ed.), *Comprehensive Review in Toxicology*. Rockville, Md.: Aspen, 1989. pp. 165–180.

Greeff, K. *Cardiac Glycosides*, Part I and II. *Heffter's Handbook of Experimental Pharmacology,* Vol. 56. Berlin: Springer, 1981.

Herzig, S., and Luellmann, H. Effects of Cardiac Glycosides at the Cellular Level. In E.M. Vaughan Williams (ed.), *Antiarrhythmic drugs. Heffter's Handbook of Experimental Pharmacology,* Vol. 89. Berlin: Springer, 1989. pp. 545–563.

Hickey, A.R., et al. Digoxin immune Fab therapy in the management of digitalis intoxication: Safety and efficacy results of an observational surveillance study. *J. Am. Coll. Cardiol.* 17:590, 1991.

Kennedy, R.H., and Seifen, E. Cardiac Toxicology of Digitalis. In S.I. Baskin (ed.), *Principles of Cardiac Toxicology*. Caldwell, N.J.: Telford, 1990.

Mahdyoon, H., et al. The evolving pattern of digoxin intoxication: Observations at a large urban hospital from 1980 to 1988. *Am. Heart J.* 120:1189, 1990.

Seifen, E., Kennedy, R.H., and Seifen, A.B. Interaction of BAY K-8644 with effects of digoxin in the dog heart-lung preparation. *Eur. J. Pharmacol.* 158:109, 1988.

Smith, T.W. *Digitalis Glycosides*. Orlando: Grune & Stratton, 1985.

Sperelakis, N. *Physiology and Pathophysiology of the Heart*. Boston: Kluwer, 1991.

25

Antianginal Drugs

Garrett J. Gross

Angina pectoris is a clinical manifestation that results from coronary atherosclerotic heart disease. An acute anginal attack (*secondary angina*) is generally thought to occur because there is an imbalance between myocardial oxygen supply and demand owing to the inability of coronary blood flow to increase in proportion to increases in myocardial oxygen requirements. Angina pectoris (*variant, primary angina*) may also occur as a result of vasospasm of large, surface coronary vessels or one of their major branches. In addition, angina in certain patients may result from a combination of coronary vasoconstriction and an increase in myocardial oxygen demand (*crescendo* or *unstable angina*).

Antianginal drugs may effectively relieve attacks of acute myocardial ischemia by increasing myocardial oxygen supply or by decreasing myocardial oxygen demand, or through a combination of these two effects. Three groups of pharmacological agents have been shown to be effective in reducing the frequency, the severity, or both, of primary or secondary angina. These agents include the *nitrates, β-adrenergic receptor antagonists, and the calcium antagonists or calcium entry blockers.* To understand the beneficial actions of these pharmacological agents, it is important to be familiar with the major factors regulating the balance between myocardial oxygen supply and demand (Table 25-1).

Oxygen Supply

The energy expenditure of the human heart in relation to its size is the greatest of any organ in the body and depends almost exclusively on aerobic metabolism. *The delivery of oxygen, then, is critical to sustained cardiac activity.* The arteriovenous (AV) oxygen difference in the coronary circulation is 10 to 12 vol%, and oxygen extraction is approximately 75 percent. In the systemic circulation, the AV oxygen difference is 4 vol% and oxygen extraction

is approximately 25 percent. These figures illustrate the efficient oxygen-extracting ability of the heart.

Although the heart is capable of extracting a small additional amount of oxygen from the blood perfusing it, this amount is limited because of the nearly maximal oxygen extraction that occurs in the resting state. Therefore, *the major determinant of myocardial oxygen supply under normal physiological conditions is the total coronary blood flow.* In normal hearts, coronary blood flow is capable of increasing four- to fivefold to meet increases in myocardial oxygen demands. The rate of coronary flow is directly related to aortic blood pressure minus left ventricular and diastolic pressure, and is inversely related to the resistance of the small coronary vessels or arterioles. The diastolic blood pressure and the duration of diastole are particularly important for coronary perfusion, because most of the blood flow to the left ventricle is supplied during diastole, when myocardial compressive forces are at a minimum.

Coronary blood flow, through changes in arteriolar resistance, is also importantly linked to the metabolic activity of the heart. An increase in oxygen demand, as occurs in physical exercise, is associated with an increase in coronary flow, whereas a decrease in oxygen demand is associated with a decrease in coronary flow. This phenomenon has been termed *metabolic autoregulation*. Vasodilator metabolites, such as adenosine, lactic acid, hydrogen ions, potassium ions, and prostaglandins, have been implicated as regulatory links between cardiac metabolic rate and myocardial blood flow. Recent evidence suggests that adenosine may be the most likely candidate as the physiological mediator in coronary autoregulation, although it does not appear to be the sole factor involved.

The autonomic nervous system also has important influences in the regulation of coronary blood flow (see Chap. 11). Stimulation of sympathetic nerves to the heart results in a marked increase in coronary blood flow, owing primarily to increased metabolic activity of the heart, which is produced by β-receptor–mediated, positive chro-

Table 25-1. Major Determinants of Myocardial Oxygen Supply and Demand

Oxygen supply	Oxygen demand
Oxygen extraction (%)	Wall tension
Coronary blood flow	Ventricular volume
Aortic diastolic pressure	Radius or heart size
Coronary arteriolar resistance	Ventricular pressure
Metabolic autoregulation	Systolic pressure
Endocardial–epicardial flow	(afterload)
Coronary collateral blood flow	Diastolic pressure
Large coronary artery diameter	(preload)
	Heart rate
	Contractility

notropic and inotropic effects of released norepinephrine. Studies with α- and β-receptor agonists and antagonists indicate the presence of α-constrictor and β-dilator receptors in the coronary vasculature. The importance of these receptors in the normal regulation of coronary blood flow is uncertain. Vagal stimulation has been demonstrated to produce coronary vasodilation through activation of muscarinic receptors. However, it is unlikely that the vagus is important in coronary blood flow regulation because of the overriding influence of metabolic autoregulation.

A third determinant of oxygen supply is the regional distribution of blood flow between the subendocardium (inner layers) and subepicardium (outer layers) of the left ventricle. Normally, blood flow is evenly distributed across the left ventricular wall over the whole cardiac cycle; however, because left ventricular pressure during systole is greatest in the subendocardium, this region receives most of its blood flow during diastole. The vasodilator reserve in the subendocardium is smaller than that in the subepicardium, and during ischemia, owing to severe hypotension or to coronary artery stenosis, subendocardial blood flow is more severely impaired than subepicardial flow. For this reason, subendocardial ischemia is very common during acute attacks of stress-induced angina pectoris.

Another determinant of oxygen supply to ischemic myocardium is the coronary collateral circulation. *The collateral circulation can be defined as an alternative system of blood vessels that substitutes for a major coronary vessel that has become occluded and nonfunctional.* In the normal human heart, there are essentially no functional collateral vessels; however, during gradual coronary artery narrowing, collateral vessels develop and may prevent or limit the extent of ultimate myocardial damage. The functional capacity of these collaterals, however, is limited and becomes inadequate during stress or severe exercise.

Oxygen Demand

The three major determinants of myocardial oxygen demand are *myocardial wall tension, heart rate,* and *contractility* (see Table 25-1).

Myocardial wall tension, according to the law of Laplace, is directly related to ventricular pressure times the radius of the ventricle and inversely related to ventricular wall thickness. The radius of the heart is directly correlated with ventricular volume. For a given heart rate and contractile state, a larger heart will use more oxygen and will need to generate greater tension to develop the same systolic pressure.

Heart rate is the second major determinant of myocardial oxygen demand. The more rapid the heart rate up to a certain point, the greater the oxygen requirements of the myocardium.

The third major determinant of myocardial oxygen demand is the contractile state of the heart. The more forcefully the heart beats, the greater the oxygen requirements for the same heart rate and wall tension.

Pathophysiology of Secondary Angina Pectoris

Coronary artery disease is the result of progressive atherosclerosis of one or more of the major epicardial or surface coronary vessels. As a result of this process, the lumen of the involved coronary arteries is narrowed and the blood supply to areas of the myocardium is limited. At rest, this marginal blood flow may be sufficient to meet the oxygen demands of the heart; however, during physical or emotional stress, an *imbalance* between oxygen supply and demand occurs. This imbalance leads to myocardial ischemia and angina pectoris.

During the classic stress-induced attack of angina, the most pronounced circulatory change observed is acute left ventricular failure. This condition is characterized by a marked increase in ventricular volume and left ventricular end-diastolic pressure (LVEDP). The resulting increase in heart size and myocardial wall tension dramatically elevates myocardial oxygen requirements. In addition, the marked increase in LVEDP reduces blood flow to the subendocardium because of the elevated intramyocardial compressive forces around the vessels in this region. This increase in oxygen requirements and reduction in blood flow to the subendocardium leads, in turn, to severe subendocardial ischemia, chest pain, and S–T segment depression of the electrocardiogram. If this situation persists, myocardial infarction and death may occur. Platelet aggregation and thrombus formation may also be important factors in this process and may result in angina and myocardial infarction.

Coronary Vasospasm (Primary Angina, Variant Angina)

Coronary vasospasm is defined as segmental or diffuse, reversible, subtotal, or total narrowing of a major epicardial coronary artery that is associated with myocardial ischemia and manifested by chest pain and S–T segment elevation in the electrocardiogram. Vasospasm occasionally occurs in patients (10–15%) at rest (*Prinzmetal's variant angina*), with no evidence of coronary atherosclerosis; however, most patients (85–90%) with variant angina have significant atherosclerotic lesions superimposed at the site of spasm.

Coronary artery spasm has been shown to occur in certain munitions workers who had been chronically exposed to nitroglycerin but were no longer exposed. Endogenous substances that have been implicated in the pathogenesis of spasm include prostaglandins, thromboxanes, endothelins, norepinephrine, serotonin, potassium, and calcium.

Therapeutic Objectives in the Treatment of Angina Pectoris

The major therapeutic objectives in the treatment of angina are to terminate or prevent an acute attack and to increase the exercise capacity of the patient by prophylactic drug therapy. *These objectives can be achieved by reducing overall myocardial oxygen requirements or by increasing oxygen supply to ischemic areas.* A decrease in myocardial oxygen demand can be attained with the organic nitrates, calcium entry blockers, and β-adrenergic receptor blocking agents. More difficult to achieve are increases in oxygen supply mediated by increases in total coronary blood flow when vessels are partially or totally obstructed. However, a redistribution of blood flow to the subendocardium of ischemic areas has been documented in experimental animals following nifedipine, diltiazem, nitroglycerin, or propranolol administration, and increases in collateral flow to ischemic areas have been observed in experimental animals and humans after treatment with calcium entry blockers and nitrates.

When coronary vasospasm occurs, the balance between oxygen supply and demand can be restored by relieving the spasm and restoring normal coronary blood flow. *Acute attacks of vasospasm can be successfully aborted by the use of nitroglycerin, whereas calcium entry blockers and long-acting nitrates have been used effectively in the chronic therapy of coronary vasospasm.*

Antianginal Drugs

Organic Nitrates

Nitroglycerin and other organic nitrates have been used routinely for over 100 years in the therapy of angina pectoris. Use of these compounds is also increasingly favored in a variety of other cardiac conditions, such as congestive heart failure and acute myocardial infarction.

The prototype of these agents is *nitroglycerin*. Other common organic nitrates are *isosorbide mononitrate* and *dinitrate, erythrityl tetranitrate,* and *pentaerythritol tetranitrate.* With the exception of nitroglycerin, which is a liquid that has a high vapor pressure, these compounds are solid at room temperature. All organic nitrates are very lipid soluble.

Mechanism of Vasodilator Action

The mechanism of action of nitroglycerin and other organic nitrates is thought to involve an interaction with nitrate receptors that are present in vascular smooth muscle. An intact vascular endothelium is not necessary for the vasodilator action of the nitrates to be produced. The nitrate receptor possesses sulfhydryl groups, which reduce nitrate to inorganic nitrate and nitric oxide. The formation of nitrosothiol has been proposed to stimulate soluble guanylate cyclase, which leads to an increase in intracellular cyclic guanosine monophosphate (GMP) formation (Fig. 25-1). The increase in GMP leads to vascular smooth muscle relaxation by several possible mechanisms, including an inhibition of calcium entry, a decreased calcium release from intracellular stores, or an increase in calcium extrusion.

Pharmacological Actions

There is little doubt concerning the effectiveness of nitroglycerin in the treatment of angina pectoris; however, controversy still exists regarding the exact mechanism by which this drug acts to reduce myocardial ischemia (Fig. 25-2). Although nitroglycerin dilates both peripheral capacitance and resistance vessels, the effect on the venous

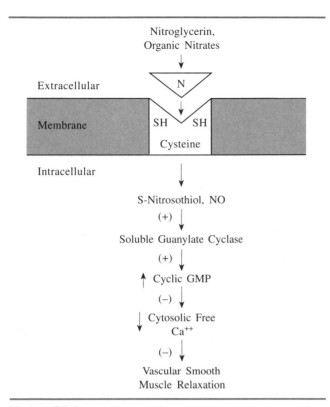

Figure 25-1. A schematic diagram showing the proposed mechanism by which nitroglycerin and the organic nitrates produce relaxation in vascular smooth muscle. Nitrates induce endothelial cells to release nitric oxide (NO) or a nitrosothiol (endothelium-derived releasing factor, EDRF). EDRF activates the enzyme, guanylate cyclase. Activation of guanylate cyclase in turn causes the generation of cyclic guanosine monophosphate (GMP), which produces a decrease in cytosolic free calcium. The end result is vascular smooth muscle relaxation. SH = sulfhydryl.

capacitance system predominates. Dilation of the capacitance vessels leads to pooling of blood in the veins and to diminished venous return to the heart (*preload*). This occurrence reduces ventricular diastolic volume and pressure, and it shifts blood from the central to the peripheral compartments of the cardiovascular system. These effects of nitroglycerin are similar to those of a mild phlebotomy, which has been shown clinically to relieve acute anginal attacks by decreasing circulating blood volume.

According to Laplace's law, a reduction in ventricular pressure and heart size results in a decrease in the myocardial wall tension that is required to develop a given intraventricular pressure and, therefore, in a decreased oxygen requirement. Since blood flow to the subendocardium occurs primarily in diastole, the reduction in LVEDP induced by nitroglycerin reduces extravascular compression around the subendocardial vessels and favors a redistribution of coronary blood flow to this area. This effect of nitroglycerin on the distribution of coronary flow is impor-

tant because the subendocardium is particularly vulnerable to ischemia during acute anginal attacks.

At higher concentrations, nitroglycerin also relaxes arteriolar smooth muscle, which leads to a decrease in both peripheral vascular resistance and aortic impedance to left ventricular ejection (*afterload*). The decreased resistance to ventricular ejection may also reduce myocardial wall tension and oxygen requirements.

Thus, *nitroglycerin relieves the symptoms of angina by restoring the balance between myocardial oxygen supply and demand*. Oxygen demand is lowered as a consequence of the reduction in cardiac preload and afterload, and this results in a decrease in myocardial wall tension. Oxygen supply to the subendocardium of ischemic areas is increased, because extravascular compression around the subendocardial vessels is reduced. In addition, nitroglycerin may also increase blood flow to ischemic areas by its direct vasodilator effect on epicardial coronary stenoses and collateral blood vessels. *Other organic nitrates are thought to exert the same beneficial actions as nitroglycerin.*

Absorption, Metabolism, and Excretion

Nitroglycerin is a lipid-soluble substance that is rapidly absorbed from the sublingual mucosa. Its onset of action occurs within 2 to 5 min, with maximal effects observed at 3 to 10 min. Little residual activity remains at 20 to 30 min. The plasma half-life of nitroglycerin is estimated to be between 1 and 3 min. Isosorbide dinitrate and erythrityl tetranitrate are also administered sublingually. These compounds have a slower onset and slightly longer duration of action than nitroglycerin.

Nitroglycerin and other nitrate esters are rapidly and efficiently metabolized in the liver by the enzyme glutathione organic nitrate reductase. Although the metabolites of nitroglycerin are virtually inactive as vasodilators, two metabolites of isosorbide dinitrate, isosorbide 2- and 5-mononitrate, do retain some vasodilator and antianginal activity. These latter compounds are generally water soluble and are readily excreted by the kidney.

Clinical Uses

Sublingual nitroglycerin is used either to terminate an acute attack of angina or for short-term prevention of angina. *Nitroglycerin is still the mainstay of therapy for relieving acute coronary vasospasm.* When taken at the onset of chest pain, the effects of nitroglycerin appear within 2 to 5 min; however, the true duration of action is difficult to establish, since the onset of pain causes patients to reduce their physical activity, and this alone can ameliorate the symptoms of angina pectoris. Isosorbide dinitrate and erythrityl tetranitrate can also be taken sublingually, shortly before anticipated physical or emotional stress, to prevent anginal attacks.

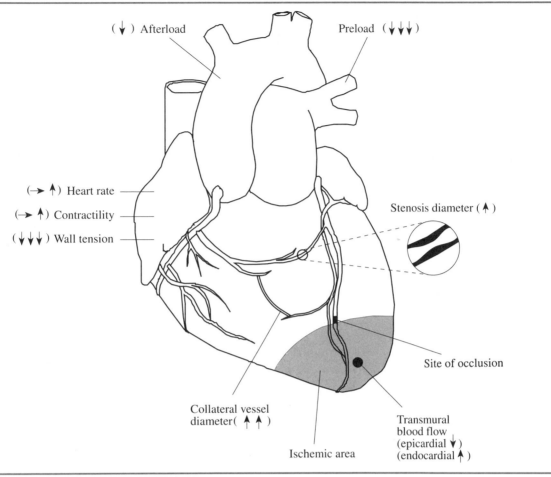

(↓) Afterload

Preload (↓↓↓)

(→ ↑) Heart rate

(→ ↑) Contractility

(↓↓↓) Wall tension

Stenosis diameter (↑)

Site of occlusion

Collateral vessel
diameter(↑ ↑)

Ischemic area

Transmural
blood flow
(epicardial ↓)
(endocardial ↑)

Figure 25-2. A schematic drawing indicating the major actions of the nitrates on the ischemic heart and peripheral circulation. ↓ = decrease; ↑ = increase; → = unchanged; ↓↑ = variable effect.

Nitroglycerin ointment applied to the skin produces its effects within 15 min and may last for 2 to 6 hr. Transdermal nitroglycerin has been shown to deliver a sustained antianginal effect for 2 to 4 hr in small doses and up to 24 hr with larger doses.

Orally administered long-acting nitrates—including nitroglycerin and various nitrate esters, nitroglycerin ointment, and transdermal and transmucosal nitroglycerin—were developed with the goal of providing a nitrate preparation that would have prolonged pharmacological activity for prophylactic therapy of angina pectoris. Considerable controversy surrounds the therapeutic use of the orally active agents, and many clinicians consider them to be ineffective.

In the past 10 years, however, numerous clinical investigations have demonstrated the efficacy of large doses of orally, transmucosally, or transdermally administered long-acting nitrates in the treatment of angina pectoris. Apparently, the large doses produce prolonged pharmacological effects by saturating hepatic nitrate reductase activity. Intermittent dosing regimens are essential to reduce the occurrence of tolerance.

Adverse Reactions

Vascular headache and postural hypotension are common side effects of organic nitrate therapy. Fortunately, tolerance to nitrate-induced headache develops after a few days of initiating therapy. Postural hypotension can be minimized by proper adjustment of the dosage and by instructing the patient to sit down when taking rapidly acting preparations. An effective dose of nitrate usually produces a fall in upright systolic pressure of 10 mm Hg and a reflex rise in heart rate of 10 beats per minute. Larger changes than these should be avoided, because a reduction in myocardial perfusion and an increase in cardiac oxygen requirements may occur that may actually exacerbate angina.

Nitrite ions oxidize the iron atoms of hemoglobin and convert it to methemoglobin, with a consequent loss in oxygen delivery to tissues. Methemoglobinemia does not occur with therapeutic doses of organic nitrates, but it can be observed after overdosage or accidental poisoning with nitrates.

Cautions

Chest pain that is not relieved by two or three tablets within 30 min may be due to myocardial infarction. Patients and their relatives should be properly instructed about this possibility. In addition, nitrate administration may result in an increase in intracranial pressure and therefore these drugs should be used cautiously in patients with cerebral bleeding and head trauma.

Tolerance and Dependence

Repeated and frequent exposure to organic nitrates is accompanied by the development of tissue tolerance to their vasodilating effects. This tolerance may occur within 24 hr when nitroglycerin formulations that produce sustained plasma and tissue levels are used, that is, transdermal patches, sustained-action oral formulations, and ointments. The mechanism underlying the phenomenon of nitrate tolerance is as yet unknown, but it may be related to nitrate-induced oxidation of sulfhydryl groups in vascular smooth muscle. The organic nitrates have less affinity for the disulfide receptor.

To help avoid nitrate tolerance, clinicians should employ the smallest effective dose and administer the compound at less frequent intervals. A daily nitrate-free period is also recommended, particularly when using the transdermal patches or ointment. A better understanding of the pharmacokinetic profile achieved with these sustained-release formulations should result in more effective dosing regimens.

Since depletion of tissue stores of sulfhydryl groups has been proposed to play an important role in nitrate tolerance, some investigators have administered sulfhydryl-containing compounds in an attempt to reverse or prevent the development of tolerance to organic nitrates. The most commonly used agent is N-*acetylcysteine* (NAC), which is hydrolyzed in vivo to cysteine. Although some investigators have shown a positive effect with NAC, the antinitrate tolerance effect of this compound has not been universally confirmed. Thus, further well-controlled clinical studies are necessary to conclusively establish the effectiveness of sulfhydryl-containing compounds at preventing or reversing nitrate tolerance.

Industrial exposure to organic nitrates induces both tolerance and physical dependence. The state of dependence becomes manifest when exposure to nitrates is withdrawn suddenly. Thus, in munitions workers who have become dependent on nitroglycerin, removal from contact with it has been reported to produce angina, myocardial infarction, or sudden death. It is important to recognize that some of these patients showed symptoms of ischemic heart disease, even though their coronary arteriography was judged to be normal. It is possible that coronary vasospasm plays a role in the pathogenesis of angina that occurs in nitrate-dependent individuals. These individuals should be cautioned to watch for symptoms of increased chest pain when they withdraw from medication or discontinue their exposure.

Preparations

Nitroglycerin (*Nitrostat, Nitro-Bid, Nitrospan, Nitrolingual,* generic nitroglycerin) is available in the form of sublingual tablets, oral capsules, and oral tablets. Nitrolingual is also available as a metered spray to be administered under the tongue. The usual dose, time of onset of action, and duration of action for nitroglycerin and the agents discussed below are described in Table 25-2.

Nitroglycerin ointment, 2% (*Nitrol, Nitro-Bid*) has been recommended for the management of nocturnal angina. The proper dose is determined by titration, using relief of symptoms or appearance of headache as the end points. The usual dose is 1 to 2 in. of ointment, squeezed from the tube and applied to the skin. Treatment should be terminated by tapering the dosage to avoid withdrawal reactions.

Transdermal nitroglycerin (*Nitro-Dur, Transderm-Nitro, Nitrodisc*) discs or patches have been developed to provide a long-acting delivery system. The discs have been designed for application once a day and are considered to be effective in the prophylaxis of angina for up to 24 hr. However, recent evidence suggests that tolerance may develop rapidly to the sustained plasma levels that result from the use of these patches and a daily drug-free interval is recommended. As with nitroglycerin ointment, treatment should be discontinued by gradually decreasing the dose.

Transmucosal nitroglycerin (*Susadrin, Nitrogard*) is a buccal tablet that is inserted under the upper lip between the buccal mucosa and gingiva. The onset of action is almost immediate and the release of nitrate is gradual and sustained for up to 5 hours.

Intravenous nitroglycerin (*Tridil, Nitro-Bid IV, Nitrostat IV*) is widely utilized for the treatment of unstable angina. This preparation has the advantage over other forms of nitroglycerin administration in its ability to maintain a steady blood level. Intravenous nitroglycerin also permits a very close titration of dose. All solutions must be diluted in sterile water or saline before administration.

Isosorbide dinitrate (*Isordil, Sorbitrate,* generic isosorbide) is available in the form of sublingual tablets and cap-

Table 25-2. Dosage Forms and Pharmacokinetics of Nitrates Most Commonly Used in Angina Pectoris

Drug and dosage form	Usual dose (mg)	Onset of action (min)	Duration of action (hr)
Nitroglycerin			
Sublingual	0.3–0.6	2–5	0.16–0.50
Transmucosal (buccal)	1–3	2–5	3–6
Oral	3–20	20–45	2–8
Ointment (2%)	1–5 (½–2″)	15–60	3–8
Transdermal	5–30 (per 24 hr)	30–60	12–24
Intravenous	5–300 mEq/min	Immediate	Transient
Isosorbide dinitrate			
Sublingual	2.5–10	3–20	1–2
Oral, chewable	5–60	30–60	2–10
Oral, sustained release	40	30–60	6–10
Isosorbide mononitrate			
Oral	20	15–30	6–12
Erythrityl tetranitrate			
Sublingual	5–10	5–15	2–3
Oral, chewable	10–30	30	2–6
Pentaerythritol tetranitrate			
Oral	10–20	30	2–6
Oral, sustained release	30–80	30–60	4–12

sules. An active metabolite of isosorbide dinitrate, isosorbide mononitrate (*Ismo*) has also been recently approved for use in the United States and is available as a 20-mg tablet.

Erythrityl tetranitrate (*Pentritol, Peritrate,* generic pentaerythritol) is available in the form of oral tablets and oral capsules.

Dipyridamole

Dipyridamole (*Persantine*) is a potent nonnitrate coronary vasodilator that is still used in long-term prophylactic therapy of certain patients with angina pectoris. Dipyridamole inhibits the uptake of adenosine into myocardial cells and also inhibits adenosine deaminase, the enzyme responsible for the breakdown of adenosine. Thus, *the coronary vasodilator properties of the drug are primarily due to its ability to potentiate the actions of adenosine at the coronary resistance vessels.* This effect of dipyridamole solely at the arterioles is in contrast to the actions of the calcium entry blockers and nitrates, which are capable of dilating the large epicardial coronary conductance vessels as well. This more limited effect of dipyridamole may account for its ineffectiveness in angina pectoris when a component of large-vessel epicardial coronary spasm is present.

In spite of the enthusiasm that initially greeted dipyridamole as an efficacious agent in the treatment of angina pectoris, it is probably no more effective than a placebo in decreasing the incidence or severity of anginal attacks. It is likely that any beneficial actions dipyridamole may have in patients with ischemic heart disease are not related to its powerful vasodilating action but to its ability to inhibit platelet aggregation in the coronary circulation.

Recently, intravenous dipyridamole has been approved for use in thallium imaging in patients unable to undergo stress testing. These include patients who are old, frail, and obese.

β-Adrenergic Blocking Agents

β-Adrenergic blockade is a rational approach to the treatment of angina pectoris, since an increase in sympathetic nervous system activity is a common feature in acute anginal attacks. Propranolol is the prototype of this class of compounds, although all other β-blockers tested are also effective in the treatment of secondary angina. Administration of these compounds results in a decrease in frequency of anginal attacks, a reduction in nitroglycerin consumption, an increased exercise tolerance on the treadmill, and a decreased magnitude of S–T segment depression on the electrocardiogram during exercise.

β-Blockers approved for this clinical use in the United States include propranolol and nadolol, compounds that block both β_1- and β_2-adrenergic receptors equally, and atenolol and metoprolol, compounds that are cardioselective β_1-receptor antagonists.

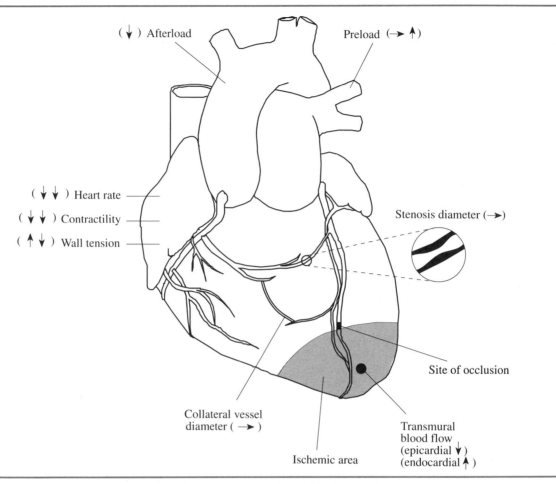

(↓) Afterload

Preload (→ ↑)

(↓ ↓) Heart rate

(↓ ↓) Contractility

(↑ ↓) Wall tension

Stenosis diameter (→)

Site of occlusion

Collateral vessel
diameter (→)

Transmural
blood flow
(epicardial ↓)
(endocardial ↑)

Ischemic area

Figure 25-3. A schematic drawing indicating the major actions of the β-blockers on the ischemic heart and peripheral circulation. For key, see Fig. 25-2.

Pharmacological Actions

The myocardial response to exercise includes an increase in heart rate and myocardial contractility. These effects are, in part, mediated by the sympathetic nervous system. Propranolol and other β-adrenergic blockers antagonize the actions of catecholamines on the heart and thereby attenuate the myocardial response to stress or exercise (Fig. 25-3). In addition, the resting heart rate is reduced by propranolol, but not to the same extent as exercise-induced tachycardia. Overall, propranolol reduces myocardial oxygen consumption for a given degree of physical activity.

Arterial blood pressure (afterload) is also reduced by propranolol (see also Chap. 22). Although the mechanisms responsible for this antihypertensive effect are not completely understood, they are thought to involve (1) a reduction in cardiac output, (2) a decrease in plasma renin activity, (3) an action in the central nervous system, and (4) a resetting of the baroreceptors. Thus, propranolol

may exert a part of its beneficial effects in angina by decreasing the three major determinants of myocardial oxygen demand, that is, heart rate, contractility, and systolic wall tension.

Propranolol has also been shown to produce an increase in oxygen supply to the subendocardium of ischemic areas. The mechanism of this effect is most likely related to the ability of propranolol to reduce resting heart rate and increase diastolic perfusion time. Because subendocardial blood flow and flow distal to a severe coronary artery stenosis occur primarily during diastole, this increase in diastolic perfusion time due to the bradycardic effect of propranolol would be expected to increase subendocardial blood flow to ischemic regions. Propranolol has no significant effect on coronary collateral blood flow.

Absorption, Metabolism, and Excretion

Propranolol is well absorbed from the gastrointestinal tract, but it is avidly extracted by the liver as the drug

Table 25-3. Doses and Pharmacokinetics of β-Receptor Antagonists Used in the Treatment of Angina Pectoris

Compound	Usual daily dose (mg)	Oral bioavailability (%)	Plasma $t_{1/2}$ (hr)	First-pass metabolism (%)
Propranolol	40–80	25–30	3–6	90
Nadolol	40	30–40	12–24	0
Metoprolol	50–100	40–45	3–4	50
Atenolol	50	50–55	5–10	0

Table 25-4. Effects of Nitrates, β-Receptor Antagonists, and Calcium Entry Blockers on Determinants of Cardiac Oxygen Supply and Demand

Determinant	Nitrates	β-Receptor blockers	Calcium entry blockers
Wall tension	↓	±	↓
Ventricular volume	↓	↑	±
Ventricular pressure	↓	↓	↓
Heart size	↓	↑	±
Heart rate	↑ (reflex)	↓	±
Contractility	↑ (reflex)	↓	±
Endocardial-epicardial blood flow ratio	↑	↑	↑
Collateral blood flow	↑	→	↑

Key: ↑ = increase; ↓ = decrease; → = no change; ± = variable effect.

passes to the systemic circulation (first-pass effect). This effect explains the large variation in plasma levels of propranolol after oral administration. For additional details on the pharmacokinetics of propranolol and other β-receptor antagonists approved for clinical use in the treatment of angina pectoris, see Table 25-3 and Chap. 13.

Because of the interindividual variations in the kinetics of propranolol, the therapeutic dose of this drug is best determined by titration. End points of titration are (1) relief of anginal symptoms, (2) increase in exercise tolerance, or (3) plasma concentrations of propranolol between 15 and 100 ng/ml.

Clinical Uses

By attenuating the cardiac response to exercise, propranolol increases the amount of exercise that can be performed before angina develops. Although propranolol does not change the point of imbalance between oxygen supply and demand at which angina occurs, this β-blocker slows the *rate* at which the imbalance point is reached.

Propranolol is indicated in the management of patients whose attacks of angina are frequent and unpredictable despite the use of organic nitrates. Therapy with propranolol is combined with the use of nitroglycerin, the latter being used to control acute attacks of angina. The combined use of propranolol and organic nitrates theoretically should enhance the therapeutic effects of each and mini-

mize their adverse effects (Table 25-4). Unfortunately, no clinical studies have demonstrated conclusively that the combination of these two drugs produces a synergistic response. Propranolol and nadolol also have been used successfully in combination with the calcium entry blockers, particularly nifedipine, for the treatment of secondary angina.

Adverse Reactions

Abrupt interruption of propranolol therapy in individuals with angina pectoris has been associated with reappearance of angina, myocardial infarction, or sudden death. The mechanisms underlying these reactions are unknown, but they may be caused by an increase in the number of β-receptors that occur as a result of chronic β-receptor blockade (upregulation). When it is advisable to discontinue propranolol administration, such as before coronary bypass surgery, the dosage should be tapered over 2 to 3 days.

Additional discussion of the adverse reactions associated with the use of β-blocking agents can be found in Chap. 13.

Preparations

See Table 25-3 and Chap. 13 for more details concerning the most commonly used β-blockers (i.e., propranolol, nadolol, atenolol, and metoprolol) in the treatment of angina pectoris.

Calcium Entry Blockers

The *calcium entry blockers* or *calcium antagonists* are a group of drugs that have been approved for use in the treatment of vasospastic and effort-induced angina. These compounds are particularly effective in the prophylaxis of coronary vasospasm or variant angina. In addition, these compounds are used in the treatment of secondary angina. Two members of this group, verapamil and diltiazem, also have been approved for use in the therapy of certain supraventricular tachyarrhythmias (see Chap. 26). Other potential clinical uses of these compounds include systemic and pulmonary hypertension, Raynaud's syndrome, and acute myocardial infarction.

A detailed discussion of the pharmacology of this important class of drugs can be found in Chap. 23.

Supplemental Reading

Abrams, J. A reappraisal of nitrate therapy. *J.A.M.A.* 259:396, 1988.

Ahlner, J., et al. Organic nitrate esters: Clinical use and mechanisms of actions. *Pharmacol. Rev.* 43:351, 1991.

Boesgaard, S. Preventive administration of intravenous *N*-acetylcysteine and development of tolerance to isosorbide dinitrate in patients with angina pectoris. *Circulation* 85:143, 1992.

Elkayam, U. Tolerance to organic nitrates: Evidence, mechanisms, clinical relevance, and strategies for prevention. *Ann. Intern. Med.* 114:667, 1991.

Frishman, W.H., and Kafka, K.R. Antianginal Agents. In R.J.H. Wang (ed.), *Practical Drug Therapy.* Milwaukee: Medstream, 1987.

Katz, R.J. Mechanisms of nitrate tolerance: A review. *Cardiovasc. Drugs Ther.* 4:247, 1990.

Rinde-Hoffman, D., Glasser, S.P., and Arnett, D.K. Update on nitrate therapy. *J. Clin. Pharmacol.* 31:697, 1991.

Smith, J.J., and Kampine, J.P. (eds.). *Circulatory Physiology* (3rd ed.). Baltimore: Williams & Wilkins, 1990.

26

Antiarrhythmic Drugs

Shawn C. Black and *Benedict R. Lucchesi*

Cardiac arrhythmias occur in many diverse forms that involve alterations in the orderly sequence of the electrical events in any region of the heart. Therefore, *cardiac arrhythmias can be defined as disturbances in heart rate, rhythm, impulse generation, or conduction of the electrical impulses responsible for membrane depolarization.* These disturbances can lead to alterations in overall cardiac function that may be life threatening.

The pharmacological approach to the management of patients with disturbances in cardiac rhythm involves the use of drugs that act on cardiac cells directly, thereby leading to a modification in their electrophysiological properties. Nonpharmacological management may employ the use of implantable electrical devices to control the cardiac rate and rhythm or to interrupt potentially life-threatening disturbances in heart rhythm, or both. Surgical removal of the offending region of abnormal electrical impulse formation and conduction has become increasingly successful under the appropriate clinical situations.

Therapeutically successful antiarrhythmic drug therapy is a combination of the correct diagnosis of the underlying cause of the arrhythmia, identification of a drug known to influence the relevant electrophysiological parameters, and careful titration of the drug's dose to correct the abnormal electrophysiological events giving rise to the arrhythmia. Knowledge of the basic electrophysiological properties of cardiac cells is essential to an understanding of antiarrhythmic drug action.

It may be helpful, therefore, to characterize major antiarrhythmic mechanisms as involving one or more of the following: (1) ability to inhibit the fast inward sodium current, (2) ability to block the electrophysiological effects of β-adrenoceptor stimulation, (3) ability to inhibit one or more repolarizing currents in ventricular myocardium, and (4) ability to inhibit the slow myocardial inward current.

This chapter initially describes the basic electrophysi-

ological events underlying the electrical activity of cardiac cells responsible for normal abnormal cardiac rhythms. Thereafter, the pharmacology of the different antiarrhythmic drugs and relevant electrophysiological mechanisms are discussed.

Cardiac Electrophysiology

The purpose of this introduction is to outline the *major features* of the transmembrane action potential of normal cardiac tissue and to serve as a basis for understanding the mechanisms of cardiac arrhythmogenesis.

Transmembrane Potential

Figure 26-1 shows the phases of the cardiac transmembrane potential, as recorded through an intracellular microelectrode. These phases result from activation and inactivation of various inward and outward ion currents. The interior of the cardiac muscle cell is electrically negative with respect to the surrounding medium. This potential difference between the exterior and interior of a myocardial cell is the result of an intracellular potassium ion concentration ($[K^+]_i$) that is greater than that in the extracellular medium. The high ($[K^+]_i$) is maintained by the activity of a membrane Na^+, K^+–adenosine triphosphatase (ATPase) that actively pumps Na^+ out of and K^+ into the cell. The ($[K^+]_i$) is approximately 150 mM tissue water, whereas the extracellular K^+ concentration ($[K^+]_o$) is 2.7 mM. The chemical gradient favors the efflux of K^+ from the inside to the outside of the cell. The resting myocardial cell tends to be highly permeable to K^+ and less so to Na^+ and Ca^{2+}. Therefore, a net diffusion of K^+ flows toward the outside of the cell, leaving behind negatively charged proteins that cannot diffuse out. The interior of

275

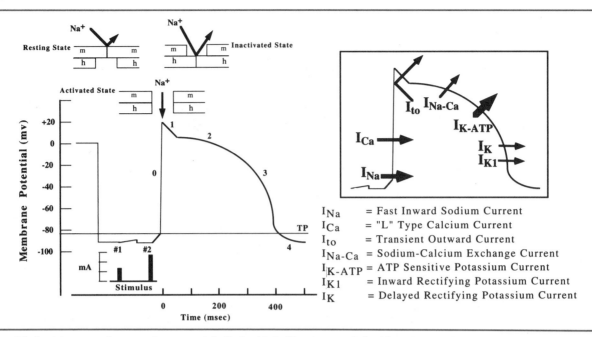

Figure 26-1. Transmembrane action potential of a Purkinje fiber as recorded with an intracellular microelectrode. When the electrode tip penetrates the fiber, a resting membrane potential of -90 mV is recorded. The application of a subthreshold stimulus (#1) produces a depolarizing current that fails to result in excitation of the myocardial cell. The application of a threshold stimulus (#2) reaches the threshold potential (TP) and results in an inward current and an action potential. Major transmembrane currents carried by specific ions entering the cell through selective ion channels are depicted to the right. Antiarrhythmic agents alter the electrophysiologic properties of the cardiac cells by modulating one or more of the transmembrane currents, especially the fast inward sodium current and the transmembrane currents carried by the potassium ion (I_K and I_K-ATP). I_{Na} = fast inward sodium current; I_{Ca} = "L"-type calcium current; I_{to} = transient outward current; I_{Na-Ca} = sodium-calcium exchange current; I_{K-ATP} = adenosine triphosphate–sensitive potassium current; I_{K1} = inward rectifying potassium current; I_K = delayed rectifying potassium current.

the cell becomes electronegative and, thus, two opposing forces are established: a *chemical force* due to a concentration gradient and a counteracting *electrostatic force* established by the negatively charged ions within the cell.

At equilibrium, the chemical and electrostatic forces will be equal, a relationship that is expressed by the Nernst equation:

$$E_K = -61.5 \; log \; ([K^+]_i/[K^+]_o)$$

in which E_K is the potassium equilibrium potential. The contribution of other ions to the overall membrane potential is smaller, since they do not penetrate membranes as easily as does K^+. It is this passive movement of K^+ that is primarily responsible for the outward current that gives rise to the *transmembrane resting potential.*

An examination of the relationship of the ($[K^+]_o$) and ($[K^+]_i$) in the Nernst equation shows that an increase in the ($[K^+]_o$) will result in a decrease (less negative potential) in the membrane resting potential. Changes in the extracellular concentrations of other ions (Na^+, Ca^{2+}, Mg^{2+}, or Cl^-) may modify a resting potential, but they will not determine its final value. *The resting transmembrane potential is primarily determined by the outward diffusion of K^+.*

In order to produce membrane depolarization, the applied stimulus must be of sufficient intensity to bring about an inward current that exceeds the outward K^+ current. The application of a depolarizing stimulus causes an inward movement of Na^+ and an inward Na^+ current (I_{Na^+}). A subthreshold stimulus will fail to produce a net inward movement of Na^+ and the membrane will return to its resting state. If, on the other hand, the applied stimulus results in a net inward movement of Na^+ (Na^+ conductance, gNa^+), there results a self-sustaining depolarization of the membrane that gives rise to a membrane action potential (Fig. 26-1). A rapid depolarization decreases the transmembrane potential to a level approximating, but never attaining, the Na^+ equilibrium potential (+25 to +35 mV).

Ionic Basis for the Membrane Action Potential

Phase 0

Depolarization results in the opening of membrane channels that permit an inward current and is responsible for the rapid upstroke (*phase 0*) of the membrane action potential (Fig. 26-1). Because of the rapidity with which this change occurs, the channels that conduct the inward Na^+ current during this phase of the excitation sequence are referred to as *fast inward channels,* in contrast to other inward current channels that have somewhat different kinetics and ion selectivity, such as the *slow inward calcium current I_{Ca}^{2+}),* carried by channels that open when the membrane is depolarized to approximately -60 mV. *The rate of recovery of the Na^+ channels from voltage-dependent inactivation determines the refractory period and thus the maximal rate at which the cardiac cells will respond to applied stimuli and propagate impulses to neighboring cells.* The increase in sodium conductance (gNa^+) has a duration of 1 to 2 msec as it undergoes voltage-dependent inactivation and curtails the upstroke of the membrane action potential. The rate at which an impulse conducts from one cell to another is dependent on the intensity or density of I_{Na} as indicated by the maximal upstroke velocity of phase 0 (V_{max}); the latter is a major determinant of the speed of impulse conduction within the ventricular myocardium.

Phase 1

At the peak of the upstroke, there occurs a phase of rapid repolarization in which the membrane potential returns toward 0 mV as a result of the rapid inactivation of the I_{Na}, and the activation of a short-lived outward current carried primarily by K^+ and referred to as the transient outward current, or I_{to}.

Phase 2 (Action-Potential Plateau)

During phase 2, conductance of all ion channels decreases rapidly so that there is a net balance between inward (depolarizing) and outward (repolarizing) ion currents. With time, however, the outward currents predominate and repolarization of the membrane is favored, thus allowing for the transition from the plateau phase (phase 2) to that late rapid phase of repolarization (phase 3). A major contributor to phase 2 of the membrane action potential is the I_{Ca}^{2+} initiated during the upstroke of the action potential. Opening of a voltage-dependent channel, selective for Ca^{2+}, occurs rapidly when the membrane is depolarized to -40 mV. The channel (*"L-type" calcium channel*) shows slow inactivation kinetics, thereby giving rise to a long-lasting current to allow calcium conductance via slow inward calcium channel. In addition, the plateau phase is influenced by the repolarizing effect of outward K^+ currents carried by several separate K^+ channels.

The effect of the inward I_{Ca}^{2+} on the plateau phase is opposed by several distinct K^+ conductances. The latter include the inwardly rectifying K^+ conductance (gK_1), the delayed outwardly rectifying K^+ conductance (gK), and the calcium-activated K^+ conductance (gK^+-Ca^{2+}). Most importantly, another channel is present, the adenosine triphosphate (ATP)-sensitive K^+ conductance (I_{K-ATP}), that is inhibited by intracellular ATP. Under conditions of myocardial ischemia, resulting in a decrease in intracellular ATP content, there is an associated opening of the ATP-dependent potassium channel. The latter leads to a sustained repolarizing K^+ current that decreases the plateau phase and hastens the onset of the late rapid repolarization phase (phase 3) of the membrane action potential.

Phase 3 (Late Phase of Repolarization)

Termination of phase 2 of the membrane action-potential plateau results from a time-, voltage-, and intracellular Ca^{2+}-dependent inactivation process plus the unopposed repolarizing effects of the outward K^+ currents. *The combination of these effects results in repolarization of the membrane action potential.* The two important membrane currents responsible for the rapid repolarization phase during the normal cardiac cycle are I_{K1}, which exhibits the property of inward rectification, and I_K (delayed outward rectifier). Opening of either I_{K1} or I_K will abbreviate the duration of the action potential and decrease the time for repolarization. Pharmacological interventions that inhibit either I_{K1} or I_K will increase the duration of the membrane action potential by delaying the process of repolarization. On the other hand, myocardial ischemia and the resulting decrease in the tissue content of ATP will result in an opening of the ATP-sensitive potassium channel thereby decreasing the duration of the membrane action potential. The transmembrane currents carried by specific ions flowing through their respective ion channels are presented schematically in Fig. 26-1.

Phase 4

Phase 4 of the membrane action potential represents electrical silence in normal atrial and ventricular muscle. *It is during phase 4 that the Na^+ channels recover from inactivation whereupon normal excitability or responsiveness to depolarizing stimuli returns.* The myocardial cell is now prepared for generation of the next action potential.

The events that have been described are characteristic for *ventricular muscle* and *Purkinje fibers.* Atrial muscle fibers have action potentials with similar characteristics, but they differ in that the resting potential, the amplitude of

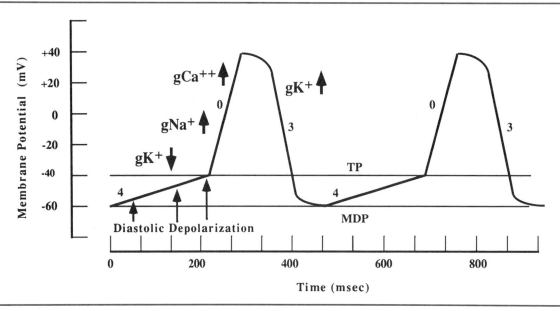

Figure 26-2. Transmembrane action potential of a sinoatrial node cell. In contrast to other cardiac cells, there is no phase 2 or plateau. The *threshold potential (TP)* is −40 mV. The maximum diastolic potential (MDP) is achieved as a result of a gradual decline in the potassium conductance (gK⁺). Spontaneous phase 4 or diastolic depolarization permits the cell to achieve the TP, thereby initiating an action potential (g = transmembrane ion conductance). Stimulation of pacemaker cells within the sinoatrial node decreases the time required to achieve the TP, whereas vagal stimulation and the release of acetylcholine decrease the slope of diastolic depolarization. Thus, the positive and negative chronotropic actions of sympathetic and parasympathetic nerve stimulation can be attributed to the effects of the respective neurotransmitters on ion conductance in pacemaker cells of the sinoatrial node. gNa⁺ = Na⁺ conductance.

the action potential, the rate of depolarization, and the total duration of the action potential are lower.

Automaticity

Automaticity can be defined as the ability of a cell to alter its resting membrane potential to the excitation threshold *without* the influence of an external stimulus. The characteristic feature of cells that possess the property of automaticity is the presence of a slow decrease in the membrane potential during diastole (*phase 4*) such that the membrane potential reaches threshold (Fig. 26-2). Diastolic depolarization in the sinoatrial node is the result of the spontaneous decline in potassium conductance. Under these conditions, the outward current is curtailed, whereas the inward current, believed to be due to calcium, continues. *The net result is a spontaneous diastolic depolarization.*

Since *the sinoatrial (S-A) node possesses the highest intrinsic automaticity,* it serves as the normal pacemaker of the heart. Specialized cells within the atria, atrioventricular (A-V) node, and His-Purkinje system also can initiate di-

astolic depolarization under special circumstances. They will become pacemakers when their own intrinsic rate of depolarization becomes greater than that of the sinoatrial node or when the pacemaker cells within the sinoatrial node are depressed. In those instances in which impulses fail to conduct across the A-V node to excite the ventricular myocardium, spontaneous depolarization within the His-Purkinje system may become the dominant pacemaker that maintains the cardiac rhythm.

The rate of pacemaker discharge within the sinoatrial node is influenced by the activity of both divisions of the autonomic nervous system. The sinoatrial node and the A-V node are innervated by sympathetic nerves, with a less dense innervation being provided to the Purkinje fibers. Increased sympathetic nerve activity to the heart, the release of catecholamines from the adrenal medulla, or the exogenous administration of adrenomimetic amines will cause an increase in the rate of pacemaker activity in the sinoatrial node through stimulation of β-adrenoceptors on the pacemaker cells (Fig. 26-3). Pacemaker cells in other regions of the heart are influenced in a similar manner, and the cardiac rhythm will be under the influence of the dominant pacemaker.

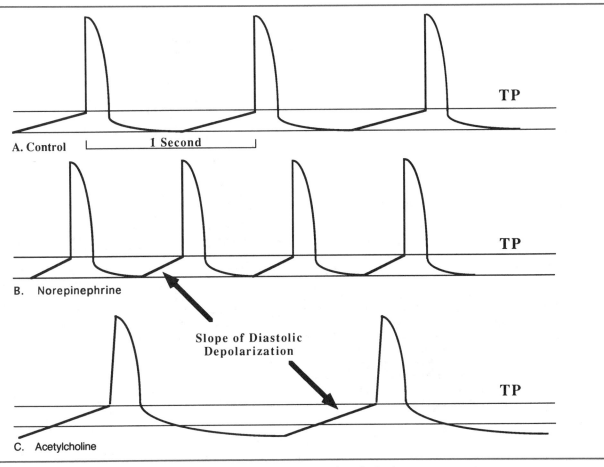

A. Control

1 Second

B. Norepinephrine

Slope of Diastolic
Depolarization

C. Acetylcholine

Figure 26-3. Effects of norepinephrine and acetylcholine on *spontaneous diastolic depolarization (automaticity)* in a pacemaker cell for the sinoatrial node. The pacemaker cell discharges spontaneously when the threshold potential (TP) is attained. The rate of spontaneous discharge is determined by the initial slope of the membrane potential and the time required to reach the threshold potential. A. Control recording showing the spontaneous diastolic depolarization. B. The effect of norepinephrine is to increase the slope of diastolic depolarization. The frequency of spontaneous discharge is increased. This effect is mediated through the activation of β-adrenoceptors in sinoatrial nodal cells. C. Acetylcholine stimulates muscarinic receptors in sinoatrial nodal cells. There is a decrease in the slope of diastolic depolarization as well as hyperpolarization of the cell. The time to reach the threshold potential is prolonged, with the net effect being a decrease in the rate of spontaneous depolarization.

The parasympathetic nervous system, through the vagus nerve, has an inhibiting effect on the spontaneous rate of depolarization of the sinoatrial node pacemaker cells. The release of acetylcholine from cholinergic vagal fibers increases potassium conductance (gK^+) in sinoatrial pacemaker cells, and this enhanced outward movement of K^+ results in a more negative potential or hyperpolarization of the sinoatrial cells. Thus, during vagal stimulation, the threshold potential of the sinoatrial node pacemaker cells is achieved more slowly and the heart rate is slowed.

Specialized atrial muscle fibers, A-V nodal cells and His-Purkinje cells, also display automaticity and can function as *subsidiary pacemakers*. Since diastolic depolarization in such subsidiary pacemakers, particularly in the His-

Purkinje cells, depends on ionic currents that differ from those of the dominant sinus pacemaker, these *distal subsidiary pacemakers discharge at inherently slower rates.* If a proximal pacemaker ceases to function or its impulse transmission is blocked, the distal subsidiary pacemakers can dominate the cardiac rate. If pathological changes occur in the electrophysiology of these distal subsidiary pacemakers, their rate of discharge may increase and cardiac arrhythmias may ensue. Myocardial ischemia, excessive myocardial catecholamine release, or cardiac glycoside toxicity has been shown to produce some of these pathological disorders in electrophysiology. A special situation arises when oscillatory afterdepolarizations develop in the early or late phase of membrane repolarization. If the af-

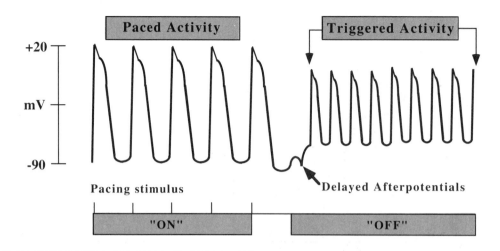

Figure 26-4. An example of *triggered activity* developing in Purkinje tissue. The appearance of a *delayed afterdepolarization (DAD)* after the fifth paced impulse is followed by a burst of triggered activity that maintains the rapid rate of impulse formation despite the cessation of electrical pacing. Triggered activity from DADs occurs in Purkinje fibers or ventricular muscle when the tissues are exposed to toxic concentrations of digitalis, catecholamines, or other interventions that increase intracellular calcium concentrations. Whereas DADs occur after the the cell has achieved its maximum diastolic potential, the phenomenon of *early afterdepolarization (EADs)* occurs before complete repolarization has taken place. EADs can occur after exposure to drugs that prolong the action-potential duration and may account for the *proarrhythmic action* (discussed in the text) of several antiarrhythmic drugs.

terdepolarizations are of sufficient amplitude, they can reach the threshold potential and initiate a series of impulses, thereby resulting in the phenomenon referred to as *triggered activity*. Triggered activity can be the result of early or delayed afterdepolarizations (Fig. 26-4). Triggered activity associated with early afterdepolarizations is observed under conditions of a decreased extracellular potassium ion concentration. Conditions that favor an increase in intracellular calcium or toxic concentrations of digitalis glycosides lead to the development of triggered activity due to delayed afterdepolarization in Purkinje tissue or ventricular muscle. Triggered activity, therefore, is of two types depending on the temporal relationship of the triggered activity to the initiating impulse. The upstroke of the triggered impulse is carried by either the fast inward sodium current or the slow inward current of the L-type calcium channel. Triggered impulses differ from automatic impulses in that they occur after one or more action potentials associated with afterdepolarizations. Early afterdepolarizations are seen most commonly at slow rates and can be suppressed by increasing the frequency of stimulation (e.g., increased pacing rate or increase in the sinus rate) or by drugs that decrease action-potential duration.

Atrial and ventricular muscle cells, in contrast to Purkinje fibers, do not possess the property of automaticity under normal physiological conditions. If, however, the resting membrane potentials of such tissues are reduced to values below −60 mV, spontaneous diastolic depolarization can give rise to regions of abnormal automaticity.

Many antiarrhythmic agents depress automaticity in pacemaker cells, *particularly in subsidiary pacemakers.* Most of the drugs depress abnormal automaticity at concentrations that exert little effect on the automaticity of the normal sinus node.

Cardiac Conduction

The major determinants of myocardial conduction velocity include the maximum rate of depolarization (V_{max}) of phase 0 of the action potential, the threshold potential, and the resting membrane potential. The ability of cardiac fibers to respond to a propagating impulse depends on the membrane potential at the moment of excitation. Conduction velocity is proportional to the rate of phase 0 depolarization; therefore, as the membrane is depolarized or the resting potential decreased due to cellular injury, conduction velocity decreases.

Like other excitable tissues, *cardiac cells become refractory to restimulation during depolarization.* The term *effective refractory period* (ERP) describes the duration of refractoriness, which includes phases 0, 1, 2, and most of phase 3. At the end of the relative refractory period, the fiber has

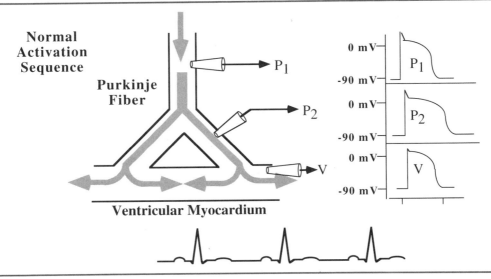

Figure 26-5. Schematic representation of normal activation and impulse transmission through the His-Purkinje system with final entry into ventricular myocardium. Intracellular recording electrodes are placed in the proximal Purkinje network (P_1), in the Purkinje branch on the right of the diagram (P_2), and in ventricular myocardium (V). The inset to the right illustrates the membrane action-potential recordings from the respective microelectrodes. The action-potential duration, and thus the effective refractory period, is longest in the more distal portion of the Purkinje branch immediately before insertion into the ventricular myocardium. Under normal conditions, the impulses within the terminal Purkinje network conduct with relatively equal velocities so as to activate the ventricular myocardium in a uniform manner. The longer duration of the effective refractory period in the terminal Purkinje fiber prevents the impulse, traversing within ventricular myocardium, from reentering the Purkinje network in the retrograde direction. The many wave fronts of excitation invading the ventricular myocardium from multiple insertions of the Purkinje network will collide in the ventricular myocardium and terminate. The net result is a homogeneous and nearly simultaneous activation of the entire ventricular myocardium within 400 msec. The electrocardiographic tracing below illustrates a normal sinus rhythm in which there is a repetitive and coordinated activation of the entire heart. One conducted sinoatrial impulse entering the ventricle from the atrioventricular node distributes over the His-Purkinje system to elicit one QRS complex indicating depolarization of the ventricular myocardium.

repolarized, and external stimulation again produces a normally conducted cardiac impulse.

A disturbance in cardiac conduction that results in arrhythmias is called *reentry*. Figures 25-5 and 25-6 are schematic representations of a normally propagated and a reentrant event in injured ventricular myocardium, respectively. As illustrated in Fig. 26-5, the wave of excitation passes through relatively homogeneous tissue involving the Purkinje system (P_1 and P_2) and enters normal ventricular myocardium. As indicated in this figure, the action-potential duration, and thus the refractory period, is longer in the distal Purkinje fibers as compared to the respective durations in ventricular myocardium (V). The intracellular action-potential recordings from the respective regions are illustrated on the right. A normally propagating impulse will enter ventricular myocardium nearly simultaneously at multiple regions where Purkinje fibers terminate in the walls of both ventricles. The sequence of

activation of the ventricular myocardium is rapid ($\sim$0.04 sec). The various wave fronts of activation entering at different points may collide within the ventricular myocardium and terminate. *The net result is an orderly activation of all ventricular myocardial fibers, giving rise to normal-appearing action potentials* in the respective tissues and a normal electrocardiogram.

In the undamaged myocardium, cardiac impulses travel in both anterograde and retrograde directions through the Purkinje fibers; the ventricular rate depends primarily on the refractory period of the Purkinje fibers. In the presence of ischemic damage, however, propagation of cardiac impulses is interfered with and a functional *unidirectional block* may occur. Impulses can no longer travel in the anterograde direction, although retrograde transmission is still possible (see impulse 1, Fig. 26-6), albeit at a slower rate. In some situations the retrograde impulse will enter an area of normal myocardium that has repolarized suffi-

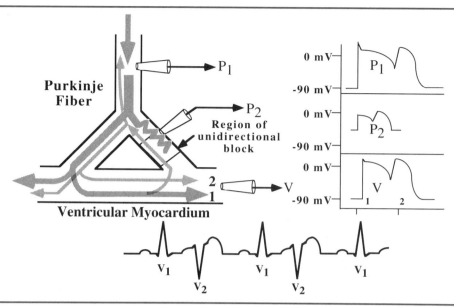

Figure 26-6. Conduction disorders due to *reentry* as might occur in the ischemic or postinfarcted myocardium. See Fig. 25-5 for a description of the format. As in the previous figure, *antegrade conduction* occurs in a normal manner over the proximal Purkinje system (P_1) and in the distal Purkinje network on the left of the diagram. However, the Purkinje network on the right (P_2) has been subjected to injury. The intracellular recordings from the respective electrodes indicate that the resting membrane potential from P_2 is decreased due to the presence of injury at this site. Therefore, the impulse conducts slowly and decrementally, and finally is blocked in the area of injury *(unidirectional block)*. The ventricular myocardium, however, has been depolarized from normally conducting Purkinje fibers at remote insertion sites. The excitatory impules traversing within the ventricular myocardium will reenter the distal portion of the Purkinje network (right side of diagram) and conduct slowly in the retrograde direction through the area of unidirectional block. The appropriate conditions are established by the conduction velocities and refractory periods in the respective tissues. The retrograde impulse can reenter the proximal Purkinje system and initiate reexcitation of the proximal and distal Purkinje network as well as the ventricular myocardium if each of these sites has recovered its excitability from the previous depolarization. The reentry impulse may give rise to a *premature coupled ventricular complex* in which the normally conducted impulse (V_1) is followed with precise timing by a *reentry ventricular complex* (V_2). The reentry impulses could occur more frequently so that the cardiac rhythm becomes dominated by the activity in the reentry pathway, thus leading to a rapid, repetitive series of ventricular complexes *(ventricular tachycardia)* in which the ventricular rate becomes rapid (>100 beats min) an may degenerate into ventricular fibrillation. The object of antiarrhythmic drug therapy is to reduce the frequency of hemodynamically disturbing premature ventricular impulses and to prevent the establishment of a sustained and rapidly conducting reentrant rhythm capable of becoming lethal.

ciently such that it is no longer absolutely refractory and an action potential will result. This generation of an action potential may produce an increased rate of ventricular firing and may become self-sustaining. The latter phenomenon is known as a reentrant, or circus, rhythm. If the speed of propagation is too rapid through the region of myocardial damage, the retrograde impulse will attempt to reenter the normal region at a time when the tissue is refractory. This will give rise to bidirectional block, thereby terminating the reentrant wave front. Therefore, in order for *reentry* to occur, there must be a region of *unidirectional block* and *slow conduction*. The delay in conduction permits the tissue ahead of the advancing wave front to regain its excitability, thereby sustaining the reentry

circuit. As shown in Fig. 26-6, the reentrant wave front gives rise to a second depolarizing impulse (#2) in the ventricular myocardium, as well as in each of the branches of the Purkinje network (P_1 and P_2). The net result of the reentrant wave is depicted in the electrocardiogram in which coupled ventricular premature complexes (V_2) follow each normal (V_1) complex.

Through their ability to interact with sodium channels, the antiarrhythmic drugs, especially those belonging to class I (see the following discussion), have the ability to increase the myocardial refractory period and to decrease conduction velocity in myocardial tissue. The latter effect becomes more pronounced in cells that are partially depolarized due to injury. *In reentrant pathways where one is*

Table 26-1. Classification of Antiarrhythmic Drugs

Antiarrhythmic class	Representative drugs	Principal pharmacological effects
IA	Quinidine Procainamide Disopyramide Moricizine[a]	Decrease V_{max} of phase O, increase refractory period, moderate decrease in conduction velocity, decrease fast inward sodium current, inhibit potassium repolarization current
IB	Lidocaine Phenytoin Tocainide Moricizine[a] Mexiletine	Minimal change in V_{max} of phase O, decrease in cardiac action-potential duration, decrease inward sodium current in ventricular muscle, increase outward potassium current
IC	Flecainide Propafenone	Marked decrease in V_{max} of phase O, profound decrease in ventricular conduction velocity, marked inhibition of inward sodium current
II	Propranolol Metoprolol Nadolol Acebutolol Atenolol Pindolol Timolol Sotalol Esmolol[b]	β-Adrenoceptor antagonist, cardiac membrane stabilization, indirectly effect the sinoatrial and atrioventricular nodes to slow conduction and increase the effective refractory period
III	Amiodarone Bretylium Sotalol	Prolong the duration of ventricular action potential, prolong refractoriness, inhibit potassium repolarization current
IV	Verapamil Diltiazem Bepridil[c]	Inhibit the slow inward calcium channel, minimal effect on ventricular action potential, major effects on the atrioventricular node to slow conduction and increase the effective refractory period

[a]A mixed-class IA/IB drug.
[b]Ultra–short-acting β-adrenoceptor blocking agent.
[c]May also show class III activity.

most likely to encounter damaged myocardial cells, antiarrhythmic drugs are prone to produce greater effects on conduction in partially depolarized cells than in normal myocardial cells. Therefore, conduction block in a reentrant pathway may lead to an interruption of the reentry circuit and an abolition of arrhythmic disturbances due to the establishment of bidirectional block. However, if the drug in question also has the ability to slow conduction velocity more than it increases refractoriness, it may facilitate the onset or maintenance, or both, of a reentry rhythm.

One mechanism whereby an antiarrhythmic agent may abolish reentry is by converting unidirectional block to bidirectional block. A second mechanism to explain the action of antiarrhythmic drugs is that they can prevent reentry by increasing the effective refractory period of the cardiac fibers within or surrounding the region of the reentry circuit.

Classification of Antiarrhythmic Drugs

Although it is possible to arrange the known antiarrhythmic agents into four classes according to their predominant electrophysiological effect (Table 26-1), in many instances an agent can be shown to possess a multitude of effects, each of which may be beneficial in controlling cardiac arrhythmias. Thus, although the grouping of antiarrhythmic agents into four classes is convenient, it should be remembered that such a classification may fall short in explaining the underlying mechanisms by which the drugs ultimately exert their therapeutic antiarrhythmic activity. There are also certain agents that do not fall neatly into the four classes; these are discussed at the end of the chapter.

Class I Drugs

Class I antiarrhythmic drugs are characterized by their ability to restrict the rate of sodium entry during cardiac membrane depolarization, decrease the rate of rise of phase 0 of the cardiac membrane action potential, require that a greater (more negative) membrane potential be achieved before the membrane becomes excitable and can propagate to its neighbors, and prolong the effective refractory period of fast-response fibers. Although many class I antiarrhythmic drugs possess local anesthetic actions and can depress myocardial contractile force, these effects are usually observed only at higher plasma concentrations.

The antiarrhythmic drugs in class I are known to suppress both normal Purkinje fiber and His bundle automaticity as well as abnormal automaticity resulting from myocardial damage. The ability to "selectively" suppress abnormal automaticity permits the sinoatrial node to once again assume the role of the dominant pacemaker.

The antiarrhythmic agents that belong to class I have been divided into three subgroups (see Table 26-1). Class IA drugs depress the rate of rise in potential and prolong the ventricular ERP. Members of class IB have a minimal effect on the rate of depolarization and are characterized by their ability to decrease the action-potential duration and ERP of Purkinje fibers. The drugs in class IC produce a marked depression in the rate of rise of the membrane action potential and have minimal effects on the duration of membrane action potential and ERP of ventricular myocardial cells.

Class II Drugs

The class II antiarrhythmic drugs are characterized by the fact that *virtually all of them can competitively block β-adrenoceptors.* They inhibit catecholamine-induced stimulation of cardiac β-receptors. In addition, some members of the group (e.g., *propranolol* and *acebutolol*) cause electrophysiological alterations in Purkinje fibers that resemble those produced by class I antiarrhythmic drugs. The latter actions have been referred to as "membrane-stabilizing" effects. Another member of this drug class, *sotalol*, possesses electrophysiological effects that resemble those of the class III group of drugs. Determining which of the actions of the β-receptor blocking drugs can explain their antiarrhythmic effects has proved to be a complex problem.

Class III Drugs

Although the class III antiarrhythmic drugs (e.g., *bretylium, amiodarone,* and *sotalol*) possess complex and unrelated pharmacological properties, they seem to share one common characteristic—*they prolong the duration of the membrane action potential without altering the phase 0 of depolarization or the resting membrane potential.* It is most likely that the antiarrhythmic actions of class III compounds can be attributed to this singular electrophysiological effect rather than to the secondary effects that involve alterations in responses of the heart to sympathetic innervation. The importance of the class III drugs is that they have been shown clinically to be effective in cases of intractable ventricular tachycardia and in reducing the likelihood of developing ventricular fibrillation.

Many class III drugs induce arrhythmias by a mechanism or mechanisms related to prolongation of the action-potential duration. The ionic basis for the proarrhythmic action may relate to the ability of the members of this class to reduce potassium ion conductance sufficiently, leading to a marked prolongation in repolarization. Under such circumstances, early afterdepolarizations may become prominent, thereby giving rise to oscillatory behavior and episodes of ventricular tachycardia. Clinically, the disturbances in rhythm mimic the electrocardiographic pattern referred to as torsades de pointes. This event is not specific for the class III agents and is noted to occur with class IA and IC.

Class IV Drugs

The members of class IV are characterized by their ability to *block the slow inward current in cardiac tissue, a current that is dependent on the inward movement of Ca^{2+}* during phases 0 to 2 of the membrane action potential. The most pronounced electrophysiological effects are exerted on cardiac fibers with slow-response action potentials, such as those found in the sinus and A-V nodes. The administration of class IV drugs slows conduction velocity and increases refractoriness in the A-V node, thereby reducing the ability of the A-V node to conduct supraventricular impulses to the ventricle. This action will terminate supraventricular tachycardias that utilize the A-V conduction of supraventricular impulses during atrial flutter or atrial fibrillation. Although many drugs are capable of blocking the slow inward calcium channel, two agents in particular, *verapamil* and *diltiazem*, are recognized for their potential as antiarrhythmic agents. A third agent, *bepridil*, while not approved as an antiarrhythmic agent, is of interest in that it has properties of both the class III and IV groups of antiarrhythmic drugs.

Class IA

Quinidine

The efficacy and long history of the use of quinidine (Fig. 26-7) in the treatment of disorders of cardiac rhythm has led to its establishment as the prototypical antiarrhythmic agent. Quinidine shares all the pharmacological properties of quinine, including antimalarial (see Chap. 57), antipyretic (see Chap. 39), oxytocic, and skeletal muscle relaxant actions.

Electrophysiological Actions

The net effect of quinidine on the electrical properties of a particular cardiac tissue depends on the extent of para-

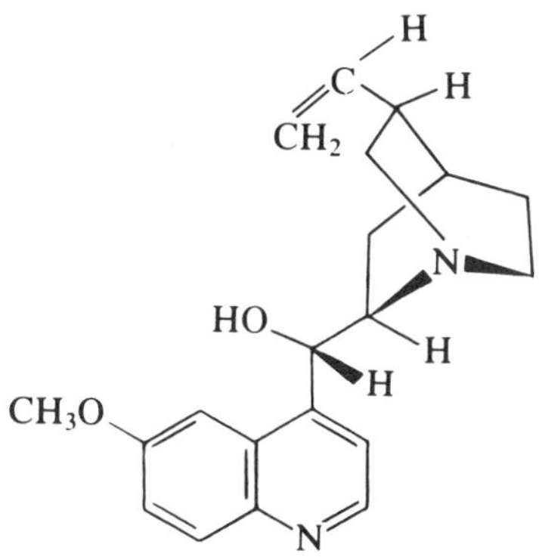

Figure 26-7. Quinidine.

are believed to be the direct result of a reduction of conduction velocity in atrial myocardium.

A-V Node

Both the direct and indirect actions of quinidine are important in determining its ultimate effect on A-V conduction. The *indirect (anticholinergic) properties* of quinidine prevent both vagally mediated prolongation of the A-V node refractory period and depression of conduction velocity. Thus, the ability of quinidine to produce cholinergic blockade leads to an enhancement of A-V transmission. Quinidine's *direct* electrophysiological actions on the A-V node are to decrease conduction velocity and increase the ERP.

His-Purkinje System and Ventricular Muscle

Quinidine can depress the automaticity of ventricular pacemakers by depressing the slope of phase 4 depolarization. Depression of pacemakers in the His-Purkinje system is more pronounced than depression of sinus node pacemaker cells.

Quinidine also prolongs repolarization in Purkinje fibers and ventricular muscle, and this results in an increase in the duration of the action potential. As in atrial muscle, quinidine administration results in *postrepolarization refractoriness*, that is, an extension of refractoriness beyond the recovery of the resting membrane potential. The indirect (anticholinergic) properties of quinidine are not a factor in its actions on ventricular muscle and the His-Purkinje system.

Serum K^+ concentrations have a major influence on the activity of quinidine on cardiac tissue. Low extracellular K^+ concentrations antagonize the depressant effects of quinidine on membrane responsiveness, whereas high extracellular K^+ concentrations increase quinidine's ability to depress membrane responsiveness. This dependency may explain why hypokalemic patients are often unre-

sympathetic innervation, the level of parasympathetic tone, and the dose. The anticholinergic actions of quinidine predominate at lower plasma concentrations and are most apparent during the initiation of oral therapy. Later, when steady-state therapeutic plasma concentrations have been achieved, the drug's direct electrophysiological actions predominate. The direct and indirect electrophysiological actions are summarized in Table 26-2.

Sinoatrial Node

Quinidine administration results in a dose-dependent depression of membrane responsiveness in atrial muscle fibers. The maximum rate of phase 0 depolarization and the amplitude of phase 0 are depressed equally at all membrane potentials. Quinidine also decreases atrial muscle excitability in such a way that a larger current stimulus is needed for initiation of an active response. These actions of quinidine often are referred to as its "local anesthetic" properties and

Table 26-2. Electrophysiological Actions of Quinidine, Procainamide, and Disopyramide at Therapeutic Plasma Concentrations

Tissue	Direct action	Indirect anticholinergic action	Net effect
Sinus node depolarization	Decrease	Increase	No change
Atrial tissue			
Conduction velocity	Decrease	Decrease	Decrease
Effective refractory period	Increase	Increase	Increase
A-V node			
Automaticity	Decrease	Increase	Increase/decrease*
Conduction velocity	Decrease	Increase	Increase/decrease*
Effective refractory period	Increase	Decrease	Decrease/increase*
His-Purkinje system–ventricular muscle			
Automaticity	Decrease		Decrease
Conduction velocity	Decrease		Decrease
Effective refractory period	Increase		Increase

*Dose dependent (low dose/high dose).

Table 26-3. Pharmacokinetic Characteristics of the Class IA Drugs

Drug	Therapeutic serum concentration (μg/ml)	Time to onset of action (hr)	Time to peak concentration (hr)	Duration of action (hr)	Elimination half-life (hr)	Percent protein bound	Volume of distribution (L/kg)
Quinidine	2–4	0.5	2–4	6–8	6–7	60–80	2.7 ± 1.2
Procainamide	4–10	0.5	0.5–1.5	3	2.5–4.5	15–20	1.9 ± 0.3
Disopyramide	2–5	0.5	2	6–7	4–10	20–60[a]	0.6 ± 0.2
Moricizine[b]	–	2	0.8–2	10–24	3–4 (9[c])	95	8.3–11.1

[a]There is dose-dependent protein binding. Increased concentrations effect decreases in the percentage of drug bound.
[b]Moricizine is a mixed-class IA/IB drug.
[c]Plasma half-life is increased in patients treated chronically for arrhythmias.

sponsive to the antiarrhythmic effects of quinidine and are more prone to development of cardiac rhythm disorders.

Electrocardiographic Changes

At normal therapeutic plasma concentrations, quinidine prolongs the P–R, the QRS, and the Q–T intervals. QRS and Q–T prolongations are more pronounced with quinidine than with other antiarrhythmic agents. The magnitude of these changes is related directly to the plasma quinidine concentration.

Hemodynamic Effects

Although quinidine is capable of producing a negative inotropic effect on atrial and ventricular myocardium, myocardial depression is not a problem in patients with normal cardiac function. However, in patients with compromised myocardial function, the drug may depress cardiac contractility sufficiently to result in a decrease in cardiac output and a significant rise in left ventricular end-diastolic pressure, and overt heart failure may ensue.

Quinidine can depress vascular smooth muscle directly and thereby bring about a decrease in peripheral vascular resistance. The peripheral vasodilation also can be attributed, in part, to blockade of α-adrenoceptors. The reduction in peripheral vascular resistance, combined with a reduction in cardiac output, can produce a decrease in arterial pressure. The depressant effects of quinidine on the cardiovascular system are more likely to occur after intravenous administration and, therefore, the drug should not be employed routinely in the emergency treatment of arrhythmias.

Pharmacokinetics

The pharmacokinetic characteristics of quinidine are summarized in Table 26-3. Quinidine is almost completely absorbed from the gastrointestinal tract after oral administration. Quinidine is bound (~80%) to serum proteins including albumin and α_1-glycoprotein. The extent of protein binding decreases with liver disease and hypoalbuminemia. It is the nonionized quinidine molecule that is preferentially bound to albumin. The binding of quinidine to plasma proteins shows significant interpatient variability. The unbound form of the drug is considered to be the biologically active species.

Therapeutic concentrations, as measured by recently developed specific assays, are 2 to 4 μg/ml. Toxic manifestations are commonly observed at concentrations above 8 μg/ml. Renal and liver disease may require a dosage reduction or an increase in the dosage interval. Renal function decreases with age, and lower doses may be necessary in elderly patients.

Clinical Uses

Primary indications for the use of quinidine include: (1) abolition of premature beats that have an atrial, A-V junctional, or ventricular origin; (2) restoration of normal sinus rhythm in atrial flutter and atrial fibrillation after controlling the ventricular rate with digitalis; (3) maintenance of normal sinus rhythm after electrical conversion of atrial arrhythmias; (4) prophylaxis against arrhythmias associated with electrical countershock; (5) termination of ventricular tachycardia; and (6) suppression of repetitive tachycardia associated with Wolff-Parkinson-White (WPW) syndrome.

Quinidine is not the drug of choice either for prophylaxis or for active treatment of ventricular flutter or ventricular fibrillation. Management of these arrhythmias often requires IV drug administration, and quinidine carries significant risk of toxicity when given by this route.

Although quinidine often is successful in producing normal sinus rhythm, its administration in the presence of a rapid atrial rate (flutter and, possibly, atrial fibrillation) can lead to a further, and dangerous, increase in the ventricular rate. For this reason, digitalis should be used before quinidine when one is attempting to convert atrial flutter or atrial fibrillation to normal sinus rhythm.

Through the combined effects of reducing the volume of distribution and the renal clearance of digoxin, quinidine can increase the incidence of digoxin-induced toxicity. Therefore, a reduction in digoxin dosage is suggested when quinidine is given concurrently.

Adverse Reactions

The most common adverse effects associated with quinidine administration are diarrhea (35%), upper-gastrointestinal distress (25%), and light-headedness (15%). Other relatively common adverse effects include fatigue, palpitations, and headache (each occurring with an incidence of 7%), and anginalike pain and rash (at 5% incidence each). These adverse effects are generally dose related and reversible with cessation of therapy. In some patients, thrombocytopenia may occur as a result of quinidine administration; it is due to the formation of a plasma protein–quinidine complex that evokes a circulating antibody directed against the blood platelet. Although platelet counts return to normal on cessation of therapy, administration of quinidine or quinine at a later date can cause the reappearance of thrombocytopenia.

The cardiac toxicity of quinidine includes A-V and intraventricular block, ventricular tachyarrhythmias, and depression of myocardial contractility. In most patients, toxicity can be controlled either by proper adjustment of the dose or by discontinuing the drug.

Large doses of quinidine can produce a syndrome known as *cinchonism,* which is characterized by ringing in the ears, headache, nausea, visual disturbances or blurred vision, disturbed auditory acuity, and vertigo. Larger doses can produce confusion, delirium, hallucinations, or psychoses.

Quinidine syncope, or sudden arrhythmic death (an uncommon but major complication of quinidine therapy), is caused by transient or irreversible ventricular tachycardia or ventricular fibrillation. This action is not necessarily due to overdosage, but it may occur at therapeutic or subtherapeutic plasma concentration. The mechanism for these arrhythmias is poorly understood, but it may be a result of slowed myocardial conduction.

Contraindications

One of the few absolute contraindications for quinidine is the presence of complete A-V block with an A-V pacemaker or idioventricular pacemaker; this may be suppressed by quinidine, thereby leading to cardiac arrest. Owing to the negative inotropic action of quinidine the drug is contraindicated in congestive heart failure and hypotension. Digitalis intoxication and hyperkalemia can accentuate the depression of conduction caused by quinidine, and the drug should be used with extreme care in these conditions. Myasthenia gravis can be aggravated severely by quinidine's actions at the neuromuscular junction.

Drug Interactions

Quinidine can increase the plasma concentrations of digoxin, which may, in turn, lead to signs and symptoms of digitalis toxicity. In most (90% or more) patients receiving quinidine and digoxin, the digoxin serum concentration is increased. Gastrointestinal, central nervous system (CNS), or cardiac toxicity associated with elevated digoxin concentrations may occur. Although this is a probable drug interaction, quinidine and digoxin can be administered concurrently; however, a downward adjustment in the digoxin dose may be required. It is important to monitor such patients with respect to signs of digoxin toxicity.

Quinidine also may interact with other drugs to produce changes in its plasma concentrations. Drugs that have been associated with elevations in quinidine concentrations include acetazolamide, certain antacids (magnesium hydroxide and calcium carbonate), and the H_2-receptor antagonist, cimetidine. Cimetidine inhibits the hepatic metabolism of quinidine. Phenytoin, rifampin, and barbiturates increase the hepatic metabolism of quinidine and reduce its plasma concentrations. To maintain antiarrhythmic efficacy when quinidine is administered concurrently with these drugs, an increase in quinidine dose may be required.

Procainamide

Procainamide is a derivative of the local anesthetic agent procaine. However, procaine is not used clinically for its antiarrhythmic properties because the drug is rapidly hydrolyzed in the blood, resulting in a very short duration of action; can produce CNS toxicity; and is ineffective orally due to its inactivation by hydrolysis in the gastrointestinal tract. Therefore, structurally similar chemicals have been synthesized and their electrophysiological and antiarrhythmic properties studied. This has led to the development of procainamide, which, compared to procaine, has a longer half-life, does not cause CNS toxicity at therapeutic plasma concentrations, and is effective orally. *Procainamide is a particularly useful antiarrhythmic drug, effective in the treatment of supraventricular, ventricular, and digitalis-induced arrhythmias.*

Electrophysiological Actions

Table 26-2 describes the direct, indirect, and net actions of procainamide on cardiac electrophysiology.

Hemodynamic Effects

The hemodynamic alterations produced by procainamide are similar to those of quinidine but are not as intense. However, the dose, route, and rate of administration determine the magnitude of the hemodynamic response to procainamide. Alterations in circulatory dynamics also vary according to the cardiovascular state of the individual.

Early hemodynamic studies with procainamide suggested that the drug produced both marked depression of myocardial contractility and vasodilation. More recent studies suggest that these effects are primarily the result of excessive dosage, too-rapid administration, or both. The hypotensive effects of procainamide are less pronounced after intramuscular administration and seldom occur after oral administration.

Pharmacokinetics

Table 26-3 describes the pharmacokinetic parameters of procainamide.

Renal failure shifts procainamide elimination from a kidney-dependent to a liver-dependent function. Renal disease causes N-acetylprocainamide (NAPA) plasma concentrations to increase, even after therapy is adjusted to maintain normal therapeutic plasma concentrations. Liver disease does not appear to alter procainamide clearance.

Congestive heart failure alters many of the pharmacokinetic values that describe procainamide disposition. The steady-state volume of distribution is reduced by 20 to 25 percent, and renal clearance is reduced, thereby increasing the plasma half-life. The extent and rate of oral and IM absorption are also reduced.

The usual target plasma concentration of procainamide is 4 to 10 μg/ml. The relatively short half-life of 3 to 4 hr requires that the oral dosing regimen be maintained on an every-4-hr schedule. This inconvenience has been overcome somewhat with the introduction of sustained-release forms of the drug that permit dosing every 6 hr. Caution must be exercised with the sustained-release form, however, since excessively high plasma concentrations may occur, thus leading to cardiac depression. The patient should be instructed that the vehicle used in the sustained-release form of procainamide may appear in the stool relatively intact.

The rate of hepatic metabolism for procainamide will show a bimodal distribution in which patients will be either fast or slow acetylators. The major active metabolite of procainamide, NAPA, has electrophysiological properties that differ from those of the parent compound, having characteristics more like those of the class III antiarrhythmic agents. Monitoring of the serum concentrations of NAPA becomes important, especially in patients with renal failure.

Clinical Uses

Procainamide is an effective antiarrhythmic agent when given in sufficient doses at relatively short (3–4 hr) dosage intervals. It is useful in the treatment of premature atrial contractions, paroxysmal atrial tachycardia, and atrial fibrillation of recent onset. Procainamide is only moderately effective in converting atrial flutter or chronic atrial fibrillation to sinus rhythm, although it has value in preventing recurrences of these arrhythmias once they have been terminated by DC cardioversion.

Procainamide can decrease the occurrence of all types of active ventricular dysrhythmias in patients with acute myocardial infarction who are free from A-V dissociation, serious ventricular failure, and cardiogenic shock. Ninety percent of patients with ventricular premature contractions, and 80 percent of patients with ventricular tachycardia, respond to procainamide administration.

Although the spectrum of action and electrophysiological effects of quinidine and procainamide are similar, the relatively short duration of action of procainamide has restricted its use to patients who are intolerant or unresponsive to quinidine. The introduction of *Procan-SR*, a sustained-release form of procainamide, allows 6-hr dosing intervals and may encourage patient compliance.

Adverse Reactions

Acute cardiovascular reactions to procainamide administration include hypotension, A-V block, intraventricular block, ventricular tachyarrhythmias, and complete heart block. The drug dosage must be reduced, or even stopped, if severe depression of conduction (severe prolongation of the QRS interval) or repolarization (severe prolongation of the Q–T interval) occurs.

Long-term drug use leads to increased antinuclear antibody titers in over 80 percent of patients; in more than 30 percent of patients receiving long-term procainamide therapy, a clinical lupus erythematosus–like syndrome develops. The symptoms may disappear within a few days of cessation of procainamide therapy, although the tests for antinuclear factor and lupus erythematosus cells may remain positive for several months.

Procainamide, unlike procaine, has little potential to produce CNS toxicity. However, CNS manifestations of toxicity have been observed after rapid IV administration. Rarely, patients may experience mental confusion or hallucinations.

Contraindications

Contraindications for procainamide are similar to those for quinidine. Because of its effects on A-V nodal and His-Purkinje conduction, procainamide should be administered with caution to patients with second-degree A-V block and bundle branch block. Parenteral administration may be hazardous in patients with compromised hemodynamic function, because further depression may occur as a result of procainamide's negative inotropic action. The drug should not be administered to patients who have shown previous procaine or procainamide hypersensitivity and should be used with caution in patients with bronchial asthma. Prolonged administration should be accompanied by hematologic studies, since agranulocytosis may occur.

Drug Interactions

The inherent anticholinergic properties of procainamide may interfere with the therapeutic effect of cholinergic agents. Patients receiving cimetidine and procainamide may exhibit signs of procainamide toxicity as cimetidine inhibits the metabolism of procainamide. Simultaneous use of alcohol will increase the hepatic clearance of procainamide. Unlike quinidine, procainamide does not alter the plasma concentration of digoxin. Procainamide may enhance or prolong the neuromuscular blocking activity of the aminoglycosides with the potential of producing respiratory depression. The simultaneous administration of quinidine or amiodarone may increase the plasma concentration of procainamide.

Preparations

Procainamide hydrochloride (Pronestyl), is available for oral as well as for IV and IM use. *Procan-SR* is procainamide in a tablet matrix designed for prolonged release.

Disopyramide

Disopyramide is capable of suppressing atrial and ventricular arrhythmias and has a longer duration of action than other drugs in its class.

Electrophysiological Actions

The effects of disopyramide on the myocardium and specialized conduction tissue (see Table 26-2) are a composite of its direct actions on cardiac tissue and its indirect actions mediated by competitive blockade of muscarinic cholinergic receptors.

Sinoatrial Node

The direct depressant actions of disopyramide on the sinoatrial node are antagonized by its anticholinergic properties, so that at therapeutic plasma concentrations, either no change or a slight increase in sinus heart rate is observed. Both the anticholinergic and direct depressant actions of disopyramide on sinus automaticity appear to be greater than those of quinidine.

Atrium

Disopyramide reduces membrane responsiveness in atrial muscle and reduces the amplitude of the action potential. Excitability of atrial muscle is decreased. These changes result in a decrease in atrial muscle conduction velocity. Action-potential duration in atrial muscle fibers is prolonged by disopyramide administration. This occurrence results in an increase in ERP. Postrepolarization refractoriness does not occur with disopyramide, and the drug appears to differ from quinidine and procainamide in this respect.

Abnormal atrial automaticity may be abolished at disopyramide plasma concentrations that fail to alter either conduction velocity or refractoriness. Disopyramide increases atrial refractoriness in patients pretreated with atropine, suggesting that the primary action of disopyramide is a direct one and not a consequence of its anticholinergic effect.

Atrioventricular Node

Disopyramide depresses conduction velocity and increases the ERP of the A-V node through a direct action. Its anticholinergic actions, however, produce an increase in conduction velocity and a decrease in the ERP. The net effect of disopyramide on A-V nodal transmission, therefore, will be determined by the sum of its direct depression and indirect facilitation of transmission.

His-Purkinje System and Ventricular Muscle

Disopyramide administration reduces membrane responsiveness in Purkinje fibers and ventricular muscle, and reduces the action-potential amplitude. Although disopyramide depresses conduction velocity in normal Purkinje and ventricular tissue, even greater depression may occur in damaged or injured myocardial cells. Action-potential duration is prolonged after disopyramide administration, and this results in an increase in the ERPs of His-Purkinje and ventricular muscle tissue. Unlike procainamide and quinidine, disopyramide does not produce postrepolarization refractoriness.

The effect of disopyramide on conduction velocity depends on extracellular K^+ concentrations. Hypokalemic patients may respond poorly to the antiarrhythmic action of disopyramide, whereas hyperkalemia may accentuate the drug's depressant actions.

Electrocardiographic Changes

The electrocardiographic changes observed after disopyramide administration are identical to those seen with quinidine and procainamide. Dose-dependent increases in the P–R, QRS, and Q–T intervals can be observed.

Hemodynamic Effects

Disopyramide directly depresses myocardial contractility. This results in an increase in left ventricular end-diastolic pressure and a decrease in cardiac output. *The negative inotropic effect may be detrimental in patients with compromised cardiac function.* In some patients, overt congestive heart failure may be produced. At usual doses, depression of myocardial function is not a problem in most patients.

Despite the decrease in cardiac output produced by disopyramide, blood pressure is well maintained, owing to a reflex increase in vascular resistance. Catecholamine administration can reverse the myocardial depression.

Pharmacokinetics

The salient pharmacokinetic features of disopyramide are summarized in Table 26-3. Disopyramide is rapidly and almost completely absorbed (83%) after oral administration, and peak plasma concentrations are obtained within 2 hr. First-pass liver metabolism is not significant and plasma disappearance is the result of both renal and hepatic clearance. The major metabolite of disopyramide, the mono-N-dealkylated metabolite, is an active antiarrhythmic agent that accumulates slowly during prolonged therapy and may accumulate even faster in the presence of decreased renal function.

The renal clearance of disopyramide exceeds the rate of creatinine clearance. This implies that disopyramide is secreted actively by the renal tubules. Urinary excretion accounts for 80 percent of the administered dose. About 50 percent appears in the urine unchanged, while about 20 percent appears as the mono-N-dealkylated metabolite. The remainder is found in the feces.

Clinical Uses

The indications for use of disopyramide are similar to those for quinidine, except that it is not approved for use in the prophylaxis of atrial flutter or atrial fibrillation after DC conversion. The indications are as follows: unifocal premature (ectopic) ventricular contractions, premature (ectopic) ventricular contractions of multifocal origin, paired premature ventricular contractions (couplets), and episodes of ventricular tachycardia (persistent ventricular tachycardia is usually treated with DC conversion).

Adverse Reactions

The major toxic reactions to disopyramide include hypotension, congestive heart failure, and conduction disturbances. These effects are the result of disopyramide's ability to depress myocardial contractility and myocardial conduction. Although disopyramide initially may pro-duce ventricular tachyarrhythmias or ventricular fibrillation in some patients, the incidence of disopyramide-induced syncope in long-term therapy is not known. Most other toxic reactions (e.g., dry mouth [xerostomia], blurred vision, constipation, etc.) can be attributed to the anticholinergic properties of the drug.

Central nervous system stimulation and hallucinations are rare. The incidence of severe adverse effects in long-term therapy may be lower than those observed with quinidine or procainamide.

Contraindications

Disopyramide should not be administered in cardiogenic shock, preexisting second- or third-degree A-V block, or known hypersensitivity to the drug. Neither should it be given to patients who are poorly compensated or those with uncompensated heart failure or severe hypotension. Because of its ability to slow cardiac conduction, disopyramide is not indicated for the treatment of digitalis-induced ventricular arrhythmias. Patients with congenital prolongation of the Q–T interval should not receive quinidine, procainamide, or disopyramide because further prolongation of the Q–T interval may increase the incidence of ventricular fibrillation.

Because of its anticholinergic properties, the drug should not be used in patients with glaucoma. Urinary retention and benign prostatic hypertrophy are also relative contraindications to disopyramide therapy. Patients with myasthenia gravis may have a myasthenic crisis after disopyramide administration owing to the drug's local anesthetic action at the neuromuscular junction. The elderly patient may exhibit increased sensitivity to the anticholinergic actions of disopyramide.

Caution is advised when disopyramide is used in conjunction with other cardiac depressant drugs, such as verapamil, which may adversely affect atrioventricular conduction.

Drug Interactions

The therapeutic efficacy of disopyramide may be influenced by the concurrent administration of phenytoin or rifampin. In the presence of phenytoin, the metabolism of disopyramide is increased (reducing its effective concentration) and the accumulation of its metabolites is also increased, thereby increasing the probability of anticholinergic adverse effects. Although coadministration is not contraindicated, changes in therapeutic response to disopyramide are possible. Rifampin also stimulates the hepatic metabolism of disopyramide, reducing its plasma concentration.

Unlike quinidine, disopyramide does not increase the plasma concentration of digoxin in previously digitalized patients. Hypoglycemia has been reported with the use of disopyramide, particularly in conjunction with moderate or excessive alcohol intake.

Preparations

Disopyramide phosphate (Norpace) is only available for oral administration as immediate-release and controlled-release capsules (*Norpace-CR*). The dosage of each of the orally administered formulations must be individualized for each patient.

Moricizine

Moricizine (*Ethmozine*) is an antiarrhythmic drug recently approved for use in the United States to treat documented life-threatening arrhythmias. It is a phenothiazine derivative that is used when the risk associated with the drug is outweighed by the benefits of its use.

Electrophysiological Actions

Moricizine exerts electrophysiological effects common with both class IA and IB agents; however, it does not belong in any of the existing drug classes.

Sinoatrial Node
No significant effect of moricizine is noted on the sinus cycle length or on automaticity within the sinoatrial node.

Atria
Moricizine does not affect the atrial refractory period or conduction velocity within atrial muscle.

Atrioventricular Node
Moricizine depresses conduction and prolongs refractoriness in the atrioventricular node as well as in the infranodal region. These changes are manifest in a prolongation of the P–R interval on the electrocardiogram.

His-Purkinje System and Ventricular Muscle
The primary electrophysiological effects of moricizine relate to its inhibition of the fast inward sodium channel. Moricizine reduces the maximal upstroke of phase 0 and decreases the duration of the cardiac transmembrane action potential. The sodium channel blocking effect of moricizine is more significant at faster stimulation rates, an action referred to as "use dependence." The phenomenon of use dependence may explain the efficacy of moricizine in suppressing rapid ectopic activity. An interesting effect of moricizine is its depressant effect on automaticity in ischemic Purkinje tissue in contrast to its inability to alter the slope of phase 4 depolarization of spontaneous automatic Purkinje fibers.

An important consideration is that moricizine prolongs ventricular conduction, thereby widening the QRS complex on the electrocardiogram. It has no significant effects on the Q–T interval.

Electrocardiographic Changes

The electrocardiographic effects of moricizine include alterations in conduction velocity without an effect on the refractoriness of heart tissue. Moricizine enhances sinus node automaticity and prolongs sinoatrial and His-Purkinje intervals and the QRS duration.

Hemodynamic Effects

The administration of moricizine is not associated with clinically significant hemodynamic effects.

Pharmacokinetics

Moricizine is almost completely absorbed from the gastrointestinal tract; however, oral bioavailability is 30 to 40 percent due to extensive first-pass hepatic metabolism. Although the elimination half-life of moricizine is 2 to 6 hr, the antiarrhythmic effects of the drug are much more prolonged, suggestive of metabolites with antiarrhythmic effects. The pharmacokinetic data are shown in Table 26-3.

Clinical Uses

Moricizine is indicated for the treatment of documented ventricular arrhythmias, particularly sustained ventricular tachycardia.

Contraindications

Patients with preexisting second- or third-degree A-V block should not be treated with moricizine. Cardiogenic shock and hypersensitivity to the drug are also contraindications. Unlike other neuroleptic phenothiazine derivatives, moricizine has not been associated with any adverse effects related to the endocrine system, such as antagonism of dopaminergic receptors. There are no clinical reports of increased serum prolactin concentrations, galactorrhea, or gynecomastia.

Adverse Reactions

The most common adverse reactions are gastrointestinal and CNS related. The principal adverse gastrointestinal effect is nausea (7%). Abdominal discomfort has also been reported. Dizziness (11%) is the most frequently reported CNS-related adverse effect. Such reactions increase in frequency with prolonged drug administration.

As with other antiarrhythmic drugs, moricizine has proarrhythmic activity, and this is the most serious adverse effect associated with its use. The proarrhythmic effects may be manifest as new ventricular ectopic beats or a worsening of preexisting ventricular arrhythmias, and are more common in patients with depressed left ventricular function and a history of congestive heart failure. Cardiovascular effects requiring drug withdrawal include conduction defects, sinus pauses, junctional rhythm, and atrioventricular block.

Drug Interactions

Clinically significant interactions with moricizine do not appear to exist.

Class IB

Lidocaine

Lidocaine was introduced as a local anesthetic and is still used extensively for that purpose (see Chap. 32). In contrast to quinidine and procainamide, *lidocaine acts primarily on disturbances of ventricular origin* and has a narrow spectrum of antiarrhythmic effects.

Electrophysiological Actions

Sinoatrial Node
When administered in normal therapeutic doses (1–5 mg/kg), lidocaine has no effect on the sinus rate.

Atria
The electrophysiological properties of lidocaine in atrial muscle resemble those produced by quinidine. Membrane responsiveness, action-potential amplitude, and atrial muscle excitability are all decreased. These changes result in a decrease in conduction velocity. However, the depression of conduction velocity is less marked than that caused by quinidine or procainamide. Action-potential duration of atrial muscle fibers is not altered by lidocaine at either normal or subnormal extracellular K^+ levels. The ERP of atrial myocardium either remains the same or increases slightly after lidocaine administration.

Atrioventricular Node
Lidocaine minimally affects both the conduction velocity and the ERP of the A-V node. It does not possess anticholinergic properties and will not improve A-V transmission when atrial flutter or atrial fibrillation is present.

His-Purkinje System and Ventricular Muscle
Lidocaine reduces action-potential amplitude and membrane responsiveness. Severe depression can be observed in Purkinje fibers in which the resting membrane potentials have been reduced (i.e., −70 to −60 mV) as a result of myocardial ischemia. This depression of phase 0 upstroke can be so severe that it will produce complete conduction block at lidocaine concentrations in the high therapeutic range. Significant shortening of the action-potential duration and ERP occurs at lower concentrations of lidocaine in Purkinje fibers than in ventricular muscle. Lidocaine, in very low concentrations, slows phase 4 depolarization in Purkinje fibers and decreases their spontaneous rate of discharge. In higher concentrations, automaticity may be suppressed, and phase 4 depolarization eliminated.

Lidocaine does not alter the resting membrane potential of isolated ventricular muscle fibers. However, the action-potential duration and ERP are both decreased. It is difficult to suggest a mechanism for lidocaine's antiarrhythmic action on the basis of its effects on normal ventricular myocardial tissue and His-Purkinje tissue. However, it is possible that lidocaine more profoundly affects damaged myocardial cells than it does normal cardiac tissue.

Electrocardiographic Changes

The P–R, QRS, and Q–T intervals are usually unchanged, although the Q–T may be shortened in some patients. These minimal electrocardiographic changes reflect lidocaine's inability to alter conduction velocity in specialized conduction tissue and myocardium.

Hemodynamic Effects

Myocardial contractility and peripheral vascular resistance are depressed only slightly, if at all, by therapeutic doses of lidocaine, but may be adversely affected by higher than therapeutic plasma concentrations.

Pharmacokinetics

Therapeutically adequate blood levels have not been achieved by the oral route because of extensive first-pass liver metabolism; lidocaine is absorbed rapidly after IM injection. The prompt action of lidocaine after IV administration is a result of rapid delivery to, and uptake in, myocardial tissue. Lidocaine then slowly redistributes to other organ systems with lower blood flows. Pharmacokinetic data for lidocaine are shown in Table 26-4.

Approximately 70 percent of the drug entering the liver from the systemic circulation is metabolized on a sin-

Table 26-4. Pharmacokinetic Characteristics of the Class IB Drugs

Drug	Therapeutic serum concentration (μg/ml)	Time to onset of action (hr)	Time to peak concentration (hr)	Duration of action (hr)	Elimination half-life (hr)	Percent protein bound	Volume of distribution (L/kg)
Lidocaine[a]	1.5–6	Very rapid	–	0.25[b]	1–2	60–80	1.1 ± 0.4
Phenytoin	10–20	0.5–1.0	12	24	6–24	87–93	0.64 ± 0.04
Tocainide	4–10	0.5–1.0	0.5–4	12	11–15	10–20	3.0 ± 0.2
Mexiletine	0.5–2.0	0.5–1.0	2–4	8–12	8–10	55–65	4.9 ± 0.5

[a]Data shown are for intravenous administration.
[b]After cessation of intravenous administration.

gle circulation through the liver. The rate of lidocaine metabolism is, therefore, critically dependent on hepatic blood flow. Reductions in liver blood flow sharply reduce lidocaine plasma clearance and, therefore, dosage must be reduced.

Two major metabolites of lidocaine are found in significant concentrations. Monoethylglycine xylidide is formed by the N-deethylation of lidocaine; it is as potent an antiarrhythmic agent as lidocaine and has similar convulsant activity. Monoethylglycine xylidide has a plasma half-life of 120 min and is eliminated from plasma primarily by a second N-deethylation to form glycine xylidide. Glycine xylidide possesses both antiarrhythmic and convulsant activity, although it is only 10 to 26 percent as potent as lidocaine. Glycine xylidide is both metabolized and excreted by the kidney. It has a plasma half-life of 10 hr.

Accumulation of metabolites during prolonged intravenous administration may help to explain why toxicity develops despite plasma lidocaine concentrations that remain in the therapeutic range. About 90 percent of an administered lidocaine dose appears in the urine as metabolites. Excretion of unchanged drug by the kidney is a minor route of elimination (10% of dose). Lidocaine readily crosses the placenta and is then broken down in the fetus or neonate at a rate comparable to that in the mother. The safety of lidocaine for use in pregnancy has not been established.

Clinical Uses

Lidocaine is much less effective than quinidine, disopyramide, and procainamide in the treatment of supraventricular arrhythmias. The observation that lidocaine usually fails to alter atrial refractoriness or conduction velocity may explain its ineffectiveness in the treatment of most supraventricular arrhythmias. It is useful in the control of ventricular arrhythmias in patients with acute myocardial infarction. Lidocaine administration carries relatively little risk for the patient with acute myocardial infarction both because it lacks significant depressant ef-

fects on the cardiovascular system and because of the reversibility and short duration of its toxic side effects. Routine lidocaine administration may be indicated for all patients with acute myocardial infarction as a result of its ability to prevent ventricular arrhythmias and ventricular fibrillation. *The clinical efficacy of lidocaine in the prevention of ventricular fibrillation during acute myocardial infarction is unquestioned.*

Lidocaine is the drug of choice for treatment of the electrical manifestations of digitalis intoxication.

Adverse Reactions

The most common toxic reactions seen after lidocaine administration are those involving the CNS. Drowsiness is common, but unless excessive, may not be particularly undesirable in patients suffering from acute myocardial infarction. Some patients experience paresthesias, disorientation, and muscle twitching. These effects may make the patient agitated or frightened, and, equally important, they forewarn of more serious deleterious effects, which may include psychosis, respiratory depression, and seizures. Focal seizures often occur just before generalized tonic-clonic seizures. Convulsions are a dose-related side effect and can be avoided by controlling the rate of infusion and keeping plasma concentrations below 5 μg/ml.

Lidocaine may produce clinically significant hypotension, but this is exceedingly uncommon if the drug is given in moderate dosage. Depression of an already damaged myocardium may result from large doses.

Contraindications

Contraindications include hypersensitivity to local anesthetics of the amide type (a very rare occurrence), severe hepatic dysfunction, a previous history of grand mal seizures due to lidocaine, and an age of 70 or older. The drug is contraindicated in the presence of second- or third-degree heart block, since it may increase the degree of block and can abolish the idioventricular pacemaker responsible for maintaining the cardiac rhythm.

Drug Interactions

The concurrent administration of lidocaine with cimetidine may cause an increase (15%) in the plasma concentration of lidocaine. This effect is a manifestation of cimetidine reducing the clearance and volume of distribution of lidocaine. An increase in lidocaine's therapeutic and adverse effects may occur. Ranitidine is not associated with alterations in lidocaine plasma concentrations. The myocardial depressant effect of lidocaine is enhanced by phenytoin administration.

Preparations

Lidocaine hydrochloride injection, USP (*Xylocaine Solution*) is supplied in ampules or prefilled syringes for IV injection and 100-mg/ml ampules for IM injection. Intramuscular lidocaine is best reserved for emergency, out-of-hospital use.

Phenytoin

Phenytoin was introduced in 1938 for the control of convulsive disorders (see Chap. 37). It was not until 1950 that it was used for the treatment of cardiac arrhythmias.

Electrophysiological Actions

Sinoatrial Node

Most clinically used concentrations of phenytoin do not significantly alter sinus rate in humans. Of the antiarrhythmic agents currently in use, phenytoin (and possibly lidocaine) produces the least alterations in nodal function, even when that function is altered by disease. However, the hypotension that may follow IV administration of phenytoin can result in an increase in sympathetic tone and, therefore, an increased sinus heart rate.

Atria

Phenytoin, like lidocaine, usually does not alter the action-potential duration or ERP of atrial tissue, except at very high concentrations. The effect of phenytoin on membrane responsiveness of atria muscle depends on the frequency of stimulation and the extracellular K^+ concentration. When extracellular K^+ is normal (3–5 mM), phenytoin depresses the rate of phase 0 depolarization. Atrial conduction velocity is either unchanged or slightly depressed.

Atrioventricular Node

Phenytoin lacks the anticholinergic properties of quinidine, disopyramide, and procainamide. However, the direct actions of phenytoin on the A-V node facilitate transmission.

In human electrophysiological studies, phenytoin decreased nodal ERPs and increased conduction velocity. Depression of conduction has not been observed. Phenytoin can return transmission toward normal in the digitalis-intoxicated patient and can reduce digitalis-induced ventricular automaticity.

His-Purkinje System

The electrophysiological effects of phenytoin on the His-Purkinje system resemble those of lidocaine; that is, *action-potential duration and ERPs are shortened.*

The effects of phenytoin on membrane responsiveness are confusing. Phenytoin can increase the maximum rate of phase 0 depolarization when it has been depressed by digitalis overdoses or hypoxia. However, normal Purkinje fibers and Purkinje fibers damaged by myocardial ischemia do not respond to phenytoin in the same manner. At normal extracellular K^+ concentrations, phenytoin produces either no change or a slight decrease in V_{max} of phase 0 depolarization.

Phenytoin decreases the rate of phase 4 depolarization in Purkinje tissue and reduces the rate of discharge of ventricular pacemakers. The effects of phenytoin on ventricular refractoriness are unknown at present.

Electrocardiographic Changes

Because phenytoin improves A-V conduction and shortens the action-potential duration of ventricular myocardium, it may decrease the P–R and Q–T intervals of the surface electrocardiogram.

Hemodynamic Effects

The effects of phenytoin on the cardiovascular system vary with the dose, the mode and rate of administration, and the presence of cardiovascular pathology. Rapid administration can produce a transient hypotension that is the combined result of peripheral vasodilation and depression of myocardial contractility. These effects are due to direct actions of phenytoin on the vascular bed and ventricular myocardium. If large doses are given slowly, dose-related decreases in left ventricular force, rate of force development, and cardiac output can be observed, along with an increase in left ventricular end-diastolic pressure.

Pharmacokinetics

Phenytoin is slowly and somewhat unpredictably absorbed after an oral dose and IM injection is not recommended. In uremic patients, a two- to threefold increase in free (unbound) phenytoin can be observed, even though total phenytoin plasma concentrations remain in the "therapeutic" range.

Phenytoin is metabolized by hepatic microsomal enzymes, primarily to 5-phenyl-5-parahydroxyphenylhydantoin. This compound is conjugated in the liver with glucuronic acid. Considerable variation in phenytoin plasma concentrations can occur in patients receiving identical phenytoin doses. Part of this variation may be a result of marked differences in the rate of hepatic metabolism. Some patients have a genetic deficiency in activity of microsomal enzymes responsible for phenytoin metabolism; others metabolize phenytoin at rates much faster than those of the normal population.

About 50 to 75 percent of a single dose of phenytoin is excreted in the urine as the parahydroxyglucuronide metabolite; less than 5 percent of the parent compound is found unchanged in the urine. Pharmacokinetic data for phenytoin are summarized in Table 26-4.

Clinical Uses

Phenytoin, like lidocaine, is more effective in the treatment of ventricular than of supraventricular arrhythmias. It has been particularly effective in treating ventricular arrhythmias associated with digitalis toxicity, acute myocardial infarction, open-heart surgery, anesthesia, cardiac catheterization, cardioversion, and angiographic studies. Three fourths of responsive cardiac arrhythmias are abolished at concentrations of 10 to 18 μg/ml. Because a nonlinear relationship exists between dose and steady-state plasma concentrations, maintenance of consistent plasma concentrations is difficult. To achieve plasma concentrations of 10 to 18 μg/ml within 24 hr, an initial loading dose of 1,000 mg of phenytoin sodium (*Dilantin*) must be given. The dose on the second day is 500 to 600 mg, with maintenance doses of 300 to 400 mg per day thereafter. Intravenous doses of 100 mg can be given every 5 min until the arrhythmia is abolished or until 1,000 mg has been given. Oral maintenance therapy should then be started.

Phenytoin finds its most effective use in the treatment of supraventricular and ventricular arrhythmias associated with digitalis intoxication. The ability of phenytoin to improve digitalis-induced depression of A-V conduction is a special feature and contrasts with the actions of other antiarrhythmic agents. Another important application of phenytoin has been as a prophylactic agent in the prevention of postconversion arrhythmias, particularly in the digitalized patient.

Most investigators believe that phenytoin is ineffective in the conversion of atrial flutter or atrial fibrillation to normal sinus rhythm. It is also ineffective in the treatment of supraventricular arrhythmias not associated with digitalis toxicity. It should be appreciated that phenytoin, by virtue of its ability to enhance A-V conduction, may increase the ventricular rate in the presence of atrial flutter or atrial fibrillation. Also, phenytoin is not a drug of choice for the treatment of complicated ventricular arrhythmias resulting from coronary artery disease. The efficacy of phenytoin in ventricular dysrhythmias may be enhanced when used in conjunction with β-receptor antagonists or with other class I agents.

Adverse Reactions

The IV administration of phenytoin can present a hazard. Respiratory arrest, arrhythmias, and hypotension have been reported. In most cases, toxicity was due to a too-rapid rate of administration (>50 mg/min).

Even though A-V block and bradycardia are occasionally associated with phenytoin administration, much of the rationale for its use in digitalis toxicity in preference to other antiarrhythmic agents is that phenytoin usually enhances, rather than depresses, A-V conduction. Depression of conduction is rare, but it may occur occasionally. Other adverse reactions and potential drug interactions are discussed in Chap. 37.

It is important to recognize that the diluent supplied with phenytoin is not pharmacologically inert, and many of the adverse hemodynamic effects attributed to phenytoin may actually be due to the administration of the diluent. Because of the high pH of the solution, IV administration of phenytoin may cause local irritation at the site of injection.

Contraindications

The contraindications to the use of phenytoin are similar to those of other antiarrhythmic drugs. The drug either should not be used or should be used cautiously in patients with hypotension, severe bradycardia, high-grade A-V block, severe heart failure, or hypersensitivity to the drug.

Because of the increase in A-V transmission observed with phenytoin administration, it should not be given to patients with atrial flutter or atrial fibrillation. Phenytoin will probably not be effective in restoring normal sinus rhythm and may produce a dangerous acceleration of the ventricular rate.

Drug Interactions

Similar to other antiarrhythmic agents, concurrent administration of phenytoin and certain drugs can increase or decrease the effective plasma concentration of phenytoin, leading to adverse effects or a decrease in therapeutic response, respectively. Plasma phenytoin concentrations are increased in the presence of chloramphenicol, disulfiram, and isoniazid, since the latter drugs inhibit the hepatic metabolism of phenytoin. In the case of the antituberculosis drug isoniazid, approximately 20 percent of patients experience some degree of phenytoin toxicity with coadministration. A reduction in phenytoin dose can alleviate the consequences of these drug-drug interactions.

Tocainide

Tocainide is an orally effective antiarrhythmic agent with close structural similarities to lidocaine.

Electrophysiological Actions

In healthy volunteers, the administration of 450 mg tocainide over a period of 45 min produced a slight depression in His-Purkinje conduction as well as a slightly delayed enhancement of A-V node conduction during atrial pacing. No significant alterations in heart rate, right ventricular ERP, or the excitation thresholds of atrial or ventricular muscle were observed in these subjects.

Hemodynamic Effects

The acute hemodynamic effects are slight and transient and are observed most often during or immediately after drug infusion. Although overall hemodynamic function is minimally altered by tocainide infusion, it has been suggested that the drug be used with caution in patients with pulmonary or systemic hypertension or with uncompensated ventricular failure.

Pharmacokinetics

Tocainide is absorbed readily after oral administration, with bioavailability exceeding 90 percent (Table 26-4).

Unlike lidocaine, tocainide does not undergo significant first-pass hepatic metabolism. The probable major pathways for the biotransformation of tocainide are oxidative deamination to form lactylxylide and hepatic conjugation of the *N*-carboxy metabolite to form tocainide carbamoyl glucuronide. Urinary excretion of unchanged tocainide has been reported to be 35 to 50 percent of the administered dose.

Clinical Uses

Currently, tocainide is indicated for the *suppression of symptomatic ventricular arrhythmias,* including frequent premature ventricular contractions and ventricular tachycardia. Like other antiarrhythmic drugs in the class I category, tocainide has not been shown to prevent sudden death in patients with serious ventricular ectopic activity.

Adverse Effects

Toxicity associated with tocainide therapy most often involves the CNS or gastrointestinal tract. Adverse effects were noted in 36 to 75 percent of patients given tocainide IV during cardiac catheterization; these effects included sensations of coolness or numbness, confusion, and dizziness or light-headedness. With oral administration of tocainide, a similar profile of adverse effects is possible. Light-headedness/dizziness or nausea occurs in approximately 15 percent of patients, paresthesias/numbness in 9 percent, and tremor in 8 percent. These adverse effects are generally mild in intensity, transient, and dose related. A reduction in dose or administering the drug with meals can alleviate these responses. Overall, however, approximately 20 percent of patients prescribed tocainide discontinue therapy because of such effects.

Leukopenia, agranulocytosis, hypoplastic anemia, and thrombocytopenia, possibly drug related, have been reported in patients receiving tocainide. Periodic blood counts are recommended, especially during the first 6 months of therapy. Tocainide may cause an acceleration of the ventricular rate in patients who have atrial flutter or atrial fibrillation.

Contraindications

Patients who are hypersensitive to tocainide or to local anesthetics of the amide type should not be exposed to tocainide. The presence of second- or third-degree heart block in the absence of an artificial pacemaker would also constitute a contraindication to the use of tocainide.

Drug Interactions

When used with other class Ib antiarrhythmic drugs, toxicity may be increased without significant gain in antiarrhythmic efficacy.

Preparation and Dosage

Tocainide (*Tonocard*) is supplied as tablets. Dosage must be individualized on the basis of antiarrhythmic response and tolerance, both of which are dose related. Electrocardiographic evaluation is needed to assess whether or not the desired antiarrhythmic effect has been achieved and as a guide to dose adjustment.

Mexiletine

Mexiletine (*Mextil*) is a class IB antiarrhythmic agent that has pharmacological properties and antidysrhythmic effects similar to those of lidocaine and tocainide.

Electrophysiological Actions

As with other members of class IB, mexiletine slows the maximal rate of depolarization of the cardiac membrane action potential and exerts a negligible effect on the phase of repolarization. Electrophysiologically, mexiletine resembles lidocaine so that its major effects from the point of producing an antiarrhythmic action will be directed against disorders of ventricular rhythm. Mexiletine shows a rate-dependent blocking action on the sodium channel that has a rapid onset and recovery, suggesting that the drug may be of greater efficacy in the control of rapid as opposed to slow ventricular tachyarrhythmias.

Hemodynamic Effects

Cardiovascular toxicity has been considered as minimal even among patients with compromised ventricular function. Despite its relative safety, the drug should be used with caution in patients who are hypotensive or who exhibit severe left ventricular dysfunction.

Pharmacokinetics

Mexiletine is effective by oral administration and is almost completely absorbed from the small intestine. The pharmacokinetic profile of mexiletine is presented in Table 26-4. Mexiletine undergoes less than 10 percent first-pass hepatic metabolism. Thus, bioavailability is about 90 percent of the administered dose. The drug is metabolized extensively by hepatic mechanisms, with the metabolites being excreted *via* the kidneys. The plasma half-life of mexiletine can be increased to 18 hr in patients with acute myocardial infarction. None of the metabolites of mexiletine are known to possess antiarrhythmic properties. Therapeutic plasma concentrations of mexiletine are in the narrow range of 0.5 to 2.0 $\mu g/ml$, thus accounting for the narrow toxic/therapeutic ratio of the drug.

Clinical Uses

Mexiletine is useful as an antiarrhythmic agent against ventricular arrhythmias associated with a wide variety of cardiac diseases. It has been reported to be effective in the *management of patients with either acute or chronic ventricular arrhythmias.* Its oral efficacy and low incidence of serious side effects suggest that the drug should find wide patient acceptance.

Adverse Effects

The first signs of toxicity are manifest by a fine tremor of the hands, followed by dizziness and blurred vision. Hypotension, sinus bradycardia, and widening of the QRS complex have been noted as the most common unwanted cardiovascular effects of intravenous mexiletine. The side effects of oral maintenance therapy include reversible upper-gastrointestinal distress (40%), tremor (12%), light-headedness (10%), and coordination difficulties (10%). These effects generally are not serious and can be reduced by downward dose adjustment or administering the drug with meals. Cardiovascular related adverse effects are less common and include palpitations (4–8%), chest pain (2–7%), and angina or anginalike pain (0.3–1.7%).

Contraindications

Mexiletine is contraindicated in the presence of cardiogenic shock or preexisting second- or third-degree heart block in the absence of a cardiac pacemaker. Caution must be exercised in administration of the drug to patients with sinus node dysfunction or disturbances of intraventricular conduction.

Drug Interactions

An upward adjustment in dose may be required when mexiletine is administered with phenytoin or rifampin, since these drugs stimulate the hepatic metabolism of mexiletine, reducing its plasma concentration.

Class IC

Flecainide

Flecainide acetate (*Tambocor;* Fig. 26-8) is a fluorinated aromatic hydrocarbon examined initially for its local anesthetic action and subsequently found to have antiarrhythmic effects.

Electrophysiologic Actions

Sinoatrial Node
Flecainide will decrease the mean sinus cycle length, but the change represents a clinically insignificant decrease in heart rate, with a maximum change of fewer than 10 beats per minute.

Atria
Flecainide, in common with class IA and other IC antiarrhythmic agents, decreases the maximal rate of depo-

Figure 26-8. Flecainide.

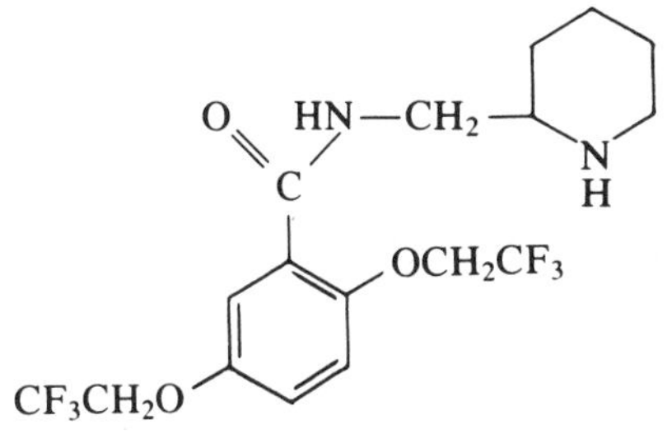

Table 26-5. Pharmacokinetic Characteristics of the Class IC Drugs

Drug	Therapeutic serum concentration (μg/ml)	Time to onset of action (hr)	Time to peak concentration (hr)	Duration of action (hr)	Elimination half-life (hr)	Percent protein bound	Volume of distribution (L/kg)
Flecainide	0.2–1.0	0.5	3–4	12	10–16 (20[a])	75–85	4.9
Propafenone	0.06–0.10	0.5–1.0	2–3	8	5–8 (10–32[b])	97	3.6

[a]Plasma half-life increases in patients with cardiac rhythm disorders.
[b]Plasma half-life increases in "slow" metabolizers of propafenone (see text).

larization in atrial tissue and shifts the membrane responsiveness curve to the right. Some evidence suggests that a dominant effect of the drug is to slow conduction by prolonging sodium-mediated, time-dependent refractoriness.

Atrioventricular Node
The atrioventricular conduction time, measured as the A–H interval, is prolonged by flecainide as is the His-Purkinje or H–V interval.

His-Purkinje Conduction and Ventricular Myocardium
Flecainide has profound effects on the inward sodium current in His-Purkinje tissue and in ventricular myocardium. Depression in the inward sodium current during depolarization decreases the upstroke velocity of the action potential of His-Purkinje tissue and ventricular muscle. Intraventricular conduction velocity is depressed.

Electrocardiographic Changes

Flecainide increases the P–R, atrioventricular nodal, and His–ventricular intervals. There is a marked increase in the QRS duration associated with the depression of conduction velocity in His-Purkinje and ventricular muscle. The rate of ventricular repolarization is not affected and any apparent prolongation of the Q–T interval is related to the increase in the QRS duration.

Hemodynamic Effects

Flecainide produces modest negative inotropic effects that may become significant in that subset of patients with compromised left ventricular function.

Pharmacokinetics

After a single IV dose, flecainide and its metabolites distribute extensively to many tissues, but less so to the brain.

As a fluorinated aromatic hydrocarbon, flecainide would have greater lipid solubility, thereby allowing it to concentrate in tissues. Cardiac muscle concentration of the drug is 11 to 12 times greater than that in the plasma, and the heart muscle concentration declines at the same rate as the plasma concentration. Thus, plasma concentrations of the drug should correlate with anticipated cardiac electrophysiological and antiarrhythmic effects. The pharmacokinetic profile of flecainide is presented in Table 26-5.

Flecainide does not undergo first-pass biotransformation after its oral administration. Most of a single oral dose of flecainide is excreted in the urine as the parent compound or its metabolites, 27 percent being unchanged. The two major metabolites of flecainide do not possess detectable antiarrhythmic activity and are not likely to contribute to any of the observed pharmacological effects.

Clinical Uses

Flecainide has an unusual *efficacy in suppressing chronic stable ventricular arrhythmias* after oral dosing; it appears to be more effective than quinidine. Repetitive episodes of ventricular tachycardia may be eliminated by the drug. The drug also has been reported to suppress ventricular tachycardia in patients at high risk of development of life-threatening ventricular tachyarrhythmias. However, because these patients are more likely to have poor left ventricular function, flecainide should be used with caution in this population. The recent warning issued by the Food and Drug Administration with regard to flecainide and encainide has changed the status of the two drugs, which are now restricted to use in patients with life-threatening arrhythmias.

Adverse Reactions

Most adverse effects occur within a few days of initial drug administration. The most frequently reported effects are dizziness (18%, which includes light-headedness, faintness, and unsteadiness), visual disturbances (15%, includes blurred vision, spots before the eyes, and difficulty in focusing), nausea (9%), headache (9%), and dyspnea (10%). Decreasing the dose may alleviate these effects without reducing the therapeutic efficacy of the drug.

Worsening of heart failure and prolongation of the P–R and QRS intervals are likely to occur with flecainide. The risk of proarrhythmic effects has been reported in 4 to 12 percent of patients and may be manifest as an increase in the frequency of premature ventricular complexes to the development of ventricular tachycardia or ventricular fibrillation. The proarrhythmic effects appear to be more likely in patients with left ventricular dysfunction and life-threatening arrhythmias.

Contraindications

Flecainide is contraindicated in patients with preexisting second- or third-degree heart block or with bundle branch block unless a pacemaker is present to maintain ventricular rhythm. The drug should not be used in patients with cardiogenic shock.

Drug Interactions

In patients whose condition has been stabilized by flecainide, the addition of cimetidine may reduce the rate of flecainide's hepatic metabolism, thereby increasing the potential for toxicity. Flecainide may increase digoxin concentrations on concurrent administration. This effect generally does not require changes in drug dose, except in patients receiving amounts of digoxin at the higher end of the dose range.

Propafenone

Propafenone possesses properties similar to those of β-adrenoceptor antagonists and exhibits class IC properties. Propafenone also has a slight potential to depress the slow inward calcium current. The effect of propafenone on β-adrenoceptor function may be of clinical significance, whereas its potency as a calcium channel entry blocker may be relatively insignificant.

Electrophysiologic Actions

As with all members of its class, propafenone has its major effect on the fast inward sodium current. The IC agents depress V_{max} over a wide range of heart rates and shift the resting membrane potential in the direction of hyperpolarization. The IC agents bind slowly to the sodium channel and dissociate slowly. Therefore, they exhibit what is referred to as a "rate-dependent block." Inhibition of the sodium channel throughout the cardiac cycle will result in a decrease in the rate of ectopy and the trigger for the initiation of ventricular tachycardia.

Sinoatrial Node

Propafenone causes sinus node slowing that could lead to sinoatrial block. It may lengthen the sinus node recovery time with minimal effects on sinus cycle length.

Atrium

The action-potential duration and effective refractory period of atrial muscle are both prolonged by propafenone. The electrophysiologic effects are of long duration and persist beyond the time when the drug is removed from the tissue.

Atrioventricular Node

The intravenous administration of propafenone prolongs the A–H and A–V intervals.

His-Purkinje System and Ventricular Muscle

The major effect of propafenone on His-Purkinje fibers and ventricular muscle is blockade of the fast inward sodium channel. Propafenone has little effect on the resting membrane potential, but increases the excitability threshold and the effective refractory period. The slow rate of dissociation from the sodium channel contrasts with the mode of action of mexiletine or lidocaine, which dissociate rapidly during the resting phase of the membrane action potential. While mexiletine and lidocaine will suppress closely coupled extrasystoles, propafenone will influence cardiac excitability and refractoriness regardless of the cycle length.

Electrocardiographic Changes

Propafenone causes dose-dependent increases in the P–R interval and QRS duration. Nonsignificant increases occur in the QTc interval and occasional slowing of the heart rate has been observed.

Hemodynamic Effects

The intravenous administration of propafenone is accompanied by an increase in right atrial, pulmonary arterial, and pulmonary artery wedge pressures in addition to an increase in vascular resistance and a decrease in the cardiac index. In patients with preexisting left ventricular dysfunction, propafenone causes a significant decrease in ejection fraction as determined with M-mode echocardiography. In the absence of cardiac abnormalities, propafenone has no significant effects on cardiac function.

Adverse Reactions and Drug Interactions

Concurrent administration of propafenone with digoxin, warfarin, or metoprolol increases the serum concentrations of the latter three drugs. Cimetidine slightly increases the propafenone serum concentrations. Additive pharmacological effects can occur when lidocaine, procainamide, and quinidine are combined with propafenone.

Overall, 21 to 32 percent of patients experience adverse effects, with 3 to 7 percent of these serious enough to warrant discontinuing therapy. The most common adverse effects are dizziness or light-headedness, metallic taste, and nausea and vomiting; the most serious adverse effects are proarrhythmic events.

Pharmacokinetics

Propafenone is well absorbed ($\sim$100%) after oral administration and its bioavailability is in the range of 3 to 40 percent due to extensive first-pass metabolism. Patients can be classified as fast (90%) or slow (10%) metabolizers of propafenone. This variability in metabolism is thought to be due to a genetically determined deficiency in a metabolic pathway.

Propafenone is metabolized extensively and undergoes oxidative metabolism to form 5-hydroxy and hydroxymethoxy metabolites, which are then conjugated to form glucuronides and sulfates. The majority of individuals are extensive metabolizers and form the active 5-hydroxy metabolite. The conjugates represent the major forms in which the drug is eliminated either by way of urinary excretion or through its appearance in the feces.

Elimination is primarily hepatic, with a mean elimination half-life after oral administration of 5.5 hr in extensive metabolizers, and 17.2 hr in poor metabolizers. The relationship between plasma propafenone concentration and clinical response varies extensively among individual patients; therefore, plasma concentrations have limited usefulness in predicting the efficacy of the drug or the anticipated electrophysiologic effects.

Preparation and Dosage

Propafenone (*Rythmol*) is available in tablets for oral administration. The dose must be titrated to the individual patient's needs.

Contraindications

Propafenone is contraindicated in the presence of severe or uncontrolled congestive heart failure; cardiogenic shock; sinoatrial, atrioventricular, and intraventricular disorders of conduction; and sinus node dysfunction such as sick sinus syndrome. Other contraindications include severe bradycardia, hypotension, obstructive pulmonary disease, and hepatic and renal failure. As a result of its weak β-blocking action, propafenone can cause possible

dose-related bronchospasm. This problem is greatest in patients who are slow metabolizers.

Indications

Propafenone is *indicated for the suppression of ventricular tachycardia and/or the suppression of ectopic ventricular rhythms,* such as premature ventricular complexes of unifocal or multifocal origin, couplets, or R-on-T phenomena when they are of sufficient severity to require treatment. Propafenone appears to have utility in pediatric patients with supraventricular tachycardia.

Propafenone is effective in reducing the frequency of premature ventricular complexes and is of special value in the management of patients with supraventricular tachyarrhythmia when the disorder is associated with the preexcitation syndrome. The efficacy and safety of propafenone in patients with life-threatening arrhythmias have not been demonstrated. Like other members of the class IC group, propafenone has not been shown to prevent sudden death in patients with serious ventricular ectopic activity. Furthermore, the potential to exert a proarrhythmic action makes it essential that each patient given propafenone be evaluated electrocardiographically and clinically before and during therapy to determine whether the response to the drug warrants its continued administration.

Class II

Table 26-6 summarizes the actions of the β-receptor blocking agents that make up the class II drugs. The complete spectrum of cardiovascular effects of these agents should be borne in mind when prescribing their use. For example, while patients with a normally functioning cardiovascular system may be able to tolerate adrenergic blockade of the heart, patients with compensated heart failure, who depend on adrenergic tone to maintain an adequate cardiac output, may experience acute congestive heart failure if prescribed any of the class II drugs. Table 26-7 summarizes the clinical use of the β-adrenoceptor blocking drugs in the treatment of cardiac arrhythmias. To fully elucidate the mode of action, uses, and broad effects of these drugs, a representative agent, propranolol, is discussed in this section.

Propranolol

Electrophysiological Actions

Unlike the other antiarrhythmic agents discussed previously, the actions of propranolol involve two separate and distinct effects. The first effect is a consequence of the

Table 26-6. β-Adrenoceptor Antagonists

Drug (trade name; form)	Description
Propranolol (*Inderal*; tablets, solution)	A prototype β-adrenoceptor antagonist that is nonselective in that it blocks both the β_1- and β_2-adrenoceptors. In addition, propranolol has membrane-stabilizing properties that can contribute to its antiarrhythmic action. Since the latter action is obtained at plasma concentrations beyond those that may be encountered clinically, it is the β-receptor blocking property that may best explain the antiarrhythmic action of propranolol.
Acebutolol (*Sectral*; capsules)	A cardioselective β_1-adrenoceptor blocking agent with partial agonist activity (intrinsic sympathomimetic activity, ISA). It is approved for use in the management of patients with premature ventricular complexes and for use in treating essential hypertension.
Atenolol (*Tenormin*; tablets)	A β_1- selective (cardioselective) adrenoceptor blocking agent. It lacks membrane-stabilizing effects and does not exhibit intrinsic sympathomimetic activity. Cardioselectivity is not absolute and β_2-adrenoceptors are blocked at higher doses. Atenolol does not undergo appreciable metabolism and has an elimination half-life of 6–7 hr.
Metoprolol (*Lopressor*; tablets)	A selective β_1-adrenoceptor blocking agent. The cardioselectivity is not absolute and at higher doses β_2-adrenoceptors are blocked as well. The drug does not possess ISA. Metoprolol undergoes extensive hepatic metabolism and has a plasma half-life of 3–7 hr. It is used primarily in the management of patients with essential hypertension and angina pectoris.
Nadolol (*Corgard*; tablets)	A nonselective β-adrenoceptor blocking agent that lacks membrane-stabilizing and ISA properties. Nadolol is not metabolized and is excreted unchanged. Therefore, the drug has a long duration of action with a pharmacologic half-life of 20–24 hr that permits once-daily administration. It is eliminated by renal mechanisms as the unchanged drug. Nadolol is used primarily for the management of patients with angina pectoris.
Pindolol (*Visken*; tablets)	A nonselective β-adrenoceptor antagonist with considerable ISA and devoid of membrane-stabilizing activity. The drug is metabolized extensively and has a plasma half-life of 3–4 hr. It is indicated primarily for the management of patients with hypertension. The ISA possessed by pindolol may exacerbate symptoms in patients with ischemic heart disease.
Timolol (*Blocadren*; tablets)	A nonselective β-adrenoceptor blocking agent without ISA, membrane-stabilizing, and local anesthetic properties. The drug is metabolized partially by hepatic mechanisms and has a plasma half-life of 4 hr. It is indicated for the management of patients with essential hypertension as well as for long-term prophylactic management of patients who have survived the acute phase of myocardial infarction who are given 10 mg twice a day.
Esmolol (*Brevibloc*; solution)	An ultra–short-acting, cardioselective β-adrenoceptor blocking agent. It is indicated for use in patients with supraventricular tachyarrhythmias where short-term management is indicated. The drug is given IV: 500 μg/kg/min initially for 1 min followed by 50 μg/kg/min for 4 min, then 100 μg/kg/min for 4 min.

Table 26-7. Efficacy of β-Adrenoceptor Blocking Agents in the Control of Cardiac Rhythm Disorders

Rhythm disorder	Efficacy of β-adrenoceptor blocking agent
Supraventricular arrhythmias Sinus tachycardia	First treat the underlying cause, e.g., hyperpyrexia, hypovolemia, etc. β-Adrenoceptor blockade is most effective in decreasing the heart rate by inhibiting S-A response to enhanced adrenergic stimulation. Do not use as the initial drug in tachycardia associated with pheochromocytoma.
Atrial fibrillation	Sinus rhythm is unlikely to be restored. However, the effect of β-adrenoceptor blockade on the A-V node will decrease the ventricular response to the atrial tachyarrhythmia. Effect is enhanced by the simultaneous use of digoxin or verapamil.
Atrial flutter/tachycardia	β-Adrenoceptor blockers will reduce the ventricular rate by inhibition of transmission through the A-V node as a result of inhibition of adrenergic influences. May be useful for the prevention of recurrent episodes of tachyarrhythmia.
Ventricular arrhythmias Premature ventricular complexes	Effective in mitral valve prolapse, hypertrophic cardiomyopathy, and digitalis-related ectopic activity as well as ventricular complexes associated with exercise or ischemia induced.
Ventricular tachycardia	Most effective against arrhythmias associated with digitalis toxicity and exercise, particularly if the latter is related to ischemia.
Ventricular fibrillation	Postmyocardial infarct patients show increased survival if treated with a β-adrenoceptor antagonist. The beneficial effect may be related to the decrease in heart rate and the antiischemic benefits of β-adrenoceptor blockade.

drug's β-blocking properties and the subsequent removal of adrenergic influences on the heart. The second is associated with the direct myocardial effects (membrane stabilization) of propranolol. The latter action, especially at the higher clinically employed doses, may account for its effectiveness against arrhythmias in which enhanced β-receptor stimulation does not play a significant role in the genesis of the rhythm disturbance.

Sinoatrial Node

The ability of propranolol to block β-receptors in the sinoatrial node and prevent adrenergic influences on this structure is the primary mechanism by which propranolol produces a bradycardia. In addition, doses in excess of those required to produce β-receptor blockade can exert a *direct* negative inotropic action on sinoatrial nodal pacemaker cells.

Atria

Propranolol possesses local anesthetic properties and exerts actions similar to those of quinidine on the atrial membrane action potential. Membrane responsiveness and action-potential amplitude are reduced, and excitability is decreased; conduction velocity is reduced. Because these concentrations are similar to those that produce β-blockade, it is impossible to determine whether the drug acts by specific receptor blockade or through an action that some have referred to as a "quinidinelike" or "membrane-stabilizing" effect.

Atrioventricular Node

The depressant effects of propranolol on the A-V node are more pronounced than are the direct depressant effects of quinidine. This is due to propranolol's dual actions of β-blockade and direct myocardial depression. Propranolol administration results in a decrease in A-V conduction velocity and an increase in the A-V nodal refractory period. Propranolol does not display the anticholinergic actions of quinidine and other antiarrhythmic agents.

His-Purkinje System and Ventricular Muscle

Propranolol decreases Purkinje fiber membrane responsiveness and reduces action-potential amplitude. His-Purkinje tissue excitability also is reduced. These changes result in a decrease in His-Purkinje conduction velocity. It should be noted, however, that these electrophysiological alterations are observed at propranolol concentrations in excess of those normally used in therapy. The most striking electrophysiological property of propranolol at usual therapeutic concentrations is a depression of catecholamine-stimulated automaticity.

Electrocardiographic Changes

Either no change or an increase in the P–R interval is usually observed. The QRS interval is prolonged only when large doses are given. The Q–T interval is usually shortened by propranolol administration.

Hemodynamic Effects

The blockade of cardiac β-adrenoceptors prevents or reduces the usual positive inotropic and chronotropic actions produced by catecholamine administration or cardiac sympathetic nerve stimulation. Blockade of β-receptors prolongs systolic ejection periods at rest and during exercise. Both alterations tend to increase myocardial oxygen consumption. However, these alterations are offset by factors that tend to reduce oxygen consumption, such as decreased heart rate and decreased force of contraction. The decrease in oxygen demand produced by a decrease in heart rate and a decrease in force of contraction is usually greater than the increase in oxygen demand that results from increased heart size and increased ejection time. *The net result is that oxygen demand is decreased.*

Clinical Uses

Propranolol is indicated in the management of a variety of cardiac rhythm abnormalities that are totally or partially due to enhanced adrenergic stimulation. In selected cases of sinus tachycardia caused by anxiety, pheochromocytoma, or thyrotoxicosis, β-blockade will reduce the spontaneous heart rate.

Propranolol alone or in conjunction with digitalis can help control the ventricular rate in patients with atrial flutter or atrial fibrillation. Patients with supraventricular extrasystoles and intermittent paroxysms of atrial fibrillation may benefit from β-receptor blockade with propranolol.

The arrhythmias associated with halothane or cyclopropane anesthesia have been attributed to the interaction of the anesthetic with catecholamines, and they have been suppressed by IV administration of 1 to 3 mg propranolol. An increase in circulating catecholamines also has been observed in patients with acute myocardial infarction and has been correlated with the development of arrhythmias.

Clinically, tachyarrhythmias associated with digitalis excess (including supraventricular and ventricular extrasystoles) and ventricular tachycardia have been suppressed by IV and orally administered propranolol. In spite of experimental studies implicating catecholamines in the genesis of digitalis-related arrhythmias, recent evidence suggests that the suppression of this group of arrhythmias is not entirely a result of β-blockade. Although propranolol has been recommended for the treatment of digitalis toxicity, it is not the agent of choice, since it depresses myocardial contractility and A-V transmission and causes bradycardia. *Even though propranolol is highly effective in the treatment of digitalis-induced arrhythmias, phenytoin and lidocaine are preferred.*

During the past several years, long-term treatment with β-adrenoceptor blocking agents has provided clear indications that several members of this class (propranolol, timolol, metoprolol) are of value in reducing mortality and morbidity in patients with ischemic heart disease who have recovered from an acute myocardial infarction.

Adverse Reactions

The toxicity associated with propranolol is, for the most part, related to its primary pharmacological action, inhibition of the cardiac β-adrenoceptors. This topic is discussed in detail in Chap. 13. In addition, propranolol exerts direct cardiac depressant effects that become manifest when the drug is administered rapidly by the IV route. Glucagon immediately reverses all cardiac depressant effects of propranolol, and its use is associated with a minimum of side effects. The inotropic agents amrinone (*Inocor*) and milrinone (*Primacor*) provide alternative means of augmenting cardiac contractile function in the presence of β-adrenoceptor blockade.

Since propranolol crosses the placenta and enters the fetal circulation, fetal cardiac responses to the stresses of labor and delivery will be blocked.

Contraindications

Propranolol is contraindicated for patients with any type of depression of cardiac contractility, particularly congestive heart failure. It may be contraindicated in the presence of digitalis toxicity because of the possibility of producing complete A-V block and ventricular asystole. Patients receiving anesthetic agents that tend to depress myocardial contractility (ether, halothane) should not receive propranolol.

Sudden abrupt withdrawal of β-blockers may be potentially dangerous for patients with ischemic heart disease. Increased incidence of angina, coronary spasm, and myocardial infarction can occur; the reason for this occurrence is unclear, but it may be related to the increased density of cardiac β-receptors noted to occur in response to chronic administration of the receptor antagonist.

Preparations and Dosage

For the treatment of supraventricular arrhythmias, 10 to 40 mg propranolol hydrochloride (*Inderal*), given orally three or four times a day, is usually sufficient. Treatment of ventricular arrhythmias may require very large doses (320 mg/day or greater). Intravenous administration of propranolol is reserved for life-threatening arrhythmias or those that occur when the patient is under anesthesia. The usual dose is 1 to 3 mg, administered under careful hemodynamic and electrocardiographic monitoring.

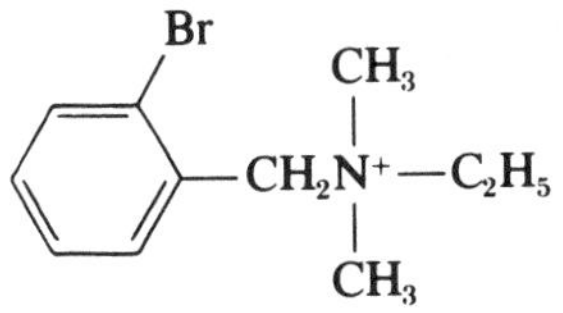

Figure 26-9. Bretylium.

Class III

Bretylium

Bretylium (Fig. 26-9) was introduced for the treatment of essential hypertension. It soon proved to be ineffective because of the development of tolerance to its antihypertensive effect. Subsequently, it was reported that bretylium suppressed the ventricular fibrillation often associated with acute myocardial infarction.

Electrophysiological Actions

The net effects of bretylium on the electrical and mechanical properties of the heart are a composite of the direct actions of the drug on cardiac tissues and indirect actions mediated through the drug's effects on the sympathetic nervous system.

Sinoatrial Node
Bretylium administration produces an initial brief increase in sinus node automaticity that is probably the result of a drug-induced release of catecholamines from sympathetic nerve terminals. No change or a slight decrease in sinus heart rate is observed after the initial phase of catecholamine release.

Atria
At therapeutic concentrations, the only significant effect of bretylium is to prolong the action-potential duration. This action results in a prolongation of the atrial muscle effective refractory periods (ERP).

A-V Node
Moderate doses increase conduction velocity and decrease the A-V nodal refractory period; this effect may result from the initial drug-induced catecholamine release. The net effect of bretylium on A-V transmission during chronic therapy is unknown.

His-Purkinje System and Ventricular Muscle
The most prominent electrophysiological action of bretylium is to raise the intensity of electrical current necessary to induce

ventricular fibrillation. This action is more prominent with bretylium than with any other currently available antiarrhythmic agent and can be observed in both normal and ischemic hearts. Spontaneous conversion of ventricular fibrillation to sinus rhythm in humans has been observed after bretylium administration. Bretylium also lowers the electrical threshold for successful defibrillation and increases the rate of success in achieving electrical defibrillation.

Hemodynamic Effects

A unique property of bretylium as an antiarrhythmic agent is its positive inotropic action. This effect is related to its actions on the sympathetic nervous system and includes an initial release of neuronal stores of norepinephrine, followed shortly by a prolonged period of inhibition of direct or reflex-associated neuronal norepinephrine release. The onset of a bretylium-induced hypotension is delayed 1 to 2 hr, because the initial catecholamine release maintains arterial pressure before this time.

Pharmacokinetics

Bretylium, a quaternary ammonium compound, has poor systemic availability after oral administration, and plasma concentrations are erratic, achieving a peak in about 3 hr with only 10 to 30 percent of an oral dose reaching the general circulation (Table 26-8). Bretylium is well absorbed after IM injection, with peak plasma concentrations being attained within 1 hr. No metabolites of bretylium have been observed, and the drug is excreted almost entirely by renal mechanisms.

Clinical Uses

Bretylium is not to be considered a first-line antiarrhythmic agent. However, because of its ability to prolong the refractory period of Purkinje fibers and to elevate the electrical threshold to ventricular fibrillation, bretylium has been found *useful in the treatment of life-threatening*

ventricular arrhythmias, principally recurrent ventricular tachycardia, ventricular fibrillation, or both, especially when conventional therapeutic agents, such as lidocaine or procainamide, prove to be ineffective. In addition, bretylium is known to facilitate the ease with which precordial electrical shock reverses ventricular fibrillation. Indications for the use of bretylium limit its administration to no longer than 5 days. Bretylium tosylate (*Bretylol*) is available for IM and IV use in 10-ml ampules containing a total of 10 mg of drug; an oral formulation is not available.

Adverse Reactions

The most important side effect associated with the use of bretylium is hypotension, a result of peripheral vasodilation caused by adrenergic neuronal blockade (a guanethidinelike action). Nausea, vomiting, and diarrhea have been reported with IV administration and can be minimized by slow infusion. Longer-term problems include swelling and tenderness of the parotid gland, particularly occurring at mealtime.

Contraindications

The associated initial release of catecholamines could result in an excessive pressor response and stimulation of cardiac force and pacemaker activity. The resulting increase in myocardial oxygen consumption in a patient with ischemic heart disease could lead to the development of ischemic pain (angina pectoris). Patients in a state of circulatory shock probably should not be administered bretylium because of its delayed sympatholytic action.

Amiodarone

Amiodarone (Fig. 26-9) is an iodine-containing benzofuran derivative that possesses cardiac electrophysiological actions that differ fundamentally from those of currently available antiarrhythmic agents. *Amiodarone is an*

Table 26-8. Pharmacokinetic Characteristics of the Class III Drugs

Drug	Therapeutic serum concentration (μg/ml)	Time to onset of action	Time to peak concentration (hr)	Duration of action (hr)	Elimination half-life	Percent protein bound	Volume of distribution (L/kg)
Bretylium	0.5–1.5	6–8 hr	3	6–8	5–10 hr	0–8	5.9 ± 0.8
Amiodarone	0.5–2.5	1–3 wk	3–7	?	25–100 days	99	66 ± 44
Sotalol	1–4	1 hr	2–3	12	7–15 hr	0	1.6–2.4

effective agent for the treatment of supraventricular arrhythmias and for ventricular tachyarrhythmias refractory to conventional antiarrhythmic therapy. Toxicity associated with amiodarone has led the FDA to recommend that the drug be reserved for use in patients with life-threatening arrhythmias.

Electrophysiologic Actions

The most notable electrophysiologic effect of amiodarone after long-term administration is a prolongation of repolarization and refractoriness in all cardiac tissues, an action that is characteristic of class III antiarrhythmic agents. The exact mechanism of action of amiodarone is unknown.

Sinoatrial Node
Amiodarone decreases the action-potential amplitude and the slope of phase 4 of the membrane action potential recorded from the sinoatrial node. The cycle length of the S-A node is increased by amiodarone as well as by its metabolite, desethylamiodarone. The depressant action of amiodarone on sinoatrial pacemaker function may be related to an inhibition of the slow inward current carried by the calcium ion.

Atria
Amiodarone causes prolongation of the action potential in atrial muscle as well as an increase in the absolute and effective refractory periods.

Atrioventricular Node
Amiodarone, as well as its major metabolite, desethylamiodarone, increases A-V nodal conduction time and refractory period.

His-Purkinje System and Ventricular Myocardium
As with many antiarrhythmic agents, the actions of amiodarone on the electrophysiology of the His-Purkinje system may be related to its direct as well as its indirect actions. (Data derived with the acute application of amiodarone may not coincide with information derived from studies in which the drug is administered over a prolonged period.) While the acute and chronic effects of amiodarone on the electrophysiology of the cardiac tissue must be distinguished, from the standpoint of its clinical application, the effects of the long-term administration of the drug would appear to be most important.

The dominant effect on ventricular myocardium chronically treated with either amiodarone or desethylamiodarone is a prolongation in the action-potential duration with an associated increase in the refractory period and a modest decrease in V_{max} as a function of stimulus frequency. Amiodarone has been reported to decrease the delayed outward potassium current, a finding consistent with the observation of a prolonged action-potential duration. Both amiodarone and its metabolite significantly decrease the action-potential duration and shorten the effective refractory period in Purkinje fibers while at the same time causing a prolongation of action potential in ventricular muscle.

Electrocardiographic Changes

The predominant electrocardiographic changes observed with the administration of amiodarone consist of a decrease in the sinus rate of 10 to 15 percent, a prolongation of the P–R and Q–T intervals, the development of U waves, and changes in T-wave contour. In rare instances Q–T prolongation has been associated with a worsening of arrhythmias.

Hemodynamic Effects

Amiodarone relaxes vascular smooth muscle; one of its most prominent effects is on the coronary circulation, thereby reducing coronary vascular resistance and improving regional myocardial blood flow. In addition its effects on the peripheral vascular bed lead to a decrease in left ventricular stroke work and myocardial oxygen consumption. Therefore, amiodarone has a beneficial effect on the relationship between myocardial oxygen demand and oxygen supply.

Toxic Reactions

Toxic reactions of most concern are hepatitis, exacerbation of arrhythmias, worsening of congestive heart failure, and pneumonitis. Pulmonary toxicity results in clinically manifest disease in 10 to 15 percent of patients who receive 400 mg per day of the drug. Hepatic toxicity manifested as elevations in liver enzyme levels is seen frequently in patients taking amiodarone.

Corneal microdeposits will develop in the majority of adults receiving amiodarone. As many as 10 percent of patients will observe halos or blurred vision. The corneal microdeposits are reversible upon stopping the drug.

Photosensitization occurs in about 10 percent of patients taking amiodarone. With continued treatment the skin assumes a blue-gray coloration. The risk is increased in patients of fair complexion. The discoloration of the skin regresses slowly, if at all, after discontinuation of amiodarone.

Amiodarone inhibits the peripheral and, possibly, intrapituitary conversion of thyroxine (T_4) to triiodothyronine (T_3) by inhibiting 5′-deiodination. The serum concentration of T_4 is increased due to a decrease in its clearance and thyroid synthesis is increased due to a reduced suppression of the pituitary thyrotropin by T_3. The concentration of T_3 in the serum decreases and reverse T_3 appears in increased amounts. Despite these changes, the majority of patients appear to be maintained in a euthyroid state. Manifestations of both hypo- and hyperthyroidism have been reported.

Tremors of the hands and sleep disturbances in the form of vivid dreams, nightmares, and insomnia have been reported in association with the use of amiodarone. Ataxia, staggering, and impaired ambulation have been noted. Peripheral sensory and motor neuropathy or severe proximal muscle weakness develops infrequently. Both neuropathic and myopathic changes are observed on biopsy. Neurologic symptoms resolve or improve within several weeks of dosage reduction.

Pharmacokinetics

Amiodarone is absorbed slowly after oral administration. Bioavailability varies widely and is estimated to be between 35 and 65 percent. The onset of antiarrhythmic action may take from 2 to 3 days but more commonly is achieved only after 1 to 3 weeks, even with the use of a loading dose (Table 26-8). The prolonged period required to obtain a consistent antiarrhythmic action relates to the extensive protein and lipid binding of the drug. As the drug accumulates in adipose tissue, the storage sites generally must be saturated before a steady-state response is obtained.

The volume of distribution of amiodarone is extremely large (60 liters/kg) in part because of the extensive deposition in adipose tissue. The plasma clearance is low with negligible renal elimination. The major metabolite is desethylamiodarone, which achieves a plasma ratio of one with respect to the parent compound after chronic administration.

Hepatic excretion into the bile is the primary route of elimination of amiodarone and its major metabolite. Neither the parent compound nor the metabolite is dialyzable. After discontinuation of amiodarone, the plasma half-life varies from 26 to 107 days, with a mean of approximately 53 days. The prolonged elimination half-life of amiodarone relates to the slow elimination of the drug from tissue storage depots, predominantly adipose tissue. The elimination half-life of desethylamiodarone is longer than that of the parent drug.

There is no apparent relationship between the plasma concentration of amiodarone and its clinical efficacy. It has been observed that concentrations below 1 mg per liter (L) are associated with lack of efficacy while plasma concentrations of less than 2.5 mg/L are needed.

Contraindications

Amiodarone is contraindicated in patients with sick sinus syndrome and may cause severe bradycardia and second- and third-degree atrioventricular block. Amiodarone crosses the placenta and will affect the fetus as evidenced by bradycardia. The drug is secreted in breast milk.

Drug Interactions

Amiodarone increases the hypoprothrombinemic response to warfarin (an oral anticoagulant) by reducing its metabolism. Amiodarone interacts with other drugs used to treat arrhythmias, including flecainide, phenytoin, and quinidine. Patients receiving digoxin may experience an increase in serum digoxin concentrations when amiodarone is added to the treatment regimen. Amiodarone interferes with hepatic and renal elimination of these drugs.

Indications

Amiodarone is indicated for the *management of patients with documented life-threatening recurrent ventricular arrhythmias that are not controlled by other therapeutic interventions.* The approved indicated uses are for recurrent ventricular fibrillation and recurrent hemodynamically unstable ventricular tachycardia. There is no evidence that amiodarone influences survival in patients subject to sudden coronary death.

Amiodarone is effective in maintaining sinus rhythm in most patients with paroxysmal atrial fibrillation and in many patients with persistent atrial fibrillation. It is also effective in preventing recurrences of A-V nodal reentry and atrial tachyarrhythmias, and in the prevention of reentrant rhythms and atrial fibrillation in patients with the WPW syndrome.

Preparation and Dosage

Amiodarone HCl (*Cordarone*) is supplied as 200-mg tablets. Amiodarone should be administered by physicians who are experienced in the treatment of life-threatening arrhythmias and versed in the risks and benefits of the therapeutic agent.

Sotalol

In addition to belonging to the class II group of antiarrhythmic agents due to its β-adrenoceptor blocking properties, sotalol also is a member of class III because it prolongs the duration of the cardiac membrane action potential. Sotalol is a nonspecific β-adrenoceptor antagonist and lacks intrinsic β-adrenoceptor agonist activity.

Electrophysiological Actions

Sinoatrial Node

Pacemaker activity in the sinoatrial node is decreased as a result of β-adrenoceptor blockade and a removal of sympathoadrenal influences on spontaneous diastolic depolarization.

Atria

Sotalol increases the refractory period of atrial muscle.

Atrioventricular Node

Sotalol would decrease conduction velocity and prolong the effective refractory period in the atrioventricular node, an action held in common with other β_1-adrenoceptor blocking agents.

His-Purkinje System and Ventricular Muscle

The actions of sotalol on the delayed rectifier potassium current result in a prolongation of the effective refractory period in His-Purkinje tissue. Like other members of class III, the electrophysiologic action of sotalol is characterized by prolongation of repolarization and an increase in the effective refractory period of ventricular muscle.

Electrocardiographic Changes

Administration of sotalol is associated with dose and concentration-dependent slowing of the heart rate and prolongation of the P–R interval. The QRS duration is not affected with plasma concentrations within the therapeutic range. The corrected Q–T interval is prolonged as a result of the increase in the effective refractory period of ventricular myocardium.

Hemodynamic Effects

The hemodynamic effects of sotalol are related to its β-adrenoceptor antagonist activity. Accordingly, a decrease in resting heart rate and in exercise-induced tachycardia is seen in patients receiving sotalol. A modest reduction in systolic pressure and in cardiac output may occur. The reduction in cardiac output is a consequence of the lowering of heart rate, since stroke volume is unaffected by sotalol treatment. In patients with normal ventricular function, cardiac output is maintained despite the decrease in heart rate due to the simultaneous increase in the stroke volume. Thus, in the absence of heart failure, sotalol is well tolerated. In long-term studies (1 year) no significant hemodynamic deterioration was observed.

Pharmacokinetics

The bioavailability of sotalol approximates 100 percent. Sotalol does not undergo biotransformation, is not protein bound, and is therefore totally bioavailable. The drug is eliminated entirely by the kidney. The maximum plasma concentration is achieved rapidly on oral administration. The relatively long elimination half-life of the drug of 11 hr may permit a once- or two-times-a-day dosing schedule. The pharmacokinetic data of sotalol are shown in Table 26-8.

Clinical Uses

Sotalol (*Betapace*) possesses a broad spectrum of antiarrhythmic effects in ventricular and supraventricular arrhythmias. It has value in the management of patients with paroxysmal supraventricular arrhythmias, in terminating the reentrant arrhythmia in which the atrioventricular node serves as the reentrant pathway, and also may terminate supraventricular tachyarrhythmias associated with an accessory pathway.

Adverse Reactions

Side effects include those attributed to both β-adrenoceptor blockade and proarrhythmic effects. Proarrhythmia has been seen in 4 to 7 percent of patients, and torsades de pointes has been documented in 1.9 percent of patients. This arrhythmia is a serious threat as it may lead to ventricular fibrillation. Other adverse effects of sotalol are attributable to its β-blocker activity. In decreasing order of frequency, these include fatigue (21%), dyspnea (19%), chest pain (17%), headache (10%), and nausea and vomiting (9.6%).

Contraindications

The contraindications that apply to other β-adrenoceptor blocking agents also apply to sotalol (see section on propranolol). In addition, however, hypokalemia as well as drugs known to prolong the Q–T interval may be contraindicated, as they enhance the possibility of proarrhythmic events.

Drug Interactions

The class III effects of sotalol may be enhanced by drugs with inherent Q–T interval–prolonging activity (i.e., thiazide diuretics, terfenadine).

Class IV

Verapamil

Verapamil, in addition to its use as an antiarrhythmic agent, has been employed extensively in the management of variant (Prinzmetal's) angina and effort-induced angina pectoris (see Chaps. 23 and 25). It produces a selective inhibition of transmembrane calcium fluxes in myocardial cells by affecting a secondary inward depolarizing current that flows through a slow channel. This current is carried primarily by calcium ions, and voltage changes due to this current are referred to as slow-channel depolarizations, or slow responses.

Electrophysiological Actions

The calcium antagonism produced by verapamil is considered to be a specific action, as opposed to nonspecific calcium-antagonistic effects obtained with high doses of barbiturates or certain β-adrenoceptor blocking agents.

Sinoatrial Node

Pacemaker activity in the sinoatrial node has an ionic mechanism that is completely different from action potentials generated in Purkinje fibers or ordinary atrial muscle cells. Spontaneous phase 4 depolarization, a characteristic of normal sinoatrial nodal cells, relies on deactivation of an outward current that is selective for K^+ ions and a slow inward current that is carried by Na^+ and Ca^{2+} ions. Verapamil produces reductions in the rate of rise and slope of the slow diastolic depolarization, the maximal diastolic potential, and the membrane potential at the peak of depolarization in the sinoatrial node.

Atria

Verapamil fails to exert any significant electrophysiological effects on atrial muscle.

Atrioventricular Node

Verapamil impairs conduction across the A-V node and prolongs the A-V nodal refractory period at plasma concentrations that show no effect on the His-Purkinje system.

His-Purkinje System and Ventricular Muscle

The most important electrocardiographic change produced by verapamil is a prolongation of the P–R interval, a response consistent with the known effects of the drug on A-V nodal transmission. Verapamil has no effect on intraatrial and intraventricular conduction. The predominant electrophysiological effect is on A-V conduction proximal to the His bundle.

Hemodynamic Effects

The usual intravenous dose of verapamil employed for antiarrhythmic effects (10 mg) is not associated with marked alterations in arterial blood pressure, peripheral vascular resistance, heart rate, left ventricular end-diastolic pressure, or contractility. The changes that do occur on intravenous administration are short lived.

Pharmacokinetics

This topic is covered in Chap. 23.

Clinical Uses

Verapamil appears to be *most valuable as an antiarrhythmic drug in the management of patients with atrial tachyarrhythmias*. Reentrant paroxysmal supraventricular tachycardia involving the sinoatrial or atrioventricular nodes has responded favorably to verapamil, both for the acute attack and for prevention of recurrences of the tachyarrhythmias. There has been limited success in reversing atrial flutter and atrial fibrillation to sinus rhythm.

A distinct advantage of verapamil in supraventricular tachyarrhythmias is its rapid onset of effect. In paroxysmal supraventricular tachycardia, the drug is 80 to 100 percent effective in restoring sinus rhythm and offers an advantage over current therapy.

In addition to its use in the management of atrial rhythm disorders, verapamil and other slow-channel antagonists (nifedipine, diltiazem, amlodipine) are known to be effective therapeutic agents in the management of patients with vasospastic angina pectoris (Prinzmetal's angina, variant angina), as well as in effort-induced angina (see Chap. 23).

Adverse Reactions

Orally administered verapamil is well tolerated by the majority of patients. Most complaints are with respect to gastrointestinal side effects of constipation and gastric discomfort. Other complaints include vertigo, headache, nervousness, and pruritus.

Contraindications

Verapamil must be used with extreme caution or not at all in patients who are receiving β-adrenoceptor blocking agents. Normally, the negative chronotropic effect of verapamil will, in part, be overcome by an increase in reflex sympathetic tone. The latter would be prevented by simultaneous administration of a β-adrenoceptor blocking agent, thus exaggerating the depressant effects of verapamil on heart rate, atrioventricular node conduction, and myocardial contractility.

Preparations

Verapamil (*Isoptin, Calan*) is provided as an intravenous formulation for use in the management of patients with atrioventricular nodal or sinus nodal reentrant tachycardia or reciprocating tachycardia in the WPW syndrome. Verapamil is contraindicated in the latter situation in the presence of atrial flutter or atrial fibrillation.

Diltiazem

The antiarrhythmic actions and uses of diltiazem are similar to those of verapamil. Diltiazem injectable is indicated for the temporary control of rapid ventricular rate during atrial flutter or atrial fibrillation. The drug rarely converts the atrial rhythm disorder to normal sinus rhythm. Therefore, as with verapamil, diltiazem is intended for the management of patients with supraventricular tachyarrhythmias. Diltiazem is administered by the intravenous route. When given orally without or with digitalis, diltiazem is effective in controlling the ventricular rate in patients with atrial flutter or atrial fibrillation.

The pharmacology of diltiazem is discussed in detail in Chap. 23.

Preparation

Diltiazem (*Cardizem*) is available as an injectable solution. It should be used only where facilities are available for continuous monitoring of the electrocardiogram and frequent blood pressure recordings can be obtained.

Miscellaneous Antiarrhythmic Agents

Digitalis Glycosides and Vagomimetic Drugs

Digitalis glycosides, especially digoxin, although used primarily for their positive inotropic action in patients with congestive heart failure, have been and continue to be used for the management of patients with supraventricular arrhythmias. Since the digitalis glycosides are discussed elsewhere (see Chap. 24), it suffices to mention that they derive their usefulness in the *management of patients with supraventricular tachyarrhythmias* where the primary goal is to slow the rate of ventricular response.

The mechanisms that give rise to the beneficial action of digoxin are twofold. By virtue of a direct effect on the heart, *digoxin slows conduction over the atrioventricular node and increases the refractory period of the atrioventricular nodal tissue.* Therefore, fewer impulses originating in the atria are able to invade the ventricular myocardium over the atrioventricular nodal pathway. Despite the continued presence of a supraventricular arrhythmia (e.g., atrial fibrillation or atrial flutter), the ventricular rate will de-

crease thereby improving cardiac hemodynamics. In addition to acting directly on the atrioventricular node, digoxin has an indirect effect whereby it also increases the refractory period and slows conduction in atrioventricular nodal tissue. The latter mechanism is due to the ability of digitalis glycosides to *increase vagal tone* to the heart. Since the effects of vagal stimulation are mediated by the release of acetylcholine at the postganglionic nerve endings, drugs that affect this neurotransmitter will have the ability to alter atrioventricular conduction velocity and refractoriness. Anticholinesterases, such as neostigmine, will potentiate the muscarinic effects of locally released acetylcholine and will be additive to the indirect actions of digoxin. The digitalis glycosides will act synergistically or additively with other agents that depress the electrophysiologic properties of the atrioventricular node.

Adenosine

Adenosine (Fig. 26-10) is an endogenous chemical, an end product of the metabolism of adenosine triphosphate. The utility of adenosine in the management of patients with supraventricular tachyarrhythmias has been known for over 50 years. It is important to realize however, that adenosine has physiological effects beyond the heart. A diverse physiological role for adenosine is suggested by the fact that specific receptors for it are present in virtually every tissue. Adenosine has been approved for use as an antiarrhythmic drug.

Electrophysiological Actions

Adenosine acts through specific receptors, α_1-receptors, to produce its electrophysiologic effects on the atrioventricular and sinoatrial nodes. The effects of adenosine are inhibited competitively by methylxanthines such as caffeine and theophylline.

The electrophysiologic actions of adenosine on the atrioventricular node resemble those of acetylcholine.

Figure 26-10. Adenosine.

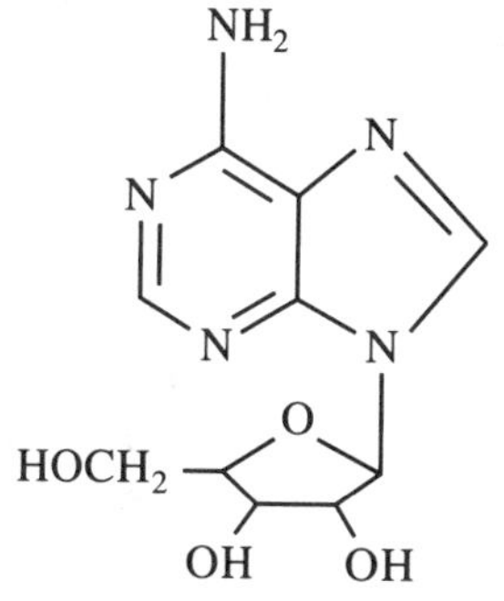

The effective refractory period is increased and conduction velocity is depressed. Therefore, adenosine has gained acceptance in the clinical management of patients with paroxysmal atrial tachycardia. Adenosine markedly affects sinoatrial and atrioventricular nodal tissues and produces transient second-degree atrioventricular block. Adenosine is not inhibited by muscarinic antagonists (atropine).

Adenosine receptor activation stimulates a time-dependent outward potassium current, hyperpolarizing the cell. This leads to a decrease of phase 4 depolarization in sinoatrial nodal cells and a decrease in the action-potential duration of atrial muscle. Adenosine also depresses the upstroke of the action potential of "N" cells in the atrioventricular node. This latter effect slows conduction through the atrioventricular node, and also can block reentry pathways through the A-V node. Adenosine does not influence ventricular action-potential kinetics because the adenosine-stimulated potassium channel is not present in ventricular myocardium.

Electrocardiographic Changes

The electrophysiological effects of adenosine relate to the action of the drug on supraventricular structures. Rapid administration of adenosine leads to sinus bradycardia within 10 to 20 sec of administration. Adenosine increases the A–H interval, but does not affect the H–V interval. The drug is ineffective on supraventricular tachycardias *when administered as an infusion.*

Hemodynamic Effects

The administration of a bolus dose of adenosine is followed by a characteristic biphasic pressor response. There is an initial brief increase in both systolic and diastolic blood pressure followed by a decrease and a secondary tachycardia.

Pharmacokinetics

The half-life of adenosine is extremely short (10 sec). The rapid metabolism of the drug accounts for its brief period of action. The action of adenosine may be intensified by the presence of dipyridamole, which delays the uptake and metabolic termination of adenosine by the red blood cells.

Clinical Uses

Adenosine is approved for the acute management and termination of supraventricular tachyarrhythmias. The supraventricular arrhythmias that may respond to adenosine include atrioventricular nodal reentrant tachycardia and atrioventricular reciprocating tachycardia. The drug is not recommended for use in the management of ventricular tachycardia. Adenosine also has a role in the diagnosis of certain arrhythmias.

Adverse Reactions

Adverse reactions to the administration of adenosine are not uncommon; however, the short half-life of the drug limits the duration of such events (usually dissipated by 5–20 sec after administration of a bolus dose). The most common adverse effects of adenosine are flushing, chest pain, and dyspnea. The vasodilator action of adenosine is responsible for the flushing (18% incidence). Chest pain may radiate to upper extremities and mimic that of myocardial ischemia. Interestingly, the chest pain associated with adenosine is not alleviated by β-adrenoceptor blocking agents, atropine, or naloxone, indicating that adrenergic, cholinergic, and opioid receptors are not involved. Dyspnea occurs because adenosine can act as a bronchoconstrictor, although the precise mechanism of this effect remains unknown. This adverse effect is of particular importance in asthmatic patients, in whom the increase in airway resistance may last for 30 min or more.

Contraindications

Patients with second- or third-degree A-V block should not be administered adenosine. As indicated previously, the use of adenosine in asthmatic patients may exacerbate the asthmatic symptoms. Known hypersensitivity to adenosine precludes its use.

Drug Interactions

The metabolism of adenosine is slowed by dipyridamole, indicating that in patients stabilized on dipyridamole the therapeutically effective dose of adenosine may need to be increased. Methylxanthines will antagonize the effects of adenosine through blockade of the adenosine receptors.

Preparation

Adenosine (*Adenocard*) is supplied as an injectable (6 mg/2 ml) for rapid intravenous administration.

Magnesium Sulfate

Magnesium sulfate is effective in terminating refractory ventricular tachyarrhythmias. Digitalis-induced arrhythmias are more likely in the presence of magnesium deficiency. Magnesium sulfate can be administered orally, intramuscularly, or, preferably, intravenously, when a rapid response is intended. The loss of deep tendon reflexes is a sign of overdose.

Conclusions

Recent years have witnessed an intensified search for new and more effective antidysrhythmic drugs that lack important side effects when administered chronically. Part of the stimulus for new investigative efforts has been the recognition that sudden coronary death constitutes a major problem and that the currently available antiarrhythmic agents either are ineffective in the prevention of sudden coronary death or are limited by serious toxicity when administered on a chronic basis.

Drugs used to treat cardiac arrhythmias are intended to control abnormal myocardial electrophysiological activity and reduce the frequency or prevent the development of ectopic ventricular complexes. However, under certain, but incompletely understood, conditions, antiarrhythmic drugs also exhibit proarrhythmic activity (i.e., drug-induced cardiac arrhythmias). It has been recently realized that efficacious antiarrhythmic drugs may exhibit proarrhythmic effects, and that the consequences of such adverse activity can be fatal.

Proarrhythmia must be considered an inherent property of antiarrhythmic drugs. It is a manifestation of inherent pharmacologic properties of the drug. However, a number of patient and medically related factors may contribute to the occurrence of proarrhythmia. Drug-drug interactions that result in an increase in the effective plasma concentration of an antiarrhythmic drug may lead to proarrhythmic events. A drug (B) that displaces only 2 percent of a highly plasma protein-bound (98% bound) drug (A) can double the effective (free) concentration of the drug (A) and increase the probability of proarrhythmia.

Other patient-related factors that contribute to the risk that a proarrhythmic event may occur include severe ventricular dysfunction, hypokalemia or hypomagnesemia, and serious underlying arrhythmias. Most important is the fact that transient ischemic events in the presence of a given antiarrhythmic agent may lead to a proarrhythmic episode terminating in ventricular fibrillation.

Supplemental Reading

Anderson, J.L. Reassessment of benefit-risk ratio and treatment algorithms for antiarrhythmic drug therapy after the cardiac arrhythmia suppression trial. *J. Clin. Pharmacol.* 30:981, 1990.

Camm, A.J., and Garratt, C.J. Drug therapy: Adenosine and supraventricular tachycardia. *N. Engl. J. Med.* 325:1621, 1990.

Campbell, R., and Loaiza, A. Class III drugs: Their effects on arrhythmias and on the QT interval. *Ann. N.Y. Acad. Sci.* 644:223, 1992.

The Cardiac Arrhythmia Suppression Trial (CAST) Investigators. Preliminary report: Effect of encainide and flecainide on mortality in a randomized trial of arrhythmia suppression after myocardial infarction. *N. Engl. J. Med.* 321:406, 1989.

The Cardiac Arrhythmia Suppression Trial Investigators. Effect of the antiarrhythmic agent moricizine on survival after myocardial infarction. *N. Engl. J. Med.* 327:227, 1992.

Carlsson, L., et al. Antiarrhythmic effects of potassium channel openers in rhythm abnormalities related to delayed repolarization. *Circulation* 82:2235, 1990.

Clyne, C.A., Estes, N.A.M., and Wang, P.J. Drug therapy: Moricizine. *N. Engl. J. Med.* 327:255, 1992.

Colatsky, T.J., Follmer, C.H., and Starmer, C.F. Channel specificity in antiarrhythmic drug action. Mechanism of potassium channel block and its role in suppressing and aggravating cardiac arrhythmias. *Circulation* 81:1151, 1990.

Hammermeister, K.E. Adverse hemodynamic effects of antiarrhythmic drugs in congestive heart failure. *Circulation* 81:1151, 1990.

Nattel, S. Antiarrhythmic drug classifications. A critical appraisal of their history, present status, and clinical relevance. *Drugs* 41:672, 1991.

Pritchett, E.L. Management of atrial fibrillation. *N. Engl. J. Med.* 326:1264, 1992.

Vaughan Williams, E.M. Significance of classifying antiarrhythmic actions since the cardiac arrhythmia suppression trial. *J. Clin. Pharmacol.* 31:123, 1991.

Woosley, R.L. Antiarrhythmic drugs. *Annu. Rev. Pharmacol. Toxicol.* 31:427, 1991.

27

Anticoagulant, Antiplatelet, and Fibrinolytic (Thrombolytic) Drugs

Jeffrey S. Fedan

Little intravascular coagulation of blood occurs under normal physiological conditions. The process of *hemostasis* involves the interplay of three phases (*vascular, platelet, and coagulation phases*) that promote blood clotting to prevent blood loss (Fig. 27-1). The *fibrinolytic phase* prevents propagation of clotting beyond the site of vascular injury and is involved in clot dissolution (lysis).

Hemostatic Mechanisms

Endothelial cells maintain a nonthrombogenic lining in blood vessels. This results from several phenomena, including (1) the maintenance of a transmural negative electrical charge, which is important in preventing adhesion of circulating platelets; (2) the release of plasminogen activators, which activate the fibrinolytic pathway; (3) the activation of protein C, which degrades coagulation factors—a process involving thrombin and its endothelial cofactor (thrombomodulin); (4) the production of heparinlike proteoglycans, which inhibit coagulation; and (5) the release of prostacyclin (PGI$_2$), a potent inhibitor of platelet aggregation. PGI$_2$ is a product of the sequential actions of phospholipase A$_2$, cyclooxygenase, and PGI$_2$ synthetase on membrane lipids. The production of PGI$_2$ increases under pathological conditions to limit the enlargement of the platelet thrombus. Vascular endothelial cells synthesize fibronectin and factor VIII–related von Willebrand polymers (factor VIII:vWF), which bind to the subendothelial matrix and also are released into the circulation.

In normal individuals, injury severe enough to cause hemorrhage initiates the coagulation process. Vasoconstriction, combined with increased tissue pressure caused by the presence of extravasated blood, results in a reduction, or stasis, of blood flow. Stasis favors the restriction

of thrombus formation to the site of injury. The extravasation of blood exposes platelets and the plasma clotting factors to subendothelial collagen and endothelial basement membranes, which results in activation of the clotting sequence. Several substances that participate in coagulation are released or become exposed to blood at the site of injury. These include adenosine diphosphate (ADP), a potent stimulus to platelet aggregation, and *tissue factor,* a membrane glycoprotein cofactor of factor VII that normally is not expressed in endothelial cells, but is present in the subendothelium.

Platelet aggregation is the most important defense mechanism against leakage of blood from the circulation. Ordinarily, unstimulated platelets do not adhere to the endothelial cell surface. Following disruption of the endothelial lining and exposure of blood to the subendothelial vessel wall, platelets come into contact with and adhere within seconds to factor VIII:vWF polymers and fibronectin. The platelets change shape and then undergo a complex secretory process termed the *release reaction.* This results in the release of ADP from platelet granules and activation of platelet phospholipase A$_2$. This enzyme, cyclooxygenase, and thromboxane synthetase sequentially convert arachidonic acid into cyclic endoperoxides and thromboxane A$_2$ (TxA$_2$). In contrast to endothelial cells, platelets lack PGI$_2$ synthetase. ADP promotes fibrinogen binding to platelet membranes, and thrombin is produced locally. Fibrinogen forms a bridge between adjacent activated platelets by binding to membrane fibrinogen receptors. ADP, endoperoxides, TxA$_2$, and thrombin in concert cause further release, resulting in the aggregation of circulating platelets to those already adherent, and amplify the release reaction.

Other substances are liberated from platelets during the release reaction, including serotonin (which may promote vasospasm in coronary vessels), platelet factor 4 (a basic glycoprotein that can neutralize the anticoagulant action

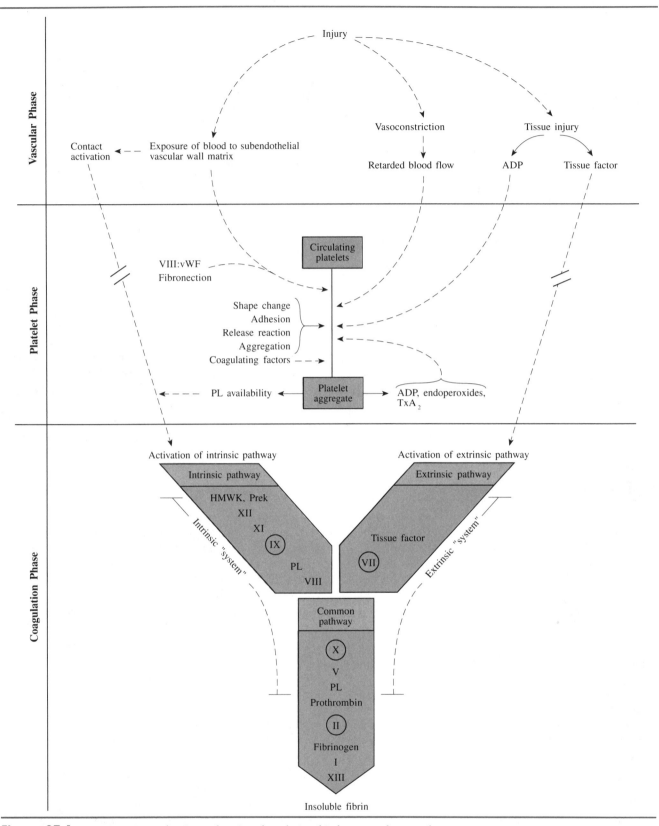

Figure 27-1. Hemostatic mechanisms, showing the relationship between the vascular, platelet, and coagulation phases. Action is denoted by dashed arrows; transformation by solid arrows. PL = platelet phospholipid; HMWK = high-molecular-weight kininogen; Prek = prekallikrein; ADP = adenosine diphosphate; vWF = von Willebrand factor; TxA$_2$ = thromboxane A$_2$. Circled factors are those that require vitamin K for activity. Proteins C and S, which also require vitamin K for activity, are not shown in this scheme. This figure is a highly simplified summary and the reader is referred to Supplemental Reading for further details. (Modified from M. M. Wintrobe et al., *Clinical Hematology* (7th ed.). Philadelphia: Lea & Febiger, 1974. Chaps. 9, p. 390, and 10, p. 422.)

of circulating heparin), platelet-derived growth factor (a mitogen that initiates smooth muscle cell proliferation and may be involved in atherogenesis), and factors that are also found in the plasma (factor V, factor VIII:vWF, and fibrinogen). During aggregation, the rearrangement of the platelet membrane makes available a phospholipid surface (*platelet factor 3*) that is required for the activation of several clotting factors. *The platelet aggregate becomes a hemostatic plug and is the structural foundation for the assembly of the fibrin network.*

Coagulation Systems

Two interrelated processes, the *intrinsic* and *extrinsic* coagulation systems (Fig. 27-1), cause the coagulation of blood in vitro and are the basis for laboratory coagulation tests. They both converge on a common pathway that leads to the activation of factor X, the formation of thrombin (factor IIa), and the conversion by thrombin of the soluble plasma protein fibrinogen into insoluble fibrin. The relative roles of these systems in coagulation in vivo is uncertain. *The extrinsic pathway appears to be important for initiating fibrin formation, while the intrinsic pathway is involved in fibrin growth and maintenance.* The extrinsic and intrinsic systems comprise the coagulation cascade. This series of linked and overlapping reactions involves factors that are proenzymes (designated by roman numerals) that are converted into serine proteases (designated by roman numeral followed by the suffix "a"), and cofactors that speed the protease reactions (factors V and VII).

Exposure of blood to tissue factors activate the extrinsic system, beginning with mild proteolytic conversion of factor VII into factor VIIa. The mechanism of activation of the intrinsic system in vivo after extravasation involves factors XI and XII, and high-molecular-weight kininogen-prekallikrein complex activation yielding factors XIa, XIIa, and kallikrein. The endogenous activator of the intrinsic system is not defined.

An acceleration in the degradation of factors V and VIII can occur following increases in the rate of coagulation reactions. This process can eventually give rise to an anticoagulant effect at locations distant from the site of vascular injury, thereby providing an additional mechanism for localization of clot formation.

The coagulation cascade is capable of tremendous amplification as the protease reactions progress. Many of the activated coagulation factors feed back positively in the extrinsic, intrinsic, and common pathways, and accelerate the formation of enzymatic products. Either deficiencies in a single clotting factor or therapy with the drugs described in this chapter will result in abnormal hemostasis. Treatment with these agents should be judicious, because

the margin of safety between insufficient therapy and hemorrhage is often small.

Anticoagulant Drugs

Anticoagulant drugs inhibit the inappropriate development and enlargement of clots by actions on the coagulation phase.

Heparin

Chemistry

Heparin is a mixture of highly electronegative acidic mucopolysaccharides that contain numerous *N*- and *O*-sulfate linkages. It is produced by, and can be released from, mast cells and is abundant in liver, lungs, and intestines. Commercial preparations are obtained by extraction from animal by-products (e.g., alimentary tract, lung).

Mechanism of Action

The anticoagulation action of heparin is dependent on the presence in normal blood of a specific *serine protease inhibitor* (serpin) of thrombin, *antithrombin III.* Heparin binds to antithrombin III and induces a conformational change that accelerates the interaction of antithrombin III with the coagulation factors. Heparin also catalyzes the inhibition of thrombin by heparin cofactor II, a circulating inhibitor. Lesser amounts of heparin are needed to prevent the formation of thrombin from prothrombin than are needed to inhibit thrombin's protease activity. This is the basis of "low-dose" prophylactic therapy.

Pharmacological Actions

The physiological function of heparin is not completely understood. It is found only in trace amounts in normal circulating blood. Heparin exerts an antilipemic effect by releasing lipoprotein lipase from endothelial cells. Heparinlike proteoglycans produced by endothelial cells have anticoagulation activity. Heparin may decrease platelet adhesiveness to endothelial cells, reduce the local release of platelet-derived growth factor, and exert an antiproliferative action on vascular smooth muscle. Heparin also possesses anticomplement and slight antihistaminic activity.

Therapy with heparin occurs in an inpatient setting. It can be used to establish anticoagulation while the delayed response to oral anticoagulants takes place. *Heparin inhibits both the in vitro and in vivo clotting of blood.* One-stage laboratory tests of coagulation (e.g., whole blood clotting time; activated partial thromboplastin time, or APTT) are prolonged in proportion to blood heparin concentrations, and can be influenced by blood levels of antithrombin III.

Absorption, Metabolism, and Excretion

Heparin is not well absorbed after oral administration and therefore must be given parenterally. Intravenous administration results in an almost immediate anticoagulant effect. There is an approximate 2-hr delay in onset of drug action after subcutaneous administration. Intramuscular injection of heparin is to be avoided because of the unpredictable absorption rates, local bleeding, and irritation that result.

After intravenous administration, heparin distribution is generally limited to the intravascular compartment; the drug is not bound to plasma proteins. Heparin is not secreted into breast milk, and it does not cross the placenta, as do orally effective anticoagulants. Depending on the route of administration, heparin is rapidly taken up by vascular and lymphatic endothelium and by cells of the reticuloendothelial system.

Heparin's action is terminated by uptake by the reticuloendothelial system, liver metabolism, and renal excretion of the unchanged drug and its depolymerized and desulfated metabolite. The relative proportion of administered drug that is excreted as unchanged heparin increases as the dose increases. Renal insufficiency reduces the rate of heparin clearance from the blood.

Adverse Reactions

The major adverse reaction resulting from heparin therapy is hemorrhage. Bleeding can occur in the urinary or gastrointestinal tracts and in the adrenal gland. Subdural hematoma, acute hemorrhagic pancreatitis, hemarthrosis, and wound ecchymosis also occur. The incidence of life-threatening hemorrhage is rather low, but variable. Heparin-induced thrombocytopenia of *immediate* and *delayed* onset may occur in 3 to 30 percent of patients and increases the risk of bleeding. The immediate type is transient during continuous therapy and may not involve platelet destruction. The delayed reaction is thought to involve the production of heparin-dependent antiplatelet antibodies and the clearance of platelets from the blood. Heparin-associated thrombocytopenia may be associated with thrombotic complications. Additional untoward effects of heparin treatment include hypersensitivity reactions (e.g., rash, urticaria, pruritus), fever, alopecia, hypoaldosteronism, osteoporosis, and osteoalgia.

Contraindications, Cautions, and Drug Interactions

Absolute contraindications that apply to therapy with heparin include serious or active bleeding; intracranial bleeding; recent brain, spinal cord, or eye surgery; severe liver or kidney disease; dissecting aortic aneurysm; and malignant hypertension. Relative contraindications include active gastrointestinal hemorrhage, recent stroke or major surgery, severe hypertension, bacterial endocarditis, threatened abortion, and severe renal or hepatic failure.

Drugs that inhibit platelet function (e.g., aspirin, dipyridamole) increase the risk of bleeding when heparin is administered. The presence of thrombocytopenia may rule out the use of heparin. *Oral anticoagulants and heparin produce synergistic effects.* Many basic drugs are chemically incompatible with the highly acidic heparin. For instance, antihistamines, quinidine, quinine, phenothiazines, tetracyclines, gentamicin, and neomycin may precipitate with heparin when placed in the same solution.

Minor hemorrhage occurring during heparin therapy is generally controlled either by dosage reduction or by discontinuing drug administration. *The specific heparin antagonist protamine can be employed to "neutralize" heparin in cases of serious hemorrhage.* Protamines are basic, low-molecular-weight, positively charged proteins that have a high affinity for the negatively charged heparin molecules. The binding of protamine to heparin is immediate and results in the formation of an inert complex. Protamine has some, albeit weak, anticoagulant activity. It is available as a powder to be dissolved. One milligram of protamine neutralizes 90 units of lung-derived heparin and 115 units of intestine-derived heparin.

Preparations and Dosage

Heparin is prescribed on a unit (IU) rather than milligram basis. It is available as *heparin sodium injection* and as *heparin calcium (Calciparine)*. Heparin sodium and heparin calcium are derived from different sources and may not be bioequivalent. The dose must always be determined on an individual basis.

Continuous IV infusions are usually given by drip or delivered with a pump. Intermittent IV therapy has been used, but it is associated with a higher risk of hemorrhagic complications. *SC administration* of the repository form of heparin is also used.

Orally Effective Anticoagulants

Chemistry

The orally effective anticoagulant drugs are fat-soluble derivatives of 4-hydroxycoumarin or of indan-1,3-dione. They bear a close structural resemblance to vitamin K (Fig. 27-2). Warfarin is the oral anticoagulant of choice. The indandione anticoagulants have greater toxicity than the coumarin drugs.

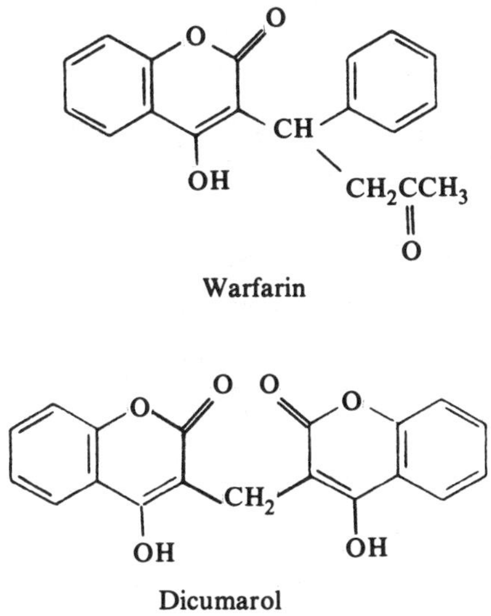

Figure 27-2. Chemical structures of two major oral anticoagulants.

Mechanism of Action

Unlike heparin, *the oral anticoagulants induce hypocoagulability only in vivo.* They are vitamin K antagonists. Vitamin K is required to catalyze the conversion of the precursors of certain vitamin K–dependent clotting factors and of proteins C and S into active forms. This involves the posttranslational γ-carboxylation of glutamic acid residues, which is an obligatory synthetic step required for the coagulation factors to bind via Ca^{2+} to membrane phospholipid surface on which the protease reactions take place. The γ-carboxylation step is linked to a cycle of enzyme reactions involving the active hydroquinone form of vitamin K (K_1H_2). The regeneration of K_1H_2 by an epoxide reductase *thus causes hypocoagulability by inducing the formation of structurally incomplete clotting factors.*

Pharmacological Actions

The oral anticoagulants are used both on an inpatient and outpatient basis when long-term therapy is indicated. The onset of anticoagulant action is delayed, the latent period being determined in part by pharmacokinetic properties of the individual drugs and in part by the half-lives of the vitamin K–dependent clotting factors. *The anticoagulant effect will not be evident until the active factors already present in the blood are catabolized;* this takes from 5 hr for factor VII to 2 to 3 days for prothrombin. Peak anticoagulation occurring after 3 days of therapy reflects reduc-

tions in the levels of all four vitamin K–dependent clotting factors. The action of these drugs will be potentiated by a reduced dietary intake of vitamin K or fat and by disorders that impair vitamin K absorption.

Absorption, Metabolism, and Excretion

Warfarin is rapidly and almost completely absorbed after oral administration, whereas the absorption of dicumarol and the other anticoagulants is erratic and delayed. These drugs are bound extensively to plasma albumin ($>$ 95%) and, therefore, have relatively long plasma half-lives. Since it is the unbound drug that produces the anticoagulant effect, displacement of albumin-bound drug by other agents may result in bleeding. Although these drugs do not cross the blood-brain barrier, they can cross the placenta and may cause teratogenicity and hemorrhage in the fetus.

Warfarin and dicumarol are inactivated by hepatic microsomal enzymes.

Adverse Reactions

The principal adverse reaction encountered during oral anticoagulant therapy is hemorrhage. Prolonged therapy with the coumarin-type anticoagulants is relatively free of untoward effects. Bleeding may be observable (e.g., skin, mucous membranes) or occult (e.g., gastrointestinal, renal, cerebral, hepatic, uterine, or pulmonary hemorrhage). Rarer untoward effects include diarrhea, small intestine necrosis, urticaria, alopecia, skin necrosis, and dermatitis.

Contraindications, Cautions, and Drug Interactions

Oral anticoagulants are ordinarily contraindicated in the presence of active or past gastrointestinal ulceration; thrombocytopenia; hepatic or renal disease; malignant hypertension; recent brain, eye, or spinal cord surgery; bacterial endocarditis; chronic alcoholism; and pregnancy. These agents also should not be prescribed for individuals with physically hazardous occupations.

Minor hemorrhage caused by oral anticoagulant overdosage can be treated by discontinuing drug administration. Vitamin K_1 (phytonadione, *AquaMEPHYTON*) administration will return prothrombin time to normal within 24 hr. Several hours are required for de novo synthesis of biologically active coagulation factors. *Serious hemorrhage may be stopped by administration of fresh frozen plasma or plasma concentrates containing vitamin K–dependent factors.*

Prior or concomitant therapy with a large number of pharmacologically unrelated drugs can either potentiate

Table 27-1. Drug Interactions Involving
Oral Anticoagulants*

Drugs that increase oral anticoagulant effects	
Alcohol (acute intoxication)	Ketoconazole
Allopurinol	Lovastatin
Amiodarone	Mefenamic acid
Anabolic and androgenic steroids	Metronidazole
Aspirin	Micolazole
Cephalosporins	Nalidixic acid
Chloral hydrate	Naproxen
Chloramphenicol	Omeprazole
Cimetidine	Oral hypoglycemics
Clofibrate	Oxyphenbutazone
Cyclophosphamide	Phenylbutazone
Diflunisal	Phenytoin
Disulfiram	Peroxicam
Erythromycin	Phenylbutazone
Fenoprofen	Propafenone
Fluconazole	Propoxyphene
Fluoroquinolones	Quinidine, quinine
Flurbiprofen	Sulfamethoxazole-
Gemfibrozil	trimethoprim
Glucagon	Sulfinpyrazone
Heparin	Sulindac
Ibuprofen	Tamoxifen
Ifosfamide	Ticlopidine
Indomethacin	Tolmetin
Isoniazid	Tricyclic antidepressants
	Vitamin E (large doses)

Drugs that decrease oral anticoagulant effects	
Alcohol (chronic abuse)	Glutethimide
Aminoglutethimide	Griseofulvin
Antacids	Meprobamate
Azathioprine	Nafcillin
Barbiturates	Oral contraceptives
Carbamazepine	Penicillins (large doses)
Cholestyramine	Primadone
Corticosteroids	Rifampin
Dextrothyroxine	Thioamides
Diuretics	Trazodone
Ethchlorvynol	Vitamin K (large doses)

*Oral anticoagulants also may potentiate hypoglycemia caused by oral
hypoglycemic agents, and may enhance phenytoin toxicity.

or inhibit the actions of oral anticoagulants. Laxatives and
mineral oil may reduce the absorption of the oral anticoagulants. The patient's prothrombin time should be monitored whenever a drug is added or removed from therapy.
Selected drug interactions involving oral anticoagulants
are summarized in Table 27-1.

Preparations and Dosage

Warfarin sodium (*Coumadin, Panwarfin*) is available in
1-, 2-, 2.5-, 5-, 7.5-, and 10-mg tablets.
Dicumarol (generic) is available as 25- and 50-mg capsules or tablets.
Anisindione (*Miradon*) is usually employed if intoler-

ance to coumarin anticoagulants is present. The drug is
long acting and potentially very toxic.

Clinical Indications for Anticoagulant Therapy

Anticoagulant therapy provides prophylactic treatment of venous and arterial thromboembolic disorders.
Anticoagulant drugs are ineffective against already
formed thrombi, although they may prevent their further
propagation. Generally accepted major indications for anticoagulant therapy with heparin and the orally effective
drugs are similar and include the following:

Deep Vein Thrombosis and Pulmonary Embolism

Venous stasis resulting from prolonged periods of bed
rest, cardiac failure, or pelvic, abdominal, or hip joint surgery may precipitate thrombus formation in the deep
veins of the leg or calf. In addition to the damage to the
venous circulation, deep vein thrombosis may lead to fatal
pulmonary embolism. Renal vein thrombosis places patients at the highest risk of pulmonary embolism.
Heparin is of *prophylactic* benefit in reducing the appearance of deep vein and pulmonary thrombosis after
surgery in low- to moderate-risk patients.

Arterial Embolism

Heparin and the oral anticoagulants are equally effective in preventing venous thrombosis formation. However, since arterial emboli formation involves platelet aggregation and leukocyte and erythrocyte infiltration into
the fibrin network, the treatment and prophylaxis of arterial thrombi are more difficult. Arterial embolism is
treated more successfully with heparin than with the oral
anticoagulants.

Prevention of Arterial Emboli Arising from Valvular Heart Disease and Prosthetic Heart Valves

Anticoagulants are useful therapy in the prevention of
systemic emboli resulting from valvular disease (rheumatic heart disease) and from valve replacement. In the
latter case, addition of antiplatelet drugs (see below) may
provide an additional therapeutic benefit.

Atrial Fibrillation

Restoration of sinus rhythm in atrial fibrillation may
dislodge thrombi that have developed as a result of stasis

in the enlarged left atrium. The risk of stroke and systemic arterial embolism is significantly decreased by achieving anticoagulation in such patients.

Myocardial Infarction and Coronary Artery Disease

The goals of anticoagulant therapy in survivors of acute myocardial infarction are the prevention of subsequent venous thrombosis, pulmonary embolism, and recurrent infarction. *Thrombolytic drugs are more effective than anticoagulants in treating coronary thromboembolism and in establishing reperfusion of occluded arteries after an infarction.* While there is a rational basis for their use, the regimens and long-term benefits of adjunctive anticoagulant therapy along with thrombolytic therapy are not yet firmly established.

Coronary Artery Bypass Grafts and Angioplasty

Anticoagulants, in combination with antiplatelet drugs, have reduced the incidence of thrombus formation and reocclusion after coronary arterial bypass surgery and percutaneous coronary angioplasty.

Disseminated Intravascular Coagulation

Disseminated intravascular coagulation is characterized by a widespread systemic activation of the coagulation system, consumption of coagulation factors, occlusion of small vessels by a coat of fibrin, and a hypocoagulable state with bleeding. In conjunction with management of the underlying etiologic factor(s) leading to the disorder, and coagulation factor and platelet replacement, bleeding may be reversed with IV heparin.

Anticoagulants in Clinical Trial

Low-molecular-weight fractions of heparin (LMWH; <6,000 molecular weight) that have fourfold greater antifactor Xa activity than antithrombin activity, and that cause less platelet aggregation and thrombocytopenia, are under evaluation. Low-molecular-weight fractions of heparin have greater bioavailability and produce longer anticoagulation than unfractionated heparin.

Hirudin, a potent anticoagulant originally obtained from leeches, but now made available through recombinant DNA technology, binds with great affinity to thrombin and inhibits its proteolytic activity, fibrin formation on platelets, and platelet aggregatory activity. Antithrombin III is not involved in hirudin's action, and bleeding time is not affected.

Antiplatelet Drugs

The formation of platelet aggregates and thrombi in arterial blood may precipitate coronary vasospasm and occlusion, and myocardial infarction, and contribute to atherosclerotic plaque development. Drugs that inhibit platelet function are administered for the relatively specific prophylaxis of arterial thrombosis and for the therapeutic management of myocardial infarction.

Antiplatelet therapy must be initiated soon after an infarction has occurred, that is, within 2 hr, for significant benefit against reinfarction and morbidity reduction to be obtained. The antiplatelet drugs are administered as adjuncts to thrombolytic therapy, along with heparin, to maintain perfusion and to limit the size of the infarction.

Aspirin is an inhibitor of platelet aggregation and prolongs the bleeding time. It is of prophylactic use in preventing coronary thrombosis in patients with unstable angina, as an adjunct to thrombolytic therapy, and in reducing recurrence of thrombotic stroke. The drug acetylates and inhibits irreversibly cyclooxygenase both in platelets, preventing the formation of TxA_2, and in endothelial cells, inhibiting the synthesis of PGI_2. While endothelial cells can synthesize cyclooxygenase, platelets cannot. *The goal of therapy with aspirin is to inhibit selectively the synthesis of platelet TxA_2 and thereby inhibit platelet aggregation.* This is accomplished with a low dose of aspirin (one 325-mg tablet every other day), which spares the endothelial synthesis of PGI_2. Aspirin-inhibited platelets can nevertheless be activated by thrombin.

Dipyridamole (*Persantine*), a coronary vasodilator, does not alter bleeding time or platelet aggregation in vitro, but decreases platelet adhesiveness to damaged endothelium. The drug is a phosphodiesterase inhibitor and increases platelet cyclic adenosine monophosphate (cAMP) concentration. It also may potentiate the effect of PGI_2, which stimulates platelet adenylate cyclase. These effects would prevent both platelet aggregation and the release reaction. However, dipyridamole itself neither prevents nor exerts a prophylactic effect on the incidence of death following myocardial infarction. A beneficial effect in antithrombotic therapy may occur when the drug is used in combination with aspirin or when it is combined prophylactically with warfarin in patients with artificial heart valves. Dipyridamole is available in 25-, 50-, and 75-mg tablets.

Ticlopidine inhibits platelet aggregation and prolongs bleeding time. Its mechanism of action is not fully understood. Ticlopidine may interfere with exposure of platelet membrane glycoprotein IIb/IIIa (GPIIb/IIIa) in response to ADP. GPIIb/IIIa is the platelet fibrinogen receptor that, through fibrinogen, links platelets together to form an aggregate. Ticlopidine has been approved for the secondary prevention of thrombotic stroke in patients with a previous history who cannot tolerate aspirin. Ticlopidine

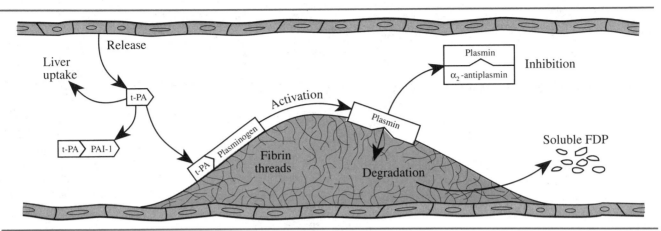

Figure 27-3. The fibrinolytic system in blood vessels, showing the mechanisms of activation of plasminogen on fibrin and the effects of physiological inhibitors of tissue-type plasminogen activator (t-PA) and plasmin. The release of t-PA from vascular endothelium is depicted. PAI-1 = plasminogen activator inhibitor-1; FDP = fibrin degradation products. (Modified and reprinted with permission from B. Wiman and A. Hamsten, *Semin. Thromb. Hemost.* 16:209, 1990, Thieme Medical Publishers, Inc.)

is well absorbed orally, binds weakly to plasma proteins, and is metabolized by the liver. Dosage with ticlopidine hydrochloride (*Ticlid*) is 250 mg twice a day with food. Gastrointestinal disturbances and agranulocytosis have been observed in patients receiving ticlopidine.

Sulfinpyrazone (*Anturane*), a nonsteroidal antiinflammatory agent, is a competitive inhibitor of cyclooxygenase, but its precise action in platelets is not known. The drug inhibits platelet adherence and the release reaction. It has no effect on platelet aggregation or on bleeding time, but it prolongs circulating platelet survival time. The effectiveness of sulfinpyrazone as primary therapy after myocardial infarction has not been established unequivocally. The drug may be useful (800 mg/day) for secondary prevention in patients who cannot tolerate aspirin.

Drugs that can inhibit platelet function but have unproven clinical efficacy include hydroxychloroquine, clofibrate, certain prostaglandins, indomethacin, phenylbutazone, tricyclic antidepressants, and some phenothiazine antipsychotic agents.

Fibrinolytic System

The fibrinolytic system (Fig. 27-3) is involved in restricting clot propagation in the blood and in the removal of fibrin as wounds heal. The fibrinolytic system is the functional antithesis of the coagulation system, but it is activated simultaneously with hemostatic mechanisms. Treatment of patients with *thrombolytic drugs* that activate the fibrinolytic system is not a substitute for the anticoagulant drugs. On the one hand, *anticoagulant and antiplatelet drugs are administered prophylactically to prevent thrombus formation and propagation, while on the other hand, the purpose of thrombolytic therapy is to rapidly lyse already formed clots. Thrombolytic drugs produce more profound alterations in the blood than are produced with anticoagulant and antiplatelet drugs.*

Fibrinolysis is initiated by the activation of the proenzyme *plasminogen* (present in clots and in plasma) to *plasmin*, a protease enzyme not normally present in blood. Plasmin catalyzes the degradation of fibrin. The conversion of plasminogen to plasmin is initiated normally by the *plasminogen activators, tissue-type plasminogen activator (t-PA) and single-chain urokinase-type plasminogen activator (scu-PA).* t-PA and scu-PA are serine protease enzymes synthesized by the endothelium and released into the circulation. The endothelium also releases *plasminogen activator inhibitor-1 (PAI-1)*, which complexes with and inactivates t-PA in the plasma.

t-PA and scu-PA bind with high affinity to fibrin on the clot surface. Circulating plasminogen binds to the plasminogen activator-fibrin complex to form a ternary complex consisting of fibrin, activator, and plasminogen. Therefore, the specificity of t-PA and scu-PA binding to fibrin normally localizes plasmin protease activity to thrombi.

Circulating plasmin is rapidly neutralized by α_2-antiplasmin, a physiological serine protease inhibitor that forms an inert complex with plasmin. In contrast, fibrin-bound plasmin is resistant to inactivation by α_2-antiplasmin. Under normal circumstances plasma t-PA is inactive because it is inhibited by PAI-1, while t-PA bound to fibrin is unaffected by PAI-1. In addition, plasma t-PA has a very rapid turnover in blood (half-life = 5–8 min). For these reasons, fibrinolysis is normally restricted to the thrombus.

Activation of the fibrinolytic system with thrombolytic drugs can disturb the balance of these regulatory mechanisms and elevate circulating plasmin activity. Plasmin has low substrate specificity and can degrade fibrinogen (*fibrinogenolysis*), plasminogen, α_2-antiplasmin, and factors V and VIII. The systemic activation of the fibrinolytic system with thrombolytic drugs causes consumption of the coagulation factors, a lytic state, and bleeding.

Thrombolytic Drugs

Mechanism of Action

Thrombolytic drugs are plasminogen activators. The ideal thrombolytic agent is one that can be administered intravenously to produce a clot-selective fibrinolysis without activating plasminogen to plasmin in plasma. The first-generation thrombolytic agents (e.g., **streptokinase** and **urokinase**) are not clot selective, and appreciable systemic fibrinogenolysis accompanies successful clot lysis. Second-generation thrombolytic agents (e.g., *t-PA*) bind selectively to fibrin and cause clot-selective fibrinolysis with less systematic fibrinogenolysis.

Pharmacological Actions and Clinical Uses

Thrombolytic agents have been shown to cause lysis of formed clots in both arteries and veins and to reestablish tissue perfusion. They are indicated in the management of severe pulmonary embolism, deep vein thrombosis, and arterial thromboembolism.

Thrombolytic drugs are especially important therapy in heart attack patients. While all of the thrombolytic agents are effective, the second-generation drugs are more efficacious at lysing coronary arterial thrombi and reestablishing myocardial perfusion. After myocardial infarction, thrombolysis in the affected coronary artery must be accomplished quickly in order to limit the size of the infarction. Clots become more difficult to lyse as they age. Recanalization after approximately 6 hr provides little benefit to the infarcted area. The incidence of rethrombosis and reinfarction is greater when thrombolytic drugs with shorter plasma half-lives are used. Concurrent therapy with heparin, followed by warfarin, as well as aspirin, has been advocated to reduce reocclusion. The ideal protocols and long-term benefit of such combination therapy have not been firmly established. Adjunctive anticoagulant and antiplatelet drugs probably contribute to bleeding accompanying thrombolytic therapy.

Early thrombolytic therapy provides a significant improvement in left ventricular function and reduction in postinfarction short-term (1 month) mortality. Whether a long-term (5 years) reduction in mortality is achieved after thrombolytic therapy is not known at present.

Thrombolytic therapy with available agents causes hypofibrinogenemia, and laboratory tests of reduced clotting activity (e.g., 2- to 2.5-fold with the APTT) are needed to monitor the induced coagulation defect. The second-generation agents, both approved and under evaluation, cause, at effective thrombolytic doses, a much less extensive fibrinogenolysis, but bleeding occurs with similar incidence for all agents.

Adverse Reactions

The principal adverse effect associated with thrombolytic therapy is bleeding, and is usually mild and common at sites of arterial or venous puncture. Bleeding may involve systemic fibrinogenolysis, but fibrinolysis of hemostatic plugs at sites of vascular injury is thought to be the primary cause. The incidence of bleeding is similar with all of the currently available thrombolytic drugs; that is, the bleeding side effect is not eliminated with fibrin-selective agents. Life-threatening intracranial bleeding has been observed in 1 percent of patients. Severe bleeding may necessitate stoppage of therapy, administration of whole blood, platelets or fresh frozen plasma, protamine (if heparin has been administered), and administration of an antifibrinolytic drug (discussed at the end of this chapter).

Contraindications

The contraindications to the use of thrombolytic drugs are similar to those for the anticoagulants. Absolute contraindications to thrombolytic therapy include active bleeding, cardiopulmonary resuscitation (trauma to thorax is possible), intracranial trauma, vascular disease, and cancer. Relative contraindications include uncontrolled hypertension, earlier central nervous system surgery, and any known bleeding risk.

Specific Thrombolytic Drugs

Streptokinase

Streptokinase, a nonenzymatic protein from Lancefield group C β-hemolytic streptococci, is an *indirectly acting* activator of plasminogen. It forms a 1:1 complex with plasminogen, which results in the exposure of an active site that can convert additional plasminogen into plasmin.

The systemic administration of streptokinase can produce significant lysis of acute deep vein and pulmonary emboli and acute arterial thrombi. Treatment is, however, usually less, or not, effective in subacute or chronic occlusions. Intravenous or intracoronary artery (IC) streptokinase is very effective in establishing recanalization after myocardial infarction and in increasing short-term survival.

Intracoronary administration delivers a high concentration of the drug at the site where it is needed, lessens the induction of a lytic state, and protects the drug from inactivation by antibodies. These theoretical advantages of the intracoronary route are offset by the limited availability of facilities for intracoronary drug delivery and the inherent delay in catheterizing the patient for therapy. The greatest benefit of streptokinase appears to be achieved by early intravenous drug administration. Intravenous streptokinase, followed by intracoronary infusion of the drug in the hospital, may be more effective than intravenous therapy alone.

Complications associated with the administration of streptokinase include hemorrhage in up to one third of treated patients, pyrexia, and allergic-anaphylactic reactions. Patients may become refractory to streptokinase during therapy due to the presence of preexisting or streptokinase-induced antibodies. Streptokinase has two half-lives. The faster one (11–13 min) is due to drug distribution and inhibition by circulating antibodies, and the slower one (23–29 min) is due to loss of enzyme activity.

Streptokinase (*Streptase, Kabikinase*) is available as a powder for reconstitution with 0.9% saline or 5% dextrose.

Urokinase

Urokinase, or two-chain urokinase-type plasminogen activator, is a two-polypeptide chain serine protease that activates plasminogen directly. It activates both circulating and fibrin-bound plasminogen. It is obtained from primary culture of human fetal kidney cells. The plasma half-life of urokinase is approximately 10 to 20 min. Urokinase is not antigenic in humans.

Clinical evaluation of urokinase has not been as extensive as that for streptokinase. Urokinase produces a significant resolution of recent pulmonary emboli. It is more effective than heparin therapy for large pulmonary emboli, especially in patients in shock. The drug is approved for intravenous and intracoronary use after myocardial infarction. Urokinase is not as widely used as streptokinase and t-PA.

Urokinase (*Abbokinase*) is available as a powder for reconstitution with water.

Second-Generation Thrombolytics

Tissue-Type Plasminogen Activator

Tissue-type plasminogen activator (t-PA) is a second-generation thrombolytic drug that has several advantages over streptokinase in its ability to lyse coronary arterial thrombi after myocardial infarction. The drug has a high binding affinity for fibrin and produces, after intravenous administration, a fibrin-selective activation of plasminogen. This selectivity is not absolute; circulating plasminogen also may be activated by large doses or lengthy treatment.

After intravenous administration, t-PA is more efficacious (70–75% patency) than streptokinase in establishing coronary reperfusion. At equieffective thrombolytic doses of t-PA and streptokinase, t-PA causes less fibrinogenolysis, but bleeding nevertheless occurs with a similar incidence.

The rate of rethrombosis after t-PA is greater than after streptokinase, possibly because of the faster clearance of t-PA from plasma. It has been suggested that reocclusion may be lessened by continued infusion with t-PA or with simultaneous administration of heparin and antiplatelet drugs. Insufficient evidence exists to ascertain the benefits of adding these drugs to thrombolytic therapy.

The t-PA available currently is a product of recombinant DNA technology and consists predominantly of the single-chain form. It is referred to as recombinant human tissue-type plasminogen activator (rt-PA), and altepase, recombinant. Single-chain rt-PA has a shorter plasma half-life (5 min) than two-chain rt-PA (8 min), and a greater dose is needed to achieve a similar thrombolytic effect. Upon exposure to fibrin, single-chain rt-PA is converted to the two-chain dimer. rt-PA (altepase; *Activase*) is available as a powder for reconstitution with water.

Anistreplase

Anistreplase (acetylated streptokinase-plasminogen activator complex, ASPAC) consists of streptokinase in a noncovalent 1:1 complex with plasminogen. Anistreplase is catalytically inert due to acylation of the catalytic site of plasminogen. It has a long catalytic half-life (90 min), and the time required for deacylation lengthens its thrombolytic effect after IV injection. Anistreplase is more effective than streptokinase in establishing coronary reperfusion, but it causes considerable fibrinogenolysis and is antigenic. It is available (*Eminase*) as a powder for reconstitution with water.

Thrombolytic Agents and Combinations in Clinical Trial

Several preparations developed to improve thrombolytic efficiency, or to increase fibrin specificity and decrease fibrinogenolytic activity, are under clinical investigation for their benefit after myocardial infarction.

Saruplase (*Sandolase;* recombinant single-chain urokinase-type plasminogen activator, rscu-PA, pro-urokinase), in contrast to urokinase (two-chain), has a high binding affinity for fibrin, where it is converted by small amounts of plasmin to two-chain urokinase. In its coronary thrombolytic effectiveness, ability to cause fibrinogenolysis, and clearance rate, saruplase is very similar to rt-PA.

t-PA Plus rscu-PA

Different mechanisms determine t-PA and rscu-PA binding to fibrin, which offers the potential of drug synergism. In early studies these agents together in one-fifth normal dosages produced reperfusion of coronary artery, with little fibrinogenolysis.

Antifibrinolytic Drugs

Hyperplasminemia resulting from thrombolytic therapy exposes fibrinogen and other coagulation factors, plasminogen, and α_2-antiplasmin to nonspecific proteolysis by plasmin, a process normally regulated by α_2-antiplasmin. Consumption of these factors and extensive fibrin dissolution may lead to hemorrhage. The binding of plasminogen to fibrin involves lysine interactions with lysine-binding sites in plasmin(ogen). These interactions are blocked by *antifibrinolytic drugs,* and plasminogen activation and plasmin proteolytic activity are inhibited.

In addition to being an antidote to thrombolytic therapy, antifibrinolytic drugs are used as adjuncts to coagulation factor replacement to control bleeding accompanying surgery (tonsillectomy) and dental procedures in hemophiliacs. Antifibrinolytic drugs are contraindicated if intravascular coagulation is present. These drugs may cause nausea.

The antifibrinolytic drug aminocaproic acid (*Amicar*) is available for IV or oral administration.

Tranexamic acid (*Cyklokapron*) is more potent and longer acting than aminocaproic acid. It is administered IV or orally.

Supplemental Reading

Cairns, J.A., et al. Antithrombotic agents in coronary artery disease. *Chest* 102:456S, 1992.
Collen, D., and Lijnen, H.R. Thrombosis and Thrombolysis. In H.A. Fozzard et al. (eds.), *The Heart and Cardiovascular System* (2nd ed.). New York: Raven, 1992. P. 275.
Davie, E.W., et al. The coagulation cascade: Initiation, maintenance, and regulation. *Biochemistry* 30:10363, 1991.
Eisenberg, P.R. Role of new anticoagulants as adjunctive therapy during thrombolysis. *Am. J. Cardiol.* 67:19A, 1991.
Fears, R. Biochemical pharmacology and therapeutic aspects of thrombolytic agents. *Pharmacol. Rev.* 42:201, 1990.
Furie, B., and Furie, B.C. Molecular and cellular biology of blood coagulation. *N. Engl. J. Med.* 326:800, 1992.
Haynes, R.B., et al. A critical appraisal of ticlopidine, a new antiplatelet agent. *Arch. Intern. Med.* 152:1376, 1992.
Mammen, E.F. Why low molecular weight heparin? *Semin. Thromb. Hemost.* 16:1S, 1990.
Mosher, D.F. Disorders of Blood Coagulation. In J.B. Wyngaarden et al. (eds.), *Cecil Textbook of Medicine* (19th ed.). Philadelphia: Harcourt Brace Jovanovich, 1992. P. 998.
Pratt, C.W., and Church, F.C. Antithrombin: Structure and function. *Semin. Hematol.* 28:3, 1991.
Verstraete, M. Heparin and thrombosis: A seventy year long story. *Haemostasis* 20:4S, 1990.
Verstraete, M. Advances in thrombolytic therapy. *Cardiovasc. Drugs Ther.* 6:111, 1992.
Wessler, S., and Gitel, S.N. Pharmacology of heparin and warfarin. *J. Am. Coll. Cardiol.* 8:10B, 1988.
Williams, W.J., et al. (eds.). *Hematology* (4th ed.). New York: McGraw-Hill, 1990.

IV

Drugs Affecting the Central Nervous System

Introduction to Central Nervous System Pharmacology

Charles R. Craig

In this section we focus principally on drugs that affect the central nervous system (CNS); that is, we are concerned with agents that have a primary action on the brain and spinal cord. The CNS is much more complex and less well understood than are other organs and, in many cases, the mechanism of action of neuropharmacological agents is not clear. However, all the agents discussed have in common the capacity to alter brain function.

Review of Basic Neuroscience

It is presumed that the functional unit of the CNS is the neuron, that most neuropharmacological agents have the neuron as their primary site of action, and that these agents act by somehow altering the normal function of that neuron.

CNS neurons, like those in the periphery, are capable of transmitting information to, and receiving information from, other neurons and peripheral end organs, such as muscle cells, glandular cells, and specialized receptors (such as those involved with proprioception, temperature sensing, etc.).

The depolarization associated with an action potential results in the release of a specific chemical substance at the synapse between two neurons. This chemical substance (or *neurotransmitter*) is released, diffuses across the synaptic cleft, and interacts with the second neuron to initiate a local change in the ionic composition and a local altered potential difference in the second neuron. This potential difference change is known as a *postsynaptic potential* and the direction of the potential change may be either *depolarizing* or *hyperpolarizing*. A depolarizing postsynaptic potential is called an *excitatory postsynaptic potential* (EPSP). If the magnitude of depolarization produced by EPSPs in the

second neuron is great enough, an action potential will be produced in the second neuron that will be transmitted in an all-or-none fashion through the neuron and its processes. If, on the other hand, a hyperpolarizing potential (known as an *inhibitory postsynaptic potential,* or IPSP) is produced, it will inhibit the formation of depolarizing action potentials.

Most cells normally receive a large excitatory input, and the net result of IPSPs will be to decrease the number of nerve impulses generated per unit of time. By these mechanisms, neurotransmitters producing either an EPSP (*excitatory neurotransmitter*) or an IPSP (*inhibitory transmitter*) are able to influence directly the number of action potentials generated by the neurons with which they interact.

Morphologically, many synapses in the CNS appear to be quite similar to those previously described for the peripheral autonomic nervous system. Electron microscopic studies have verified the similarities and, additionally, have shown the presence of several types of vesicles in the areas of synapses. It is generally accepted that the vesicles serve as storage sites for transmitter substances. Neurons may synthesize, store, and release one or more transmitters.

The major difference between neurons in the peripheral autonomic nervous system and those in the CNS is the complexity of the circuitry of the latter. It is clear that many more synapses exist in the CNS, that many more neurotransmitters are involved, and that very precise self-regulatory processes occur within and between nerve endings.

It should be apparent that several ways exist in which neuropharmacological agents could act to modify neurotransmission. The agent could effectively increase the amount of transmitter at the synapse and thereby produce an exaggerated effect. This can be accomplished by increasing the rate of transmitter synthesis, by increasing the rate of transmitter release, by prolonging the time the transmitter is in the synapse, or by decreasing the transmitter's enzymatic breakdown. Since the actions of several CNS transmitters are terminated by an active neuronal uptake mechanism (similar to that established for norepinephrine in the peripheral sympathetic nervous system), drugs could produce an exaggerated neuronal response by inhibiting the reuptake of a previously released transmitter.

On the other hand, a drug could cause a diminished response by decreasing synthesis of transmitter, by increasing transmitter metabolism, by promoting an increased neuronal uptake, or by blocking access of the transmitter to its receptor. As has been discussed in previous chapters, agents are presently available that possess most of these capabilities at norepinephrine or acetylcholine (ACh) synapses in the peripheral autonomic nervous system. Many of the same drugs function similarly at noradrenergic and cholinergic sites in the CNS. Likewise, there is evidence that some drugs can interfere with other CNS transmitter systems in some of the above-mentioned ways to produce their effects.

In the mammalian CNS, unlike the peripheral autonomic nervous system, there are powerful inhibitory systems that function continually. The effects of stimulating an excitatory pathway can appear to be exaggerated if normal inhibitory influences to that region are diminished. Correspondingly, the effects of activation of an inhibitory pathway can appear exaggerated if part of the excitatory influence to that system has been removed.

Central Nervous System Neurotransmitters

A large number of CNS neurotransmitters have been either tentatively or positively identified. While a detailed discussion of the various central neurotransmitters and the criteria for their identification is beyond the scope of this text, a summary of the most important mammalian central neurotransmitters is considered worthwhile.

Acetylcholine

The discovery that acetylcholine (ACh) was a transmitter in the peripheral nervous system formed the basis for the theory of neurotransmission. It is now known that acetylcholine is also a neurotransmitter in the mammalian brain. Due to technical difficulties, only a few cholinergic

tracts have been clearly delineated. ACh is an excitatory neurotransmitter in the mammalian CNS.

Dopamine

In the peripheral sympathetic nervous system, norepinephrine and epinephrine are the most important biogenic amine neurotransmitters. Quantitatively, in the CNS, dopamine is the most important. Large concentrations of dopamine are found in the basal ganglia (particularly in the caudate nucleus), as well as in other areas of the midbrain. The concentration of dopamine in the brain of patients with Parkinson's disease is markedly reduced (see Chap. 38). Several classes of drugs (notably the antipsychotics, Chap. 35) are capable of interacting with dopaminergic transmission. Dopamine appears to be exclusively an inhibitory neurotransmitter.

Norepinephrine

Most central noradrenergic neurons are located in the nucleus locus coeruleus of the pons and in neurons of the reticular formation. Fibers from these nuclei innervate a large number of cortical, subcortical, and spinomedullary fields. Many functions have been ascribed to the central noradrenergic neurons, including a role in affective disorders (see Chap. 36), in learning and memory, and in sleep-wake cycle regulation. The mammalian CNS contains both α- and β-adrenoceptors.

Epinephrine

Epinephrine is found only in very low concentration in the mammalian CNS, and it has been questioned whether or not it has any role to play in CNS function. However, enzymes for the synthesis of epinephrine are present in the CNS and, therefore, it is possible that epinephrine may serve as a central neurotransmitter, possibly in blood pressure regulation.

Serotonin

Serotonin (5-hydroxytryptamine) is present in the brain as well as in the periphery. In humans, about 90 percent of the total serotonin in the body is in enterochromaffin cells in the gastrointestinal tract; the remaining 10 percent is primarily in the platelets and brain. The physiological significance of the vast amounts of serotonin constantly synthesized and metabolized in the periphery still remains an enigma. Brain serotonin, on the other hand,

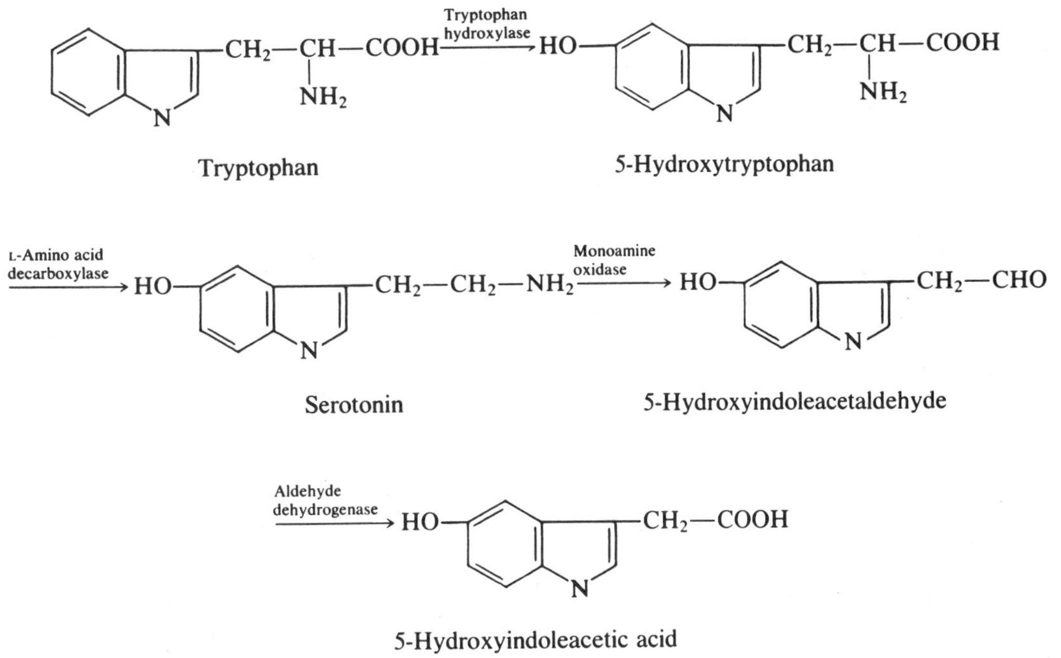

Figure 28-1. Steps involved in the synthesis and metabolic degradation of serotonin.

has been implicated as a potential neurotransmitter in the mediation of a wide variety of phenomena (see Actions).

Synthesis

Dietary tryptophan serves as the source for the formation of serotonin within the body. Enzymes and cofactors necessary for serotonin synthesis are present in both the enterochromaffin cells of the gastrointestinal tract and the brain. Tryptophan is initially hydroxylated to form 5-hydroxytryptophan. Decarboxylation of the latter compound results in the formation of serotonin (Fig. 28-1).

Distribution

Like the enterochromaffin cells and central neurons, platelets also contain storage granules for serotonin. Although platelets cannot synthesize serotonin, these cells do have the capacity for its uptake by both passive and active mechanisms. Normally, release of serotonin from platelets appears to occur only during the thrombin-induced release reaction and during platelet destruction.

Metabolism

The enzymes responsible for the metabolism of serotonin are present in all of the cells containing this amine

and in the liver as well. Serotonin is initially oxidatively deaminated to form 5-hydroxyindoleacetaldehyde; this compound is subsequently rapidly oxidized to the major metabolite 5-hydroxyindoleacetic acid (see Fig. 28-1), which is then excreted in the urine.

Actions

Most of the serotonin in the brain is localized in the raphe nuclei; considerable amounts also are present in areas of the hypothalamus, the limbic system, the brainstem, and the pituitary gland. Current evidence indicates that serotonin is involved in the regulation of several aspects of behavior, including sleep, pain perception, depression, sexual activity, and aggressiveness. Some newer antidepressant agents are believed to prevent the reuptake of serotonin (see Chap. 36). Serotonin also appears to be involved in temperature regulation and in the hypothalamic control of the release of pituitary hormones.

In addition to its presumed role as a neurotransmitter within the brain, serotonin indirectly affects the activity of the CNS. It is synthesized locally in the pineal gland, where it serves as a precursor for the synthesis of melatonin, a hormone that influences endocrine activity, presumably by an action within the hypothalamus.

Most of the serotonin that escapes from the enterochromaffin cells of the gastrointestinal tract into the cir-

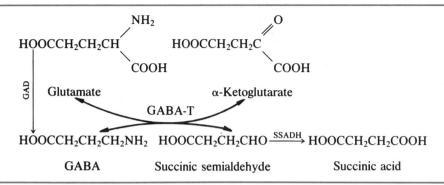

Figure 28-2. Steps involved in the synthesis and metabolism of γ-aminobutyric acid (GABA).

culation either is taken up by the platelets or is metabolized. However, if large amounts of serotonin are released, as occurs from enterochromaffin cell tumors (carcinoid tumors), peripheral physiological effects can occur.

Amino Acid Neurotransmitters

It is now well accepted that several amino acids function as neurotransmitters.

γ-Aminobutyric Acid

γ-Aminobutyric acid (GABA) is the major inhibitory neurotransmitter in the mammalian CNS. GABA is primarily synthesized (Fig. 28-2) from glutamate by the enzyme L-glutamic acid-1-decarboxylase (GAD); it is subsequently transaminated with α-oxoglutarate by GABA-α-oxoglutarate transaminase (GABA-T) to yield glutamate and succinic semialdehyde.

Two types of GABA receptors have been identified in mammals, a $GABA_A$ and a $GABA_B$ receptor. The $GABA_A$ receptor (or recognition site), when coupled with GABA, induces a shift in membrane permeability (primarily to chloride ions), causing a hyperpolarization of the neuron. This GABA receptor appears to be part of a macromolecule that contains, in addition to the $GABA_A$ receptor, a benzodiazepine receptor and the chloride ionophore (chloride channel) (Fig. 28-3).

A number of drugs are thought to exert their CNS effect by altering $GABA_A$ receptor activity. The 1,4-benzodiazepines, β-carbolines, barbiturates, alcohols, and general anesthetics appear to facilitate GABA transmission by interacting at this macromolecular complex. Several CNS convulsants including bicuculline, picrotoxinin, and pentylenetetrazol are antagonists at the GABA receptor. There are also several GABA agonists that have been

studied including muscimol, isoguvacine, and THIP. At the present time, there are no clinical uses for these compounds. Since GABA agonists have been shown to be anticonvulsants and GABA antagonists are convulsants, there is much current interest in the role of GABA in epilepsy (see Chap. 37). The $GABA_B$ receptor is present at lower concentrations than is the $GABA_A$ receptor, is not modulated by benzodiazepines, is not linked to chloride movement, and is not nearly as well characterized as is the $GABA_A$ receptor.

Glycine

Glycine is another inhibitory CNS neurotransmitter. Whereas GABA is located primarily in the brain, glycine is found predominantly in the ventral horn of the spinal cord. Relatively few drugs are known to interact with glycine; the best-known example is the convulsant strychnine, which appears to be a relatively specific antagonist of glycine.

Glutamic Acid and Aspartic Acid

These two excitatory amino acids are widely distributed throughout the mammalian CNS. Their administration leads to a rapid depolarization of neurons and an increase in firing rate. It has been extremely difficult to study the role of glutamate and aspartate as neurotransmitters, since these compounds are involved directly in intermediary metabolism of neural tissue; that is, it has been difficult to separate "transmitter glutamate" (or aspartate) from "metabolic glutamate."

The role of excitatory amino acids (EAA) has only recently been clarified. There are now at least five distinct EAA receptors (Table 28-1). The best characterized is a receptor known as the NMDA (N-methyl-D-aspartate) receptor. The NMDA receptor-ionophor complex is an-

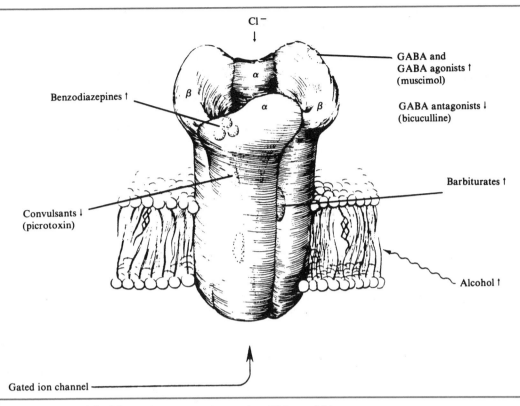

Figure 28-3. Schematic model of the GABA_A receptor complex. This model is not meant to indicate the subunit assembly or the location and stoichiometry of the various recognition sites associated with the subunits. Arrows indicate the enhancement (↑) or inhibition (↓) of GABAergic function by various agents. (Reprinted with permission from R. D. Schwartz, The GABA_A receptor-gated ion channel: Biochemical and pharmacological studies of structure and function. *Biochem. Pharmacol.* 37:3370, 1988, copyright 1988, Pergamon Press plc.)

Table 28-1. Receptors for Excitatory Amino Acids

Receptor designation	Function
NMDA	Produces excitation by increasing Ca^{2+} conductance; generates slow component of EPSP
AMPA	Generates fast component of EPSP
Kainate	Specific distribution, similar pharmacologically to AMPA
L-AP4	May function presynaptically to decrease transmitter release
ACPD	Linked to IP_3 formation

NMDA = *N*-methyl-D-aspartate; AMPA = α-amino-3-hydroxy-5-methyl-isoxazole-4-propionic acid; L-AP4 = L-2-amino-4-phosphonobutanoic acid; ACPD = 1-amino-cyclopentane-1,3-dicarboxylic acid; iP_3 = inosine triphosphate.

alogous to the GABA-benzodiazepine receptor previously discussed. In the case of the NMDA complex, the ion channel is a Mg^{2+} gated cation channel that is permeable to Ca^{2+} and Na^+. There are a number of sites on the complex where compounds can interact pharmacologically to alter the activity of the receptor. Compounds that block the NMDA receptor complex may attenuate the neuronal damage seen following anoxia, such as occurs during a stroke; much of the neuronal damage associated with strokes may be related to the release of glutamic or aspartic acids, or both. Similarly, neuronal damage can occur as a result of seizures, and this also may be related to excessive EAA release. Antagonists of the NMDA-receptor complex are being studied for possible uses in seizure disorders and in the treatment of recent strokes and other types of hypoxia.

Histamine

Histamine occurs in the brain, particularly in certain hypothalamic neurons, and evidence is strong that histamine is a neurotransmitter. Depolarization of hypothalamic slices causes a calcium-dependent release of histamine. There is a nonuniform distribution of histamine, its synthetic enzyme (histidine decarboxylase), and methyl histamine (the major brain metabolite). An ascending histamine-containing neural tract has recently been visualized using immunohistochemical techniques. A possible role for histamine in the regulation of food and water intake, thermoregulation, and hormone release has been suggested. Additional information on histamine can be found in Chap. 72.

Other Potential Amino Acid Neurotransmitters

Several additional amino acids are considered to be neurotransmitter candidates. Either they have not been as extensively studied or the evidence for a transmitter role is not as secure as it is for GABA, glycine, glutamic acid, or aspartic acid.

Taurine, a sulfur-containing amino acid, is considered to be a possible inhibitory neurotransmitter, particularly in the retina.

There also is evidence that amino acids such as *α-* and *β-alanine, cysteine, 2-phenylethylamine*, and *imidazole-4-acetic acid* may have neurotransmitter properties, but no conclusion can be reached at this time.

Peptides

An exciting area of research at the present time concerns the elucidation of the role played by a variety of peptides that are present in the CNS. A large number of these endogenous peptides are produced by neurons. They appear to possess the essential characteristics of neurotransmitters (i.e., their release is Ca^{2+} dependent, they are localized in specific neurons, their release induces changes in postsynaptic neuronal systems, etc.). Since several dozen substances are known now and more are being discovered all the time, no attempt is made to cover them all in this chapter. A few of the most important are discussed briefly. The interested reader can refer to the supplemental readings at the end of the chapter.

Endogenous Opioid Peptides

It is fair to say that interest in endogenous peptides increased dramatically when it was shown that two brain peptides had pharmacological properties similar to those of morphine and other narcotic analgesics. It is now known that there are several endogenous peptides that pharmacologically mimic opioid action and that bind to "morphine receptors." The most prominent of these are met-enkephalin, leu-enkephalin, β-endorphin, and dynorphin (see Chap. 39 for further details).

Substance P

The first neuropeptide to be isolated and characterized is known as substance P. It is believed to function within certain nerves in a transmitter capacity. It is an undecapeptide (Arg-Pro-Lys-Pro-Gln-Glin-Phe-Phe-Gly-Leu-Met-NH₂) that has been isolated and purified from hypothalamic tissue. This polypeptide is present in higher quantities in spinal dorsal roots than in ventral roots and is particularly concentrated in the dorsal horn region, where large numbers of primary afferent nerve fibers terminate and form synapses. It is presumed that substance P is formed in spinal ganglia and then transported through the dorsal root until it reaches its spinally located nerve terminals. Substance P is, in all likelihood, stored within granular structures in the nerve terminals in a manner analogous to other putative neurotransmitters. Substance P can directly depolarize motor neurons and, therefore, appears to be an excitatory transmitter. It may also affect motor neurons indirectly through activation of excitatory interneurons that synapse with motor neurons. Based on these observations, *substance P has been proposed as an excitatory transmitter of primary sensory neurons.* It has also been suggested that substance P may serve as a transmitter of axon vasodilation after its release from the peripherally located nerve terminal of sensory neurons. In addition to its effects on neurons, direct application has revealed a powerful smooth muscle–stimulating action as well as a vasodilator effect.

Neurotensin

This peptide is located in largest amounts in the hypothalamus, in the nucleus accumbens, and in the septum. Following intracisternal administration, neurotensin lowers body temperature and stimulates the release of growth hormone and prolactin.

Neuropeptide Y

This compound is a 36 amino acid residue peptide that occurs in highest concentrations in the hypothalamus, limbic system, and neocortex. Neuropeptide Y coexists with either norepinephrine or epinephrine and increases the sensitivity of smooth muscle to norepinephrine. By itself, it is a very potent vasoconstrictor. Its role in the CNS is not known.

Somatostatin

Somatostatin is a 28 amino acid peptide that is widely distributed in the gastrointestinal tract and pancreatic islets in addition to being concentrated in the mediobasal hypothalamus of the CNS. Somatostatin-reactive cells and fibers are also present in many other locations in the brain and spinal cord. Its most important action appears to be its ability to enhance responsiveness to acetylcholine. In certain types of Alzheimer's disease, the content of both acetylcholine and somatostatin is markedly reduced. Somatostatin frequently coexists in neurons with GABA.

Other Peptides

There are other peptides present in the brain, and in the gut as well, that appear to possess neurotransmitter properties. These peptides include *vasoactive intestinal peptide* (VIP) and *gastrin*. In addition, there is growing evidence that the peptides that were originally termed hypothalamic-releasing hormones are actually functioning as neurotransmitters. Since our understanding of the role played by these peptides is just beginning to emerge, these substances are not presently useful as drugs.

Central Nervous System Methodology

The actions and cellular locations of many neurotransmitters have become established through the appropriate use of a wide variety of neurochemical and neuroanatomical techniques. For example, anatomically well-defined dopamine pathways have been demonstrated in the basal ganglia (among other areas) by histochemical fluorescence methods. Likewise, histofluorescence procedures have demonstrated the presence of norepinephrine pathways that originate from cell bodies located primarily in the nucleus locus ceruleus. Both ascending and descending serotoninergic pathways from cell bodies originating in the raphe nuclei and reticular systems of the brainstem have also been demonstrated using similar methods. Acetylcholine pathways likewise have been demonstrated histochemically.

Unfortunately, histofluorescent methods are not available to delineate the pathways and distribution of most other suspected CNS neurotransmitters. Much of our present information is obtained from determining the concentration of the agent in discrete sections of brain from experimental animals; from determining how single neurons respond to the administration of minute quantities of the suspected transmitters (e.g., ejected from micropipettes by pressure or by means of very small electrical currents [microiontophoresis]); from studying the effects of agents that have known pharmacological actions (i.e., compounds that inhibit transmitter synthesis, metabolism, etc.), and from isolation and characterization of specific receptors for the suspected transmitter.

The use of "receptor-binding" techniques is particularly useful in this regard. If one assumes that neurotransmitters function by binding to a specific cellular receptor macromolecule, then it should be possible, using either radioactively labeled neurotransmitter or some chemically similar substance (ligand), to specifically label a particular receptor and to isolate the resulting receptor-ligand complex. To date, receptors have been identified in the brain for most of the putative neurotransmitters that have been mentioned in this chapter.

There is evidence that receptors for neurotransmitters play more than the strictly passive role of serving as a place to which neurotransmitters may attach; they may, in fact, form a part of the regulative process to increase or decrease synthesis of the transmitter. The chronic use of drugs also may modify the responsiveness of a receptor. For example, the chronic administration of high doses of antipsychotic drugs leads to the development of tardive dyskinesias. The mechanism by which this occurs is presumed to involve an alteration of dopaminergic receptors in the striatonigral system as a consequence of long-term blockade of these receptors by the antipsychotic drugs (see Chap. 35).

It is believed that *most neurons possess receptors for several different neurotransmitters.* The network of relationships among neurons in all the various nuclei and fiber tracts of the brain and spinal cord is like a very large and infinitely complicated jigsaw puzzle. Unfortunately, very few pieces are yet in place. Each correctly identified piece makes the next one easier to fit, however, and it is reasonable to expect much progress in the near future.

Blood-Brain Barrier

It has been appreciated for over a century that not all substances present in the bloodstream can readily gain entry into the brain. Initially, it was shown that organic dyes, when injected intravenously into animals, could stain all tissues except the brain, which remained *schneeweiss* (snow-white). There appeared to be a barrier to the passage of drugs from the systemic circulation to the parenchyma of the brain. However, this apparent barrier to drugs and other chemicals is relative rather than absolute,

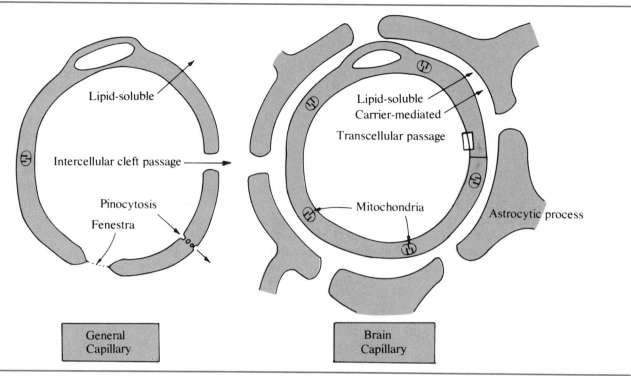

Figure 28-4. Major differences between a general (nonneural) and a brain capillary. In the brain capillary, the intercellular clefts are sealed shut by tight junctions. There are also reduced pinocytosis and no fenestrae. Exchange of compounds between the circulation and the brain must take place through the cells of the capillary wall, the major barriers of which are the plasma membranes (inner and outer) of the capillary endothelial cells. (From W. H. Oldendorf, Permeability of the Blood-Brain Barrier. In D. B. Tower [ed.], *The Nervous System.* New York: Raven, 1975. Vol. 1.)

and, in fact, there are several barriers to substances entering the brain from the systemic circulation. The term *blood-brain barrier* is usually applied to the lack of passage of certain drugs or other exogenously administered chemicals into the brain (see also Chap. 3).

Drugs or Compounds Excluded From The Brain

An important property that determines entry to the brain from the systemic circulation is molecular weight. Compounds with molecular weights of about 60,000 and above tend to remain within the circulatory system. Furthermore, that portion of administered drugs that is bound to plasma proteins will be unavailable for distribution to the brain (as well as to other tissues and organs), in part because of the high molecular weight of the plasma protein-drug complex.

Two physicochemical factors are of particular importance in allowing a drug to enter the CNS. First, for compounds that are mainly un-ionized at plasma pH (pK_a 7.4 or higher), the drug's *solubility in lipids is an important determinant.* Lipid solubility is generally expressed as a fat-to-water partition coefficient. A more lipid-soluble agent can more easily penetrate lipid membranes, such as those found in the CNS. The other important factor appears to be the proportion of drug that is un-ionized. These two properties cannot be completely separated from each other, however, since un-ionized drugs are generally more lipid soluble than ionized ones.

Location of the Blood-Brain Barrier

The capillaries of the brain are the most likely location of the blood-brain barrier. Brain capillaries appear to differ in several important respects from capillaries in other body locations (Fig. 28-4). For example, the endothelial cells of brain capillaries are so closely joined to each other that passage of substances cannot readily occur through the intercellular clefts located between adjacent cells; fur-

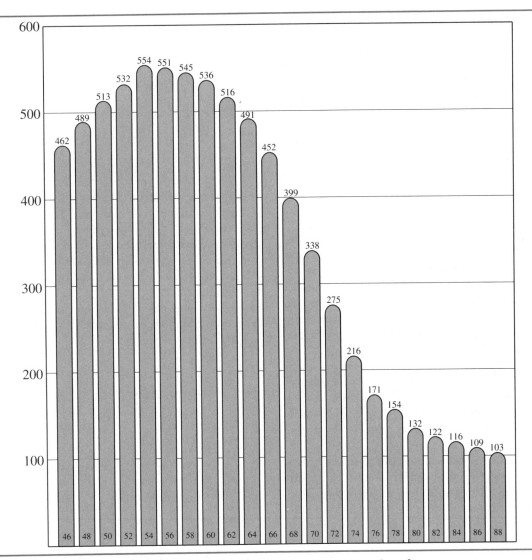

Figure 28-5. Influence of widespread use of the first antipsychotic drugs on the number of hospitalized mental patients in state and local hospitals in the United States (USPHS statistics). Graph illustrates number of patients in mental hospitals in the US in thousands from 1946 through 1988. (Provided by Virginia R. Hannon, Sc.D., Principal Research Scientist, The Nathan S. Kline Institute for Psychiatric Research, Orangeburg, N.Y.)

thermore, brain capillaries do not contain fenestrae (pores). Fenestrae are very prominent in many capillaries, especially those in renal glomeruli and in the choroid plexus. The number of capillary pores appears to be directly related to the ability of a drug to leave a capillary by diffusion. Compared to capillaries at other sites, brain capillaries also appear to possess very few pinocytotic vesicles. Pinocytotic vesicles are believed to play a role in the transport of large molecules through capillary walls.

Several enzymes are present in much greater amounts in cerebral endothelium. These enzymes include pseudo-cholinesterase, alkaline phosphatase, aromatic L-amino-acid decarboxylase, α-glutamyl transpeptidase, and Na$^+$, K$^+$–adenosine triphosphatase (ATPase). Brain capillaries contain many more mitochondria than do other capillaries, and it is probable that the mitochondria function to supply energy for active transport of water-soluble nutrient substances into the brain. A large number of lipid-insoluble endogenous substances are known to be taken up by the brain. These substances include glucose, amino acids, simple carboxylic acids, and purines.

Significance of the Blood-Brain Barrier

It is doubtful that the barrier evolved solely in response to the potential toxicities of drugs or other exogenous materials that might have entered the systemic circulation, although certain constituents of foods and other natural products have significant effects on the CNS. Rather, it is likely that the blood-brain barrier serves primarily to preserve the internal environment of the brain and prevent sudden increases in concentration of a variety of water-soluble, ionized substances, including many circulating neurotransmitters such as norepinephrine, epinephrine, ACh, serotonin, and dopamine. The concentration in the brain of these bioactive substances appears to be very carefully regulated. On the other hand, the biochemical precursors of the above-mentioned transmitters can pass relatively easily, although usually by active transport, from the blood to the brain, and this ensures an adequate supply of locally synthesized transmitters. By and large, the precursors are inactive biologically or, at best, have only minimal biological activity. The amino acid transmitters GABA, glycine, glutamic acid, and aspartic acid are actively taken up by the brain capillaries, but ordinarily the transport system for these amino acids is close to being saturated. Therefore, a sudden increase in blood concentration of these substances would have little effect on subsequent brain levels.

The blood-brain barrier is not found in all parts of the brain. Certain small areas, including the *area postrema* beneath the floor of the fourth ventricle, an area in the *preoptic recess,* and portions of the floor of the third ventricle surrounding the stalk of the pituitary appear to be devoid of this barrier.

The ability of the blood-brain barrier to exclude entry of a number of drugs into the brain has several therapeutic implications. Many drugs, most notably certain antibiotics, are relatively excluded from the brain. In the treatment of infectious diseases of the CNS, the physician must, in addition to establishing the organism's drug sensitivity, either select an agent that can get to the site of the infection or use a route (intrathecal) that bypasses the barrier. In the human fetus and newborn, the barrier is not as well developed as it is in later life. This fact also must be taken into consideration when one is prescribing drugs during pregnancy and the neonatal period.

Practical Consequences of Neuropharmacological Drug Use

One quantifiable consequence of the development and widespread use of neuropharmacological agents has been a steady decline in the number of hospitalized psychotic patients (Fig. 28-5). Although antipsychotic drugs do not usually provide a permanent cure, their use in conjunction with supportive treatment has allowed many patients who would otherwise be permanently hospitalized to resume functioning in the community. It should be noted, however, that the needs of some individuals who have been released might have been better served by remaining in a hospital setting.

Supplemental Reading

Brown, A.G. *Nerve Cells and Nervous Systems.* Heidelberg: Springer-Verlag, 1991.

Cooper, J.R., Bloom, F.E., and Roth, R.H. (eds.). *The Biochemical Basis of Neuropharmacology* (6th ed.). New York: Oxford, 1991.

Hall, A.K., and Rao, M.S. Cytokines and neurokines: Related ligands and related receptors. *TINS.* 15:35, 1992.

Leonard, B.E. *Fundamentals of Psychopharmacology.* New York: Wiley-Liss, 1992.

Olney, J.W. Excitotoxic amino acids and neuropsychiatric disorders. *Annu. Rev. Pharmacol. Toxicol.* 30:47, 1990.

29

Inhalational Anesthetics

David J. Smith

Inhalational anesthetic agents are drugs that exist either in a gaseous form or as volatile liquids that are transformed into vapors by vaporizers on anesthesia machines. The anesthetics can produce a degree of unconsciousness that is adequate to eliminate the awareness of surgical manipulation. The manner in which drugs produce this state of interruption of central nervous system (CNS) function is unknown. However, a *unitary theory of narcosis* has been advanced suggesting that all inhaled anesthetics have a similar interaction with specific cellular macromolecules. Meyer and Overton theorized that anesthetic molecules dissolve into membrane lipids and interact at hydrophobic sites. An extension of the Meyer-Overton hypothesis is that the association of anesthetic molecules with lipids causes an expansion of the membrane and a disorganization of its functional components, that is, the so-called *critical volume hypothesis.* Ultimately, the alterations lead to a failure of synaptic transmission and nerve conduction.

Regardless of the specific mechanisms involved in the production of anesthesia, the pharmacological effect (unconsciousness) results when a specific concentration of the agent is achieved at the site of action. This chapter deals with concepts related to the achievement of this effective concentration of anesthetic in the brain. The elimination of anesthetics is essentially a reverse of the processes discussed.

Henry's Law

Henry's law describes the behavior of gases in solutions and body tissues. Inhalational anesthetic agents appear to be inert gases that interact with tissues and liquids physically rather than chemically. Therefore, laws governing the physical association of gases and liquids are of paramount importance to an understanding of the pharmacokinetics of these drugs. Anesthesiologists must appreciate the factors responsible for the establishment of the anesthetic concentration in a tissue in order to adequately control anesthetic delivery and to adjust for physiological and pathological influences on anesthetic concentration.

Henry's law describes the regulation of gas concentration in a liquid when the association of these two phases is through physical interaction alone. The law states that *at equilibrium, the concentration of gas physically dissolved in a liquid is directly proportional to the partial pressure (or tension) of the agent and its affinity for the molecules of the liquids (or its solubility in the liquid).*

Concentration of gas in a liquid = partial pressure of the gas × affinity of gas molecules for liquid molecules

Partial pressure is defined by Dalton's law as the individual pressure (P) exerted by a gas in a mixture of gases:

$$P_t \text{ (total pressure)} = P_1 + P_2 + P_3 + P_4 + P_n$$

For a clear understanding of Henry's law, it is important to consider each of the component parts individually.

Development of the Partial Pressure of a Gas in Solution

Inherent in Henry's law is the concept that when a liquid is exposed to a gas, a partial pressure equilibrium will be achieved between the gas and liquid phases. Thus, *molecules of the gas that are physically dissolved in the liquid will exert a tension that is equal to the partial pressure of the gas above the liquid.* It is not necessary that a defined gas space, such as a bubble, exist before pressure can be generated. Individual molecules of gas become surrounded and separated by liquid or tissue molecules. Furthermore, since they are inert and do not combine chemically with the solvent, the gas molecules remain independent and therefore are free to undergo random molecular motion and exert a pressure equal to that in the gas phase.

Practically speaking, this concept explains the basis for the establishment of a partial pressure equilibrium of anesthetic gas between the lung alveoli and the arterial blood. *Gas molecules will move across the alveolar membrane until those in the blood, through random molecular motion, exert a pressure equal to their counterparts in the lung.* Similar gas-tension equilibria also will be established between the blood and other tissues. For example, gas molecules in the blood will diffuse down a tension gradient into the brain until equal random molecular motion (equal pressure) occurs in both tissues.

Affinity of Gas Molecules for Solvent Molecules

A primary force opposing random molecular motion is the *affinity* of gas molecules for the tissue in question (a second factor in Henry's law that expresses the degree of solubility of the agent in the tissue). The affinity of a gas for a solvent results essentially from weak intermolecular attractions, such as van der Waal's forces. Consequently, *affinity is a function of the molecular composition of both the gas and the solvent medium.* If a particular gas has a strong affinity for the molecules of a solvent, its random molecular motion will be impeded by a greater number of collisions with the solvent molecules. Therefore, *a greater volume of an agent of high affinity (or greater solubility) will be required to enter a tissue to generate the same partial pressure as does an agent of low affinity.*

Concentration of Anesthetic Gas in a Tissue

The concentration of an anesthetic at its site of action or, for that matter, in any body tissue, is a function of the partial pressure delivered to the lung and the affinity of gas molecules for the particular tissue. *The anesthesiologist can control brain concentration of a gas only by modifying the partial pressure of the agent that is delivered to the alveoli.* The gas then diffuses across the alveolus to the blood and ultimately into the CNS. Of course, since *gases diffuse from areas of high partial pressure to areas of low partial pressure*, a series of pressure equilibria will have to be achieved from the alveolus to the blood and to the brain. Subsequently, tension in other body tissues, such as muscle, fat, and bone, will also come into equilibrium with the alveolar tension.

The second factor in Henry's equation, affinity of the gas for molecules of the solvent medium, is a function of the molecular nature both of the tissue and of the inhalational agent and, as such, is not under direct control of the anesthesiologist. It is, however, an important factor in de-

termining the final concentration (partial pressure × affinity: Henry's law) of anesthetic at the site of action.

A Concept of Anesthetic Dose Based on Partial Pressure–Minimum Alveolar Concentration

Since the anesthesiologist has control over the partial pressure of anesthetic delivered to the lung, it can be manipulated to control the anesthetic gas concentration in the brain and hence the level of unconsciousness. For this reason, *anesthetic dose is usually expressed in terms of the alveolar tension required at equilibrium to produce a defined depth of anesthesia.* The dose is determined experimentally as the partial pressure needed to eliminate movement in 50 percent of patients challenged with a standardized skin incision. The tension required is defined as the *minimum alveolar concentration (MAC)* and is usually expressed as the percentage of inhaled gases that is represented by anesthetic gas at 1 atm.

Various anesthetic agents require widely different partial pressures to produce the same depth of anesthesia (Table 29-1). Methoxyflurane, for example, with a MAC of 0.16 percent, would be the most potent agent listed in the table. Only 0.16 percent of the molecules of inspired gas need be methoxyflurane. Nitrous oxide (N_2O), on the other hand, is the least potent agent, with a MAC that exceeds 100 percent. Thus, a level of unconsciousness needed to eliminate movement is seldom achieved with N_2O.

MAC is a valuable index for clinical anesthesia, but it is seldom employed without taking other factors into consideration. For example, inhibiting movement in only 50 percent of patients is not acceptable. Consequently, if an

Table 29-1. Minimum Alveolar Concentration in Humans

Anesthetic gas	Minimum alveolar concentration[a]
Nitrous oxide	>100
Cyclopropane	9.2
Desflurane *(Suprane)*	6.0
Diethyl ether	1.92
Sevoflurane[b]	1.7
Enflurane *(Ethrane)*	1.68
Isoflurane *(Forane)*	1.15
Halothane *(Fluothane)*	0.75
Methoxyflurane *(Penthrane)*	0.16

[a]Measured as percent of total gases in the inspired air.
[b]Not yet marketed in U.S.
Source: Data taken from E. I. Eger II (ed.), *Anesthetic Uptake and Action.* Baltimore: Williams & Wilkins, 1974. P. 5; and E. I. Eger, Isoflurane: A review. *Anesthesiology* 55:559, 1981.

inhalational agent is being used alone—that is, without the administration of other anesthetics or analgesic drugs—the anesthesiologist would employ a multiple of its MAC value to ensure a reasonable level of unconsciousness in all patients. MAC is frequently multiplied by a factor of 1.3 to achieve nearly 100 percent clinical efficacy.

Anesthetics are infrequently used without the administration of other drugs. Many of these drug combinations may interact to alter MAC requirements. For example, inhalational anesthetics used in combination appear to have an additive effect on the level of unconsciousness achieved in patients. Therefore, when a combination of inhalational agents is used (e.g., N_2O with halothane), MAC values for the individual agents can be reduced appropriately. In this regard, an acceptable anesthetic maintenance tension for N_2O and halothane in the inspired air may be 40 percent and 0.5 percent, respectively.

The MAC requirement also is reduced by the coadministration of other CNS depressants (such as barbiturates that can be used as preanesthetic medications) or narcotic analgesics. On the other hand, CNS stimulants, such as amphetamine, may elevate the partial pressure needed for anesthesia.

Factors Affecting the Rate of Development of Anesthetic Concentration in the Lung

The depth of anesthesia depends on the concentration of anesthetic agent in the brain; concentration, in turn, is directly proportional to the partial pressure of the agent in brain tissue. However, since gases diffuse from areas of high partial pressure to areas of low partial pressure, the tension of anesthetic in the alveoli must provide the driving force to establish brain tension. In fact, the tension of anesthetic in all body tissues will tend to rise toward the lung tension as equilibrium is approached. Consequently, factors that control or modify the rate of accumulation of anesthetic in the lung (e.g., rate of gas delivery, uptake of gas from the lung into the pulmonary circulation) will simultaneously influence the rate at which tension equilibria in other body compartments is established.

It is of value to consider the development of alveolar tension in an uncomplicated hypothetical model. We assume in this model that anesthetic gas is delivered in an inspired mixture of gases at a constant rate and that no uptake of gases into the pulmonary circulation occurs. The anesthetic tension in the lung will begin at zero and cannot, of course, accumulate to exert a pressure greater than the inspired tension. Graphs of the alveolar tension plotted against time are used in this chapter to illustrate the changes in lung partial pressure as anesthetic is inhaled. It

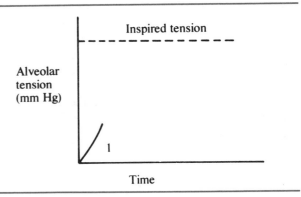

Figure 29-1. Alveolar tension of an anesthetic gas, with time, after a single breath.

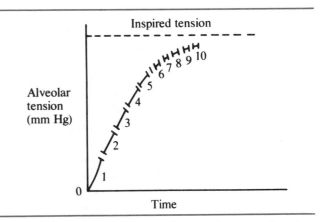

Figure 29-2. Alveolar tension of an anesthetic gas after 10 breathing cycles. Note that the alveolar tension approaches the inspired tension.

is important to realize that only a fraction of total lung gases are exchanged during one breathing cycle. Therefore, the first breath containing anesthetic will be diluted by the volume of gases already present in the lung. Consequently, after the gases from the first breath have mixed with lung gases, the alveolar tension will still be considerably lower than the inspired tension (Fig. 29-1).

In subsequent breathing cycles, the alveolar tension will continue to rise toward the inspired level along an exponentially declining curve (Fig. 29-2). The shape of the curve is dictated by the fact that each breathing cycle brings a constant amount of fresh gas to the lung; after mixing with anesthetic already present in the alveoli, however, an increasingly greater amount is lost during expiration. Consequently, the net change of anesthetic tension becomes smaller with each breathing cycle, and the curve of alveolar tension will approach the inspired level more slowly.

The alveolar tension–time curve always declines in an exponential manner, but the position of the curve can be affected greatly by the rate of delivery of anesthetic gases and the rate of their uptake into the pulmonary circulation. For this reason, it is important to consider factors that modify or regulate input (delivery) and uptake. In this discussion, uptake of gases from the lung are considered first, and it is assumed that the anesthetics are delivered at a constant rate.

Alveolar Uptake of Anesthetic Gases

Effect of the Alveolar-Arterial Tension Gradient

Uptake of anesthetics from the alveolus into the pulmonary circulation is a factor that retards the rate of development of alveolar tension. However, uptake is not constant. As body tissues become saturated with anesthetic molecules, blood returning to the lung will have an increasingly higher anesthetic tension, and the alveolar-arterial tension gradient will be reduced. Since the gradient controls the rate of diffusion across the alveolar capillary membrane, uptake is also reduced.

The saturation of body tissues occurs in at least three phases as major tissue groups, *distinguished by their blood flow*, equilibrate with the alveolar tension of an anesthetic. These major tissue groups include a vessel-rich group with a high blood flow per unit of mass (brain, heart, liver, and kidney), a group of tissues with an intermediate blood flow per unit of mass (skin and muscle), and those with a lower blood flow per unit of mass (fat, bone, tendon, and connective tissue).

The effect of uptake and saturation of different body tissues may be reflected in the shape of the alveolar tension–time curve. In Fig. 29-3 the line from a to b represents the time during which fresh anesthetic gas is being brought into the lung, before significant uptake begins. Point b represents the moment that input (delivery of gas) is matched by uptake into the pulmonary circulation. Rather than flattening at point b, the curve continues to rise since uptake is changing. At point c on the curve, a "knee," or bend, is produced as the vessel-rich group of tissues becomes saturated and stops removing anesthetic from the blood. The line from c to d, then, would represent the time required to saturate the muscle and skin, and so on.

Theoretically, uptake should eventually become zero when the alveolar tension and inspired tension are equal. Practically, however, this never happens. Anesthetic evaporates from the skin surface and, additionally, fat deposits, which have a high affinity for anesthetic agents, may continue to take up anesthetic for hours or days.

Effect of Solubility of Various Agents

The inhalational anesthetics available to the clinician in modern practice have distinctly different solubility (affinity) characteristics in blood as well as in other tissues (Table 29-2). These solubility differences are usually expressed as partition coefficients and indicate the number of volumes of a particular agent distributed in one phase as compared to another, when the partial pressure is at equilibrium. For example, ether has a blood-to-gas partition

Table 29.2 Partition Coefficients of Some Anesthetic Gases at 37°C

Anesthetic gas	Blood/gas	Tissue/blood
Cyclopropane	0.41	1.16 muscle 0.76 brain
Desflurane	0.42	2.0 muscle 1.3 brain
Nitrous oxide	0.47	1.15 muscle 1.06 brain
Sevoflurane	0.69	3.1 muscle 1.7 brain
Isoflurane	1.4	4.0 muscle 2.6 brain
Enflurane	1.8	1.7 muscle 1.45 brain
Halothane	2.3	3.4 muscle 3.5 brain (white) 2.3 brain (gray) 2.6 liver
Diethyl ether	12.1	1.14 brain 0.98 muscle
Methoxyflurane	12.0	2.3 brain (white) 1.7 brain (gray) 1.3 muscle

Source: Adapted from E. I. Eger II (ed.), *Anesthetic Uptake and Action.* Baltimore: Williams & Wilkins, 1974. P. 82.

Figure 29-3. Alveolar tension, with time, of an anesthetic gas. The various points along the curve are explained in the text.

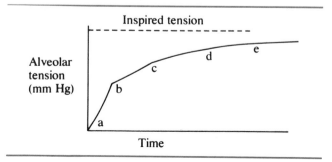

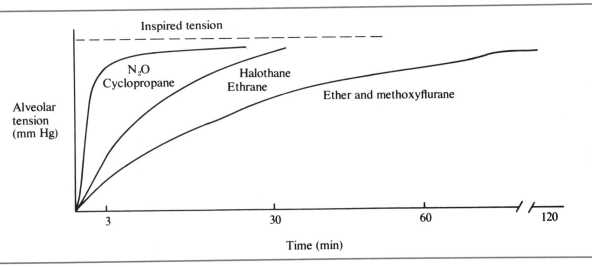

Figure 29-4. The rate of rise in alveolar tension of several anesthetic agents.

coefficient (often referred to as the *Ostwald solubility coefficient*) of approximately 12.0. Thus, when the partial pressure has reached equilibrium, 12 vol of ether will be dissolved in blood for every 1 vol in the alveolus.

The volume of the various anesthetics required to saturate blood is similar to that needed to saturate other body tissues (Table 29-2); that is, the blood-tissue partition coefficient is usually not more than 2 (with the exception of that of adipose tissues, which is higher). Therefore, an estimate of the volume of gas required for total body saturation can be roughly derived from the blood-gas partition coefficient.

The solubility of anesthetic agents is a factor of major significance for the rate of induction of anesthesia or the time required to establish a level of unconsciousness adequate for surgery. If an agent is highly soluble in plasma (e.g., ether, methoxyflurane), the rate of rise of its alveolar tension to the inspired level will be delayed by a higher initial uptake into plasma from the alveoli. Since the partial pressure of the anesthetic in tissues also is dependent on the alveolar tension, high plasma solubility also delays the time necessary for an anesthetic partial pressure in the brain to be reached. On the other hand, agents with limited plasma solubility and a lower rate of uptake (e.g., N_2O, cyclopropane, and desflurane) will equilibrate more rapidly with tissues.

To illustrate the effect of solubility on the rate of induction of anesthesia, we can consider a situation in which individual agents are delivered to patients at their equivalent MAC values. Under these conditions, regardless of the agent being employed, a similar level of anesthesia will be achieved. In contrast, induction rates, illustrated as the time required for the alveolar tension to rise to the inspired level (Fig. 29-4), can be seen to be quite different.

A patient receiving a MAC of either N_2O, cyclopropane, or desflurane will be unconscious within 3 min. However, halothane or enflurane, which both have significant blood and tissue solubilities, will require at least 30 min before surgical anesthesia is established. Ether and methoxyflurane, which are highly soluble agents, will require several hours and may be clinically impractical if used in this way.

Effect of Pulmonary Perfusion

The rate of pulmonary perfusion (in healthy individuals, essentially equivalent to the cardiac output) also has an effect on the rate of induction of anesthesia. Since more blood will pass through the pulmonary capillary bed when the cardiac output is high, it follows that a greater total transfer of any anesthetic agent across the alveolus will occur. Thus, in a manner similar to the influence of higher solubility of gases on alveolar tension, the greater uptake will slow the rate of rise of the alveolar tension-time curve. Therefore, *anesthetic induction with an individual agent may be slower when the cardiac output and perfusion of the lung are high.* In low cardiac output states, the reverse is true. The rate of uptake will be lower, and the alveolar tension will rise toward the inspired tension more quickly.

The effect of the perfusion of the lung on the rate of anesthetic induction is much less significant for agents of low solubility. Since the rate of uptake of these agents is minimal, factors that alter uptake are less important. Therefore, *if it is desirable clinically to minimize the effect of cardiac output on the rate of induction of anesthesia, agents of lower solubility would be preferred.*

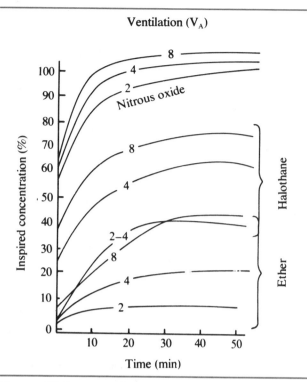

Figure 29-5. The alveolar rate of rise toward the inspired concentration (F_A/F_I) is accelerated by an increase in alveolar ventilation from 2 to 4 and from 4 to 8 liters per minute (constant cardiac output). The ratio of lowest to highest anesthetic dose produced by these differences in ventilation is greatest with the most soluble anesthetic, ether; less with the anesthetic of intermediate solubility, halothane; and smallest with the least soluble anesthetic, nitrous oxide. (From E. I. Eger II [ed.], *Anesthetic Uptake and Action.* Baltimore: Williams & Wilkins, 1974.)

Effect of the Rate of Ventilation and Inspired Gas Concentration

Frequently, it is desirable to overcome the slow rate of rise of the alveolar tension associated with such factors as the high solubility of some anesthetics or increased pulmonary blood flow. Since both these factors retard tension development by increasing the uptake of anesthetic, the most effective way to alleviate the problem is to accelerate the input of gas to the alveoli.

A technique used to increase the input of anesthetic to the lung is to elevate the minute alveolar ventilation. This maneuver will effectively cause a greater quantity of fresh anesthetic gas to be delivered to the patient *per unit of time* (Fig. 29-5). The anesthesiologist can control the initial rate of ventilation either by using a ventilator or by manually assisting the patient's breathing with a breathing bag. It should be remembered that hypoventilation,

which may be encountered when patients are breathing spontaneously, will result in a reduced input of anesthetic gases and a slower rise of the alveolar tension to the inspired level.

Increasing the inspired tension of an anesthetic gas above the maintenance tension (near the MAC value) is also an effective means of more quickly establishing an effective alveolar tension. This maneuver parallels the concept of loading dose, which is effectively used in the other areas of pharmacology (e.g., digitalis therapy). Beginning the anesthetic administration with high inspired tensions will cause a more rapid rate of induction with any agent, but it is particularly useful for overcoming the slow rate of induction (development of an effective alveolar tension) with highly soluble drugs. However, as the desired depth of anesthesia or level of alveolar tension is achieved, the delivered tension of anesthetic must be returned to the maintenance (MAC) level to avoid overdosing the patient. Anesthesiologists commonly use high inspired tensions to rapidly produce the desired partial pressure in the brain. For example, 50% N_2O and 0.5% halothane in the inspired air represent an effective maintenance tension for these agents when they are used in combination. Frequently, however, 3% halothane will be used at the onset of administration until the desired anesthetic level is obtained.

Other Factors Affecting the Alveolar Tension of Anesthetic Agents

Concentration Effect

When anesthetics are delivered in high concentration, the alveolar tension will rise more rapidly to the inspired level than if they were delivered in low concentrations. Thus, if 75% N_2O is being delivered in the inspired air, the 75% tension in blood will be established more quickly than if 40% N_2O were being inhaled and a 40% N_2O tension were desired in blood. This phenomenon is illustrated in Fig. 29-6. One explanation is that when high inspired tensions of anesthetics are used, particularly if they are highly soluble, a large uptake will occur from the alveoli. Consequently, the lung volume may tend to shrink, causing negative pressure. However, the shrinkage is opposed by the pulling in of fresh gases from nonrespiratory, conducting airway passages between inspirations, thus effectively increasing the total ventilation. Since greater uptake will occur with 75% N_2O than with 40%, the effect will be greater at higher inspired anesthetic tensions.

An additional or modifying influence on gas delivery is

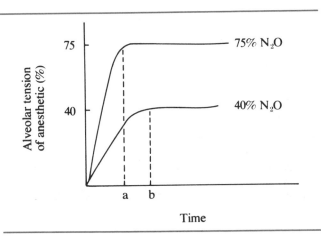

Figure 29-6. The effect of two concentrations of N_2O on the alveolar tension of anesthetic, with time.

also embodied in the concentration effect. One should remember that if a lung contains 80% N_2O and 20 percent of diluent gases (O_2, CO_2, N_2, and H_2O vapor) and one half of the N_2O is taken up, the remaining N_2O now represents 40 vol (40 were taken up) in a total gas volume of 60 (40 vol of N_2O and 20 vol of diluent gas). In this example, one half the total N_2O presented in the inspired air is transferred to the pulmonary circulation, with limited net exchange of diluent gases. Thus, after one half the original N_2O is taken up, the remaining N_2O (40 vol/60 vol) is actually 67 percent of the total lung gases. When concentrations of N_2O in the inspired air are low, the difference between the percentage of N_2O delivered and that remaining after partial uptake is progressively smaller. For example, when a mixture of 40% N_2O and 60% diluent gas is used and one half of the N_2O is taken up, the percent remaining is 25 percent (20 vol/80 vol) and not the expected value of 20 percent. In both of the examples, the shrinkage in lung volume is, of course, opposed by the pulling in of fresh gases between inspirations, as discussed previously.

Second Gas Effect

The alveolar tension of other gases that are being transferred to the blood also rises more rapidly when an anesthetic such as N_2O is present in high concentration. These gases are subject to the increased inflow (pulling in of fresh gases) as N_2O is taken up into the blood in large volume. If one of the diluent gases is halothane, for example, the increase in the tension of the second gas (i.e., halothane) during a breathing cycle will be greater than if it were being administered alone—the *second gas effect*.

Diffusion Hypoxia

Diffusion hypoxia is a condition that may be encountered at the end of an anesthetic administration with N_2O. The mechanism underlying diffusion hypoxia is essentially the reverse of the concentration effect; that is, when anesthetic administration is stopped, large volumes of N_2O move from the blood into the alveolus, diluting oxygen and expanding lung expiratory volume. The expansion of lung volume may restrict the inflow of fresh gases because the elasticity of the tissue tends to cause excessive outflow of gas. Carbon dioxide tension is also reduced in a similar manner, thus reducing the stimulus to ventilation.

To avoid diffusion hypoxia, the anesthesiologist may employ 100% oxygen, rather than room air, after discontinuing administration of the anesthetic gas mixture. A few minutes of inhalation of pure oxygen is sufficient time to allow N_2O levels in the blood and alveoli to drop to low levels and to eliminate the chance of reduced arterial O_2 tension.

Anesthetic Apparatus

With the exception of N_2O and cyclopropane, which are supplied as gases, inhalational anesthetics are volatile liquids that must be converted to a gaseous form by vaporizers attached to the anesthesia machines. The concentration of an anesthetic vapor that will develop over its liquid phase will vary, depending on the temperature of the liquid, the vapor pressure of the liquid anesthetic, the volume of gas passing over the liquid, the surface area exposed to the gas, and the volume of gas diluting the anesthetic vapor. Anesthetic machines can help control many of these potential sources of variability in anesthetic gas delivery. Some vaporizers are lined with a metal, such as copper, that conducts heat to the vaporizing liquid, thus partially compensating for changes in temperature that will occur as a result of the latent heat of vaporization.

If a nonrebreathing technique is used, the patient inspires the same anesthetic concentration as that delivered by the machine. With a rebreathing apparatus, such as the circle absorption system, there is early dilution of the anesthetic during induction, owing to the large internal capacity of the system. Also, with a circle system, there is some rebreathing of the patient's expired air and therefore more dilution of the anesthetic during induction. Some anesthetics are quite soluble in rubber (ether, halothane, methoxyflurane) and therefore the rubber in the gas delivery system must be saturated before equilibrium can be achieved.

A rapid increase in ventilation will occur if there is a change from spontaneous to controlled positive pressure ventilation. This increase will lead to a rise both in the alveolar and arterial blood tension of the anesthetic agent. This action is much more pronounced with an anesthetic that is highly soluble in blood.

Upper Airway, Dead Space, and the Lung

The airway above the area of alveolar-capillary gas exchange comprises *dead space ventilation,* and it must be saturated with the anesthetic vapor before the alveolar concentration will approximate the inspired concentration. If there is partial obstruction of the airway, a decrease in the alveolar anesthetic concentration will occur. A decreasing alveolar-capillary gas exchange will decrease the uptake of the anesthetic (e.g., as occurs in emphysema, tumor, fibrosis, atelectasis, hypovolemia, and other conditions).

Supplemental Reading

Miller, R.D. (ed.). *Anesthesia* (3rd ed.). New York: Churchill Livingstone, 1990.

Morgan, G.E., and Mikhail, M.S. (eds.). *Clinical Anesthesiology.* Norwalk, Conn.: Appleton & Lange, 1992.

30

General Anesthetics: Gases and Volatile Liquids

Frank G. Zavisca

Anesthetic agents affect every organ. The physician, no matter what his or her specialty, must know something about these anesthetic agents, since patients with every conceivable illness may require anesthesia and surgery. Because the response to anesthetics is modified by patient disease, surgical stress, drug therapy, and many other factors, anesthesiology has become a complex medical specialty that requires expertise in clinical pharmacology and the use of sophisticated monitoring equipment, as well as general medicine.

The primary emphasis of this chapter is on *general anesthesia* as compared to *regional* (or *local*) *anesthesia,* which is discussed in Chap. 32. The commonly accepted characteristics of general anesthesia include *unconsciousness, amnesia,* and *analgesia.* Analgesia encompasses the inability to feel or remember pain as well as the blockade of motor and autonomic reactions to painful stimuli. An expanded definition of anesthesia would also include muscular relaxation.

An ideal anesthetic agent (see Chap. 29) would produce minimal disturbances of cardiovascular and respiratory functions, would allow adequate oxygenation, and would be chemically stable, nonflammable, nontoxic, easy to administer, and be inexpensive. Because no such agent exists, the search for new, better anesthetic agents continues.

Signs and Stages of Anesthesia

Classic (Ether) Anesthesia

Diethyl ether has been used extensively for over a century; therefore, its properties are well known, making it a classic anesthetic agent to which newer agents are compared. Because the use of ether illustrates basic principles

so well, it is discussed in some detail in this chapter, despite its present-day limited use.

Because ether is relatively soluble in blood and tissues, it is rapidly taken up into muscle and fat storage depots, thus resulting in a moderately slow increase in its blood and brain concentration. Therefore, it produces a readily observed sequence of signs and stages during anesthetic induction and emergence. Ether is a *complete* anesthetic and thus can be used without additional drugs that might otherwise obscure these events. In the 1920s, these signs and stages were used as a guide in teaching technicians to administer ether. Guedel arbitrarily divided the sequence of events seen during the induction of ether anesthesia into stages (Table 30-1). Unfortunately, the "cookbook" method of ether administration led to a number of tragedies when unskilled individuals, unaware of the potential hazards, used the agent improperly. A critical evaluation of these tragedies has led to the development of the modern medical specialty of anesthesiology.

Stage I: Analgesia

Stage I lasts until consciousness is lost and, provided supplemental muscle relaxation is used, allows surgery in a relatively awake patient. Analgesia persists postoperatively because ether, being lipid soluble, is released slowly from tissue stores.

Stage II: Excitement

Stage II begins with the loss of consciousness and ends with the beginning of rhythmical respiration. This stage is the most difficult one to manage, since patients may move, vocalize, salivate, cough, retch, and vomit. Vomiting can result in the aspiration of the stomach contents into the lungs, which may produce pneumonia and, occasionally, death. Modern drugs allow patients to pass through this stage rapidly, reducing the hazards.

Table 30-1. The Stages and Signs of Ether Anesthesia

Stage	Respiration			Pupils		Reflex depression
	Rhythm	Volume	Pattern	Size	Position	
Stage I (analgesia)						
Analgesia to loss of consciousness	Irregular	Small		Small	Divergent	Nil
Stage II (excitement)						
Loss of consciousness to rhythmical respiration	Irregular	Large		Large	Divergent	Eyelash Eyelid
Stage III (surgical anesthesia)						
Plane 1						
Rhythmical respiration to cessation of eye movement	Regular	Large		Small	Divergent	Skin Vomiting Conjunctival Pharyngeal Stretch from limb muscles
Plane 2						
Cessation of eye movement to start of respiratory muscle paresis (excl. diaphragm)	Regular	Medium	(*)	½ dilated	Fixed centrally	Corneal
Plane 3						
Respiratory muscle paresis to paralysis	Regular Pause after expiration	Small		¾ dilated	Fixed centrally	Laryngeal Peritoneal
Plane 4						
Diaphragmatic paresis to paralysis	Jerky Irregular Quick inspiration Prolonged expiration, i.e., "seesaw"	Small		Fully dilated	Fixed centrally	Anal sphincter Carinal
Stage IV Apnea						

*If the respiration is slow, an expiratory pause may be seen in plane 2.
Source: W. D. Wylie and H. C. Churchill-Davidson (eds.), *A Practice of Anaesthesia* (4th ed.). London: Lloyd-Luke, 1978. P. 264.

Stage III: Surgical Anesthesia

Stage III, arbitrarily divided into four planes, begins with the appearance of rhythmical respirations and ends with the cessation of respiration (apnea).

Plane 1

The plane begins with the reappearance of regular respiration. Patient behavior is characterized by loss of automatic eyelid closure as well as by loss of reflex closure of the eyelids on conjunctival stimulation. Most muscular and airway reflexes are obtunded. This plane ends with the cessation of eye movement.

Plane 2

This plane begins with the cessation of eye movement and ends with the beginning of paralysis of the respiratory muscles (except the diaphragm).

Plane 3

This plane begins with increased abdominal excursions (evidence of beginning paralysis of the intercostal and other respiratory muscles, with subsequent domination by diaphragmatic respiration) and ends with paralysis of all of the respiratory muscles except the diaphragm.

Plane 4

This plane begins with the cessation of intercostal muscle movements and ends with diaphragmatic paralysis.

Stage IV: Apnea

Stage IV begins with complete respiratory paralysis and ends with failure of the circulation.

Modern anesthetics act more rapidly than ether, and their actions are more difficult to observe.

Volatile Liquids

Ether

Ether (diethyl ether [$(C_2H_5)_2O$]) has been used more than any other anesthetic agent and has been studied extensively in humans and animals. Because its use illustrates some basic principles, it is discussed here in some detail.

Chemistry

Diethyl ether is a clear, volatile liquid with a pungent odor. It boils at 36.5°C and has a vapor pressure of 425 torr at 20°C. The minimum alveolar concentration (MAC) (see Chap. 29) in humans is 1.9 percent. At low concentrations, ether will burn; at higher concentrations, in the presence of oxygen, it may explode.

Pharmacological Actions

Ether is a general central nervous system (CNS) depressant. The observed signs of anesthesia result from a differential suppression of facilitative and inhibitory neurons, as well as from some peripheral effects. The high solubility of ether in blood and tissues leads to a slow induction and emergence.

Respiration

Ether increases the rate and minute volume of ventilation *directly* through stimulation of the brainstem respiratory center and *indirectly* through an irritation of the sensory receptors of the airways. Although ventilation is maintained, the sensitivity of the respiratory center to elevated CO_2 is reduced; this suggests the simultaneous presence of some degree of respiratory depression.

The ability of ether to stimulate respiration permits surgical anesthesia to be maintained with the patient breathing spontaneously. Too deep a level of anesthesia will depress respiration, thereby slowing the uptake of additional ether.

Ether is a respiratory irritant associated with a high incidence of nausea and vomiting during induction and emergence, and in the postoperative period. It also has an unpleasant aftertaste. Atropine and other cholinergic muscarinic blocking drugs are used to decrease excessive secretions.

Circulation

Ether is a direct myocardial and peripheral vascular depressant. However, a simultaneous augmentation of central sympathetic outflow and adrenal catecholamine secretion, combined with a vagolytic effect, results in an increased heart rate and relatively stable cardiac output and blood pressure at surgical levels of anesthesia. At very deep levels, however, the depressant effect predominates, leading to failure of the circulation. Ether does not sensitize the myocardium to catecholamine-induced arrhythmias as does halothane.

Metabolism

A small fraction of inhaled ether is metabolized to relatively nontoxic products, such as ethanol and acetaldehyde.

Clinical Uses

Ether is a "complete" anesthetic, producing unconsciousness, amnesia, analgesia, and muscular relaxation at concentrations that permit adequate oxygenation.

Drug Interactions

Because ether is a direct vascular depressant, its administration may lead to severe hypotension in patients who are taking drugs that interfere with sympathetic nervous system reflexes. For instance, ganglionic blockade, catecholamine synthesis or storage inhibitors, and spinal anesthesia all can prevent the compensatory responses to the depressant effects of ether on the peripheral circulation.

Adverse Reactions

Despite its desirable properties, ether is seldom used today. Its high solubility in blood and tissues makes induction and emergence inconveniently prolonged and occasionally hazardous. It produces a high incidence of nausea and vomiting and an unpleasant aftertaste. Furthermore, flammability makes this agent unsuitable for safe use in many modern operating rooms.

Since ether produces such clear signs and stages of anesthesia, it remains a valuable teaching aid. It also is used fairly often in the laboratory to anesthetize animals safely and is frequently the standard to which newer anesthetic agents are compared.

Halothane

Halothane (CF_3-CHClBr) was the first practical, nonflammable volatile anesthetic agent, and its use has allowed the introduction of newer and more complex surgical techniques. Because of halothane's relatively narrow margin of safety, however, complex equipment has been necessary to administer the drug safely.

Chemistry

Halothane is a volatile, nonflammable, and relatively nontoxic fluorinated hydrocarbon. It has a sweet odor, boils at 50.2°C, and has a vapor pressure of 241 torr at

20°C. Halothane is slightly more soluble in tissues than is ether, but it is considerably less soluble in blood.

Pharmacological Actions

Since it produces little analgesia or neuromuscular blockade, as compared to ether, halothane is a complete anesthetic only in high doses. *Because it is much less soluble in blood than is ether, it reaches equilibrium more rapidly, and hence induction and emergence occur more quickly.* Its rapid action makes signs and stages of anesthesia difficult to observe. Therefore, overdosage may occur rapidly and with little warning.

Respiration

Halothane depresses respiration at all levels of anesthesia, leading to a decreased tidal volume and an increased respiratory rate. In contrast to ether, spontaneous ventilation with halothane cannot be used safely for very deep levels of anesthesia. If profound analgesia and neuromuscular relaxation are needed, respiration must be controlled and, therefore, a valuable sign of anesthetic depth is lost. Since other signs of anesthesia are less clear with halothane than with ether, dangerous overdosage can readily occur when ventilation is controlled.

Halothane is not a respiratory irritant and is, therefore, a desirable agent for use in asthmatic patients.

Halothane does not produce significant neuromuscular blockade at clinical levels of anesthesia. Relaxation is produced primarily by CNS depression of muscle activity.

Circulation

Like ether, halothane is a myocardial and peripheral circulatory depressant. Unlike ether, however, halothane does not produce a compensatory increase in central sympathetic tone; therefore, the depressant actions are unopposed. By a direct action on smooth muscle, halothane causes dilation of cerebral blood vessels, which, in patients with intracranial pathology, can, in turn, result in an increased intracranial pressure, at times with disastrous consequences.

Halothane, especially in the presence of hypoxia or hypercarbia, sensitizes the myocardium to the arrhythmogenic actions of catecholamines.

Halothane produces a rather predictable lowering of blood pressure, partly due to vasodilation but mainly as a result of myocardial depression. In patients with severe coronary artery disease, severe hypotension may prevent adequate myocardial perfusion. On the other hand, since the myocardium that is depressed by halothane requires less oxygen than in the basal state, there could be some benefit from this myocardial depression. The end result of course, depends on the balance between myocardial oxygen supply and oxygen demand. This balance is the subject of much controversy.

Clinical results to date suggest that the myocardial depression, as well as the lower blood pressure and heart rate, produced by halothane may be preferable to the hypertension and tachycardia seen with ether and some other anesthetic techniques.

Clinical Use

Halothane is pleasant smelling, nonirritating, and nonflammable. It is also potent enough to allow adequate oxygenation of severely ill patients. Because of these advantages, halothane has been widely used. Lack of analgesia and muscular relaxation have been compensated for by administration of analgesic drugs and muscular relaxants, thereby resulting in balanced anesthesia.

At present, halothane remains a versatile anesthetic agent and has accumulated an impressive safety record. However, because of fear that it is toxic to the liver (see the following section), its use has greatly declined.

Potential Toxicity

Halothane has been suspected of causing hepatic necrosis in a few patients who were previously healthy and had only minor surgery. It is believed that a hypersensitivity mechanism may be responsible, since the necrosis occurred more often after multiple anesthetic use. A few anesthesiologists who have been repeatedly exposed to trace concentrations of halothane also have had a hepatitislike syndrome (confirmed by liver biopsy).

Much of the evidence, however, is anecdotal and is based on reports involving single patients. It has been thought that some patients had an undetected viral hepatitis, and when they received halothane the appearance of the hepatitis was attributed to the drug rather than to the virus. Controversy continues to be associated with a possible halothane-related hepatitis.

Metabolism

Despite the presence of relatively stable carbon-fluorine bonds, halothane is readily metabolized to many products, some of which may be detected several weeks after administration. Although the metabolites may be nontoxic in the healthy individual, prior exposure to drugs that induce drug-metabolizing enzymes, as well as hypoxia, may increase the toxicity by modifying pathways of biotransformation and excretion.

Adverse Reactions

An increased incidence of spontaneous abortions and fetal malformations has been demonstrated in animals exposed to trace amounts of halothane for prolonged periods of time. Although operating room personnel also may be exposed to small amounts of halothane, there is no conclusive evidence that this type of exposure has any long-term harmful effects. However, modern operating rooms have been equipped with gas evacuation systems to prevent possible harm from trace amounts of these gases.

Preparations and Dosage

Halothane (*Fluothane*) is a liquid and is available in 125- and 250-ml containers. A 1% to 4% concentration (vaporized by a flow of oxygen or nitrous oxide and oxygen) is used for induction, whereas for maintenance of anesthesia, a 0.5% to 2.0% concentration is given.

Enflurane

Enflurane (*Ethrane*; CHF_2-O-CF_2CHFCl) is a nonflammable halogenated ether anesthetic. It produces some neuromuscular blockade (by a mechanism similar to that of ether). Its administration results in a rapid induction with little or no evidence of excitement, and recovery is rapid. An occasional case of hepatitis has been reported, but enflurane has not had the degree of adverse publicity that halothane has received. Enflurane produces a dose-dependent decrease in cardiovascular and respiratory function, but it does not sensitize the heart to catecholamines as much as does halothane. Higher concentrations are associated with seizurelike electroencephalographic (EEG) changes.

It is used today as an alternative to halothane. However, because it is also extensively metabolized, fear of toxicity has caused a decrease in its use as well.

Isoflurane

Isoflurane (*Forane*; CF_3CHCl-O-CHF_2), an isomer of enflurane, is a pungent nonflammable liquid. Because it is less soluble in tissues than either halothane or enflurane, emergence is more rapid. However, its pungent odor limits the speed of induction. Isoflurane maintains cardiac output, increases heart rate, and produces a peripheral vasodilation. These effects result from a combination of central sympathetic stimulation and peripheral depression. Isoflurane also potentiates the action of neuromuscular blocking agents. It does not sensitize the heart to catecholamines as greatly as does halothane.

Isoflurane is metabolized much less extensively than either halothane or enflurane, and thus it has less theoretical potential for hepatotoxicity. Only a few cases of hepatitis after isoflurane have been reported. These characteristics have caused isoflurane to overtake halothane as the most-used volatile anesthetic agent in many institutions, despite its much higher cost.

Methoxyflurane

Methoxyflurane (*Penthrane*; $CHCl_2CF_2$-O-CH_3) is a sweet-smelling, nonflammable halogenated ether whose high solubility in blood and tissues makes induction and emergence slow. It produces profound analgesia and depresses the myocardium, but it does not cause an increased arrhythmogenic effect in the presence of catecholamines. Unfortunately, methoxyflurane may cause irreversible renal failure as a result of toxic amounts of fluoride ion produced during the drug's metabolism by microsomal enzymes. Methoxyflurane is no longer used clinically.

Chloroform

Chloroform ($CHCl_3$) was used extensively as an anesthetic from the 1840s onward and was used in England even before ether. It thus has an important place in the history of anesthesia. It is a rapidly acting agent, with many similarities to halothane. Because many deaths from cardiac arrhythmias resulted from its sensitization of the heart to catecholamines, and because it produced a dose-related hepatotoxicity, it is no longer used clinically.

Sevoflurane

Sevoflurane (($CF_3)_2$-CH-O-CH_2F) is a fluorinated anesthetic that is currently being tested in the United States. It is half as soluble in blood as is halothane, and is not pungent. Therefore, induction and emergence are rapid and pleasant. Its cardiovascular and respiratory effects are similar to those of other fluorinated agents. Sevoflurane is extensively metabolized to inorganic fluoride and alkylating agents. Although it has been used safely in Japan for several years, its potential for toxicity may delay or prevent its introduction in the United States.

Desflurane

Desflurane (*Suprane*; CF_3-CHF-O-CF_2H) is another new fluorinated agent under clinical evaluation. It is even less soluble in blood than sevoflurane. Although emergence is rapid, its extreme pungency severely limits its use as an induction agent. Desflurane is a direct myocardial and respiratory depressant, but sustained sympathetic activity helps to preserve cardiac output. It is very stable chemically. Desflurane's extreme volatility makes administration difficult without special vaporizer technology.

Gases

The agents discussed in the following sections are gases at room temperature and atmospheric pressure; they are liquids when stored under pressure. Because these substances require more elaborate apparatus for their administration than do volatile liquids, their extensive use was delayed. Nitrous oxide is discussed in some detail because it is one of the most widely used general anesthetics. Cyclopropane also is discussed briefly because it was once a popular agent, and because its use illustrates some important pharmacological principles.

Nitrous Oxide

History

Nitrous oxide (N_2O) was first prepared by Joseph Priestley in 1772; its anesthetic properties were demonstrated in 1800.

Chemistry

Nitrous oxide is a colorless, relatively odorless gas that is available as a liquid under pressure in metal cylinders. Its vapor pressure at 20°C is 50 atm. Since its MAC is greater than 100 percent (see Chap. 29, Table 29-1), *it is incapable of producing surgical anesthesia in most patients*. It is used, therefore, as a supplement to other agents. N_2O is relatively insoluble in blood and tissues and thus induction and emergence are rapid. Although it is not itself flammable, it supports combustion and can lead to explosion when used with flammable agents.

Pharmacological Actions

Usually, 60 to 80% N_2O (with 20–40% oxygen) is needed to produce unconsciousness. Analgesia may be produced by concentrations of N_2O in the 25 to 50% range. For example, 40% N_2O in oxygen can be used in obstetrics to relieve the pain of labor. Higher concentrations induce excitement (hence the term *laughing gas*), nausea and occasional vomiting, and unconsciousness. That *analgesia is profound* is evident from the decrease in the MAC of other agents that occurs when N_2O is used in conjunction with them; the effect on MAC seems to be additive to that of the other agents.

Respiration

While N_2O stimulates respiration, after the use of barbiturates and narcotics, the addition of N_2O may further depress respiration. N_2O is not an irritant, and induction is pleasant.

Circulation

Blood pressure is well maintained with N_2O, although the gas is a mild, direct myocardial depressant. Stimulation of the sympathetic nervous system as well as an increased responsiveness of vascular smooth muscle to norepinephrine contributes to the maintenance of blood pressure. N_2O does not sensitize the heart to the arrhythmogenic effects of catecholamines. When it is used with halothane, a reduction in cardiac output and an increase in peripheral resistance result, the latter effect helping to maintain blood pressure.

Interpretation of the effects produced by N_2O are difficult, because N_2O must be used with other agents.

Clinical Uses

Nitrous oxide is an *incomplete anesthetic*. When it is used along with other agents, a summation of MACs occurs; that is, the amount of intravenous or volatile agents needed to produce anesthesia is decreased as the concentration of N_2O is increased. This reduced requirement for other agents is desirable because the use of lesser amounts of these other agents allows more rapid awakening and a decreased incidence of cardiovascular side effects. Nitrous oxide is commonly employed as an adjunct to the use of volatile anesthetics.

Adverse Reactions

Chronic exposure of animals to trace amounts of N_2O may be teratogenic and may produce bone marrow depression; however, significant toxicities have not been apparent in humans. N_2O is not metabolized.

Preparation

This gas is available in sealed, blue metal cylinders as *nitrous oxide.*

Cyclopropane

Although cyclopropane was synthesized in 1882, it was not used clinically until 1934.

Chemistry

Cyclopropane (C_3H_6) is a sweet-smelling gas with a relatively high boiling point (-33°C). The MAC in humans is 9.2 percent, which allows maintenance of adequate oxygenation. Its solubility in blood is relatively low, and thus induction of anesthesia in 1 or 2 min is possible. *Cyclopropane is explosive,* giving off a large amount of energy when its strained ring structure is broken.

Table 30-2. Summary of Major Characteristics of Important Anesthetics

Anesthetic	Analgesia	Blood pressure	Respiration	Muscle relaxation	Prominent adverse effects	MAC (%)	Blood-gas partition coefficient at 37°C	Vapor pressure at 20°C (torr)
Ether	4+	↑	↑	3+	Flammable; slow action	1.9	12	425
Halothane	2+	↓	↓↓	+.	Myocardial depression; hepatotoxicity?	0.77	2.3	243
Methoxyflurane	3+	↓	↓↓	+	Renal toxicity	0.16	12	23
Enflurane	2+	↓	↓↓	2+	Respiratory and cardiovascular depression	1.68	1.8	175
Isoflurane	2+	↓	↓↓	2+	Respiratory and cardiovascular depression	1.15	1.4	239
Chloroform	2+	↓	↓↓	+	Hepatotoxicity; narrow margin of safety	0.77 in dogs		160
Sevoflurane	2+	↓	↓↓	2+	Respiratory and cardiovascular depression	1.71	0.6–0.7	160
Desflurane	2+	↓	↓↓	2+	Respiratory and cardiovascular depression	6–7	0.42	669
Nitrous oxide	4+	Little change	Little change	None	Weak anesthetic—need other agents as well	105	0.47	Gas
Cyclopropane	2+	↑	↓	2+	Flammable; expensive	9.2	0.4	Gas

Key: MAC = minimum alveolar concentration; ↑ = increases; ↓ = decreases; + = slight change; 4 + = large change.

Pharmacological Actions

Cyclopropane decreases the tidal volume and increases the rate of ventilation, producing an overall decrease of alveolar ventilation. It is not a respiratory irritant and therefore induction is generally rapid, easy, and pleasant.

The mechanism by which cyclopropane maintains cardiac output and blood pressure in the presence of myocardial depression remains controversial. CNS sympathetic outflow is increased, leading to an increased peripheral sympathetic tone and an increased level of circulating catecholamines. An additional factor may be an increase in vascular sensitivity to the action of circulating catecholamines.

Cyclopropane can maintain blood pressure even in the presence of severe hypovolemia. This effect may lead to a false belief that the patient's blood volume is adequate. Termination of cyclopropane administration after prolonged anesthesia may then result in a severe hypotension (i.e., "cyclopropane shock").

Clinical Uses

Cyclopropane produces a rapid, pleasant induction, rapid emergence, and good muscle relaxation; it has a wide margin of safety, even when ventilation is spontaneous. On the other hand, it is expensive and explosive. Its use has markedly diminished in recent years.

Balanced Anesthesia

The adverse effects of anesthetic agents (Table 30-2) can be minimized by combining these agents with other drugs in *balanced anesthesia*. For example, while halothane-oxygen can be used to produce surgical anesthesia and muscular relaxation, the concentrations of halothane needed may produce unacceptable cardiovascular depression as well as prolonged awakening. N_2O is a profound analgesic and produces minimal cardiovascular depression; therefore, addition of N_2O to the anesthetic decreases the amount of halothane needed for anesthesia. In addition, nitrous oxide is less soluble in tissues than is halothane, so awakening is rapid. If neuromuscular blockers are added, even less halothane is needed. Finally, addition of small amounts of narcotics to provide supplementary analgesia, and benzodiazepines to provide supplementary sedation and amnesia, can reduce the halothane requirement even further. Similar considerations apply to N_2O-narcotic techniques.

Supplemental Reading

Baden, J.M., and Rice, S.A. Metabolism and Toxicity in Anesthesia. In R.D. Miller (ed.), *Inhaled Anesthetics* (3rd ed.). New York: Churchill Livingstone, 1990. P. 135–170.

Pavlin, E.G., and Su, J.Y. Cardiopulmonary Pharmacology in Anesthesia. In R.D. Miller (ed.), *Inhaled Anesthetics* (3rd ed.). New York: Churchill Livingstone, 1990.

Stevens, W.C., and Kingstone, H.G.G. Inhalation Anesthesia. In P.G. Barash, B.F. Cullen, and R.K. Stoelting (eds.), *Clinical Anesthesia* (2nd ed.). Philadelphia: Lippincott, 1992. Pp. 439–465.

Stoelting, R.K., and Dierdorf, S.F. (eds.). *Anesthesia and Co-Existing Disease* (2nd ed.). New York: Churchill Livingstone, 1988. Pp. 105–134.

Tinker, J. H. (ed.) Clinical pharmacology of desoflurane. *Anesth. Analg.* 75(Suppl.):S1–S54, 1992.

31

General Anesthetics: Intravenous Drugs

Michael B. Howie and *David J. Smith*

Contemporary anesthetic management of the average surgical patient is so structured that unconsciousness is achieved rapidly, intraoperative analgesia and muscle relaxation are easily maintained, and awakening is comfortable. Furthermore, it is desirable to have complete patient recovery from the residual psychomotor influences of the anesthetics and adjunctive drugs soon after emergence from unconsciousness. Thus, from a practical point of view, the anesthesiologist must be concerned with four major phases of patient management: *induction, maintenance, emergence,* and *recovery.* Throughout these phases, a primary clinical concern is that the drugs used be safe both for the patient and the operating room personnel. Therefore, pharmacological agents are chosen that do not severely or irreversibly compromise vital physiological functions and are not hazardous (e.g., flammable).

If most of the requirements of contemporary anesthetic management could be met by a single drug, its list of pharmacological credits would read as follows:

1. *It should induce anesthesia rapidly and safely.* Onset of anesthesia should occur within one arm-to-brain circulation time. The anesthetic used should not interact with other drugs, or irritate veins or injure tissues on injection.
2. *It should have limited effects on vital functions and protective reflexes.* Major physiological processes, such as the respiratory and cardiovascular systems, should not be dangerously affected. Minimal alterations may be acceptable on induction of anesthesia, but they should be transient.
3. *It should possess analgesic activity.* The relief of pain is a primary concern during surgery. A hypnotic agent that is also an analgesic would minimize reflex activities that occur in response to pain, such as movement or alterations in the cardiovascular or respiratory systems.

4. *It should produce neuromuscular relaxation.* Relaxation of skeletal muscle is particularly advantageous in facilitating intubation of the trachea to provide a manageable and safe airway. It may also be a prerequisite for the surgeon's access to the operating field.
5. *It should present no safety hazard.* The anesthetic agent must not be teratogenic, allergenic, flammable, or explosive. It should also not sensitize the myocardium to arrhythmias, induce vomiting, or cause elevated intracranial pressure.
6. *It should allow pleasant emergence from unconsciousness and a rapid return to psychomotor competence.* Recovery must be progressive and quick, with no lingering anesthetic depression. Metabolism to pharmacologically inactive metabolites should be so rapid that repeated dosing does not cause drug accumulation. Prompt recovery should facilitate the clinician's assessment of the patient and the patient's ability to become physiologically self-supporting.

As one critically evaluates the currently available intravenous (IV) anesthetics, it is apparent that none of these drugs possesses all these characteristics. Consequently, the anesthesiologist must employ a *combination* of drugs to take advantage of each drug's beneficial effects and minimize each agent's adverse qualities.

The choice of IV agents and anesthetic technique for a particular clinical situation is not simple. Although the patient's disease state may largely dictate the drugs to be used, it is rare that only one anesthetic technique or combination of drugs will meet the needs of a particular patient or operation. Furthermore, secondary factors, including the strong personal preference of the patient and the requirements of the surgeon, may modify the approach to anesthesia. In addition, the individual anesthesiologist's professional background may play a role, since the technique used will be performed best when the practitioner is confident.

Pharmacokinetic Properties of Intravenous Anesthetic Agents

Distribution

The *IV* anesthetic agents are drugs that are uniquely suited to accomplish the first requirement of anesthetic management—a rapid induction of unconsciousness. These agents induce anesthesia within one or two circulation times after their administration because they quickly achieve high concentrations in the central nervous system (CNS). The reason for their rapid appearance in the brain is twofold. First, they are very lipid soluble and, consequently, they diffuse rapidly through biological membranes, including the blood-brain barrier. Second, since the tissue accumulation of IV-administered lipid-soluble drugs is initially proportional to the distribution of cardiac output, a large proportion of the total dose of an IV anesthetic will be distributed to those tissues that have a high blood flow per unit of mass (e.g., brain, heart, liver, and kidney). Tissues with lower blood flows receive and remove proportionally less anesthetic during the initial phase of distribution. This concept is illustrated for thiopental in Fig. 31-1. All currently used IV anesthetic drugs show this pattern of initial distribution. The use of these agents permits the patient to pass rapidly through the initial stages of anesthesia, and sleep is induced quickly.

The initial unequal tissue distribution of the drugs that is responsible for the rapid induction of anesthesia cannot persist. Physicochemical forces eventually dictate the establishment of concentration equilibria throughout the body. Therefore, as the drug continues to be removed from the blood by the less richly perfused tissues or eliminated by metabolism and excretion, or both, plasma levels will fall, and the concentration of anesthetic in the brain will decline precipitously. The rate of decline from a single intravenous bolus of drug is defined by the half-life ($t_{1/2}$) (see Chap. 6).

Tissues with an intermediate blood flow per unit of mass, such as skeletal muscle and skin, are among the first to participate in the drug redistribution process. In fact, it is the patient's skeletal muscle tissue groups that will contain the largest proportion of the initial dose of anesthetic when the patient awakens (Fig. 31-2). *The majority of the IV drugs used to induce anesthesia are slowly metabolized and excreted, and depend on redistribution to terminate their pharmacological effects.* It can be said, therefore, that redistribution of IV anesthetics to skeletal muscle accounts for the

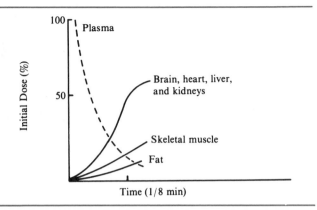

Figure 31-1. The initial distribution of thiopental in different body tissues and organs following its IV injection. (From H. L. Price et al., The uptake of thiopental by body tissues and its relation to the duration of narcosis. *Clin. Pharmacol. Ther.* 1:16, 1960.)

return to consciousness after a single "sleep dose" of these agents. Patients generally awaken 15 to 30 min after a single IV injection of most of the commonly used IV anesthetics.

Poorly perfused tissues (adipose tissue, connective tissue, and bone) require hours to come into equilibrium with plasma drug concentrations (see Fig. 31-2). Since the accumulation of anesthetic in body fat is relatively small soon after IV administration, it is common clinical practice to calculate drug dosage on the basis of *lean body mass* rather than on total body weight. Thus, an obese patient may receive the same dose of IV anesthetic as a patient of normal body weight.

Since the distribution of blood flow is the dominant factor controlling both tissue drug levels and the accumulation of IV anesthetics, changes in cardiac output can be expected to influence the pharmacological effects of the IV anesthetics.

Because the body restricts blood flow to muscle and fat to preserve perfusion of the brain, *a greater proportion of the total dose of anesthetic will be delivered to the brain during times of diminished cardiac output,* such as in congestive heart failure or hemorrhage. At such times, smaller doses of anesthetic must be administered to avoid excessive CNS depression. The use of significantly lower doses of IV anesthetic drug also should be a consideration in elderly patients. They have lower cardiac output, less lean body mass, and often a reduced capacity for drug clearance.

The effect of increased cardiac output on the administered dose is opposite that discussed for a reduction in cardiac output. Patients who exhibit intense anxiety or who suffer from such diseases as thyrotoxicosis usually require greater amounts of anesthetic drug.

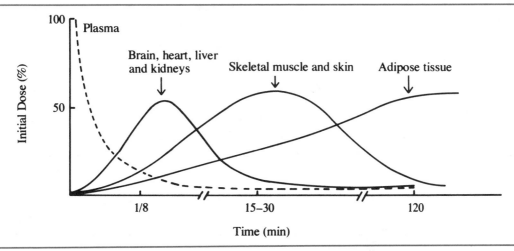

Figure 31-2. The distribution of thiopental in different body tissues and organs following its IV injection. Note the redistribution of the drug, with time, to tissues with lower rates of blood flow. (From H. L. Price et al., The uptake of thiopental by body tissues and its relation to the duration of narcosis. *Clin. Pharmacol. Ther.* 1:16, 1960.)

Metabolism and Excretion

The clearance of IV anesthetics from the body eventually requires metabolism and excretion. Specific characteristics of the biotransformation and elimination of these drugs are presented elsewhere in this text. Only those aspects of clearance that bear directly on clinical application are discussed in this chapter. In this regard, most of the IV agents, including ketamine, methohexital, midazolam, droperidol, highly potent phenylpiperidine narcotics, etomidate, and propofol, have elimination half-lives of 1 to 4 hr. The half-life of thiopental, however, is long (6.2 hr); diazepam has a half-life of about 30 hr.

Since the long half-lives of these drugs dictate that clearance will be slow, their use by repeated IV bolus to maintain anesthesia has been restricted. Repeated application, with limited concern for the pharmacokinetics of the agents, leads to delayed awakening, as tissues such as skeletal muscle and fat contain large quantities of these drugs. Thus, after lengthy anesthetic administration, drug plasma levels will remain high as the compound diffuses from these tissue reservoirs. Patients, therefore, may awaken quite slowly (hours) and psychomotor competence may be impaired for prolonged periods.

On the other hand, with the recent advent of computer-assisted intravenous drug administration, maintenance of anesthesia with IV anesthetics that have relatively shorter half-lives (1–4 hr) is more practical. *The loading and maintenance doses of each agent can be programmed taking their individual pharmacokinetic profiles into consideration.* Thus, dosage is automatically adjusted to maintain a plasma level that is just adequate for the proper depth of anesthesia. This approach prevents inadvertently overdosing the patient with repeated IV boluses, which may yield concentrations in excess of the therapeutic range.

In addition to the control derived from computer-assisted drug delivery, evolving methods of processing the electroencephalogram (EEG) may help quantify anesthetic depth and drug dose requirement. One of the more promising techniques is the bispectral index, which is derived by quantifying relationships that exist between the various frequencies that make up the EEG. Initial studies have found it to predict accurately movement responses to a skin incision independent of the type of anesthetic administered.

General Uses of Intravenous Anesthetic Agents

The rapid onset of action of IV anesthetics makes them ideally suited for the induction of anesthesia. However, some of the agents with shorter half-lives such as propofol and midazolam assume a greater role as maintenance anesthetics, since delayed recovery is limited. This is particularly true for operative procedures of shorter duration. As will be apparent later in this chapter, IV anesthetics can also be administered in combination for the maintenance of anesthesia when both hypnosis and analgesia (a characteristic that is achieved predominantly by the IV narcotic anesthetics) are necessary. They are also used to intermittently supplement inhalational anesthesia. Furthermore, infusions of the drugs can be used to provide sedation of either short duration during topical or regional anesthesia, or for longer periods as may be encountered in intensive care.

Ultra–Short-Acting Barbiturates

Among the barbiturates (see Chap. 33), three compounds, thiopental sodium (*Pentothal Sodium*), thiamylal sodium (*Surital*), and methohexital sodium (*Brevital Sodium*), are useful either as induction agents or as maintenance hypnotics for short surgical procedures. These drugs are called *ultra–short-acting agents,* since their rapid entry into the CNS is followed by a relatively quick redistribution of the drug to indifferent tissues, such as skeletal muscle. Because of their slow rate of metabolism, these agents, when used in large repeated doses or by continuous infusion, will cause a persistent hypnosis or a subtle mental cloudiness.

Chemistry

The rapid entry of the ultra–short-acting barbiturates into the brain is related to their high lipid solubility. The structural characteristic responsible for the high lipid-water partition coefficient of these weak acid drugs is a sulfur substitution (thiobarbiturates) at the C2 position on the oxybarbituric acid ring (thiopental and thiamylal) or a methyl substitution on the nitrogen ring adjacent to the C1 or C3 position (methohexital, an oxybarbiturate).

Pharmacological Actions

All three IV barbiturates rapidly produce unconsciousness after IV administration. Since *unconsciousness is attended by amnesia without analgesia or skeletal muscle relaxation,* anesthetized patients may react to painful stimuli but are unaware of, and do not remember, the procedure. For example, patients undergoing short surgical procedures with thiopental alone would respond to surgical maneuvers with facial grimaces or arm and leg movements as well as with potentially dangerous changes in blood pressure and heart rhythm. Consequently, induction of anesthesia may be nearly the only indication for thiopental. However, should it be used as a maintenance anesthetic for short operative procedures, analgesia should be supplemented with a narcotic or with the inhalational anesthetic nitrous oxide (N_2O).

Thiopental is currently the most popular IV induction agent. Among the reasons for its high acceptance rate by both the patient and the practitioner is its rapid and pleasant induction of anesthesia. Additionally, it does not induce obstructive secretions in the airway, produces little or no emesis, and does not sensitize the myocardium to endogenous catecholamines that may be released in response to the stress of surgery.

Although the pharmacological actions of the IV barbiturates are similar, methohexital may provide some advantages in selected situations. Methohexital is about three times more potent than thiopental; its duration of action is only half as long, and thus it exerts fewer cumulative effects. The occasional requirement of intraoperative communication between the patient and surgeon is easily satisfied with methohexital because of its short duration of action. For example, it can be used for basal sedation in the few moments that a very painful stimulus is applied, and then, as consciousness is quickly regained, the surgeon can assess the results by talking to the patient.

Adverse Reactions

Cardiovascular depression may occur after the administration of barbiturates by IV bolus. The hemodynamic changes are transient in the healthy patient with good cardiovascular reserve, but they may be prolonged and/or not well tolerated in elderly patients or those with poorly compensated myocardial function. For example, thiopental decreases myocardial contractility and also dilates capacitance vessels, thereby reducing venous return to the heart. The healthy, normovolemic patient may compensate for these changes by an increase in heart rate to maintain stroke volume and blood pressure. The patient with myocardial disease or hypovolemia may not be capable of an appropriate compensation. In fact, the combination of decreased contractility, hypotension, reduced myocardial blood flow, and increased heart rate may cause serious ischemic impairment of the myocardium in those patients with coronary artery disease.

Respiratory depression may also occur after the administration of barbiturates by IV bolus. Respiration may be further compromised by barbiturate-induced laryngospasm, as it is with most anesthetics.

Since the ultra–short-acting barbiturates are weak acids that are poorly soluble in aqueous acidic media, they are marketed as injectable solutions that are maintained at pH 11.0. There is some tendency for the drugs to precipitate at biological pH once they are injected, especially if the injection solution is not given slowly enough to allow the drug to be diluted by the venous blood. If inadvertent intraarterial injection occurs and drug precipitates are formed, arterial thrombosis, vasospasm, local ischemia, and possibly tissue sloughing may occur. Methohexital precipitation is less common, since it is a more potent barbiturate and can be provided in a more dilute solution. To avoid drug precipitation in the IV lines, the commercially available barbiturate solutions must not be coadministered with acidic solutions such as those containing meperidine, morphine, or ephedrine.

Most of the adverse reactions are predictable and therefore can be controlled or avoided. There are also reactions, such as hypersensitivity reactions, that are entirely unpredictable. Patients, particularly those with asthma, urticaria, or angioedema, may acquire an allergic hypersensitivity to the barbiturates. Therefore, the ultra–short-acting barbiturates should be used with caution in patients who have a history of hypersensitivity reactions.

An absolute contraindication to the use of barbiturates is acute intermittent porphyria (see Chap. 33).

Benzodiazepines

The benzodiazepine derivatives diazepam (*Valium*) and midazolam hydrochloride (*Versed*) have gained popularity as IV anesthetic agents because of their limited effects on the cardiovascular and respiratory systems. IV doses, delivered slowly, produce little change in blood pressure and only a transitory depression of respiratory minute volume. As a consequence, benzodiazepines may be logical substitutes for barbiturates in poor-risk patients who cannot tolerate respiratory depression. In other respects, they appear pharmacologically similar to the barbiturates (see Chap. 33), although they produce a more intense anesthetic effect that extends into the postoperative period. *IV administration causes unconsciousness without analgesia;* skeletal muscle relaxation is inadequate for intubation or short surgical procedures.

Midazolam is currently the most popular benzodiazepine used for IV anesthesia. Its aqueous solubility is one of the reasons for its popularity. In contrast, diazepam has limited water solubility and must be formulated in special solvents that consist mainly of propylene glycol, ethyl alcohol, and sodium benzoate (*Valium Injectable*). Because of the formulation's viscosity, injection must be performed slowly, and induction is delayed. Diazepam also may precipitate on injection and cause pain and vascular irritation. These disadvantages are minimized by the aqueous solution of midazolam, although some irritation at the injection site is still reported.

Midazolam has a shorter half-life ($t_{1/2}$ = 1.3–2.2 hr) than diazepam ($t_{1/2}$ = 30 hr) and is not converted to active metabolites by microsomal oxidation in the liver. Thus, a more rapid return to psychomotor competence is achieved. The recommended dosage of midazolam for induction of anesthesia is 0.3 to 0.35 mg/kg IV. Doses may need to be lowered by at least 30 percent in older patients or in those premedicated with narcotics or other sedative drugs.

A benzodiazepine drug that is used extensively in cardiac surgery is lorazepam (*Ativan*). It produces profound amnesia and is particularly useful during cardiopulmonary bypass to ensure unawareness of the procedure during that initial period when anesthetics become diluted in the fluid in the bypass circuit, before the adjustment of dosage. If the operation is to be short, lorazepam may not be the benzodiazepine of choice because of its prolonged duration of action. In this instance, midazolam might be used.

Recently, benzodiazepine antagonists have been developed.

Ketamine

Ketamine (Fig. 31-3), a cyclohexanone derivative, is a nonbarbiturate compound whose pharmacological actions are distinctly different from those of the other IV anesthetics. The state of unconsciousness it produces is trancelike (eyes may remain open until deep anesthesia is obtained) and cataleptic in nature; it has frequently been characterized as dissociative (the patient may appear awake and reactive but does not respond to sensory stimuli). The action is quite different from that of any other compound used in anesthesia, and the term *dissociative anesthesia* is used to describe these qualities of profound analgesia, amnesia, and a superficial level of sleep.

Pharmacological Actions

The clinical signs seen during anesthesia with ketamine can be contrasted with those produced by the barbiturates. Slow IV administration of ketamine causes neither gradual loss of airway reflexes, nor apnea, nor generalized relaxation, which are seen with the barbiturates. The onset of the ketamine-induced "anesthetic state" is accompanied by a gradual, mild increase in muscle tone (which greatly resembles catatonia), a continued maintenance of pharyngeal and laryngeal reflexes, and opening of the eyes (usually accompanied by nystagmus). Although muscle tone may be maintained, the airway still deserves protection, since ketamine sensitizes laryngeal

Figure 31-3. Ketamine.

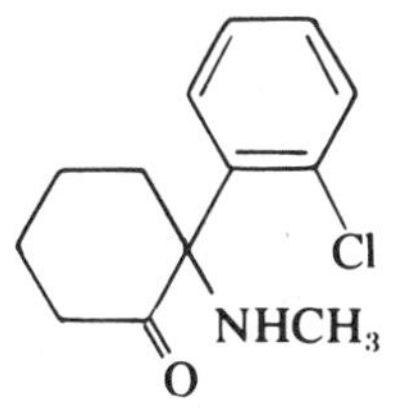

and pharyngeal muscles to mucous or foreign substances and laryngospasms may occur.

Ketamine also can be contrasted with the barbiturates in its ability to cause cardiovascular stimulation rather than depression. The observed increases in heart rate and blood pressure appear to be mediated through a stimulation of the autonomic nervous system. In a healthy, normovolemic, and unpremedicated patient, the initial induction dose of ketamine *maintains or stimulates cardiovascular function*. Additional doses of ketamine, however, are less predictable in this regard.

Patients with poor cardiac reserve, compromised autonomic control, or hypovolemia may experience a precipitous fall in blood pressure after induction of anesthesia with ketamine. However, if patient selection and preoperative preparation are carefully done, ketamine may be an excellent drug for the induction of anesthesia in individuals who cannot tolerate a compromise of their cardiovascular system.

The analgesia induced by ketamine also is a property that separates it from other IV anesthetic drugs. The analgesia is obtained without the induction of deep levels of anesthesia. When subdissociative doses of ketamine are given either IV or intramuscularly, they provide adequate analgesia for postoperative pain relief as well as analgesia for brief operations on the skin, such as debridement of third-degree burns.

A most important advantage of ketamine over other anesthetic agents is its potential for administration by the intramuscular route. This is particularly useful in anesthetizing children, since anesthesia can be induced relatively quickly in a child who resists an inhalation induction or the insertion of an IV line.

Clinical Use

Ketamine has a limited but useful role as an IM induction agent and/or in pediatrics. Because it is such a good analgesic, it is used for the repeated need for anesthesia in burn patients, especially during the changing of dressings.

Because it can be regarded as nearly a complete anesthetic (hypnosis and analgesia), does not require anesthesia equipment, and is relatively protective of hemodynamics, ketamine can be very useful outside of normal operating room conditions. It has a great value in developing countries and under military conditions.

Adverse Reactions

The most serious disadvantage to the use of ketamine as an IV anesthetic agent is the drug's *propensity to evoke excitatory and hallucinatory phenomena* as the patient emerges from anesthesia. Patients in the postoperative re-

covery period may be agitated, scream and cry, hallucinate, or experience vivid dreams. These episodes may be controlled to some extent by maintaining a quiet reassuring atmosphere in which the patient can awaken or, if necessary, by administering tranquilizing doses of diazepam. Adults appear more likely to experience terrifying reactions postoperatively. Although children probably have such reactions, they are less likely to report them.

Other reported side effects include vomiting, salivation and lacrimation, shivering, skin rash, and an interaction with thyroid preparations that may lead to hypertension and tachycardia. Ketamine may also raise intracranial pressure and elevate pulmonary vascular resistance, especially in children with trauma or congenital heart disease. Increases in intraocular pressure also may occur and vigilance is required if ketamine is used in ocular surgery.

Preparations and Dosage

Ketamine hydrochloride (*Ketaject, Ketalar*) is available in the form of injectable solutions containing 10 mg/ml, 50 mg/ml, or 100 mg/ml. Induction by the IV route usually requires a dose of 1 to 2 mg/kg, whereas IM induction commonly employs 10 mg/kg. Injections of one-half the induction dose are used for maintenance.

Etomidate

Etomidate (Fig. 31-4) is a carboxylated derivative of imidazole. Its pharmacological properties are similar to those of the barbiturates, although it may have a greater margin of safety because of its limited effects on the cardiovascular and respiratory systems. Since the drug has a relatively short elimination half-life ($t_{1/2} = 2.9$ hr), in addition to its use as an induction agent etomidate has been used as a supplement to maintain anesthesia in some crit-

Figure 31-4. Etomidate.

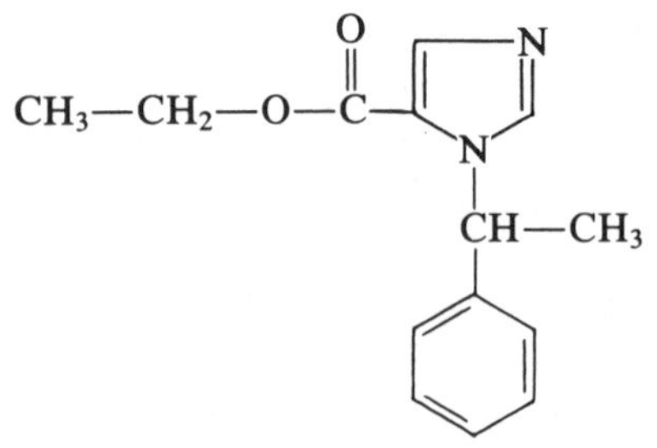

ically ill patients. Etomidate is rapidly hydrolyzed in the liver.

Pharmacological Actions

A primary advantage of etomidate is its ability to preserve cardiovascular and respiratory stability; cardiac output and diastolic pressure are well maintained. Use of etomidate may offer some advantage to the patient with compromised myocardial oxygen or blood supply, or both, since it appears to be capable of producing mild coronary vasodilation. Preservation of diastolic perfusion pressure may be particularly important when myocardial blood supply cannot be increased by autoregulation.

Adverse Reactions

Etomidate may cause pain on injection; the incidence is minimized by formulating it in 35% propylene glycol and using a slow injection into large veins. The drug can also produce myoclonic muscle movements in approximately 40 percent of patients during its use as an induction anesthetic.

An important adverse effect of etomidate is suppression of the adrenocortical response to stress. This suppression may last up to 10 hr if etomidate is used for induction of anesthesia. In fact, it has been suggested that patients at risk due to unexpected stress perioperatively may benefit from supplementation with glucocorticoids and mineralocorticoids.

Preparation and Dosage

Etomidate (*Amidate*) is available in an injectable solution: 2 mg of etomidate/1 ml of 35% propylene glycol. The recommended induction dose is 0.3 mg/kg administered IV. Smaller increments can be administered to adult patients to supplement the maintenance of anesthesia for short procedures.

Propofol

Propofol (*Diprivan*) (Fig. 31-5), an alkylphenol, is a rapidly acting compound, has a short recovery time, and is associated with less nausea and vomiting than some other IV anesthetics. It is very lipid soluble and enters the brain quickly. It is, however, nearly insoluble in aqueous solution and has to be solubilized in an emulsion formulation.

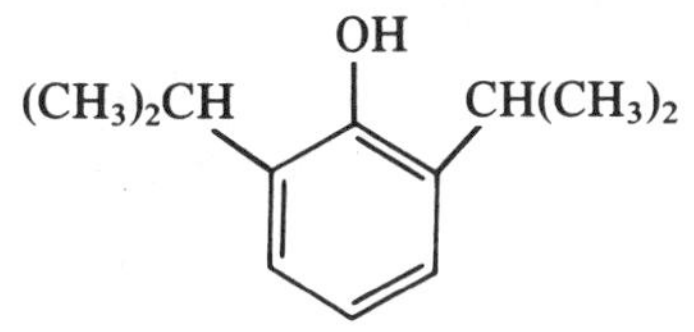

Figure 31-5. Propofol.

A rapid onset of anesthesia (50 sec) is achieved with 1.5 to 3.0 mg/kg IV of propofol and, if no other drug is administered, recovery will take place in 4 to 8 min. The recovery is attributed to a rapid redistribution of the drug to many tissues, including those where elimination processes take place.

Rapid recovery from propofol anesthesia makes the drug very popular in ambulatory anesthesia. Propofol can also be used to supplement inhalational anesthesia in longer procedures, and the continuous infusion of this drug is now an acceptable technique.

Propofol lacks analgesic properties but lowers the dose of opioid needed when used in combination. Logically, shorter-acting narcotics (e.g., alfentanil) are appropriate for use in matching the short duration of action of propofol, and in ensuring rapid recovery from anesthesia. In principle, the use of two or three drugs in combination, to decrease the total dose of each and yet still achieve the desirable properties of a good anesthetic agent, may be the most appropriate application of propofol in anesthesia.

The dose of propofol should be reduced in older patients; however, the drug does have a relatively linear dose-response characteristic, and it can be safely titrated. There is pain on injection especially through small veins. The pain can be reduced considerably if a small dose of lidocaine (20 mg) is administered first into the vein.

Anesthesia induction with propofol causes a significant reduction in blood pressure that is proportional to the severity of cardiovascular disease or the volume status of the patient, or both. However, in healthy patients a significant reduction in systolic and mean arterial blood pressure still occurs.

Although systemic vascular resistance is decreased by propofol, a reflex tachycardia is not observed. This is in contrast to thiopental, with which a reduction of cardiac output is accompanied by a slight heart rate increase. It is likely that the heart rate stabilization of propofol relative to other agents is the result of increased vagal tone. Propofol does not affect the pressor and depressor baroreflexes. Since propofol does not depress the hemodynamic response to laryngoscopy and intubation, its use may permit wide swings in blood pressure to occur at the time of induction of anesthesia. Propofol should be used with utmost caution in patients with cardiac disease.

Intravenous Anesthetic Techniques Managed With Narcotics

Narcotic analgesics have always been important for the control of pain in the pre- and postoperative periods. They also have been used during anesthesia to provide supplemental analgesia when pain reactions are not adequately controlled by other anesthetic drugs (see Balanced Anesthesia, in Chap. 30). Recently, the more potent and rapidly acting narcotics have been used as induction agents when hemodynamic stability is essential, as it is for cardiovascular surgery. High doses are required to induce unconsciousness, but hemodynamic responses to intubation are inhibited with minimal depression of cardiovascular function.

The narcotics most commonly used are the highly potent, short-acting phenylpiperidine compounds (see Chap. 39), such as fentanyl (25–150 μg/kg), sufentanil citrate (*Sufenta*, 5–15 μg/kg), and alfentanil (*Alfenta*, 130–245 μg/kg).

The phenylpiperidine narcotics also can be used in supplemental doses or by continuous infusion to maintain anesthesia (*opioid anesthesia*). This technique is particularly useful in patients with compromised myocardial function. However, the narcotics depress respiration by inhibiting the responsiveness of the medullary respiratory center to pCO_2 and alter the rhythm of breathing. Consequently, it is necessary to be prepared to assist ventilation intraoperatively. Since respiratory depression may extend into the postoperative period as a result of drug accumulation in the tissues, *the use of opioid anesthesia remains most appropriate for patients who are expected to require postoperative ventilatory care.* Alfentanil has been used to minimize this postoperative complication because of its shorter elimination half-life and reduced accumulation in tissues. There also are ultra–short-acting phenylpiperidines currently in development.

Less potent narcotics have fallen into disfavor because of the prominence of untoward effects they produce when given in high doses. Meperidine hydrochloride (*Demerol*) causes tachycardia and morphine produces hypotension and brochoconstriction as a consequence of its histamine-releasing action.

Opioid-induced muscle rigidity is a frequent complication of this form of anesthesia. It is most common with phenylpiperidine drugs and occurs even after low doses of fentanyl, such as those needed for neuroleptanalgesia. Rigidity involves the chest wall and abdomen and thus significantly interferes with breathing. The problem may result from a narcotic-induced stimulation of spinal reflexes or interference with basal ganglia integration; the rigidity can be controlled through the use of neuromuscular blocking agents (e.g., pancuronium) and ventilatory support.

One of the most serious drawbacks of opioid anesthesia is the possibility of inadequate anesthetic depth. Signs of inadequate anesthesia include sweating, pupillary dilation, wrinkling of the forehead, and opening of the eyes. Most importantly, however, awareness or incomplete amnesia may occur. Consequently, additional doses of the narcotics are appropriate when signs of light anesthesia are manifest. Furthermore, many clinicians supplement the "high-dose" narcotic technique with either inhalational anesthetics or hypnotics such as benzodiazepines (midazolam for shorter cases; the longer-acting drug lorazepam for cases > 4 hr in duration) or, more recently, propofol. Unfortunately, the use of many of these supplemental drugs may result in some loss of cardiovascular stability; even when used alone, the supplemental agents may cause minimal hemodynamic alterations.

Supplemental Reading

Bovill, J.G., Sebel, P.S., and Stanley, T.H. Opioid analgesics in anesthesia: With special reference to their use in cardiovascular anesthesia. *Anesthesiology* 61:731, 1984.

Miller, R.D. (ed.). *Anesthesia.* New York: Churchill Livingstone, 1981.

Reves, J.G., et al. Midazolam: Pharmacology and uses. *Anesthesiology* 62:310, 1985.

Vernon, J. EEG bispectrum predicts movement at incision during isoflurane or propofol anesthesia. *Anesthesiology* 77:502, 1992.

White, P.F., Way, W.L., and Trevor, A.J. Ketamine—its pharmacology and therapeutic uses. *Anesthesiology* 56:119, 1982.

32

Local Anesthetics

J. David Haddox and *Patricia L. Baumann*

The first clinical use of a local anesthetic agent occurred in 1884, when German physician Carl Koller used cocaine as a topical agent for eye surgery. That same year, in the United States, Halsted used cocaine for a nerve block. These events inaugurated a new era of anesthesia, that of regional anesthesia. Regional anesthesia was adapted for a wide variety of surgical procedures. New applications were developed, including spinal, epidural, and caudal anesthesia. There were problems, however; cocaine was found to be extremely toxic and addictive. The search for a better local anesthetic led to the chemical synthesis of a number of other local anesthetics, which have more selective local anesthetic properties and few systemic side effects when used in therapeutic doses.

Properties of Local Anesthetics

An important property of the ideal local anesthetic is low systemic toxicity at an effective concentration. Onset of action should be quick, and duration of action should be sufficient to allow adequate time for the surgical procedure. The local anesthetic should be soluble in water and stable in solution. It should not deteriorate by the heat of sterilization. It should be effective both when injected into tissue or when applied topically to mucous membranes, and the effects it produces should be completely reversible.

Although the characteristics of an ideal local anesthetic are easily identifiable, synthesis of a compound possessing all these properties has not been accomplished. The compounds discussed in the following sections fall short of the ideal in at least one aspect. However, the judicious choice of a particular agent for a particular need will permit the practitioner to employ local anesthesia effectively and safely.

Chemistry

The basic components in the structure of local anesthetics are the lipophilic aromatic portion (a benzene ring), an intermediate chain, and the hydrophilic amine portion (see Fig. 32-1). In the intermediate chain, there is either an *ester linkage* from the combination of an aromatic acid and an amino alcohol (Fig. 32-1A) or an *amide linkage* from the combination of an aromatic amine and an amino acid (Fig. 32-1B). The commonly used local anesthetics can be classified as *esters* or *amides* based on the structure of this intermediate chain. Since the amide local anesthetics are chemically stable in vivo and in vitro, our current knowledge of the pharmacokinetics of local anesthetics is mostly derived from a study of these compounds. Esters, on the other hand, are rapidly hydrolyzed by plasma cholinesterase, and in vivo measurements of these compounds have been more limited.

Mechanism of Action

The application of a local anesthetic to a nerve that is actively conducting impulses will inhibit the inward migration of Na^+ ions. This results in elevation of the threshold for electrical excitation, reduction in the rate of rise of the action potential, slowing of the propagation of the impulse, and, if the drug concentration is sufficiently high, complete block of conduction. *The local anesthetics interfere with the process fundamental to the generation of the action potential, namely, the large transient, voltage-dependent rise in the permeability of the membrane to Na^+ ions.*

In addition to their effects on Na^+, local anesthetics also can reduce the increase in K^+ conductance that occurs in response to a voltage change. However, this effect is much smaller than that on Na^+ conductance and is not of major significance in blocking nerve conduction. *The effect*

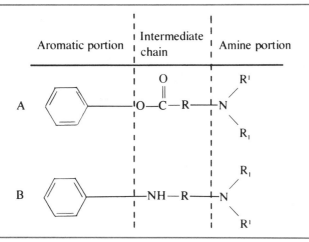

Figure 32-1. Model structure of local anesthetics, showing aromatic portion, intermediate chain, and amine portion.

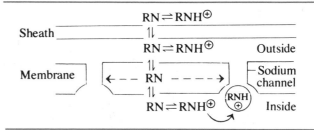

Figure 32-2. A diagrammatic representation of the proposed mechanism of action of local anesthetics. The ionized form (RNH^+) is required for binding to sites on sodium channels *(solid arrow)*, while the un-ionized form (RN) is necessary for the drug to reach its intracellular site of action and to cause membrane expansion *(dashed arrows)*. (Modified from J. M. Ritchie, Mechanism of action of local anesthetic agents and biotoxins. *Br. J. Anaesth.* 47:191, 1975.)

on K^+ conductance is manifest chiefly as a slowing of repolarization; the action-potential duration is lengthened.

Local anesthetics also can reduce the permeability to Na^+ and K^+ in a resting nerve, that is, one that is not actively generating action potentials. Because K^+ distribution and transmembrane movement are chief contributors to resting membrane potential, one might assume that local anesthetics would produce depolarization. This does not generally occur, however, because higher concentrations of drug are required to produce these effects on resting nerves than are needed for active nerves. This accounts for the fact that *nerve conduction can be blocked without any large or consistent change in resting membrane potentials.*

While the physiological basis for the local anesthetic action is known, the precise molecular nature of the process is not completely clear. At present, two theories enjoy considerable experimental support.

One proposal, the *membrane expansion theory,* is that the local anesthetics, by virtue of their lipophilic nature, become incorporated into the nerve cell membrane and disrupt the normal integrity of the membrane. This theory suggests that either a conformational change occurs in a critical macromolecule associated with the Na^+ conducting channels or that the lateral pressure in the membrane is increased because of the presence of the drug, or both. If lateral pressure is increased, the channels become constricted and, therefore, unable to accommodate the passage of ions.

Another hypothesis of local anesthetic action, the *specific receptor theory,* arises from knowledge that almost all local anesthetics can exist as either the uncharged base or as an ionized cation. *The uncharged base is important for adequate penetration to the site of action, and the charged form of the molecule is required at the site of action.*

In a nerve denuded of its sheath, and thus in the absence of a barrier to diffusion, local anesthetic activity was found to be greatly enhanced at low pH (i.e., under conditions favoring the formation of the cation). The cation appears to be required for binding to specific sites in or near the Na^+ channels. The presence of the local anesthetic at these sites interferes with the normal passage of Na^+ through the cell membrane. *In a sense, the local anesthetic "plugs" the Na^+ channel.*

Additional studies suggest that the receptor for the local anesthetic is near the inner (axoplasmic) surface of the cell membrane, because quaternary analogues of local anesthetics are quite effective when applied to the inside, but are inactive when placed on the outside of the membrane. These permanently charged molecules cannot penetrate to the receptor sites.

In summary, studies such as those just described have led to a proposal of a schematic model that incorporates elements of both the membrane expansion theory and the specific receptor theory to explain local anesthetic action. This model is shown in Fig. 32-2.

Differential Blockade

It is apparent from clinical observation that peripheral nerve functions are not affected equally by local anesthetics. Loss of sympathetic function usually occurs first, followed by loss of pin-prick sensation, touch, and temperature, and, lastly, motor function. This phenomenon is called *differential blockade.* Differential blockade may be related to the size of the nerve or the presence of myelin. These structural differences among the nerves that subserve different functions are summarized in Table 32-1. Nerve fibers are categorized into three major classes based on conduction velocity: A, B, and C. Myelinated somatic

Table 32-1. Classification of Nerve Fibers by Conduction Velocity

Classification	Location	Myelin	Relative diameter	Relative conduction velocity	Function
A fibers					
A-α	Efferent: Motor control	Yes	Large	Fast	Motor function
	Afferent: Muscle spindles				
A-β	Afferent: Muscle and skin	Yes	Large	Fast	Touch, pressure, vibration
A-γ	Efferent: Muscle spindles	Yes	Intermediate	Intermediate	Muscle tone
A-δ	Afferent: Skin	Yes	Intermediate	Intermediate	Pain, temperature, touch
B fibers	Efferent: Preganglionic	Yes	Small	Intermediate	Vasomotor, visceromotor, sudomotor
C fibers	Afferent: Skin and viscera	No	Small	Slow	Pain, temperature

nerves are A fibers, thinly myelinated preganglionic sympathetic nerves (white rami) are B fibers, and nonmyelinated nerves are C fibers. The nonmyelinated C fibers subserve pain and temperature transmission as well as postganglionic sympathetic efferent functions. The thinnest A fibers, the δ group, also subserve pain and temperature. Humans, therefore, have two separate systems that convey pain-related messages. The myelinated A-δ fibers convey sharp well-localized pain messages rapidly. The nonmyelinated C fibers are slowly conducting and convey diffuse, deep, pain messages.

Pharmacological Actions

Central Nervous System (CNS)

Local anesthetics given in initially high doses produce CNS stimulation characterized by restlessness, disorientation, tremors, and, at times, clonic convulsions. Continued exposure to high concentrations results in generalized CNS depression; *death occurs from respiratory failure* secondary to medullary depression. Treatment requires ventilatory assistance and drugs to control the seizures. The ultra–short-acting barbiturates and the benzodiazepine derivatives, such as diazepam, are effective in controlling these seizures. Respiratory stimulants are not effective.

Local anesthetics in therapeutic doses have anticonvulsant properties and have been administered to control status epilepticus. The presence of a convulsive disorder, such as epilepsy, does not contraindicate the use of local anesthetics. *The amygdala is the site of origin of convulsions produced by local anesthetics,* in contrast to the presumed cortical origin of idiopathic epilepsy.

Cardiovascular System

A high concentration of a local anesthetic in the systemic circulation will cause direct myocardial depression and, with the exception of cocaine, arteriolar dilation. Hypotension and cardiovascular collapse can ensue. The

effects on the myocardium include a decrease in contractile force as well as a decrease in electrical excitability and rate of conduction. The refractory period is prolonged and the threshold for stimulation is elevated. *Procainamide and lidocaine are, in fact, used extensively as antiarrhythmic agents* (see Chap. 26), but lidocaine has the advantage over procainamide of producing less depression of ventricular contractility.

The high incidence of hypotension associated with spinal and epidural anesthesia is related not to the direct effects of local anesthetics on the heart and blood vessels, but to the blockade of sympathetic outflow from the spinal cord. The degree of the sympathetic depression is proportional to the extent of the block. For example, a subarachnoid block (*spinal anesthetic*) given at the level of the fourth thoracic segment (T4) results in a higher incidence and more profound drop in blood pressure than does a block that only anesthetizes segments up to T10.

Neuromuscular System

Local anesthetics will inhibit or depress the actions of Ca^{2+} necessary to permit skeletal muscular excitation and contractility. Twitch response and the effects of tetanic stimulation are reduced along with the response of skeletal muscle to acetylcholine. Local anesthetics potentiate the effect of curare and other muscle relaxants.

Pharmacokinetic Properties

Absorption and Distribution

The rate of absorption of a local anesthetic into the bloodstream is affected by the dose administered, the vascularity at the site of injection, and the specific physicochemical properties of the drug itself. Local anesthetics gain entrance into the bloodstream by absorption from the injection site, direct intravenous injection, or absorption across the mucous membranes after topical application. Direct intravascular injection occurs accidentally when the needle used for infiltration of the local anesthetic lies within a blood vessel, or it occurs intentionally when lidocaine is used for the control of cardiac arrhythmias.

All tissues will be exposed to local anesthetics after their absorption, but the concentration achieved will vary among the different organs. Although the highest concentrations appear to occur in the more highly perfused organs (i.e., brain, kidney, and lung), factors such as degree of protein binding and lipid solubility also affect drug distribution. The lung requires special consideration because it has been shown to absorb as much as 90 percent of a local anesthetic drug during the first pass. Consequently, it acts as a buffer to prevent higher and, therefore, more toxic concentrations than would occur otherwise.

Chemical substitution in the aromatic or amine portion of the molecule will alter the compound's lipid-water partition coefficient. Etidocaine, for example, is highly lipid soluble and therefore is found in higher concentration in body fat than are most of the other local anesthetics.

Placental transfer of local anesthetics is known to occur rapidly, and fetal blood concentrations generally reflect those found in the mother. However, the quantity of drug crossing to the fetus is also related to the time of exposure, that is, from the time of injection to delivery. Subtle neurobehavioral changes in the neonate are detectable for as long as 8 hr after mepivacaine administration to the mother, but are absent following the use of bupivacaine, lidocaine, and chloroprocaine. In general, minimal amounts of chloroprocaine reach the fetus because of its rapid hydrolysis by serum cholinesterase; this feature is its principal advantage in obstetrics.

Metabolism

The metabolic degradation of local anesthetics depends on whether the compound has an ester or an amide linkage. Esters are extensively and rapidly metabolized in plasma by pseudocholinesterase, whereas the amide linkage is resistant to hydrolysis. The rate of local anesthetic hydrolysis is important, since a slow biotransformation may lead to drug accumulation and toxicity when repetitive doses are required. In patients with atypical plasma cholinesterase, the use of ester-linked compounds, such as chloroprocaine, procaine, and tetracaine, has an increased potential for toxicity. The hydrolysis of all ester-linked local anesthetics leads to the formation of para-aminobenzoic acid (PABA), which is known to be allergenic in nature. Therefore, some people experience allergic reactions to the ester class of local anesthetics.

Local anesthetics with an amide linkage (and one ester drug, cocaine) are almost completely metabolized by the liver before excretion. However, the total dose administered and the degree of drug accumulation resulting from the initial and subsequent doses are still of concern. For example, the repetitive doses of mepivacaine that are re-

quired for lumbar epidural anesthesia may lead to drug accumulation and toxicity.

Clinical Uses

Local anesthetics are extremely useful in a wide range of procedures, varying from needle insertion to extensive surgery under regional block. For minor surgery, the patient can remain awake; this is an advantage in emergency surgery, because protective airway reflexes remain intact. Many operative procedures in the oral cavity are facilitated by regional block of specific nerves. If surgery permits, the patient can return home because he or she is less sedated than would be the case after general anesthesia.

Topical Anesthesia

Local anesthetics are used extensively on the mucous membranes in the nose, mouth, tracheobronchial tree, and urethra. *The vasoconstriction produced by some local anesthetics adds a very important advantage to their use in the nose by preventing bleeding and inducing tissue shrinkage.* Topical anesthesia permits many diagnostic procedures in the awake patient, and when it is combined with infiltration techniques, excellent anesthesia may be obtained for many surgical procedures in the eye and nose. The practitioner should be cautious when higher volumes are required, since systemic reactions may occur from overdosage. Additionally, when the tracheobronchial tree and larynx are anesthetized, normal protective reflexes, which prevent pulmonary aspiration of material, such as blood from surgery or regurgitated gastric contents, are lost.

Infiltration

Infiltration (i.e., the injection of local anesthetics under the skin) of the surgical site provides adequate anesthesia if contiguous structures are not stimulated. Since the onset of local anesthesia is rapid, the surgical procedures can proceed with little delay. Minimally effective concentrations should be used, especially in extensive procedures, so that toxicity from overdosage may be avoided.

Regional Block

Regional block, a form of anesthesia that *includes spinal and epidural anesthesia,* involves the injection near a nerve or nerve plexus proximal to the surgical site. It provides excellent anesthesia for a variety of procedures. Brachial plexus block is commonly used for the upper extremity. Individual blocks of the sciatic, femoral, and obturator nerves can be used for the lower extremity. An amount that is close to the maximally tolerated dose is required to produce blockade of a major extremity.

Spinal Anesthesia

Spinal anesthesia (subarachnoid block) produces extensive and profound anesthesia with a minimum amount of drug. *The local anesthetic solution is introduced directly into the spinal fluid* where the nerves are not protected by a perineurium. This produces, in effect, a temporary cord transection such that no impulses are transmitted beyond the level that is anesthetized. The onset is rapid, and with proper drug selection, the anesthesia may last from 1 to 4 hr. With careful technique, neurological complications are extremely rare. Procedures as high as upper-abdominal surgery can be performed under spinal anesthesia. Arterial hypotension produced by the local anesthetic is proportional to the degree of interruption of sympathetic outflow. The blood pressure is easily controlled and hypotension is not usually a deterrent to its use. The sites of action of spinal anesthesia are the spinal nerve roots, spinal ganglia, and (perhaps) the spinal cord. Respiration remains adequate with blocks as high as T4.

Lumbar Epidural Anesthesia

This procedure involves the same area of the body as does spinal anesthesia. As the name implies, *the drug is deposited outside the dura;* in contrast to spinal anesthesia, this method requires a much larger amount of drug. This procedure makes segmental anesthesia possible, whereby the anesthetized area is bordered caudally and cephalad by unaffected dermatomes.

The concentration and volume of the local anesthetic solution will affect the extent of the cephalad and caudad spread of the block. The anesthesia can be made continuous by maintaining a small catheter in the epidural space; prolonged effects are obtained by periodically injecting supplemental doses through the catheter. The site of anesthetic action is on the nerves as they leave the intervertebral foramina. However, effective drug concentrations may be found in the spinal fluid, probably gaining entrance through the arachnoid villi. Arterial hypotension occurs by the same mechanism and is managed as in spinal anesthesia. Inadequate respiration may occur if there is a block of both the thoracic nerves and the components of the phrenic nerve.

Epidural anesthesia is especially useful in obstetrics. Excellent analgesia occurs and the patient remains awake. Analgesia can be provided for labor and delivery or for cesarean section by the epidural route. Bupivacaine in lower concentrations has the advantage of providing excellent analgesia while minimally reducing motor strength.

Caudal Anesthesia

In this form of extradural anesthesia, the agent is introduced through the sacral hiatus above the coccyx. *It is particularly applicable to perineal and rectal procedures.* Anesthetization of higher anatomical levels is not easily obtained, because the required injection volume may be excessive.

Although caudal anesthesia has been used extensively in obstetrics, lumbar epidural blockade is now more commonly used because of the lower dose of drug required; in addition, the sacral segments are spared until their anesthesia is required for the delivery.

Intravenous Extremity Block

Excellent and rapid anesthetization of an extremity can be obtained easily. A rubber bandage is used to force blood out of the limb, and a tourniquet is applied to prevent the blood from reentering; a dilute solution of local anesthetic, most commonly lidocaine, then is injected intravenously. This technique fills the limb's vasculature and carries the anesthetic solution to the nerve by means of the blood supply. Because of the pain produced by a tourniquet after a period of time, this procedure usually is limited to a duration of less than 1 hr. The systemic blood levels of drug achieved after tourniquet release generally remain below toxic levels.

Although it is more easily and, therefore, more commonly used on the upper extremity, intravenous extremity anesthesia can be used on the leg and thigh.

Sympathetic Block

Blockade of the sympathetic nervous system can be more selectively accomplished than that which occurs during spinal or epidural anesthesia. Cell bodies for preganglionic sympathetic nerves originate in the intermediolateral cell column of the spinal cord, from the first thoracic to the second lumbar segments. The myelinated axons of these cells travel as white communicating rami before joining the sympathetic chain and synapsing with the ganglia. The best location for a sympathetic block is at the sympathetic ganglia since a block at this level will affect only the sympathetic nerves. For example, local anesthetic blockade of one stellate ganglion (which includes T1) blocks sympathetic innervation to all of the upper extremity and head on the injected side. A block of the sympathetic chain at L2 affects all of the lower extremity. This form of local anesthesia is particularly useful during treatment of a variety of vasospastic diseases of the extremities and for some pain syndromes.

Control of Cardiac Arrhythmias

Procainamide and lidocaine are two of the primary drugs that are used in treating cardiac arrhythmias. Since lidocaine has a short duration of action, it is common to administer it by continuous infusion. Procainamide, because of its amide linkage, has more prolonged action than does its precursor, procaine. Orally active analogues of local anesthetics (e.g., mexiletine) also are used as antiarrhythmics. These drugs are more effective in treating ventricular arrhythmias than those of atrial origin (see Chap. 26 for further details).

Use of Vasoconstrictors

The most commonly used vasoconstrictors, the *adrenomimetic drugs, are often added to local anesthetics to delay absorption of the anesthetic after its injection.* By slowing absorption, these drugs reduce the anesthetic's systemic toxicity and keep it in contact with nerve fibers longer, thereby increasing the drug's duration of action. Administration of lidocaine 1% with epinephrine results in the same degree of blockade as that produced by a 2% lidocaine solution without the vasoconstrictor.

Many vasoconstrictors are available, but *epinephrine is by far the most commonly employed.* Because epinephrine can have systemic effects, precaution is needed when local anesthetics containing this amine are given to a patient with hypertension or an irritable myocardium. Epinephrine-containing solutions should be used cautiously in persons taking tricyclic antidepressants, since those drugs may enhance the systemic pressor effects of adrenomimetic amines (see Chap. 36). Epinephrine is most commonly used with local anesthetics in a 1:200,000 concentration (5 μg/ml).

Levonordefrin (*Neo-Cobefrin*) is an active optical isomer of nordefrin that has α_1-adrenergic activity and possesses little or no β-agonist properties. It is used exclusively in some dental anesthetic cartridges as a vasoconstrictor. Its theoretical advantage is that it causes less hypertension and tachycardia than does epinephrine. It is used in a 1:20,000 concentration.

Phenylephrine hydrochloride (*Neo-Synephrine Hydrochloride*) is a pure α-agonist that is occasionally used in performing a subarachnoid block, and is marketed with procaine for use in dentistry in a 1:2,500 concentration. Systemic absorption can cause hypertension, but it has little direct cardiac effect. A reflex bradycardia, mediated by baroreceptors, may occur in response to the increased systolic and diastolic pressures.

Adverse Reactions

The central nervous and cardiovascular systems are most commonly affected by high plasma levels of local anesthetics. CNS toxicity is manifested initially by uneasiness, tremors, tinnitus, and shivering. Higher doses may result in convulsions, followed by respiratory depression and eventually coma. CNS manifestations generally occur before cardiovascular collapse.

Cardiac toxicity is generally the result of a drug-induced depression of cardiac conduction (e.g., atrioventricular block, intraventricular conduction block) and sys-

temic vasodilation. These effects may progress to severe hypotension and cardiac arrest.

Allergic reactions, such as a red and itchy eczematoid dermatitis or vesiculation, are of concern when administering the ester-type local anesthetics. True allergic manifestations have been reported with procaine. *The amides are essentially free of allergic properties,* but suspected allergic phenomena may be caused by methylparaben, a parahydroxybenzoic acid derivative used as an antibacterial preservative in multiple-dose vials and some dental cartridges. Because of the possibility of cross-sensitivity among the esters, they probably should be avoided in favor of an amide when the patient has a history of allergy to a local anesthetic or a PABA-containing preparation such as certain cosmetics or sunscreens.

Individual Agents

Esters

Cocaine hydrochloride (Fig. 32-3) is obtained from the leaves of the *Erythroxylon coca* and other species of *Erythroxylon*, trees indigenous to Peru and Bolivia. It is an ester of benzoic acid and ecgonine, an amino alcohol that is related to atropine. It remains useful primarily because of the vasoconstriction it provides with topical use. *Toxicity prohibits its use for other than topical anesthesia.*

Cocaine has a rapid onset of action (1 min) and a duration of up to 2 hr, depending on the dose or concentration used. Concentrations employed vary from 1 to 10 percent; the lower concentrations are used for the eye, while the higher ones are used on the nasal and pharyngeal mucosa. The combination of epinephrine with cocaine, although still used occasionally, is hazardous because the catecholamine potentiates the cardiovascular toxicity (e.g., arrhythmia, ventricular fibrillation) of cocaine.

Cardiovascular effects are related both to central and peripheral sympathetic stimulation. An initial bradycardia

Figure 32-3. Cocaine.

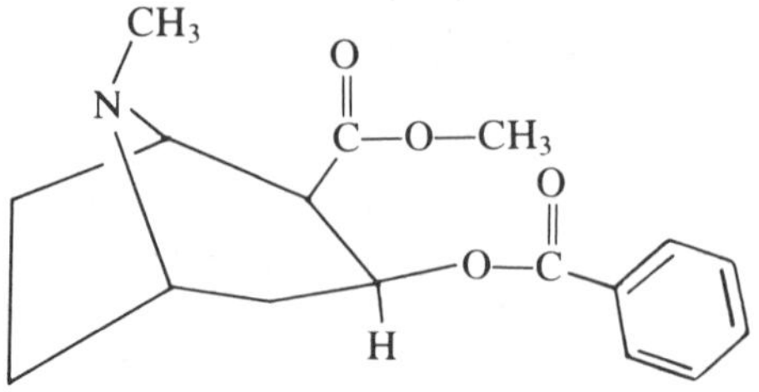

appears to be related to vagal stimulation; this is followed by tachycardia and hypertension. Larger doses are directly depressant to the myocardium, and death results from cardiac failure.

Cocaine is readily absorbed from mucous membranes and therefore the potential for systemic toxicity is great. The CNS is stimulated, and euphoria and cortical stimulation (e.g., restlessness, excitement) frequently result. Overdosage leads to convulsions followed by CNS depression. The cortical stimulation it produces is responsible for the drug's abuse (see Chap. 41), and because of its addictive potential the drug is controlled by federal regulation. It is available as crystalline powder; the hydrochloride readily dissolves in water.

Benzocaine is a PABA derivative used primarily for topical application to skin and mucous membranes. Its low aqueous solubility allows the drug to stay at the site of application for long periods. Its minimal rate of absorption after topical administration is associated with a low incidence of systemic toxicity. Benzocaine is contraindicated in patients with known sensitivity to ester-linked anesthetics or PABA-containing compounds. It is available in liquids, sprays, and ointments in concentrations ranging from 6 to 20 percent.

Chloroprocaine hydrochloride (*Nesacaine*) is obtained from the addition of a chlorine atom to procaine, which results in a compound of greater potency and less toxicity than procaine itself. This local anesthetic is hydrolyzed very rapidly by cholinesterase and therefore has a short plasma half-life. Because it is broken down rapidly, chloroprocaine is commonly used in obstetrics. It is believed that the small amount that might get to the fetus continues to be rapidly hydrolyzed, so there can be no residual effects on the neonate. It is used as a 1 to 3% solution, with the higher concentration used for epidural anesthesia.

Procaine hydrochloride (*Novocain*) was first synthesized in 1905 and continues to be useful today. It is readily hydrolyzed by plasma cholinesterase, although hepatic metabolism also occurs. It is not effective topically, but is employed for infiltration, nerve block, and spinal anesthesia. It has a relatively slow onset and short (1 hr) duration of action. Preparations are available from 0.25 to 2.0%; higher concentrations are used for nerve block, while lower concentrations are employed for infiltration anesthesia. For spinal anesthesia, up to 200 mg procaine can be used in a concentration as high as 10 percent. All concentrations can be combined with epinephrine. It is available in dental cartridges with phenylephrine as the vasoconstrictor.

Tetracaine hydrochloride (*Pontocaine Hydrochloride*) is an ester of PABA that is an effective topical local anesthetic agent at concentrations of 0.5 to 2.0 percent. It is quite commonly used for spinal (subarachnoid) anesthesia at doses from 5 to 20 mg, depending on the extent of the

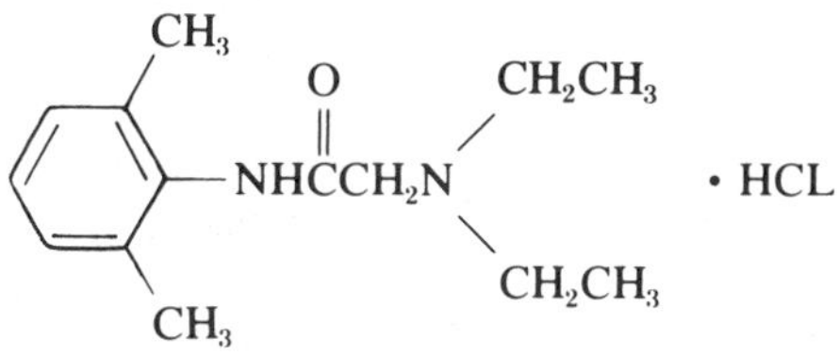

Figure 32-4. Lidocaine hydrochloride.

desired block. Epinephrine is frequently added to prolong the anesthesia. Tetracaine is considerably more potent and more toxic than procaine and cocaine. It has, approximately, a 5-min onset and a 2- to 3-hr duration of action.

Amines

Lidocaine hydrochloride (*Xylocaine*) is the most commonly used local anesthetic. Structurally, it is an amide type (Fig. 32-4). Lidocaine is well tolerated, and, in addition to its use in infiltration and regional nerve blocks, it is commonly used for spinal and topical anesthesia, and as an antiarrhythmic agent (see Chap. 26). It has a more rapidly occurring, more intense, and more prolonged duration of action than does procaine. Concentrations for surface anesthesia vary from 2 to 4 percent. Injectable concentrations are available in a range of 0.5 to 2.0 percent and contain epinephrine 1:50,000 to 1:200,000.

Bupivacaine hydrochloride (*Marcaine Hydrochloride*) has a particularly prolonged duration of action, and some nerve blocks last more than 24 hr; this is often an advantage for postoperative analgesia. Its use for epidural anesthesia in obstetrics has attracted interest, because it can relieve the pain of labor at concentrations as low as 0.125 percent while permitting some motor activity of abdominal muscles to aid in expelling the fetus. The lower concentration minimizes the possibility of cardiac toxicity. Fetal drug concentrations remain low and drug-induced neurobehavioral changes are not observed in the newborn. It also is approved for spinal anesthesia. It is approximately four times more potent and more toxic than mepivacaine and lidocaine. Bupivacaine is available in concentrations of 0.25 to 0.75 percent, with and without epinephrine (1:200,000).

Etidocaine hydrochloride (*Duranest*), although chemically similar to lidocaine, has a more prolonged action. It is used for regional blocks, including epidural anesthesia. It exhibits a preference for motor rather than sensory block; its use in obstetrics, therefore, is limited, although fetal drug concentrations remain low. It is available in 0.5 to 1.5% solutions, with or without epinephrine (1:200,000).

Mepivacaine hydrochloride (*Carbocaine Hydrochloride*) has a more prolonged action than that of lidocaine and a more rapid onset of action (3–5 min). Topical application is not effective. The drug has been widely used in obstetrics, but its use has declined recently because of the early transient neurobehavioral effects it produces. Adverse reactions associated with mepivacaine are generally similar to those produced by other local anesthetics. It is available in 1 to 2 percent concentration for injection and can be used with epinephrine or levonordefrin (dental use only).

Prilocaine hydrochloride (*Citanest*) is an amide anesthetic whose onset of action is slightly longer than that of lidocaine; its duration of action is comparable. Prilocaine is 40 percent less toxic acutely than lidocaine, making it especially suitable for regional anesthetic techniques. It is metabolized by the liver to orthotoluidine which, when it accumulates, can cause conversion of hemoglobin (Hb^{2+}) to methemoglobin (Hb^{3+}). When methemoglobinemia occurs, oxygen transport is impaired. Treatment involves the use of reducing agents, such as methylene blue, given intravenously, to reconvert methemoglobin to hemoglobin.

Ropivacaine is a recently developed long-acting, amide-linked local anesthetic. Its duration of action is similar to that of bupivacaine, but it is slightly less potent, requiring higher concentrations to achieve the same degree of block. Its primary advantage over bupivacaine is its lesser degree of cardiotoxicity.

New Directions

EMLA

A new type of topical anesthetic preparation is currently undergoing clinical trials. It is a formulation consisting of a *eutectic mixture of local anesthetics* (EMLA) prepared by mixing high concentrations of local anesthetics in an oil–water emulsion. It is used to provide topical anesthetic to intact skin. Currently available topical preparations are effective only on mucosal surfaces.

An EMLA containing lidocaine and prilocaine has been shown to provide reduced pain on venipuncture and substantial anesthesia for skin graft donor sites. No significant local or systemic toxicity has been demonstrated.

TAC

TAC (tetracaine, Adrenalin [epinephrine], and cocaine) is a combination topical anesthetic frequently used in pediatric emergency rooms for repair of minor lacerations. The usual mixture is 0.5% tetracaine, 1:2,000 epinephrine, and 11.8% cocaine. Because of potential complications (seizures), lower concentrations of cocaine and epinephrine in a 1% tetracaine solution have been suggested (TAC III).

Supplemental Reading

Arthur, G.R., and Covino, B.G. What's New in Local Anesthetics? In J.L. Benumuf and R.J. Fragen (eds.), *Anesthesiology Clinics of North America.* Philadelphia: Saunders, 1988. P. 357.

Butterworth, J.F., et al. Molecular mechanisms of local anesthesia: A review. *Anesthesiology* 72:4, 1990.

Carpenter, R.L., and Mackey, D.C. Local Anesthetics. In P.G. Barash, B.F. Cullen, and R.K. Stoelting (eds.), *Clinical Anesthesia* (2nd ed.). Philadelphia: Lippincott, 1992. P. 509.

Covino, B.G. Clinical Pharmacology of Local Anesthetic Agents. In M.J. Cousins and P.O. Bridenbaugh (eds.), *Neural Blockade in Clinical Anesthesia and Management of Pain* (2nd ed.). Philadelphia: Lippincott, 1988. P. 111.

Denson, D.D., and Mazoit, J.X. Physiology, Pharmacology and Toxicity of Local Anesthetics: Adult and Pediatric Considerations. In P. Prithvi Raj (ed.), *Clinical Practice of Regional Anesthesia.* New York: Churchill Livingstone, 1991. P. 73.

DiFazio, C.A., and Woods, A.M. Drugs Commonly Used for Nerve Blocking. In P. Prithvi Raj (ed.), *Practical Management of Pain* (2nd ed.). St. Louis: Mosby, 1992.

Lee-Son, S., et al. Stereoselective inhibition of neuronal sodium channels by local anesthetics. *Anesthesiology* 77:2, 1992.

Malamed, S.F. *Handbook of Local Anesthesia.* St. Louis: Mosby, 1980.

Smith, S.M., and Barry, R.C. A comparison of three formulations of TAC (tetracaine, Adrenalin, cocaine) for anesthesia of minor lacerations in children. *Pediatr. Emerg. Care* 6:4, 1990.

Tucker, G.T., and Mather, L.E. Properties, Absorption, and Disposition of Local Anesthetic Agents. In M.J. Cousins and P.O. Bridenbaugh (eds.), *Neural Blockade in Clinical Anesthesia and Management of Pain* (2nd ed.). Philadelphia: Lippincott, 1988. P. 47.

33

Sedative-Hypnotic and Anxiolytic Drugs

John W. Dailey

The primary use of drugs classified as sedative-hypnotics and anxiolytics is to encourage calmness (*anxiolytics or sedatives*) or to produce sleep (*sedative-hypnotics*). States of emotional tension and uneasiness are experienced by all people. For otherwise healthy individuals, these occasions are usually sufficiently mild and of such short duration that pharmacological intervention is unnecessary. However, at times, the symptoms of anxiety become quite discomforting and can interfere with a person's ability to function effectively. Anxiety almost invariably accompanies many medical and surgical conditions, and it is often a symptom of psychiatric illness. When the symptoms become intolerable or interfere with the treatment of the underlying disease and if counseling is not sufficiently effective, drug treatment can be considered as a means of helping patients cope with their anxiety.

All central nervous system depressants have some ability to relieve anxiety. However, most of these drugs relieve symptoms of anxiety only at doses that produce noticeable sedation. Drugs used to produce sedation and relieve anxiety are consistently among the most commonly prescribed drugs. Whether they are prescribed too frequently remains a matter of controversy.

Insomnia is also a very common problem. It includes a wide variety of sleep disturbances, such as difficulty in falling asleep, early or frequent awakenings, and remaining unrefreshed after sleep. Use of sedative-hypnotic drugs is one approach to the therapy of insomnia. Nonpharmacological measures can include advice to avoid stimulants before retiring, maintenance of a proper diet, initiation of an exercise program, and avoidance of stressful or anxiety-provoking situations.

Most anxiolytic and sedative-hypnotic drugs produce a dose-dependent depression of central nervous system function, and consequently various drugs in these categories are employed to relieve anxiety, produce muscle relaxation, induce or facilitate sleep, treat epilepsy (see Chap. 37), produce amnesia, and produce or facilitate general anesthesia (see Chap. 31).

The ideal anxiolytic drug should calm the patient without causing too much daytime sedation and drowsiness and without producing physical or psychological dependence. Similarly, the ideal hypnotic drug should allow the patient to fall asleep quickly and should maintain sleep of sufficient quality and duration so that the patient awakes refreshed without a "drug hangover." Also, both types of drugs should have very low toxicity and should not interact with other medications in such a way as to produce unwanted or dangerous effects.

Benzodiazepines

The benzodiazepines constitute the most commonly used group of anxiolytics and sedative-hypnotics. Since the first member of this group, *chlordiazepoxide,* was introduced into therapeutics, many congeners have been marketed. Most of these drugs possess anxiolytic, sedative-hypnotic, and anticonvulsant properties. Thus, the clinical indications for specific benzodiazepines are not absolute and considerable overlap exists in their use.

Chemistry

The basic chemical structure of the benzodiazepines consists of a benzene ring coupled to a seven-membered heterocyclic structure containing two nitrogens (diazepine) at positions 1 and 4 (Fig. 33-1). Of the 2,000 benzodiazepines that have been synthesized, there are approximately 15 clinically useful compounds on the market in the United States.

Mechanism of Action

The benzodiazepines bind with high affinity to specific macromolecules within the central nervous system. These

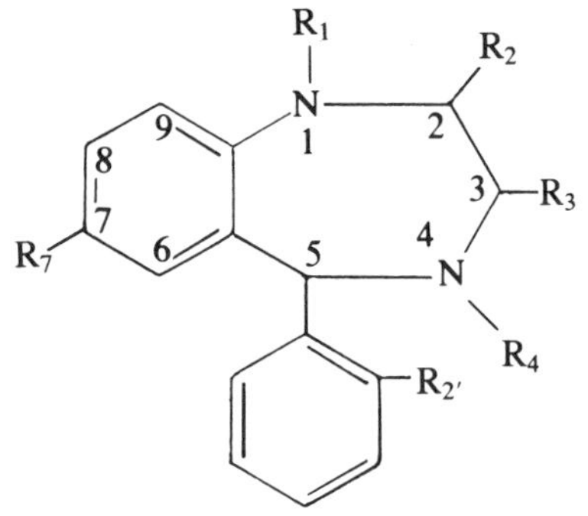

1,4-Benzodiazepine nucleus

Figure 33-1. General structure for 1,4-benzodiazepines.

benzodiazepine-binding sites (receptors) are closely associated with the receptors for γ-aminobutyric acid (GABA), which is the major inhibitory neurotransmitter in the mammalian brain. Extensive experimental evidence suggests that benzodiazepines potentiate GABAergic neurotransmission in essentially all areas of the central nervous system. This enhancement is thought to occur indirectly at the postsynaptic $GABA_A$ receptor complex.

The functional significance of this drug-receptor interaction is that the receptor complex regulates the entrance of chloride into the postsynaptic cells. It is thought that the increase in chloride conductance mediated by GABA is intensified by the benzodiazepines. This facilitation of GABA-induced chloride conductance results in a relatively greater hyperpolarization of these cells and therefore leads to diminished synaptic transmission.

Another chemical class of sedative-hypnotic drugs, the barbiturates, also bind to receptors associated with the GABA-chloride ionophore but these drugs appear to prolong rather than intensify GABA effects. For a schematic depiction of the presumed drug receptor–GABA–chloride ionophore relationship, see Fig. 28-3.

In addition to the clinically useful benzodiazepines, which act as agonists at the benzodiazepine receptor, at least two other types of ligands also interact with this binding site. These are the benzodiazepine receptor antagonists and the inverse agonists. For example, flumazenil is a receptor antagonist that selectively blocks the effects of other benzodiazepines at their binding sites; it has clinical application in the treatment of benzodiazepine overdose and in the reversal of benzodiazepine-induced sedation.

The inverse agonists are compounds that interact with benzodiazepine receptors and decrease, rather than increase, GABA-mediated changes. They also can antagonize the effects of benzodiazepine agonists and, when administered alone, can be anxiogenic and proconvulsant.

Pharmacological Actions

Although it is widely claimed that the benzodiazepine drugs have a specific calming or anxiolytic effect, their most prominent and easily quantifiable action is central nervous system depression. In very low therapeutic doses, this depression is manifest by relief of anxiety that is often accompanied by a feeling of sluggishness or drowsiness. As the dose is increased, the degree of depression is intensified such that muscle relaxation, hypnosis, and a more intense central nervous system depression occur. This depression is thought to be related to the ability of these drugs to facilitate the inhibitory actions of GABA.

A significant advantage of the benzodiazepines over other central nervous system depressants (e.g., the barbiturates) is that they possess a much greater separation between the dose that produces sleep and the dose that produces death. This increased margin of safety has been one of the major reasons why benzodiazepines have largely replaced the barbiturates and other types of sedative-hypnotics in the treatment of anxiety and insomnia. In addition, benzodiazepine administration is associated with few side effects. The lack of GABA neurons in the periphery may explain the minimal direct peripheral effects produced by these compounds.

Absorption, Distribution, and Metabolism

Benzodiazepines are usually given orally and are well absorbed by this route. Since the benzodiazepines are weak bases, they are less ionized in the relatively alkaline environment of the small intestine and, therefore, most of their absorption takes place at this site. For emergency treatment of seizures or when used in anesthesia, the benzodiazepines also can be given parenterally. However, the absorption of several of these compounds is unreliable after intramuscular injection.

The distribution of the benzodiazepines from blood to tissues and back again is a dynamic process and has a considerable influence on the onset and duration of the therapeutic effects produced by these compounds. Those having greater lipid solubility tend to enter the central nervous system more rapidly and thus tend to produce their effects more quickly. Several of the benzodiazepines have therapeutic effects that are much shorter in duration than would be predicted based on their rates of metabolism and excretion; redistribution away from the central nervous system is of primary importance in terminating their therapeutic effects.

Although tissue redistribution of benzodiazepines may be an important means of terminating the actions of selected members of this class of drugs, many benzodiazepines do undergo extensive biotransformation. Metabo-

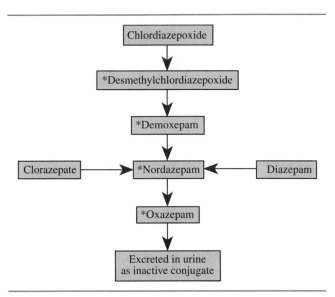

Figure 33-2. The metabolism of some benzodiazepines. Note that in some cases, several active metabolites are formed. A result is very long apparent half-lives. In many cases, the ultimate product is oxazepam. * = an active metabolic product.

lism takes place both by dealkylation (phase 1) and conjugation (phase 2) reactions. In many instances, dealkylation can result in the formation of pharmacologically active compounds. Indeed, *the majority of clinically available benzodiazepines are converted in the liver to one or more active metabolites.* In several cases the active metabolites have a much longer half-life than the parent compound. In one case, acid hydrolysis in the stomach converts an inactive compound (clorazepate) to an active drug (nordazepam). Figure 33-2 shows the biotransformation reactions involved in the metabolism of representative benzodiazepines. The water-soluble metabolites of the benzodiazepines are excreted primarily in the urine.

Since most of the benzodiazepines do undergo biotransformation, it is possible that changes in liver function may alter the duration of the therapeutic effect produced by these drugs. Despite the fact that few clinical studies have demonstrated serious toxicities associated with benzodiazepine administration in individuals with compromised liver function, prudence in the use of these compounds in the elderly and in individuals with liver disease seems advisable.

One of the great disadvantages associated with many of the sedative and hypnotic drugs (e.g., barbiturates, propanediol carbamates), which have now largely been replaced by the benzodiazepines, is the fact that those drugs are very effective inducers of hepatic drug-metabolizing enzymes. Since the benzodiazepines are only weak inducers of hepatic microsomal enzymes, they cause relatively few clinically significant drug interactions related to metabolism.

Clinical Uses

Anxiety

Anxiety disorders are among the most common form of psychiatric illness. Anxiety also often accompanies other psychiatric diseases as well as such medical illnesses as angina pectoris, gastrointestinal disorders, and hypertension. Anxiety that results from fear caused by an acute illness, or a stressful event such as a divorce or the loss of a loved one, is usually self-limiting and can be of relatively short duration. Other disorders that have anxiety as a component are not necessarily associated with a life event, and may persist for considerable periods, even throughout the individual's life span.

Both acute and chronic anxiety can be treated with benzodiazepines, although it is anticipated that for most anxiety disorders counseling will also play an important role. As with any medication, benzodiazepines employed in the treatment of anxiety should be used in the lowest effective dose for the shortest duration. Use of the drugs in this way will provide maximum benefit to the patient while minimizing the potential for adverse reactions. For most types of anxiety, none of the benzodiazepines is therapeutically superior to any other. Choice of a particular agent is usually made on the basis of pharmacokinetic rather than pharmacodynamic considerations. A benzodiazepine with a long half-life should be considered if the anxiety is intense and sustained. A drug with a short half-life may have advantages when the anxiety is provoked by clearly defined circumstances and is likely to be of short duration. Table 33-1 shows pharmacokinetic data for selected benzodiazepines.

One possible exception to the general rule that benzodiazepines are pharmacodynamically equivalent is in the treatment of anxiety associated with a major depression. In this disorder, alprazolam may be preferred over other benzodiazepines because it appears to have antidepressant as well as anxiolytic properties.

Insomnia

All of the benzodiazepines will produce sedative-hypnotic effects of sufficient magnitude to induce sleep, provided that the dosage employed is high enough. However, the aim in the treatment of sleep disorders is to induce sleep that is as close as possible to natural sleep so that the patient falls asleep quickly, sleeps through the night, and has sleep of sufficient quality to awake refreshed.

Extensive sleep studies have been conducted with a variety of sedative-hypnotic drugs, and all of these drugs appear to alter the normal distribution of rapid eye movement (REM) and non-REM sleep. Most of the older sedative-hypnotic agents, such as the barbiturates, pro-

Table 33-1. Pharmacokinetic Properties
of Selected Benzodiazepines

Drug	Time to peak (hr)	Elimination half-life (hr)*
Chlordiazepoxide	0.5–2.0	8–20
Diazepam	0.5–1.5	20–60
Flurazepam	0.5–1.0	24–120
Alprazolam	1.0–2.0	12–15
Oxazepam	2.0–4.0	4–12
Triazolam	1.5–2.0	3–5

*Includes parent compounds and active metabolites.

duce a marked depression of REM sleep. In contrast, when the benzodiazepines are used in appropriate doses, they depress REM sleep to a much smaller extent. As was the case with treatment of anxiety, the choice of a particular benzodiazepine to treat a sleep disturbance is again generally based on pharmacokinetic criteria. While longer-acting compounds may assure that a patient will sleep through the night, they also may cause cumulative effects resulting in a daytime sluggishness or drug hangover. Shorter-acting compounds avoid the hangover problem, but their use may be associated with an early awakening and increase in daytime anxiety.

Epilepsy and Seizures

Nearly all central nervous system depressants have some capacity to suppress seizures by virtue of their depressant activity on the brain and spinal cord. *Clonazepam* and *diazepam* are two benzodiazepines that depress epileptiform activity and are currently used in the treatment of epilepsy and seizure disorders.

Sedation, Amnesia, and Anesthesia

Benzodiazepines have the capacity to produce a calming effect and to cause *anterograde amnesia.* Anterograde amnesia is a condition in which the patient is unable to recall events that took place for a period of time after the drug was administered. Benzodiazepine-induced sedation and amnesia are deemed useful in the preparation of patients for anesthesia and surgery as well as in preparation for frightening or unpleasant medical and dental procedures and diagnostic tests.

Muscle Relaxation

Benzodiazepines have the capacity to depress polysynaptic reflexes. They have been shown to decrease decerebrate rigidity in cats and spasticity in patients with cerebral palsy. What is not clear is whether they can, in humans, cause relaxation of voluntary muscles in doses

that do not cause considerable central nervous system depression. Nevertheless, benzodiazepines, such as diazepam, are often prescribed for patients who have muscle spasms and pain as a result of injury. In these circumstances, the sedative and anxiolytic properties of the drug also may promote relaxation and relieve tension associated with the condition.

Alcohol and Sedative-Hypnotic Withdrawal

Withdrawal from long-term high-dose use of alcohol or sedative-hypnotic drugs can be life threatening if physical dependence is present. Benzodiazepines, such as *chlordiazepoxide* and *diazepam,* are sometimes used to lessen the intensity of the withdrawal symptoms when alcohol or sedative-hypnotic drug use is discontinued. Benzodiazepines are also employed to help relieve the anxiety and other behavioral symptoms that may occur during the rehabilitation process.

Adverse Effects and Toxicities

Most adverse effects associated with use of the benzodiazepines are related to their ability to produce central nervous system depression. The most common undesirable effects are drowsiness, excessive sedation, impaired motor coordination, confusion, and memory loss. These effects are most troublesome during the initial week or two of treatment. Subsequently, the patient becomes tolerant and these effects produce less difficulty. Although for most individuals these symptoms are mild, patients should be cautioned against engaging in potentially dangerous tasks such as operating machinery or driving a car during the initial treatment period.

Other, less common adverse effects include blurred vision, hallucinations, and paradoxical reactions consisting of excitement, stimulation, and hyperactivity. Also, a variety of gastrointestinal complaints occur, and blood dyscrasias have been reported, but these are rare. Benzodiazepine administration during pregnancy, delivery, or lactation has the potential to have adverse effects on the fetus or newborn.

As with other central nervous system depressants, the effects of benzodiazepines are additive with those of ethanol. Patients should be warned that *ethanol-containing beverages may produce a more profound depression when taken simultaneously with a benzodiazepine.*

One of the major reasons for the popularity of the benzodiazepines is their relative safety. Overdoses with the benzodiazepines occur commonly, but fatal toxic occurrences are rare. Fatal intoxications are more likely in children, in individuals with respiratory difficulties, and in individuals who have consumed another central nervous

Table 33-2. Doses for Common Sedative-Hypnotics and Anxiolytics

Generic name	Trade name	Usual doses	Major use
Alprazolam	Xanax	0.25–0.5 mg, 2–3 times daily	Anxiety
		1–2 mg, 2–3 times daily	Depression
Chloral hydrate	Noctec, Somnos	500–1,000 mg, before bed	Insomnia
Chlordiazepoxide hydrochloride	Librium	10–20 mg, 2–3 times daily	Anxiety
		50–100 mg, IM or IV	Alcohol withdrawal
Clorazepate dipotassium	Tranxene	5.0–7.5 mg, twice daily	Anxiety
Diazepam	Valium	2–5 mg, twice daily	Anxiety
		2–10 mg, 2–4 times daily	Muscle relaxation
		5–30 mg, IV	Status epilepticus
Flurazepam hydrochloride	Dalmane	15–30 mg, before bed	Insomnia
Lorazepam	Ativan	1–2 mg, once or twice daily	Anxiety
Oxazepam	Serax	15–30 mg, 3–4 times daily	Anxiety
Prazepam	Centrax	10–20 mg, 2–3 times daily	Anxiety
Temazepam	Restoril	15–30 mg, before bed	Insomnia
Triazolam	Halcion	0.25–0.5 mg, before bed	Insomnia

system depressant such as alcohol. After an overdose, the patient begins a deep sleep that may last for 24 to 48 hr depending on the dose. However, even with large overdoses the patient can usually still be aroused.

Tolerance and dependence do occur with the use of benzodiazepines (see Chap. 41). Discontinuation of drug administration, particularly an abrupt withdrawal, can be associated with a variety of symptoms including rebound insomnia and rebound anxiety. The level of insomnia or anxiety may even exceed that which preceded the treatment. Usually, a gradual tapering of the dose until it is eventually discontinued lessens the likelihood of a withdrawal reaction, although in some individuals even this method of drug removal can result in anxiety, apprehension, tension, insomnia, and loss of appetite. More severe symptoms may occur when an individual withdraws from a supratherapeutic dose, particularly if the drug has been taken for months or years. These symptoms can include, in addition to those already mentioned, muscle weakness, tremor, hyperalgesia, nausea, vomiting, weight loss, and possibly convulsions.

Drug Interactions

When used with other sedative-hypnotics or alcohol, the benzodiazepines will produce additive central nervous system depression. The benzodiazepines have been shown to be weak inducers of the cytochrome P450 drug-metabolizing system and therefore have the potential for accelerating the metabolism of other drugs. In addition, cimetidine has been reported to increase the elimination half-life of diazepam, presumably through its interference with the hepatic metabolism of the coadministered benzodiazepine. Clinically significant interactions between the benzodiazepines and other drugs, however, are rare.

Preparations and Dosage

The trade names, usual doses, and major clinical use for the most commonly employed benzodiazepines can be found in Table 33-2.

Azapirones

Buspirone is the first example of a relatively new class of anxiolytic agents that can relieve some symptoms of anxiety in doses that do not cause sedation. Buspirone is structurally unrelated to existing psychotropic drugs (Fig. 33-3).

Mechanism of Action

Although buspirone has been shown to interact with a number of neurotransmitter systems within the brain, it appears that its clinically relevant effects are mediated through interactions at the serotonin (5-hydroxytryptamine, 5-HT) 5-HT$_{1A}$ receptor, where it acts as a partial agonist.

Figure 33-3. Structure of buspirone hydrochloride.

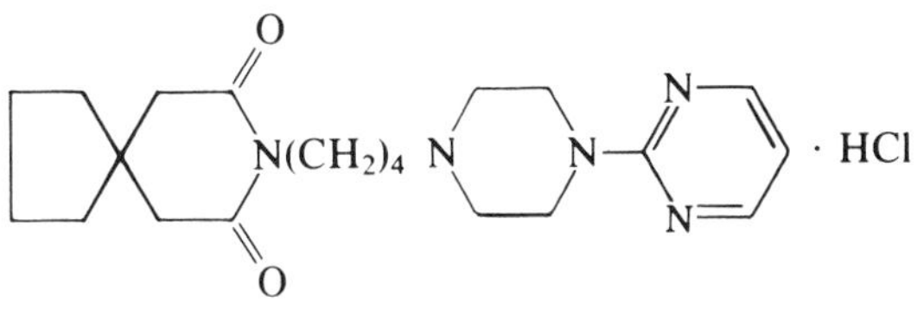

Pharmacological Actions

Several clinical trials have shown that buspirone is as effective as the benzodiazepines in the treatment of generalized anxiety. However, the full anxiolytic effect of buspirone takes several weeks to develop whereas the anxiolytic effect of the benzodiazepines is maximal after a few days of therapy. In therapeutic doses, buspirone has little or no sedative effect and also lacks the muscle relaxant and anticonvulsant properties of the benzodiazepines. In addition, buspirone does not potentiate the central nervous system depression caused by sedative-hypnotic drugs or by alcohol, and it does not prevent the symptoms associated with the benzodiazepine withdrawal syndrome.

Absorption, Distribution, and Metabolism

Buspirone is well absorbed from the gastrointestinal tract and peak blood levels are achieved in 1 to 1.5 hr; the drug is more than 95 percent bound to plasma proteins. Buspirone is extensively metabolized, with less than 1 percent of the parent drug excreted into the urine unchanged. At least one of the metabolic products of buspirone is biologically active. The parent drug has an elimination half-life of 4 to 6 hr.

Clinical Uses

Buspirone is effective in generalized anxiety and in anxiety with depression. It may also have specific antidepressant properties. Its effectiveness in other anxiety disorders, such as panic disorder or posttraumatic stress disorder, remains to be established.

Adverse Reactions

Like the benzodiazepines, buspirone appears to be safe even when given in very high doses. The most common side effects reported by patients using buspirone are dizziness, light-headedness, and headache. Abuse, dependence, and withdrawal symptoms have not been reported and buspirone administration does not produce any cross-tolerance to the benzodiazepines. Buspirone has been reported to increase blood pressure in patients taking monoamine oxidase inhibitors, and it also may increase plasma levels of haloperidol if coadministered with that agent.

Preparation and Dosage

Buspirone hydrochloride (*BuSpar*) is available as 5- and 10-mg tablets.

Sedatives and Anxiolytics with Other Major Uses

Antihistamines

Several H₁ histamine antagonists (e.g., diphenhydramine, promethazine, hydroxyzine) have been used as sedative-hypnotics, since they produce some degree of sedation. While this sedation is usually considered a side effect of their antihistaminic activity, in some cases the sedation is of sufficient magnitude to allow the drugs to be used in the treatment of anxiety and sleep disturbances. For these drugs, their anxiolytic properties are thought to be a direct consequence of their ability to produce sedation.

Hydroxyzine hydrochloride (*Atarax, Vistaril*) is the antihistamine with the greatest use in the treatment of anxiety. It is often used to reduce the anxiety that is associated with anesthesia and surgery. It also produces sedation, dries mucous membranes, and has antiemetic activity. A more extensive discussion of the pharmacology of the H₁-receptor antagonists is found in Chap. 72.

β-Adrenergic Blocking Agents

β-Adrenergic antagonists such as propranolol have been widely used in the treatment of cardiovascular diseases. These β-blockers also are useful in some forms of anxiety, particularly those that are characterized by somatic symptoms or by performance anxiety (stage fright). There is general agreement that β-blockers can lessen the severity and perhaps prevent the appearance of many of the autonomic responses associated with anxiety. These symptoms include tremors, sweating, tachycardia, and palpitations. There is some controversy about whether the β-blockers can do more than control some of the peripheral symptoms of anxiety. This controversy stems, in part, from the fact that some of those compounds do not cross the blood-brain barrier readily.

A discussion of the β-blockers in the treatment of cardiovascular disease, their side effects, and information about commercial products and doses is found in Chap. 13.

Antipsychotics and Antidepressants

Antipsychotic drugs (neuroleptics) such as chlorpromazine have been used in the treatment of anxiety for many years. These drugs are more toxic and produce many more side effects than do the benzodiazepines or azapirones. However, they have been used in selected patients for treatment of anxiety. Chapter 35 has a more detailed description of the pharmacology of these drugs.

Tricyclic antidepressants such as amitriptyline produce considerable sedation and are used to treat some forms of anxiety such as phobic disorder and panic disorder. Similar to the antipsychotic drugs, the tricyclic antidepressants are much more toxic and produce many more side effects than do the benzodiazepines or azapirones. Their use should be reserved for those situations in which the patient does not respond to or cannot tolerate the safer anxiolytics. Chapter 36 describes the pharmacology of the antidepressant drugs.

Older Sedative-Hypnotic and Anxiolytic Agents

Before the introduction of the benzodiazepines, a number of drugs from different chemical and pharmacological classes were used in the treatment of anxiety and insomnia. However, these drugs are more toxic and produce more serious side effects than do the benzodiazepines. Many also have significant abuse potential (see Chap. 41). Consequently, most of these compounds are no longer widely used. Nevertheless, the properties of selected examples from each class will be briefly described so that the reader can develop an understanding of the shortcomings that have caused these compounds to fall into disfavor.

Barbiturates

The barbituric acid derivatives, or barbiturates, were the mainstays in the treatment of anxiety and insomnia for almost 50 years. During this time, they were also used in many suicides and have been implicated in thousands of deaths due to accidental ingestion. In spite of their serious central nervous system toxicity, the barbiturates have been and continue to be chronically abused by a surprisingly large number of people (see Chap. 41). Additionally, the barbiturates produce a number of serious and potentially lethal interactions with other drugs. For these reasons, drugs such as the benzodiazepines have largely replaced the barbiturates for the treatment of anxiety and insomnia.

Besides their use in the treatment of sleep disorders and anxiety, selected barbiturates are employed in the treatment of convulsive disorders (see Chap. 37) and in general anesthesia (see Chap. 31).

Chemistry

The general chemical structure for the barbiturates is shown in Fig. 33-4. With a few exceptions involving the anticonvulsant drugs, substitutions on the structural nucleus produce pharmacokinetic rather than pharmacody-

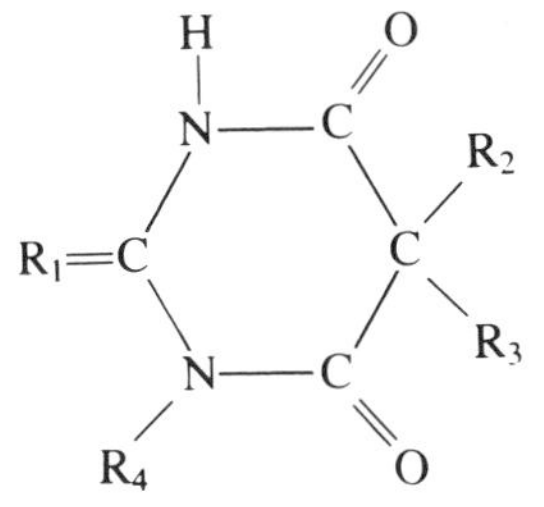

Figure 33-4. General structure of the barbiturates.

namic differences among these drugs. That is, the substitutions influence the duration of action more than they influence therapeutic effectiveness. For example, the substitution of a sulfur for an oxygen atom at the R_1 position produces *thiobarbiturates* that are classified as ultra–short-acting. Alternatively, substitution of a phenyl group at R_3 produces compounds that are classified as long-acting. Other substitutions produce compounds whose effects are short- to intermediate-acting.

Mechanism of Action

Like the benzodiazepines, the barbiturates are thought to bind to receptors associated with the GABA-chloride ionophore. In the case of the barbiturates, this binding prolongs the effects of GABA on the chloride channel, whereas the benzodiazepines intensify the effects of GABA. See Fig. 28-3 for a diagrammatical depiction of these interrelationships.

Pharmacological Action

Barbiturates produce a central nervous system depression that can range from slight sedation to surgical anesthesia, depending on the dose. At usual therapeutic doses, other organs are little affected; cardiovascular collapse can occur following large overdoses. Despite the fact that the barbiturates depress most areas of the central nervous system and are used in anesthesia, they have no analgesic properties. Even though the barbiturates were long used to treat insomnia and sleep disturbances, they commonly produce a "barbiturate hangover" that has been associated with their ability to cause substantial depression of REM sleep.

Absorption, Distribution, Metabolism, and Excretion

The barbiturates are weak organic acids (pK_a 7.3–8.0). Binding to plasma albumin varies from compound to compound, and the barbiturates can compete with, displace, or be displaced from binding sites by other organic acids such as aspirin.

The *thiobarbiturates,* which are used for anesthesia and are administered primarily by intravenous injection, are distributed rapidly to those organs that have the highest blood flow. Thus, they are distributed rapidly to the brain and are capable of producing a loss of consciousness in a matter of seconds after intravenous administration. They also are rapidly distributed away from the brain such that recovery from an anesthetic dose also is rapid and is dependent on the rate of the redistribution process. Since metabolism and excretion of the thiobarbiturates are relatively slow processes, *the duration of the therapeutic effect of these compounds is quite dependent on drug redistribution.*

An important aspect of barbiturate administration, particularly long-term use, is their ability to cause significant induction of drug-metabolizing enzymes (see also Chap. 4). This process is of therapeutic importance because the duration of effect of several drugs can be altered in ways that interfere significantly with their effectiveness.

Since the barbiturates are organic acids, the rate at which they are excreted into urine can be influenced by the pH of the urine. These drugs are more soluble in an alkaline urine and alkalinization of the urine, therefore, will result in a higher concentration of the ionized and nonreabsorbable form of the drug being present in the urine. For example, phenobarbital, which has a long half-life (80–120 hr), low pK_a, and is not extensively metabolized, will have its renal excretion accelerated through alkalinization of the urine by administration of sodium bicarbonate; this procedure can be an effective adjunct to the treatment of toxic overdoses of this compound. Since other barbiturates are more extensively metabolized, this procedure does not speed their elimination to nearly the same extent.

Clinical Use

Insomnia and Anxiety

At one time, low or sedative doses of the barbiturates were a mainstay in the treatment of anxiety while larger or hypnotic doses were used extensively to treat sleep disturbances. However, for reasons of safety and efficacy, the barbiturates have been replaced almost entirely for both of these uses.

Epilepsy and Seizures

Phenobarbital (*Luminal*) was one of the first effective drugs to be used in the treatment of epilepsy. It can help a significant percentage of patients to achieve a reduction in the incidence of seizures in doses that do not produce an intolerable degree of central nervous system depression. Its place in the pharmacology of seizure disorders is discussed in more detail in Chap. 37.

Anesthesia

The ultra–short-acting barbiturates such as thiopental sodium (*Pentothal Sodium*) are used extensively in the induction of surgical anesthesia. This use is described more extensively in Chap. 31.

Adverse Reactions

Many, but not all, of the adverse reactions associated with barbiturate administration are the result of their ability to depress the central nervous system and produce undesirable levels of sedation. Laryngospasm is a relatively common complication seen when ultra–short-acting compounds such as thiopental are given intravenously to induce anesthesia. In overdoses, death is usually attributed to respiratory depression, although pulmonary edema and pneumonia are frequently contributory factors.

As is the case with most drug overdoses, with the exception of that caused by the narcotic-analgesics, *no specific antidotes are available to counteract the effects of excessive barbiturate intake.* Treatment is aimed at supporting the respiratory and cardiovascular systems until the drug can be eliminated. Alkalinization of the urine may speed the elimination of the long-acting barbiturates such as phenobarbital. Chapter 41 contains a description of the general considerations applicable to chronic barbiturate abuse and the treatment of drug overdose.

Drug Interactions

Barbiturates participate in an impressive list of clinically significant drug interactions. Most of these interactions result from the induction of hepatic microsomal enzymes. There can be a considerable acceleration of the disappearance of a variety of drugs including oral contraceptives, phenytoin, digitoxin, quinidine, β-adrenergic blockers, and oral anticoagulants. This acceleration of metabolism can result in lower drug levels and a need for increased doses in order to maintain the desired response to the drug. With the combined use of barbiturates and anticoagulants, a dangerous change can take place if the barbiturate is discontinued. During combined use, induction of drug-metabolizing enzymes takes place and more anticoagulant is required in order to produce the desired degree of anticoagulation. If the barbiturate is stopped, drug-metabolizing enzyme levels will return to normal and the barbiturate-induced increase of metabolism decreases. Thus, blood levels of the anticoagulant rise and the patient is at risk for a severe hemorrhage.

Preparations and Dosage

There is a wide variation in individual response to the barbiturates, and the dosage range is relatively great. In general, the hypnotic dose is three to four times the sedative dose. Preparations and average sedative doses are indicated below for the most commonly employed barbiturates.

Amobarbital (*Amytal*) is supplied in various-sized tablets and is available as amobarbital sodium (*Amytal Sodium*) in an elixir and as capsules. As a sedative, the usual adult dosage is from 20 to 30 mg two to four times a day.

Pentobarbital sodium (*Nembutal Sodium*) is available in a variety of dosage forms. The sedative dose is usually 30 to 60 mg.

Propanediol Carbamates

Meprobamate, the most widely used of these compounds, was originally synthesized in 1951 during efforts to develop long-acting muscle relaxants. Its sedative-anxiolytic properties were recognized and it was soon introduced into therapeutics for that purpose.

The pharmacological profile of the propanediol carbamates places them somewhere between the benzodiazepines and the barbiturates. All three classes of drugs produce sedative-hypnotic effects and have been used to relieve anxiety. The popularity of the benzodiazepines for the treatment of anxiety and insomnia has resulted in a considerable decline in the use of the propanediol carbamates. Meprobamate (*Equanil, Miltown*) is used occasionally to treat insomnia and anxiety in geriatric patients.

Chloral Hydrate

Chloral hydrate (*Noctec, Somnos*) was developed in the late 1800s. It is still used and is an effective sedative-hypnotic agent. It is a hydrated aldehyde [$CCl_3CH(OH)_2$]

with a disagreeable smell and taste. It is rapidly reduced in vivo to trichloroethanol (CCl_3CH_2OH), which is considered to be the active metabolite. It produces a high incidence of gastric irritation and allergic responses, occasionally causes cardiac arrhythmias, and is unreliable in patients with liver damage.

Nonprescription Drugs

A wide variety of sedative-hypnotic products that do not require a prescription are available. Most of these over-the-counter products have antihistamines, such as pyrilamine, diphenhydramine, or promethazine, as the active ingredient. In most cases, the dose of the active ingredient is low and the preparations are safe.

Supplemental Reading

Curran, H.V. Benzodiazepines, memory and mood: A review. *Psychopharmacology* 105:1, 1991.

Dahl, R.E. The pharmacologic treatment of sleep disorders. *Psychiatr. Clin. North Am.* 15:161, 1992.

Doble, A., and Martin, I.L. Multiple benzodiazepine receptors: No reason for anxiety. *TIPS* 13:76, 1992.

Enkelmann, R. Alprazolam versus buspirone in the treatment of outpatients with generalized anxiety disorder. *Psychopharmacology* 105:428, 1991.

Huybrechts, I. The pharmacology of alprazolam: A review. *Clin. Ther.* 13:100, 1991.

Piekarski, J.M., Rossmann, J.A., and Putman, J. Benzodiazepine reversal with flumazenil—a review of the literature. *J. Can. Dent. Assoc.* 58:307, 1992.

Sheikh, J.I. Anxiety disorders and their treatment. *Clin. Geriatr. Med.* 8:411, 1992.

34

Central Nervous System Stimulants

David A. Taylor

Central nervous system (CNS) stimulation is the primary action of a diverse group of pharmacological agents; in addition, it is an adverse effect associated with the administration of an even larger and more diverse group of drugs. Manifestations of CNS stimulation can be observed in a range of behaviors that include mild elevation in alertness, increased nervousness and anxiety, and convulsions. The intensity of the CNS stimulation associated with the administration of a particular agent appears to depend, in large part, on both the CNS region that is primarily affected by the compound and the molecular mechanism underlying the increased excitability.

In most instances, the "hyperexcitability" associated with any drug administration (either as a desired or undesired effect) results from an alteration in the fine balance normally maintained in the CNS between excitatory and inhibitory influences. Thus, at the regional level, a compound may produce stimulation in one of two ways: through a reduction in the net inhibitory information in the region or by an enhancement in the output from other brain regions that provide excitatory influences.

The molecular and cellular bases for CNS stimulation also reside in the fine adjustment of integration of excitatory and inhibitory influences at the level of the individual neuron. An agent that induces CNS stimulation appears to act by one or more of the following mechanisms: (1) potentiation or enhancement of excitatory neurotransmission (e.g., doxapram), (2) depression or antagonism of inhibitory neurotransmission (e.g., strychnine), or (3) presynaptic control of neurotransmitter release (e.g., picrotoxin antagonism of presynaptic inhibition of excitatory transmitter release).

Although the use of CNS stimulants (also known as *analeptics* or *convulsants*) has declined steadily through the years, certain compounds within this category do possess some clinical utility. Historically, general CNS stimulants were used primarily as respiratory stimulants in the treatment of acute overdosage with CNS depressants (e.g., barbiturates). Several factors are likely to have contributed

to the reduction in the use of CNS stimulants in this clinical situation. First, the stimulants were not specific antagonists of the depressant agents and therefore were not particularly effective in reversing severe pharmacologically induced CNS depression. Second, the duration of action of the CNS stimulant was generally shorter than that of the CNS depressant that they were meant to antagonize. Thus, the physiological antagonism subsided before the elimination of the action of the depressant agent, which led to a false sense of success in the amelioration of the crisis. In addition, the dose of most CNS stimulants required to reverse severe CNS depression was quite close to the dose that produced convulsions and cardiac arrhythmias. In such cases, therefore, the CNS stimulant often exacerbated the clinical picture by producing severe life-threatening complications in the face of an already compromised clinical situation.

Another major factor contributing to the decline in CNS stimulant use for drug-induced CNS depression has been the development of alternate, more conservative, and generally safer procedures for managing the patient. Under these circumstances, supportive measures (e.g., maintenance of a patent airway, elevation of low blood pressure, etc.) provided greater benefit to the patient than the use of analeptic drugs. With the psychomotor stimulants (amphetamine and many congeners), tolerance and abuse potential represent continuing problems. However, this particular class of CNS stimulants enjoys the greatest clinical utility for weight control, treatment of minimal brain dysfunction, and hyperactivity in children. The cholinesterase inhibitor, physostigmine, is also used to counteract the CNS depression associated with anticholinergic drugs such as the tricyclic antidepressants.

Compounds that possess as their primary action the stimulation of the CNS can be divided roughly into three major categories (Table 34-1) based either on their proposed mechanism of action (analeptic stimulants and psychomotor stimulants) or their chemical classification (methylxanthine derivatives). Each class of compounds is

379

Table 34-1. Classification of CNS Stimulants

Analeptic stimulants	Psychomotor stimulants	Methylxanthines
Doxapram	Amphetamine	Caffeine
Nikethamide	Methamphetamine	Theophylline
Pentylenetetrazol	Methylphenidate	Theobromine
Strychnine	Pemoline	
Picrotoxin	Ephedrine	
Bicuculline	Phentermine	
	Fenfluramine	
	Phenylpropanolamine	

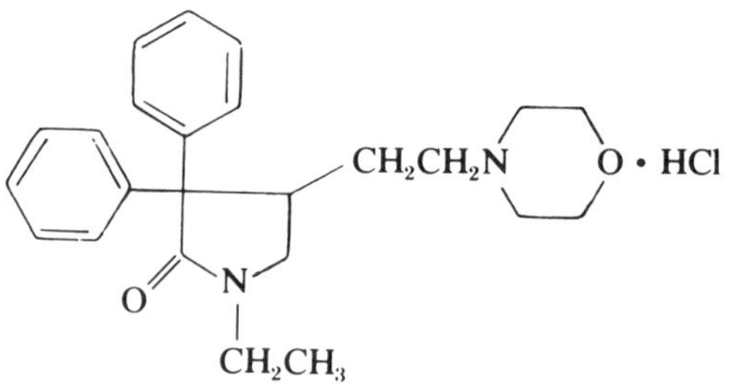

Figure 34-1. Doxapram.

discussed in general terms and individual drugs are mentioned only as appropriate.

Analeptic Stimulants

Chemistry and Pharmacokinetics

The analeptic stimulants comprise a diverse chemical class of agents ranging from plant alkaloids, such as picrotoxin and strychnine, to synthetic compounds, such as pentylenetetrazol and doxapram (Fig. 34-1). The wide range of chemical structures makes this particular class somewhat difficult to categorize with respect to absorption, distribution, and metabolism. However, the majority of analeptic stimulants can be absorbed orally and have short durations of action. The pharmacological effect of most of these compounds is terminated through hepatic metabolism rather than renal excretion of unchanged drug.

Mechanism of Action

Perhaps the most unifying concept concerning the mode of action of these agents comes from recent studies of the γ-aminobutyric acid (GABA)-receptor-chloride ionophore interaction. It has long been recognized that the inhibitory action of many amino acid neurotransmitters (e.g., GABA) involves an increase in chloride conductance. Thus, GABA and other inhibitory amino acids actively promote an increase in chloride influx through an interaction with the chloride channel in the neuronal membrane. Such an increase in chloride conductance generally leads to a membrane *hyperpolarization* and a reduction in the probability of action-potential generation (i.e., inhibition of neuronal activity). With GABA, in particular, the interaction appears to occur through protein molecules (receptors) with specific affinity for the amino acid.

Recently, the chloride channel has been shown to contain at least one regulatory subunit, the GABA receptor (see Chap. 28). Interestingly, the chloride channel appears to contain regulatory sites in addition to those specific for GABA. These additional binding sites possess high affinity for such agents as the benzodiazepines, picrotoxin, alcohol, and the barbiturates.

Chloride movement across neuronal membranes can be regulated at this ion channel by at least three distinct molecular entities: (1) a GABA binding site, (2) a benzodiazepine binding site, and (3) a picrotoxin binding site. GABA and other agonists have the ability to open the chloride channel (i.e., increase chloride conductance). Benzodiazepine-induced facilitation of GABA-mediated increases in chloride conduction are antagonized by pentylenetetrazol and possibly by the methylxanthines, while picrotoxin closes the chloride channel. Agents that appear to promote chloride conductance through the picrotoxin site include the barbiturates and possibly phenytoin.

Although this hypothesis may ultimately prove to be too simplistic, it does offer the advantage of ascribing to a single molecular event (control of chloride ion movement) the mechanism of action of a diverse class of agents. Utilizing such a scheme may, in fact, be beneficial to a greater understanding of CNS mechanisms underlying excitation or inhibition.

Strychnine is an analeptic stimulant with a well-defined mechanism of action that is unrelated to an interaction with either GABA receptors or other binding sites that modulate the activity of the chloride ionophore. Strychnine appears to be a specific, competitive, postsynaptic antagonist of glycine in the CNS. Glycine, like GABA, is a known inhibitory transmitter in the mammalian CNS. Whereas GABA is likely to be more important in the brain, glycine is more important in the spinal cord. Glycine mediates inhibition of spinal cord neurons and is intimately involved in the regulation of spinal cord and brainstem reflexes. Strychnine directly antagonizes this inhibition, allowing excitatory impulses to be greatly exaggerated.

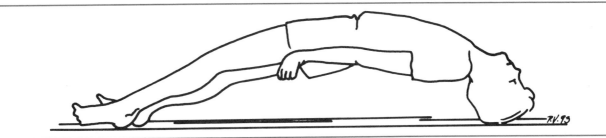

Figure 34-2. Patient in opisthotonos.

Therapeutic Uses

As indicated, most of the analeptic stimulants were used as pharmacological treatments for overdosage of CNS depressants. *Doxapram and nikethamide are sometimes used to counteract postanesthetic respiratory depression and as an aid in chronic obstructive pulmonary disease.* Pentylenetetrazol is used clinically on rare occasions to "activate" the electroencephalogram in order to aid in the differential diagnosis of epilepsy or latent epileptic tendencies. It is also used experimentally to screen compounds for their possible anticonvulsant activity. Strychnine is used almost exclusively in animal studies as a tool for studying CNS mechanisms because of its relatively specific action as a glycine antagonist.

Adverse Reactions

Most of the CNS stimulants produce adverse reactions that are extensions of their therapeutic effect. These agents produce convulsions that can be followed by coma and death. Convulsions produced by this class of agents (with the exception of strychnine) are usually tonic-clonic in nature and are uncoordinated. In some cases, the convulsions may be preceded by marked stimulation of respiration, tachycardia, and excessive pressor effects.

The uncontrolled excitation that occurs after strychnine administration (in the absence of normal inhibition) results in very characteristic convulsions. In humans, in whom extensor muscles are normally dominant, tonic extension of the body and all limbs is observed. This hyperextension is known as *opisthotonos* and, at its extreme, consists of a characteristic posture in which the back is arched and only the back of the head and the heels are touching the surface on which the victim is lying. Figure 34-2 illustrates a patient in opisthotonos.

In the presence of strychnine, all sensory stimuli produce exaggerated responses, and even slight sensory stimulation may precipitate convulsions. The primary therapeutic consideration after strychnine poisoning is to prevent convulsions, which may be fatal. Diazepam or clonazepam (see Chap. 33) appear to be moderately effec-

tive in preventing strychnine convulsions and are the agents of choice. Barbiturates are often used to treat overdoses of all of the analeptic stimulants. Generally, however, antidotal therapy is not required, but mechanical resuscitation equipment should be available.

Preparations and Dosage

Doxapram hydrochloride (*Dopram*) is available as a solution in multidose vials. The drug can be used to hasten arousal from anesthesia by a single, slow intravenous injection of 0.5 to 1.5 mg/kg body weight or by slow sustained infusion of 1.5 to 2.0 mg/ml at an initial rate of 5 mg/min followed by a maintainence infusion of 1 to 3 mg/min. Other uses for doxapram include reversal of drug-induced depression.

Nikethamide (*Coramine, Nikorin*) is available as ampules for injection or for oral use.

Pentylenetetrazol (*Metrazol*) is available as 100-mg tablets or as solutions of various concentrations.

Psychomotor Stimulants

Pharmacokinetics

Many of the compounds in this category possess activities similar to those of amphetamine. Several of these drugs have been discussed previously in Chap. 12. Of primary importance to our discussion of the psychomotor stimulants are *amphetamine, methamphetamine,* and *methylphenidate* (Fig. 34-3).

All of these compounds are well absorbed after oral administration, leaving injectable forms with few legitimate applications. Although the amphetamines are metabolized by several catabolic pathways, a considerable portion of untransformed drug is excreted in the urine. Thus, it is possible to "ion-trap" this weak organic base and hasten its clearance by acidifying the urine, thereby reducing its reabsorption in the renal tubules.

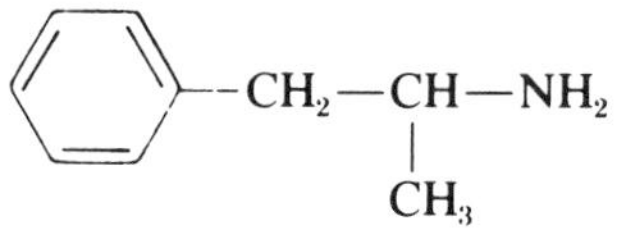

Figure 34-3. Psychomotor stimulants.

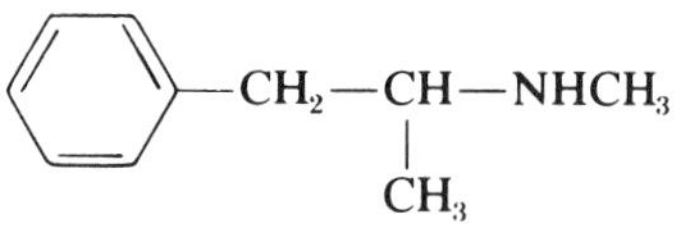

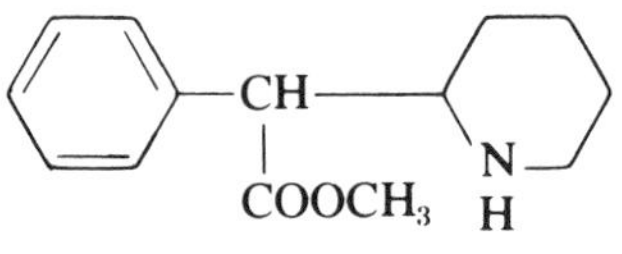

Mechanism of Action

There is good evidence that the facilitation of peripheral sympathetic nervous system transmission that has been demonstrated for the amphetamines extends to the CNS. The possibility that amphetamines act indirectly (i.e., by releasing monoamines) at monoaminergic synapses in the brain and spinal cord seems likely. However, amphetamine has multiple effects beyond displacement of catecholamines; these effects include the ability to inhibit neuronal amine uptake and to act as direct agonists at dopamine and serotonin receptors. Furthermore, amphetamine has been shown to act as an antagonist at certain α-adrenoceptors and may inhibit monoamine oxidase. Interestingly, none of these actions has successfully explained the therapeutic benefit of the amphetamines in hyperkinetic children.

Clinical Uses

The therapeutic indications for the psychomotor stimulants are quite limited. They are of benefit in the treatment of the *hyperkinetic syndrome* (minimal brain dysfunction, attention deficit disorder). This is a childhood disease characterized by hyperactivity, inability to concentrate, and a high degree of impulsive behavior. Amphetamines, and the more extensively used methylphenidate, paradoxically, are quite effective in calming a large proportion of

children with this disorder. The mechanism by which these compounds are effective in this disorder is not known.

Narcolepsy is another medically recognized indication for the psychomotor stimulants. This is a disorder characterized by sleep attacks (particularly during the daytime), *cataplexy* (sudden loss of muscle tone), sleep paralysis, and vivid visual and auditory nightmares that may persist into the waking state. Narcolepsy is remarkably affected by drugs that influence adrenomimetic amines centrally. Monoamine oxidase inhibitors and amphetamines are both quite effective in preventing sleep attacks and improving cataplexy. Amphetamines or methylphenidate are considered the drugs of choice in this disorder.

An additional use of the amphetamines and other related centrally acting adrenomimetics is in obesity and weight reduction. Although the amphetamines have a significant anorexic effect, tolerance to this action develops within a few weeks. In addition, insomnia restricts their use during the latter part of the day. The combined drawbacks of the development of tolerance and potential for drug abuse have convinced much of the medical community that the use of amphetamines in weight control is no longer valid.

Fenfluramine is an anorexigenic drug that produces *depression* of the CNS and may offer an alternative to the amphetamine-like compounds in the treatment of obesity.

Adverse Effects

The acute effects of psychomotor stimulant overdosages are related to their CNS stimulant properties and may include euphoria, dizziness, tremor, irritability, and insomnia. At higher doses, convulsions and coma may ensue. These drugs are cardiac stimulants and may cause headache, palpitation, cardiac arrhythmias, anginal pain, and either hypotension or hypertension. Dextroamphetamine produces somewhat less cardiac stimulation.

Chronic intoxication, in addition to the above symptoms, commonly results in weight loss and a psychotic reaction that is often diagnosed as schizophrenia.

Addiction, including psychological dependence, tolerance, and physical dependence, is produced by these agents. A psychic dependence also has been seen following high doses of methylphenidate. The abstinence syndrome seen after abrupt discontinuation of amphetamines is neither as dramatic nor as predictable as that observed during withdrawal after chronic use of barbiturates or narcotics. With the amphetamines, the abstinence syndrome consists primarily of prolonged sleep, fatigue, and extreme hunger (*hyperphagia*). These symptoms may be accompanied by a profound and long-lasting depression. Amphetamine abuse is discussed more completely in Chap. 41.

Preparations

Amphetamine sulfate (*Benzedrine*) is available in tablets and slow-release capsules. The *d* isomer is available separately as dextroamphetamine sulfate (*Dexedrine*). In addition to their use in narcolepsy and the hyperkinetic syndrome, the amphetamines have been used to treat depression and fatigue.

Methamphetamine hydrochloride (*Desoxyn, Methedrine*) is available in tablets and in sustained-release and elixir preparations.

Methylphenidate hydrochloride (*Ritalin Hydrochloride*) is supplied as tablets. Its abuse potential is somewhat less than that of the amphetamines.

Pemoline (*Cylert*) is available as regular and chewable tablets for use in children with hyperkinetic behavioral syndrome.

Phentermine hydrochloride (*Adipex-P, Fastin*) is available in tablets or in cation exchange resin capsules.

Fenfluramine hydrochloride (*Pondimin*) is available in tablets.

Phenylpropanolamine hydrochloride is available in numerous over-the-counter (OTC) formulations either alone or in combination with caffeine. Care should be exercised in treating patients who are currently taking monoamine oxidase inhibitors. In addition, patients should generally avoid an evening dosage schedule. The prevalence of phenylpropanolamine in OTC preparations should also be a concern of the physician when prescribing other CNS stimulants of this class.

Xanthines

The series of compounds known as xanthines, methylxanthines, or xanthine derivatives constitutes a particularly interesting class of drugs. Since the xanthines possess diverse pharmacological properties, there is always a question of where most appropriately to discuss them in a pharmacology text. The xanthines are clearly CNS stimulants, although not all drugs in this class possess this characteristic equally. Although the xanthines have legitimate therapeutic uses, by far the greatest public exposure to them is in xanthine-containing beverages, including coffee, tea, cocoa, and cola-flavored drinks. The popularity of xanthine-containing drinks appears to be related to the subtle CNS stimulant effect realized. It is primarily for this reason, therefore, that xanthines are included under CNS stimulants in this text.

Chemistry and Pharmacokinetics

Currently, there are three pharmacologically important xanthines: *caffeine, theophylline,* and *theobromine.* Their

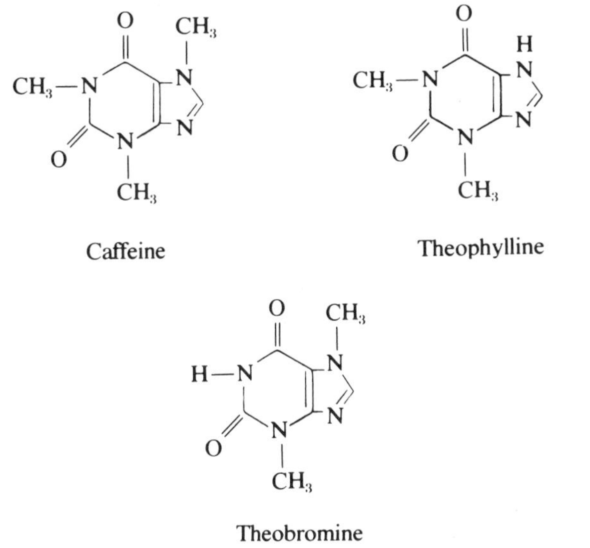

Figure 34-4. Pharmacologically important xanthines.

structures are given in Fig. 34-4. All three alkaloids, which occur naturally in certain plants, are widely consumed in the form of beverages (infusions or decoctions) derived from these plants. Coffee contains primarily caffeine (about 100–150 mg per average cup); tea contains caffeine (30–40 mg per cup) as well as theophylline; cocoa contains caffeine (15–18 mg per cup) and theobromine. Cola drinks also contain significant amounts of caffeine (about 40 mg/12 oz). *The CNS stimulation associated with these beverages in all cases is due predominantly to caffeine.* Theophylline has some CNS stimulant properties, although much less than caffeine, and theobromine possesses very little stimulant activity.

These drugs are readily absorbed by the oral and rectal route of administration. Although these agents can be administered by injection (*aminophylline* is a soluble salt of theophylline), intravascular administration is indicated only in status asthmaticus and apnea in premature infants. Intramuscular injection generally produces considerable pain at the injection site.

The compounds are extensively metabolized, primarily to uric acid derivatives. There is, however, no indication that methylxanthines aggravate gout.

Mechanism of Action

The mechanism of action of methylxanthine-induced stimulation of the CNS has been the subject of much investigation. Initial, now no longer widely held, proposals focused on the ability of these agents to inhibit the action of the enzyme phosphodiesterase.

At least two other possibilities for the mechanism of action of the methylxanthines have been raised. The first derives from the ability of the methylxanthines to act as antagonists of the naturally occurring compound adenosine, a substance that can inhibit both neuronal activity and behavior through a direct action at postsynaptic sites on neurons as well as through an indirect action involving a presynaptic inhibition of neurotransmitter release. These actions of adenosine are mediated by the A_1 type of purine receptor. Thus, as an equilibrium-competitive antagonist of adenosine, the methylxanthines may produce excitation either by a direct blockade of an inhibitory effect of adenosine at the neuron, or by an antagonism of the presynaptic inhibitory effect of adenosine on the release of an excitatory substance (e.g., acetylcholine).

A final suggested mechanism of action involves the chloride channel. As discussed previously (see Analeptic Stimulants), the chloride channel is intimately associated with neuronal inhibition and appears to be modulated by at least three different sites. Caffeine can compete for binding at the benzodiazepine site and would, therefore, be expected to reduce chloride conductance. Thus, caffeine may act functionally like pentylenetetrazol or biculline and limit chloride channel activation.

Therapeutic Uses

Methylxanthines possess some significant clinical utility in a variety of situations. In some instances, these actions are discussed in much greater detail in other chapters, as indicated.

Central Nervous System

Xanthines, primarily as the intramuscularly administered combination of *caffeine and sodium benzoate,* have been used in the treatment of CNS depressant overdosage. In some cases, black coffee is used physiologically to antagonize alcohol intoxication. Many physicians, however, believe that this is ineffective therapy and simply produces a "wide-awake drunk."

Many OTC preparations are aimed at improving or relieving fatigue through CNS stimulation. Such compounds take the form of either "wake-up" tablets or imitations of controlled substances. It should be emphasized that wake-up tablets do little to offset physical fatigue, thereby placing individuals using such methylxanthine products at risk for accidental injuries.

Diuresis

All the xanthines are capable of producing some degree of diuresis in humans. In this regard, theophylline is the most effective compound. This specific action of the methylxanthines is discussed in greater detail in Chap. 21.

Bronchial Asthma

Theophylline is used frequently as a bronchodilator in the treatment of asthma. The importance of the methylxanthines in the management of bronchial asthma is discussed in Chap. 45.

Cardiac Uses

Theophylline, given as the soluble ethylenediamine salt aminophylline, is of some help in relieving paroxysmal dyspnea associated with left heart failure, although a major portion of its efficacy may be due to the relief of bronchospasm that develops secondarily to pulmonary vascular congestion. Theophylline increases myocardial contractile force and has been used in the treatment of refractory forms of congestive heart failure. Theophylline also has shown some benefit in the treatment of neonatal apnea syndrome.

Miscellaneous Uses

Xanthines (usually caffeine) are frequently combined with aspirin and are used widely in the treatment of headaches. In combination with an ergot derivative, methylxanthines have been used to treat migraine. These effects are likely due to vasoconstriction of cerebral blood vessels. Aminophylline (a soluble salt of theophylline) is useful in the relief of pain due to acute biliary colic.

Adverse Reactions

Toxicity associated with the methylxanthines usually takes the form of nervousness, insomnia, and, in more severe cases, delirium. Cardiovascular stimulation is seen as tachycardia and extrasystoles. Excessive respiratory stimulation may occur and diuresis may be prominent.

The intravenous administration of aminophylline (or theophylline) may present some problems if the drug is given too rapidly. In such cases, drug administration is accompanied by severe headache, hypotension, and palpitation. Subsequently, the patient may show signs of excessive CNS stimulation, shock, and even death. Since children appear to be more prone to this toxicity, it is suggested that the dose of aminophylline be no greater than 5 to 7 mg/kg every 6 to 8 hr in infants and young children regardless of the route of administration.

Abuse of Xanthines

The use of some xanthine-containing beverages appears to be customary in most cultures, and moderate use of such beverages does not appear to cause problems in most people. There is little question, however, that such use is habituating, and it has been observed that chronic coffee drinkers who suddenly abstain frequently experience a higher incidence of headaches and a general feeling of fatigue that may last for several days. Although it has not been established that these symptoms constitute any kind of abstinence syndrome, it remains a possibility. There is no good evidence for the development of tolerance to the CNS stimulant effects of caffeine.

The CNS stimulant effects are thought to be diffuse in the brain rather than directed toward any particular brain area. Large parenteral doses of caffeine and theophylline can stimulate directly the respiratory center in the medulla and cause an increase both in respiratory rate and depth.

Drug Interactions

An interaction of potential clinical significance involves the xanthines and the coumarin anticoagulants. Xanthines, by themselves, shorten clotting time by increasing tissue prothrombin and factor V and, in this regard, it might be expected that xanthines would tend to antagonize the effectiveness of oral anticoagulants. However, the usual therapeutic doses of xanthines probably have no significant effect on the patient's response to oral anticoagulants.

Preparations

The most common preparations are given in Table 34-2. It should be noted that a wide variety of OTC preparations contain methylxanthines (usually caffeine) and adrenomimetic agents. The combination of such agents

Table 34-2. Preparation and Dosage of Some Commonly Available Xanthines

Preparation	Usual adult dose and route
Caffeine	200 mg, orally
Caffeine and sodium benzoate	500 mg in 2 ml, IM
Aminophylline (Somophyllin)[a]	200–400 mg, orally
	300 mg, rectally
	500 mg, slowly, IV
Theophylline	200 mg, orally
Theophylline SR[b]	500 mg, orally
Theophylline sodium glycinate	300–600 mg, orally
Theophylline in ethanol (Elixophyllin)	400 mg, orally
Oxytriphylline	200 mg, orally
Dyphylline (Neophyl)[c]	500 mg in 2 ml, IM

[a]Ethylenediamine salt of theophylline; soluble salt.
[b]A sustained-release preparation.
[c]Dyphylline is stable in gastric juice and produces minimal gastric irritation.

could lead to CNS stimulation either as a desired or undesired effect.

Supplemental Reading

Biggio, G., Concas, A., and Costa, E. (eds.). *GABAergic Synaptic Transmission.* New York: Raven, 1992.

Leibowitz, S.F. The role of serotonin in eating disorders. *Drugs* 39 (Suppl. 3):33, 1990.

Linden, J. Structure and function of A$_1$ adenosine receptors. *FASEB J* 5:2668, 1991.

Silverstone, T. Appetite suppressants: A review. *Drugs* 43:820, 1992.

Williamson, D.A. Assessment of eating disorders: Obesity, anorexia and bulimia nervosa. New York: Pergamon, 1990.

35

Antipsychotic Drugs

Brenda K. Colasanti

A diagnosis of *psychosis* is made when the mental functioning of an individual is impaired enough to grossly interfere with the handling of the ordinary demands of life. Behavior is markedly impaired, and the patient has a marked inability to think coherently and comprehend reality. Delusions and hallucinations may exist as well.

The symptoms associated with the psychoses are usually sufficiently distinct to allow differentiation between several major forms. *Organic conditions* usually have a definable toxic, metabolic, or neuropathologic origin, and clinical features of confusion, disorientation, and memory disturbances are apparent. The underlying causes of the remaining conditions are unknown, and they are considered functional. One such condition is *schizophrenia*. Symptoms common to all forms of schizophrenia include chronically disordered thinking, blunted affect, and emotional withdrawal. Paranoid delusions and auditory hallucinations may also be present. The *major affective* and *manic-depressive psychoses* form a second group of functional disorders. In these conditions, alterations in mood and emotion are the predominant symptoms. These may be either unipolar or bipolar, with recurrent episodes fluctuating irregularly between mania or depression. Delusional and paranoid ideation may or may not be present.

The treatment of psychotic conditions was revolutionized by the introduction of *chlorpromazine* into medical therapy in 1952. The success with this drug in ameliorating psychotic symptoms led to the development of a variety of structurally diverse antipsychotic drugs over the next three decades. Unfortunately, virtually all of these compounds have simultaneously produced a high incidence of adverse extrapyramidal motor effects. The recent introduction of clozapine, an antipsychotic drug that exerts minimal motor effects, has spurred a search for similarly acting drugs.

The antipsychotic drugs are effective in reducing symptomatology associated with both organic and functional psychotic states. They are indicated for the treatment of the manic phase of manic-depressive psychosis and for the treatment of psychotic symptoms occurring during major depression as well. The treatment of depression is considered in Chap. 36.

Biochemical Bases of Psychoses

The presence of abnormal substances in the tissues of schizophrenics has long been proposed to be responsible for the individual's psychotic symptoms. For example, since the methylation of several naturally occurring brain biogenic amines results in the formation of compounds that are hallucinogenic, interest has arisen in this as a possible biochemical basis for schizophrenia.

Another possible biochemical basis for schizophrenia comes from studies on the mechanism of action of antipsychotic drugs. A common feature shared by all known antipsychotics is their ability to block the effects of dopamine. This finding suggests that an abnormality in the regulation of brain dopamine could be involved in schizophrenia.

Genetic studies also support the contention that there is a biochemical basis for schizophrenia. The most solid evidence has been provided by experiments in which offspring of both schizophrenic and nonpsychotic patients were reared by foster parents. A higher incidence of schizophrenia occurred in the former group of offspring, and an involvement of genetic factors in the etiology of this mental disorder was strongly suggested. Much support also comes from studies of identical twins; such studies show that the incidence of schizophrenia in both monozygotic individuals, when reared in different environments, is about the same as that for those reared together.

The possible biochemical bases for affective disorders are discussed in Chap. 36.

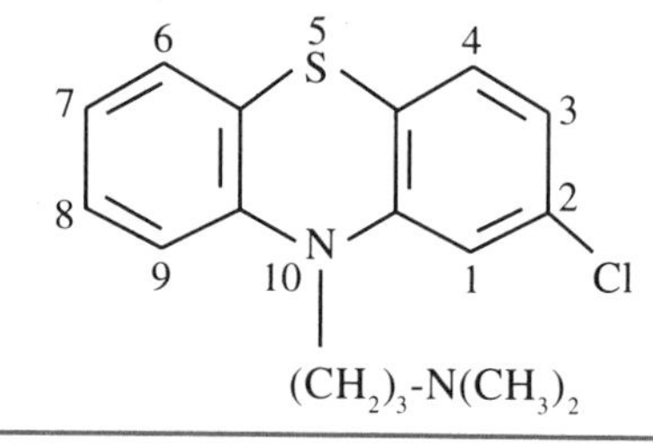

Figure 35-1. Chlorpromazine.

Phenothiazine Derivatives

Chlorpromazine (Fig. 35-1) was the forerunner of a large number of phenothiazine derivatives, approximately two dozen of which are used in medical therapy. Of these, one dozen are employed specifically for psychiatric disorders. Three major chemical groups of phenothiazines possessing similar pharmacological profiles exist: the *aliphatic phenothiazines* (e.g., chlorpromazine and triflupromazine), the *piperidine phenothiazines* (e.g., thioridazine and mesoridazine), and the more potent *piperazine phenothiazines* (e.g., trifluoperazine and congeners). A comparison of the principal properties of some of the most common antipsychotic phenothiazines is provided in Table 35-1.

Chemistry

All the phenothiazines possessing antipsychotic activity have a three-carbon bridge between the nitrogen atom of the middle ring and that of the side chain (see Fig. 35-1). Substitutions at positions 2 and 10 modify pharmaco-logical activity. For example, the presence of a chloride or methoxy group in position 2 increases muscle-relaxing potency. A CF_3 substitution in this position greatly increases antipsychotic and antiemetic potency. Placement of a piperidine moiety in the side chain at position 10, as occurs in the thioridazine and mesoridazine molecules, reduces the incidence of extrapyramidal effects. Substitution of a piperazine group at this position, as found in perphenazine, fluphenazine, prochlorperazine, and trifluoperazine, markedly increases antipsychotic activity.

Mechanism of Action

The brainstem reticular system has been suggested as one site of action of the phenothiazines. Chlorpromazine may *increase reticular activity;* such an action would result in the stimulation of information-filtering mechanisms in the reticular formation and thereby *reduce the inflow of stimuli* reaching higher brain centers. Because of the close correlation that exists between the functions of the limbic system and the emotional disturbances of the schizophrenic, this area of the brain also has been suggested as a possible site of drug action.

Limbic system dopamine receptors are blocked after phenothiazine administration, and the turnover rate of dopamine in this area is increased, presumably through feedback mechanisms. Antipsychotic drugs other than the phenothiazines also block limbic dopamine receptors. Additional findings suggest that dopaminergic sites in the cortex also may be involved in antipsychotic drug action.

Unfortunately, the phenothiazines as well as most other antipsychotic drugs exert major motor side effects by action at dopaminergic receptors within the extrapyramidal system. Figure 35-2 depicts the main neuroanatomical sites of action of the antipsychotic drugs.

Table 35-1. A Comparison of the Main Properties of Some Antipsychotic Phenothiazine Derivatives

Compound (trade name)	Pharmacological property		
	Sedation	Hypotension	Extrapyramidal effects
Chlorpromazine *(Thorazine)*	Marked	Moderate	Moderate
Fluphenazine *(Permitil)*	Slight	Slight	Marked
Mesoridazine *(Serentil)*	Marked	Moderate	Slight
Perphenazine *(Trilafon)*	Moderate	Slight	Marked
Prochlorperazine *(Compazine)*	Slight	Slight	Marked
Thioridazine *(Mellaril)*	Marked	Moderate	Slight
Trifluoperazine *(Stelazine)*	Slight	Slight	Marked
Triflupromazine *(Vesprin)*	Moderate	Moderate	Marked

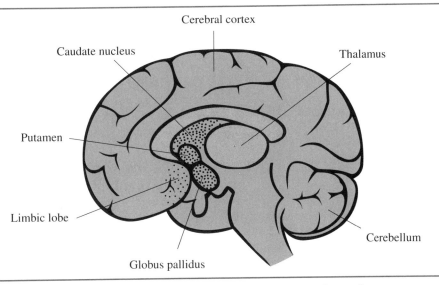

Figure 35-2. Major sites of action of antispychotic drugs within the brain. Antipsychotic effects are presumably mediated by limbic dopaminergic receptors, while the motor side effects are mediated by dopaminergic receptors within the striatum.

Pharmacological Actions

Central Nervous System

Initial doses of chlorpromazine and most other phenothiazine derivatives produce a considerable degree of tranquilization, or quieting. This action differs from that seen after hypnotic drug administration, in that the individual still can be easily aroused. Three noteworthy exceptions are *prochlorperazine, fluphenazine,* and *trifluoperazine,* drugs that possess very little sedative-like effect.

Normal individuals who are given a phenothiazine generally sit quietly and display no interest in surrounding external events; stimuli that ordinarily arouse emotion evoke no response. This drug-induced behavior, which consists of psychomotor slowing, emotional quieting, and affective indifference, is known as a *neuroleptic syndrome.* Subjectively, the normal individual experiences dysphoria.

Acute administration of a phenothiazine to the *psychotic patient* results in an immediate calming effect that is most conspicuous in the agitated patient. Several weeks of drug administration are required, however, for the antipsychotic effect to develop fully.

Chlorpromazine and other phenothiazines exert an antiemetic effect by virtue of their action within the *chemoreceptor trigger zone* of the medulla. However, emesis produced by the action of drugs on either the nodose ganglion or the gastrointestinal tract is not prevented. Emesis due to vestibular stimulation is similarly unaffected by phenothiazine administration.

The phenothiazines interfere with temperature-regulating mechanisms, presumably by an action within the hypothalamus. The direction of change in body temperature is dependent on the prevailing ambient temperature. Hypothermia is produced under conditions of low environmental temperatures, whereas high environmental temperatures result in hyperthermia.

Drug administration has complex effects on the excitability of various brain structures. Small doses of chlorpromazine elevate the pentylenetetrazol seizure threshold, whereas large doses lower it. In humans, a chlorpromazine-induced facilitation of seizure activity has most often been observed either in patients with a history of a seizure disorder or in those who have a condition that predisposes them to seizures. However, chlorpromazine is not usually contraindicated in epileptics who are adequately controlled by anticonvulsant drug therapy, since drug control of the seizures usually can be maintained. The occurrence of convulsive phenomena after administration of piperazine and piperidine phenothiazines is rare.

A variety of changes in the endocrine system are produced as a result of the central actions of the phenothiazines. These are summarized in Table 35-2. Most of these drugs depress the release of *prolactin release inhibiting hormone* from the hypothalamus and thereby induce lactation. They also interfere with *pituitary gonadotropin* output, resulting in an inhibition of ovulation and, occasionally, the development of amenorrhea. Secretion of pituitary growth hormone and neurohypophyseal hormones is also inhibited. Chlorpromazine additionally re-

Table 35-2. Endocrine Effects of the Phenothiazines

Hormonal change	Effect
Prolactin release inhibiting hormone	Increased lactation
Gonadotropins	Inhibition of ovulation
Corticotropins	Decreased adrenal corticosteroid secretion

duces *corticotropin* release, resulting in a decreased secretion of adrenal corticosteroids. Chlorpromazine also enhances *melanocyte-stimulating hormone* (MSH) release from the pituitary, while simultaneously inhibiting the biotransformation of *melatonin*, a pineal hormone that has effects opposite to those of MSH.

Autonomic Nervous System

The phenothiazines exert weak anticholinergic activity, which may result in dry mouth, blurring of vision, decreased gastric secretion and motility, constipation, and diminished sweating and salivation. Thioridazine is the most potent muscarinic antagonist, while the piperazine phenothiazines are much weaker. The inhibition of ejaculation that occurs in men taking chlorpromazine may be due, in part, to α-adrenoceptor blockade. Thioridazine also produces this effect with regularity, while the piperazine phenothiazines do not.

Cardiovascular System

The phenothiazines exert complex effects on the cardiovascular system. These agents depress vasomotor reflexes controlled by the hypothalamus and the brainstem. This action results in a centrally mediated lowering of blood pressure and in orthostatic hypotension. More direct effects on the cardiovascular system itself also occur. Mild hypotension and reflex tachycardia are produced as a result of both peripheral nerve blockade and an interference with central reflexes. Chlorpromazine and thioridazine more frequently cause orthostatic hypotension, whereas the piperazine phenothiazines are less likely to do so.

Chlorpromazine has antiarrhythmic properties, possibly as a result of a local anesthetic effect or a quinidine-like action. In addition, this drug is directly depressant to the myocardium. Chlorpromazine may cause Q- and T-wave distortions. Thioridazine has frequently caused changes in the T wave of the electrocardiogram (ECG). Such changes have rarely been seen in response to the piperazine phenothiazines.

Miscellaneous Peripheral Effects

A diuresis is sometimes seen after chlorpromazine administration. Whether this action is caused by an inhibition of water and electrolyte reabsorption by the renal tubule or is the result of an inhibition of secretion of antidiuretic hormone, possibly by an action on the hypothalamus, is not known. All the phenothiazines promote appetite increase and weight gain.

Tolerance and Abrupt Drug Discontinuance

Tolerance to the sedative-like effects of the phenothiazines develops during a period of time ranging from a few days to several weeks. Although tolerance to the hypotensive effect is seen after several weeks of chronic administration, some degree of orthostatic hypotension may persist. In contrast, *there is no tolerance to the antipsychotic action* of the phenothiazines. After abrupt cessation of long-term administration, muscular discomfort and motor hyperactivity have been reported. Difficulty in sleeping also has occurred.

Absorption, Metabolism, and Excretion

Most of the phenothiazines exhibit erratic and unpredictable absorption from the gastrointestinal tract and thus rates of drug absorption differ considerably from one individual to another. Intramuscular administration increases the bioavailability by as much as tenfold. The phenothiazines are highly lipophilic and highly bound to both membranes and proteins. Elimination half-lives have ranged from 20 to 40 hr. This agrees with the observed 24-hr pharmacological effect of single doses after patient stabilization. Metabolism occurs primarily by oxidative processes. Hydroxylation and subsequent conjugation with glucuronic acid represent the principal metabolic pathway. Metabolites of some of the phenothiazines have been detected in the urine for as long as several months after drug discontinuation.

Clinical Uses

The phenothiazines alleviate the wide array of symptoms associated with the various forms of psychosis. There is no evidence that any one drug more selectively influences a given symptom than does another. Drug choice should be made after considering both the patient's medical history and the more prominent side effects associated with the use of a particular phenothiazine. If patient compliance is a problem, parenteral fluphenazine, administered biweekly, can be used once an orally effective dose has been established. Patients with a known history of cardiovascular disease are best treated with a piperazine phenothiazine, which reduces the incidence of hypotension.

Certain medical conditions, as well as advancing age, may predispose the patient to extrapyramidal side effects. In these cases, thioridazine would be the agent of choice. If sedative-like effects are undesirable, a piperazine phenothiazine may be preferred.

Dosage and duration of therapy must be determined on an individual basis. A low dose should be used initially, which can be increased gradually until acute symptoms are controlled. Because *the onset of an antipsychotic effect may take 3 weeks or longer,* rapid increases in dose should be undertaken judiciously. In general, drug treatment is continued for 6 months to 1 year after a psychotic episode. If subsequent episodes occur, longer maintenance therapy may be indicated. Patients with a history of chronic relapsing schizophrenia often are maintained on antipsychotic therapy indefinitely.

The antiemetic properties of the phenothiazines have been used to control the vomiting associated with a number of disorders, including uremia, gastroenteritis, and radiation sickness. Drug-induced emesis (e.g., that caused by narcotics, estrogens, cancer chemotherapeutic agents, and disulfiram) is also relieved. Additional discussion of the use of phenothiazines in the treatment of emesis is found in Chap. 73. Chlorpromazine also can be used in the control of intractable hiccup.

Adverse Reactions

Table 35-3 summarizes the primary adverse peripheral effects of the phenothiazines. Most side effects are direct extensions of their pharmacological actions. Common adverse effects include faintness, palpitation, nasal stuffiness, dry mouth, and orthostatic hypotension. The endocrine changes described previously are also frequently observed.

The most disturbing side effects commonly produced

Table 35-3. Adverse Peripheral Effects of Phenothiazines

Mechanism	Effect
Anticholinergic activity	Dry mouth
	Blurred vision
	Constipation
α-Adrenoceptor blockade	Orthostatic hypotension
	Inhibition of ejaculation
Endocrine	Appetite increase
	Weight gain

Table 35-4. Extrapyramidal Side Effects of Phenothiazines

Syndrome	Symptoms
Acute dystonia	Spasm of muscles of face, tongue, neck, and back
Akathisia	Motor restlessness
Parkinsonism	Rigidity, tremor, shuffling gait
Tardive dyskinesia	Oral-facial involuntary movements, choreiform movement of extremities

by chronic administration of the phenothiazines are the result of their actions on the extrapyramidal system. Three syndromes may be differentiated during the period of drug use, while a fourth may occur either during prolonged treatment or after cessation of use. These are summarized in Table 35-4.

One syndrome, whose most prominent signs are rigidity and tremor at rest, is indistinguishable from idiopathic parkinsonism. This disorder may respond to benztropine, an anticholinergic antiparkinsonian drug. It is reversible on discontinuance of the drug or lowering of the dosage.

A second syndrome typically seen is *akathisia,* a condition in which the patient feels compelled to move about continuously. Although benztropine can sometimes alleviate this symptom, a reduction of the antipsychotic drug dosage also is necessary.

A third group of symptoms (*acute dystonic reaction*) is characterized by facial grimacing, and torticollis is seen occasionally. These symptoms are dramatically reversed by anticholinergic antiparkinsonian drugs.

The fourth syndrome, *tardive dyskinesia,* may appear either during or after prolonged chlorpromazine treatment. This disorder is less common and occurs most frequently in older patients. Stereotyped involuntary movements, such as sucking and smacking the lips, lateral jaw movements, and darting of the tongue, are characteristic signs. Choreiform and purposeless, quick movements of the extremities also may occur. In contrast with the other syndromes, tardive dyskinesia does *not* respond favorably to antiparkinsonian drugs (see also Chap. 38).

Opinion is divided as to the best means of controlling extrapyramidal side effects induced by antipsychotic drug therapy. Some clinicians recommend the simultaneous administration of antiparkinsonian drugs, such as benztropine, whereas others feel strongly that the dosage of the antipsychotic medication should be reduced immediately.

Chlorpromazine causes jaundice in approximately 2 to 4 percent of individuals taking the drug; it usually occurs during the second to fourth week of therapy and is thought to be the result of a hypersensitivity reaction. Jaundice is seen much less frequently after administration of the other phenothiazines. Symptoms include bile in the urine and abnormally high plasma levels of both alkaline phosphatase and bilirubin. Clinically, this complication resembles obstructive jaundice.

Blood dyscrasias, including eosinophilia, agranulocytosis, and leukopenia, constitute a second hypersensitivity reaction to phenothiazine administration. The incidence is relatively low and has been estimated at 1 in 10,000 patients. This complication usually appears during the first 6 weeks of therapy with chlorpromazine or other low-potency agents and occurs more often in females.

Less serious adverse effects sometimes associated with phenothiazine therapy include such skin reactions as urticaria, contact dermatitis, photosensitivity, and abnormal pigmentation. The last-named is usually seen only after long-term, high-dosage treatment regimens. Regions of the skin exposed to sun take on a gray-blue pigmentation. Deposits also may form in the lens and retina, leading to impairment of vision and retinopathy.

Drug Interactions

The phenothiazines alter the effects of a variety of drugs. The actions of CNS depressants, such as alcohol, the narcotics, and the sedative-hypnotics, are enhanced. Thioridazine is an exception in that it causes little potentiation of hypnotic drug action. In contrast, the antihypertensive effects of guanethidine are blocked by the phenothiazines.

Preparations

Chlorpromazine hydrochloride (*Thorazine*) is available for oral use as tablets, as sustained-release capsules, and as a syrup or concentrate.

Thioxanthenes

The replacement of the nitrogen at position 10 of the phenothiazine molecule (Fig. 35-1) by a carbon atom linked by a double bond to the side chain yields a compound known as a thioxanthene. Although four thioxanthene derivatives are used as antipsychotics clinically, only two of these, chlorprothixene and thiothixene, are available in the United States.

The spectrum of pharmacological activity of each of these agents is quite similar to that of its corresponding phenothiazine derivative. Chlorprothixene resembles chlorpromazine, an aliphatic phenothiazine, while thiothixene corresponds to thioproperazine, a piperazine phenothiazine used clinically abroad.

Chlorprothixene

Pharmacological Actions

Like chlorpromazine, initial doses of chlorprothixene produce considerable sedation and drowsiness. Anticholinergic effects and postural hypotension also occur as frequently as with chlorpromazine. Galactorrhea and menstrual changes may also be produced as a result of actions within the central nervous system (CNS); weight gain also may occur. Chlorprothixene produces changes in central nervous system excitability similar to those of chlorpromazine, and convulsions have occurred in susceptible individuals. In the periphery, chlorprothixene causes ECG abnormalities similar to those seen after chlorpromazine.

Clinical Uses

As in the case of the phenothiazines, choice of a particular agent within the thioxanthene group of neuroleptics is based primarily on avoidance of side effects for the individual patient. As with chlorpromazine, usage of chlorprothixene can be considered in younger patients free of cardiovascular and neurological disease in whom a sedative effect is desirable.

Adverse Reactions

Side effects commonly produced by chlorprothixene include faintness, palpitation, nasal stuffiness, dry mouth, and orthostatic hypotension. Endocrine changes also are frequently observed. Extrapyramidal side effects occur as frequently as with chlorpromazine. Cholestatic jaundice likewise has the same high incidence. Skin rash, photosensitivity, lenticular deposits, and blood dyscrasias also have occurred.

Preparations

Chlorprothixene (*Taractan*) is available for oral use as tablets and as a concentrate.

Thiothixene

Pharmacological Actions

Like the piperazine phenothiazines, thiothixene possesses only mild to moderate sedative activity. As with the piperazine compounds, extrapyramidal effects occur with high frequency. Anticholinergic activity appears to be greater than that of most of the piperazine phenothiazines. The incidence of orthostatic hypotension, however, appears to be about the same and is less than that occurring after chlorpromazine. As with most neuroleptics, galactorrhea and menstrual changes may be produced.

Clinical Uses

Thiothixene is indicated in patients in whom sedative effects are not desired. It is also useful in patients with cardiovascular disease.

Adverse Reactions

The frequency of occurrence of extrapyramidal effects, akathisia, and dystonia is quite high after treatment with thiothixene. Tardive dyskinesia also occurs after long-term continued use. Endocrine changes are likely to occur. Skin rash, blood dyscrasias, and lenticular deposits also have been observed.

Preparations

Thiothixene hydrochloride (*Navane Hydrochloride*) is available for oral administration as capsules and as a concentrate.

Haloperidol

A search for meperidine analogues with increased analgesic potency fortuitously led to the discovery of the phenothiazine-like properties of the butyrophenones. *Haloperidol* (Fig. 35-3) is the only agent from this group used as an antipsychotic in the United States today.

Pharmacological Actions

Central Nervous System

Although the basic structure of haloperidol shows little resemblance to that of the phenothiazines, the pharmacological properties of this agent are remarkably similar to those of the piperazine phenothiazines. The tranquilizing properties of haloperidol, like those of the piperazine phenothiazines, are less prominent than those of chlorpromazine.

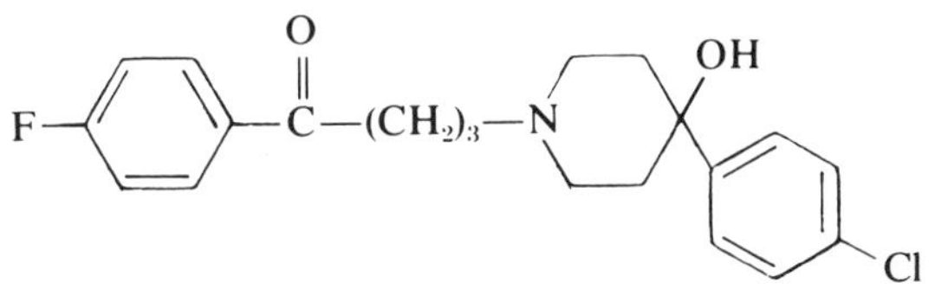

The antipsychotic effects of haloperidol are useful not only in the treatment of schizophrenia but also in the management of the manic phase of the manic-depressive syndrome. Haloperidol also possesses antiemetic activity. The centrally mediated changes in the endocrine system seen after phenothiazine therapy also occur in response to haloperidol administration. The convulsive threshold may be lowered by haloperidol.

Peripheral Effects

The anticholinergic activity and α-adrenergic blockade associated with the use of haloperidol are less prominent than those produced by the phenothiazines. Hypotension similarly is less severe, but tachycardia still can occur. Weight gain does not appear to be significant.

Absorption, Metabolism, and Excretion

Absorption of haloperidol following oral administration is quite good, and peak plasma levels are achieved within 2 to 6 hr after its ingestion. Since the rates of haloperidol metabolism and elimination are very slow, drug blood levels remain near their peak for up to 72 hr; this agent, therefore, has a relatively long duration of action. About 15 percent of a single dose is excreted in the bile. It takes approximately 5 days for 40 percent of a single dose to be excreted by the kidney.

Clinical Uses

Several factors should be considered before selecting haloperidol for use as an antipsychotic medication. If medical conditions predispose the patient to the development of extrapyramidal syndromes, this agent is contraindicated. On the other hand, haloperidol is very useful in situations in which sedation or hypotension is undesirable. The choice of this drug rather than one of the phenothiazines is particularly desirable in patients with impaired hepatic function, since the risk of jaundice may be avoided.

Adverse Reactions

The most prominent side effect occurring after chronic haloperidol therapy is the production of extrapyramidal syndromes. The incidence is high, and the symptoms are pronounced, even in younger patients. Leukopenia is frequent, but jaundice is rare.

Figure 35-3. Haloperidol

Drug Interactions

The actions of CNS depressants are potentiated by haloperidol.

Preparations

Haloperidol (*Haldol*) is available for oral use as tablets and as a concentrate.

Loxapine

Loxapine (Fig. 35-4) is an antipsychotic drug indicated for the treatment of diverse psychotic conditions.

Most of the effects of loxapine on the CNS resemble those produced by the phenothiazines. Sedation and weight gain appear to occur less frequently than when chlorpromazine is used; extrapyramidal signs also occur less frequently. On the other hand, lowering of the convulsive threshold appears to be more marked, and seizures have occurred when loxapine was added to the treatment regimen of previously well-controlled epileptics. Although an antiemetic effect has been demonstrated in experimental animals, comparable human data are not available.

The peripheral effects of loxapine resemble those of the phenothiazines. However, its hypotensive and anticholinergic effects are somewhat milder, whereas the occurrence of sinus tachycardia is similar both in degree and frequency to that produced by phenothiazines.

The absorption of loxapine from the gastrointestinal tract is virtually complete; the drug is then rapidly distributed to the tissues. Almost all the loxapine administered is metabolized in the liver and subsequently excreted by the kidneys. Virtually all of a single dose is eliminated within 24 hr of its ingestion.

The production of an extrapyramidal syndrome constitutes the most serious side effect of loxapine therapy. Dermatitis and photosensitivity also occur occasionally.

Figure 35-4. Loxapine

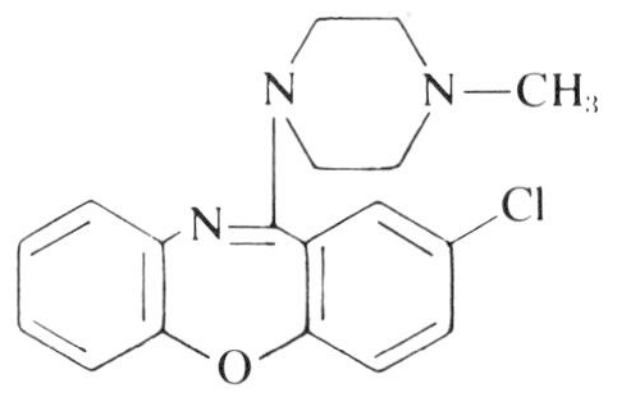

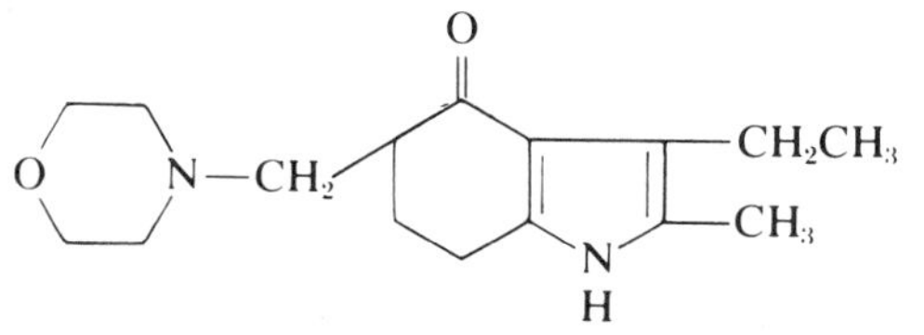

Figure 35-5. Molindone

To date, no instances of blood dyscrasias or jaundice have been reported.

Loxapine succinate (*Loxitane*) is given orally, either as tablets or as a concentrate.

Molindone

The indole derivative molindone is an antipsychotic drug that has been on the market for a decade (Fig. 35-5). It has been used most frequently in the treatment of schizophrenia. It produces moderate sedation, increased activity, and possibly euphoria. Molindone does not appear to induce weight gain. The anticholinergic activity of molindone is comparable to that of the phenothiazines; the hypotension it induces is milder, but tachycardia does occur.

Molindone is rapidly absorbed from the gastrointestinal tract, with peak blood levels being reached within 60 to 90 min after ingestion. The drug is almost completely metabolized in the liver and is then excreted in the urine.

The emergence of extrapyramidal syndromes constitutes the most prominent adverse reaction to molindone. Skin rashes, apparently of allergic origin, and some instances of leukopenia have occurred. In contrast to other antipsychotic drugs, molindone does not appear to potentiate the effects of CNS depressants. It does decrease the seizure threshold in experimental animals, but the degree of lowering is not as marked as that caused by other antipsychotic drugs.

Molindone hydrochloride (*Moban, Lidone*) is marketed as 5-, 10-, and 25-mg tablets.

Clozapine

Clozapine (*Clozaril*) is the most recent antipsychotic drug to be introduced into therapy. It is the first of a group of new drugs classified as *atypical* antipsychotics. Unlike previous agents, these drugs exert few extrapyramidal side effects. They correspondingly exhibit a different profile with regard to binding to dopamine receptors and effects on dopamine-mediated behaviors. Their antipsychotic efficacy is presumed to be due to preferential action at limbic dopaminergic receptors.

The oral bioavailability of clozapine averages around 50 to 60 percent. About 95 percent of the drug is bound to plasma proteins. The half-life is about 12 hr. Clozapine is virtually completely metabolized before excretion.

Clozapine exerts antagonistic activity at central adrenergic, serotonergic, histaminergic, and cholinergic receptor sites. Sedation and weight gain may occur. However, elevation of serum prolactin concentrations, typically produced by most other neuroleptics, does not occur. There is a relatively high risk of grand mal seizures at increasing doses.

Peripherally, clozapine causes orthostatic hypotension and exerts strong anticholinergic activity. Associated with the latter is sustained mild sinus tachycardia. Paradoxically, excessive salivation, particularly during sleep, occurs frequently. Agranulocytosis is a serious toxic effect of clozapine, and this limits the clinical utility of the drug. Clozapine is used only for the treatment of severely ill schizophrenic patients who have failed to respond adequately to standard antipsychotic therapy. Monitoring of the white cell count is done on a weekly basis.

Lithium Carbonate

Lithium is a monovalent cation that is a member of the same family of elements as sodium and potassium. Although this mood-stabilizing drug has been administered with widely varying degrees of effectiveness to patients with a variety of mental illnesses, including schizophrenia and depression, its sole Food and Drug Administration (FDA)-approved therapeutic use is for the treatment of *mania* accompanying manic-depressive disorders. The pharmacology, clinical usefulness, and toxicity of lithium are discussed in Chap. 36.

Supplemental Reading

Baldessarini, R.J. Clozapine. A novel antipsychotic agent. *N. Engl. J. Med.* 324:746, 1991.

Casey, D.E. Neuroleptic drug-induced extrapyramidal syndromes and tardive dyskinesia. *Schizophr. Res.* 4:109, 1991.

Deutch, A.Y., et al. Mechanisms of action of atypical antipsychotic drugs. Implications for novel therapeutic strategies for schizophrenia. *Schizophr. Res.* 4:121, 1991.

Gerlach, J. New antipsychotics: Classification, efficacy and adverse effects. *Schizophr. Bull.* 17:289, 1991.

Holland, D., Watanabe, M.D., and Sharma, R. Atypical antipsychotics. *Psychiatr. Med.* 9:5, 1991.

Krishel, S., and Jackimczyk, K. Cyclic antidepressants, lithium, and neuroleptic agents. Pharmacology and toxicology. *Emerg. Med. Clin. North Am.* 9:53, 1991.

Levinson, D.F. Pharmacologic treatment of schizophrenia. *Clin. Ther.* 13:326, 1991.

Marks, R.C., and Luchinsi, D.J. Antipsychotic medications and seizures. *Psychiatr. Med.* 9:37, 1991.

Meltzer, H.Y. The mechanism of action of novel antipsychotic drugs. *Schizophr. Bull.* 17:263, 1991.

Ryan, P.M. Epidemiology, etiology, diagnosis and treatment of schizophrenia. *Am. J. Hosp. Pharm.* 48:1271, 1991.

Van Kammen, D.P. The biochemical basis of relapse and drug response in schizophrenia: Review and hypothesis. *Psychol. Med.* 21:881, 1991.

36

Drugs Used in Mood Disorders

Albert J. Azzaro and *Herbert E. Ward*

Throughout the course of history, disorders of mood (or affect) have been recorded and noted as a pathological condition. Presently, the American Psychiatric Association has established diagnostic criteria for the mood disorders (DSM-IIIR) that permit clinicians to consistently distinguish between pathological states and normal changes in emotion in everyday life. In this regard, epidemiological studies would indicate that as many as 5 percent of the US adult population, at any point in time, suffers from a mood disorder.

The most common mood disorders are *major depression* (unipolar disorder) and *manic-depressive illness* (bipolar disorder). Each of these disorders is characterized by exaggerated mood associated with physiological, cognitive, and psychomotor disturbances. For example, major depression generally presents as depressed mood, diminished interest in normal activities, anorexia with significant weight loss, insomnia, fatigue, and inability to concentrate. By contrast, manic episodes associated with manic-depressive illness are characterized by expansive mood, grandiosity, inflated self-esteem, pressured speech, flight of ideas, and poverty of sleep (generally 3 hr/night). While each condition is a diagnostic entity unto itself, it can also be secondary to specific medical problems (e.g., hypothyroidism), neurological disease (e.g., Parkinson's disease), and chronic administration of specific medications (e.g., antihypertensives). Attempts to rule out these latter possibilities are essential before additional treatment of the mood disorder.

In this chapter, the basic and clinical pharmacology of each class of agents that demonstrates efficacy in the treatment of individual mood disorders is discussed. Some distinctions can be made between agents that are effective in major depression as opposed to those useful for the treatment of manic-depressive illness. However, the major distinguishing features among agents for the treatment of individual illnesses (i.e., depression) are their side-effect profiles and relative toxicity. Physicians should have an understanding both of the appropriate agent for the treatment of specific mood disorders and of pharmacological factors that allow for the individualization of medication to meet the patient's needs.

Treatment of Major Depression

Tricyclic Antidepressants

In the late 1950s, by serendipity, the drug imipramine hydrochloride was noted to be effective for the symptomatic treatment of depression. Over the years, a number of chemical congeners of imipramine have been synthesized and tested for antidepressant properties. These substances have come to be known by the trivial name of *tricyclic antidepressants* (TCA) as a result of their basic chemical structures (i.e., a three-ring core) (Fig. 36-1). Presently, these agents are the most widely used substances for the treatment of major depression. Accordingly, their pharmacology is discussed here in detail.

Chemistry

Currently, seven TCA drugs are available in the United States for the treatment of major depression. They are generally categorized as tertiary or secondary amines, based on the degree of chemical substitution that exists on the terminal nitrogen of the side chain. Hydrochloride salts of the tertiary amines have been synthesized and include imipramine, amitriptyline, trimipramine, and doxepin. Desipramine hydrochloride (HCl), nortriptyline HCl, and protriptyline HCl are classified as secondary amines. Clomipramine HCl is also a member of the tricyclic family, with similar pharmacology and antidepressant efficacy. However, this agent has Food and Drug Administration (FDA) approval only for obsessive-compulsive disorder and is not included in this discussion of antidepressant drugs.

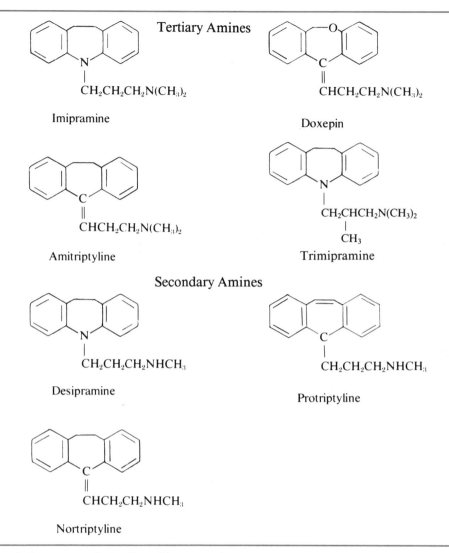

Figure 36-1. Chemical structures of tricyclic antidepressant drugs.

Maprotiline HCl and amoxapine are two other heterocyclic antidepressant agents that are not chemically members of the tricyclic family. However, their pharmacology is so similar to the tricyclic secondary amines that they are included for discussion purposes with this class of agents. Desipramine and nortriptyline (see Fig. 36-1) are major metabolites of imipramine and amitriptyline, respectively.

Pharmacological Actions in the Central Nervous System

While imipramine-like agents produce biological changes in a number of organ systems of the body, the most relevant to their therapeutic effects in depression are those associated with actions in the central nervous system (CNS). In this regard, it is always surprising for the student to learn that mood-elevating agents *do not* act as stim-

ulants of the CNS. With the exception of some degree of mild sedation, associated with alterations of the sleep cycle (especially with the tertiary amines), and perhaps some mild cognitive difficulty, these agents have little effect on behavior early in treatment. Patients will, however, experience side effects during this period that are generally associated with peripheral actions of these agents (see below).

Only after a period of 2 to 3 weeks of chronic dosing will a therapeutic benefit on depression emerge. At this point the patient begins to demonstrate an elevation in mood and self-esteem. In addition, many of the vegetative signs of the illness (e.g., insomnia, anorexia) abate, and the patient regains an interest in daily activities. Failure to continue the medication, however, will result in an immediate relapse into the depressive state. Therefore, *maintenance therapy must be continued for at least 6 months.*

All of the TCA drugs demonstrate full efficacy as antidepressant agents. However, the literature indicates that secondary amines (e.g., desipramine) are more potent than tertiary amines (e.g., imipramine). This is reflected in the higher serum concentration of the latter agents necessary for effective treatment of major depression. This finding, coupled with the lower toxicity generally associated with secondary amines (see below), suggests a preferential role in the treatment of depression for these agents.

Mechanism of Action

The precise molecular mechanism responsible for the antidepressant action of the TCA drugs is unknown. Soon after their discovery, it was shown that imipramine and imipramine-like drugs could alter the normal physiology of neurotransmission at norepinephrine and serotonin synapses of the brain. These actions resulted from an inhibitory effect of the TCA drugs on neuronal membrane transport mechanisms (neuronal reuptake) present at the nerve terminal; reuptake serves to terminate biological activity of these amine transmitter substances. Accordingly, a number of hypotheses have been generated to account for the antidepressant actions of the tricyclic compounds that involve alterations in neurotransmission of norepinephrine or serotonin, or both.

β-Adrenoceptor "down-regulation" at central noradrenergic synapses is one popular theory used to explain the antidepressant properties of TCA drugs and other antidepressants. This theory focuses on a cascade of adaptive changes occurring at the noradrenergic synapse that appears to be triggered by inhibition of norepinephrine neuronal reuptake by TCA drugs (see Fig. 36-2 for sequence of adaptive changes). Animal studies clearly demonstrate a time-dependent reduction in the density of the CNS β-adrenoceptor population with corresponding functional changes (subsensitivity) in the β-adrenoceptor–coupled adenylyl cyclase system at noradrenergic synapses. The adenylyl cyclase system is thought to act as the effector coupling system for β-adrenoceptors. Accordingly, chronic treatment with TCA drugs produces a time-dependent reduction in the flow of synaptic information through β-adrenoceptors of the brain.

Subsensitivity in the β-adrenoceptor–coupled adenylyl cyclase system and associated reductions in β-adrenoceptor density appear to be common features of all clinically effective antidepressant drugs (with the exception of fluoxetine) and electroconvulsant treatment. Moreover, the time-dependent changes in β-adrenoceptor function parallel the time delay associated with clinical efficacy of these drugs (2–3 weeks). These latter findings have added to the attractiveness of this theory.

It should be noted, however, that at those noradrenergic synapses where multiple adrenoceptors are present (i.e., α_1-, α_2-, and β-adrenoceptors), synaptic transmission through α_1-adrenoceptors will likely be enhanced at the same time that synaptic transmission through α_2- and β-

Inhibition of nerve terminal NE neuronal uptake system

Increase in synaptic concentrations of NE

Desensitization of nerve terminal α_2-adrenoceptors

Increase of neuronal NE release during normal rates of neuronal firing

Further increase in synaptic concentrations of NE

Desensitization of postsynaptic β-adrenoceptors with no change in postsynaptic α_1-adrenoceptor sensitivity

Figure 36-2. Cascade of adaptive changes occurring at norepinephrine (NE) synapses following chronic TCA drug treatment.

adrenoceptors is reduced (Fig. 36-3). This conclusion is based on more recent studies on the electrophysiology of norepinephrine synaptic transmission after long-term TCA drug treatment. It is presently unclear why postsynaptic α_1-adrenoceptors do not become subsensitive (down-regulated) under conditions of TCA drug-induced elevations in synaptic norepinephrine. It is conceivable that these receptors are protected by the α_1-adrenoceptor antagonist properties of the TCA drugs. In any event, the role of enhanced synaptic transmission through α_1-adrenoceptors in the therapeutic action of TCA drugs will undoubtedly be the subject of future studies in this field.

While much emphasis has been placed on alterations in noradrenergic neurotransmission as the basis for clinical efficacy of TCA drugs, these same agents are not without effect on central serotonin (5-HT) neurotransmission. In this regard, long-term studies with TCA drugs in animals have demonstrated a postsynaptic supersensitivity to certain serotonin (5-HT$_{1A}$) receptor agonists at serotonin synapses, with an associated enhancement of serotonergic neurotransmission. The sensitization phenomena to 5-HT$_{1A}$ agonists is mediated in part by an increase in the density of postsynaptic 5-HT$_{1A}$ receptors. *Enhancement of transmission through 5-HT$_{1A}$ receptors appears to be a common phenomenon after chronic administration of all clinically effective antidepressants and electroconvulsive treatment.* In addition, the occurrence of this 5-HT$_{1A}$ supersensitivity parallels the delayed onset of the therapeutic actions of these agents (2–3 weeks). These observations lend strong support to the hypothesis that enhanced serotonergic neuro-

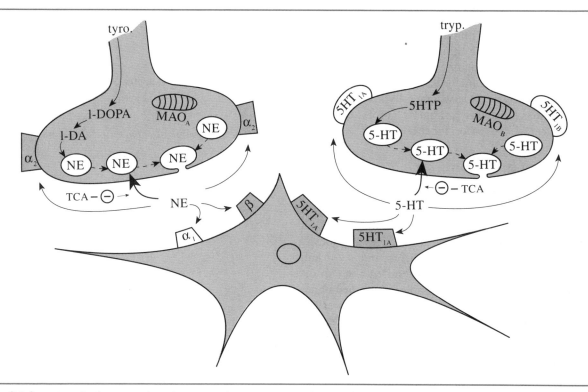

Figure 36-3. *Flow of information through receptor subtypes at norepinephrine and serotonin synapses following chronic TCA drug administration.* A cascade of events leads to altered receptor-mediated physiology of the norepinephrine (NE) and serotonin (5-HT) synapses of the brain following long-term TCA drug administration. The adaptive changes in synaptic physiology are triggered by selective inhibition of the NE and/or 5-HT neuronal reuptake systems. Responses at β- and α_2-adrenoceptors are depressed, whereas responses at 5-HT$_{1A}$ receptors are enhanced. Responses at α_1-adrenoceptors and 5-HT$_{1B}$ receptors remain unchanged. Accordingly, the postsynaptic flow of information at NE and 5-HT synapses will be reduced through β-adrenoceptors but enhanced through 5-HT$_{1A}$ receptors. Although the responsiveness of α_1-adrenoceptors remains unchanged, it is likely that transmission through these postsynaptic sites will be enhanced. In this regard, desensitization of α_2-adrenoceptors will provide greater concentrations of synaptic NE to activate normosensitive, postsynaptic α_1-adrenoceptors.

transmission is required for therapeutic benefit from TCA drugs.

It is likely that TCA drugs produce their therapeutic benefits by acting at both serotonin and norepinephrine synapses. The literature would also support the notion of an interdependence of these two monoamine systems in the treatment of depression. In this regard, destruction of serotonergic neurons in animals prevents the down-regulation of β-adrenoceptors following chronic TCA drug treatment. In addition, the acute administration of lithium (Li$^+$) carbonate to TCA-resistant patients produces a rapid (within 24–48 hr) and profound antidepressant action. It is interesting that such patients would respond in this fashion since acute administration of Li$^+$ is without antidepressant effects in untreated depressed patients. However, Li$^+$ can also enhance synaptic transmission at central serotonin synapses (mechanism unknown), following acute administration. Therefore, it is possible that

in this group of TCA-resistant patients, a combination of the actions of the TCA agent and Li$^+$ at the serotonin synapse provides an added amount of enhancement to serotonin synaptic transmission to allow for the expression of the β-adrenoceptor down-regulation.

Clearly, additional research in this field will be required to determine the nature of the neurotransmitter interaction in affective states and its role in the actions of TCA drugs. The time-dependent changes in the flow of synaptic information through individual receptor subtypes within the norepinephrine and serotonin synapses following chronic TCA administrations are summarized in Fig. 36-3.

Adverse Reactions

Toxic reactions and side effects of TCA drugs are primarily the result of the actions of these agents on the au-

Table 36-1. Side Effects and Toxic Reactions Associated with TCA Drugs

Effect	Comment
Antimuscarinic (tachycardia, blurred vision, constipation, dry mouth, urinary retention, etc.)	Less common with secondary TCAs, maprotiline or amoxapine; some tolerance will develop
Orthostatic hypotension	Special concern for elderly; some tolerance will develop
Arrhythmias	Can be life threatening; common at toxic serum levels; less common with amoxapine
Sedation	Can be therapeutic for insomnia associated with depression; less common with secondary TCAs
Toxic delirium	Cognitive, affective, motor, and psychotic features; common at toxic serum levels (seizures may occur); can be mistaken as worsening of the depression
Seizures	More common with maprotiline
Weight gain	
Involuntary movements; lactation; gynecomastia; neuroleptic malignant syndrome	Only with amoxapine; related to dopamine receptor antagonist properties

tonomic, cardiovascular, and central nervous system (Table 36-1). In the autonomic nervous system, TCA drugs are effective inhibitors of norepinephrine neuronal reuptake at the noradrenergic, sympathetic nerve terminal. In addition, these agents are weak α_1-adrenoceptor antagonists but potent cholinergic, muscarinic receptor antagonists. The combined effect of these actions produces an imbalance in the autonomic nervous system that favors the sympathetic innervation of autonomically innervated tissues. Accordingly, side effects, such as blurred vision, tachycardia, constipation, urinary retention, dry mouth, palpitation, and so forth, are normally seen even with subtherapeutic doses of TCA drugs. Generally, these anticholinergic side effects are not dangerous to the patient but are a nuisance and may contribute to a lack of compliance. Some patients may be unable to tolerate such effects and may require a change in medication. In this regard, it can be generally accepted that tertiary TCAs (e.g., imipramine) are more likely to produce anticholinergic side effects than are the secondary TCAs (e.g., desipramine).

Cardiovascular effects of TCA drugs are numerous and can be life threatening. The most common of the cardiovascular effects are orthostatic hypotension and/or tachycardia. Both of these actions occur at therapeutic doses. Tachycardia results from actions of these agents on the autonomic nervous system (see above). Orthostatic hypotension is caused by a combination of the weak antagonist properties of these agents at α_1-adrenoceptors in vascular smooth muscle and a blunting of the carotid sinus reflex.

Tricyclic antidepressant drugs have potent membrane-stabilizing properties similar to those of quinidine, which produces rhythm disturbances in a dose-related fashion. Conduction is slowed throughout the heart and serious ventricular arrhythmias may develop. Fortunately, such actions are dose dependent and rarely occur at therapeutic plasma levels (Fig. 36-4).

The CNS is also a target of TCA drug toxicity. At subtherapeutic doses these agents can produce mild sedation. However, this action is generally viewed in a positive sense by the physician and the patient, for it assists in allowing for natural sleep in the depressed patient. Sedation is thought to result from the antagonist properties of TCA drugs at α_1-adrenoceptor and H_1-histaminergic receptor sites of the brain. Tertiary TCA drugs (e.g., amitriptyline) generally cause greater sedation than do secondary agents (e.g., nortriptyline). If daytime sedation is a problem, a change to a secondary amine agent may be in order.

High serum concentrations of TCA drugs are generally associated with more severe forms of CNS toxicity. These toxicities can be the result of a purposeful overdose in an attempt at suicide, or may be due to an overtitration of the patient by the physician in an attempt to produce a therapeutic effect. CNS toxicity presents as a delirium with affective, cognitive, motor, and psychotic symptoms that can be clinically difficult to manage. Often, the treating physician may misinterpret the delirium as a worsening of the depression and further increase the dose of the TCA, leading to life-threatening seizures. Fortunately, TCA-induced toxicity of the CNS, like that seen for the cardiovascular system, is dose dependent and is unlikely to occur at therapeutic serum levels (see Fig. 36-4).

Weight gain is a common feature of treatment with TCA drugs. The cellular mechanism for this action is unknown but is generally unpopular with patients and may lead to a lack of compliance.

Tolerance will develop to the anticholinergic effects and orthostatic hypotension associated with TCA medication. To assist the patient with these annoying side effects enroute to the therapeutic maintenance dose, patients are typically titrated with increasing increments of the TCA drugs over a 2- to 3-week period. Such an approach has proved successful in reducing the severity of side effects.

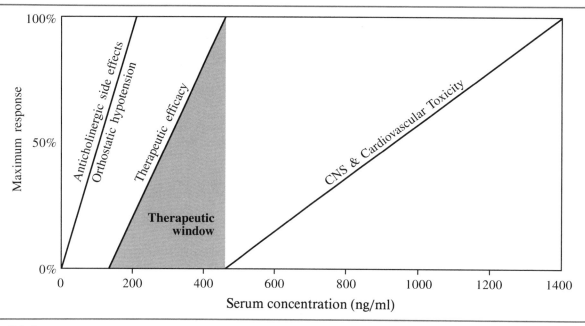

Figure 36-4. Pharmacological actions of TCA drugs at different serum concentrations. The "therapeutic window" represents the concentration of TCA drug whose optimal efficacy can be achieved with minimal risks of severe and even fatal CNS and cardiovascular toxicities. Below the "therapeutic window" patients experience only annoying side effects (such as blurred vision, constipation, tachycardia, etc.) with no therapeutic benefit. Therapeutic window concentrations will differ for each of the TCA drugs administered (see Table 36-2 for individual drug values).

Finally, most antidepressants, including the TCA agents, cause a reduction in the seizure threshold. Therefore, patients with a history of seizures must be dosed cautiously.

Maprotiline HCl and *amoxapine* are much less likely to produce anticholinergic side effects than are TCA drugs. Maprotiline, however, has demonstrated a high incidence of seizures that occur over a broad range of doses. This latter effect can occur in as many as 25 percent of the patients receiving a maprotiline overdose. Therefore, this agent should not be used in patients with a neurological history of epileptic seizures.

Tachycardia and rhythm disturbance have been reported less frequently with amoxapine than with TCA drugs. However, this agent has been associated with reports of extrapyramidal involuntary movement, gynecomastia, lactation, and neuroleptic malignant syndrome. Each of these actions may result from amoxapine's structural similarity to the antipsychotic agent loxapine. In this regard, amoxapine and loxapine demonstrate dopamine receptor antagonist properties that most likely account for many of these side effects (see Chap. 35). Because of these side effects, amoxapine is generally reserved for patients with psychotic depression who may benefit from its weak antipsychotic properties as well as its potent antidepressant action.

Therapeutic Drug Monitoring

The monitoring of serum levels of TCA drugs in the treatment of major depression has become the standard of care in psychiatry today. The importance of this monitoring is based on the relatively narrow range between therapeutic and toxic doses (therapeutic index of 3) of each agent. Figure 36-4 demonstrates the relationships between therapeutic and toxic effects of the TCA drugs. While annoying side effects (anticholinergic; orthostatic hypotension) begin to occur at subtherapeutic serum concentrations, life-threatening cardiac and CNS effects develop at the upper limit of the therapeutic range. This creates a narrow "therapeutic window" where optimal antidepressant efficacy can be obtained without serious or dangerous toxicity. (Note that below therapeutic concentrations of the TCA drugs, the patient experiences annoying side effects and no therapeutic benefit.)

If the pharmacokinetic parameters for each TCA agent were reproducible in individual patients, a simple knowledge of the therapeutic index for each agent would be sufficient to avoid clinical difficulties. However, 10- to 30-fold differences exist in the metabolism and elimination rates of individuals taking TCA drugs. For this reason, it is estimated that only 50 percent of the patients receiving a standard dose of a TCA drug would achieve an optimal

Table 36-2. Typical Doses and Serum Therapeutic Concentrations of Antidepressant Drugs

Drug (trade name)	Oral dose (mg/day)	Half-life (hr)	Serum therapeutic concentration (ng/ml)
Tricyclics			
Amitripytyline HCl *(Elavil)*	75–200	16–26	100–250[a]
Nortriptyline HCl *(Pamelor)*	50–100	19–45	50–150
Imipramine HCl *(Tofranil)*	75–200	11–25	150–250[a]
Desipramine HCl *(Norpramin)*	75–200	20–25	100–200
Protriptyline HCl *(Vivactil)*	15–40	67–89	50–100
Trimipramine maleate *(Surmontil)*	75–150	8	200–300[a]
Doxepin HCl *(Sinequan)*	75–200	11–23	110–250[a]
Maprotiline HCl *(Ludiomil)*	75–200	27–58	200–300
Amoxapine *(Asendin)*	200–300	8	150–500
SSRI			
Fluoxetine HCl *(Prozac)*	20–80	48–72[b]	100–300
Sertraline HCl *(Zoloft)*	50–200	25	32–190[a]
MAO inhibitors			
Phenelzine HCl *(Nardil)*	30–90	1.5–4.0	NA
Tranylcypromine sulfate *(Parnate)*	10–60	1.5–3.5	NA
Isocarboxazid *(Marplan)*	10–30	-------	NA
Miscellaneous agents			
Trazodone HCl *(Desyrel)*	150–300	5–9	800–1,600
Bupropion HCl *(Wellbutrin)*	300–450	10–20	25–100

Key: SSRI = selective serotonin reuptake inhibitors; MAO = monoamine oxidase.
[a]The serum concentration is for the parent agent and its demethylated metabolite.
[b]Active metabolite; $t_{1/2}$ = 7–15 days.

therapeutic serum concentration, and 3 to 5 percent of the remaining patients would have serum concentrations in the life-threatening range. Therefore, to avoid serious toxicity, monitor compliance, and optimize the therapeutic response in the patient, steady-state serum levels of TCA drugs are monitored as a matter of good practice. The typical therapeutic serum concentration range of each TCA drug is summarized in Table 36-2. Note that therapeutic ranges for tertiary amines are always expressed as total TCA (i.e., also includes any tertiary and secondary amine metabolite).

Pharmacokinetics

The TCA drugs are well absorbed from the gastrointestinal tract. Therefore, these agents are typically given by the oral route. In extreme circumstances parenteral (intramuscular) administration can be used. Once absorbed, TCA drugs generally have a large volume of distribution (average = 35 liters/kg); this results from their extreme lipid solubility and extensive binding to plasma proteins and other tissue-binding sites.

Tricyclic antidepressant drugs possess half-lives that range from 8 to 89 hr (see Table 36-2). Thus, several days are required for complete elimination of these agents from the body. Long biological half-lives make most of these agents amenable to once-a-day dosing, generally at bedtime.

Inactivation occurs through oxidative metabolism by hepatic microsomal enzymes. Tertiary amines are converted to secondary amines, which generally possess biological activity and are frequently found in serum at levels equal to or greater than the parent tertiary amine. A second route of inactivation includes conjugation of hydroxylated metabolites with glucuronic acid.

Multiple drug interactions can occur with TCA drugs. For example, because of their high degree of binding to plasma proteins, competition for binding sites can exist between TCAs and phenytoin, aspirin, phenothiazines, and other agents that also display avid plasma protein-binding characteristics. Elevation in the serum level of TCAs (with corresponding toxicity) can occur following the administration of one of these second drugs to the patient. Elevations in the serum TCA level also can occur following inhibition of hepatic TCA metabolism by antipsychotics, methylphenidate, and oral contraceptives.

Tricyclic antidepressant drugs can prevent the action of antihypertensive agents such as guanethidine or clonidine. This antagonistic action appears to be related to the primary (inhibition of neuronal reuptake) and secondary (adaptive changes) effects of TCA drugs at noradrenergic synapses (see Fig. 36-2). A more serious, but rare, interaction exists between TCA drugs and monoamine oxidase (MAO) inhibitor agents. While both are effective in the treatment of major depression, simultaneous administration with these two classes of antidepressants can result in

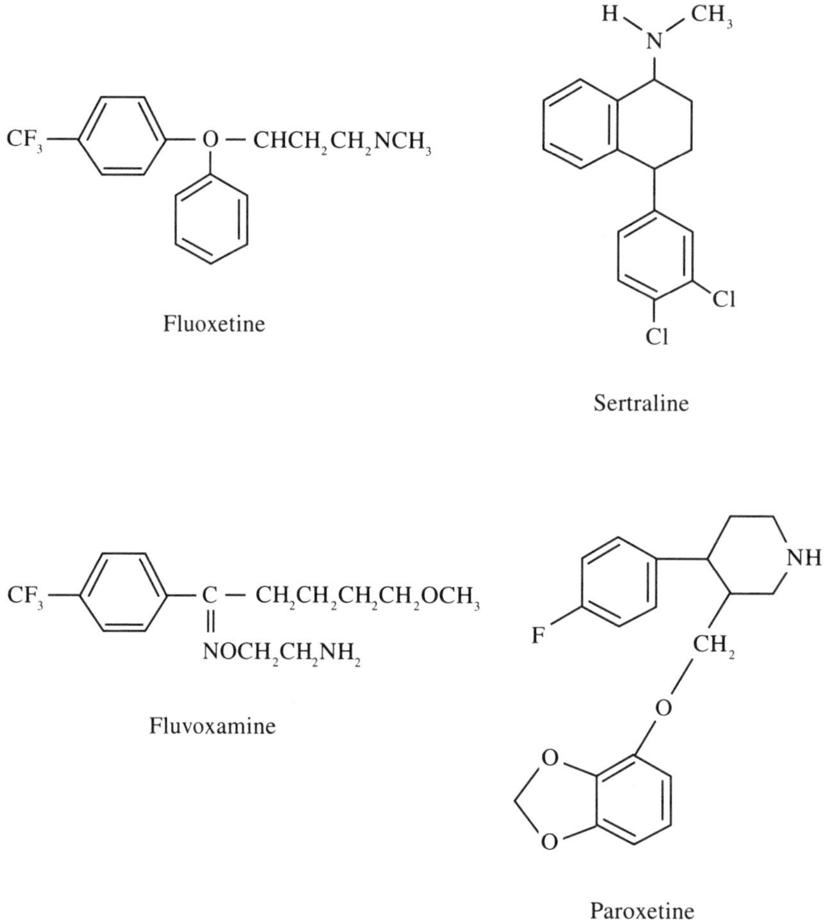

Figure 36-5. Chemical structures of selective serotonin reuptake inhibitor agents.

severe CNS toxicity (hyperpyrexia, convulsions, and coma). In TCA-resistant patients, it is advisable to discontinue the TCA drug for 2 to 3 weeks before initiation of a MAO inhibitor agent. Finally, TCA drugs potentiate the sedative effects of alcohol, and patients must be cautioned about this interaction.

Selective Serotonin Reuptake Inhibitors

In 1987, the FDA approved the drug fluoxetine HCl (*Prozac*) for use in the treatment of major depression. Fluoxetine belongs to a class of agents referred to as *selective serotonin reuptake inhibitors* (SSRI); all members of this class of drugs share this neuronal action. Fluoxetine is the first of what would appear to be many SSRI agents to be marketed in the United States. Others include sertraline HCl, fluvoxamine HCl, and paroxetine HCl. These agents differ significantly in chemical structure (Fig. 36-5).

Mechanism of Action

The high degree of selectivity of SSRI for the nerve terminal serotonin reuptake system has supported the hypothesis that these agents produce their therapeutic action through an ability to modulate serotonin neurotransmission in the brain. Chronic studies in animals have provided evidence for a cascade of altered synaptic events, which include desensitization of 5-HT_{1A} somatodendritic receptors (responsible for regulation of neuronal firing rate) and desensitization of 5-HT_{1B} nerve terminal autoreceptors (responsible for the regulation of neuronal 5-HT release). These events, triggered by a sustained inhibition of the nerve terminal serotonin reuptake system, ultimately cause a potentiation of serotonin neurotransmission at central synaptic sites. The development of these synaptic events shares the same time frame as that observed for the delayed appearance of the therapeutic benefit of these agents in depression. Accordingly, it is currently believed that these biochemical actions of the SSRI

Table 36-3. Common Side Effects Seen with Therapeutic Doses of Antidepressants

Agent	Central nervous system			Cardiovascular		Nausea, vomiting, diarrhea	Weight gain	Autonomic NS anticholinergic
	Sedation	Stimulation	Seizures	Hypotension	Hypertension			
Tricyclic antidepressants	+++	o	+	+++	o	+	++	++++
Selective serotonin reuptake inhibitors	o	+++	o	o	o	++++	o	o
Monoamine oxidase inhibitors	o	+++	+	+++	+++*	+	++	+
Misc. agents Trazodone	++++	o	+	++	o	+	++	++
Bupropion	o	+++	++	+	o	o	o	+

Key: O = no effect; +, ++, +++ indicate increasing effect.
*Only seen in patients who do not comply with dietary restrictions.

are associated with their mechanism of action in major depression.

Clinical Pharmacology and Pharmacokinetics

Fluoxetine was the first of the SSRI to be marketed in the United States. Controlled, multicentered efficacy studies in 540 depressed patients revealed fluoxetine to be as effective as imipramine and superior to placebo over a 4-week period of treatment. Similar results were obtained when fluoxetine was compared to doxepin or amitriptyline.

The major pharmacological difference between fluoxetine and the TCA agents is found in their side effect profile (Table 36-3). While TCA agents commonly cause anticholinergic and cardiovascular side effects, the SSRI, as a group, are devoid of these properties. They are more likely to cause gastrointestinal effects (nausea and diarrhea), tremor, CNS stimulation (nervousness, anxiety), and sexual dysfunction (anorgasmia and ejaculatory delay). In addition, a small weight loss is often seen with chronic fluoxetine treatment, as compared to the weight gain associated with the TCA agents.

The pharmacokinetic profile of fluoxetine is favorable for the long-term treatment of major depression. Fluoxetine is well absorbed from the GI tract independent of the presence of food. This favorable absorption makes oral administration a reliable method for dosing. Elimination studies have demonstrated a plasma half-life of 2 to 3 days for fluoxetine and 7 to 15 days for norfluoxetine, its biologically active metabolite. These elimination half-lives make it possible for once-a-day dosing to enhance compliance. Caution is required when fluoxetine is administered with other CNS active agents, since an increase in the plasma levels of other antidepressants, neuroleptics,

benzodiazepines, and carbamazepine has been noted following the addition of fluoxetine to the treatment plan. These drug interactions are based on alterations in a variety of cellular properties, including hepatic metabolism, renal clearance, and plasma protein binding. Ethanol metabolism is not affected by fluoxetine. Finally, elderly volunteers appear to demonstrate similar pharmacokinetic profiles, making this a reliable drug for the treatment of depression in the elderly.

Sertraline HCl (*Zoloft*) is a highly specific and effective serotonin reuptake inhibitor; it is 10 times more potent than fluoxetine. Sertraline is the second of the SSRI to be approved by the FDA for the treatment of major depression. Controlled clinical studies demonstrate sertraline to be as effective as TCA agents and more effective than placebos in alleviating the symptoms of major depression. Sertraline has an elimination half-life of 25 hr and is metabolized by brain microsomes to desmethylsertraline, a metabolite that lacks antidepressant activity.

Sertraline, unlike fluoxetine, will also produce a downregulation of β-adrenoceptors following chronic administration. Thus, the mechanism of action of sertraline in the treatment of depression may be related to a dual action at both serotonin and norepinephrine synapses of the brain.

Like fluoxetine, the most common side effects of sertraline are associated with the GI tract (nausea and diarrhea). However, because of its high potency, therapeutic concentrations are less likely to cause CNS stimulation. The reduced incidence of CNS toxicity, coupled with a shorter elimination half-life and reliable pharmacokinetics in the elderly, makes sertraline an attractive alternative to fluoxetine in this patient population.

Paroxetine (*Paxil*) is also approved in the United States. It appears to be very similar to both fluoxetine and sertraline.

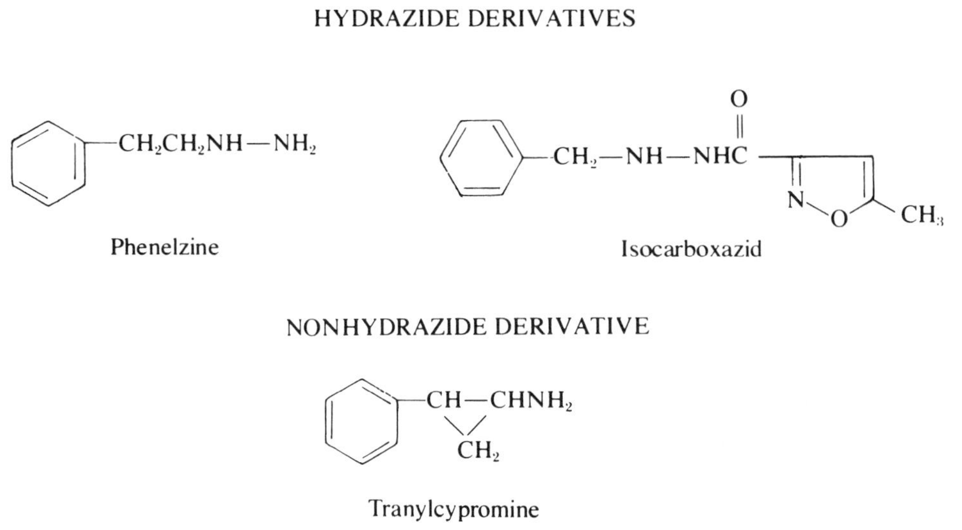

HYDRAZIDE DERIVATIVES

Phenelzine   Isocarboxazid

NONHYDRAZIDE DERIVATIVE

Tranylcypromine

Figure 36-6. Monoamine oxidase inhibitors (MAOI).

Monoamine Oxidase Inhibitors

The mood-elevating properties of a class of drugs that have now come to be known as *monoamine oxidase inhibitors* (MAOI) were recognized in the early 1950s. **Iproniazid,** a drug originally developed for the treatment of tuberculosis, exhibited mood-elevating properties during clinical trials in tuberculosis sufferers with depression. The distinguishing biochemical feature between iproniazid and other chemically similar antituberculosis compounds was the ability of the former to inhibit MAO. Thus, a series of hydrazine and nonhydrazine-related MAOI agents was synthesized and tested for antidepressant properties. To date, three clinically effective MAOI agents have been approved for use in major depression. These drugs are isocarboxazid, phenelzine and tranylcypromine (Fig. 36-6).

Several major, double-blind, randomized antidepressant trials have demonstrated MAOI to be as effective in major depression as the TCA agents. However, at least two forms of life-threatening toxicity (hepatotoxicity and hypertensive crisis) have been associated with the chronic use of MAOI. For this reason, these agents are generally reserved for use in TCA-resistant depression, when electroconvulsive therapy (ECT) is inappropriate, or in atypical depressions (i.e., those associated with increased appetite, phobic anxiety or panic attacks, hypersomnolence, fatigue but no melancholia). In other words, with the exception of atypical depressions, MAOI would not be considered as primary medications.

Mechanism of Action

Monoamine oxidase exists in the human body as two molecular forms known as type A and type B MAO. Each of these isozymes has selective substrate and inhibitor characteristics. Transmitter amines, such as norepinephrine or serotonin, are preferentially metabolized by MAO-A in brain tissue. Type B MAO is more likely to be involved in the catabolism of human brain dopamine, although dopamine is also a good substrate for MAO-A.

Isocarboxazid, phenelzine, and tranylcypromine are irreversible, nonselective inhibitors of MAO-A and MAO-B. However, in clinical trials where newer selective MAOI have been tested, only the selective MAO-A inhibitors demonstrate potent antidepressant properties that are superior to placebo. It appears that inhibition of MAO-A, not MAO-B, is important to the antidepressant action of these agents.

Therapeutic efficacy by selective MAO-A inhibitors in major depressions strongly suggests that MAO inhibition at central serotonin or norepinephrine synapses, or both, is responsible for the antidepressant properties of these agents. However, complete MAO-A inhibition is achieved clinically within a few days of treatment, while the antidepressant effects of MAOI are not observed for 2 to 3 weeks. This apparent discrepancy has become the topic of many recent studies.

Similar to observations made with TCA and SSRI, MAOI induce adaptive changes in CNS synaptic physiology over a period of 2 to 3 weeks. These changes result in both a *down-regulation* of synaptic transmission mediated through noradrenergic α_1- and β-adrenoceptors and an *up-regulation* or enhancement of synaptic transmission at serotonin synapses (at 5-HT$_{1A}$ receptors). This action on serotonin neurotransmission is the result of desensitized somatodendritic autoreceptors responsible for the regulation of the firing rate of serotonin-containing neurons of the forebrain. Accordingly, these neurons fire at elevated rates, releasing large quantities of serotonin into the synapse; this serotonin is protected from degradation by the inhibition of synaptic MAO-A.

It is currently believed that the development of these physiological changes at norepinephrine and serotonin synapses, which parallel the time delay associated with the antidepressant properties of MAOI, is the mechanism of action for these agents in the treatment of major depression. These findings reinforce the corrective nature of antidepressant therapy in general on these two monoaminergic neuronal systems, and their interaction in the expression of normal affective function.

Side Effects and Toxicities

The potential toxicities of MAOI restrict their use in major depression. These toxicities involve the cardiovascular system and the liver. Hepatotoxicity is especially likely to occur with isocarboxazid or phenelzine since hydrazine compounds can cause damage to hepatic parenchymal cells. This is particularly true for those patients identified as slow acetylators of hydrazine compounds. Fortunately, the incidence of hepatotoxicity is low with the currently available agents.

Of greater concern is the potentially lethal cardiovascular effects that can occur in patients who do not comply with their dietary restriction. When patients receive MAO inhibitor drugs, their diets should not contain food rich in tyramine or other biologically active amines. Normally, these substances are rapidly metabolized by MAO-A present within the cells of the intestinal wall and MAO-A and MAO-B in the liver parenchyma. If each isozyme of MAO is inhibited, circulating levels of tyramine will be elevated. Tyramine is then free to interact with the sympathetic, noradrenergic nerve terminals innervating smooth muscle cells of the blood vessels to act as an indirectly acting sympathomimetic amine. With the inhibition of synaptic MAO, this norepinephrine-releasing action of tyramine can cause an elevation in blood pressure, leading to a hypertensive crisis. This potentially lethal clinical situation must be emphasized to the patient taking MAOI. Cheese, beer, wine, and a whole host of other foods rich in tyramine must be avoided.

A number of reversible MAO-A inhibitors have been developed and tested recently for antidepressant efficacy, and agents such as brofaramine, moclobemide, and toloxatone have shown clinical promise. These agents are less likely to be associated with hypertensive crisis since foodborne tyramine could effectively compete for intestinal and hepatic MAO-A sites with the reversible inhibitor. Moreover, liver MAO-B would be available to terminate any tyramine that escaped the actions of intestinal or hepatic MAO-A.

A number of minor side effects, such as tremors, orthostatic hypotension, ejaculatory delay, mild anticholinergic effects, fatigue, and weight gain, are common at therapeutic doses of MAOI (see Table 36-3). Serious hyperpyrexia is likely, however, with concomitant administration of meperidine, dextromethorphan, or TCA drugs. Before replacing an MAOI with a TCA, a drug-free period of 2 weeks should be observed in order to allow for the regeneration of tissue MAO and the elimination of the MAOI.

Miscellaneous Antidepressants

Trazodone

Trazodone HCl is a relatively new agent for the treatment of major depression (Fig. 36-7). It was introduced in the early 1980s as a *second-generation* antidepressant medication. It was thought of as safer, less toxic, and faster-acting than the traditional TCA drugs. Multicenter clinical trials have demonstrated trazodone to be effective in major depression and to possess anxiolytic properties. When compared to the TCA drugs, trazodone is relatively free of antimuscarinic and cardiovascular side effects.

Animal studies have demonstrated that trazodone can act as a selective serotonin neuronal reuptake inhibitor as well as a partial agonist at postsynaptic 5-HT$_{1A}$ receptors. However, these actions may be due to a hepatic metabolite (*m*-chlorophenylpiperazine) that has similar pharmacological properties at serotonin synapses. Acute studies directed at norepinephrine metabolism demonstrate a potentiation of the neuronal release of norepinephrine, presumably caused by antagonist properties of trazodone at α_2-adrenoceptors. After chronic dosing, these actions of trazodone at the norepinephrine synapse cause a β-adrenoceptor down-regulation (subsensitivity) that parallels the time delay required for antidepressant efficacy. Actions at both serotonin and norepinephrine synapses probably account for antidepressant and anxiolytic efficacy of trazodone.

Common side effects associated with trazodone administration include marked sedation, dizziness, hypotension, and nausea (see Table 36-3). Because of its sedative properties, a large percentage of the daily dose is often admin-

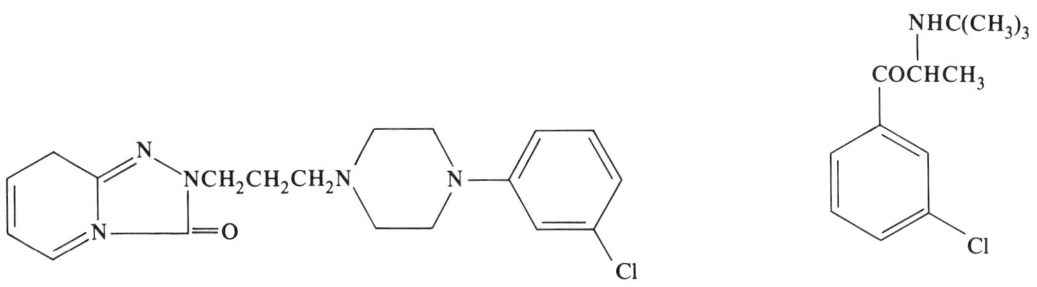

Figure 36-7. Trazodone and bupropion.

istered at bedtime. Priapism is an uncommon but serious side effect, and surgical intervention is required in one third of the cases reported. Drug administration should be immediately discontinued in patients who experience prolonged erections after the initiation of trazodone therapy.

Bupropion

Bupropion HCl is a structurally and pharmacologically unique antidepressant agent (see Fig. 36-7). Little is known about its antidepressant mechanism of action. Unlike other antidepressant agents, bupropion is devoid of inhibitory actions on both norepinephrine and serotonin neuronal reuptake systems. It does not inhibit MAO, but is a potent inhibitor of the dopamine neuronal reuptake system and down-regulates β-adrenoceptor function in about 40 percent of the animals tested following chronic dosing.

Because of a low incidence of side effects (see Table 36-3), bupropion is well tolerated by patients of all ages, including the elderly. It is essentially free of antimuscarinic and cardiac actions and, in addition, is far less likely to cause orthostatic hypotension compared to TCA drugs. However, bupropion is prone to cause CNS stimulation including nervousness and insomnia; higher doses may cause seizures (4/1,000 patients). Fortunately, these actions can be minimized through administration of lower and divided doses over a 24-hr period, which argues against a single dose at bedtime. Aside from dose, predisposing factors contribute significantly to the risk of seizures. Thus, bupropion is contraindicated in patients with a history of seizures or head trauma, or those who are taking medications that lower the seizure threshold (antipsychotics, TCA drugs, etc.).

Treatment of Manic-Depressive Illness

Lithium Carbonate

In 1949, Cade introduced the world to lithium (Li^+) salts in the treatment of behavioral disorders. In a group of manic individuals, he observed that Li^+ carbonate seemed to abate many of their symptoms. It was not until 1970, however, that general acceptance by US physicians was established for Li^+ in the treatment of bipolar illness. This reluctance was based on the potential for lethal reactions in patients taking this medication (see Adverse Reactions). We now have learned to use Li^+ salts safely in behaviorally disturbed patients. Li^+ carbonate (*Eskalith*) is presently the drug of choice for the treatment of manic-depressive illness.

Pharmacological Actions in the CNS

For more than 30 years, Li^+ has been used to treat mania. While it is relatively inert in the normal individual with regard to psychotropic actions, this monovalent cation is effective in 60 to 80 percent of all acute manic episodes within 5 to 21 days of beginning administration. Because of its delayed onset of action in the manic patient, Li^+ is often used in conjunction with low doses of high-potency anxiolytics (e.g., lorazepam) and antipsychotics (e.g., haloperidol) to initially stabilize the behavioral state of the patient. Over time, increased therapeutic responses to Li^+ allow for a gradual reduction in the amount of anxiolytic/neuroleptic required, so that eventually Li^+ is the sole agent controlling the patient's behavior.

In addition to its acute actions, Li^+ also can reduce the frequency of manic or depressive episodes in the bipolar patient and is considered a *mood-stabilizing* agent. Accordingly, bipolar patients are maintained on low, stabilizing doses of Li^+ indefinitely as a prophylaxis to future mood disturbances. Under these circumstances, antidepressant medication may occasionally be required for the treatment of breakthrough depression.

Mechanism of Action

The cellular mechanism(s) associated with the psychotropic actions of Li^+ are not well understood. Lithium is a monovalent cation that can replace Na^+ in some biological processes. It could be argued that competition by Li^+ for active Na^+ sites might lead to altered neuronal function that could account for its antimanic and mood-stabilizing actions. In this regard, the failure of Li^+ to maintain a normal membrane potential because of its lower affinity for the Na^+ pump has been demonstrated. However, this action of Li^+ would not explain its relatively selective effects on the CNS, while sparing comparable excitable tissues (e.g., cardiac muscle) in the periphery. Moreover, an action on membrane polarity would be so generalized that the entire pool of brain neurons would be affected by Li^+. It would seem more reasonable for Li^+ to produce its psychotropic actions by perturbation of molecular events common to a few CNS synapses that might be disturbed during the course of the manic-depressive illness.

Recently, attention has focused on the actions of Li^+ on receptor-mediated, second-messenger signaling systems of the brain. In this regard, interactions between Li^+ and guanine nucleotide (GTP) binding proteins (G-proteins) have been the target of many studies, since G-proteins play a pivotal role in the function of many second-messenger signaling systems. These proteins couple the agonist-induced changes of the receptor recognition site to intracellular biochemical events through activation of regulatory enzymes, such as adenylyl cyclase or phospholipase C, leading to the formation of individual second-messenger substances. Moreover, they are a heterogeneous family of proteins that confer stimulatory or inhibitory properties to receptor function. Molecular cloning techniques suggest the existence of several G-proteins.

Lithium is capable of altering G-protein function. It can diminish the coupling between the receptor recognition site and the G-protein. The molecular mechanism involves the competition for Mg^{2+} sites on the G-protein, which are essential for GTP binding. Guanine nucleotide acts as the G-protein activator. Accordingly, in the presence of Li^+, receptor-mediated activation of the G-protein is attenuated. This property of Li^+ is shared by other mood-stabilizing agents, such as carbamazepine, but not by traditional antidepressant agents.

Presently, this action of Li^+ has been selectively demonstrated for G-proteins associated with β-adrenoceptors and M_1 muscarinic receptors of the CNS (Fig. 36-8). It is likely that future experiments will demonstrate a down-regulation of other receptor systems that share these Li^+-sensitive G-proteins in their second-messenger signaling systems. While it is not possible at present to assign a therapeutic role to this action of Li^+, it is a positive step toward explaining the stabilizing actions of this drug. Since several neurotransmitter receptors share common G-protein–regulated, second-messenger signaling systems, Li^+ could simultaneously correct the alterations at individual synapses associated with depression and mania by a single action on the function of specific G-proteins.

An additional action of Li^+ involves the interruption of the phosphatidylinositide cycle, through an inhibitory action on inositol phosphate metabolism. Through this mechanism, a depletion of membrane inositol and the phosphoinositide-derived second-messenger products (diacylglycerol and inositol triphosphate) ultimately reduces signaling through those receptor systems dependent on the formation of these products. While this action of Li^+ provides a high degree of selectivity at the neurotransmitter level, it is presently unclear to what extent inhibition of inositol phosphate metabolism contributes to the therapeutic properties of Li^+ in bipolar patients.

Pharmacokinetics

Lithium is readily absorbed from the GI tract, reaching a peak plasma level in 2 to 4 hr. Distribution occurs throughout the extracellular fluid with no evidence of protein binding. Passage through the blood-brain barrier, however, is limited so that cerebrospinal fluid (CSF) levels are 50 percent of plasma levels at steady state.

The elimination half-life of Li^+ is estimated at 24 hr, and greater than 90 percent of the dose of Li^+ is excreted into the urine. Renal clearance, however, is only 20 percent, since Li^+ is actively reabsorbed in the proximal tube at sites normally used for the conservation of Na^+. Thus, competition between Li^+ and Na^+ for uptake sites can alter the elimination of Li^+ and its concentration in total body water. *Na^+ loading enhances Li^+ clearance while Na^+ depletion promotes Li^+ retention.* This important relationship explains the appearance of Li^+ toxicity (see below) associated with diet (low Na^+), drugs (diuretics), medical conditions (diarrhea), or physical activities (those that induce sweating) that deplete the body of Na^+.

The elimination rate of Li^+ from the body is variable. It is quite rapid during the first 10 hr after ingestion, and accounts for about 40 percent of the total Li^+ excretion. However, the remaining portion of the Li^+ dose is excreted very slowly over a 14-day period. Because of this biphasic elimination rate, clinically useful serum Li^+ concentrations are usually determined 12 hr after the last dose. This time period assures a more accurate reflection of the Li^+ concentration, since it is beyond the most vari-

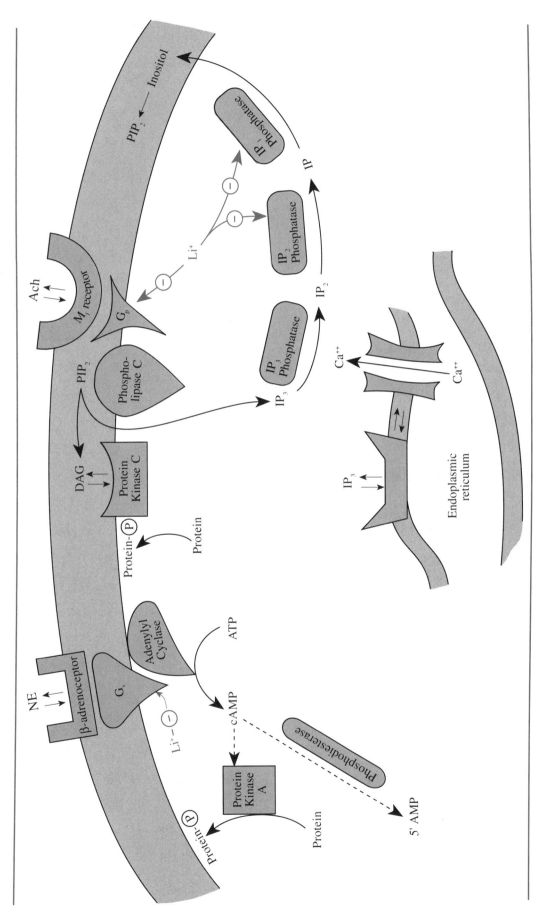

Figure 36-8. *The actions of Li⁺ on postsynaptic receptor-mediated, second-messenger signaling systems.* Lithium can simultaneously alter the flow of synaptic information through several receptor-mediated systems by diminishing coupling between the receptor recognition site and its specific G-proteins. This model provides an explanation for the stabilizing actions of Li⁺ at both ends of the mood spectrum through a single action at the G-protein level. Presently, attenuating actions of Li⁺ have been demonstrated through G-protein interactions at the β-adrenoceptor and the acetylcholine M₁ muscarinic receptor systems of the CNS. A second action of Li⁺ as an inhibitor of inositol diphosphate (IP₂) phosphatase may further attenuate the flow of synaptic information through the M₁ muscarinic receptor by the eventual depletion of membrane phosphatidyl inositol-bis-phosphate (PIP₂). IP₃ = inositol triphosphate; DAG = diacylglycerol; ATP = adenosine triphosphate; cAMP = cyclic adenosine monophosphate; 5′-AMP = 5′-adenosine monophosphate; NE = norepinephrine; ACh = acetylcholine.

able portion (rapid elimination phase) of the Li^+ elimination profile.

Adverse Reactions

The frequency and severity of adverse reactions associated with Li^+ therapy are directly related to serum Li^+ levels. Since Li^+ exhibits a low therapeutic index (approximately 3) and a narrow therapeutic window (0.5–1.5 mEq/liter), the frequent measurement of serum steady state Li^+ concentrations is standard practice in the treatment of bipolar patients.

Adverse reactions occurring at serum trough levels (12 hr after the last dose) of Li^+ below 1.5 mEq per liter (L) are generally mild, whereas those seen above 2.5 mEq/L are usually quite severe. Mild toxicity is usually represented by nausea, vomiting, abdominal pain, diarrhea, polyuria, sedation, and fine tremor. These reactions are sometimes associated with absorption peaks of Li^+ following acute oral ingestion. However, if the serum concentration of Li^+ progressively rises above 2.0 mg/L, frank neurological toxicity appears, beginning with mental confusion and progressing to hyperreflexia, gross tremor, dysarthria, focal neurological signs, seizures, progressive coma, and even death.

Chronic maintenance of bipolar patients on Li^+ is occasionally associated with hypothyroidism or acquired, nephrogenic diabetes insipidus, or both. Although both conditions are generally benign, should hypothyroidism or alterations in renal function develop, both conditions are readily reversible by discontinuation of Li^+.

No specific antidotes are available to treat an acute Li^+ intoxication; treatment is supportive. In life-threatening cases, however, osmotic diuresis or hemodialysis is effective in assisting the removal of Li^+ from the body.

Miscellaneous Mood-Stabilizing Agents

While Li^+ is the drug of choice for the treatment of bipolar affective illness, a number of patients have inadequate responses to Li^+. Many of these patients demonstrate atypical, bipolar illness characterized by *rapid cycling*. For these patients additional or alternative medications are necessary.

Over the past 10 years, selective anticonvulsant agents have shown their antimanic effectiveness. These agents include carbamazepine, valproic acid, and clonazepam; the latter two are generally used in combination with Li^+. (The pharmacology of these agents is covered in Chap. 37.) However, it is interesting that each of these anticonvulsant medications has the selective ability to retard the *kindling* of seizures and the expression of the kindled epileptic focus in experimental animal models of epilepsy. These experimental observations have led to some interesting theoretical aspects on the pathogenesis of the recurrence of bipolar, affective disease. This is not to suggest that epileptiform activity is responsible for the occurrence of manic-depressive episodes on a periodic basis; however, it is conceivable that initial affective cycles, if left untreated, lead to additional or more frequent cycles, such that the development of rapid cycling could occur. These patients may be regarded as "behaviorally kindled," requiring selective "antikindling" medication (e.g., carbamazepine) to abort the rapid cycling of affective states.

Supplemental Reading

Avissar, S., and Schreiber, G. The involvement of guanine nucleotide binding proteins in the pathogenesis and treatment of affective disorders. *Biol. Psychiatry* 31:435, 1992.

Baldessarini, R.J. Current status of antidepressants: Clinical pharmacology and therapy. *J. Clin. Psychiatry* 50:117, 1989.

Ballenger, J.C. The clinical use of carbamazepine in affective disorders. *J. Clin. Psychiatry* 49 (Suppl. 4):13, 1988.

Berridge, M.J., Dorones, L.P., and Hanley, M.R. Neural and developmental actions of lithium: A unifying hypothesis. *Cell* 59:411, 1989.

Blier, P., DeMontigny, C., and Chaput, Y. A role for the serotonin system in the mechanism of action of antidepressant treatments: Preclinical evidence. *J. Clin. Psychiatry* 51 (Suppl. 4):14, 1990.

DeVane, C.L. Pharmacokinetics of selective serotonin re-uptake inhibitors. *J. Clin. Psychiatry* 53 (Suppl. 2):13, 1992.

Feighner, J.P. The new generation of antidepressants. *J. Clin. Psychiatry* 44:49, 1983.

Heym, J., and Koe, B.K. Pharmacology of sertraline: A review. *J. Clin. Psychiatry* 49 (Suppl. 8):40, 1988.

Judd, L. Psychiatric Disorders (Section 1). In J.D. Wilson et al. (eds.), *Harrison's Principles of Internal Medicine* (12th ed.). New York: McGraw-Hill, 1991. pp. 2124–2128.

Lacroix, D., et al. Effects of long-term desipramine administration on noradrenergic neurotransmission: Electrophysiological studies in the rat brain. *J. Pharmacol. Exp. Ther.* 257:1081, 1991.

Preskorn, S.H., and Fast, G.A. Therapeutic drug monitoring for antidepressants: Efficacy, safety, and cost effectiveness. *J. Clin. Psychiatry* 52 (Suppl. 6):23, 1992.

Sulser, F. Mode of action of antidepressant drugs. *J. Clin. Psychiatry* 44:14, 1983.

37

Anticonvulsant Drugs

Charles R. Craig

Not all seizures or convulsive states indicate the presence of the syndrome known as *epilepsy*. Seizures may occur as a toxic manifestation of the use of central nervous system (CNS) stimulants and other drugs, and are sometimes observed in eclampsia, uremia, hypoglycemia, hyperthermia (febrile seizures are common in infants), pyridoxine deficiency, and as a part of the abstinence syndrome of individuals physically dependent on CNS depressants. However, by far the largest number of convulsive disorders is grouped under the heading of epilepsy (or, more correctly, the epilepsies, since markedly different clinical entities are well recognized). Table 37-1 illustrates the major types of epileptic seizures. It is important to consider the type of epilepsy to be treated, since drugs may be more or less specific for a particular seizure type. Many patients exhibit a mixture of more than one type, which poses additional therapeutic problems.

A Consideration of Epilepsy

Epilepsies have been present throughout recorded history and are not restricted to humans. Epilepsy is fairly common in dogs as well as in other species. The incidence of epilepsy in humans is not clearly established but probably occurs in about 0.5 percent of the population. Some known causes are meningitis, childhood fevers, brain tumors, head trauma, and degenerative diseases of the cerebral circulation. In most cases, however, the cause is not known (*idiopathic epilepsy*). Trauma during the birth process is suspected of being one cause. Nontraumatic epilepsy commonly appears before the age of 10 years, although it can begin at any age. It is estimated that about 70 to 75 percent of patients with epilepsy can have their seizures controlled with the drugs currently available. Pa-

tients with a diagnosis of partial seizures with complex symptomatology are more difficult to treat with available drugs than are those with other types of epilepsy.

Epileptic seizures are chronic, spontaneous, recurrent, and paroxysmal, with a discontinuity of symptoms and widely varying intervals between seizures (*interictal period*). The primary defect in epilepsy is in the brain and, characteristically, predictable abnormal electroencephalographic (EEG) tracings are obtained, particularly during a seizure (*ictal period*).

The salient feature of epilepsy is excessive electrical discharge of certain neurons in the brain, which "spreads" to other neurons. The cause of this excessive electrical activity is not known, but evidence is accumulating implicating abnormal levels of certain central neurotransmitters or hyperactivity of certain central neurons.

Since both effective and toxic blood level ranges have been established for the major anticonvulsant drugs, it is possible to titrate individual patients so that drug levels fall within the therapeutic range. The laboratory monitoring of blood concentrations can allow for individualization of a dosage regimen, can measure patient compliance, and can be used to identify the responsible agent in patients on multiple drug therapy who show toxic responses. Blood level determinations also serve as indicators of drug interaction, especially enzyme induction, and of efficiency of absorption—a major variable with these relatively insoluble drugs. Monitoring of blood levels has, therefore, increased the efficiency and safety of anticonvulsant drug therapy, but it should be used only in conjunction with sound clinical judgment since each patient will have an individual optimal drug concentration.

In recent years, therapy of epilepsy has been aimed at single-drug use, rather than multiple-drug therapy. In many cases, a single drug is as effective as several drugs and is usually safer for the patient. It is not likely that the use

Table 37-1. Major Seizure Types*

Clinical seizure type	Key ictal EEG manifestations	Major clinical manifestations
I. Partial (focal, local) seizures A. Simple partial seizures	Local contralateral discharge	Seizures may be limited to a single limb or muscle group; may show sequential involvement of body parts (epileptic "march"); consciousness usually preserved; may be somatosensory (hallucinations, tingling, gustatory sensations); may have autonomic symptoms or signs such as epigastric sensations, sweating, pupillary dilation, etc.
B. Complex partial seizures (psychomotor epilepsy, temporal lobe epilepsy)	Unilateral or bilateral asynchronous focus; most often in temporal region	Impairment of consciousness, may have automatisms, flashback (déjà vu, terror); autonomic activity such as pupil dilation, flushing, piloerection, etc.
C. Partial seizures evolving to secondary generalized seizures		May generalize to tonic, clonic, or tonic-clonic
II. Generalized seizures A. Absence seizures (petit mal epilepsy)	3-Hz polyspike and wave	Brief loss of consciousness, with or without motor involvement; occurs in childhood with a tendency to disappear following adolescence
B. Myoclonic seizures		Sudden, brief, shocklike contractions of musculature (myoclonic jerks)
C. Clonic seizures	Fast activity (10 Hz or more; slow waves)	Repetitive muscle jerks
D. Tonic seizures	Low-voltage, fast activity	Rigid, violent muscular contraction with limbs fixed
E. Tonic-clonic seizures (grand mal epilepsy)	Fast activity (10 Hz or more) increasing in amplitude during tonic phase; interrupted by slow waves during clonic phase	Loss of consciousness; sudden sharp tonic contractions of muscles, falling to ground, followed by clonic convulsive movements; often postictal depression and incontinence
F. Atonic seizures (astatic)	Polyspikes and wave	Sudden diminution in muscle tone affecting isolated muscle groups, or loss of all muscle tone; may have extremely brief loss of consciousness

*Modified from the International Classification of Epileptic Seizures. It should be noted that various methods of seizure classification are used by different authors.

of drugs in combination for the treatment of epilepsy will cease, however, since there is good clinical evidence demonstrating the utility of certain combinations in some patients.

Search for Better Anticonvulsants

In the 1850s bromides were discovered to be effective in the treatment of epilepsy, although the side effects and low level of therapeutic activity limited their usefulness. The introduction of phenobarbital and, later, phenytoin (diphenylhydantoin), made bromide use obsolete.

Until the basic biochemical abnormality, or abnormalities, responsible for seizure activity in epileptics is established, new drugs will continue to be sought, either through animal experimentation or serendipitous clinical observation. Much present research is being devoted to basic studies of possible etiological factors in seizure disorders.

Anticonvulsant Drugs

Phenytoin

Phenytoin (formerly known as diphenylhydantoin) is still one of the most widely used anticonvulsant drugs. *Phenytoin (Fig. 37-1) was the first anticonvulsant drug without sedative activity.* This drug marked a milestone in the therapy of epilepsy by showing that it was not necessary to produce generalized CNS depression to alleviate seizures.

Mechanism of Action

Phenytoin suppresses seizures by reducing the spread of the seizure process from an active, abnormally firing epileptic focus into adjacent normal brain tissue. It has no apparent effect on the seizure threshold. The major mechanism of anticonvulsant action of phenytoin in excitable tissue involves a decrease in sodium influx into neurons. When a neuron is fired, sodium enters the cell and phe-

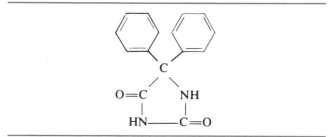

Figure 37-1. Phenytoin.

nytoin binds to the sodium channel in such a manner as to block further sodium entry (Fig. 37-2). This is called a "use-dependent" blockade of sodium channels.

Phenytoin appears to have a stabilizing effect on all neuronal membranes and probably on all excitable and nonexcitable membranes as well.

Clinical Uses

Phenytoin (Dilantin) is a valuable agent for the treatment of generalized tonic-clonic seizures and for the treatment of partial seizures with complex symptomatology. Phenytoin has other therapeutic uses in addition to its use in epilepsy. It is of some value in treating disturbed psychotic patients without epilepsy, useful in the treatment of trigeminal neuralgia, and useful as an antiarrhythmic agent, particularly in the treatment of digitalis-induced arrhythmias (see Chap. 26).

Pharmacokinetics

An understanding of absorption, binding, metabolism, and excretion is more important for phenytoin than it is for most drugs. One reason for this is that phenytoin, like most other antiepileptic drugs, is commonly administered for a long time, frequently for years. Phenytoin also possesses unique pharmacokinetic properties. Following oral administration, the absorption of phenytoin is slow and usually complete, and takes place primarily in the duodenum. Simultaneously ingesting an antacid significantly decreases the absorption of phenytoin. The intravenous route is sometimes used to terminate seizures in status epilepticus (see below).

Phenytoin is highly bound (about 90%) to plasma proteins, primarily plasma albumin. Since several other substances can also bind to the same protein, phenytoin administration can displace (and be displaced) by such agents as thyroxine, triiodothyronine, valproic acid, sulfafurazol, and salicylic acid.

Phenytoin is one of very few drugs that displays zero-order (or saturation) kinetics in its metabolism (see Chap. 6). It is metabolized and bioinactivated in the liver by microsomal enzymes. At low blood levels the rate of metab-

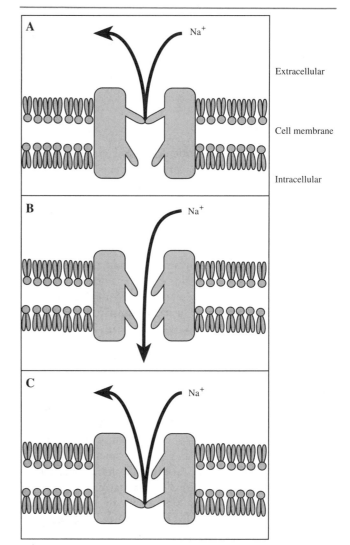

Figure 37-2. Mechanism of action of phenytoin on sodium channels. The sodium channel can normally exist in either a *closed* (panel A), *open* (panel B), or *inactivated* (panel C) state. In panel A, an *activation gate* is closed and sodium ions cannot get through the channel. In panel B, the channel is open during depolarization and sodium enters freely. During the inactivated state shown in panel C, an *inactivation gate* closes, thereby preventing the further entry of sodium ions into the cell. Phenytoin prolongs the existence of the inactivated state and, therefore, sodium entry is impeded for a longer time than occurs in the absence of the drug.

olism of phenytoin is proportional to the drug's blood levels (i.e., first-order kinetics). However, at the blood levels usually required to control seizures, the maximum capacity of drug-metabolizing enzymes is often exceeded (i.e., the enzyme is saturated), and further increases in the dose of phenytoin may lead to a disproportionate increase in the drug's blood concentration. Since the plasma levels continue to increase in such a situation, steady-state levels are not attained and toxicity may ensue. Calculation of half-life ($t_{1/2}$) values for phenytoin often is meaningless since the apparent $t_{1/2}$ varies with the drug blood level. At average therapeutic blood levels of 10 to 12 μg/ml, the $t_{1/2}$ is ordinarily about 24 hr, but this may vary considerably.

Adverse Reactions

At normal oral therapeutic doses, phenytoin is a relatively safe drug, although several side effects have been reported. Gingival hyperplasia, or overgrowth of the gums, is the most common side effect in children (20% of patients). This condition may be minimized by good oral hygiene, but it is a cosmetic problem and can be embarrassing.

CNS effects, including nystagmus, ataxia, vertigo, and diplopia, can occur. These side effects may result from an action of the drug on the cerebellum and are dose related. Behavioral abnormalities, usually consisting of slight CNS stimulation, may also be seen. Peripheral neuropathy is more common in elderly patients.

A variety of poorly understood side effects has been reported, although their incidence is quite low. These include hyperglycemia, osteomalacia, and lymphadenopathy. A variety of rashes have been noted, including Stevens-Johnson syndrome. Hematological reactions, including leukopenia, megaloblastic anemia, thrombocytopenia, agranulocytosis, and aplastic anemia, have all been recorded. Hematological effects, rashes, and other allergic manifestations require discontinuation of the drug. Hirsutism is an annoying side effect of phenytoin in young females. Phenytoin has been reported to cause fetal abnormalities. Since long-term treatment with many antiepileptic drugs including phenytoin, is associated with a deficiency of folate, and since folate deficiency is associated with the production of fetal abnormalities, folic acid deficiency may be an important factor in the teratogenic potential of phenytoin. A discussion of anticonvulsant therapy during pregnancy is presented at the end of this chapter. Cardiovascular collapse is the most serious effect following intravenous administration of phenytoin.

Although the list of untoward effects reported after phenytoin administration appears extensive, it should be remembered that the drug has been available for over 50 years, it is widely employed as an anticonvulsant, and individual patients have received the drug over a period of years.

Drug Interactions

Most of the drug interactions associated with phenytoin administration are related to effects on its metabolism. Some drugs increase phenytoin's metabolism by inducing hepatic microsomal enzymes (chronic drug administration), while other drugs decrease it, apparently by competitively inhibiting phenytoin's metabolism (acute drug administration). Both of these interactions can occur between phenytoin and phenobarbital. Phenobarbital can induce microsomal enzymes as well as acutely compete with phenytoin for the enzymes. If phenobarbital is added to the regimen of a patient receiving phenytoin, careful blood level determinations of phenytoin must be made to determine which metabolic effect is predominant.

Agents that decrease phenytoin blood levels include carbamazepine and chronic alcohol administration. Agents that elevate blood levels of phenytoin include phenylbutazone, chlordiazepoxide, phenothiazines, estrogens, propoxyphene, halothane, ethosuximide, diazepam, disulfiram, cimetidine, and isoniazid.

The coadministration of valproate and phenytoin may lead to increased phenytoin toxicity due to valproate displacing phenytoin from binding sites on serum proteins. The efficacy of coumarin anticoagulants is impaired by coadministration of phenytoin. It is not clear whether the effects are due to a competition for microsomal metabolism or to an altered plasma protein binding. It is best not to use these drugs together.

Other Anticonvulsant Hydantoins

Mephenytoin (*Mesantoin*) and ethotoin (*Peganone*) are not used to any extent. Mephenytoin is considered to be more toxic than phenytoin, while ethotoin has a very low efficacy.

Carbamazepine

Carbamazepine (Fig. 37-3) has recently become a major drug in the treatment of seizure disorders. Its structure is unlike that of other anticonvulsants, but does resemble that of the phenothiazines or tricyclic antidepressants.

Absorption, Metabolism, and Excretion

The oral absorption of carbamazepine is quite slow and often erratic. Its half-life is reported to vary from 12 to 60 hr in humans. The development of blood level assays has markedly improved the success of therapy with this drug, since serum concentration is only partially dose related. The therapeutic blood level is 5 to 8 μg/ml. Carbamazepine is metabolized in the liver, and there is evidence that its continued administration leads to hepatic enzyme induction. Only 2 percent is excreted unchanged, and about 70 percent is recovered as the 10,11-epoxide, 10,11-dihydroxide, and other metabolites.

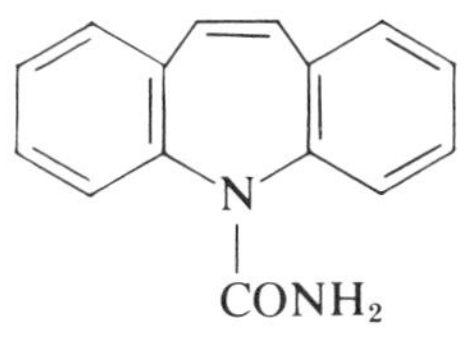

Figure 37-3. Carbamazepine.

Clinical Uses

Carbamazepine (Tegretol) is an effective anticonvulsant for the treatment of generalized tonic-clonic seizures and particularly for the treatment of partial seizures with complex symptomatology. It may well be more effective and produce fewer adverse effects than phenytoin in these conditions. Carbamazepine resembles phenytoin very closely in its spectrum of anticonvulsant activity. It is likely, therefore, that they both share a common mechanism of action.

Both carbamazepine and phenytoin are effective in relieving pain associated with trigeminal neuralgia. Phenytoin also can be given concurrently with carbamazepine if either drug alone is not fully effective. Both compounds are ineffective in absence seizures and might even make these seizures worse.

Adverse Reactions

The overall incidence of toxicity seems to be fairly low at usual therapeutic doses. Aplastic anemia, agranulocytosis, thrombocytopenia, and leukopenia have been reported, but the incidence of serious blood dyscrasias seems to be quite low. Other, more common, side effects include gastrointestinal complaints, dizziness, diplopia, and blurred vision. Additionally, visual hallucinations, peripheral neuritis, tinnitus, abnormal involuntary movements, rashes (including Stevens-Johnson syndrome), congestive heart failure, hypotension, syncope, and cholestatic and hepatocellular jaundice have been reported.

Drug Interactions

Most of the drug interactions that are seen after the use of carbamazepine are related to its effects on microsomal drug metabolism. Carbamazepine can induce its own metabolism (*autoinduction*) after prolonged administration; its clearance rate, half-life, and serum concentrations may all be decreased. *The possibility of autoinduction requires the clinician to reevaluate the patient's blood levels after a month of carbamazepine therapy.*

Carbamazepine also can induce the enzymes that metabolize other anticonvulsant drugs including phenytoin, primidone, pentobarbital, valproic acid, clonazepam, and ethosuximide, as well as the metabolism of other drugs that the patient may be taking. Similarly, other drugs may induce the metabolism of carbamazepine; the end result is the same as for autoinduction and the dose of carbamazepine must be readjusted. A common drug-drug interaction that has been recognized is that between carbamazepine and the macrolide antibiotics (erythromycin and troleandomycin). After a few days of antibiotic therapy, symptoms of carbamazepine toxicity develop; this is readily reversible if either the antibiotic or carbamazepine is discontinued.

Cimetidine, propoxyphene, and isoniazid also have been reported to inhibit the metabolism of carbamazepine. *It is essential to monitor blood levels and adjust the dose, if necessary, whenever additional drugs are given to patients taking carbamazepine.*

Phenobarbital

Phenobarbital is a long-acting barbiturate, the structure of which is shown in Fig. 37-4.

Mechanism of Action

The mechanism of action of phenobarbital in alleviating seizures is poorly understood, although there is evidence that phenobarbital's mechanism of action is due, in part, to its ability to enhance γ-aminobutyric acid (GABAergic) inhibition. Phenobarbital increases the threshold for neuronal firing and inhibits the spread of seizure activity from a discrete focus. As a generalized CNS depressant, however, it tends to depress all neuronal activity. Although phenobarbital is not unique among barbiturates in displaying anticonvulsant activity in humans, it does possess a reasonable separation between the dose that is effective in preventing convulsions and a dose that produces an intolerable amount of CNS depression.

Figure 37-4. Phenobarbital.

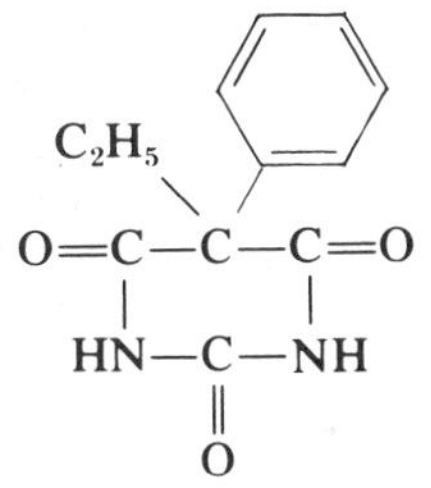

Absorption, Metabolism, and Excretion

Phenobarbital is effective orally and is distributed widely throughout the body. Approximately 40 percent of the phenobarbital in the blood is bound to plasma proteins, but a significant amount is still distributed to the brain. It is metabolized by microsomal drug-metabolizing enzymes, primarily to p-hydroxyphenobarbital, although a certain amount (usually 10–20%, but up to 50% in some cases) of the parent drug is excreted unchanged by the kidneys. Phenobarbital is one of the classic inducing agents for microsomal drug-metabolizing enzymes (see Chap. 4), and this fact must be considered when using this agent singly or in combination with other drugs. Phenobarbital may initially inhibit the metabolism of other drugs, presumably by competitive inhibition of microsomal enzymes. This may be followed by an enhanced metabolism as a result of enzyme induction. Both situations have been encountered, which emphasizes the value of routine blood level determinations in patients receiving anticonvulsant drug therapy.

Clinical Uses

Phenobarbital is most effective in the treatment of generalized tonic-clonic epilepsy and cortical focal seizures. It also has some value in the treatment of complex partial seizures. Phenobarbital has been used prophylactically or as a treatment for febrile convulsions in young children, but this use should be reserved only for those individuals at highest risk for subsequent development of epilepsy.

Adverse Reactions

The major untoward effect of phenobarbital, when used as an anticonvulsant, is sedation, although tolerance often develops to this effect on continued administration. Rashes, usually scarlatiniform or morbilliform, occur in 1 to 2 percent of patients. The occurrence of rashes after anticonvulsant therapy can be taken as evidence of an allergic reaction and should be considered a basis for withdrawal of the drug. Nystagmus, ataxia, and osteomalacia have been seen, as has hemorrhage in babies born to mothers receiving phenobarbital. Megaloblastic anemia also has been reported.

Interactions with Other Drugs

Most interactions between phenobarbital and other drugs are related to the previously mentioned effects of phenobarbital's inhibiting and, subsequently, inducing hepatic microsomal drug-metabolizing enzymes. It is necessary to monitor anticonvulsant blood levels to ensure that therapeutic levels of all administered drugs are being maintained. Phenobarbital administration is known to alter blood phenytoin levels.

The enzymes responsible for metabolizing the coumarin anticoagulants are induced by phenobarbital to the extent that an increase in the anticoagulant dosage may be required. Additionally, these microsomal enzymes rapidly fall to normal levels after withdrawal of phenobarbital, and the patient may risk hemorrhage if the anticoagulant dosage also is not reduced. In addition to effects on microsomal enzymes, additive CNS depression may be seen with the concomitant use of any other CNS depressant. If valproic acid is coadministered with phenobarbital, striking increases in phenobarbital blood levels are frequently observed.

Mephobarbital and Metharbital

Mephobarbital (*Mebaral*) is the *N*-methyl analogue of phenobarbital. Mephobarbital is demethylated in the body to phenobarbital, and available evidence indicates that most of the salutary effects of mephobarbital after prolonged administration are due to its metabolic conversion to phenobarbital. There appears to be no justification for its use.

Although metharbital (*Gemonil*) continues to be listed as an anticonvulsant drug, it is infrequently used.

Primidone

Primidone (*Mysoline*) is chemically similar to phenobarbital and, as with mephobarbital, a portion is converted in vivo to phenobarbital. However, primidone appears to differ somewhat from phenobarbital in its anticonvulsant spectrum (see below). Primidone is adequately absorbed following oral administration and is converted in the liver to two active metabolites: phenobarbital and phenylthylmalonamide (PEMA).

In order to establish optimal therapeutic benefits, it is necessary to measure serum levels of both primidone and phenobarbital. *Optimal blood levels of phenobarbital derived from the metabolism of primidone are similar to those found when phenobarbital itself is given.* Concentrations of unchanged primidone should be maintained below 10 μg/ml to prevent overt CNS depression.

Clinical Uses

Primidone appears to be more effective than phenobarbital in the treatment of partial seizures with complex symptomatology. This result is presumably due to the activity of its metabolite, PEMA. Primidone is also effective in generalized tonic-clonic seizures and cortical focal epilepsy. It is frequently combined with phenytoin, but since it is, in part, converted to phenobarbital, combination with phenobarbital makes little sense.

Adverse Reactions

Rashes, leukopenia, thrombocytopenia, and systemic lupus erythematosus have been reported. Some personality changes, megaloblastic anemia, and osteomalacia also have occurred. As with phenobarbital, the most common side effects associated with primidone therapy are related to CNS depression.

Interactions with Other Drugs

Drug interactions described for phenobarbital also can occur following primidone administration.

Valproic Acid

Valproic acid (*Depakene*) may prove to be one of the more important anticonvulsant drugs both from the standpoint of its usefulness in the treatment of epilepsies and because its reported mechanism of action may shed some light on basic seizure mechanisms. Valproic acid (Fig. 37-5) contains no nitrogen or aromatic moiety. In this regard, its structure is unique among anticonvulsants.

It was early hypothesized that the mechanism of action of valproic acid involved an elevation of brain levels of GABA through an inhibition of the neurotransmitter's breakdown. There is little doubt that valproic acid can accomplish this in experimental animals, but only at very high doses. It is unlikely that such a simple explanation can account for the antiepileptic action of this agent. Valproate can enhance GABAergic tone in certain brain areas, however, and this action might be related to its ability to inhibit seizures. It is probable that valproic acid acts through more than a single mechanism, since it has a very broad spectrum of anticonvulsant activity.

Clinical Uses

Valproic acid has become a major antiepileptic drug against several seizure types. It was originally approved for use in absence seizures, particularly in myoclonic types that had been difficult to treat with other drugs, and this is still its major indication when it is used alone. In addition, valproic acid can be used either alone or in combination with other drugs for the treatment of generalized tonic-clonic epilepsy and for partial seizures with complex symptomatology.

Adverse Reactions

The most serious adverse effect associated with valproic acid is hepatic failure resulting in fatality. Fatal hepatotoxicity is much more likely to occur in children under the age of 2 years, especially those with severe seizures who are given multiple anticonvulsant drug therapy. The hepatoxicity is not dose related and is considered an idiosyncratic reaction; it can occur in individuals in other age groups and, therefore, valproic acid should not be administered to patients with hepatic disease or significant hepatic dysfunction, or to those who are hypersensitive to it.

Valproic acid causes hair loss (alopecia) in about 5 percent of patients, but this effect is reversible. Transient gastrointestinal effects are common, and some mild behavioral effects have been reported. Metabolic effects, including hyperglycemia, hyperglycinuria, and hyperammonemia, have been reported. An increase in body weight has been noted. Valproic acid is not a CNS depressant, but its administration may lead to increased depression if it is used in combination with certain other anticonvulsants (see Drug Interactions). At present, valproic acid is not recommended for use during pregnancy; it is teratogenic in animals.

Drug Interactions

Valproic acid administered concomitantly with phenobarbital leads to an increase in serum phenobarbital levels, presumably by impairing the nonrenal clearance of phenobarbital. This increase may be accompanied by indications of barbiturate toxicity (severe CNS depression). An elevation of primidone levels also has been observed when primidone is combined with valproic acid. This is not surprising since primidone is metabolized, in part, to phenobarbital. On the other hand, it has been reported that in patients receiving *phenytoin,* valproic acid administration leads to increased phenytoin toxicity as a result of competition between the two agents for binding sites on plasma proteins, with a resultant increase in unbound phenytoin. The dosage of phenytoin should be adjusted as required. The concomitant use of valproic acid and clonazepam may produce absence status. *These examples reinforce the need to determine serum anticonvulsant levels in epileptic patients.*

Figure 37-5. Valproic acid.

$$\overset{\text{H}}{\underset{|}{(CH_3CH_2CH_2)_2\,C\,COOH}}$$

Ethosuximide

Ethosuximide (*Zarontin*) *appears to be effective only in the treatment of absence seizures;* it is still generally considered to be the drug of choice for this condition, but many clinicians prefer to use valproic acid. Although ethosuximide is an older drug that has been investigated extensively, its mechanism of action is still unexplained. The favored concept is that ethosuximide enhances central inhibitory processes.

Absorption, Metabolism, and Excretion

Ethosuximide is absorbed well following oral administration; a single dose achieves peak plasma concentrations in about 3 hr. Plasma steady-state levels are reached after about 9 days of once-daily dosing. The plasma half-life of ethosuximide is about 30 to 40 hr. Up to 80 percent of a single dose is recovered in the urine as either unchanged ethosuximide or its major metabolite, 2-(1-hydroxyethyl)-2-methylsuccinimide.

Clinical Uses

The only indication for ethosuximide is in the treatment of uncomplicated absence epilepsy. However, it can be combined safely with other anticonvulsants in patients with absence as well as other types of epilepsy (multiple seizure types). The optimal plasma ethosuximide levels are from 40 to 100 μg/ml; these levels provide practical control in 80 percent of patients with absence epilepsy.

Adverse Reactions

The most common adverse reactions are gastrointestinal irritation, CNS depression, and rashes. A variety of blood dyscrasias, including pancytopenia and aplastic anemia, have occurred. Eosinophilia develops in about 10 percent of patients. Systemic lupus erythematosus and Stevens-Johnson syndrome also have been reported.

Clonazepam

Clonazepam (*Klonopin*) is a benzodiazepine and is a useful antiepileptic agent in some situations.

Absorption, Metabolism, and Excretion

Maximal blood levels are achieved in 1 or 2 hr after oral administration. Clonazepam has a long and variable half-life (18–50 hr). The major metabolic pathways are oxi-

dative hydroxylation and reduction of the 7-nitro function.

Clinical Uses

Clonazepam is used in myoclonic, absence, atonic, and akinetic seizures, especially as an adjunct with other drugs. Clonazepam is generally less effective than valproate or ethosuximide in absence seizures.

Adverse Reactions

Tolerance to its anticonvulsant effects is a major disadvantage associated with clonazepam use. Tolerance develops rapidly in a large proportion of patients. Clonazepam is also a CNS depressant, and sedation and drowsiness are the most common side effects; they occur in up to 50 percent of patients receiving the drug. Ataxia is also commonly seen. Behavioral problems (such as confusion, depression, hysteria, increased libido, and suicidal attempts) may be noted in approximately 25 percent of patients. Among a wide variety of other side effects that have been reported, hypersecretion in the upper-respiratory tract has been a major problem. Physical and psychological dependence may develop; an abstinence syndrome, including the occurrence of convulsions, similar to those seen after withdrawal from other CNS depressants, has been reported. Periodic blood counts and liver function tests should be carried out during long-term therapy.

Interactions

The CNS depression may be exaggerated if other CNS depressants, antipsychotic agents, narcotic analgesics, tricyclic antidepressants, or monoamine oxidase (MAO) inhibitors are given at the same time. When clonazepam is used in combination with valproic acid, a profound depression may result.

Other Benzodiazepines

Diazepam (*Valium*) is relatively ineffective when used orally for its anticonvulsant effect; tolerance also develops. Furthermore, it produces drowsiness, ataxia, and dizziness in up to 40 percent of patients. *Its use is reserved for the treatment of status epilepticus,* for which it is administered either intravenously or rectally.

Nitrazepam (*Mogadon*) use is generally *restricted to the treatment of myoclonic seizures, infantile spasms, and Lennox-Gastaut syndrome.* It appears to be effective in the treatment of reflex epilepsies, but tolerance develops on continued use.

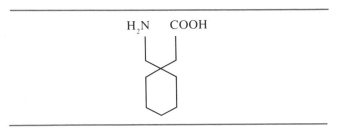

Figure 37-6. Gabapentin.

Chlorazepate dipotassium (*Tranxene*) is occasionally employed as an anticonvulsant as an adjunct to other antiepileptic drugs in the management of partial seizures.

New Drugs

Two new antiepileptic drugs have been tentatively approved (in the United States) for the treatment of epilepsy: gabapentin and felbamate.

Gabapentin (*Neurontin*) is an amino acid, chemically related to GABA (Fig. 37-6); however, there is little evidence that it works by a GABAergic mechanism. So far, few major side effects have been observed. The major use of gabapentin will probably be as an adjunct for the treatment of intractable partial complex seizures.

The second new agent is felbamate (*Felbatol*). Felbamate is chemically related to meprobamate; it will most likely be used in patients with Lennox-Gastaut syndrome (a syndrome characterized by multiple types of seizures beginning in early childhood that is difficult to treat with presently available drugs) and in patients with partial and secondarily generalized seizures. Felbamate has also been remarkably free of serious side effects to date.

Two other drugs that are considered promising are lamotrigine (*Lamictal*) and vigabatrin (*Sabril*).

Other Rarely Used Anticonvulsants

Methsuximide (*Celontin*) is chemically very similar to ethosuximide, but is not as effective.

Trimethadione (*Tridione*) is little used today and is important only from a historical viewpoint. Trimethadione was the first anticonvulsant useful specifically against absence epilepsy. It is neither as effective nor as safe as ethosuximide or valproic acid for this indication.

Paramethadione (*Paradione*) is used less often than trimethadione, a compound that it resembles structurally.

Phenacemide (*Phenurone*) is effective in the treatment of partial seizures with complex symptomatology (temporal lobe epilepsy). However, it has such a high incidence of adverse effects associated with its administration that it should only be used by trained neurologists who are fully aware of the risks involved. The adverse effects include serious psychological changes in 15 to 20 percent of patients. These effects include acute psychosis, paranoid and depressive reactions, and aggressive behavior. In addition, aplastic anemia and hepatitis occur in approximately 2 percent of patients.

Acetazolamide (*Diamox*) has been used occasionally in absence epilepsy, although it is not a particularly effective drug. It was postulated that its mechanism of action as an antiepileptic drug was exerted through its inhibition of carbonic anhydrase (see Chap. 21), but the evidence for this is not convincing.

Sulthiame (*Conadil*) is also a carbonic anhydrase inhibitor and, at best, is marginally effective. It may be useful in combination with other agents.

Therapeutic Indications of Primary Agents

Table 37-2 gives a quick appraisal of the indications for use of the agents discussed to this point. It must be kept in

Table 37-2. Therapeutic Indications for Use of Primary Anticonvulsant Agents

Agent	Generalized tonic-clonic seizures	Partial seizures with complex symptomatology	Absence	Akinetic and atonic
Phenytoin	3	3	−1	
Phenobarbital	1	1	1	
Primidone	1	1	0	
Carbamazepine	3	3	−1	
Valproic acid	2	1	3	3
Ethosuximide	0	0	3	
Clonazepam	0	0	2	2

Key: 3 = treatment of choice; 2 = recommended separately or in combination as alternate; 1 = usually of benefit, but not as good as categories above; 0 = usually little or no benefit; −1 = usually makes condition worse.

Table 37-3. Some Properties of the Most Commonly Used Anticonvulsant Drugs

Agent	Trade name	Degree of protein binding (%)	$t_{1/2}$ (hr)	Therapeutic blood levels (μg/ml)	Most frequent adverse effect	Most serious adverse effect
Phenytoin	Dilantin	90	15–24[a]	10–20	Gingival hyperplasia	
Carbamazepine	Tegretol	75	6–12	5–8	Dizziness Nausea	Aplastic anemia Agranulocytosis[b]
Phenobarbital	Luminal	60	70–100	15–30	Sedation	
Valproic acid	Depakene	90	8–10	50–100	Transient hair loss	Hepatic toxicity[c]
Ethosuximide	Zarontin	0	30–70	40–100	Sedation	
Primidone	Mysoline		9–20	5–12[d]	Sedation	
Clonazepam	Klonopin		25–50	<0.1	Sedation	

[a]May be markedly increased with higher doses due to saturation kinetics (see text).
[b]Incidence is low, but fatality is frequent.
[c]Especially in patients under 2 yr of age.
[d]Primidone, as well as its metabolites phenobarbital and PEMA, has antiepileptic properties.

mind that many patients present with mixed types of epilepsies and the choice of drug(s) to be employed must be made carefully. Table 37-3 provides essential information about the most widely used antiepileptic drugs.

General Principles of Anticonvulsant Therapy

The successful management of convulsive disorders presents a formidable challenge even to experienced neurologists. Some general principles of anticonvulsant therapy are outlined as follows:

1. Patients who are suspected to be epileptic should be referred promptly to a specialist for evaluation and treatment.
2. Before initiating drug therapy, a complete neurological examination, history, and EEG data should be obtained. If possible, the incidence of seizures over a reasonable period of time also should be determined.
3. The choice of the initial drug to be used should be considered carefully in light of EEG, clinical presentation, and history of any previous drug sensitivity.
4. The physician must be prepared to continue with the initial drug for several weeks or months unless significant side effects dictate otherwise. Many patients experience seizures at infrequent intervals, and it may take several months to establish whether any improvement has occurred.

Furthermore, it may take weeks before a plateau is reached with regard to drug blood levels. If possible, serum levels of the drug should be monitored at regular intervals. This procedure will check on patient compliance and will allow the physician to know when the drug plateau is reached. A careful record of seizure incidence should be maintained as should follow-up EEG recordings.
5. If adequate control of seizures is not achieved, the physician must decide whether to add a second drug to the first or whether to discontinue the initial drug and substitute a second. Too often in the past, additional drugs have been added indiscriminately until the patient was taking as many as six or more drugs simultaneously. If the decision is made to discontinue the first drug, it should be *withdrawn gradually* to avoid a possible abstinence syndrome, since many anticonvulsants cause physical dependence. If the decision is to add a second drug, it should be *added gradually*. Serum levels of both the first and second drug should be measured regularly, since, as we have seen previously, certain anticonvulsant drugs may alter the blood levels of other drugs given concurrently.
6. On finding a drug (or combination) to be effective in preventing seizures in a given patient, the physician must follow the patient's progress routinely to ensure that the medication is taken regularly, that serious side effects do not appear, that serum levels remain within the therapeutic range, and that tolerance does not develop.
7. The question of withdrawing medication from a patient who has been seizure-free for a significant period of time poses certain problems. If the EEG

is normal and the patient is relatively young, and if the patient can be followed regularly, a gradual reduction in medication is probably warranted. It should be kept in mind that, as far as we know, the drugs available are prophylactic only, not curative. Although certain seizures types (particularly absence) tend to disappear spontaneously, in most patients the basic abnormality probably is still present even though no seizures occur.

Anticonvulsant Drugs and Pregnancy

The treatment of epileptic pregnant women poses particularly difficult questions for the physician. There is clear evidence that most anticonvulsant drugs produce teratogenic effects in laboratory animals, and, presumably, also in humans. There is a small elevation in the incidence of birth defects in children of drug-treated epileptic women, although the great majority of such women give birth to normal infants. The most common abnormality is cleft palate although valproic acid is known to cause spina bifida in a small percentage of cases. Trimethadione should not be given to women of childbearing age since it is clearly teratogenic.

Withdrawal of medication from an epileptic, pregnant woman is not without its hazards, both to the patient and possibly to the fetus. It is not clear whether maternal seizures can directly affect the fetus, but this occurrence is possible. Certainly, during severe motor seizures or status epilepticus, the danger of hypoxia to the fetus is present. The decision concerning whether to discontinue or decrease dosage in a pregnant patient must be carefully considered and account must be taken of a number of factors, including seizure type, severity of the epilepsy, drugs involved, and dosage levels. If it seems warranted, a reduction in dosage during pregnancy might be considered a prudent measure. Monotherapy is preferred to polytherapy if at all possible.

Deficiency of folate during gestation has been associated with abnormal growth and development, and most antiepileptic drugs cause some degree of folate deficiency. It is, therefore, considered worthwhile to administer folate daily as a supplement during the period of organogenesis in the first trimester.

Another concern in infants of mothers with epilepsy is a serious hemorrhagic disorder that is associated with a high (25–35%) mortality. Many antiepileptic drugs can act as competitive inhibitors of vitamin K–dependent clotting factors. The competitive inhibition can be overcome by the administration of oral vitamin K supplements to the mother during the last week or 10 days of pregnancy.

Treatment of Febrile Seizures

Febrile seizures are convulsions that are associated with fever and generally occur in children between 3 months and 5 years of age. Epilepsy later develops in approximately 2 to 3 percent of children who exhibit one or more febrile seizures. There still remains some question concerning whether or not to prescribe anticonvulsant drugs prophylactically to such patients in order to prevent additional febrile seizures, the later development of epilepsy, or both.

Most authorities now recommend prophylactic treatment only to those patients at highest risk for the subsequent development of epilepsy or those who experience multiple recurrent febrile seizures. If prophylactic treatment is given, phenobarbital is the drug usually employed although diazepam is also effective. Phenytoin and carbamazepine are ineffective and valproic acid may cause hepatotoxicity in very young patients.

Treatment of Status Epilepticus

Status epilepticus is a continuous seizure state that can prove fatal unless the convulsions are terminated. It is a leading cause of death in epileptic patients and must be considered a medical emergency. Virtually any generalized CNS depressant, including general anesthetics, can be used to terminate the seizure state. The pharmacological treatment of choice at present consists of the intravenous infusion of either diazepam or lorazepam (the only benzodiazepines available in the United States for parenteral administration) followed by the IV administration of phenytoin, in a dose of 20 mg/kg, to provide a long-term anticonvulsant effect. Phenytoin will stop most status epilepticus episodes and long-term control will be provided without any decreased level of consciousness. If the patient's condition is refractory to the combined benzodiazepine and phenytoin treatment, phenobarbital is generally chosen as the agent to employ next. A loading dose of 20 mg/kg phenobarbital is usually given IV; this can be followed by additional maintenance amounts, if necessary. The drugs should be administered slowly to avoid respiratory depression and the development of apnea.

In addition to terminating the seizures, it is important that the systemic consequences of prolonged seizures are recognized and treated as well. It is vital to maintain an adequate airway and correct any fluid and electrolyte imbalances. The cause of the seizures also must be determined.

Supplemental Reading

Brodie, M.J. Drug interactions in epilepsia. *Epilepsia* 33 (Suppl. 1):S13, 1992.

Dansky, L.V., Rosenblatt, D.S., and Andermann, E. Mechanisms of teratogenesis: Folic acid and antiepileptic therapy. *Neurology.* 42 (Suppl. 5):32, 1992.

De Lorenzo, R.J. Phenytoin Mechanisms of Action. In R. Levy et al. (eds.), *Antiepileptic Drugs,* (3rd ed.) New York: Raven, 1989. Pp. 143–158.

Faingold, C.L., and Fromm, G.H. (eds.). *Drugs for Control of Epilepsy: Actions on neuronal networks involved in seizure disorders.* Boca Raton, Fla.: CRC, 1992.

Fariello, R., and Smith, M.C. Valproate Mechanisms of Action. In R. Levy et al. (eds.), *Antiepileptic Drugs* (3rd ed.). New York: Raven, 1989. Pp. 567–582.

Levy, R.H., et al. (eds.). *Antiepileptic Drugs* (3rd ed.). New York: Raven, 1989.

Macdonald, R.L. Carbamazepine Mechanisms of Action. In R. Levy et al. (eds.), *Antiepileptic Drugs* (3rd. ed.). New York: Raven, 1989. Pp. 447–455.

Pitlick, W.H. (ed.). *Antiepileptic Drug Interactions.* New York: Demos, 1989.

Ramsay, R.E. Treatment of status epilepticus. *Epilepsia* 34 (Suppl. 1): S71, 1993.

Rogawski, M.A., and Porter, R.J. (eds.). *Antiepileptic drugs: Pharmacological mechanisms and clinical efficacy with consideration of promising developmental stage compounds. Pharmacol. Rev.* 42:223, 1990.

Treiman, D.M. The role of benzodiazepines in the management of status epilepticus. *Neurology,* 40 (Suppl. 2):32, 1990.

Trimble, M.R. (ed.). *Chronic Epilepsy, Its Prognosis and Management.* New York: Wiley-Liss, 1989.

Tunnicliff, G.K., and Raess, B.U. (eds.). *GABA Mechanisms in Epilepsy.* New York: Wiley-Liss, 1991.

Yerby, M.S. Risks of pregnancy in women with epilepsy. *Epilepsia* 33 (Suppl. 1):S23, 1992.

Drugs Used in Parkinsonism and Other Basal Ganglia Disorders

Charles O. Rutledge

Parkinson's Disease

The careful observations of James Parkinson on six patients with "shaking palsy" resulted in the publication in 1817 of an essay that has become a classic in the history of medicine. He differentiated a triad of symptoms, including involuntary tremor of the limbs, rigidity of muscles, and slowness of movement, that has since been called *Parkinson's disease,* or *parkinsonism.* There are almost 1 million cases of Parkinson's disease in the United States, with 50,000 new cases being diagnosed each year. The disease is almost exclusively seen in patients 50 to 70 years of age. Most cases of parkinsonism are of unknown origin (*idiopathic parkinsonism*). Idiopathic parkinsonism has been considered to be a part of the aging process that is associated with the loss of neurons. There appears to be a threshold number of neurons required for smooth functioning of the muscles. Clinical symptoms of parkinsonism appear when neuronal loss exceeds this threshold number.

There are a few types of Parkinson's disease for which the cause is known. *Postencephalitic parkinsonism* is most commonly the result of the pandemic of *encephalitis lethargica,* a viral encephalitis that began in the winter of 1916–1917 and lasted for about 10 years. In some patients, the parkinsonism appeared within a few weeks of the infection, while in others the onset was delayed for as long as 30 years. *Iatrogenic parkinsonism* is a frequent adverse side effect of most antipsychotic drugs. One of the primary goals in developing new antipsychotic drugs is the avoidance of parkinsonism and other motor disorders. Parkinsonism is also known to result from arteriosclerosis, manganese poisoning, carbon monoxide poisoning, and hepatolenticular degeneration (Wilson's disease). A toxic intermediate in the synthesis of meperidine analogues, 1-methyl-4-phenyl-1,2,5,6-tetrahydropyridine (MPTP), can induce the symptoms of Parkinson's disease within a few days after its intravenous injection. This observation has led to the search for other environmental factors.

Clinical Findings

The onset of symptoms of Parkinson's disease is usually quite gradual; therefore, the disease may be difficult to diagnose. The most prominent features of parkinsonism are *tremor, rigidity,* and *bradykinesia.* All of these symptoms usually are present, but the relative severity of each may markedly differ in individual patients. The tremor often begins in one hand; less frequently, it begins in one foot. The hand tremor often involves all of the fingers and the thumb. Tremors are usually present at rest and cease during voluntary movement. Rigidity is characterized by increased muscle tone. It may be detected by passively moving the arm of the patient, which will produce a jerky resistance that has been likened to the movement of a cogwheel (*cogwheel rigidity*). Bradykinesia, extreme slowness of movement, is the most disabling feature because it prevents the patient from performing routine daily activities. It may occur in the absence of rigidity. Bradykinesia diminishes all movements, including facial movements, which leads to a typical "masklike" facies. It also results in a typical stooped posture when standing or walking and a characteristic shuffling gait marked by the absence of normal arm-swinging movements. The inability to swallow leads to drooling, while bradykinesia of the muscles in the larynx results in changes in voice quality. Patients with Parkinson's disease may have a hyperactive blink reflex, which is sometimes helpful in making the diagnosis. Orthostatic hypotension is also frequently observed; it constitutes a significant therapeutic problem since hypotension is also a frequent side effect of drug therapy for this condition.

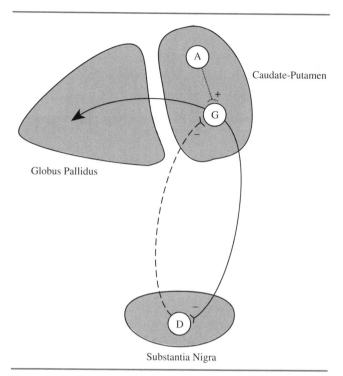

Figure 38-1. Some possible relationships between acetylcholine (A), dopamine (D), and GABA (G) in the caudate putamen and substantia nigra. + = excitatory; − = inhibitory.

Pathology

Parkinson's disease is one of the few neurological disorders in which knowledge of the pathology involved led directly to the rational development of drugs to treat the disease. It is now generally recognized that *Parkinson's disease is characterized by a progressive and selective degeneration of neurons that originate in the substantia nigra of the midbrain and terminate in the basal ganglia* (caudate nucleus, putamen, and pallidum). These neurons utilize the neurotransmitter dopamine and interact with short cholinergic interneurons in the basal ganglia. Although the precise neuronal network that controls basal ganglia function is quite complex, it is clear that γ-aminobutyric acid (GABA) and substance P neurons originating in the basal ganglia send axons back to the substantia nigra, thereby participating in the regulation of the activity of the dopamine neurons (Fig. 38-1). These *feedback loops* help control the rate of impulse flow to skeletal muscle and provide for smooth, coordinated motor movements.

When the dopamine neurons have degenerated beyond a threshold number, the inhibitory influence of dopamine is reduced and the activity of the cholinergic neurons is increased. Thus, *the principal goal of drug therapy is to decrease the activity of cholinergic neurons in the basal ganglia, either by activating the inhibitory dopamine receptors or by antagonizing the stimulatory action of acetylcholine.* The most

important evidence supporting the existence of such a pathological mechanism is the finding that brains taken at autopsy from parkinsonism patients have markedly reduced levels of dopamine and its major metabolite, homovanillic acid.

Drug-induced (or iatrogenic) parkinsonism has similar biochemical features to Parkinson's disease. Butyrophenone and phenothiazine antipsychotic drugs (see Chap. 35) commonly produce parkinsonism, and although levels of dopamine are not reduced after their administration, they do produce a functional decrease in dopamine activity by blocking postsynaptic dopamine receptors. The amine-depleting drug reserpine produces parkinsonism through a depletion of dopamine in the basal ganglia; it interferes with the vesicular storage of dopamine. Regardless of the cause, *a reduced functional role of dopamine is characteristic of all types of parkinsonism.*

Therapy of Parkinsonism

Levodopa

The administration of the immediate precursor of dopamine, l-dopa (levodopa, Fig. 38-2) is used to elevate brain dopamine levels in patients with parkinsonism. Dopamine itself does not cross the blood-brain barrier in sufficient concentrations after systemic administration to be useful clinically. Since levodopa is an amino acid, it is accumulated in the brain by amino acid transport systems. In the presence of l-aromatic amino-acid decarboxylase, levodopa is converted to dopamine.

When levodopa is used alone for the treatment of parkinsonism, it is necessary to give large doses, up to several grams per day. Most of the levodopa administered does not reach its intended site of action in the brain because of its metabolism to dopamine by l-aromatic amino-acid decarboxylase, which is present in the liver, kidney, and gastrointestinal tract. This decarboxylation in peripheral tissues can be markedly reduced if levodopa is given in combination with a peripheral decarboxylase inhibitor. However, it is important that the decarboxylase inhibitor not enter the brain so that the needed decarboxylation of levodopa to dopamine can occur at the site of its therapeutic action. This is achieved through the administration of the decarboxylase inhibitor *carbidopa,* which is ionized at physiological pH and therefore cannot readily penetrate the blood-brain barrier.

Levodopa is routinely given in combination with carbidopa, thereby permitting lower doses of levodopa to be given. Such a drug combination also enhances therapeutic effectiveness by decreasing the frequency of drug administration and by shortening the onset of drug action. The discussion of levodopa in the following sections also applies to the carbidopa/levodopa combination, except where indicated.

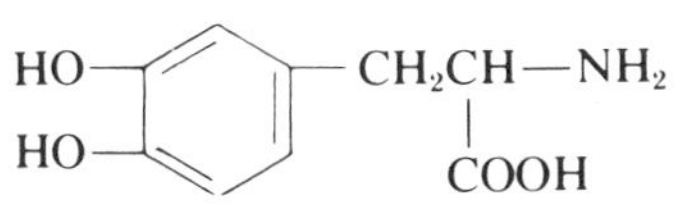

HO—⟨benzene ring⟩—CH₂CH—NH₂
HO—⟨benzene ring⟩ |
                          COOH

Figure 38-2. Levodopa.

Pharmacological Actions

Most of the pharmacological effects seen after levodopa administration appear to be due to newly formed dopamine. Drug-mediated effects appear to result from stimulation of both central and peripheral dopamine receptors. The best-characterized peripheral dopamine receptors are located in the kidney. The therapeutic effects of levodopa, as well as most of the prominent side effects associated with its use, are due to activation of dopamine receptors in the central nervous system.

Clinical Uses

Levodopa is widely used for the treatment of all types of parkinsonism except those associated with antipsychotic drug therapy. Levodopa therapy is not usually begun until all signs of the disease become clearly manifest. Approximately 75 percent of patients with parkinsonism respond favorably to levodopa, with some experiencing a dramatic improvement of all signs and symptoms. Improvements in rigidity and bradykinesia are generally more complete and appear sooner than do improvements in tremor. However, there are considerable individual differences in the long-term response to levodopa therapy. In one study, after 6 years of treatment with levodopa, half the patients failed to maintain benefit or could not tolerate the drug's side effects. In about 25 percent of the patients, substantial or moderate benefit was still obtained, and survival in this smaller group was enhanced to almost normal life expectancy. However, *parkinsonism is a chronic, progressive disease.*

There is no question that levodopa enhances the quality of life for most patients with this disease. The primary benefits are increased mobility, a decreased incidence of pulmonary infections leading to pneumonia, and a marked reduction in fractures due to falls. Epidemiological studies have shown that the mortality of patients with Parkinson's disease has been halved since the advent of levodopa therapy; the average life expectancy of the newly diagnosed patient is now probably about 20 additional years, compared to 10 years before the introduction of levodopa.

Adverse Reactions

Adverse reactions to levodopa therapy can be grouped into two classes. In the first class are those that occur early in therapy and to which tolerance develops; the most common of these are the gastrointestinal symptoms of anorexia, nausea, and vomiting. These side effects are thought to be caused by direct stimulation of the chemoreceptor trigger zone of the area postrema in the medulla oblongata by the newly formed dopamine. Gastrointestinal symptoms occur in up to 80 percent of patients taking levodopa, but tolerance to these effects usually develops within a few weeks. Orthostatic hypotension also occurs early in therapy and is thought to be caused by an accumulation of dopamine in norepinephrine nerve terminals. Although orthostatic hypotension tends to disappear with continued drug administration, its onset can be minimized by beginning with low doses and then gradually increasing the dose to the desired therapeutic level. If these side effects still occur, they can be reduced by temporarily reducing the dose. Cardiac arrhythmias may occur in some patients and are attributed to the stimulation by dopamine of β-adrenoceptors in the heart. These peripheral side effects are usually less prominent with administration of carbidopa/levodopa as compared to levodopa alone.

A second class of adverse side effects all increase with increasing duration of levodopa therapy and result from the central stimulation of dopamine receptors. The most common and serious of these side effects are abnormal choreiform movements of the limbs, hands, trunk, and tongue. These *dyskinesias* eventually occur in 40 to 90 percent of patients receiving long-term high-dosage levodopa therapy. The mechanism by which these abnormal movements are produced appears to be related to the presence of hypersensitive dopamine receptors. It is not clear whether this occurs as a result of denervation supersensitivity or from continuous stimulation by dopamine for long periods of time. Dyskinesias can be reduced by lowering the dosage; however, the symptoms of parkinsonism then reappear. Most patients prefer to tolerate a certain degree of dyskinesia if their mobility can be improved by levodopa therapy.

Serious mental disturbances occur in 10 to 15 percent of patients receiving levodopa. It is important to distinguish between the dementia and depression that accompany the disease and that which are drug induced. When a psychosis occurs early in the course of therapy, the patient usually had a past history of mental illness, often diagnosed as schizophrenia. Otherwise, psychosis usually occurs after several years of levodopa therapy. A large percentage of patients receiving long-term levodopa therapy experience vivid dreams, delusions, and visual hallucinations. If serious psychiatric problems develop, the dosage can be decreased or the patient can be put on a "drug holiday" during which all medication is removed for at least 5 days. Following such a period, the medication can be gradually reintroduced.

Levodopa therapy in parkinsonism is frequently characterized by a high day-to-day and within-day variation in effectiveness. However, in a few patients, this phenomenon becomes marked and is called the *on-off phenomenon*. In a matter of minutes, a patient enjoying normal or near-normal mobility may suddenly develop a severe degree of parkinsonism. The tremor reappears, normal postural reflexes disappear, and bradykinesia suddenly develops; such symptoms may persist from 30 min to 3 to 4 hr. These on-off cycles may occur anywhere from once a day to 10 or more times daily during the waking hours. This problem usually develops after 2 years of levodopa treatment. There is no completely satisfactory explanation for it, although the abrupt nature of the oscillation suggests an imbalance in physiological regulatory mechanisms. Although the cycles are not clearly related to blood levels of either levodopa or dopamine, the on-off phenomenon usually occurs when the blood levels are in the lower region of the therapeutic range.

One approach taken in an attempt to deal with this problem has been to utilize a sustained-release preparation of carbidopa/levodopa (*Sinemet CR*). In this dosage form, the dissolution of levodopa is slower and its absorption is more gradual, resulting in more sustained plasma levels of levodopa and less pronounced pharmacokinetic plasma troughs. In patients with moderately severe disease, the benefits of Sinemet CR include less of an "off" effect and some increase in the "on" effect; often, fewer daily doses are required. It is important to carefully adjust the dose with each patient as there is considerable variation in response among patients.

Contraindications and Drug Interactions

Certain drugs are known both to interfere with the clinical effectiveness and to exacerbate the adverse reactions of levodopa therapy. For instance, because of the pathways involved in levodopa metabolism, administration of peripheral (type A) monoamine oxidase (MAO) inhibitors and levodopa would result in a massive buildup of dopamine and, to a lesser extent, norepinephrine and epinephrine, with the possibility of a hypertensive crisis and hyperpyrexia. Levodopa should not be given to patients with narrow-angle glaucoma, since it can produce severe mydriasis that would markedly aggravate the glaucoma. Because of its tendency to produce psychoses, levodopa should not be given to patients with a history of significant psychiatric disturbances. The additive effects of levodopa and adrenomimetic amines suggest that extreme care should be exercised in treating the symptoms of asthma or emphysema in patients with Parkinson's disease. Patients with a history of cardiac arrhythmias or recent cardiac infarction should receive levodopa only when absolutely necessary.

Pyridoxine, a cofactor for the decarboxylation of levodopa to dopamine, rapidly reverses the therapeutic effectiveness of levodopa by promoting a more rapid conversion of levodopa to dopamine in the periphery. This process makes less levodopa available for transport into the brain.

Since levodopa utilizes the amino acid transport system to cross biological membranes, meals rich in protein may produce sufficient amino acids to compete effectively with levodopa transport both in the gastrointestinal tract and in the brain. If a drug-associated gastrointestinal upset occurs, patients should take levodopa with a light snack that is low in protein. Otherwise, levodopa should be taken 30 min before meals.

The phenothiazines, butyrophenones, and reserpine can produce the extrapyramidal symptoms of parkinsonism as adverse reactions. Coadministration of these drugs will antagonize the therapeutic effects of levodopa.

One of the major side effects of antidepressant drug therapy is orthostatic hypotension. This effect could be additive if the antidepressant is given concomitantly with levodopa. The hypotension can be minimized, however, by administering the antidepressant once a day at bedtime.

Preparations and Dosage

Levodopa (*Dopar, Larodopa*) is available for oral use as capsules or tablets; the maximal therapeutic dosage should not exceed 8 gm/day. When levodopa is used in conjunction with a peripheral decarboxylase inhibitor, its dosage is decreased.

Decarboxylase Inhibitors

Carbidopa (Fig. 38-3) is sold either as a single agent (*Lodosyn*) or in fixed combination with levodopa (*Sinemet*). Sinemet is available in the following combinations (mg carbidopa/mg dopa): 10/100, 25/100, 25/250. A sustained-release preparation (*Sinemet CR*) is available as a 50/200 combination. Although the fixed-dosage combinations offer the advantage of being more convenient to administer, prescribing each drug separately allows the physician to modify the proportions of carbidopa and levodopa and thereby individualize therapy. It should be noted that both therapeutic and adverse responses occur more rapidly with combined therapy than with levodopa alone. A reduction in dosage may be required if dyskine-

Figure 38-3. Carbidopa.

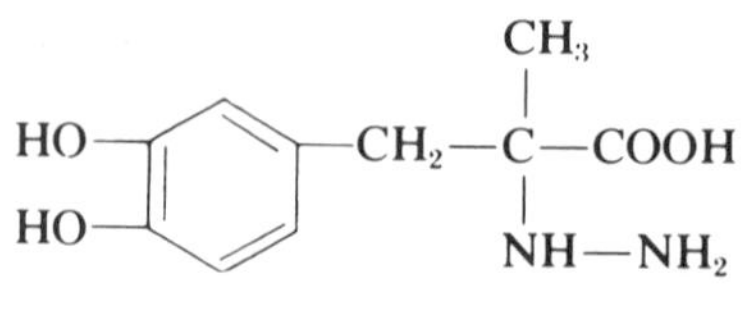

sias appear; an increased blink reflex may be an early sign of excess dosage.

Anticholinergic Drugs

For more than 100 years, the *belladonna alkaloids* (e.g., atropine and scopolamine) were the primary agents used in the treatment of parkinsonism. The effectiveness of anticholinergic drugs in parkinsonism gave support to the theory that acetylcholine as well as dopamine is involved in the maintenance of basal ganglia function. Anticholinergic drugs are most commonly used in mild cases of parkinsonism and during the early stages of the disease.

Although in the severe stages of parkinsonism these agents are definitely inferior to levodopa, symptoms are further alleviated by the addition of anticholinergics to a levodopa regimen. When given alone, the anticholinergic drugs seem to be more effective in combating tremor and rigidity than bradykinesia. Anticholinergic compounds also help in the treatment of drug-induced parkinsonism and dystonias. There is, however, a risk that their use may mask the side effects of excessive antipsychotic medication.

The limiting factor in the treatment of parkinsonism with anticholinergic therapy is usually the appearance of drug-associated side effects. These antimuscarinic side effects include cycloplegia, dry mouth, urinary retention, and constipation. Confusion, delirium, and hallucinations may occur at higher doses.

The belladonna alkaloids have been replaced by anticholinergic agents with more selective CNS effects. Trihexyphenidyl (*Artane*) and benztropine mesylate (*Cogentin*) are useful in most types of parkinsonism, including those produced by antipsychotic drugs. They are especially useful in preventing the tremors.

The antihistamine diphenhydramine (*Benadryl*), which also has marked anticholinergic properties, is used for mild parkinsonism and with the elderly, who may not be able to tolerate levodopa or dopamine agonists.

Amantadine

Amantadine was originally introduced as an antiviral compound (see Chap. 54; Fig. 54-1). Although less effective than levodopa, amantadine does produce an initial improvement in about two thirds of patients. Unfortunately, the improvement is usually not sustained, and tolerance appears to develop. Amantadine is often used in combination with levodopa, especially in patients who cannot tolerate high doses of levodopa.

Selegiline

Selegiline (formerly deprenyl) inhibits MAO_B, which catalyzes the metabolism of dopamine in the brain. It has been suggested that toxic products formed in the oxidation of brain dopamine may be responsible for the neuronal damage seen in parkinsonism. Thus, inhibition of dopamine metabolism by selegiline not only increases the half-life of dopamine available to stimulate dopamine receptors but also may decrease the rate of degradation of dopamine neurons. Clinical trials have shown that selegiline is of benefit in the treatment of parkinsonism. There are indications that selegiline alone can slow the progression of Parkinson's disease, when taken in the early stages of the disease.

Dopamine Agonists

Since a hallmark of Parkinson's disease is degeneration of dopamine neurons, considerable effort is being put forth to discover drugs that act directly on postsynaptic dopamine receptors.

Bromocriptine

The therapeutic efficacy of bromocriptine (*Parlodel*) is thought to be equal to that of levodopa. An improved therapeutic response results in some patients when bromocriptine and levodopa are combined; however, such side effects as the levodopa dyskinesias and the on-off phenomenon are not eliminated by bromocriptine. It is suggested that bromocriptine be tried in patients who have been treated for several years with levodopa and who are experiencing "end-of-dose failure." Bromocriptine may permit a reduction of the maintenance dose of levodopa and thus reduce the occurrence and severity of adverse reactions associated with long-term levodopa therapy. The long-term benefit from bromocriptine has not been firmly established.

Pergolide

Another ergoline derivative, pergolide (*Permax*), is now available for adjunctive treatment with levodopa/carbidopa in the management of the signs and symptoms of Parkinson's disease.

One advantage of dopamine agonists such as pergolide is their ability to reduce the dose of levodopa administered and thus avoid the complications associated with high-dose levodopa therapy.

Tissue Transplantation

Transplantation of human fetal adrenal medullary tissue into the caudate nucleus has been shown to lead to improvement in motor function in Parkinson's disease. The improvement seen is attributable to the capability of the grafted fetal tissue to synthesize dopamine. The ultimate success of this procedure will depend on future research and adequate resolution of the ethical and moral issues surrounding the use of human fetal tissue.

Other Basal Ganglia Disorders

Chorea

The clinical features of *chorea* consist of rapid, irregular, involuntary jerky movements that tend to be more pronounced during activity. The muscles of the face, tongue, and extremities are most commonly involved, although trunk and respiratory muscles may also be affected. Most types of chorea begin in childhood; the condition is frequently related to perinatal brain damage, encephalitis, or hypoparathyroidism. A chorea appearing as a late sequela of rheumatic fever is designated as *Sydenham's chorea* (St. Vitus' dance).

Huntington's chorea is an autosomal dominant inherited disorder of the central nervous system. Each child of a Huntington's disease-affected parent has a 50 percent chance of inheriting the disorder. The disease usually appears when patients are in their early forties. Choreiform movements first appear as involuntary movements of the extremities and twitching of the face, progressing over a 15- to 20-year period to involve more muscle groups, until the patient is immobile and unable to speak. Huntington's chorea is associated with progressive dementia and possibly a psychosis resembling paranoid schizophrenia. *The pathology of Huntington's chorea involves a degeneration of acetylcholine and GABA neurons, with dopamine neurons relatively unaffected.*

Most drugs that alleviate the signs and symptoms of parkinsonism appear to produce or exacerbate chorea. Levodopa in optimal dosage produces choreiform movements in many, if not most patients with Parkinson's disease and worsens the clinical symptoms of individuals with Huntington's chorea. Amantadine and anticholinergic drugs also exacerbate the symptoms. Drug treatment of Huntington's chorea has not, in general, been successful. Drugs used to treat this condition are antipsychotic medications of the phenothiazine and butyrophenone class that are known to antagonize dopamine receptors, and drugs, including tetrabenazine and reserpine, that deplete dopamine in the basal ganglia region. *Perphenazine has been viewed as the drug of choice in treating this disorder* because of its positive effect in reducing the abnormal movements, its relatively low price, and its infrequent side effects. Haloperidol and reserpine have been used as alternative agents. The most common side effects of these agents include drowsiness, depression, and, at high doses, parkinsonism.

Therapy aimed at increasing cholinergic influence in the basal ganglia has been disappointing. Administration of choline or choline precursors does not significantly improve the abnormal movements. Physostigmine and other cholinesterase inhibitors produce a transient improvement in patient symptoms, but this improvement is not sustained. Likewise, GABA agonists also have not proved helpful.

Tardive Dyskinesia

Tardive (late-appearing) *dyskinesia* is frequently associated with long-term antipsychotic drug treatment, especially phenothiazine therapy. It is most commonly characterized by choreoathetoid movements involving the mouth, lips, tongue, and, to a lesser degree, the trunk and extremities. Tardive dyskinesia was reported to be present in 36 percent of patients chronically confined in mental hospitals. Tardive dyskinesia usually occurs after many months or even years of continuous therapy with antipsychotic drugs. The tragic nature of this condition is that often the psychotic symptoms are controlled, but the patient is left with the disfiguring consequences of tardive dyskinesia. Often, symptoms cannot be eliminated by withdrawal of the drug. The underlying cause of the disorder is not known, but it has been postulated that prolonged blockade of dopamine receptors in basal ganglia neurons by antipsychotic drugs may result in the development of a receptor supersensitivity.

The dyskinesia can be treated by increasing the dose of the antipsychotic, but it is believed that this will eventually further exacerbate the condition, and it is not recommended. Early detection of abnormal movements of the tongue as well as low-dose and intermittent-dose therapy are generally recommended as the best way to prevent the occurrence of these dyskinesias.

Supplemental Reading

Collier, D.S., Berg, M.J., and Fincham, R.W. Parkinsonism treatment: Part III,—Update. *Ann. Pharmacother.* 26:227, 1992.

King, D.B. The place of the dopaminergic agonists in the treatment of Parkinson's disease: The view from the trenches. *Can. J. Neurol. Sci.* 19:156, 1992.

Koller, W.C. Initiating treatment of Parkinson's disease. *Neurology* 42 (Suppl. 1):33, 1992.

Pfeiffer, R. Optimization of levodopa therapy. *Neurology* 42 (Suppl. 1):39, 1992.

Pleet, A.B. Newly-diagnosed Parkinson's disease: A therapeutic update. *Geriatrics* 47:24, 1992.

Robertson, H.A. Dopamine receptor interactions: Some implications for the treatment of Parkinson's disease. *Trends Neurosci.* 15:201, 1992.

Rodnitzky, R.L. The use of Sinemet CR in the management of mild to moderate Parkinson's disease. *Neurology* 42 (Suppl. 1):44, 1992.

Wessel, K., and Szelenyi, I. Selegiline—an overview of its role in the treatment of Parkinson's disease. *Clin. Invest.* 70:459, 1992.

39

Opioid and Nonopioid Analgesics

Billy Martin

Pain serves the useful function of alerting an individual that some component of a physiological system has gone awry. The consequences of pain can range from mild discomfort to debilitation. Although pain is most effectively eliminated by removal of the underlying cause, the stimulus for pain is usually not easily defined or is not readily susceptible to removal. Therefore, the physician is often faced with the necessity of treating pain as a symptom.

The concept of pain can be divided into acute and chronic categories. The occurrence of chronic pain can endure long after healing, such as in the case of phantom limb pain, and need not be related to any physical pathology. On the other hand, acute pain is directly related to a noxious stimulus and is further distinguished into phasic and tonic components.

Phasic pain is produced by the presence of a noxious stimulus that threatens to injure tissue. This superficial pain often involves the skin and usually produces an intense, sharp sensation. Initiation of pain likely involves interaction of endogenous substances, such as bradykinins and prostaglandins, with their receptors in the free nerve endings. This fast, precise pain is transmitted through fast-conducting, lightly myelinated A-δ fibers that enter the spinal cord through the dorsal horn. The major ascending pain pathways for phasic pain are in the well-myelinated, fast-conducting lateral spinothalamic tract.

Tonic pain is evoked either by tissue damage occurring in the skin or in the viscera. It has a more gradual onset than phasic pain and is described as a dull, throbbing, aching pain. Tonic pain is generally conducted through the unmyelinated, slow-conducting C-fiber pathways and also enters the spinal cord through the dorsal horn. Located more medially in the ventral cord are the spinoreticular and paleospinothalamic tracts, which relay tonic pain information much more slowly, frequently forming synapses at many sites along the entire neuraxis from the spinal cord to the thalamus.

The perception of acute pain can be categorized into two qualitatively different subjective measures, a sensory/ discriminative component and an affective/motivational component. The sensory/discriminative component of pain reflects the perception of noxious sensory information. In contrast, the affective/motivational component of pain reflects the cognitive and emotional aspects of pain. This facet, which involves a psychic constituent or the suffering of pain, varies greatly from one person to another and depends on such individual factors as idiosyncrasy, previous experience with pain, and awareness of the significance of pain.

The processing of both components of pain can be further distinguished by the fact that they are mediated by distinct neuroanatomical substrates. Areas of the neocortex and diencephalon that are believed to play important roles in the integration of the affective/emotional aspect of pain include the postcentral gyrus of the cerebral cortex, the cingulum, the habenula, and thalamic nuclei. For example, individuals who have undergone prefrontal lobotomies no longer experience the aversive emotions that are typically associated with pain; however, they can perceive the sensory/discriminative aspects of pain. On the other hand, brain areas that are critical for blocking the sensory components of pain are located throughout the midbrain and medulla. Critical brain structures of this descending system, including the periaqueductal gray and nucleus raphe magnus, contain opioid receptors that may be responsible for activation of this pain control system. This descending system transcends the spinal cord via the dorsolateral funiculus to the dorsal horn, where it inhibits neurons activated by painful stimuli.

Drugs can alter the pain experience in several ways. Since pain is both a sensation and an emotion, drugs may act as analgesics by altering either of these two aspects. The first step that can be interrupted is peripheral pain reception at the nerve endings, such as salicylate blockade of prostaglandin synthesis. Neuronal conduction is susceptible to the effects of local anesthetics. In the central nervous system (CNS), nonopioid as well as opioid analgesics can interfere with both the affective/motivational and sensory/discriminative components of pain integration. The route of drug administration can be used to selectively block the components of pain. For example, the emotional component of pain is much more sensitive to systemically administered opioid analgesics than are the sensory aspects of pain. Conversely, epidural administration of opioids or local anesthetics at the spinal level has been very effective in blocking the sensory components of pain, consequently preventing the affective/motivational dimensions of pain.

Chronic pain presents an entirely different clinical picture than acute pain. It persists beyond the normal expected healing time, may not be associated with a specific injury, and by definition is refractory to traditional analgesic therapy. The sufferers of chronic pain may exhibit severe depression as well as changes in both mental and physiological states. Often, emotional, environmental, and psychological factors are major contributors to this painful state. Although these patients are frequently treated with numerous drugs including antidepressants, treatment goes beyond traditional pharmacotherapy to include whatever means will enable the patient to resume a normal lifestyle.

Nonopioid Analgesics

Preparations and dosages for the agents discussed below are listed in Table 39-1.

Salicylates and Derivatives

The salicylates were discovered following the extraction of a naturally occurring substance, the glycoside salicin, from willow bark. The compound isolated from salicin in 1838 and later synthesized was *salicylic acid.* Shortly thereafter, a salt of salicylic acid, sodium salicylate, was prepared and used therapeutically. In 1853, acetylsalicylic acid (aspirin) was synthesized.

Chemistry

The salicylic acid portion of the salicylate molecule (Fig. 39-1) is the pharmacologically active moiety. It is essential that the hydroxyl group of this molecule remain in the ortho position. Substitutions on either the hydroxyl or the carboxyl group will result in changes in the potency or toxicity (or both) of the compound. Addition of a difluorophenyl group to the salicylate structure, as in diflunisal, markedly alters the symptoms of toxicity. Condensation of two salicylic acid molecules results in salsalate, which is hydrolyzed to salicylic acid during and after absorption.

Mechanism of Action

The analgesic effects of salicylates were long thought to be mediated strictly through their central actions. However, more recent studies have demonstrated that *these agents produce analgesia through both central and peripheral mechanisms.* The salicylates interfere with pain perception centrally by an action within the hypothalamus. Since the cortex is not affected by the salicylates, analgesic doses do not cause mental disturbances or drowsiness. These agents alter pain reception peripherally by interfering with the input to peripheral nerve endings. This interference occurs by inhibiting cyclooxygenase, the enzyme that converts arachidonic acid to prostaglandins E and F. It is these latter substances that are thought to sensitize nerve endings to pain.

The *antipyretic effect* (i.e., the reduction of an elevated body temperature by administration of clinical doses of the salicylates) is also centrally mediated. In contrast, toxic doses increase temperature. The hypothalamus is the anatomical site involved in the antipyresis produced by the salicylates. In the normal individual, a coordinating center in the hypothalamus maintains the body temperature within narrow limits by balancing and integrating heat-producing and heat-dissipating mechanisms. In a person with fever, salicylates promote the loss of heat by vasodilation of the small vessels of the skin and through an enhancement of sweating. These agents also prevent the temperature-elevating effects of leukocytic pyrogens, presumably by competing with the pyrogens for receptor sites in the thermoregulatory centers of the hypothalamus. Fever typically arises from a disease state in which cytokine production is increased. Cytokines, such as IL-1 and tumor necrosis factor, stimulate the synthesis of prostaglandin E_2 (PGE_2), which acts to elevate body temperature. Cyclooxygenase blockade by salicylate-like drugs may also reduce fever by decreasing PGE_2 production. Salicylates have no influence on the mechanisms subserving the production of heat.

Pharmacological Actions

Central Nervous System

Two of the main therapeutic effects of the salicylates, production of *analgesia* and *antipyresis,* result from actions within the CNS. These agents produce other important central effects as well. Large doses, such as those used for the treatment of rheumatoid arthritis (see Chap. 43), increase the depth of respiration. This effect is caused by a salicylate-induced increase in oxygen consumption, primarily in skeletal muscle, with a subsequent augmentation of carbon dioxide production and respiratory stimulation. Because increased alveolar ventilation balances the increased CO_2 production, plasma CO_2 tension does not change. If even larger doses of salicylate are administered,

Table 39-1. Analgesics Used for Mild to Moderate Pain

Drug	Trade name	Dose (mg)*	Dosing intervals (hr)	Preparation	Comments
Salicylates					
Aspirin		650	4	65- to 650-mg tablets 300-mg capsules 65- to 1,300-mg suppositories	
Sodium salicylate		325–1,000	3–4	300- and 600-mg tablets	Children: 10–20 mg q6h
Diflunisal	Dolobid	500	8–12	250- to 500-mg tablets	Because of long half-life, an initial loading dose, 1 gm, should be used
					Maintenance doses should not exceed 1.5 gm/day
					More effective than aspirin, lacks antipyretic effects
Salsalate	Disalcid, Mono-Gesic, Salflex	500–750			Maximum daily dose of 3 gm in 2–4 doses
Aniline derivatives					
Acetaminophen	Tempra, Tylenol	325–650	4	120- and 325-mg tablets Elixir and syrups contain 24 mg/ml	Children: 60–120 mg depending on age and weight
					Analgesic and antipyretic effects similar to those of aspirin but exerts weak antiinflammatory effects
Indomethacin and related compounds					
Indomethacin	Indocin	25	8–12	25- to 75-mg capsules 75-mg sustained-release capsules 50-mg suppositories 25 mg/5 ml elixir	Loading dose is usually 25 mg 2 or 3 times daily
					Doses can be increased to 150–200 mg/day
Sulindac	Clinoril	150–200	12	150- and 200-mg tablets	Similar to indomethacin
Tolmetin	Tolectin	400	8	200- and 400-mg tablets	Approved for osteoarthritis, rheumatoid arthritis
					Usually better tolerated than aspirin
Fenamates					
Mefenamic acid	Ponstel	250–500	6	250-mg capsules	Therapy should not be continued longer than 7 days
Meclofenamate sodium	Meclomen	50	4–6	50- and 100-mg tablets and capsules	Should not exceed 400 mg/day
Arylalkanoic acids					
Ibuprofen	Advil, Medipren, Nidol, Motrin, Nuprin, Rufen	200–400	4–6	200-mg tablets	Maximum daily dose should not exceed 1,200 mg
Fenoprofen	Nalfon	200	4–6	200- and 300-mg capsules 600-mg tablets	Similar to ibuprofen
Flurbiprofen	Ansaid	200–300	6–12		Similar to ibuprofen
Naproxen	Naprosyn	250	6–8	250-, 375-, and 500-mg tablets 125 mg/5 ml suspension	Loading dose of 500 mg is recommended
					Total daily dose should not exceed 1,250 mg
Ketoprofen	Orudis	25–50	6–8	25-, 50-, and 75-mg capsules	Daily dose should not exceed 300 mg
Pyrazolone					
Phenylbutazone	Butazolidin	100	4	100-mg tablets and capsules	Loading dose is usually 400 mg
					Inferior to salicylates for treating nonrheumatic pain
					Toxicity precludes its routine use as an analgesic
Oxicam					
Piroxicam	Feldene	10	12	10- and 20-mg capsules	Approved for osteoarthritis, rheumatoid arthritis
Acetic acid derivatives					
Diclofenac	Voltaren	50–75	6–8	25-, 50-, and 75-mg tablets	Approved for osteoarthritis, rheumatoid arthritis
					Has been used for selected cases of acute muscle injury

Table 39-1. *Continued*

Drug	Trade name	Dose (mg)*	Dosing intervals (hr)	Preparation	Comments
Opioids					
Codeine phosphate and sulfate		30–60	4–6	15-, 30-, and 60-mg tablets	Also used as an antitussive
					Less addicting than morphine
				15-, 30-, and 60-mg/ml injectable solution	About 12 times less potent than morphine
Oxycodone	Roxicodone	5–10		5-mg tablets	Potency equivalent to morphine
Meperidine	Demerol, Pethadol	50–100		50- and 100-mg tablets	Effects similar to those of morphine with some minor differences.
d-Propoxyphene	Darvon, Darvon-N	30–60	2–4	32- and 65-mg capsules of the hydrochloride salt	Analgesic potency similar to codeine
					Little addiction potential
				100-mg tablets of the napsylate salt	
Pentazocine	Talwin-NX	30	3–4	Tablets containing 50 mg pentazocine base and 0.5 mg naloxone base	Shorter duration but faster onset than morphine

*Oral doses for adults.

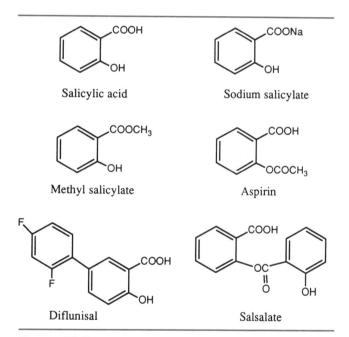

Figure 39-1. Representative salicylates.

respiration is increased in rate as well as depth. This occurrence results from a direct stimulating action of these drugs on the medullary respiratory center.

The chemoreceptor trigger zone (CTZ) of the medulla is also directly stimulated by salicylates. It is this central action that leads, in part, to the nausea and vomiting that can accompany salicylate administration.

CNS disturbances, such as confusion, delirium, tinnitus, dizziness, and, occasionally, psychosis, may develop in patients maintained chronically on large doses of salicylates. The term *salicylism* is generally applied to these characteristic symptoms, which arise from long-term salicylate therapy.

Absorption, Metabolism, and Excretion

The salicylates are among the most rapidly absorbed drugs after oral administration. Although pH can influence their rate of absorption (increased absorption at lower pH), it is nevertheless rapid at all H^+ concentrations within the physiological range. Appreciable blood levels are usually attained within 30 min, with a peak value being reached within 2 to 3 hr. From 50 to 90 percent of an ingested dose of salicylate is bound to plasma proteins. Free salicylate is distributed rapidly throughout body tissues.

Biotransformation of salicylates takes place mainly in the liver. Almost all of an ingested dose is ultimately excreted in the urine. The glycine conjugate (salicyluric acid) accounts for 75 percent of the amount of aspirin and sodium salicylate found in the urine, while the monoglucuronides and diglucuronides constitute 15 percent. The remaining 10 percent consists of free salicylate. Urinary excretion of salicylate itself, but not the metabolites, is increased three- to fivefold by alkalinization of the urine (Fig. 39-2).

The glucuronide conjugates account for 90 percent of an ingested dose of diflunisal. Metabolism of this compound does not result in the production of salicylic acid, whereas the hydrolysis of salsalate does.

Clinical Uses

Aspirin, sodium salicylate, and diflunisal are used systemically for the relief of mild to moderate pain, such as

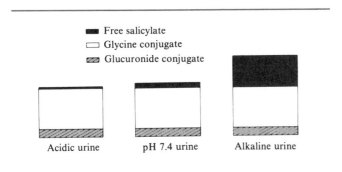

Figure 39-2. Relative changes in the excretion of salicylate and metabolites after alteration of urinary pH.

that found in patients suffering from headache, dysmenorrhea, neuralgia, myalgia, and postoperative discomfort due to surgery for dental or selected orthopedic procedures. The antiinflammatory action of higher doses of these compounds is quite useful in the treatment of rheumatic fever and rheumatoid arthritis (see Chap. 43).

Aspirin has recently been shown conclusively to be of benefit in both the primary and secondary prevention of myocardial infarction as well as in the treatment of early infarcts. Aspirin blocks production of thromboxane A, which is thought to be the physiological inducer of platelet aggregation. A dose of one standard aspirin tablet (325 mg) every other day is effective.

Salicylic acid is employed only for external use in the removal of warts and corns. Methyl salicylate likewise is reserved for topical use, but as a counterirritant. It is applied as an ointment or liniment for the treatment of painful muscles or joints. These salicylates are extremely toxic if ingested.

Adverse Reactions

The usual therapeutic doses of salicylate employed for analgesia and antipyresis have relatively few side effects. However, accidental ingestion of large amounts of aspirin, particularly by children, results in considerable toxicity. On a symptomatic level, one sees extreme thirst, sweating, blurred vision, tinnitus, nausea, vomiting, and marked changes in acid-base balance.

Several factors contribute to the salicylate-induced alterations in body pH. The early changes stem from a direct stimulation of the medullary respiratory center. The resulting increased alveolar ventilation leads to a decrease in plasma CO_2 tension and an increase in arterial pH; respiratory alkalosis ensues. There is a subsequent partial renal compensation characterized by an increased bicarbonate, sodium, and potassium ion excretion; the bicarbonate loss tends to return the plasma pH toward normal. The alkalosis is now compensated, but at the expense of a

diminished buffering capacity of the plasma (due to bicarbonate ion loss).

Salicylate-induced metabolic changes also contribute to the production of acid-base imbalances. Metabolic rate is increased as a result of uncoupling of oxidative phosphorylation; the resulting increase in plasma CO_2 tension stimulates the respiratory center further. The pyresis seen after toxic doses of salicylates is explained by this metabolic effect. The oxidatively derived energy normally used for the conversion of inorganic phosphate to adenosine triphosphate (ATP) is dissipated, principally as heat.

By the time a child who is suffering from salicylate intoxication is seen by a physician, the resultant changes in acid-base balance usually have led to the development of acidosis. Several factors contribute to this occurrence. Salicylates cause a reduction in the aerobic metabolism of glucose, leading to an accumulation of lactic and pyruvic acids. Increased fat catabolism results in the accumulation of acetone and ketone bodies; the net effect of these biochemical changes is a *metabolic acidosis*. The respiratory depression induced by the continued presence of toxic concentrations of salicylate results in a *respiratory acidosis*. The final factor contributing to the generalized acidosis is the acidic nature of the salicylate molecule itself.

The major objectives of the *therapeutic approach* are (1) prevention of further salicylate absorption either by provoking emesis, if the patient is conscious, or by gastric lavage; (2) symptomatic therapy to correct existent water and electrolyte deficits through the judicious use of Ringer's solution and isotonic sodium bicarbonate; and (3) reduction of serum and tissue salicylate levels through alkalinization of the urine, thereby limiting passive renal tubular reabsorption and promoting drug excretion. Hemodialysis also can be employed if necessary.

In contrast with other salicylates, diflunisal does not cause acid-base imbalances after overdosage. To date, drowsiness, disorientation, and stupor have been the most common symptoms reported after ingestion of toxic doses.

Contraindications, Cautions, and Drug Interactions

Because of their effects on the gastrointestinal tract, the salicylates are contraindicated in patients with peptic ulcer. These compounds should be used with special caution in children with high blood pressure, heart disease, diabetes, or thyroid disorders.

The salicylates can alter the pharmacological activity of a wide variety of drugs. The effects of methotrexate, penicillin, phenytoin, and the sulfonylurea hypoglycemics are all enhanced, owing to their displacement from plasma protein—binding sites by the salicylates. The dosage of oral anticoagulants may need to be adjusted when the salicylates are given concomitantly. Because of their biphasic effect on uric acid excretion, salicylates interfere with the action of uricosuric agents, such as probenecid. It is not yet known whether diflunisal adversely affects the activity of other uricosuric agents.

Salicylates also interfere with a number of clinical laboratory tests. Measurements of plasma proteins may show either spurious elevations or reductions, depending on the method used. Levels of serum glucose, calcium, catecholamines, and vanillylmandelic acid (VMA) also may be inaccurate because of the presence of salicylates.

Aniline Derivatives

Several chemical derivatives of the dye aniline serve as useful therapeutic alternatives to the salicylates for the production of analgesia and antipyresis. These compounds are also known as coal-tar analgesics or *p*-aminophenal additives.

Chemistry

Acetanilid, the first aniline derivative prepared, is no longer employed because of its extreme toxicity. Acetophenetidin (phenacetin) was subsequently synthesized and became widely used for fever reduction. Acetaminophen (paracetamol), the major active metabolite of both acetanilid and phenacetin (Fig. 39-3), became available about 1950.

It is the aminobenzene portion of the aniline derivatives that confers pharmacological activity. Introduction of a hydroxyl group in the para position (as occurs in acetaminophen) as well as the addition of an alkyl function on the hydroxyl moiety (as occurs in phenacetin) reduces toxicity. Acetylation of the amino group also lowers toxicity.

Pharmacological Actions

Central Nervous System

Both acetaminophen and phenacetin have *analgesic* and *antipyretic* properties comparable to those of the salicylates. The mechanism by which these agents reduce fever is similar to that of the salicylates, that is, through a hypothalamically mediated increase in heat dissipation. Whether there is a peripheral as well as a central component to the analgesic effects of the coal-tar compounds has not yet been established. In contrast to the salicylates, neither acetaminophen nor phenacetin has any effect on respiration.

Peripheral Effects

As with the salicylates, therapeutic doses of acetaminophen and phenacetin have essentially no cardiovascular effects. In contrast to the salicylates, however, these aniline derivatives do not cause gastric irritation or bleeding, *do not possess antiinflammatory activity,* and cannot be used

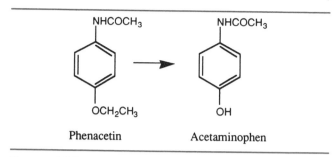

Figure 39-3. Conversion of phenacetin to acetaminophen.

in the treatment of rheumatic fever and arthritis. They only weakly inhibit prostaglandin synthesis in the periphery; their central effects may be greater. Neither acetaminophen nor phenacetin has any effect on platelet aggregation or uric acid excretion.

Absorption, Metabolism, and Excretion

After oral administration, both acetaminophen and phenacetin are rapidly absorbed from the gastrointestinal tract. Plasma concentrations peak 30 min to 1 hr after ingestion. About 75 percent of an ingested dose of phenacetin is rapidly metabolized to acetaminophen. Although peak plasma levels of unchanged phenacetin are reached within 1 hr, peak levels of the acetaminophen subsequently formed occur only after 2 hr. Both compounds are distributed relatively uniformly throughout the body. Acetaminophen is metabolized in the liver, predominantly to the glucuronide conjugate, which is then excreted in the urine. Several metabolites result from the biotransformation of phenacetin, including *N*-deacetylated and hydroxylated derivatives.

Clinical Uses

The analgesic and antipyretic effects of acetaminophen and phenacetin are very useful in patients who cannot tolerate aspirin because of allergy, gastrointestinal problems, or the possibility of aggravation of gout. Acetaminophen is generally preferred over phenacetin since it has less overall toxicity. The use of phenacetin has been confined to analgesic mixtures. In recent times it has been replaced with acetaminophen.

Adverse Reactions

Therapeutic doses of acetaminophen and phenacetin cause few side effects. Allergic phenomena, such as skin rash, occur infrequently. In contrast, overdosage with these compounds can have serious consequences. The principal toxicity associated with acetaminophen overdosage is the production of a potentially fatal hepatic necrosis. Liver damage occurs primarily in the centrolobular region, whereas the periportal area is relatively unaffected. The mechanism of toxicity appears to involve covalent binding of a toxic alkylating metabolite to liver macromolecules. The probability of occurrence of hepatotoxicity after acetaminophen overdosage can be predicted on the basis of serum concentrations. Serum levels greater than 200 μg/ml at 4 hr or 50 μg/ml at 12 hr after drug ingestion are associated with increased risk. Toxicity can be prevented by intravenous administration of sulfhydryl donors such as *N*-acetylcysteine (*Mucomyst*) and L-methionine if treatment is initiated within the first 12 hr.

Phenacetin causes some degree of methemoglobin formation, presumably by an action of its hydroxylated metabolites. Lethality results from cyanosis and cardiac arrest. Chronic use of high doses of phenacetin is frequently followed by the appearance of hemolytic anemia. Nephrotoxicity is associated with the chronic ingestion of various analgesic mixtures containing either phenacetin or acetaminophen.

Indomethacin and Related Derivatives

As with the salicylates, indomethacin, sulindac, and tolmetin have analgesic, antipyretic, and antiinflammatory activity. Toxicity, however, precludes use of these agents as general analgesics or antipyretics. They do have therapeutic usefulness for relief of pain associated with rheumatoid arthritis, gout, and other disorders of inflammatory origin when aspirin is ineffective or poorly tolerated. Sulindac is about one-half as potent as indomethacin and produces somewhat fewer side effects. Still, adverse reactions to sulindac are common.

Tolmetin, on the other hand, is approximately equipotent to aspirin in producing analgesic, antipyretic, and antiinflammatory effects, although it is usually better tolerated. Tolmetin is approved in the United States for the treatment of osteoarthritis and rheumatoid arthritis, and has been used for treating ankylosing spondylitis. The antiinflammatory effects of indomethacin and related derivatives are discussed in Chap. 43.

Fenamates

Mefenamic acid and meclofenamate are analgesics that also have antipyretic and antiinflammatory properties. They are derivatives of anthranilic acid, the amine analogue of salicylic acid. Serious toxicity is associated with their administration, however, and therefore their analgesic uses have been limited to treating pain arising from rheumatic diseases and dysmenorrhea. Severe diarrhea is commonly produced. Gastrointestinal ulceration and bleeding, as well as hematological changes (including megaloblastic anemia and agranulocytosis), have also been reported. Because of this toxicity, they should be used only when other drugs are not effective.

Arylalkanoic Acids

Arylalkanoic acid compounds currently marketed in the United States include ibuprofen, naproxen, fenoprofen, ketoprofen, and flurbiprofen. The pharmacological properties of these drugs are quite similar. All five agents can cause analgesia, antipyresis, and antiinflammatory effects. Gastrointestinal side effects are also produced, but these are usually less severe than those caused by aspirin. Similar to aspirin, these compounds prolong bleeding time by inhibition of platelet aggregation.

In the past the arylalkanoic acids were used predominantly for their antiinflammatory activity. In 1984, ibuprofen was approved by the Food and Drug Administration (FDA) for over-the-counter use as an analgesic, primarily because of its effectiveness in dysmenorrhea. For this indication, the compound appears to be superior to aspirin. Moreover, adverse effects after overdosage are clearly less than those induced by either aspirin or acetaminophen, the only other analgesic preparations available over the counter.

Naproxen, fenoprofen, ketoprofen, and flurbiprofen, compounds already on the market for the treatment of arthritis, were subsequently approved by the FDA for the relief of mild to moderate pain.

Piroxicam

Piroxicam (*Feldene*) was introduced into medical therapy several years ago. Although this drug exhibits analgesic, antipyretic, and antiinflammatory activity, at present piroxicam is used principally for its antiinflammatory properties (see Chap. 43). It has also been used for postoperative pain.

Diclofenac

Diclofenac has a pharmacological profile similar to that of the salicylates in that it possesses analgesic, antipyretic, and antiinflammatory activity. It is more potent than several other analgesic agents in blocking cyclooxygenase activity. Diclofenac produces most of the side effects common to antiinflammatory agents.

Opioid Analgesics

Although nonopioid analgesics are capable of alleviating mild to moderate pain, the opioid analgesics afford relief from the entire spectrum of pain. Unfortunately, the administration of opioid analgesics also may result in physical dependence; no opioid yet synthesized is completely free of this effect.

Morphine, the first narcotic analgesic used therapeutically, comes from the unripe seed capsules of *Papaver somniferum,* the opium poppy. Opium contains two series of alkaloids, the pharmacological properties of which differ markedly. It is the *phenanthrene series* from which morphine and a second narcotic analgesic, codeine, are derived. The second series of alkaloids obtained from opium is the *benzylisoquinoline series.* The two agents of medicinal interest in this group are papaverine and noscapine. Papaverine has a spasmolytic, or relaxing, effect on cardiac and smooth muscle and is used clinically as a vasodilator. The sole therapeutic use of noscapine is as an antitussive.

Opioid analgesics displaying only agonistic activity have long been the mainstay of medicine. In addition, compounds that are completely devoid of agonistic activity when administered alone, but which are capable of promptly reversing the effects of opioid agonists, play an important role in the pharmacology of opioids. These agents are referred to as *pure opioid antagonists.* A third group, referred to as *agonist-antagonists,* when administered alone are capable of antagonizing the agonist actions of other opioids. Further development of such compounds offers hope of divorcing the analgesic actions of opioids from their physical dependence–producing properties.

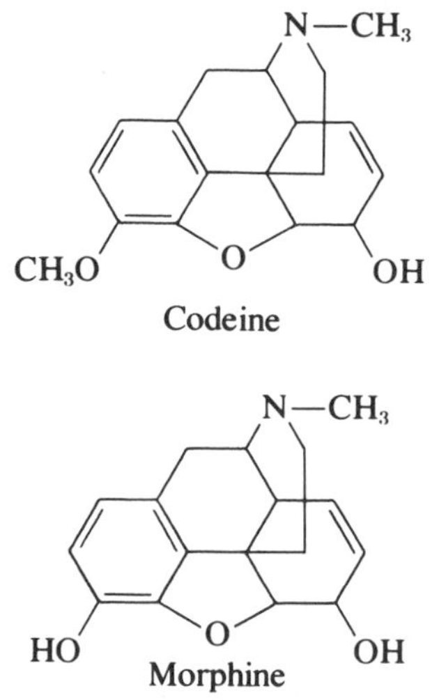

Chemistry

The structures of the main opium alkaloids are depicted in Fig. 39-4. By slight modification of the basic structure of the morphine molecule, semisynthetic derivatives of morphine that retain a five-ring nucleus have been produced. Two such derivatives are heroin, which is simply diacetylmorphine, and hydromorphone. Removal of the furan ring from morphine yields a fully potent, synthetic four-ring narcotic analogue, levorphanol. In addition, several groups of narcotic analgesics retain only two of the original five rings of the morphine structure. Phenylpiperidines, such as meperidine and fentanyl, make up one such group; methadone and its congeners form a second chemically distinct group (Fig. 39-5).

Since narcotic analgesic drugs possess such diverse molecular structures, it may, at first glance, appear difficult to conceive of any molecular basis for the analgesic action of these compounds. Closer examination, however, has pointed toward several common structural requirements for narcotic analgesic activity. Although the phenanthrene nucleus of morphine can be modified or even eliminated, the piperidine ring is essential. The nitrogen atom of this ring, which is about 80 percent cationic at physiological pH, also is necessary. The oxygen atom of the

Figure 39-4. Morphine and codeine.

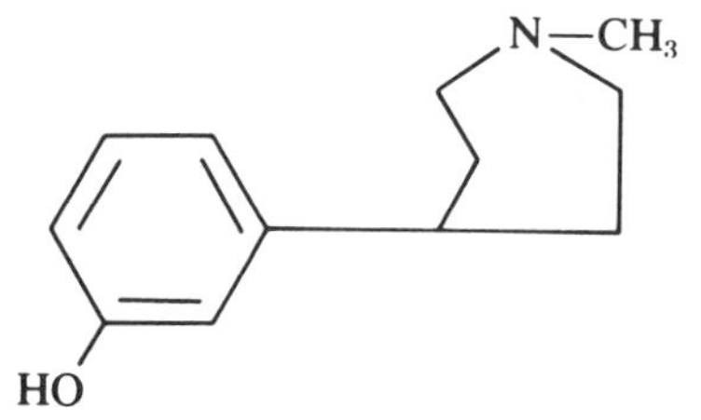

Figure 39-5. Selected synthetic opioids.

phenolic hydroxyl group attached to the piperidine ring likewise cannot be eliminated without loss of activity. Thus, the *N*-methylpiperidine portion of morphine and other opioids appears to be most essential.

A number of endogenous opioid peptides are known to exist. The enkephalins, leucine-enkephalin (leu-enkephalin) and methionine-enkephalin (met-enkephalin), were the first peptides discovered. They are pentapeptides that differ from each other at their C-terminal position. The other two families of opioid peptides are the endorphins and dynorphins. Dynorphin A(1-17), dynorphin B(1-13), dynorphin (1-8), and α- and β-endorphins, constitute the latter family. One of the striking features of the larger peptides is that they contain either a leu- or met-enkephalin at the amino terminus. Although all of these peptides are distributed widely throughout the CNS, they are present in areas closely associated with pain pathways. Despite firm evidence that the opioid peptides are involved in pain processes, their precise physiological functions remain to be elucidated.

Mechanism of Action

The discovery of specific opioid receptors in brain through in vitro binding studies prompted the successful search for endogenous opioids. Since a good correlation exists between the distribution of these receptors and anatomical areas that respond to morphine, *it is assumed that the opioids exert their analgesic activity by stimulating endogenous opioid receptors.* An excellent correlation between the in vivo potencies of opioids and their in vitro affinities for receptor binding sites supports such a hypothesis.

A variety of endogenous receptors specific for the narcotics and the endogenous opioid peptides have been identified and characterized pharmacologically. The three major classes of opioid receptors in the CNS are designated mu (μ), kappa (κ), and delta (δ).

Morphine, its congeners, and endogenous opioid peptides produce supraspinal analgesia by action at μ-receptors. These sites are localized primarily in the periaqueductal gray, the medial thalamus, and the nucleus raphe magnus. Both the narcotics and endogenous opioids produce spinal analgesia after intrathecal or epidural administration. Analgesia mediated by the narcotics occurs by an action at spinal μ-receptors. The analgesic effects of both endogenous and synthetic peptides, on the other hand, are mediated by δ- and κ-receptors. Enkephalins and several synthetic peptides act at δ recognition sites, whereas dynorphin acts more selectively at κ sites. Although all three receptor types are found throughout the gray matter of the spinal cord, the highest levels of all three occur in the dorsal horn, the substantia gelatinosa, and the intermediolateral cell column of the thoracic cord. In animals and in humans, the opioid peptides are more potent analgesics at the spinal cord level than is morphine.

Two important side effects produced by morphine and other narcotics—respiratory depression and constipation—appear to be mediated by a receptor different from the μ recognition site primarily responsible for morphine analgesia. Two subtypes of the μ-receptor have thus become recognized. The μ_1-*receptor,* localized at the anatomical sites important for pain, presumably mediates both analgesia and euphoria. The μ_2-*receptor,* found also in the brain and in the gastrointestinal tract of animals, appears to be involved in the production of respiratory depression and constipation.

Dysphoric and psychotomimetic effects are produced by some opioids, particularly benzomorphans such as pentazocine. It has been proposed that a distinct receptor, designated sigma (σ), is responsible for these unwanted effects. However, a great deal of confusion has resulted from attempts to characterize the σ-receptor. Benzomor-

phans bind to two sites. Their low-affinity site is tightly bound by phencyclidine whereas their high-affinity site appears to accommodate several classes of drugs and hormones. Unfortunately, both sites have been referred to as σ. The benzomorphans also appear to share some common behavioral properties with phencyclidine. The phencyclidine receptor has been generally well characterized and appears to inhibit glutamate-gated calcium channels, whereas the other site, more appropriately termed the σ site, is much less understood. It remains to be determined whether these two sites are responsible for the psychotomimetic effects of the benzomorphans.

Tolerance and Physical Dependence

A direct cellular tolerance develops to a number of the pharmacological actions produced by the opioids. For example, tolerance develops quite readily to analgesia and euphoria. Tolerance develops at a slower rate to respiratory depression as well. On the other hand, there is little tolerance to the stimulant and gastrointestinal effects of these compounds. Once tolerance to one drug has become manifest, cross-tolerance to other opioid analgesics, *but not to other classes of CNS depressants,* will also occur.

Because multiple opioid receptors mediate analgesia, development of selective narcotics showing no cross-tolerance is now a possibility. Preliminary evidence indicates that patients tolerant to μ_1-selective drugs can be switched to a δ-selective compound with restoration of analgesia.

The continued use of narcotic analgesics frequently results in physical dependence in the patient taking the drug; thus, the cessation of drug intake will produce a characteristic *abstinence syndrome.* The symptoms of withdrawal from opioids differ from those observed during withdrawal from other CNS depressants. Signs of autonomic nervous system hyperactivity, including diarrhea, vomiting, chills, fever, lacrimation, and rhinorrhea, are quite prominent. Tremor, abdominal cramps, and abdominal pain also may be pronounced. Withdrawal from opioids is usually not life threatening.

The onset and duration of the abstinence syndrome that follows opioid withdrawal are determined by the pharmacokinetic profile of the particular agent being used. Signs indicating abstinence from *morphine* appear 8 to 12 hr after the last dose and reach peak intensity in 36 to 72 hr. In contrast, the abstinence syndrome associated with withdrawal from meperidine, a shorter-acting drug, usually develops within 3 hr after the last dose, peaks within 8 to 12 hr, and then declines. The abstinence syndrome develops more slowly after abrupt withdrawal of methadone, a long-acting analgesic. Its onset is seen after 24 to 48 hr; withdrawal is generally more prolonged but less intense.

During abstinence from any of the opioids, drug-seeking behavior is quite prominent. Diagnosis and treatment of opioid dependence are discussed in detail in Chap. 41.

Opioid Analgesics: Individual Agents

Preparations and dosages for the agents discussed below are described in Table 39-2.

Morphine

Pharmacological Actions

Although morphine was the first opioid analgesic to be introduced into medicine, it still remains the standard for comparative studies in the evaluation of new analgesics. While many of the recently developed opioids may be considered its equal, it is doubtful that any of them are clinically superior. Extensive consideration is given here to the pharmacological spectrum of activity of morphine. The properties of the other narcotic analgesics are then compared and contrasted with those of morphine.

CENTRAL NERVOUS SYSTEM In most people, morphine produces sedation and drowsiness, although excitation occasionally occurs. The level of sedation is not as deep as that produced by sedative-hypnotic agents, however, and although patients may doze, they can be aroused readily. The feeling frequently described as "mental clouding" is experienced in individuals receiving morphine, whether or not pain is present. This sensation accompanies the drowsiness and is characterized by inability to concentrate, difficulty in formulating thoughts, apathy, and lethargy. In patients experiencing pain, mood changes, such as euphoria, are sometimes produced. In pain-free individuals, however, either euphoria or a *dysphoric* state characterized by mild anxiety or fear may follow the administration of initial doses.

A prominent effect of initial doses of morphine is nausea. Two actions of the drug contribute to the production of this unpleasant effect. The first is a direct stimulation of the CTZ of the medulla oblongata, and the second is an increase in vestibular sensitivity. The latter action, in particular, contributes to the nausea, more in ambulatory than in sedentary patients. Nausea generally subsides as morphine therapy is continued or higher doses are used because the vomit center is then depressed.

Morphine is an effective antitussive agent. It interrupts the cough response by blocking the medullary integration of this reflex. It is generally not used for this purpose, however.

Morphine produces several centrally mediated endocrinological effects. By an action within the hypothalamus, this narcotic causes a release of antidiuretic hormone, the result of which is decreased urinary output. The slight elevation of blood sugar occurring after morphine administration is also centrally mediated. Although secretion of epinephrine from the adrenal medulla ultimately produces the hyperglycemia, an intact pathway from the brain to the adrenal medulla is necessary.

EYE Morphine produces pupillary constriction by an action on the Edinger-Westphal nucleus of the oculomotor nerve. This miotic effect can be counteracted by atropine. Unless asphyxia intervenes, large doses of morphine produce extreme miosis ("pinpoint pupils").

RESPIRATORY SYSTEM Through a direct action on the respiratory centers in the pons and medulla, morphine produces respiratory depression even at therapeutic dosages. All phases of respiratory activity, including rate, minute volume, and tidal exchange are depressed. Irregular breathing is often seen. These effects on respiration are due primarily to a reduction in respiratory center responsiveness to increases in the CO_2 tension. As the dosage of morphine is increased, progressively greater respiratory depression is produced. This occurrence may indirectly increase cerebrospinal fluid (CSF) pressure and cause cerebral vasodilation by producing an elevation in serum CO_2 tension. Hypoxic drive of respiration is also depressed, and probably by this mechanism patients with pulmonary edema lose their feeling of shortness of breath. The loss of this air hunger and fostering of greater subjective comfort may mask the more hypoxic state of the arterial blood.

Although respiratory depression is generally cited as an unfavorable aspect of narcotics, this property is useful in managing postoperative or trauma patients who obviously are suffering pain and yet require artificial ventilation. Administration of narcotics to such patients readily permits unimpeded mechanical ventilation.

CARDIOVASCULAR SYSTEM At therapeutic dosages, morphine has essentially no direct effect on the cardiovascular system. After high dosages, however, the sympathetic activity on capacitance veins of the abdomen and lower extremities is decreased as a result of an effect on brainstem centers that control sympathetic efferent activity. In patients with congestive heart failure, this response can be used to decrease acutely the venous return to the heart and thus permit a more efficient contractile state, because preload and myocardial fiber tension are reduced.

GASTROINTESTINAL SYSTEM The resting tone of the smooth muscle of the stomach, small intestine, and large intestine is increased by morphine. In the stomach, this increase in tone is associated with decreased motility and delayed passage of the gastric contents to the small intestine. In both the small and large intestines, morphine induces spasm and markedly decreases propulsive peristaltic contractions; the latter effect slows the passage of material through the intestines and results in more complete reabsorption of water from the bowel contents. Constipation is the result of these actions of morphine.

Morphine also produces spasm of the smooth muscle lining the biliary tract. Biliary secretion is diminished, and biliary tract pressure markedly increases. The resulting symptoms range from epigastric distress to acute biliary colic.

GENITOURINARY SYSTEM Therapeutic dosages of morphine increase the tone and produce spasm of the smooth muscle in the genitourinary tract. This action and a centrally mediated, morphine-induced release of antidiuretic hormone contribute both to a decrease in urine volume and to urinary retention.

Therapeutic dosages of morphine do not affect normal uterine contractions appearing during labor. However, morphine will reverse uterine hyperactivity.

Absorption, Metabolism, and Excretion

Although morphine can be absorbed from the gastrointestinal tract after oral administration, a significant amount fails to reach the general circulation because of the *first-pass effect* (i.e., intestinal and hepatic metabolism). After entering the bloodstream, morphine is rapidly distributed throughout the body. Because of its basic character and its limited ionization at blood pH, it readily enters intracellular sites.

As is true of many other agents with marked central actions, morphine shows no special affinity for the brain; however, only small amounts are required to elicit pharmacological effects. In this regard, morphine administered to a pregnant woman before delivery readily passes the placenta and the immature blood-brain barrier of the fetus, thus causing more respiratory depression in the newborn than in the adult.

Metabolic transformation occurs primarily in the liver. Some morphine is converted to normorphine, and both compounds are then conjugated either as the monoglucuronide or the diglucuronide. Both metabolites are excreted in the urine.

Clinical Uses

The primary therapeutic use of morphine, of course, is in the abatement of moderate to severe pain. Morphine is more effective in relieving continuous dull pain than sharp intermittent pain, but at higher doses even the severe pain accompanying renal or biliary colic can be alleviated.

Consideration of the possibility of the development of tolerance and physical dependence (see the previous discussion) should not deter the physician from prescribing morphine to the terminally ill patient when indicated. For the drug to remain effective, dosages should not be increased more than is necessary to keep the patient comfortable. However, at the terminal stages of a disease,

when pain may become more severe, such procedures as nerve block by alcohol or neurosurgical intervention may be required.

The mode of administration of analgesics can be crucial to their effectiveness. The usual adult parenteral dose of morphine sulfate either intramuscularly (IM) or subcutaneously (SC) for moderate to severe pain is 10 mg per 70 kg of body weight every 4 to 5 hr. To relieve the dyspnea of congestive heart failure, morphine is usually given intravenously (IV) in increments of 2 to 4 mg while monitoring arterial blood gas tension to ensure adequate ventilation and oxygenation. It can also be given IV for severe postoperative pain, cardiac pain, and renal colic. Morphine can be taken orally in doses up to 30 mg, but its effectiveness as an analgesic is considerably less than that following parenteral administration. However, orally administered morphine is effective in controlling diarrhea because of its direct actions on the gastrointestinal tract to delay transit. Several opioids, including morphine, are administered either intrathecally or epidurally for postoperative pain and in situations in which pain is not controlled by traditional modes of administration. Other nontraditional procedures in the administration of analgesics have yielded promising results in the treatment of pain. First, a procedure in which the patient self-administers opiates through an infusion pump when needed, called *patient-controlled analgesia* (PCA), has been particularly useful in relieving pain. In addition to allowing the patient access to the analgesic when needed, the effectiveness of PCA is believed to be the result of the patient gaining perceived control over the pain. Second, the practice of administering analgesics and anesthetics before invasive procedures dramatically reduces both postsurgical pain and the need for additional analgesics.

Adverse Reactions

Most unwanted effects of morphine are a direct extension of its pharmacological actions. These include respiratory depression, nausea, vomiting, dizziness, mental clouding, constipation, and biliary spasm. Although allergic phenomena, predominantly skin rashes, may appear in some instances, their incidence is quite low.

Acute morphine poisoning is most frequently the result either of clinical overdosage or of accidental overdosage by addicts. *The cardinal toxic effect of morphine is respiratory depression.* This effect far outweighs all other adverse effects. The triad of coma, pinpoint pupil, and marked depression of respiration is generally diagnostic of morphine overdosage. Soon after the appearance of toxicity, the skin is clammy and pale, later becoming cyanotic. Respiration is slow, shallow, and irregular. Heart rate is slow, and blood pressure is somewhat low, but shock usually occurs only as a terminal event.

The pure narcotic antagonist naloxone (see the following discussion) rapidly reverses morphine poisoning.

Table 39-2. Analgesics Used for Moderate to Severe Pain

Drug	Trade name	Route	Dose (mg)	Dosing intervals (hr)	Preparation	Comments
μ-Opioids						
Morphine sulfate		IM, SC po	10 10–30	4–5 4–7	Injectable concentrations of 8, 10, 15 and 30 mg/ml	Standard for comparison of μ-opioid analgesics
Codeine		IM po	130 200	4–6	30- and 60-mg tablets	Traditionally used to treat moderate pain Higher doses produce more side effects than morphine
Hydromorphone	Dilaudid	IM, SC po	1.2 7.5	4–5 3–4	The hydrochloride is available as 1-, 2-, 3-, and 4-mg tablets and ampules containing 2, 3, and 4 mg	Like morphine but shorter duration of action Better oral absorption than morphine
Levorphanol	Levo-Dromoran	IM, SC po	2–3 4	4–6 4–6	2-mg tablets and 2 mg/ml for injection	Pharmacology like morphine May accumulate like methadone
Heroin		IM, SC	3–5	4–5	Not available	Not approved for use in the US
Hydrocodone	Hycodan	po	5–10	4–5	Used in combination with other agents for analgesia, antitussive and antipyretic effects	Morphine-like Traditionally used to treat moderate pain
Oxymorphone	Numorphan	IM, SC	1–1.5		Injectable and suppository forms	Morphine-like
Meperidine	Demerol Pethidine	IM, SC po	75–100 75–100	3–4 3–4	Tablets contain 50 or 100 mg Ampules contain 50 or 100 mg/ml Disposable syringes contain 50, 75, or 100 mg/ml	Less constipating than morphine
Fentanyl	Sublimaze	IM	0.1	1–2	50 μg/ml	*Innovar* represents a combination of fentanyl citrate (50 μg/ml) and droperidol (2.5 mg/ml) Fentanyl has also been used intrathecally, epidurally, and postoperatively

		Route	Dose	Duration (hr)	Preparation	Comments
Sufentanil	Sufenta				50 µg/ml	Has also been used intrathecally, epidurally, and postoperatively
Alfentanil	Alfenta				500 µg/ml	Has also been used intrathecally, epidurally, and postoperatively
Methadone	Dolophine HCl	IM po	2.5–10 20	4–6	5- and 10-mg tablets 10-mg/ml ampules	Highly effective orally Like morphine, may accumulate with continual dosing, causing sedation Oral doses of 40–100 mg used daily for maintenance therapy of opioid addicts
Opioid Agonist-Antagonists and Partial Agonists						
Pentazocine	Talwin	IM, SC po	50–60 180	4–6 4–7	Ampules containing 30 mg/ml See Table 39-3 for mixtures	Shorter duration but faster onset than morphine
Pentazocine/naloxone	Talwin Nx	po	180	4–7	50 mg pentazocine base and 0.5 mg naloxone base	Naloxone is added to minimize the possibility of abuse
Nalbuphine	Nubain	IM, SC, IV	10	4–6	10- or 20-mg/ml injectable solution	May precipitate withdrawal in opioid-dependent individuals
Butorphanol	Stadol	IM	2	4–6	1- and 2-mg/ml injectable solutions	May precipitate withdrawal in opioid-dependent individuals
Buprenorphine	Temgesic, Buprenex	IM Sublingual	0.3–0.4 0.8	4–6 5–6	0.3-mg/ml injectable solution	A partial agonist
Indole derivative						
Ketorolac tromethamine	Toradol	IM	15	6		Loading dose is 30 mg

Key: IM = intramuscular; po = by mouth; IV = intravenous; SC = subcutaneous.

Drug Interactions

Several groups of centrally acting drugs alter the effects of therapeutic doses of morphine. Monoamine oxidase (MAO) inhibitors, barbiturates, alcohol, tricyclic antidepressants, and the phenothiazines can enhance the CNS depressant effects of morphine. The degree of analgesia produced by morphine also may be increased by these drugs, although coadministration of certain phenothiazines will result in a reduction of morphine-induced analgesia.

Preparations and Dosage

Morphine is most commonly prescribed in the form of its water-soluble salt, morphine sulfate. Both preparations and doses according to route of administration are presented in Table 39-2. Precise dosage should be determined on an individual basis. Several formulations containing morphine are available for the treatment of diarrhea, including paregoric (camphorated opium tincture). However, these preparations are no longer recommended. As discussed later, meperidine congeners have largely replaced these opium preparations.

Codeine

As with morphine, codeine occurs naturally in opium and is an alkaloid of the phenanthrene series. This narcotic is much less potent than morphine; a parenteral dose of 120 mg is required to produce analgesia equivalent to that of 10 mg morphine. The oral-parenteral potency ratio of codeine, however, is much higher than that of other narcotics.

Codeine is one of the few narcotics used therapeutically for suppressing cough. Effective dosages are usually somewhat lower than those required for analgesia. The highest dose found in prescription cough preparations amounts to 20 mg; for less severe cases, over-the-counter liquid preparations can be obtained by signing a registry.

Parenteral use of codeine for pain relief offers no advantages over morphine. It does have good oral efficacy for the abatement of mild to moderate pain, as shown in Table 39-1.

Acute overdose with codeine is more commonly seen in children than adults. As is true of morphine, respiration is depressed and the patient may become comatose. In contrast to morphine, poisoning by codeine occasionally leads to the production of seizures. As in the case of morphine, overdose is treated with an opioid antagonist.

Preparations of codeine phosphate and codeine sulfate are described in Table 39-1. Since opioids and nonopioids exert different actions on pain pathways, combinations have proved to be highly effective in producing analgesia with reduced side effects. Numerous preparations containing codeine phosphate and a nonopioid analgesic are available (Table 39-3). For example, a 65-mg dose of codeine alone is equivalent to approximately 32 mg codeine in combination with 325 mg aspirin.

Heroin

Although heroin is still used clinically in England, it was banned in the United States in 1906, only 8 years after its introduction. Heroin's pharmacological actions resemble those of morphine in that it is rapidly hydrolyzed to morphine after administration. Heroin is more lipid soluble than morphine, penetrates the CNS more rapidly, and is approximately twice as potent as morphine. However, heroin does not appear to have any therapeutic advantages over other opioids.

Hydromorphone

Hydromorphone is a semisynthetic derivative of morphine that has clinical usefulness. It is 10 times more potent than morphine as an analgesic, and its respiratory depressant effect is correspondingly greater. In equieffective doses, the pharmacological actions of hydromorphone are similar to those of morphine.

Levorphanol

Levorphanol is about five times more potent than morphine, both as an analgesic and as a respiratory depressant. The pharmacology of levorphanol closely resembles that of morphine. The only advantages this narcotic has over morphine are its ability to produce less nausea and vomiting and its greater oral-parenteral potency ratio.

Meperidine

Meperidine is primarily a μ-agonist, so that its pharmacological profile resembles that of morphine. Although it is 10 times less potent than morphine, equieffective doses produce the same degree of analgesia, sedation, and respiratory depression. The spasmogenic effect of meperidine on the gastrointestinal and biliary tracts, however, is much less pronounced than that of morphine. In contrast to morphine, meperidine has no antitussive effect.

Although morphine administration reverses the hyperactivity of uterine contractions produced by oxytocics, meperidine increases the force of oxytocic-induced contractions. Unlike morphine, meperidine given during labor or before delivery produces no more respiratory depression in the newborn than in the mother. The principal disadvantages associated with its clinical use for relief of pain are its short duration of action and poor therapeutic ratio.

In contrast to morphine, meperidine toxicity may be characterized by signs of tremor, delirium, hyperactive reflexes, and possibly convulsions in addition to coma and

Table 39-3. Nonopioid and Opioid Analgesic Mixtures

Ingredients	Quantity (mg)	Common trade names
Acetaminophen +	300–650	Empracet with Codeine Phosphate, Phenaphen with Codeine\Phenaphen-650
Codeine	7.5–60	with Codeine, Tylenol with Codeine
Acetaminophen +	325–700	Lortab, Lortab 5, Lortab 7, Vicodin
Hydrocodone bitartrate	2.5–7	
Acetaminophen +	300	Demerol APAP
Meperidine hydrochloride	50	
Acetaminophen +	325–500	Percocet, Percodan, Percodan-Demi, Tylox
Oxycodone hydrochloride	2.25–5	
Acetaminophen +	650	Talacen
Pentazocine hydrochloride	28	
Acetaminophen +	325–650	Darvocet-N, Dolene AP-65, Lorcet, Propacet 100, Wygesic
Propoxyphene salt	32–100	
Aspirin +	325	Ascriptin with Codeine, Aspirin with Codeine, Empirin with Codeine,
Codeine	15–60	
Aspirin +	325	Percodan, Percodan-Demi
Oxycodone	≈2.5–5	
Aspirin +	325	Talwin Compound
Pentazocine hydrochloride	14	
Aspirin +	325–389	Darvon Compound, Darvon and Dolene Compound-65, Darvon-N
Caffeine	32.4	with ASA
Propoxyphene salt	32–100	

respiratory depression. These toxic symptoms are reflective of meperidine's greater central excitatory component; meperidine is similar to codeine in this regard. The severity of the symptoms is related to the duration of exposure to the drug. The presentation of mixed symptoms (e.g., stupor and convulsions) in addicts taking large doses of meperidine is quite common. As with morphine, meperidine overdosage can be reversed by naloxone.

Two meperidine congeners have gained widespread acceptance for managing diarrhea. Diphenoxylate salts are highly insoluble in aqueous solutions, which diminishes their abuse potential. However, they are effective orally as antidiarrheal agents because of their direct actions on the gastrointestinal tract. *Lomotil* represents a combination of diphenoxylate hydrochloride and atropine sulfate, and is available in both tablet (2.5 mg diphenoxylate and 25 μg atropine sulfate) and liquid forms. Loperamide (*Imodium*), also a meperidine derivative, is an effective antidiarrheal agent and is poorly absorbed after oral administration. It is available as capsules and as a liquid.

Fentanyl

Fentanyl is a synthetic μ-opioid that is structurally related to meperidine. It is approximately 80 times more potent than morphine as an analgesic. Its duration of action, however, is shorter than that of either morphine or meperidine.

Fentanyl is used to aid the induction and maintenance of inhalational anesthesia and to supplement regional and spinal anesthesia. It is administered either alone or in combination with the butyrophenone droperidol (see Chap. 31) or a benzodiazepine, such as diazepam. When used alone, its greatest advantage over either morphine or meperidine is the very short plasma half-life ($t_{1/2}$: 20 min), and hence the ease of safely titrating the drug intravenously to counter the patient's perception of pain.

Adverse reactions to fentanyl administration are similar to those caused by morphine. In addition, fentanyl has been known to produce muscular rigidity and apnea.

Sufentanil

Sufentanil is a synthetic opioid related to fentanyl. This opioid is about seven times more potent than fentanyl and has a slightly more rapid onset of action. Although there have been claims that recovery from anesthesia and ventilatory depression after sufentanil is more rapid than after fentanyl, in clinical use there appears to be no real difference. Sufentanil Citrate (*Sufenta*) is sold in ampules containing 50 μg/ml of drug.

Alfentanil

Alfentanil is a slightly more potent congener of fentanyl and has a shorter duration of action. Although the incidence of nausea and vomiting appears to be less after administration of alfentanil, other common adverse reactions appear to occur just as frequently.

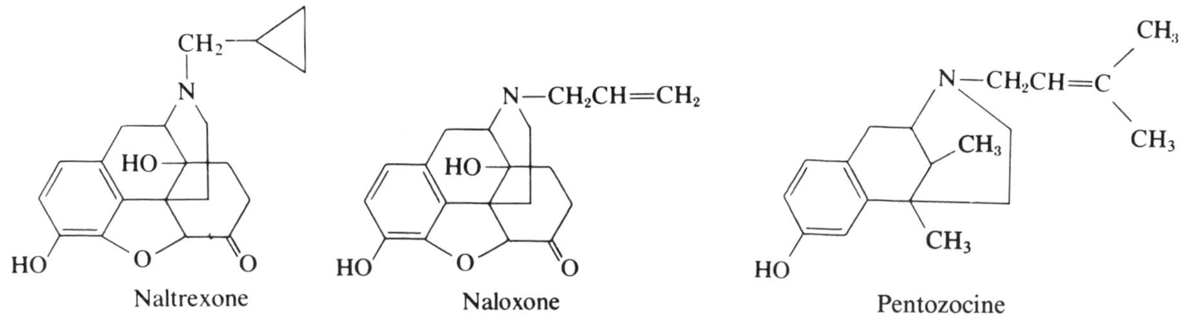

Figure 39-6. Opioid antagonists.

Methadone

The pharmacological activity and toxicity of methadone are very similar to those produced by morphine since it is primarily a μ-agonist. The principal differences between these two narcotics reside in their physicochemical properties. *Unlike morphine, methadone is highly effective after oral administration.* This agent also has a much longer duration of action than morphine. Because subcutaneous administration may cause local irritation, intramuscular injection is preferred when repeated doses are required.

Dextropropoxyphene

Although related structurally to methadone, dextropropoxyphene (*d*-proxyphene) is effective only in alleviating mild to moderate pain (see Table 39-1). Its spectrum of activity is similar to codeine's. Equieffective doses produce essentially the same degree of nausea, drowsiness, and gastrointestinal side effects as is found with codeine. Overdosages of dextropropoxyphene, like those of codeine, may cause convulsions and marked respiratory depression. The abuse liability of dextropropoxyphene is qualitatively similar to that of codeine.

Dextropropoxyphene is available as hydrochloride and napsylate salts either alone or in combination with acetaminophen, caffeine, or aspirin (Table 39-3).

Opioid Antagonists

General Characteristics

Chemistry

One structural change that converts a narcotic agonist to an antagonist is alkylation of the piperidine nitrogen. For example, when the methyl group on the piperidine nitrogen of morphine is replaced by an unbranched three-carbon side chain (e.g., propyl, allyl, or isopropyl), the compound becomes a narcotic antagonist. The *N*-ethyl and *N*-butyl compounds, however, have little agonistic or antagonistic activity. As the length of the chain increases to amyl or hexyl substituents, agonistic activity is restored.

The two narcotic antagonists currently used clinically, naloxone and naltrexone, are the *N*-allyl and methylcyclopropyl analogues of oxymorphone, respectively. The weak antagonist pentazocine has a dimethylallyl group on the nitrogen atom. See Fig. 39-6 for the structures of these three agents.

A second structural change considered necessary in order to produce compounds completely devoid of agonistic narcotic activity is the presence of a 14-hydroxyl group in the molecule. Both naloxone and naltrexone exhibit this change.

Mechanism of Action

The narcotic antagonists were formerly thought to act through their ability both to combine with the same receptor as do the narcotics and to displace the agonist from the receptor. However, it is now recognized that the effects of the narcotics are mediated by multiple opioid receptors (see above). Narcotic antagonists that are completely devoid of agonistic activity, such as naloxone and naltrexone, are capable of antagonizing the effects produced by narcotics at μ_1-, μ_2-, κ-, and δ-receptors. The affinity of these antagonists for the μ-receptors is 10- to 20-fold greater than for the κ- and δ-receptor sites. Some of the effects of narcotics at σ-receptors are antagonized by naloxone, while others are not.

Pure Narcotic Antagonists

Naloxone

When administered *alone* over a wide dose range, either acutely or chronically, naloxone produces no major physiological or subjective effects. When given *after* a narcotic analgesic has been administered, however, the effects produced by the narcotic (e.g., analgesia, respiratory depression) are promptly reversed. In this regard, naloxone is much more effective parenterally than orally since its onset of action is often noted within a few minutes after intravenous administration. After both oral and parenteral administration, its duration of action is relatively short and therefore several doses may be necessary to effectively treat narcotic toxicity. *Naloxone is the drug of choice for narcotic overdosage.*

Naloxone hydrochloride injection (*Narcan*) is available both as single ampules and as multiple-dose vials containing 400 μg/ml.

Naltrexone

As with naloxone, *naltrexone is virtually devoid of agonistic activity* when administered alone. It also promptly abolishes the actions of a narcotic analgesic when administered either before or after the narcotic. Naltrexone is effective orally and has a duration of action that is much longer than that of naloxone.

Naltrexone has recently been approved for use in the long-term treatment of addiction to heroin or other narcotics. The rationale for its use is discussed in Chap. 41.

Naltrexone hydrochloride is marketed under the trade name of *Trexan*. To avoid narcotic withdrawal symptoms, addicts must first be detoxified from opioids. In clinical practice large doses are usually administered three times a week to enhance compliance.

Nalmefene

Nalmefene is a new antagonist that is more potent than naloxone.

Opioid Agonist-Antagonists and Partial Agonists

Pentazocine

Pentazocine is one of the many compounds synthesized as part of a deliberate effort to develop an effective analgesic with little or no abuse potential. This agent presumably produces narcotic analgesia and sedation by an interaction with κ-receptors. It also exerts weak opioid antagonistic activity by an interaction with μ-receptors, for which it has low affinity. The morphine-like euphoria seen after low doses is presumably also due to an interaction with μ-receptors. Pentazocine may thus be a weak partial agonist at the μ-receptor. The dysphoric and psychotomimetic-like side effects observed after higher doses are produced by an action at σ-receptor sites.

Pharmacological Actions

The pattern of central effects produced by pentazocine is generally similar to that of the narcotics and includes analgesia, sedation, and respiratory depression. Unlike morphine, increasing the dosage does not produce proportionately as great a degree of respiratory depression. Nausea and vomiting also are less marked than after morphine administration.

Pentazocine does not antagonize the respiratory depression produced by narcotics, but it does reduce the analgesia. However, after its administration to patients regularly treated with narcotics, acute withdrawal symptoms occur.

The cardiovascular responses to pentazocine differ somewhat from those seen after narcotic administration. Therapeutic dosages generally cause an increase in blood pressure and heart rate. The effects of pentazocine on the gastrointestinal tract are qualitatively similar to those of morphine. Constipation, however, is less marked.

Absorption, Metabolism and Excretion

Pentazocine (*Talwin*) is absorbed well after oral administration. Intramuscular administration produces an effective analgesia in 30 to 60 min that lasts 2 to 3 hr. The duration of action of pentazocine is shorter than that of morphine. Inactivation occurs by hepatic metabolism, with the production of a glucuronide that is then excreted in the urine.

Clinical Uses

Pentazocine is most effective in treating moderate pain and is less effective than morphine for severe pain. It has been used in obstetrics as a preoperative analgesic and sedative and to relieve pain associated with rheumatoid arthritis and myocardial infarction. The last-named is not a preferred use since pentazocine may simultaneously increase pulmonary arterial and central venous pressure and thus increase cardiac work.

Adverse Reactions

Clinical use of pentazocine at prescribed dosages occasionally may produce psychotomimetic-like effects. These range from uncontrollable or weird thoughts, anxiety, and nightmares to actual hallucinations. Such symptoms occur more regularly after higher doses.

The clinical picture of pentazocine overdosage has not been well defined, but it is generally similar to that of other analgesics. High dosages produce marked respiratory depression, increased blood pressure, and tachycardia. Because some formulations of pentazocine contain significant amounts of either aspirin or acetaminophen, symptoms characteristically accompanying overdosages with these agents may also be observed.

Tolerance and Physical Dependence

After continued use, some degree of tolerance develops to both the analgesic and the subjective effects of pentazocine. The withdrawal syndrome seen after cessation of chronic pentazocine administration has some of the characteristics of narcotic withdrawal, including autonomic signs that are milder in degree. Other unique signs of withdrawal are seen as well, including sensations of itching and light-headedness. Abstinence from pentazocine prompts drug-seeking behavior.

When pentazocine was originally released for general use, it was not considered to have significant abuse potential. After some time, however, instances of its abuse by *parenteral* administration were reported. However, pentazocine is still not included in the list of agents subject to control under the narcotic laws.

Nalbuphine

Nalbuphine (*Nubain*) (Fig. 39-7) is a compound that is structurally related to both the potent narcotic oxymorphone and the widely used narcotic antagonist naloxone. This agent appears to interact at opioid receptors within the brain in a manner similar to pentazocine, although its effects at σ-receptors appear to be lesser in degree.

Pharmacological Actions

Nalbuphine is equipotent with morphine in the production of analgesia, and has the same time of onset and duration of action as morphine. As with pentazocine, increasing the dose does not proportionately increase the degree of respiratory depression. Indeed, in the case of nal-

Figure 39-7. Nalbuphine and butorphanol.

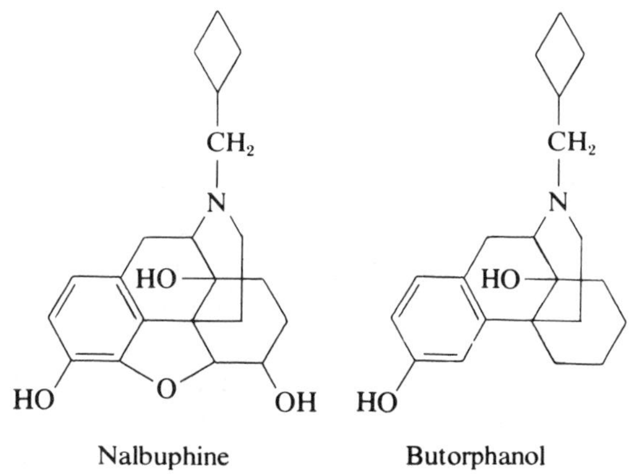

Nalbuphine   Butorphanol

buphine, a ceiling effect on respiratory depression is reached after about three times the analgesic dose. As with pentazocine, low doses produce morphine-like euphoria, while high doses cause dysphoric effects.

Nalbuphine is 10 times more potent than pentazocine in terms of narcotic antagonistic activity. Similar to pentazocine, nalbuphine may precipitate withdrawal signs in patients taking morphine-like narcotics.

Unlike pentazocine, nalbuphine does not produce increased blood pressure and tachycardia. The most frequent adverse reaction is sedation. Nausea and vomiting may occur less frequently.

Nalbuphine, like pentazocine, has a low abuse potential, but after abrupt discontinuation of long-term use withdrawal symptoms may appear.

Clinical Uses

Nalbuphine is indicated for the relief of moderate to severe pain. It also is used as a supplement to balanced anesthesia, for analgesia preoperatively and postoperatively, and for obstetrical analgesia.

Butorphanol

Butorphanol (*Stadol*) (Fig. 39-7) is a member of the phenanthrene series. This agent acts as an agonist at κ- and σ-receptors and as a weak antagonist at μ-receptors.

Pharmacological Actions

Butorphanol is five times more potent than morphine in the production of analgesia, but has the same onset and duration of action as morphine. A ceiling effect on the degree of respiratory depression occurs after about twice the usual therapeutic dose. The duration of respiratory depression, on the other hand, is dose related. Butorphanol does not produce morphine-like euphoria.

Butorphanol is 30 times more potent than pentazocine in exerting antagonistic activity. Butorphanol may precipitate withdrawal from morphine-like narcotics.

Like pentazocine, butorphanol may produce increases in blood pressure and heart rate. The most frequently observed adverse effect is sedation; nausea and vomiting occur less frequently.

Butorphanol has a low abuse liability that is probably less than that of pentazocine. Ex-narcotic addicts offered butorphanol do not like it.

Clinical Uses

Butorphanol is indicated for the relief of moderate to severe pain. This agent is used in balanced anesthesia and for both preoperative and postoperative analgesia.

Buprenorphine

Buprenorphine is the latest narcotic derived from the phenanthrene series. This agent acts as a partial agonist at μ-receptors. It appears to possess no κ- or σ-activity.

Pharmacological Actions

Buprenorphine (*Buprenex*) is highly lipophilic and is 20 to 30 times more potent than morphine in the production of analgesia. Although the duration of analgesia is only slightly longer than that of morphine after comparable doses, effects such as miosis and respiratory depression persist well after analgesia has disappeared. As with some of the above agents, however, respiratory depression reaches a ceiling at relatively low doses. Buprenorphine differs from other agonist-antagonists in that the subjective effects associated with its use resemble those of morphine at all analgesic doses.

As a partial agonist, buprenorphine does possess antagonistic activity. Following buprenorphine administration, withdrawal symptoms may occur in patients maintained on morphine or related narcotics for only several weeks. Buprenorphine dissociates quite slowly from μ-receptors and this may partially explain why large doses of naloxone are needed to antagonize the respiratory depression produced by buprenorphine.

Buprenorphine does not increase blood pressure or heart rate. Sedation appears to be the major adverse effect, and nausea and vomiting may occur.

Buprenorphine has been abused by the intravenous route and is included among schedule IV controlled substances. After discontinuation of treatment with high doses of buprenorphine, a morphine-like abstinence syndrome of mild to moderate intensity appears.

Clinical Uses

Buprenorphine is indicated for the treatment of moderate to severe pain. In addition to traditional IM and SC administration, sublingual doses of 0.4 to 0.8 mg also produce effective analgesia. Sublingual doses of 6 to 8 mg buprenorphine are effective in maintenance therapy of opioid dependence.

Antitussives

From a physiological standpoint, *cough* is a mechanism whereby the respiratory passages are cleared of excess secretions and foreign material. The cough reflex is initiated through chemical or mechanical stimulation of receptors located in many parts of the respiratory tract. These receptors communicate with cough centers in the medulla by way of the vagus nerve.

Most of the drugs used for the suppression of cough act by blocking the central component of the cough reflex. Narcotics are particularly effective in this regard. The dosages required to suppress cough are generally lower than those required to produce analgesia. Codeine is the most widely used narcotic for this purpose, and it is still the standard for comparison in assessing the usefulness of new antitussives.

Dextromethorphan

Although considerable progress has been made in separating the analgesic actions of narcotics from abuse liability, antitussive activity has been completely separated from analgesic and addictive properties. Dextromethorphan, which is the *d* isomer of the methyl ether of levorphanol, is one such compound that has antitussive but not analgesic activity. It acts centrally to elevate the cough threshold and in controlled studies has been found to be as effective as codeine. In contrast to codeine, side effects such as drowsiness and gastrointestinal disturbances do not occur. The overall toxicity of dextromethorphan is low. Extremely high dosages, however, may produce CNS depression.

Dextromethorphan is widely available in over-the-counter medications. Official preparations include dextromethorphan hydrobromide, a syrup containing 3 mg/ml, and terpin hydrate and dextromethorphan hydrobromide elixir, which contains 2 mg/ml. The usual adult dose is 15 to 30 mg every 4 to 6 hr.

Levopropoxyphene

Levopropoxyphene is also a narcotic derivative with, at best, weak antitussive properties. Unlike the *d* isomer dextropropoxyphene, it is devoid of analgesic activity. Side effects associated with its use are mild and may include drowsiness, dizziness, nausea, and urticaria. The drug is available as *levopropoxyphene napsylate* (*Novrad*). Both capsules and suspensions are supplied. The average adult dosage is 50 to 100 mg every 4 hr.

Noscapine

Noscapine, one of the nonnarcotic benzylisoquinoline alkaloids present in opium, has antitussive properties but no other significant effects on the CNS in therapeutic dosages. This compound is the principal antitussive ingredient in several proprietary mixtures. The usual adult dosage is 15 to 30 mg every 4 to 6 hr.

Benzonatate

Benzonatate is a nonnarcotic antitussive compound. It is chemically related to the local anesthetic tetracaine. The antitussive effect of benzonatate appears to be mediated by an action on both central and peripheral respiratory mucosal stretch receptors. It is somewhat less effective than codeine in suppressing cough. The drug is supplied as benzonatate (*Tessalon*). The usual adult dosage is 100 mg every 4 to 6 hr.

Supplemental Reading

American Pain Society. Principles of analgesic use in the treatment of acute pain and chronic cancer pain. *Clin. Pharmacol.* 6:523, 1987.

Beaver, W.T. Nonsteroidal Antiinflammatory Analgesics and Their Combination with Opioids. In G.M. Aronoff (ed.), *Evaluation and Treatment of Chronic Pain* (2nd ed.). Baltimore: Williams & Wilkins, 1992.

Basbaum, A.I., and Fields, H.L. Endogenous pain control: Brainstem-spinal pathways and endorphin circuitry. *Ann. Rev. Neurosci.* 7:309, 1984.

Goldstein, A., and Naidu, A. Multiple opioid receptors: Ligand selectivity profiles and binding site signature. *Mol. Pharmacol.* 36:265, 1989.

Martin, W.R. Pharmacology of opioids. *Pharmacol. Rev.* 35:283, 1984.

Pasternak, G.W. Multiple morphine and enkephalin receptors and the relief of pain. *J.A.M.A.* 259:1362, 1988.

Wagner, J.C., et al. Management of chronic cancer pain using a computerized ambulatory patient-controlled analgesia pump. *Hosp. Pharm.* 24:639, 1989.

Yaksh, T.L. Opioid receptor systems and the endorphins: A review of their spinal organization. *J. Neurosurg.* 67:157, 1987.

Ethanol and Other Aliphatic Alcohols

Walter A. Hunt

Several of the aliphatic alcohols are of toxicological interest because of their use in commercial applications. Ethanol is of particular interest because of the extensive consumption of alcoholic beverages; it only has limited use as a drug.

Ethanol

Ethanol is the most widely abused drug in the world today. There are more than 10 million alcoholics in the United States alone. Excessive consumption of alcoholic beverages has been linked to as many as one half of all traffic accidents, two thirds of homicides, and three fourths of suicides and is a significant factor in other crimes, in family problems, and in personal and industrial accidents. The annual cost to the American economy has been estimated to be in excess of $86 billion in lost productivity, medical care, and property damage.

Alcoholism has been difficult to define because of its complex nature. However, a person is generally considered an alcoholic when his or her lifestyle is dominated by the procurement and consumption of alcoholic beverages and when this behavior interferes adversely with personal, professional, social, or family relations.

For the purposes of this chapter, a *light drinker* is defined as an individual who consumes an average of one drink or less per day, usually with the evening meal; a *moderate drinker* is one who has approximately three drinks per day; and a *heavy drinker* is one who has five or more drinks per day (or in the case of binge drinkers, at least once per week with five or more drinks on each occasion).

Chemistry

Ethanol (ethyl alcohol, alcohol) is a simple organic molecule composed of a single hydroxyl group and a short, two-carbon aliphatic chain, CH_3CH_2OH. The hydroxyl and ethyl moieties confer both hydrophilic and lipophilic properties on the molecule. Therefore, ethanol is an *amphophile*, a property important to its pharmacological activity.

Ethanol occurs naturally as a product of sugar oxidation by yeast (fermentation). Although the history of the introduction of ethanol is lost, it was probably discovered quite early in our history from the accidental fermentation of fruit. Most of the alcoholic beverages available today, including wines and beers, are naturally fermented beverages and are low in ethanol content. Since concentrations greater than 12 percent are toxic to yeast, fermentation is self-limiting. Beverages of higher ethanol content are produced by distillation of fermentation products. Practically all the effects produced by drinking alcoholic beverages are due to their ethanol content.

Absorption, Distribution, Metabolism, and Excretion

Absorption

After oral administration, ethanol is almost completely absorbed throughout the gastrointestinal tract. The rate of absorption is largely determined by the quantity of ethanol consumed, the concentration of ethanol in the beverage, the rate of consumption, and the composition of the gastric contents. Eating food before or during drinking retards absorption, especially if the food has a high lipid content, as occurs in some dairy products. Since ethanol is volatile, it can be absorbed by inhalation. However, this would be relevant mostly in situations where the ethanol concentration is very high, such as in a laboratory or industrial setting.

Distribution

After absorption, ethanol is distributed throughout body water. The rate of distribution to specific parts of the body depends on the degree of vascularization. In organs with high blood flow, such as the brain, liver, lungs, and kidney, equilibrium occurs rapidly. Conversely, in organs with low blood flow, such as muscle, equilibrium occurs more slowly. Although the concentration of ethanol in the blood can be quite predictable, measurements of blood ethanol, especially when the concentrations are rising, may lead to erroneous conclusions, since the values obtained can underestimate the concentration of ethanol in the brain. This fact can confound legal proceedings in drunk driving cases where blood ethanol concentrations are considered an accurate and legally acceptable determinant of the amount of ethanol consumed.

Ethanol readily passes through the blood-placenta barrier into the fetal circulation.

Metabolism

The metabolism of ethanol has been studied widely, although some steps are still incompletely understood. Ethanol is primarily metabolized in the liver by at least two enzyme systems. The best-studied and most important enzyme is zinc-dependent, alcohol dehydrogenase. Salient features of the reaction can be seen in Fig. 40-1.

Acetaldehyde is metabolized further to acetate by the enzyme acetaldehyde dehydrogenase. In combination with coenzyme A (CoA), acetate is metabolized further to carbon dioxide and water through the many reactions involved in intermediary metabolism. *The rate of metabolism catalyzed by alcohol dehydrogenase is generally linear with time, except at low ethanol concentrations, and is relatively independent of the ethanol concentration (i.e., zero-order kinetics).* The rate of metabolism after ingestion of different amounts of ethanol is illustrated in Fig. 40-2. In adults, ethanol is metabolized at about 10 to 15 ml/hr. Since the metabolism of ethanol is slow, ingestion must be controlled to prevent accumulation and intoxication. *There is little evidence that chronic ingestion of ethanol leads to a significant induction of alcohol dehydrogenase, even in heavy drinkers.*

Some populations, most notably East Asians, exhibit an unusual response after drinking ethanol. The symptoms produced are characterized by facial flushing, vasodilation, and tachycardia. These individuals apparently have a genetic deficiency in the enzyme aldehyde dehydroge-

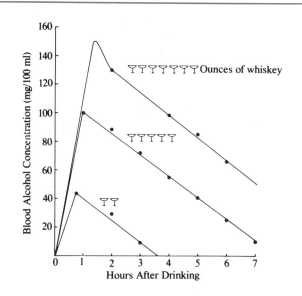

Figure 40-2. Blood alcohol concentration (mg/dl) after the consumption of different amounts of alcohol (for an adult of about 150 lb).

nase, which leads to an accumulation of acetaldehyde even after they drink relatively small amounts of ethanol.

In addition to alcohol dehydrogenase, *ethanol also can be oxidized to acetaldehyde by the microsomal mixed-function oxidase system (cytochrome P450IIEI).* Although this microsomal ethanol-oxidizing system probably has minor importance in the metabolism of ethanol in humans, it may be involved in some of the reported interactions that occur between ethanol and other drugs that are also metabolized by this system. *Microsomal mixed-function oxidases may be induced by chronic ethanol ingestion.*

Because ethanol is metabolized in the liver, it can interfere with the metabolism of other drugs by blocking microsomal hydroxylation and demethylation reactions. Drug classes whose metabolism is most affected include the barbiturates, coumarins, and anticonvulsants, such as phenytoin. *Liver damage resulting from chronic abuse of ethanol can impair the metabolism of a variety of drugs.*

Excretion

Normally, 90 to 98 percent of an ingested dose of ethanol is metabolized by the liver. Most of the remaining 2 to 10 percent is excreted unchanged in the urine and expired air. The ethanol content in the urine is normally about 130 percent of the blood concentration and is quite constant; the expired air contains about 0.05 percent of the blood ethanol level, a concentration that also is remarkably consistent. Measurements of ethanol in the breath are commonly used in legal proceedings. However, the measurements can be erroneously high as an indicator

Figure 40-1. The action of alcohol dehydrogenase. NAD = nicotinamide adenine dinucleotide; NAD H = reduced form of nicotinamide adenine dinucleotide.

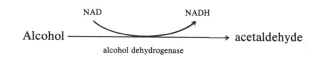

of blood ethanol concentrations if they are made shortly after consumption of an alcoholic beverage.

Mechanism of Action

Ethanol probably exerts its action on the brain by dissolving in neuronal plasma membranes rather than by acting on a specific receptor. Ethanol, because of its amphiphilic properties, can readily partition into lipids and hydrophobic portions of proteins, despite its high aqueous solubility. This property is quite similar to that described for many anesthetics (see Chap. 29). Once present in the neuronal membrane, ethanol will disorder the lipid environment, thus disrupting important cellular functions. These activities mediate the processes of electrical conduction and chemical transmission. Ethanol alters the normal movement of chloride and calcium ions involved in the regulation of electrical impulses and the release of neurotransmitters. The movement of chloride ions stimulated by γ-aminobutyric acid (GABA) is enhanced by ethanol and involves its interaction with the GABA-benzodiazepine-chloride ionophore complex (see Chap. 33). In contrast, the movement of Ca^{2+} through membranes following stimulation of N-methyl-D-aspartate (NMDA) receptors is impaired by ethanol. *Alterations in the release of specific transmitters in particular areas of the brain are presumed to underlie the manifestations of ethanol intoxication.*

Pharmacological Actions

Central Nervous System

Alcohol is primarily a central nervous system (CNS) depressant, and the degree of depression produced is directly proportional to the quantity of ethanol consumed. However, behavioral stimulation can be found after ingestion of small amounts of ethanol. This stimulation is expressed as decreased social and psychological inhibition and is most likely the result of a depression of inhibitory pathways in the brain, with a subsequent release of cortical activity. The behavioral and physiological effects associated with different blood ethanol concentrations are listed in Table 40-1.

As the blood ethanol concentration begins to increase, behavioral activation, characterized by euphoria, talkativeness, aggressiveness, and a loss of behavioral control, generally precedes the overt CNS depression induced by ethanol. At progressively higher blood ethanol concentrations, the stage of relaxation is transformed into decreased social inhibitions, slurred speech, ataxia, decreased mental acuity, decreased reflexive responses, coma, and, finally, death resulting from respiratory arrest. In moderation, however, there is no evidence that the judicious use of

Table 40-1. Behavioral and Physiological Effects of Ethanol Associated with Increasing Blood Ethanol Concentrations

Concentration	Nature of effect
<50 mg/dl	Increased sociability; euphoria
50–100 mg/dl	Disturbances in gait
	Lack of concentration
	Increased reaction time
100–150 mg/dl	Ataxia
	Impaired mental and motor skills
	Impaired short-term memory
	Slurred speech
200 mg/dl	No response to sensory stimuli
250 mg/dl	Coma
500 mg/dl	Death

small amounts of alcoholic beverages (e.g., a glass of wine with meals) is permanently harmful.

Other Body Systems

In general, ethanol, in low to moderate amounts, is relatively benign to most body systems. A moderate amount of ethanol causes peripheral vasodilation, especially of cutaneous vessels, and stimulates the secretion of salivary and gastric fluids; the latter action may aid digestion. On the other hand, ethanol consumption in high concentrations, as found in undiluted spirits, can induce hemorrhagic lesions in the duodenum, inhibit intestinal brush border enzymes, inhibit the uptake of amino acids, and limit the absorption of vitamins and minerals. In addition, ethanol can reduce blood testosterone levels, resulting in sexual dysfunction.

Ethanol is a fairly effective diuretic. This effect is believed to be caused by its ability to inhibit secretion of antidiuretic hormone from the posterior pituitary, thereby leading to a reduction in renal tubular water reabsorption. The large amount of fluid normally consumed with ethanol also contributes to increased urine production.

Therapeutic Uses

Although ethanol has little therapeutic value, it has been suggested as being useful in the treatment of almost every conceivable ailment. Certainly, its value as an aphrodisiac has been overrated, as this passage from Shakespeare correctly concludes:

> *Macduff:*   *What three things does drink especially provoke?*
> *Porter:*   *Marry, sir, nose-painting, sleep, and urine. Lechery, sir, it provokes, and unprovokes; it provokes the desire, but it takes away the performance.*
>
>   *(Macbeth, Act 2, Scene 3)*

Ethanol has frequently been used as a lay remedy for insomnia, as an analgesic, and for the relief of "head colds." The following treatment for a cold has survived for centuries: "At the first inkling of a cold, hang your hat on a bed post, drink from a bottle of good whiskey until two hats appear, and then get into bed and stay there."

There are certain accepted medical uses of ethanol, although they generally do not involve its oral consumption. By virtue of its rapid evaporation, *externally applied* ethanol cools the skin and is useful in alleviating high fever. The injection of dehydrated (absolute) ethanol in close proximity to nerves or ganglia may provide relief of pain in such conditions as trigeminal neuralgia and inoperable carcinomas through direct damage to the sensory nerve. Alcoholic beverages, in low concentrations, can stimulate appetite. This use may be valuable in alleviating anorexia, especially in geriatric patients, but it is contraindicated in patients with peptic ulcers. Finally, the inhalation of ethanol mist has been used to collapse the foam obstructing the tracheobronchial airway in acute pulmonary edema secondary to left heart failure.

Adverse Reactions

Acute Ethanol Intoxication and Hangover

Ethanol intoxication (inebriation, drunkenness) is probably the best-known form of drug toxicity. Fortunately, most patients recover with only residual hangover. While intoxicated, the individuals are threats to themselves and others, particularly if they attempt to drive or operate machinery. Although death can occur as a result of ethanol overdosage per se, it is a relatively rare occurrence. Usually the patient lapses into a coma, which prevents further intake of ethanol. Ethanol intoxication is sometimes mistakenly diagnosed as diabetic coma, schizophrenia, overdosage of other CNS depressant drugs, or skull fracture.

A diagnosis of intoxication involves legal as well as medical considerations. Most states currently use a blood ethanol concentration of 100 mg/dl or less as evidence of legal intoxication. It has been shown that persons with a blood ethanol concentration of this amount or more are six to seven times more likely to have an automobile accident than are persons who have consumed no alcohol. The approximate ethanol content of three commonly consumed beverages is shown in Fig. 40-3.

An additional feature commonly associated with excessive ethanol consumption is difficulty in regulating body temperature. *Hypothermia* frequently results, with body temperature falling toward that of the ambient environment. This problem can be particularly severe in the elderly, who normally have difficulties in regulating their body temperature.

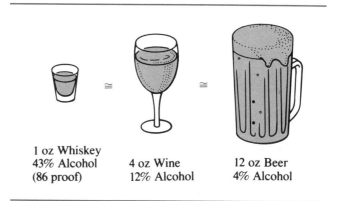

1 oz Whiskey
43% Alcohol
(86 proof)

4 oz Wine
12% Alcohol

12 oz Beer
4% Alcohol

Figure 40-3. Equivalent amounts of alcohol in three common alcoholic beverages.

One of the consequences of ethanol intoxication is the hangover. This condition is characterized by headache, nausea, sweating, and tremor. Although unpleasant, a hangover is not dangerous, even though the person having one might feel otherwise. The definitive cause of hangover is unknown; two theories have been advanced to explain it. Alcoholic beverages may contain, in addition to ethanol, small amounts of congeners of ethanol as well. These additional compounds are generally other aliphatic alcohols and aldehydes that can have their own toxic properties. A second cause, discussed in more detail below, suggests that the hangover reflects the appearance of a mild withdrawal syndrome.

Treatment

Generally, no treatment is required for acute ethanol intoxication. Allowing the individual to sleep off the effects of ethanol ingestion is the usual procedure. Hangovers are treated similarly; that is, no effective remedy exists for a hangover, except for controlling the amount of ethanol consumed. There are occasions when ethanol overdosages become medical emergencies. For example, prompt treatment is required if the patient is in danger of dying from respiratory arrest, is comatose, has dilated pupils, is hypothermic, or displays tachycardia.

Treatment for severe ethanol overdosage is generally supportive. Increased intracranial pressure can be relieved by intravenous administration of hypertonic solutions of mannitol. Hemodialysis can be helpful in accelerating the removal of ethanol from the body. Stimulants of ethanol metabolism, such as fructose, are not sufficiently effective, and *use of analeptics is not recommended because of the possibility of precipitating convulsions.*

A promising area of research involves experimental drugs that block the action of ethanol on the GABA-benzodiazepine-chloride ionophore complex. The use of these drugs is controversial because while the intoxicating properties of ethanol may be reduced in the presence of an antagonist, an individual might continue to drink and risk development of other complications of ethanol abuse.

Chronic Ethanol Abuse (Alcoholism)

Alcoholism is among the major health problems in most countries. Why alcoholism develops and why it is more prevalent in some individuals than in others is not known. There is evidence that alcoholism may be, in part, genetically determined.

Tolerance to the effects produced by ethanol frequently develops as a result of heavy consumption; both psychological and physical dependence can occur. *Dependence on ethanol, as with other addictive drugs, is expressed as drug-seeking behavior and is associated with a withdrawal syndrome that occurs after abrupt cessation of drinking.* The ethanol withdrawal syndrome is characterized by tremors, seizures, hyperthermia, hallucinations, and autonomic hyperactivity.

A number of organs are affected adversely by chronic ethanol use, the result of a *direct cytotoxic action.* Hepatic fatty infiltration and cirrhosis are common in alcoholics; cancer may develop in advanced stages of hepatic disease. Although the role of ethanol as a direct cause of liver damage has been debated for years, it appears that chronic consumption of moderate to large amounts of ethanol does lead to increased deposition of fat in liver cells. Malnutrition and vitamin deficiency, both of which often coexist in the chronic alcoholic, also may contribute to cirrhosis.

Although recent studies have not shown an association between modest ethanol consumption and an increased risk of myocardial infarction, significant alterations in myocardial contractility and muscle ultrastructure have occasionally been reported in persons who have consumed only small amounts of ethanol. A more serious clinical entity, *alcoholic cardiomyopathy,* has also been described. This condition is characterized by nonspecific electrocardiographic (ECG) abnormalities, enlarged heart, biventricular heart failure, and associated mural thrombi.

A high rate of ethanol consumption can lead to inhibition of gastric secretion and irritation of the gastric mucosa (one of every three heavy drinkers suffers from chronic gastritis). Ethanol may also cause congestive hyperemia and gastrointestinal inflammation. Since ethanol is a significant source of calories for heavy drinkers, it is not surprising that alcoholics may have several nutritional problems associated with the substitution of ethanol for food. Ethanol irritates the entire gastrointestinal tract, which may lead to constipation and diminished absorption of nutrients. Other pathological effects include pancreatitis and peripheral neuropathy. Severe gonadal failure is often found in both men and women, accompanied by low blood levels of sex hormones.

A variety of pathological problems involving the CNS have been described in chronic alcoholics, the main ones being *Wernicke's encephalopathy* and *Korsakoff's psychosis.* Wernicke's encephalopathy is characterized by mental confusion, ataxia, abnormal ocular mobility, and polyneuropathy and is a result of a thiamine deficiency. Thiamine treatment reverses this disorder. Patients with Korsakoff's psychosis have learning and memory disabilities. Cerebellar cortical degeneration can be found in some alcoholics and is characterized by spasticity, tremor, and ataxia. Lesions of the hippocampus and cerebellum are believed to be involved in these diseases. Brain damage from chronic ethanol consumption can be especially severe in the elderly and may accelerate the aging process.

Ethanol readily passes across the placenta and into the fetal circulation. The *fetal alcohol syndrome* has three primary features: *microcephaly, prenatal growth deficiency,* and *short palpebral fissures.* Other characteristics include postnatal growth deficiency, fine motor dysfunction, cardiac defects, and anomalies of the external genitalia and inner ear. Significant mental retardation, which is found in a high proportion of children born to alcoholic women, has been linked to malformation of the hippocampus. A definite risk of producing fetal abnormalities occurs when ethanol consumption by the mother exceeds 3 oz daily, the equivalent of about six drinks. The best way to ensure against the development of fetal alcohol syndrome is for women not to drink during pregnancy.

Treatment

The immediate concern in the treatment of alcoholics is detoxification and management of the ethanol withdrawal syndrome. It is frequently necessary to also treat for concomitant abuse of other drugs. *Benzodiazepines are the drugs of choice for the suppression of the withdrawal syndrome.* Other drug classes showing promise include β-adrenergic antagonists, α-adrenergic agonists, and dopaminergic antagonists. Generally, patients require multivitamin supplements because of dietary deficiencies. Long-term treatment of alcoholism requires complete abstinence, psychiatric treatment, and frequently support from lay organizations such as Alcoholics Anonymous.

Two approaches to preventive pharmacological treatment include aversion therapy and anticraving drugs. Aversion therapy uses drugs such as disulfiram (discussed below) to associate drinking ethanol with unpleasant consequences. Anticraving drugs are currently being developed and include serotonin uptake inhibitors, dopaminergic agonists, and opioid antagonists.

Interactions With Other Drugs

Ethanol can interact with other drugs in four distinct ways. It may (1) produce additive pharmacological actions (e.g., CNS depression); (2) inhibit the metabolism of a second, coadministered drug; (3) have its own metabolism inhibited by a coadministered compound; and (4) induce cross-tolerance to other drugs, particularly after chronic use.

Disulfiram

The action of disulfiram is a classic example of drug interaction. Disulfiram, by itself, is relatively innocuous. However, if ethanol is taken after disulfiram administration, vasodilation, pulsating headache, nausea, vomiting, severe thirst, respiratory difficulties, chest pains, orthostatic hypotension, syncope, and blurred vision may result. In certain cases, marked respiratory depression, cardiac arrhythmias, cardiovascular collapse, myocardial infarction, acute congestive heart failure, unconsciousness, convulsions, and sudden death have been reported.

Despite these potentially severe consequences, disulfiram is prescribed for some alcoholic patients and serves as an effective deterrent to ethanol intake. It is not, however, a therapeutic regimen to pursue without considerable care. *The patient must be informed of the risks involved in drinking any type of alcohol after taking disulfiram.* Not only alcoholic beverages but also cough syrups, certain sleep-inducing preparations, tonics, fermented vinegar, and certain sauces must be avoided. Obviously, given the consequences of disulfiram-ethanol interactions, patients cannot invariably be relied on to continue their drug therapy. Better derivatives are currently being developed to avoid the noncompliance problem.

The mechanism of action of disulfiram is well understood. *It interferes with the metabolism of acetaldehyde by inhibiting acetaldehyde dehydrogenase.* Thus, when ethanol is given to an individual who has previously taken disulfiram, blood acetaldehyde concentrations are increased 5 to 10 times. Most clinical signs presumably can be attributed to the accumulation of acetaldehyde.

Other drugs, such as metronidazole, griseofulvin, quinacrine, the hypoglycemic sulfonylureas, phenothiazines, and phenylbutazone can exert effects similar to those of disulfiram.

Central Nervous System Depressants

Additive pharmacological effects are seen after administration of all CNS depressants, narcotics, antianxiety agents, and antihistamines. A greater than additive effect (*potentiation*) has been reported between ethanol and the phenothiazine and butyrophenone antipsychotic drugs. Many deaths have occurred as a result of the combined ingestion of ethanol and CNS depressants.

One of the responses to chronic ethanol ingestion is the development of tolerance. Tolerance can occur not only at the cellular level but also at the metabolic level through an induction of the hepatic microsomal mixed-function oxidase system. Cellular cross-tolerance can develop be-

tween ethanol and other alcohols, barbiturates, paraldehyde, and general anesthetics. If induction of liver metabolism has occurred, the actions of some barbiturates, meprobamate, warfarin, and phenytoin may be reduced. Drugs that in themselves can induce hepatic drug metabolism or tolerance will, at least partially, reduce ethanol sensitivity.

Salicylates

Ethanol may increase gastrointestinal bleeding produced by the salicylates. It is probably advisable to restrict ethanol intake in patients who must take salicylates regularly.

Methanol

Methanol (methyl alcohol, wood alcohol, CH_3OH) is the simplest aliphatic alcohol. Although it has no therapeutic indications, methanol is widely used commercially as an industrial solvent, as an ethanol denaturant, and as a fuel. Since methanol has pharmacological properties similar to those of ethanol, it is sometimes consumed accidentally or as a substitute for ethanol, often with disastrous results (blindness, coma, or death).

Methanol is readily absorbed and distributed throughout body water. *It is metabolized at about one-seventh the rate of ethanol and is largely oxidized to formic acid.* In humans, methanol is metabolized predominantly by alcohol dehydrogenase, although other systems may play a role. Methanol poisoning appears to be primarily due to the formation of a metabolic product, such as formic acid, or possibly formaldehyde.

Methanol itself is a generalized CNS depressant that is very similar to ethanol, although it is less potent than ethanol. After an initial acute intoxication, there typically follows a period of 8 to 36 hr during which the patient is asymptomatic. A severe *acidosis* then develops. This is followed by optic damage that can lead to partial or total blindness. The ocular toxicity is caused by damage to the optic nerve. The likely agent of this toxicity is some by-product of methanol metabolism, probably formic acid.

Treatment of methanol poisoning involves counteracting the acidosis. This can be accomplished best by the infusion of sodium bicarbonate (about 3 gm/hr) until the urine pH reaches 7.5.

Since ethanol and methanol are metabolized by the same enzyme and since the toxicity of methanol is apparently related to the appearance of its metabolites, *ethanol administration has been used in the treatment of methanol poisoning.* Ethanol has a higher affinity for alcohol dehydrogenase than does methanol and therefore is preferentially metabolized by the enzyme. This reaction prevents the formation of the toxic metabolites of methanol, while allowing time for the methanol to be excreted unchanged.

Isopropanol and Other Alcohols

Isopropanol (isopropyl alcohol) is widely used as a rubbing alcohol and is readily available commercially. Although deaths have occurred following its ingestion, it is not abused to any appreciable extent.

Higher-chain alcohols, including the *butanols* and *pentanols,* are more toxic than ethanol, but these alcohols are rarely involved in poisoning.

The *dihydroxyalcohols* (glycols, diols), especially propylene glycol, are used as solvents for several drugs and cosmetics. Although the glycols can cause CNS depression as well as other toxicities, they also are not a frequent source of poisoning. *Ethylene glycol* was formerly used as a solvent for drugs, and before its toxicity was appreciated

it caused several deaths. Ethylene glycol is much more toxic than propylene glycol and should not be employed in the practice of medicine. Death has occurred from drinking antifreeze containing ethylene glycol.

Supplemental Reading

Cox, W.M. (ed.). *Why People Drink.* New York: Gardiner, 1990.

Eighth Special Report to the U.S. Congress on Alcohol and Health from the Secretary of Health and Human Services. Rockville, Md., 1993.

Hunt, W.A. *Alcohol and Biological Membranes.* New York: Guilford, 1985.

Hunt, W.A., and Nixon, S.J. (eds.). *Alcohol-induced Brain Damage.* Research Monograph #22. Rockville, Md.: National Institute on Alcohol Abuse and Alcoholism, 1993.

Litten, R.Z., and Allen, J.P. Pharmacotherapies for alcoholism: Promising agents and clinical issues. *Alcohol. Clin. Exp. Res.* 15:620, 1991.

Contemporary Drug Abuse

Brenda K. Colasanti and *Billy Martin*

History

Humans have always sought pleasure, abatement of anxiety, and other alterations in states of consciousness through the ingestion of various natural and chemical substances: Opium, eaten or smoked, has been a source of balm and nepenthe to generations; the flowering tops of hemp, the source of marijuana, were extolled for their psychotomimetic effects 6,000 years ago; coca leaves, the source of cocaine, have been harvested and chewed for their stimulant and euphoric effects for at least 12 centuries. Today, both the active ingredients and numerous synthetic preparations of these same classes of compounds are still widely used for their central nervous system (CNS) effects. In addition, a vast array of relatively new psychotropic agents, including the sedative-hypnotics and antianxiety drugs, have been found desirable.

Concern over the self-administration of drugs for their central effects did not arise until the late eighteenth century, at which time opium smoking in China came to be viewed as an economic problem because the country's silver reserves were being drained by the purchase of opium from India. The resulting effort to prevent opium importation into China by confiscation of the product culminated in the two Opium Wars of the mid-1800s.

In the United States, during the nineteenth century, the increased prevalence of opium smoking and the widespread use of morphine injected with a hypodermic needle (after the American Civil War) came to be viewed as both economic and social problems.

Characteristics of Drug Abuse

The term *drug abuse* refers to the inappropriate, and usually excessive, self-administration of a drug for nonmedical purposes. Inherent in this concept is the notion that harm is done both to the individual and society. Almost all abused drugs exert their primary effect on the CNS. Drugs with a high abuse potential have the capacity to induce compulsive drug-seeking behavior. Preoccupation with the procurement and use of a drug may become so demanding that the productivity of the user is decreased. In addition, prolonged abuse may cause chronic toxicity.

Continued use of some drugs leads to the development of physical dependence, or *addiction*, a condition in which the body needs the drug for physiological functions to remain normal. In addiction, drug-seeking behavior is pronounced. Physical dependence is revealed on cessation of drug use. This results in the manifestation of a *withdrawal*, or *abstinence*, *syndrome*, during which various physiologically abnormal signs and symptoms appear. The constellation of signs and symptoms produced is characteristic for a particular pharmacological class of drugs.

Whereas physical dependence may not develop to some abused drugs, a strong compulsion to resume use to maintain a feeling of well-being may still exist. This subjective need for a drug has been termed *psychological dependence*, or *habituation*.

There are conflicting opinions as to why progression from initial experimentation with drugs of abuse to continued reliance on them for optimal physiological and psychological functioning occurs in some individuals but not in others. It has been suggested that drug dependence reflects the existence of an underlying personality disorder. The contrasting opinion is that the drug effect itself induces a personality disorder, which then leads to continuing preoccupation with use of the drug. This latter viewpoint is based on the observation that animals given continuous access to various drugs show patterns of self-administration remarkably similar to those of human users of the same drugs. Although drug abuse has always been considered a serious problem, these concerns have been heightened in recent times because of several factors. The realization that drug abuse is not confined to a particular socioeconomic group, but is pervasive throughout society, has changed our perception of vulnerability. It is now more evident than ever that the consequences of drug abuse extend beyond the users themselves and exert direct adverse effects on the non–drug-abusing population. These effects range from impairment of mass transit operators to the spread of communicable diseases. It is now estimated that intravenous drug abuse accounts for 30 percent of all new cases of human immunodeficiency virus (HIV) and represents the primary mode of introducing this virus into the heterosexual population. The emergence of a less tolerant view of drug abuse has resulted in increased testing for the presence of illegal drugs as well as evaluation of impairment by alcohol.

While some drugs, particularly alcohol and marijuana, are used by a large segment of the population on a regular basis, the popularity of many other drugs is cyclical in nature. LSD enjoyed considerable popularity and notoriety in the 1970s, experienced a decline in use during the 1980s, but has recently reemerged in popularity. Many factors (cost, availability, desire to experiment with different agents, etc.) contribute to drug abuse. Frequently, the physician in the emergency room is first confronted with the resurgence in abuse of a particular drug. Regardless of the genesis of drug abuse or attitudes toward it, the physician is faced with the necessity of treating the associated problems of overdose, chronic toxicity, and various medical complications. The responsibility to point the way toward adequate rehabilitation and restoration to a more normal life likewise falls on the physician as well as on the other health professionals.

The complexity of understanding and treating drug abuse is further complicated by the fact that the user rarely relies on a single drug. Typically, alcoholics smoke cigarettes and almost all illicit drugs are coabused with marijuana, to name just a few common examples. Pharmacological intervention plays a very important role in treating the addict. However, the concurrent use of multiple drugs from different pharmacological classes illustrates the need to extend treatment to include behavioral modification. Likelihood of successful treatment outcome is frequently improved when pharmacotherapy is combined with some form of psychotherapy.

Controlled Substances Act

The Controlled Substances Act of 1970 was passed by the United States Congress as an attempt to decrease the incidence of drug abuse by regulating the manufacture, prescribing, dispensing, and general availability of drugs with abuse potential. To prescribe controlled substances, the physician must register annually with the Drug Enforcement Administration of the US Department of Justice. The individual physician's federal registration number must be indicated on all prescription orders for controlled substances.

Drugs considered to have abuse potential are divided into five *schedules*. Requirements for inventory control, security, and record keeping as well as for prescribing and dispensing the drugs in the various schedules are clearly spelled out in regulations. The drugs that come under the jurisdiction of the Controlled Substances Act are divided as follows:

Schedule I Substances

Drugs in schedule I are those that have *no accepted medical use* in the United States and have a high abuse potential. Schedule I substances may be used only in certain experimental situations. Some examples are heroin, marijuana, LSD, peyote, mescaline, psilocybin, and phencyclidine and its analogues.

Schedule II Substances

The drugs in schedule II have a *high abuse potential* and severe psychic or physical dependence liability. Most narcotic analgesics and preparations containing either amphetamine-like stimulants or barbiturate-like depressants fall into this class. Examples of schedule II controlled substances are opium, morphine, codeine, hydromorphone (*Dilaudid*), methadone (*Dolophine*), meperidine (*Demerol*), cocaine, oxycodone (*Percodan*), and oxymorphone (*Numorphan*). Also included under schedule II are the amphetamines, phenmetrazine (*Preludin*), methylphenidate (*Ritalin*), and certain short- to intermediate-acting barbiturates (e.g., amobarbital, pentobarbital, and secobarbital). Δ^9-Tetrahydrocannabinol (THC), the active constituent in marijuana, is also in this schedule.

Prescriptions for schedule II substances must be signed by the practitioner and may not be refilled. In the case of a bona fide emergency, an oral prescription may be accepted by the pharmacist. The practitioner must later furnish the pharmacist with a written and signed prescription order.

Schedule III Substances

The drugs in schedule III have an abuse potential that is lower than those in schedules I and II, and include compounds containing limited quantities of certain narcotic as well as nonnarcotic drugs. This group includes derivatives of barbituric acid (except those listed in another schedule), glutethimide (*Doriden*), methyprylon (*Noludar*), benzphetamine, and chlorphentermine. Paregoric is also in this schedule.

Schedule IV Substances

Schedule IV substances have an abuse potential that is lower than that listed in schedules II or III, and include the long-acting barbiturates (e.g., barbital, phenobarbital, methylphenobarbital), chloral hydrate, ethchlorvynol (*Placidyl*), ethinamate (*Valmid*), meprobamate (*Equanil, Miltown*), diazepam, chlordiazepoxide, paraldehyde, fenfluramine, diethylpropion, and phentermine.

Schedule V Substances

Although the drugs listed in schedule V may be distributed without a prescription, records pertaining to their sale must be kept by the pharmacist. These preparations usually are used for their antitussive (e.g., terpin hydrate and codeine elixir) and antidiarrheal (e.g., *Donnagel PG*) properties and contain limited quantities of certain narcotic drugs.

Opioid Abuse

The term *opioid* refers to all narcotic analgesics, both natural and synthetic, that possess morphine-like pharmacological activity. *The most abused opioid in the United States is heroin.* This agent is used by about 90 percent of all narcotic abusers. Terms commonly used by the addict to refer to heroin include "dope," "smack," and "horse." A newer form of heroin is "black tar" (also known as "tootsie roll" and "Mexican mud"), a smelly, dark-colored version of the drug that is more potent and much cheaper than conventional heroin. Preference for heroin is probably based on the ease with which it can be procured through illegal channels. The number of heroin addicts in the United States is estimated to be around 500,000 to 750,000. The annual prevalence of heroin use among high school seniors has remained at about 0.5 percent since 1979. The rate among young adults and college students has remained in the range of 0.1 to 0.2 percent.

Morphine, codeine, and hydromorphone (*Dilaudid*) rank next in frequency of abuse. Although not nearly as frequent, abuse of methadone has increased as a result of its greater availability. Similarly, dextropropoxyphene is now one of the more commonly abused narcotics. Synthetic fentanyl analogues produced by clandestine laboratories have become increasingly popular (see Designer Drugs).

A certain percentage of patients receiving narcotics for relief from pain become physically dependent on these drugs. These individuals, however, are not considered addicts and the number of such cases is not included in federal registries. *A number of physicians, nurses, and related health professionals likewise become dependent on narcotics,* and the incidence of narcotic abuse is indeed much higher in this group than in others of comparable educational background.

Patterns of Abuse

The majority of heroin users are introduced to the drug during their teens and early twenties. Over half of recorded addicts are under the age of 30. Most users are exposed to the drug initially by other users. The effects of a narcotic in the neophyte user are often quite unpleasant, with the production of nausea and vomiting and an associated dysphoria. It is estimated that fewer than half of the individuals who have tried heroin continue using it regularly.

Some people taking a narcotic for the first time experience feelings of tranquility and euphoria. Some may respond favorably only after several experiments with the drug. After rapid intravenous injection of the narcotic, users experience a warm flushing of the skin and sensations in the lower abdomen, which have been described as similar in intensity and quality to sexual orgasm. This initial effect is known most frequently as a "rush." Feelings of relaxation, contentment, and cheerfulness subsequently predominate, and a sense of tranquility and immunity from danger prevails. This second, more prolonged, euphoric effect is known as "the nod." The pharmacological properties of morphine and heroin are the same with the exception that heroin is more potent.

Frequent use of narcotics leads quite rapidly to the development of tolerance to many of the pharmacological effects (see Chap. 39), including the subjective changes. Cases in which addicts have taken up to 5 gm of heroin daily by the IV route have occasionally been reported. These data contrast sharply with the usual 3-mg SC dose of heroin given medically in England for analgesia.

The typical heroin addict, of necessity, usually supports his or her habit on less than 100 mg daily. Imported pure heroin is generally "cut" up to 24 times, by as many dealers, with such adulterants as milk sugar, mannose, and quinine, before the buyer on the street uses it. The resulting unit for purchase, a "bag," consequently contains 90 mg of material, of which an average of only 3 mg is heroin. After long-term use, most addicts will settle sooner or later on some constant daily amount of the drug. This amount, however, is usually divided into one large dose that is sufficient to achieve a high and several much smaller doses that serve only to prevent the user from feeling "down." Eventually, however, users build up such a tolerance to heroin that they can no longer finance the habit. The addict may then enter a hospital for detoxification, only to leave a week later to resume heroin use with a much lower level of tolerance.

Physical Dependence

Within 4 to 6 hr after the last parenteral dose of morphine or heroin, users who are physically dependent on these drugs become aware of the first signs of impending illness. At this time, episodes of yawning, perspiration, anxiety, and craving for the drug appear. By 8 to 12 hr after the last dose, the first clinical manifestations of withdrawal are usually noted. If further doses of the drug are not available, these signs progress and reach a peak intensity by 36 to 48 hr (see Chap. 39). The degree and intensity of the withdrawal symptoms are related to the magnitude of narcotic intake. Rhinitis, lassitude, and minor gastrointestinal discomfort are the usual symptoms. Many of the symptoms seen in more severe cases, including mydriasis, hyperthermia, and diarrhea, are the reverse of those seen following the pharmacological use of narcotics in nonaddicted patients.

Administration of a *narcotic antagonist,* such as naloxone, to individuals physically dependent on opioids results in the precipitation of an *acute abstinence syndrome.* Signs and symptoms of withdrawal develop within a few minutes after injection of the antagonist, reach a peak intensity in 30 to 45 min, and then subside within 2 to 3 hr. Such induced withdrawals in users dependent on long-acting narcotics, such as methadone, are more severe than those seen in addicts to shorter-acting agents, such as heroin. If the abstinence syndrome is brought about by lack of availability of the narcotic drug, administration of any narcotic during the withdrawal period will immediately suppress most symptoms of narcotic abstinence. However, if the abstinence is precipitated by narcotic antagonists, narcotic administration will be less effective in suppressing withdrawal signs and symptoms, since the antagonist will still be in the individual's system.

Twenty-four milligrams of heroin per day, taken over several weeks, has been considered to be the minimal amount necessary for the production of physical dependence. Clinical studies indicate that morphine dependence is maximal after doses that amount to 500 mg/day for several weeks, inasmuch as the intensity of withdrawal symptoms does not increase after higher doses.

Recently, many patients who have been admitted to detoxification facilities have not shown significant signs and symptoms of withdrawal. They evidently have had to maintain themselves on less than 24 mg/day owing to the escalating cost of drugs. Thus, the dependence on heroin in these cases is purely psychological.

With the decline in the quality of heroin, other opioids, such as hydromorphone, have become more subject to abuse. The withdrawal syndrome in hydromorphone addicts appears to be more severe than that in heroin addicts.

Concurrent Drug Abuse

In the past, heroin addicts have resorted to the use of drugs other than narcotics when heroin was not available. Today, the concurrent use of other groups of drugs on a daily basis is fairly common. Specific agents most frequently employed include alcohol, barbiturates, and glutethimide. Various antianxiety drugs also are commonly used. Simultaneous use of stimulant drugs has been reported as well.

Diagnosis

If a suspected narcotic addict is still under the influence of the last dose of the drug, diagnosis of opioid dependence cannot be made with certainty on the basis of a physical examination. Physical findings, such as miotic pupils and "needle tracks," however, may be suggestive of narcotic abuse. Chemical analysis of urine specimens for the presence of opioids or quinine may provide evidence of use. Administration of the narcotic antagonist naloxone serves as a rapid diagnostic test for physical dependence on opioids, but can be dangerous. The emergence of piloerection on the thorax, mydriasis, and simultaneous diaphoresis (profuse sweating) within 15 min is diagnostic of opioid dependence.

One of the main problems associated with opioid abuse is the high incidence of *relapse,* or return to narcotic use after a period of abstinence. For example, on the return of ex-addicts to their former environment after detoxification, conditioned patterns of behavior are again experienced and give rise once again to drug-seeking behavior.

A second factor thought to be involved in relapse is the phenomenon of *protracted,* or *secondary, abstinence.* Approximately 1 to 2 months after drug withdrawal, subtle abnormalities in various physiological characteristics appear, and these persist for 4 to 6 months. During this period, blood pressure, pulse rate, and body temperature remain slightly lowered, and the respiratory center remains hyposensitive to carbon dioxide. Subtle behavioral manifestations, such as inability to tolerate stress and overconcern for personal discomfort, are also evident.

Treatment

Two major strategies used in treating opioid addiction are withdrawal and maintenance regimens. In the case of withdrawal, the goal is to get the patient completely drug free within a relatively short time. A main consideration for the use of withdrawal therapy is whether the patient is highly motivated toward the goal of abstinence. Other indications for this treatment modality include absence of a previous history of relapse after medically supervised withdrawal, a short period of addiction (<1 year), and use of relatively low doses of the addicting drug. Ideally, withdrawal therapy should be carried out in a hospital setting.

During withdrawal therapy, methadone is usually substituted for the narcotic the patient has been taking. Methadone is used orally because it effectively suppresses opioid withdrawal, has a long duration of action, and allows the user to dissociate from the reinforcing properties of the needle. The initial dose of methadone, given orally, should be sufficient to suppress most of the abstinence symptoms. One milligram of methadone is the equivalent of approximately 1.5 mg heroin or 4 mg morphine. After stabilization of the patient on an appropriate amount of methadone, the dosage is reduced by one-half every other day. By the sixth to tenth day, the drug can be discontinued totally. If methadone is the drug the patient was initially abusing, reduction of the dose should be undertaken much more gradually (e.g., over a period of 2–3 weeks).

The α_2-adrenergic agonist clonidine is useful in treating mild dependence because of its ability to suppress the sympathetic nervous system hyperactivity that accompanies withdrawal. Clonidine can be used in patients maintained on moderate doses of methadone. It is substituted for methadone, and after 7 to 10 days of stabilization the patient is withdrawn from clonidine over a 3- to 4-day period. Clonidine has also been useful in methadone-maintained patients undertaking naltrexone treatment. A combination of clonidine and naltrexone is substituted for methadone and then clonidine is withdrawn, leaving the patient solely on naltrexone.

In patients who are dependent on a barbiturate in addition to a narcotic, simultaneous withdrawal of both drugs should be undertaken cautiously. Maintenance of the patient on methadone until barbiturate withdrawal is completed may be preferable.

The major signs of withdrawal in the *neonate* are a unique type of coarse, flapping tremors and irritability. Gastrointestinal symptoms of diarrhea and vomiting also may be present. Unusually rapid respiration, which is presumably related to an increased sensitivity of the respiratory center to CO_2, as in the adult addict, is also a very frequent sign. Treatment is aimed at alleviating the major neuromuscular symptoms. The use of paregoric in progressively decreasing doses has been advocated. Alternatively, phenobarbital or diazepam may be administered in initial dosages that are sufficient to control symptoms, with a subsequent reduction in dosage over a period of 6 to 10 days.

A second means for the treatment of narcotic addiction is *methadone maintenance.* The rationale underlying methadone maintenance therapy comprises two factors: (1) Administration of doses of oral methadone prevents the onset of withdrawal symptomatology while not affording the "rush" or euphoriant effects of intravenous heroin, and (2) methadone has a long duration of action. With this treatment modality, narcotic addicts are stabilized on a single daily oral dose of methadone, ranging from 50 to 100 mg. Initially, a dose that is just sufficient to relieve signs of withdrawal from heroin is administered. This dose is gradually increased over several weeks as tolerance develops until the maintenance dose of 50 to 100 mg is reached.

At the maintenance dose, signs of abstinence do not appear and the effects of intravenously injected heroin or other narcotics are blocked. The patient thus does not experience the alternating periods of euphoria and abstinence that are so commonly associated with the use of street heroin. Relief from the continuous necessity of procuring the drug—it is averred by proponents of methadone maintenance—allows the patient to participate in rehabilitation programs and to work.

Several problems have arisen as a result of the widespread use of the methadone-maintenance program. Because the requirement to attend a methadone-dispensing clinic daily to receive and consume medication was burdensome, some patients who demonstrated satisfactory adherence to the program regulations were permitted larger quantities and fewer clinic visits. A market subsequently developed for the illicit sale and redistribution of methadone, and the phenomenon of primary methadone abuse *without* prior heroin addiction emerged. To circumvent the problems created by methadone maintenance programs, longer-acting agents are being sought. LAAM (l-α-acetylmethadol, methadyl acetate), a long-acting μ-opioid that is metabolized to active metabolites, is currently undergoing clinical trials. It is active up to 3 days after oral administration, obviating take-home medication. It appears to be similar to methadone in all other respects. Another long-acting agent that has promise is buprenorphine. This partial μ-agonist is active by the sublingual route in some patients for as long as 48 hr. Its relatively long duration of action allows for the slow onset of a relatively mild withdrawal. Buprenorphine is preferred over agonist/antagonists, such as pentazocine, because it lacks antagonist properties that tend to precipitate withdrawal.

A treatment modality recently introduced for narcotic addiction is the chronic administration of naltrexone hydrochloride (*Trexan*), a long-acting pure narcotic antagonist (see Chap. 39), to former addicts. An oral dose of 50 mg is effective for up to 24 hr. Trials are under way with a depot formulation that will maintain the patients up to 60 days. With such treatment, the former user who subsequently succumbs to the desire to inject heroin intravenously has the anticipated drug "high" pharmacologically blocked. Theoretically, this therapy should lead to extinction of the drug-seeking behavior. Not too surprisingly, many addicts are reluctant to undergo antagonist treatment. This therapy has been most successful with highly motivated patients, such as medical professionals, and in work release programs.

Traditional psychiatric treatment has done little in the rehabilitation of former addicts. Recently, several types of therapeutic communities that involve both professionals and ex-addicts in the treatment of recently detoxified users have evolved. Some of the better known of these communities include Day-Top Lodge, Synanon, and Odyssey House. At these facilities, an attempt is made to restructure the lifestyle and orientation of the recent heroin user through leadership, self-help, and group help.

Medical problems related to drug use occur commonly in the heroin-addict population. Because women generally obtain money for the drug through prostitution, a high incidence of venereal disease is seen among women addicts. Infections frequently arising from shared needles and unhygienic procedures include septicemia, endocarditis, hepatitis, acquired immunodeficiency syndrome (AIDS), and pulmonary abscesses. Other medical complications are granulomas caused by injection of contaminants and a variety of neurological and musculoskeletal lesions that may be due to hypersensitivity reactions.

Abuse of Sedative-Hypnotics and Antianxiety Drugs

Abuse of drugs belonging to the sedative-hypnotic (Chap. 33) and antianxiety (Chap. 33) drug groups is a widespread phenomenon. It is estimated that over 2 million Americans are using such compounds without a prescription. Both older drugs, such as the barbiturates and glutethimide, and newer ones, such as the benzodiazepines, can be procured readily from illicit (street) sources. In addition, the number of prescription abusers who obtain inordinate amounts of these drugs by visits to different physicians has risen rapidly. Methaqualone was one of the most commonly abused sedative-hypnotics in the United States until its manufacture was discontinued.

Patterns of Abuse

Many people are introduced to illicitly obtained sedative-hypnotics and antianxiety drugs by friends. Initial exposure of many ultimate abusers also frequently occurs by way of a physician's prescription. In the latter case, the drug is usually taken over prolonged periods either for anxiety reduction or insomnia. The dosage is then progressively increased by the user to obtain the desired effects, and preoccupation with procurement and use of the drug ensues.

Barbiturates are known in the argot of the drug subculture as "goofballs" or "downs." Street names for individual sedative-hypnotics have been coined on the basis of the color of the dosage form. Thus, pentobarbital capsules are known as "yellow jackets," secobarbital as "red devils," phenobarbital as "purple hearts," and amobarbital as "blue angels."

Patients who take regular doses of barbiturates or benzodiazepines may exhibit no signs other than rebound insomnia or anxiety on cessation of treatment. However, individuals who abuse barbiturate-like drugs engage in intermittent sprees of gross intoxication, each spanning a period of a few days. Others ingest large quantities on a daily basis and remain chronically intoxicated. In both cases, the physiological effects resemble those of intoxication with alcohol. Signs of motor incoordination, including ataxia, nystagmus, and slowness of speech, predominate. The user exhibits a general sluggishness, difficulty in thinking, and a narrowed attention span. Emotional lability, irritability, and quarrelsomeness are also evident. The subjective effects experienced range from feelings of remarkable capability in coping with anxiety and distress to sensations of well-being, euphoria, and stimulation. The latter effects are considered to be caused by depression of CNS inhibitory pathways.

Chronic use of barbiturate-like hypnotics and antianxiety drugs results in the development both of metabolic and direct cellular tolerance to the physiological and subjective effects. *In contrast to the narcotics,* tolerance to these CNS depressants develops very slowly and is only partial. The lethal dose for chronic users is not much greater than that for the general population, and there is an upper limit of intake of these agents. In the case of the barbiturates, this limit ranges from 1.0 to 2.5 gm orally per day. Ingestion of as little as 100 mg additional barbiturate by an individual tolerant to 1 to 2 gm/day results in signs of gross intoxication.

When tolerance to the effects of a specific sedative-hypnotic agent has developed, there is also *cross-tolerance* to the effects of all other hypnotics, antianxiety agents, and alcohol. Because of the narrow margin between tolerance and toxicity, however, cross-tolerance only is apparent in the absence of high blood levels of the drug originally ingested chronically. *There is no cross-tolerance between these general CNS depressants and the narcotics.*

Physical Dependence

In contrast to withdrawal from narcotics, the withdrawal syndrome that follows termination of the chronic intake of high doses of hypnotics and antianxiety drugs is quite severe. In the case of *short-acting* agents, signs and symptoms first appear between 12 and 24 hr after the last dose. During this period, the user experiences feelings of anxiety and weakness, shows a loss of appetite, and exhibits coarse tremors. Deep reflexes may be hyperactive. Within the next 24 to 48 hr, the syndrome reaches peak intensity. Emerging symptoms include vomiting, hypotension, tachycardia, fever, fasciculations, tremor, and generalized tonic-clonic convulsions. Between the fourth and seventh day, delirium may develop, in which visual and auditory hallucinations occur. During this period of delirium, agitation and hyperthermia can lead to exhaustion and cardiovascular collapse.

With *longer-acting* hypnotics and antianxiety drugs, such as chlordiazepoxide, the onset of the withdrawal syndrome is delayed, and symptoms peak more slowly. Convulsions may not appear until the seventh day after the last dose. During abstinence from any of the hypnotics and antianxiety compounds, the signs and symptoms can be suppressed only by readministration of the agent *before* the appearance of delirium. Once delirium develops, the symptoms are relatively irreversible.

The severity of the abstinence syndrome associated with the chronic use of hypnotics and antianxiety drugs is related to the dose and duration of use. The minimal dose of the short-acting barbiturates required to produce a clinically significant degree of physical dependence is 400 mg/day for 2 to 3 months. After withdrawal from this dosage, 30 percent of subjects exhibit paroxysmal electroencephalographic (EEG) changes with few other symptoms. After withdrawal from a dosage of 600 mg/day for 2 months, 50 percent of subjects exhibit EEG changes and tremor, and 10 percent experience seizures. After withdrawal from dosages ranging from 900 mg to 2 gm/day for several months, seizures are manifested by 75 percent, and delirium by 66 percent of subjects.

Dependence on barbiturates and benzodiazepines can also occur in utero. The withdrawal syndrome, which is seen with varying severity in the newborn, is similar to that produced by the opioids but is treated with either benzodiazepines or other CNS depressants.

Concurrent Drug Abuse

People who primarily abuse sedatives and antianxiety agents also may abuse alcohol, but they are not likely to abuse narcotics. However, a large number of narcotic addicts simultaneously abuse hypnotic agents, many to the point of becoming physically dependent. A drug combination popular among this group is glutethimide and codeine. The effects of this mixture, which is known as "loads" or "hits" and is taken orally, are purportedly similar to those of injected heroin.

Sedative-hypnotics are commonly used simultaneously with amphetamine-like drugs to counteract the prolonged wakefulness produced by the latter agents. The two groups of drugs are also taken simultaneously, since the euphoric effects of amphetamine-like compounds are enhanced by certain sedatives, such as the barbiturates.

Diagnosis

The presence of the characteristic neurological signs produced by chronic intoxication with hypnotics and antianxiety drugs (see the previous discussion), together with a history of intake, should suggest to the physician the possibility of dependence on these agents. Early signs of withdrawal, such as nervousness, tremor, and weakness, might be seen instead and a positive blood or urine test for one of these agents may help support the diagnosis.

A useful diagnostic test in case of doubt consists of oral administration of two 200-mg doses of pentobarbital 6 hr apart. Diagnosis of hypnotic or antianxiety drug dependence is made if this dose fails to induce CNS depression. A high level of drug tolerance is assumed to have preexisted.

Treatment

Because of the possibility of life-threatening complications, withdrawal from hypnotics and antianxiety drugs should be carried out in a hospital setting. After diagnosis of chronic intoxication with hypnotics or antianxiety drugs, pentobarbital is administered at a dosage of 200 to 400 mg orally every 4 to 6 hr until the patient exhibits a mild state of barbiturate intoxication. After the patient has been stabilized on this initial dosage for 1 or 2 days, it can be reduced by 100 mg/day. Alternatively, the patient may be stabilized on the longer-acting barbiturate phenobarbital (90–120 mg/hr until the patient becomes slightly intoxicated), and the dosage is reduced by 30 mg/day. If withdrawal signs occur at any point during reduction of the dosage, the patient should be maintained again in a mild state of barbiturate intoxication by increasing the dosage before further reduction. Seizures constitute a medical emergency. If they occur, 100 or 200 mg pentobarbital should be given immediately and over the next several days, before further dosage reduction. Phenytoin is *ineffective* in controlling withdrawal seizures.

Rehabilitation of the abuser of hypnotics should begin during detoxification and should be continued afterward. Psychotherapy and participation in therapeutic communities formed by professionals and ex-users may be helpful.

Alcohol Abuse

Alcoholism is probably the most serious drug problem in the United States. Costs due to alcohol-related accidents, crime, damaged health, and loss of productivity have been estimated at $86 billion annually.

Most Americans have their initial experience with drinking alcohol during adolescence. Ninety percent of high school seniors have tried alcohol during their lifetimes and 30 percent report daily use. Chronic abuse of alcohol usually does not occur until much later. Several distinct patterns of alcohol abuse have become recognized. These differ mainly in the amount and frequency of alcohol consumption, the resulting degree of psychological and physical dependence, and the existence of associated physical disabilities.

The degree of physical dependence produced by chronic use of alcohol correlates only partially with the daily amount of alcohol consumed and the duration of use. Because of the constant rate of alcohol metabolism (see Chap. 40), intake over the course of the day may be distributed in such a manner that blood concentrations remain relatively low and constant. On the other hand, ingestion of only slightly higher amounts exceeds the body's metabolic capacity and results in much higher blood levels and a correspondingly greater degree of physical dependence.

The *withdrawal syndrome* occurring after cessation of alcohol intake is similar to that seen with sedative-hypnotics. In severe cases of dependence, *delirium tremens* may appear around the third day of withdrawal. Treatment of the alcohol withdrawal syndrome is best undertaken in a hospital setting.

Because the detoxified alcoholic shows a great tendency to resume alcohol abuse, plans for rehabilitation should be made before he or she leaves the hospital. Alcoholics Anonymous has probably been the most effective organization for the rehabilitation of alcoholics. Some individuals, however, may prefer the more personalized approach afforded by special clinics and communal treatment centers. The periodic drinker, in particular, may be aided by the use of disulfiram under close medical supervision.

Further details on the pharmacological effects of short-term and chronic use of alcohol are found in Chap. 40.

Abuse of Central Nervous System Stimulants

It is estimated that 6 million Americans are using cocaine and another 3 million are using other stimulants. As a result of numerous factors, the use of several of these agents has been on the decline. On the other hand, street supplies are still quite large, generated by diversion of drug company products, by importation (as with cocaine), and by illegal manufacture in home laboratories. In 1990, 8.6 percent of young adults reported use of some form of cocaine in the prior year and 1.6 reported the use of "crack," a form of free-base cocaine processed from the salt with the use of baking soda.

Street terms commonly used for oral amphetamine preparations include ".357 magnums," "20/20," "black beauties," "copilots," and "ups." Methamphetamine for intravenous use is known as "speed" or "crystal." Cocaine is commonly referred to as "coke" or "snow." Administration of cocaine through smoking the free base has been termed "baseballing" or "free-basing"; the resulting experience has been deemed "having a white tornado."

Patterns of Abuse

Some chronic abusers of CNS stimulants take the drug orally. The stimulants most widely abused in this manner are the amphetamines, methylphenidate, and phenmetrazine. The subjective effects produced after oral intake of these agents are feelings of mood elevation and euphoria and a sense of increased energy and alertness. Task performance that was affected by boredom or fatigue is markedly improved. With time, tolerance to these effects develops, and larger, more frequent, doses are taken. At this point, activity ceases to be channeled into useful task performance, and stereotyped repetitive behavior emerges. Hyperirritability, jumpiness, bruxism (grinding or gnashing movements of the teeth), touching and picking of the face and extremities, and suspiciousness become quite common. Further increase in the dose by the user at this time results in the development of a toxic paranoid psychosis.

A second group of stimulant abusers frequently take the drug parenterally. The agents most commonly abused in this manner are *methamphetamine* and *cocaine*. Some abusers of cocaine administer the drug intranasally through sniffing or "snorting." The discovery that conversion of cocaine hydrochloride to its free base, such as "crack," resulted in a product that could be smoked or volatilized had a dramatic impact on the abuse pattern of cocaine. Either "crack" or methamphetamine ("ice") is smoked in special glass pipes or in cigarettes mixed with marijuana, parsley, or tobacco.

Intravenous administration of either methamphetamine or cocaine as well as free-base cocaine smoking rapidly produces a euphoric state of great intensity. The constellation of effects is qualitatively similar to that seen after the oral route. An additional effect, known as the "rush" or "flash," occurs seconds after introduction of the solution into the vein. The sensation produced is one of intense pleasure during heightened awareness, which has been described as "an orgasm of the entire body." Physical hyperactivity subsequently ensues, and the user is unable to sit still. Stereotypical compulsive behavior, such as taking mechanical objects apart, occupies the individual for hours at a time. If the drugs are taken around the clock for 1 to 3 days, the resulting drug experience is called a "run." The user remains wide awake, and food intake is severely reduced; weight losses of 10 to 20 lb during a single run are not uncommon. The run is terminated by the "crash," which includes 24 to 36 hr of sleep. After awakening, irritability, hunger, and lethargy are intense. Another run may then be initiated. With continued runs, higher and higher doses are used to counteract tolerance, and periods of paranoia sometimes culminating in a toxic psychosis frequently intervene.

Although methamphetamine injected intravenously has a duration of action of about 2 to 3 hr, the effects of intravenous cocaine or smoked "crack" are quite brief; to maintain its euphoric effects, users must inject cocaine about every half-hour. At comparable doses, smoked free-base cocaine and intravenously administered cocaine have a similar onset and duration. In contrast, *intranasally* administered cocaine has a longer onset of action, with peak plasma concentrations reached only after about 1 hr. Use of the last-named route does not produce as intense a euphoric effect as does either the intravenous route or free-base smoking. It has accordingly been assumed that the rate of change of plasma cocaine concentrations, rather than actual blood levels, is a contributing factor to the intensity of the euphoria.

As a result of its capacity to cause profound vasoconstriction, the nasal inhalation of cocaine frequently leads to perforation of the nasal septum due to prolonged constriction of local blood vessels and subsequent tissue necrosis.

The stimulant effects of cocaine and amphetamines result from increased dopaminergic activity as a result of blockade of presynaptic reuptake. In addition, amphetamine can directly stimulate the release of dopamine. The actions of cocaine and amphetamine are most likely not confined to dopamine in that they also exert similar actions on norepinephrine and serotonin.

Dependence

Although *physical dependence does not develop after long-continued use of CNS stimulants,* a characteristic drug dependence of the amphetamine type has been recognized. A main component is the development of a strong *psychological dependence* on the subjective effects of these drugs. Other characteristics include a desire to continue taking the drug and consumption of increasing amounts to obtain greater excitatory and euphoric effects or to combat

depression or fatigue, or both. The use of increasing amounts is accompanied by the development of some degree of tolerance.

Some experts believe that the prolonged sleep, lassitude, fatigue, and hyperphagia, and the rebound increase in rapid eye movement (REM) sleep that follow discontinuance of the use of amphetamine or cocaine constitute an abstinence syndrome. If this is the case, the appearance of these symptoms is indicative of the development of physical dependence.

Concurrent Drug Abuse

Many CNS stimulant abusers simultaneously consume large amounts of barbiturates, antianxiety agents, and alcohol either to combat insomnia or to reduce sensations of jumpiness. Barbiturates, in particular, are taken in combination with amphetamine-like agents to enhance the subjective effects of the latter. Cocaine is commonly mixed with an opioid, and is either injected intravenously or smoked.

Diagnosis and Treatment

Excessive dosages of CNS stimulants taken acutely usually lead to the production of a state of excitation. Signs of autonomic hyperfunction, including increased blood pressure, tachycardia, hyperthermia, pupillary dilation, and various degrees of motor unrest, are prominent. Convulsions and cerebrovascular accidents have occurred. These constitute a medical emergency and should receive prompt supportive treatment and pharmacological intervention. The central excitatory effects are readily controlled by either barbiturate or diazepam administration.

Although cases of stimulant-induced *paranoid psychosis* have been reported to result from single injections of amphetamine-like drugs, this syndrome is more frequently seen after chronic abuse. The drug-induced psychosis closely resembles variants of acute paranoid schizophrenia, and differentiation can be difficult. Identification of a stimulant in the urine and disappearance of the psychosis within 7 days after drug withdrawal are considered satisfactory criteria for a diagnosis. Patients suspected to suffer from this form of stimulant intoxication should be treated on a closed psychiatric ward. Such patients usually exhibit symptoms of emotional blunting and delusions of persecution and grandeur. Combative behavior is common. Hallucinations, if present, are more likely to be auditory after oral abuse of the stimulant. Vivid visual hallucinations, however, have occurred after intravenous abuse. Irritability, restlessness, and agitation may or may not be evident.

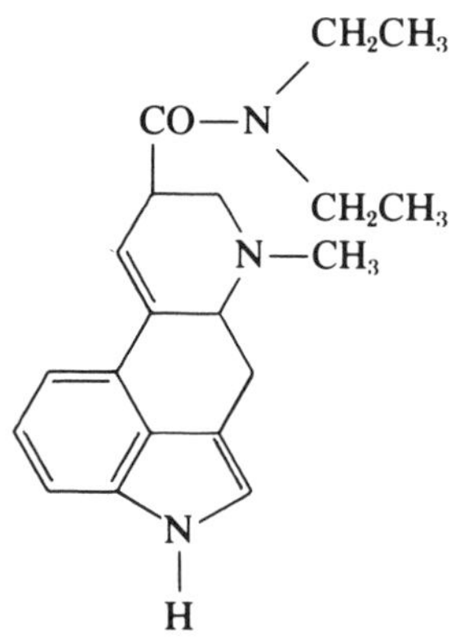

Figure 41-1. LSD-25, a representative indolealkylamine, and mescaline, a representative phenethylamine.

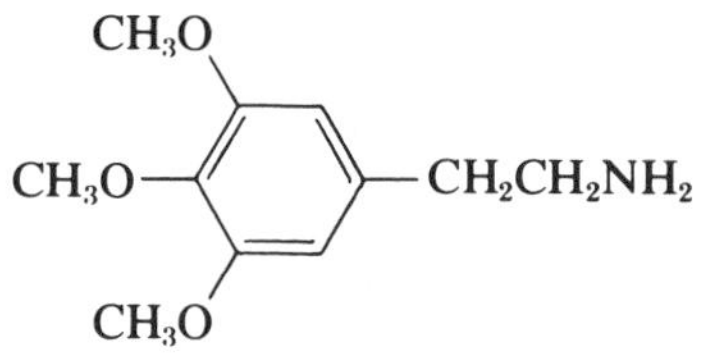

Treatment is directed toward elimination of the drug from the body. Acidification of the urine hastens the excretion of amphetamine and its metabolites. If the patient is agitated as a result of frightening hallucinations, marked improvement can be achieved by the administration of an antipsychotic agent, such as chlorpromazine or haloperidol. Because these patients may have impaired postural vasomotor compensatory mechanisms, however, the dose should be adjusted judiciously. The antipsychotics do not appear to affect the paranoia. The use of barbiturates in patients not showing signs of stimulation is not advised. The patient intoxicated with amphetamine-like drugs is difficult to sedate with these agents and may instead become belligerent and abusive.

Attempts to rehabilitate stimulant abusers have generally been made solely with the use of psychotherapy. The prognosis for such patients, however, has been poor. Emotional depression appears to persist for months, and recurrent stimulant abuse is quite common. Although withdrawal from stimulant abuse does not require medical treatment, the possibility that pharmacological treatment may reduce "craving" has been explored. Abusers have been treated with desipramine (a potent inhibitor of monoamine neurotransmitter uptake), lithium, and buprenorphine, a partial μ-opioid agonist; the success of these treatments, however, has been inconclusive.

Abuse of Hallucinogens

Although naturally occurring hallucinogens have been used since antiquity, the abuse of this group of compounds did not become widespread in the United States until the 1960s. These agents, also known as psychedelics, psychotomimetics, and psychotogens, have no accepted use in medicine and are therefore classified as schedule I drugs. At present, 100,000 people per year in the United States are estimated to engage in periodic or regular use of these drugs.

LSD-Like Hallucinogens

The pharmacological properties of the hallucinogens most frequently used are remarkably similar. Structurally, two main groups of hallucinogens exist: the *indolealkylamines* and the *β-phenethylamines* (Fig. 41-1). Agents related to the indolealkylamines include lysergic acid diethylamide (LSD), psilocybin, psilocin, dimethyltryptamine (DMT), and diethyltryptamine (DET). Agents related to the phenethylamines include mescaline, 2,5-dimethoxy-4-methylamphetamine (DOM), 3,4-methylenedioxyamphetamine (MDA), 3,4-methylenedioxymethamphetamine (MDMA), and 5-methoxy-MDA (MMDA).

LSD has long been referred to as "acid" in street jargon. DOM has been labeled "STP," while MDA has been called the "love pill" because of its purported aphrodisiac effects. Recently, large quantities of MDMA have appeared on the street scene. This drug has been dubbed "ecstasy."

The LSD-like hallucinogens all produce CNS stimulation and, after sufficient doses, convulsions. A variety of physiological changes are produced, most of which are adrenomimetic in nature. These include increases in blood pressure and respiratory rate, tachycardia, hyperthermia, pupillary dilation, and hyperreflexia. Sweating, salivation, lacrimation, and nausea and vomiting may also occur.

Changes in sensory perception are a prominent feature

of the drug effect. Perceptions of size and distance are very often distorted. Distortions of body image also occur, and there are feelings of separation of parts of the body. Time sense is lost, and time seems either extraordinarily contracted or expanded. There is a heightened awareness of sensory input. This results in the production of vivid visual illusions and hallucinations. The visual images usually comprise intensely colored geometric patterns taking on honeycomb, cobweb, cone, or spiral shapes. These images appear to move kaleidoscopically and have an iridescent quality. Oral doses of LSD as low as 25 μg can produce these CNS effects.

The *mechanism of action* of the LSD-like hallucinogens is a topic that is still being debated. It has been proposed that the hallucinations produced by LSD are a result of a repression of central serotonin neuronal (raphe nuclei) activity. This conclusion is supported by the observation that reduction of brain serotonin by other drugs increases the hallucinogenic potency of LSD. Evidence for the existence of both tryptaminergic and phenethylaminergic receptors within the CNS has recently been forthcoming, and LSD could also exert its effects by interacting with these systems.

Patterns of Abuse

LSD-like hallucinogens are abused more by college students and the affluent than by poorer and less-educated groups. The commonest form of abuse is "tripping"; that is, the user takes the drug for purposes of intensifying his or her environment and having a novel experience. Repeated trips are usually separated in time by intervals of weeks or months. The experience tends to become less interesting eventually, and use of hallucinogens is then discontinued.

In contrast to the sensory changes, the subjective effects and changes in mood after hallucinogen intake are quite variable. Euphoria may be produced, and this effect has consistently been seen after low doses in clinical studies. A dreamlike state with feelings of good humor, relaxation, and a sense of wonderment may predominate. On the other hand, dysphoria may be produced, and feelings of nervousness and anxiety may prevail. There may be a fear of fragmentation or disintegration of the self. This may lead to a *panic reaction* with severe disorientation. Such experiences, known as "bum trips," are more likely to occur after large doses. Instead of taking on any one pattern, mood also may be labile and shift frequently from depression to gaiety and from elation to fear.

Tolerance to both the physiological and behavioral effects of LSD-like hallucinogens develops quite rapidly. A high degree of tolerance may be present after only three or four daily doses. Cross-tolerance between the various hallucinogens acting similarly to LSD also exists. There is no cross-tolerance, however, between any of these agents

and CNS stimulants, such as amphetamine. Once hallucinogen use is discontinued, tolerance is lost rapidly.

Dependence

Withdrawal symptoms are *not* produced by abrupt discontinuation of chronic hallucinogen use. These agents, therefore, do not produce physical dependence. Craving for the drug after cessation of use is not great, and no marked degree of psychological dependence develops.

Concurrent Drug Abuse

Those who take hallucinogens rarely dilute the experience by simultaneous intake of drugs of another group. Between trips, however, these individuals may use marijuana.

Diagnosis and Treatment

Adverse reactions after intake of hallucinogens have been seen most commonly after the use of LSD. The margin of safety between the effective dose and the lethal dose of LSD is exceedingly high. Indeed, the LSD-related deaths that have resulted from suicide and accidents are a consequence of drug-distorted judgment rather than drug toxicity. However, a great number of panic reactions and psychotic episodes have been produced by LSD. These reactions endure for about 24 hr and differ from naturally occurring psychoses in that the hallucinations are visual rather than auditory. The symptoms respond readily to treatment with the phenothiazines.

Prolonged psychotic episodes, lasting from several days to several months, also have been precipitated by LSD. These episodes tend to resemble schizophrenic states with paranoid delusions or hallucinations. Large doses of a phenothiazine are needed for their control. An unexplained phenomenon sometimes seen is the spontaneous recurrence of the adverse LSD effects many months after the drug was last taken. These "flashbacks" are likewise responsive to the phenothiazines.

Phencyclidine

Abuse of phencyclidine (PCP) (Fig. 41-2), a psychotomimetic possessing pharmacological properties markedly different from those of LSD and related drugs, is still quite prevalent. This compound was originally considered for use as an anesthetic agent. Because of a high incidence of emergence delirium, however, the compound was found undesirable. Initial cases of abuse were identified only after treatment of victims of acute intoxication and overdosage. The popularity of phencyclidine is currently waning.

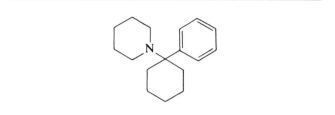

Figure 41-2. Phencyclidine.

With regard to *mechanism of action,* phencyclidine appears to interact with several central neurohumoral systems. This anesthetic both inhibits dopamine uptake and enhances dopamine release; it thus acts as an indirect dopaminergic agonist. In addition, the compound appears to possess some anticholinergic properties. Phencyclidine shares some of the dysphoric properties of σ-opioids. The subsequent identification of binding sites for both phencyclidine and σ-opioids has led to considerable confusion regarding nomenclature.

The site at which phencyclidine binds has been referred to as both the phencyclidine- and the σ-receptor. Regardless of terminology, phencyclidine binds to a receptor that appears to reside within the NMDA-gated calcium channel, which is consistent with its noncompetitive antagonism of NMDA. There are numerous therapeutic potentials for NMDA antagonists, one of the most noteworthy of which is prevention of excessive calcium entry, which occurs with brain ischemia caused by stroke, head injury, or convulsions.

Patterns of Abuse

One of the reasons for the initial surge in phencyclidine abuse was that this drug is cheap and readily available. Street sources of phencyclidine have almost all been generated by synthesis of the compound in illicit home laboratories.

Phencyclidine is used in powder, liquid, tablet, and capsule forms. The powder is either snorted or mixed with marijuana or other vegetable matter, such as parsley or oregano, and smoked. The liquid is either sprayed on organic matter and subsequently smoked, or is injected intravenously. The tablets and capsules are taken orally. The powder form of phencyclidine is most commonly known as "angel dust" in user slang. Tablets or capsules for oral ingestion have received a variety of names, the most common of which are "peace pill," "hog," and "elephant tranquilizer." Preparations combined with organic matter have been dubbed "superjoint" and "rocket fuel."

After low doses of phencyclidine, the user has a sense of thinking and acting swiftly. Mood may range from euphoria and a sense of "bouncing" to depression. Visual hallucinations may be entertained. With large doses,

changes in mood are even more unpredictable and may vacillate. A sense of unreality predominates, and bizarre sensations, such as the feeling of walking on clouds, ensue. Irrational and violent actions may be produced by single doses, but these phenomena more often emerge after chronic use.

Phencyclidine often may be misrepresented to the purchaser—usually as THC, but sometimes as LSD or cocaine. Thus, the user may not even be aware that he or she has taken phencyclidine. Street drugs with bizarre names have also been found to contain phencyclidine in varying amounts.

Diagnosis and Treatment

Acute phencyclidine intoxication produces a confusional state, during which unpredictable and violent behavior may occur. The individual initially may be unresponsive, but behavior may change rapidly to excitation and combativeness. Physical symptoms include gross ataxia, rigidity, motor restlessness, nystagmus, and repetitive movements.

After phencyclidine overdosage, the patient usually lapses into stupor or coma. Motor seizures also may be manifested. Respiratory depression, intracerebral hemorrhage, hyperpyrexia, and cardiac arrest have been observed in cases of overdosage.

Treatment is mainly symptomatic. Gastric lavage may prevent further absorption if the drug was taken orally. Vital signs should be monitored and adequate ventilation should be maintained. Diazepam has been found effective in controlling seizures. Phencyclidine can be detected through blood or urine analysis. After sensory isolation of the patient, vital signs should be observed and monitored. Precautions should be taken against the possibility of suicide. Use of antipsychotic drugs, particularly the phenothiazines, is contraindicated because hypertension may ensue. This occurrence is presumably due to the summed anticholinergic effects of the two drugs.

In some individuals, phencyclidine produces an *acute toxic psychosis* that is often indistinguishable from an acute schizophrenic episode. This psychosis may not become evident until several days after ingestion of the drug. The individual may have symptoms of stupor, unresponsiveness, and catatonia. On the other hand, tension, hyperactivity, and unexpected bizarre and violent behavior may be exhibited instead. There is difficulty with visual perception, and persistent auditory hallucinations are experienced. Affect may be blunted. Thoughts are disorganized and paranoid ideation is common. The patient should be treated under close observation in a psychiatric ward. Sensory stimulation should be kept minimal. Antipsychotic drugs have been found to be helpful in reducing the agitated state.

Ketamine, an anesthetic closely related to phencycli-

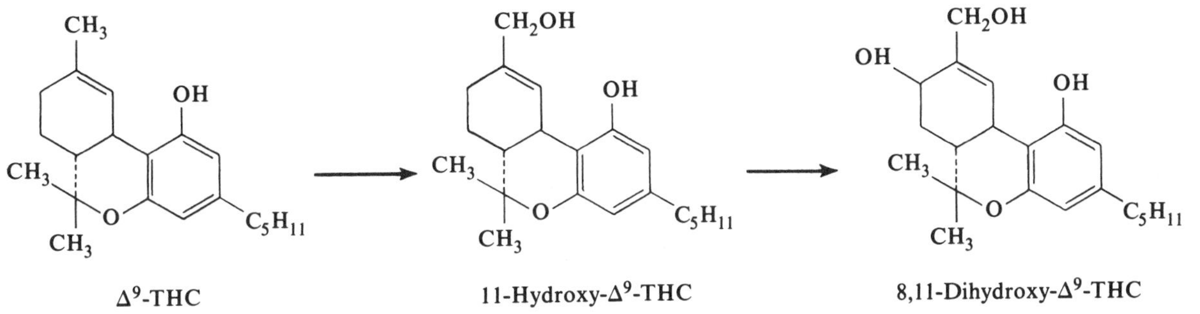

Figure 41-3. Δ^9-Tetrahydrocannabinol (THC) and its two principal metabolites, 11-hydroxy-Δ^9-THC, which is pharmacologically active, and 11-*nor*-carboxy-Δ^9-THC, which is inactive.

dine (see Chap. 31), produces effects quite similar to those of phencyclidine. This agent is abused mainly by physicians.

Abuse of Marijuana

Marijuana is derived only from the hemp species, *Cannabis sativa.* All portions of both the male and female plant contain the psychoactive principle to varying degrees, with the highest concentrations occurring in the flowering tops, and the least in the seeds. Other names for cannabis include hashish, chasra, bhang, dagga, and marijuana. Most familiar to Americans is *marijuana,* which refers to the chopped and dried entire plant, and the more potent *hashish,* the dried resinous exudate of the flowering tops. The primary constituent conferring psychoactive properties on marijuana is Δ^9-tetrahydrocannabinol (Δ^9-THC; Fig. 41-3). An average marijuana cigarette delivers a dose of Δ^9-THC ranging from about 2.5 to 5.0 mg.

In the United States, marijuana abuse first emerged in the 1920s, a time when the abuse potential of other drugs such as heroin and cocaine was realized. As a consequence, marijuana was thought to be similarly dangerous and addicting, which led to its erroneous classification as a narcotic. However, marijuana has defied most classification schemes for centrally acting drugs because of its unique behavioral profile. While the acute subjective effects that users derive from marijuana are quite variable, the most prominent behavior produced by one or two cigarettes is characterized as a period of euphoria or "high" followed by sedation. Perception of time is frequently altered; hearing becomes less discriminate but visual stimuli may be enhanced. Cannabinoids have no effects on pupil size and respiratory rate.

Short-term memory is impaired, and performance of tasks requiring multiple mental steps to reach a specific goal is impeded. Whereas simple motor tasks may be performed normally, more complex tasks, including those involved in driving, are impaired. At higher doses, abstract thinking is markedly affected. It is at these doses that illusions and vividly colored hallucinations occur. Depersonalization and paranoid feelings may predominate, and euphoria may be converted into anxiety, reaching panic proportions.

Δ^9-THC produces consistent effects on the cardiovascular system. A dose-related increase in heart rate occurs, typically 20 to 50 beats per minute following one or two cigarettes. Blood pressure remains relatively unchanged, although high doses can produce orthostatic hypotension. Peripheral vasodilation leads to a marked reddening of the conjunctivae and the appearance of bloodshot eyes.

The route of administration affects both time course and intensity of effects. The systemic availability of Δ^9-THC after smoking is approximately 25 percent. Pharmacological effects are perceived within minutes after smoking. Plasma concentrations of Δ^9-THC peak after 10 to 30 min. The duration of the entire effect is about 2 to 3 hr. Although Δ^9-THC is absorbed almost completely from the gastrointestinal tract after oral administration, its systemic availability is only about 6 percent when administered in a cookie and 10 to 20 percent if given in sesame oil. The onset of its CNS effects is delayed for 30 min to 1 hr. Peak plasma concentrations are reached within the second or third hour, and the duration of effects extends for 4 to 5 hr. The effectiveness of Δ^9-THC after oral ingestion is less than that after smoking.

Δ^9-THC is converted quite rapidly to 11-hydroxy-Δ^9-THC, a pharmacologically active metabolite. Further metabolism leads to the production of 11-*nor*-9-carboxy-Δ^9-THC, the major metabolite of Δ^9-THC. This inactive metabolite is then excreted in the urine. Very little of administered Δ^9-THC remains unchanged. The terminal half-life for Δ^9-THC in plasma is roughly 13 days and the urinary elimination half-life for 11-*nor*-9-carboxy-Δ^9-THC is approximately 10 days. The slow urinary elimination of this acid has made it an ideal marker for detecting marijuana use. However, neither plasma concentrations of Δ^9-THC nor urinary concentrations of 11-*nor*-9-carboxy-Δ^9-THC correlate well with Δ^9-THC's effects, making them poor predictors of behavioral impairment or intoxication.

Anecdotal reports of self-medication with marijuana have led to the therapeutic use of Δ^9-THC. Δ^9-THC is currently approved only for the treatment of nausea and vomiting caused by cancer chemotherapy. It is known generically as dronabinol and is marketed as *Marinol* capsules (2.5, 5.0, and 10 mg) for oral use in patients who are nonresponsive to conventional antiemetics. Older patients have some difficulty in tolerating dronabinol. It is not very effective in patients receiving cisplatin. Despite the lack of well-controlled clinical trials demonstrating a positive effect of cannabinoids on appetite and weight gain, there has been considerable pressure to approve Δ^9-THC or marijuana for treating the wasting syndrome associated with AIDS.

Patterns of Abuse

Criminalization of marijuana in 1937 led to a decline in its use until the 1960s and 1970s, when it reemerged as the most popular illegal drug of abuse, a status it enjoys today. It is estimated that 18 million people in the United States use marijuana at least occasionally. Of this number, a small percentage use the drug on a daily basis. Adolescents and young adults continue to form the majority of the population of users. Forty percent of high school seniors have tried marijuana at least once and 14 percent reported use within the past 30 days. As for young adults, 75 percent have tried marijuana at least once and 13 percent reported use during the past 30 days.

Marijuana use is usually a group activity. About 90 percent of users have their first experience with the drug in the company of at least one person who has already smoked it. Subsequent episodes of "turning on" likewise occur in intimate groups. Frequent users of marijuana (i.e., from 3 days/wk to daily) are likely to be involved in the selling of marijuana because of the cost of making large purchases.

Many street names have been given to marijuana. The commonest of these are "pot", "grass", "weed", "joint", "reefer", and "Mary Jane." The words *Bo* and *Colombian gold* refer to marijuana harvested in Colombia. According to users, this source has a higher percentage of active constituents than other preparations more widely available in the United States.

Adverse Effects

The pattern of use, age, and sex are critical factors in the production of adverse effects. Most marijuana users are able to titrate the dose taken so that the unpleasant effects emerging after acute high doses do not occur. Psychiatric emergencies resulting from the use of marijuana are quite rare. In contrast to most other drugs of abuse, almost no deaths have been attributed to marijuana use, most likely because it is devoid of respiratory depressant properties.

Despite considerable clinical and preclinical data suggestive of adverse effects of marijuana, most have been difficult to prove. It does appear that marijuana may aggravate existing psychoses or other severe emotional disorders. Marijuana has been shown to decrease luteinizing hormone levels in both men and women, but proof of decreased fertility is lacking. Marijuana smoking produces bronchitis and chronic cough with heavy use. Attributing lung damage to marijuana smoking has been confounded by its concomitant use with tobacco in many individuals.

A great deal of attention has been devoted to establishing a link between the amotivational syndrome and marijuana use. Motivation, or the lack thereof, is not a behavior that can be easily reduced to a set of parameters for study. However, it is highly likely that regular use of marijuana is detrimental to the normal psychosocial development of juveniles.

Tolerance to the effects of marijuana develops quite slowly. Only a moderate degree of tolerance is evident after daily use of low doses. Perceptual and motor functions may be less impaired in experienced users, and there may be smaller increases in heart rate. The subjective effects, however, do not appear to be reduced.

Recently, cannabinoid receptors were identified in brain, with the highest concentrations reported in basal ganglia, hippocampus, and cerebellum. Activation of this receptor leads to inhibition of adenylate cyclase. The receptor has been cloned, which confirms that it is a member of the G-protein coupled receptors.

Abuse of Inhalants

Volatile chemicals and gases that produce behavioral effects are subject to abuse. These agents represent a broad range of chemical classes, but in general can be classified as gases, volatile organic solvents, and aliphatic nitrites. Inhalant abuse differs from that of many other drugs in that it is confined primarily to juveniles and young adults. Reports of their abuse by children whose siblings consider them too young to be introduced to marijuana or heroin are common. Additionally, inhalant abuse has been rising during the past decade, whereas there is a general downward trend for most other drugs. Almost 20 percent of high school seniors have tried inhalants at least once in their lifetimes. The use of gases is primarily confined to nitrous oxide abuse by young medical professionals who have ready access to this agent. It produces a short-lived mild intoxication that typifies the early stages of anesthesia. Deaths occur occasionally by individuals who inhale nitrous oxide alone. Volatile organic solvents are usually aliphatic and aromatic hydrocarbons, and include substances such as gasoline, paint and lacquer thinners, lighter fluid, degreasers (methylchloroform and methylene chloroform), and the solvents in airplane glue, typewriter correction fluid, bathroom deodorizers, and so forth. These agents produce a sense of exhilaration and light-headedness. Judgment and perception of reality are impaired, and hallucinations may be produced. The mechanisms by which inhalants produce their behavioral effects are poorly understood, but there are some indications that their actions are similar to those of other centrally acting depressants, including alcohol. Toxicity depends on the properties of the individual solvents. The consequences of inhaling these substances can be severe, for they have been implicated in producing cancer, cardiotoxicity, neuropathies, and hepatotoxicity.

Miscellaneous Drugs of Abuse

A wide variety of drugs and chemical substances sporadically attract the attention of individuals seeking to obtain a new dimension of feeling by drug intake. Some of the agents more commonly abused are described in the following section.

Designer Drugs

In an effort to avoid federal regulation and control, chemists in clandestine laboratories adopted the strategy of synthesizing analogues of drugs that are scheduled. Although these drugs are technically not illegal until scheduled, the consequences of their abuse have often been unpredictable and in some instances lethal. Efforts to make "synthetic heroin" led to the synthesis of at least six chemicals that are structurally similar to fentanyl. These agents gained considerable attention because their increased potency over fentanyl and heroin led to a rash of overdoses and numerous deaths. The two derivatives, α-methyl fentanyl and 3-methyl fentanyl, both referred to as "China White," are 900 and 1,100 times more potent than morphine. Meperidine has also been used as a template for preparing "synthetic heroin," the end product being 1-methyl-4-propionoxy-4-phenylpiperidine (MPPP). However, MPPP is sometimes contaminated with the side reaction product 1-methyl, 4-phenyl-1,2,3,6-tetrahydropyridine (MPTP), which produces a parkinsonian syndrome through nigrostriatal lesions. Several substituted derivatives of amphetamine have also been referred to as "designer drugs." The most widely known of this group is the hallucinogen MDMA ("ecstasy").

The relatively easy synthesis of highly potent dangerous drugs illustrates another difficulty in combating drug abuse by attempting to control supply. The medical community is faced with dealing with the consequences of failed pharmacological and toxicological evaluations of these agents in the drug abuser. Diagnosis and appropriate treatment are hampered in cases of highly potent drugs that are used in trace quantities because drug detection and identification are difficult.

Nutmeg

When taken in sufficient amounts, the household spice nutmeg produces marked subjective effects. Onset of action after oral ingestion requires several hours. Nutmeg produces feelings of depersonalization and unreality, and vivid visual hallucinations. Intoxication is long-lasting. Anticholinergic symptoms such as dry mouth, thirst, rapid heart rate, and flushing of the face are common. Patients presenting in emergency rooms may show agitation and apprehension. Treatment is primarily symptomatic.

Parachlorophenylalanine

Abuse of the serotonin synthesis inhibitor, p-*chlorophenylalanine,* came into vogue shortly after reports of its production of long-lasting sexual excitation in male rats. Abusers soon became aware that high doses of the drug can induce a prolonged psychotic reaction, however, and more wary subsequent users have given it the street name of "steam."

Supplemental Reading

Abood, M.E., and Martin, B.R. Drugs of abuse: Marihuana. *Trends in Pharmacological Sciences* 13:201, 1992.

Clouet, D.H. (ed.). *Phencyclidine: An Update.* NIDA Research Monograph #64. DHHS Publication No. (ADM) 86-1443, 1986.

Gawin, F.H., and Ellingwood, E.H., Jr. Cocaine and other stimulants: Actions, abuse, and treatment. *N. Engl. J. Med.* 318:1173, 1988.

Goldstein, A. (ed.). *Molecular and Cellular Aspects of the Drug Addictions.* Secaucus, N.J.: Springer-Verlag NY, 1989.

Hollister, L.E. Health aspects of cannabis. *Pharmacol. Rev.* 38:1, 1986.

Jacobs, B.L. (ed.). *Hallucinogens: Neurochemical, Behavioral and Clinical Perspectives.* New York: Raven, 1984.

Johnston, L.D., O'Malley, P.M., and Bachman, J.B. *Drug Use Among American High School Seniors, College Students and Young Adults, 1975–1990,* Vols. 1 and 2. DHHS Publication

Nos. (ADM) 91-1813 and (ADM) 19-1835. Washington, DC: US Department of Health and Human Services, 1991.

Martin, W.R. (ed.). *Handbook of Experimental Pharmacology 45/I. Drug Addiction I: Morphine, Sedative-Hypnotic and Alcohol Dependence.* New York: Springer-Verlag, 1977.

Martin, W.R. (ed.). *Handbook of Experimental Pharmacology 45/II. Drug Addiction II: Amphetamine, Psychotogen, and Marihuana Dependence.* New York: Springer-Verlag, 1977.

Nahas, G.G., et al. *Marihuana in Science and Medicine.* New York: Raven, 1984.

Redda, K.K., Walker, C.A., and Barnett, G. *Cocaine, Marihuana, Designer Drugs: Chemistry, Pharmacology, and Behavior.* Boca Raton, Fla.; CRC, 1989.

Woods, J.H., Katz, J.L., and Winger, G. Benzodiazepines: Use, abuse and consequences. *Pharmacol. Rev.* 44:151, 1992.

V

Drugs Used to Treat Inflammatory Disorders

42

Lipid Mediators of Homeostasis and Inflammation

Eric P. Brestel and *Knox Van Dyke*

Membrane lipids are a source of important compounds involved in normal physiology and the inflammatory response. Two groups of compounds are considered in this chapter: (1) the *eicosanoids,* so called because of their derivation from a 20-carbon unsaturated fatty acid, arachidonic (or eicosatetraenoic) acid, and (2) *platelet-activating factor* (PAF). The eicosanoids and PAF are derived from membrane phospholipids and are synthesized de novo at the time of cellular stimulation.

The Eicosanoids

Biosynthesis

In the 1930s, von Euler coined the name *prostaglandin* (PG) for a factor found in the prostate gland that could cause smooth muscle contraction. It is now known that cells from many tissue types can synthesize prostaglandins and that these compounds are used both in normal physiological homeostasis and to help generate an inflammatory response. The pathways involved in the biosynthesis of the eicosanoids are outlined in Fig. 42-1.

Cellular stimulation results in the activation of the enzyme phospholipase A_2, which can cleave arachidonic acid from its location on the second carbon position of membrane-bound phosphatidylcholine. Alternatively, arachidonic acid also may be derived by the sequential actions of the enzymes phospholipase C and diacylglyceryl lipase. More recently, it has been found that arachidonic acid can be produced from alkyl-acyl-glycerophosphocholine, the membrane precursor of PAF.

Once arachidonic acid is released from membrane phospholipids, it can be oxygenated by *cyclooxygenase* to form prostaglandin G_2 (PGG_2). The peroxidase component of this enzyme reduces PGG_2 to PGH_2, which is the precursor in the production of several specific prostaglandins (cyclooxygenase and peroxidase are often collectively referred to as *prostaglandin synthase*). *The particular final product that is produced is tissue specific.* For example, platelets produce thromboxane A_2 (TxA_2), the vascular endothelial cell produces prostacyclin (PGI_2), the mast cell produces PGD_2, and PGE_2 is produced by a variety of tissues, including the vasculature, the gastrointestinal tract, and the lung.

Other eicosanoids are synthesized by the action of a variety of *lipoxygenases.* These enzymes oxygenate unsaturated fatty acids at double-bonded carbon atoms to form lipid peroxides. In the typical Western diet of humans, the major fatty acid that participates in this reaction is usually arachidonic acid, but other unsaturated fatty acids may be oxygenated if the dietary intake is large enough. The oxygenation products of the lipoxygenases are hydroperoxyeicosatetraenoic acids, often abbreviated HPETEs. Oxygenation at C15 of arachidonic acid produces 15-HPETE. Peroxidases reduce HPETEs to hydroxyeicosatetraenoic acids (HETEs).

Oxygenation of arachidonic acid at the C5 position results in the formation of 5-HPETE. Epoxidation of this product results in the formation of leukotriene A_4 (LTA_4). *Leukotrienes* are so called because of their conjugated triene structure and the fact that they were first isolated from leukocytes. Addition of the tripeptide glutathione to LTA_4 results in leukotriene C_4 (LTC_4). Removal of glutamate forms the compound leukotriene D_4 (LTD_4) and, finally, the removal of glycine (leaving only cysteine attached) forms leukotriene E_4 (LTE_4). LTA_4 also can be metabolized through other pathways to a variety of dihydroxylated compounds, including leukotriene B_4 (LTB_4).

There are many other oxygenation products of arachidonic acid and other unsaturated fatty acids produced in biological tissues. At present, however, evidence is not suf-

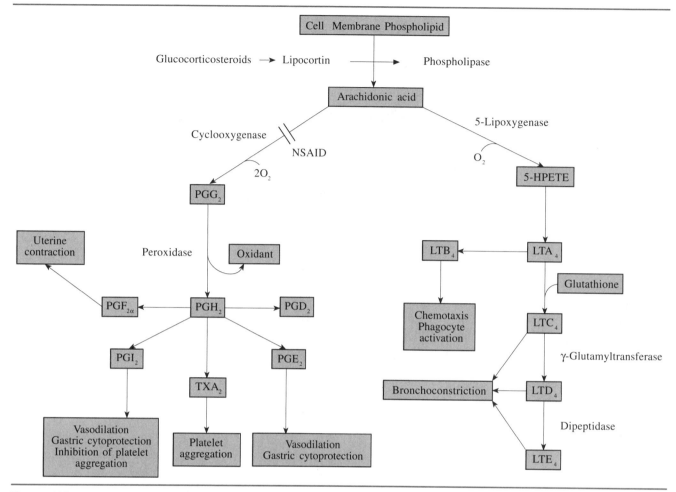

Figure 42-1. Biosynthetic pathways for synthesis of eicosanoids. The binding of a stimulant to a membrane receptor results in the activation of phospholipase A_2 (PLA_2). PLA_2 cleaves arachidonic acid from membrane phosphatidylcholine (see text for alternative pathways for arachidonic acid liberation). Liberated arachidonic acid is then metabolized through the action of membrane and microsomal enzymes (cyclooxygenase and lipoxygenases) to biologically active end products. The nature of the product(s) formed depends on the tissue. The nonsteroidal antiinflammatory agents (NSAIDs) inhibit cyclooxygenase, thus inhibiting oxygenation of arachidonic acid. The peroxidase component of cyclooxygenase generates a potentially inflammatory oxidant. Metabolism through the 5-lipoxygenase pathway results in the formation of leukotrienes (LT). LTC_4 and LTD_4 are potent bronchoconstrictors. LTB_4 is chemotactic for phagocytes and can stimulate them to produce inflammatory compounds. The glucocorticosteroids may act to induce the synthesis of lipocortin, an inhibitor of PLA_2, thus preventing the release of arachidonic acid and the formation of proinflammatory eicosanoids. PG = prostaglandin; TxA_2 = thromboxane A_2; HPETE = hydroperoxyeicosatetraenoic acid.

ficient to indicate that these other compounds play a significant role in homeostasis or pathological states.

Biological Effects

Inflammation

The classical signs of an inflammatory process are *rubor* (redness), *tumor* (swelling), *calor* (heat), *dolor* (pain), and *functio laesa* (loss of function). The actual expression of these processes depends on the site of inflammation. For example, a skin abscess may result in the appearance of all of these features; pneumonia, because of the inaccessibility of the lung to examination, may present only with loss of function (shortness of breath and hypoxia). Nevertheless, similar pathological processes are occurring in both sites.

Several classes of compounds have been associated with the inflammatory response. Early investigators emphasized vasoactive amines, such as histamine and serotonin. In the 1960s and 1970s, much research on inflammation emphasized the importance of plasma proteins and peptides such as products of both the complement and the kinin systems. Also during that period, a number of enzymes capable of digesting tissues were discovered in proinflammatory phagocytes such as polymorphonuclear leukocytes, macrophages, and eosinophils. These enzymes included proteases, hyaluronidase, collagenase, and elastase. Simultaneously, it became apparent that the prostaglandins were involved in the inflammatory process.

Biologically derived oxidants are a major contributing factor in tissue injury that results from the inflammatory response. These oxidants include the superoxide anion (O_2^-), hydrogen peroxide (H_2O_2), nitric oxide, peroxynitrate, hypochlorous acid (HOCl), peroxidase-generated oxidants of undefined character, probably the hydroxyl radical ($\cdot OH$), and possibly singlet oxygen ($^1O_2$). These oxidants, largely generated by phagocytic cells such as neutrophils and macrophages, are capable of inducing tissue injury beyond that produced by digestive enzymes and eicosanoids.

In 1971, Vane discovered that *the prostaglandin biosynthetic pathway is sensitive to inhibition by the nonsteroidal antiinflammatory drugs (NSAIDs) such as aspirin and indomethacin.* These compounds inhibit cyclooxygenase preventing the oxygenation of arachidonic acid to form PGG_2. Since the NSAIDs were known for their ability to inhibit inflammation, it was proposed that their effects were the result of the inhibition of the synthesis of prostaglandins. There is evidence that the oxidant generated by the peroxidase component of cyclooxygenase may have a proinflammatory effect as well.

It is likely that plasma proteins, vasoactive amines, tissue-digestive enzymes, biologically derived oxidants, and eicosanoids all participate in the process that we call inflammation. It is yet to be defined which, if any, of these systems is most important.

None of the products of cyclooxygenase metabolism (Table 42-1) can account for all of the features of the inflammatory response. PGE_2 can cause redness and warmth by acting as a vasodilator, but its ability to induce plasma exudation and swelling is minimal. PGE_2 can, however, greatly potentiate the plasma exudation produced by other autacoids (i.e., substances formed by one type of cell that then diffuse or are transported to produce effects on other cells) such as bradykinin and histamine, which also might be released during the inflammatory response. Similarly, PGE_1 produces hyperalgesia by itself and accentuates the effects of histamine and bradykinin on pain.

Various HETEs have been implicated in the inflammatory response. Many are *chemotactic* and *chemokinetic* (i.e., substances that enhance directed and random phagocyte migration, respectively) thereby increasing the number of proinflammatory cells at the site of inflammation.

Table 42-1. Biological Effects of Eicosanoids

Eicosanoid	Primary biological effects
PGE_2	Vasodilation, pain sensitization, gastric cytoprotection
$PGF_{2\alpha}$	Bronchoconstriction, uterine contraction
PGI_2	Inhibition of platelet aggregation, gastric cytoprotection
TxA_2	Platelet aggregation
LTC_4, D_4, E_4	Bronchoconstriction
LTB_4	Neutrophil chemotaxis and activation

LTB_4 (a di-HETE) deserves special mention since it is chemotactic as well as being capable of stimulating phagocytes to produce inflammatory substances including O_2^-, H_2O_2, and HOCl.

The glucocorticosteroids are antiinflammatory in several pathological states, especially dermatoses (such as psoriasis and eczemas) (see Chap. 46), allergic states and asthma (see Chap. 45), and chronic allograft rejection (see Chap. 63). Although the mechanism(s) by which glucocorticosteroids function as antiinflammatory drugs is unknown, it is known that they can induce the biosynthesis of a specific inhibitor of phospholipase A_2 called *lipocortin*. Thus, glucocorticosteroids may inhibit the formation of *all* eicosanoids by reducing the phospholipase A_2–associated release of arachidonic acid from membrane phospholipid. *Glucocorticosteroids seem especially effective in conditions in which eosinophils and lymphocytes predominate as the inflammatory cells.*

Asthma and Allergic States

It has long been known that histamine, an autacoid stored in the granules of tissue mast cells and circulating basophils, is capable of causing smooth muscle relaxation in the peripheral vasculature (see Chap. 72) and bronchial smooth muscle constriction. These actions result in hyperemia and plasma exudation from peripheral vessels and bronchospasm in the lung. It is also known that tissues from immunosensitized animals can, when stimulated with allergen, release leukotrienes C_4, D_4, and E_4. These compounds are synthesized when mast cells are challenged with allergen to which they are sensitized. These leukotrienes can induce bronchospasm and peripheral vascular permeability in humans. The bronchoconstrictive properties of LTC_4 and LTD_4 are far more potent than those possessed by histamine.

Leukotrienes may be more important mediators of asthma than are any of the products of the cyclooxygenase pathway. PGD_2 is the major cyclooxygenase product of the mast cell. It, too, produces bronchospasm and peripheral vasodilation. However, it is not likely to play a major role in asthma since the ingestion of NSAIDs, compounds that inhibit the cyclooxygenase pathway, is usually ineffective for this condition. In contrast, leukotriene synthesis inhibitors and leukotriene receptor blocking drugs are effective in biological models of asthma.

Prostaglandin $F_{2\alpha}$ probably does not play a significant role in the pathophysiology of asthma. Bronchospasm may occur, however, when this compound is used therapeutically to terminate pregnancy.

Surprisingly little attention has been given to the role played by 15-HETE in asthma and other obstructive lung diseases. It is the major arachidonic acid metabolite of human tracheal epithelium and is capable of causing small airway bronchoconstriction. 15-HETE also is produced by nasal polyps and human eosinophils, both of which are associated with asthma. Furthermore, this compound can sensitize the mast cell to enhance mediator release. It is hoped that further research will delineate the relative importance of the various eicosanoids in the pathophysiology of asthma.

Fever

Although eicosanoids do not seem to be involved in normal temperature homeostasis, their role in fever has been suggested. Fever results when *interleukin-1,* produced by macrophages during an inflammatory response, is released into the circulation; other cytokines have also been implicated as mediators of fever. Interleukin-1 acts on the hypothalamus to stimulate a rise in PGE in the cerebrospinal fluid. The NSAIDs may have an antipyretic effect as a result of their ability to inhibit production of PGE in response to interleukin-1; however, other humoral factors also may be involved.

Reproduction

Since early work on prostaglandin distribution demonstrated that large amounts of these compounds are present in prostate tissue and seminal vesicles, there has been an assumption that eicosanoids were involved in the physiology of reproduction. Because some of the following information is derived from animal studies, its direct application to human reproductive physiology can only be implied.

In men, prostaglandins appear to be necessary for fertility. Low concentrations have been found in the semen of infertile men, with and without normal sperm count. Fertility also may be affected by the action of prostaglandins on cervical mucus, fallopian tubal motility, ovum transport, graafian follicle development, and ovulation.

Prostaglandins probably play a role in the initiation and progression of labor. Arachidonic acid levels in amniotic fluid rise during labor and its injection into the amniotic space can initiate labor. Furthermore, treatment of premature labor with *isoxsuprine,* an adrenomimetic-like drug, results in a drop in free arachidonic acid concentrations in maternal serum and the interruption of premature labor. Ethanol has a similar effect. Further evidence supporting a role for the prostaglandins in labor is the observation that PGE_1, PGE_2, and $PGF_{2\alpha}$ are effective abortifacients when administered in the first trimester of pregnancy.

Prostaglandins E_2 and $F_{2\alpha}$ are present in menstrual discharge, and blood levels of these substances rise during menstruation. $PGF_{2\alpha}$ is elevated in endometrial tissue and is believed to cause the uterine smooth muscle contractions that result in dysmenorrhea. NSAIDs can significantly reduce the discomfort of dysmenorrhea, probably by inhibiting prostaglandin biosynthesis.

Women in whom hypertension develops during pregnancy are at increased risk for fetal growth retardation and fetal death. Data indicate that such women produce relatively high levels of TxA_2 in comparison to PGI_2. Therapeutic trials of low-dose aspirin have demonstrated a reduction in pregnancy-induced hypertension, preeclamptic toxemia, and severely low-birth-weight infants. Aspirin therapy in high-risk women resulted in decreased excretion of TxA_2 metabolites and increased excretion of PGI_2 metabolites, indicating the importance of arachidonic acid metabolites in the pathogenesis of pregnancy-induced hypertension. Hypertension may result when this imbalance in arachidonate metabolites produces heightened sensitivity to circulating angiotensin II and catecholamines.

Hemostasis

Platelets are essential for normal hemostasis. Activation of the clotting cascade (see Chap. 27) by trauma results in platelet activation, which is followed by aggregation. These aggregates, together with a fibrin network, entrap erythrocytes and result in a hemostatic plug. *The major cyclooxygenase metabolite in platelets is TxA_2.* TxA_2 and its precursors (arachidonic acid, PGG_2, PGH_2) are capable of initiating aggregation. TxA_2 is quickly converted to a more stable but far less active compound, thromboxane B_2. It is this product that is usually measured as a sign of in vivo platelet activation.

NSAIDs inhibit TxA_2 production. Aspirin irreversibly inhibits platelet cyclooxygenase by acetylating the enzyme. Since platelets cannot manufacture new cyclooxygenase, hemostasis is partially impaired until new platelets are released from the bone marrow's megakaryocytes. This property does not usually result in a clinically significant hemostatic defect unless the patient is thrombocytopenic or has another coagulation deficit such as hemophilia or von Willebrand's disease.

PGI$_2$, a cyclooxygenase product of vascular endothelial cells, antagonizes the proaggregant properties of TxA$_2$. This natural inhibition is believed to be important in preventing spontaneous thrombosis in the normal physiological state. A number of clinical trials in humans have demonstrated aspirin to be effective in transient ischemic attacks in the central nervous system, occlusion of coronary artery bypass grafts, and prevention of myocardial infarction and death in subjects with active myocardial ischemia. Aspirin also may reduce mortality and morbidity in spontaneous myocardial infarction, although the results from several studies are conflicting. The dosage of aspirin used in most of these studies was much higher than that necessary to inhibit platelet aggregation. Thus, with lower dosages of aspirin, the platelet cyclooxygenase may be inhibited without inhibiting the cyclooxygenase of the endothelial cell, thereby maintaining PGI$_2$ levels that further the antithrombotic effect.

A thromboxane synthase inhibitor combined with a thromboxane receptor antagonist may be the most selective means for suppressing the thrombogenic effects of platelets while sparing the antithrombotic effects of prostacyclin. At the present time, however, these drugs are not currently available for human use.

The Vasculature

Some members of the E series of prostaglandins cause vasodilation with hyperemia in the skin and a drop in vascular resistance and blood pressure when administered systemically. PGI$_2$, because of its synthesis by vascular endothelium, is also likely to play a role in tissue perfusion. Additionally, PGI$_2$ counterbalances the platelet-aggregating effect of TxA$_2$.

Following birth the rise in the partial pressure of oxygen normally stimulates closure of the ductus arteriosus. In some infants (especially premature infants), the ductus does not close and an inappropriate shunt occurs. Naturally produced prostaglandins maintain the vessel's patency in utero. Infants with a persistence of patent ductus arteriosus can be treated with NSAIDs, which inhibit the production of prostaglandins and thereby facilitate ductus closure.

The Kidney

Prostaglandins normally do not play an important role in the control of blood flow, and inhibition of cyclooxygenase with NSAIDs does not alter perfusion in the kidney, heart, brain, or muscle. Exceptions occur, however, in certain pathological states in which impaired blood flow to an organ already exists. *Congestive heart failure, cir-*

rhosis, nephrotic syndrome, nephritis due to systemic lupus erythematosus, and any illness affecting sodium conservation may result in a deterioration of renal function following the administration of NSAIDs. For reasons that are not known, *sulindac* does not seem to share the same renal toxicity as do the other NSAIDs.

Bartter's syndrome (juxtaglomerular hyperplasia, hypokalemic alkalosis, and elevated renin and aldosterone with normal blood pressure) has responded to NSAIDs. It is presumed that the features of the syndrome are caused by excessive tissue levels of prostaglandins because increased urinary excretion of prostaglandins has been noted in affected individuals.

The Gastrointestinal System

Prostaglandins inhibit gastric acid secretion and promote the integrity of the gastric mucosa. One of the most common complications of NSAID therapy is gastrointestinal hemorrhage. This effect is likely to be caused by a diminished production of PGE$_2$ and PGI$_2$, the major cyclooxygenase metabolites of human gastric mucosa.

A process known as *adaptive cytoprotection* has been discovered recently whereby a gastric mucosal irritant, administered at a low concentration, can protect the mucosa from a subsequent administration of the irritant even at a dose that would normally cause mucosal injury. Adaptive cytoprotection can be inhibited by NSAIDs, thus implying the importance of naturally produced prostaglandins in this phenomenon. *Aluminum sucralfate* (see Chap. 73), a medication that can protect the gastric mucosa from irritant-induced injury and can enhance the rate of healing of peptic ulcers, is believed to operate through adaptive cytoprotection by inducing the production of endogenous prostaglandins in intestinal mucosa.

NSAIDs are capable of inducing hepatotoxicity, especially during the first few months of therapy. The risk for toxicity is increased in alcoholism and coexisting chronic liver disease, and by the administration of other hepatotoxic drugs, such as methotrexate. Serum hepatic enzymes should be monitored during the first few months of NSAID administration, especially if a coexisting risk factor exists.

Bone Metabolism

PGE$_2$ can enhance bone resorption. Such an action appears to play an important pathological role in some cases of hypercalcemia due to malignancy. It appears that some tumors secrete a humoral substance that is capable of inducing calcium release from bone via a prostaglandin-dependent mechanism. In these cases administration of NSAIDs may be beneficial in controlling the hypercalce-

Table 42-2. Prostaglandins and Prostaglandin Analogues Available for Pharmacological Use

Drug	Effects	Common side effects
Alprostadil (PGE₁)	Maintains patency of ductus arteriosus	Fever, flushing, apnea, diarrhea, cortical proliferation of long bones
Dinoprost tromethamine (PGF₂ₐ)	Abortifacient	Bronchospasm
Dinoprostone (PGE₂)	Abortifacient, benign hydatidiform mole treatment, evacuation of uterine contents for missed abortion	Nausea, vomiting, fever, diarrhea, headache
Misoprostol	Gastric cytoprotection	Diarrhea, abdominal pain

mia. This therapy is not beneficial for hypercalcemia associated with bony metastases.

Therapeutic and Potentially Therapeutic Eicosanoids

Several eicosanoids are currently available for pharmacological use in humans. Alprostadil (PGE₁, *Prostin VR Pediatric*) is approved for the temporary maintenance of patency of the ductus arteriosus in infants with congenital heart anomalies until appropriate surgical correction can be performed. This drug works best in infants with severe hypoxia due to pulmonary outlet obstruction. Maintenance of a patent ductus allows bypass of the obstruction and improves blood oxygenation by improving pulmonary blood flow.

Dinoprost tromethamine (PGF₂ₐ, a component of *Prostin F2 Alpha*) is an abortifacient when administered by means of an intraamniotic injection. Dinoprostone (PGE₂, *Prostin E2*) is available as a vaginal suppository for use as an abortifacient to assist in evacuation of the uterus in missed abortion; it also can be used in the treatment of benign hydatidiform mole.

Analogues of the E and F series of prostaglandins (e.g., *Carboprost tromethamine, Prostin/15M*) either will be or have been marketed for similar uses as dinoprostone. Analogues of the prostaglandin E series are being developed as therapeutic agents for peptic ulcer disease. Misoprostol (*Cytotec*) is approved for use in the prevention of gastric ulcer in patients at high risk (e.g., those receiving NSAIDs).

Properties of therapeutic eicosanoids are summarized in Table 42-2.

Platelet-Activating Factor

While PAF is produced by a wide variety of tissues and is present in normal secretions, its role in homeostasis has not yet been determined. Rather, most research has focused on its role as a mediator of the inflammatory response.

PAF is actually a family of compounds that differ in the length of the alkyl group that is attached by an ether to the C1 of the glycerol portion of the molecule.

PAF is produced by platelets, phagocytes (neutrophils, eosinophils, basophils, and macrophages), and vascular endothelial cells. Some cells may make *lyso*-PAF, which can be exported to other cells for synthesis to PAF.

Biological Effects of Platelet-Activating Factor

PAF can induce platelet aggregation, bronchoconstriction, cutaneous vasodilation, chemotaxis of phagocytes, hypotension, and the release of inflammatory compounds (enzymes and oxidants) from phagocytes. The intravenous administration of PAF results in a state with features highly reminiscent of anaphylaxis. Because of these effects intense research is currently being focused on PAF.

In humans, PAF results in bronchoconstriction when administered by aerosol and produces a wheal-and-flare response in the skin. Additionally, in the skin of allergic individuals, there seems to be a selective accumulation of eosinophils, some of which appear to have undergone degranulation. Thus, *PAF can mimic many of the features seen in the allergic response.*

Pharmacological Antagonism of Platelet-Activating Factor

At present, no specific therapeutic antagonists of PAF are available for human use. Synthetic analogues of PAF, however, are being developed and most of these compounds are designed to be PAF receptor antagonists; *gingkolide B* (also called BN 522021), derived from the gingko tree, has received the most attention.

Supplemental Reading

Guslandi, M. Gastric cytoprotection: What does it really mean for the prescriber? *Drugs* 41:507, 1991.

Holtzman, M.J. Arachidonic acid metabolism. *Am. Rev. Respir. Dis.* 143:188, 1991.

Imperiale, T.F., and Petrulis, A.S. A meta-analysis of low-dose aspirin for the prevention of pregnancy-induced hypertensive disease. *J.A.M.A.* 266:260, 1991.

Sebaldt, R.J., et al. Inhibition of eicosanoid biosynthesis by glucocorticoids in humans. *Proc. Natl. Acad. Sci. USA* 87:6974, 1990.

Spencer, D.A. An update on PAF. *Clin. Exp. Allergy* 22:521, 1992.

Toto, R.D. Role of prostaglandins in NSAID-induced renal dysfunction. *Adv. Prostaglandin. Thromboxane Leukotriene Res.* 21:967, 1990.

43

Antiinflammatory and Antirheumatic Drugs

Donald C. Kvam

Antiinflammatory drugs are prescribed in most cases for rheumatic disease. Few, if any, drugs are recognized as "antirheumatic" in the sense that they can reverse or arrest the rheumatic disease process (gold preparations and certain immunosuppressants may be exceptions); they can, however, be shown convincingly to be antiinflammatory. Prescriptions for these agents are most commonly written for treatment of rheumatoid arthritis, osteoarthritis, or acute gouty arthritis. All these conditions are characterized by some degree of inflammation and tissue damage at joints, which become more prominent as the diseases progress. By reducing pain and inflammation, antiinflammatory drugs allow continued use of the joints, helping to preserve their mobility.

With the exception of gouty arthritis, for which the precipitating agent (urate crystals) is well known, the etiology of these diseases has not been elucidated. Osteoarthritis, the most common of the articular diseases, was formerly thought of as a degenerative joint disease without an inflammatory component. It is now recognized that an inflammatory component exists, particularly in the latter phases of the disease.

Rheumatoid Arthritis

Rheumatoid arthritis is a chronic inflammatory disease that occurs in about 1 percent of the population, affecting women two to three times more commonly than men. The synovium is primarily involved; an inflammatory process initially produces tenderness, soreness, stiffness, and eventually destruction of cartilage and bone. The pathogenesis is not understood, but aspects of the immune response appear to be involved. The hypothesis that an autoimmune reaction to cartilaginous collagen (type II collagen) is an important determinant in the pathogenesis of rheumatoid arthritis is consistent with an immune or possibly an infectious etiology. The documented immunopathological events that occur in rheumatoid arthritis

have been interpreted to be a consequence of an initiating infection. Many years of searching for the infectious agent that is responsible for rheumatoid arthritis have yielded no unequivocal candidate.

Management

The conservative treatment of rheumatoid arthritis includes rest, proper diet, physical therapy, and salicylates; further additions to the therapy carry added risks. The objectives in the management of rheumatoid arthritis are reducing pain and inflammation, preserving function of the joints, and preventing deformities. No available drug therapy is curative. It is unrealistic to expect to relieve the patient's discomfort completely with the currently available drugs, although this might be possible for a certain period of time with dangerous dosages of corticosteroids. *The aim is to produce a measure of relief with which the patient can live but not to precipitate iatrogenic disease.* There seems to be general agreement among rheumatologists that the initial treatment of the patient with "uncomplicated" rheumatoid arthritis should be conservative.

The inflammatory response is a stereotyped, homeostatic, and usually beneficial reaction by the organism to injury. *The need for antiinflammatory drugs arises when the inflammatory response is inappropriate, aberrant, or sustained, and when it causes destruction of tissue.* The complexity of the inflammatory response explains why substances of diverse chemical structure constitute a pharmacological class of agents, termed *antiinflammatory*. An *antihistamine* may be antiinflammatory in certain circumstances because of its ability to suppress a minor component of the inflammatory response. An *immunosuppressant* might be considered to have antiinflammatory activity if it prevents the inflammatory response to an interaction of antigen and antibody from developing. The various antiinflammatory drugs affect different components of the inflammatory response, certainly have different mechanisms of action, and after their administration, do not always lead to the same end

Table 43-1. Indications for Antiinflammatory Drugs

Disease	Antiinflammatory drugs used
Rheumatic	
Rheumatoid arthritis	Salicylates, other NSAIDS,[a] gold preparations, steroids, antimalarials, cytostatics
Rheumatoid variants[b]	Other NSAIDS, salicylates
Degenerative joint disease (osteoarthritis)	NSAIDs
Systemic lupus erythematosus	Salicylates, antimalarials, steroids, cytostatics
Gout	Colchicine, other NSAIDs
Nonrheumatic	
Psoriasis	Steroids (topical), cytostatics
Contact dermatitis	Steroids (topical)
Polyarteritis	Steroids
Dermatomyositis	Steroids
Ulcerative colitis	Steroids
Multiple sclerosis	Steroids
Dysmenorrhea	Ibuprofen, naproxen, ketoprofen

[a]Nonsteroidal antiinflammatory drugs (e.g., ibuprofen, indomethacin).
[b]Ankylosing spondylitis, Reiter's syndrome, psoriatic arthritis.

result. Some may prevent components of the early inflammatory response from manifesting themselves (e.g., antagonists of endogenous vascular permeability factors), others may interfere with the proliferative connective tissue phase of inflammation (e.g., cytotoxic agents), while others may aid in the elimination of the noxious stimulus (e.g., antibiotics in bacterial inflammation, uricosurics in urate crystal-induced inflammation).

Some of the more important rheumatic and nonrheumatic diseases for which therapy with antiinflammatory drugs is indicated are listed in Table 43-1. Only drugs used primarily for their antiinflammatory activity are listed. Table 43-2 lists some of the ancillary pharmacological properties of antiinflammatory drugs that are used in therapeutics.

Mechanism of Nonsteroidal Antiinflammatory Drug Action

At present, the most tenable hypothesis to explain the antiinflammatory actions of salicylates and other nonsteroidal antiinflammatory drugs (NSAIDs) is that they exert their effects through inhibition of prostaglandin synthesis. The primary site of action of these drugs is the cyclooxygenase enzyme that catalyzes the conversion of arachidonic acid to the prostaglandin and thromboxane precursor cyclic endoperoxide (see Chap. 42, Fig. 42-1). It has been shown that prostaglandins of the E and F series are capable of evoking some of the local and systemic manifestations of inflam-

mation (vasodilation and hyperemia, increased permeability, swelling and pain, increased leukocyte migration) as well as intensifying the effects of such chemical mediators of inflammation as histamine, bradykinin, and 5-hydroxytryptamine. Inhibition of prostaglandin synthesis also may account for certain toxicities that are common to all acidic NSAIDs.

All of the acidic NSAIDs studied to date are capable of inhibiting prostaglandin synthesis in vitro at concentrations that are readily achieved in vivo. Furthermore, the rank order of the inhibitory potencies of the nonsteroidal drugs agrees surprisingly well with their potencies as antiinflammatory agents. It is possible, however, that other mechanisms are involved in the antiinflammatory activity of the NSAIDs as well. For example, leukocyte adhesion may be a target for antiinflammatory drugs. The antiinflammatory doses of many NSAIDs for rheumatoid arthritis are, in some cases, much higher than those required to inhibit prostaglandin synthesis. The fact that a number of these drugs inhibit neutrophil adhesion or function at micro- or millimolar concentrations has been offered as an alternative explanation for their antiinflammatory effects.

Toxicity of Nonsteroidal Antiinflammatory Drugs

A list of the more frequently encountered side effects associated with NSAID therapy, thought to be related to prostaglandin inhibition, is given in Table 43-3. Adverse effects for which a relationship to inhibition of prostaglandin synthesis has not been unequivocally demonstrated include hepatic effects (hepatitis, hepatic necrosis, cholestatic jaundice, increased serum aminotransferases), dermal effects (photosensitivities, Stevens-Johnson syndrome, toxic epidermal necrolysis, onycholysis), central nervous system effects (headaches, dizziness, tinnitus, deafness, drowsiness, confusion, nervousness, increased sweating, aseptic meningitis), ocular effects (toxic amblyopia, retinal disturbances), and certain renal effects (acute interstitial nephritis, acute papillary necrosis).

Increasing attention has been focused on the potential of the NSAIDs to produce gastrointestinal and renal toxicities. The Food and Drug Administration (FDA) now requires a class labeling added to the package insert of each NSAID warning of the risk of serious gastrointestinal injury associated with its use. The inclusion of a similar warning for high-risk renal patients has been proposed.

A further indication of the heightened concern over gastrointestinal injury associated with NSAID therapy is the use of misoprostol (*Cytotec*), a synthetic prostaglandin E₁ analogue, for the prevention of NSAID-induced gastric ulcers in high-risk patients. Additional information is

Table 43-2. Additional Pharmacological Activities of Antiinflammatory Drugs

Drug	Activity	Use
Salicylates	Analgesic*; antipyretic; uricosuric	Headache, neuralgia, myalgia; febrile states; hyperuricemia
Corticosteroids	Endocrine; antiallergic; lympho-cytolytic; immunosuppressive	Adrenal insufficiency; asthma; leukemia; transplantation
Gold preparations	Antibiotic	None
Chloroquine	Antiplasmodial	Malaria
Cyclophosphamide, azathioprine	Cytostatic	Cancer, immunosuppression
Methotrexate	Antimetabolite	Leukemia, psoriasis, immunosuppression

*Fenoprofen, ibuprofen, ketoprofen, etodolac, and naproxen also have approved analgesic indications.

Table 43-3. Adverse Effects of Nonsteroidal Antiinflammatory Drugs—Relationship to Inhibition of Prostaglandin (PG) Synthesis

System affected	Effects	Prostaglandin synthesis
Gastrointestinal	Erosive gastritis; peptic ulceration	Inhibition of PGE_2, which suppresses gastric acid secretion, helps maintain mucosal barrier and regulate microcirculation
Antiplatelet	Prolonged bleeding time, GI blood loss	Inhibition of synthesis of thromboxane A_2 by platelets
Renal	Fluid retention, diminished sodium excretion, prerenal azotemia, hyperkalemia, oliguria, anuria	Inhibition of synthesis of renal PG involved in regulation of renal blood flow, glomerular filtration, and renal sodium and water excretion; also involved in mediation of renin release
Allergic	Bronchospasm, urticaria, rhinitis, nasal polyposis	Inhibition of cyclooxygenase pathway, allowing lipoxygenase pathway to dominate in susceptible individuals
Uterine	Delayed parturition, dystocia	Loss of contractile effects of PGs on uterine muscle

given in Chap. 73. Misoprostol is given at a dose of 200 μg four times a day concurrent with NSAID therapy.

Adverse effects that are associated with particular drugs are listed later in this chapter in the discussions of individual agents.

Agents

Acidic Nonsteroidal Antiinflammatory Agents

This class of antiinflammatory drugs includes the salicylates and an increasing number of other acid compounds. The latter agents, as a group, share many common properties; they have similar toxicities, are highly protein bound, and have the potential for interacting with other protein-bound drugs, and many have effects on platelets and the clotting process. The choice of a particular agent for an individual patient is not always easy.

Salicylates

This chemical class has been discussed previously (see Chap. 39). Only observations that are relevant to their use as antiinflammatory agents are discussed in this chapter. Among the salicylates, *aspirin* and *sodium salicylate* are by far the most commonly used. Although aspirin itself is pharmacologically active, it is rapidly hydrolyzed to salicylic acid after its absorption, and *it is the salicylate anion that accounts for most of the antiinflammatory activity* of the drug (Fig. 43-1). The superior analgesic activity of aspirin compared with sodium salicylate implies that aspirin has an intrinsic activity that is not totally explainable by its conversion to salicylic acid. Aspirin can acetylate proteins, and this property might account for some of the therapeutic and toxicological differences that exist between aspirin and the other salicylates.

Absorption, Metabolism, and Excretion

Without exception, the acidic NSAIDs in use today are well absorbed after their oral administration. Certain claims alleging enhanced aspirin absorption resulting from changes in product formulation or by buffering seem to relate to the *rate* rather than the extent of absorption. Trivial increases in the rate of absorption of a drug from a particular preparation should be of little consequence for drugs used in treating rheumatic conditions, since these drugs are prescribed on a chronic dosage schedule.

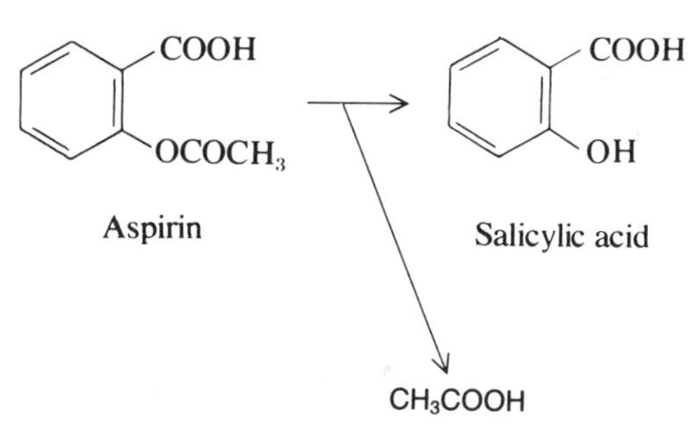

Figure 43-1. Breakdown of aspirin to salicylic acid.

The plasma concentration of salicylate that is associated with antiinflammatory activity (200–300 μg/ml) is about six times that needed to produce analgesia. At these higher concentrations, salicylate metabolism is reduced, resulting in a longer half-life for the drug. This reaction is a consequence of the capacity-limited (saturable) enzyme systems in humans that are responsible for the metabolism of salicylates. The plasma half-life for salicylate has been estimated to be 3 to 6 hr at the lower (analgesic) dosage and 15 to 30 hr at the higher (antiinflammatory) dosages. The rate of hydrolysis of aspirin to salicylic acid is not dose limited, and no differences in the absorption of aspirin have been observed between arthritic patients and normal individuals.

Clinical Uses

The salicylates are undoubtedly the drugs of choice in the treatment of the milder forms of inflammatory disease. These forms include acute rheumatic fever, rheumatoid arthritis, osteoarthritis, mild systemic lupus erythematosus, and certain rheumatoid variants, such as ankylosing spondylitis, Reiter's syndrome, and psoriatic arthritis. When antiinflammatory dosages are given, the salicylates both reduce inflammatory signs and provide an adequate degree of analgesia. However, salicylates do not affect the progress of any of the inflammatory diseases or alter in any way the proliferative reactions. They are also useful in the treatment of more trivial musculoskeletal disorders such as bursitis, synovitis, tendinitis, myositis, and myalgia, and as adjuvants to corticosteroids and other measures in more serious or severe inflammatory conditions.

Adverse Reactions

The most common adverse effects produced by the salicylates are gastrointestinal disturbances (heartburn, indigestion), which may be decreased by adjusting the dosage, using antacids, or administering the drugs after meals. Occult loss of blood from the gastrointestinal tract can result from salicylate use. Severe gastrointestinal hemorrhage after aspirin intake also has been reported, but this

is an infrequent event. The blood loss occurring during chronic therapy with aspirin is a common cause of iron deficiency anemia. Peptic ulcers may also be precipitated or reactivated. The nonacetylated salicylates have greatly reduced effects on blood loss and produce less adverse gastrointestinal effects. In addition, they may be somewhat "renal sparing." Tinnitus, hearing impairment, blurred vision, and light-headedness also may occur and are indications of toxic dosages. If these occur, a reduction in dosage is indicated.

Hypersensitivity reactions may occur in some individuals and are recognized as urticaria, rhinorrhea, purpura, pancytopenia, aggravation of asthma, or, rarely, as anaphylactic shock. These reactions may occur even in those individuals who have previously used aspirin without suffering any ill effects.

Cautions

Aspirin inhibits platelet aggregation and prolongs bleeding time. It should, therefore, be used with caution in individuals receiving coumarin anticoagulants. It should be avoided in patients receiving heparin or in those with severe bleeding disorders (see also Chap. 39).

Preparations

Aspirin is available for oral administration as capsules, tablets, enteric-coated tablets (*Ecotrin*); timed-release tablets (*Measurin, Zorprin*), chewable tablets, and buffered tablets (component of *Ascriptin; Bufferin*). It is also supplied as rectal suppositories.

Sodium salicylate is available for oral use as tablets, either plain or enteric coated, and is marketed under its generic name.

Other salicylates include choline salicylate (*Arthropan*), salsalate (salicylsalicylic acid, *Disalcid*), choline magnesium trisalicylate (*Trilisate*), and magnesium salicylate (*Mobidin*).

A summary of suggested dosages of salicylates and other NSAIDs in the treatment of rheumatoid arthritis is provided in Table 43-4.

Phenylbutazone-Type Drugs

Four members of this class have been used for their antiinflammatory effects: phenylbutazone, oxyphenbutazone, antipyrine, and aminopyrine. Only phenylbutazone is used to any extent today, and that use is declining. Because of its propensity to cause blood dyscrasias, phenylbutazone has been withdrawn from the market in some countries.

Absorption, Metabolism, and Excretion

Phenylbutazone is rapidly absorbed from the gastrointestinal tract, with peak plasma concentrations achieved in about 2 hr; its elimination half-life is about 85 hr. Phen-

Table 43-4. Usual Dosages of Nonsteroidal Antiinflammatory Drugs in Rheumatoid Arthritis

Drug	Usual dose	Comment
Salicylates (aspirin, sodium salicylate)	3.6–5.4 gm/day in divided doses; 90–130 mg/kg/day[a]	Dosage should be increased until antiinflammatory effect or ototoxic level is reached
Phenylbutazone	300–400 mg/day in 3–4 divided doses[b]	Response should occur within 1 week; maintenance doses of 100–200 mg daily may be possible and allow longer-term therapy
Piroxicam	20 mg once a day[c]	Steady-state blood levels reached in 7–12 days
Meclofenamic acid	200–400 mg/day in 3–4 divided doses[b]	Dose should be individualized; do not exceed 400 mg/day
Indomethacin	25 mg 2–3 times a day[c]	Can be increased in daily increments of 25 mg at weekly intervals to maximum of 150–200 mg
Sulindac	150 mg twice a day	Adjust dose according to response; 400 mg/day maximum
Ibuprofen	300 mg 4 times a day; 400, 600, or 800 mg 3–4 times a day	Variations in response; optimal dose must be determined individually
Fenoprofen	300–600 mg 3–4 times a day[b]	Dosage should be adjusted to patient after response has been attained; 3,200 mg maximum
Naproxen	275–550 mg twice a day[d]	Long-term dose should be individualized; dosage in juvenile arthritis is 10 mg/kg in 2 divided doses
Tolmetin	600–1,800 mg in 3–4 divided doses[d]; 15–30 mg/kg/day[a]	Long-term dose should be individualized; 600–1,800 mg/day is usually sufficient
Diclofenac	150–200 mg/day in 2–4 divided doses[b]	Maintenance dose should be lowest dose consistent with satisfactory response
Ketoprofen	150–300 mg/day in 3–4 divided doses[b]	Doses higher than 300 mg/day not recommended; reduce dose by one-half in elderly and renal-impaired patients
Flurbiprofen	200–300 mg/day in 2–4 divided doses[b]	Recommended starting dose is 100 mg twice daily
Etodolac	600–1,200 mg/day in 2–4 divided doses	Indicated for osteoarthritis only; initiate therapy at 800–1,200 mg/day and adjust to indicated range; do not exceed 1,200 mg/day
Nabumetone	1,000–2,000 mg once a day	Recommended starting dose is 1,000 mg/day

[a]Children's dose.
[b]No children's dose has been established; not recommended in children under 14 years of age.
[c]Contraindicated in children under 14 years of age.
[d]Not recommended in children under 2 years of age.

ylbutazone is metabolized to oxyphenbutazone and another metabolite. Oxyphenbutazone itself is effective as an antiinflammatory compound and also has a long elimination half-life (about 70 hr).

Clinical Uses

Although phenylbutazone is effective in the therapy of acute gout and other rheumatoid disorders, *its use should be reserved primarily for the relief of acute exacerbations of rheumatoid disease that are not controlled by other drugs,* such as salicylates. There is a risk of serious effects that frequently occur during long-term therapy with phenylbutazone, particularly in the elderly. Owing to the potential for serious side effects, its use in other less serious musculoskeletal disorders is not to be condoned.

Adverse Reactions

Phenylbutazone (and oxyphenbutazone) produce gastrointestinal disturbances (mild irritation or ulcerogenesis), hepatitis, dermatitis, stomatitis, headache, vertigo,

and sodium and water retention. With prolonged use, these drugs may depress the bone marrow and cause leukemia, leukopenia, agranulocytosis, and aplastic anemia. Caution dictates that hematological analyses be performed regularly during long-term therapy with these drugs. Patients over 40 years of age seem to be particularly prone to suffer adverse reactions from the use of the phenylpyrazolone drugs.

Because of its ability to displace other drugs from their plasma protein-binding sites, phenylbutazone can potentiate the effects of oral hypoglycemics, sulfonamides, coumarin-type anticoagulants, and other antiinflammatory agents. It may confound tests of thyroid function by displacing bound thyroid hormone from protein-binding sites.

Preparations

Phenylbutazone (*Azolid, Butazolidin*) is available as 100-mg tablets and 100-mg capsules. Generic versions are available.

Oxicam-Type Drugs

Piroxicam is the only member of this class currently available in the United States. Tenoxicam, another drug of this type, is available outside the United States.

Piroxicam is well absorbed and peak plasma levels of the drug are reached 3 to 5 hr after its oral administration. The plasma half-life of the drug is about 50 hr (range, 30–86 hr). Steady-state levels are reached in 7 to 12 days. Piroxicam is extensively metabolized to inactive compounds and excreted in the urine (two-thirds) and feces (one-third). Concurrent administration of aspirin has resulted in an approximate 20 percent reduction in plasma levels of piroxicam. *The use of piroxicam or any other NSAID in conjunction with aspirin is not recommended* because of the lack of evidence that such combinations increase efficacy and because of the increased potential for an adverse reaction.

About 30 percent of patients receiving long-term therapy with piroxicam have reported side effects. Adverse gastrointestinal reactions have been the most frequently reported side effect, but edema, dizziness, headache, rash, and changes in hematological parameters have also occurred in 1 to 6 percent of patients. *Piroxicam can cause serious gastrointestinal toxicity, particularly in the elderly,* if the recommended dosage is exceeded, or if aspirin is being taken concurrently. Bleeding, which is sometimes severe, peptic ulceration, and perforation have been associated with the use of piroxicam. Some deaths attributable to piroxicam therapy have been reported.

Piroxicam (*Feldene*) is available as 10- and 20-mg capsules. Generics are also available.

Fenamate-Type Drugs

Two compounds of this class of antiinflammatory drugs are marketed in the United States. Mefenamic acid (*Ponstel*) is indicated only for analgesia and primary dysmenorrhea when therapy will not exceed 1 week. Meclofenamate sodium (*Meclomen*) is prescribed for rheumatoid arthritis and osteoarthritis. In addition to inhibition of the cyclooxygenase enzyme, the mechanism of action of meclofenamic acid may involve direct inhibition of the effects of prostaglandins.

Administration of single oral doses of meclofenamate sodium results in peak plasma levels of drug in 0.5 to 1.0 hr. The plasma half-life is about 2 hr following a single dose and 3.3 hr with multiple dosing. About 70 percent of the administered dosage is excreted in the urine and the remainder in the feces. In general, the urinary metabolites are eliminated as glucuronide conjugates and the fecal metabolites as free acids.

Meclofenamic acid has a propensity to produce gastrointestinal side effects. In long-term studies, one-third of patients had at least one episode of diarrhea during therapy. In controlled studies, the diarrhea was severe enough

to necessitate discontinuation of meclofenamic acid in 4 percent of the patients. Diarrhea generally subsides with a reduction in dosage or termination of the drug. Other adverse gastrointestinal reactions associated with therapy with meclofenamic acid include nausea, vomiting, abdominal pains, bleeding, and peptic ulceration.

Decreases in the hematocrit or hemoglobin values occur in approximately one-sixth of patients taking meclofenamic acid, but these do not usually require discontinuation of therapy. Hematological analyses should be performed on patients receiving long-term therapy with the drug if anemia is suspected.

Aryl and Heteroarylalkanoic Acid–Type Drugs

The prototypes of this large class of NSAIDs are indomethacin and ibuprofen (Fig. 43-2). Indomethacin was the first of the new generation of NSAIDs introduced beginning in the 1960s. These drugs were the successors to phenylbutazone as the second step in antirheumatic therapy—that is, for use when salicylates were no longer effective or tolerated. They are indicated for the relief of acute and chronic rheumatoid arthritis and osteoarthritis. In addition, a number of drugs of this class are also useful in ankylosing spondylitis, acute gouty arthritis, and bursitis/tendinitis. For chronic conditions, they should be considered only after salicylates have been tried and found to be lacking in efficacy or are not well tolerated.

Adverse reactions are common with the use of these drugs but usually do not result in serious morbidity. In most cases, they disappear rather promptly after the drugs are discontinued. Gastrointestinal and central nervous system (CNS) effects (e.g., dizziness) are frequently reported. Fluid retention and skin rashes also occur, but with much lower frequency. None of the agents seems to be clearly preferable to the others. All should be used with caution in patients receiving oral anticoagulants, anticonvulsants, sulfonamides, or sulfonylureas, and all should be regarded as having the potential for producing ophthalmological problems. All these agents should be considered to have the potential to produce cross-sensitivity to aspirin and other antiinflammatory drugs. *These drugs produce less gastrointestinal blood loss than does aspirin,* and the overall incidence of adverse reactions may be lower with these drugs than with aspirin.

Indomethacin

Indomethacin is used primarily as an antiinflammatory agent when salicylates are ineffective or not well tolerated. It is used in the treatment of acute gouty arthritis, rheumatoid arthritis, ankylosing spondylitis, and degenerative joint disease of the hip. It is not recommended for use as a simple analgesic or antipyretic because of its potential for toxicity.

Administration of a single oral dose of 50 mg to fasting individuals results in peak plasma indomethacin levels of

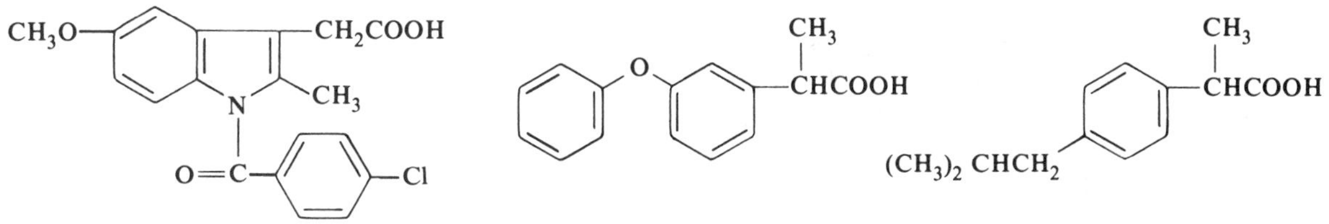

Figure 43-2. Indomethacin, fenoprofen, and ibuprofen.

1.8 to 2.0 μg/ml in approximately 1 hr. Serum half-life for elimination under these circumstances is 1.8 hr. Indomethacin is highly bound to plasma proteins (90%). After 48 hr, approximately 60 percent of the total dose may be accounted for in the urine, and about 30 percent in the feces.

Toxicity

The use of indomethacin in arthritic patients is associated with a higher incidence of CNS side effects than is found with most of the other NSAIDs. Headache, vertigo, confusion, and psychic disturbances occur with some regularity. Gastrointestinal symptoms also are frequent and include nausea, vomiting, anorexia, indigestion, epigastric distress, diarrhea, and ulcerogenesis. Side effects related to the hematopoietic system (e.g., leukopenia, hemolytic anemia, aplastic anemia, purpura, thrombocytopenia, and agranulocytosis) also are known to occur.

Ocular effects (blurred vision, corneal deposits) have been observed in patients receiving indomethacin, and regular ophthalmological examinations are necessary when the drug is used for prolonged periods. Hepatitis, jaundice, pancreatitis, and hypersensitivity reactions also have been noted.

Preparations

Indomethacin is marketed under the trademark *Indocin* as sustained-release capsules, suppositories, and a suspension. Generic versions are also available.

Sulindac

Sulindac is chemically related to indomethacin. The sulfide metabolite appears to be responsible for its pharmacological activity. Although clinical experience with sulindac has not been as extensive as that with indomethacin, the two drugs are generally used for the same indications.

Fate

After its absorption, sulindac is metabolized in two major ways. It is reversibly reduced to the sulfide (the active moiety) and is irreversibly oxidized to an inactive sulfone metabolite. Peak plasma levels of the active metabolite are achieved in 3 to 4 hr after oral administration. The plasma half-life of sulindac is about 8 hr, whereas that of its sulfide metabolite is twice that time. Significant enterohepatic recycling of sulindac and its metabolites is assumed to occur.

Toxicity

The most frequently reported side effects result from gastrointestinal irritation and include pain, nausea, diarrhea, and constipation. As with indomethacin, a rather high incidence of CNS side effects also occurs (dizziness, headache).

Preparation

Sulindac (*Clinoril*) is marketed as 150- and 200-mg tablets.

Ibuprofen

This compound displays analgesic and antipyretic activities in addition to its antiinflammatory effects. It is useful in patients with rheumatoid arthritis and degenerative joint disease. Its use as an analgesic is described in Chap. 39.

Fate

Peak plasma levels of 15 to 20 μg/ml occur about 1 hr after administration of a single 200-mg oral dose. The serum half-life after a single 200-mg oral dose in fasting subjects is estimated to be 1.9 hr. No evidence has been found for significant accumulation of ibuprofen, and no drug can be detected 24 hr after cessation of a continuous regimen of 200 mg of drug three times a day. As with other drugs of its class, ibuprofen is extensively bound (in excess of 90%) to plasma proteins. In humans, approximately 45 percent of an administered daily dose is excreted, primarily as metabolites and their conjugates, in the urine within 24 hr.

Toxicity

The most frequently observed side effects are nausea, heartburn, epigastric pain, rash, and dizziness. Blurred or diminished vision including color vision changes also have been reported. Cross-sensitivity has been reported to aspirin, and ibuprofen is contraindicated in individuals sensitive to aspirin. Ibuprofen inhibits platelet aggregation, but the duration is shorter and the effect quantitatively lower than with aspirin. The drug prolongs bleeding times toward high normal values and should be used with caution in patients with coagulation deficits or those receiving anticoagulant therapy. No interaction with coumarin-type anticoagulants has been reported.

Preparations

Ibuprofen (*Motrin, Rufen*) is available as high-strength tablets by prescription and also without prescription as 200-mg tablets under several brand names (e.g., *Advil, Nuprin*). Suspensions for pediatric use are marketed.

Fenoprofen

This drug is chemically and pharmacologically similar to ibuprofen and is used in the treatment of rheumatoid arthritis.

Fate

Fenoprofen, either as the calcium or sodium salt, is readily absorbed from the gastrointestinal tract, and a single 300-mg dose to fasting individuals yields peak plasma concentrations in the range of 23 to 31 $\mu g/ml$ in approximately 0.5 to 1.5 hr. The drug is almost totally bound to plasma albumin. The plasma half-life after a dose of 600 mg has been estimated to be 2.5 to 3.0 hr, and only small amounts of drug are present in the plasma 12 hr after dosing.

Most of an administered dose is excreted in the urine, and only about 2 percent can be detected in the feces. Since considerable amounts can be found in the bile after oral administration, the drug must undergo enterohepatic cycling.

Concomitant administration of aspirin decreases the biological half-life of fenoprofen by increasing the metabolic clearance of hydroxylated fenoprofen. Chronic administration of phenobarbital also decreases the half-life of this agent.

Toxicity

Gastrointestinal bleeding, sometimes severe, has been reported with use of this drug. Adverse effects referable to the gastrointestinal tract are most common (14% of patients) although dizziness, pruritus, and palpitations also are reported (3–9% of patients).

Preparation

Fenoprofen calcium (*Nalfon*) is available as tablets and capsules. Generic formulations are available.

Naproxen

Naproxen also is a phenylpropionic acid analogue with pharmacological properties and clinical uses similar to ibuprofen.

Fate

It is well absorbed after oral administration, and doses of 200 to 300 mg produce peak plasma levels of 30 to 40 $\mu g/ml$ in about 2 hr. Repeated dosing produces steady-state conditions after four or five doses. The plasma half-life in humans is approximately 14 hr. At therapeutic levels, naproxen is highly bound (99%) to serum albumin.

Humans excrete naproxen and its metabolites predominantly in the urine, with only 1 percent of an administered dose found in the feces.

Toxicity

Adverse reactions related to the gastrointestinal tract occur in about 14 percent of all patients and severe gastrointestinal bleeding has been reported. CNS complaints (headache, dizziness, drowsiness), dermatological effects (pruritus, skin eruptions, ecchymoses), tinnitus, edema, and dyspnea also occur.

Preparations

Naproxen (*Naprosyn*) is marketed as tablets and as a suspension. Naproxen sodium (*Anaprox*) is also marketed.

Tolmetin

This compound also is an NSAID and is rapidly absorbed from the gastrointestinal tract. After an oral dose of 400 mg, peak plasma levels of 40 $\mu g/ml$ are reached within 30 to 60 min. The drug is rapidly excreted in the urine, and its plasma half-life is approximately 60 min. At therapeutic plasma concentrations, 99 percent of the drug is bound to plasma proteins. The major route of excretion is through the urine, and essentially all of an administered dose can be recovered within 24 hr as inactive metabolites.

The most frequently reported side effects are gastrointestinal disturbances and CNS reactions (e.g., headache, asthenia, and dizziness). These effects, however, are less frequently observed than after aspirin or indomethacin use. Blood pressure elevation, edema, and weight gain or loss have been associated with tolmetin administration. No effect on the anticoagulant actions of warfarin was noted in controlled studies. In addition, no interaction appears to occur with insulin or the sulfonylureas. Tolmetin metabolites in urine have been found to produce a pseudoproteinuria in laboratory tests that utilize acid precipitation.

Tolmetin sodium (*Tolectin*) is available as tablets and capsules (*Tolectin DS*).

Ketoprofen

Ketoprofen is indicated for use in rheumatoid and osteoarthritis, for mild to moderate pain, and in dysmenorrhea.

Fate

Ketoprofen is rapidly and completely absorbed, and is 90 percent bioavailable by the oral route. Peak plasma levels occur from 0.5 to 2.0 hr after oral administration; the mean plasma elimination half-life ranges from 2 to 4 hr. Sixty percent of an administered dose is excreted in the urine, primarily as the glucuronide, within the first 24 hr. The drug is 99 percent bound to serum proteins, mainly albumin.

Toxicity

The most frequently reported side effects are gastrointestinal (dyspepsia, nausea, abdominal pain, diarrhea, constipation, and flatulence) and CNS related (headache, excitation). Edema and increased blood urea nitrogen (BUN) have also been noted in greater than 3 percent of patients. Ketoprofen decreases platelet adhesion and aggregation; bleeding time is prolonged 3 to 4 min over baseline. Other clotting measurements are not affected.

Preparation

Ketoprofen (*Orudis*) is available as 25-, 50-, or 75-mg capsules.

Diclofenac

Diclofenac is approved for use in rheumatoid arthritis, osteoarthritis, and ankylosing spondylitis.

Fate

Diclofenac is completely absorbed after oral administration, although the presence of food in the gastrointestinal tract will delay its absorption from 1 to 10 hr. Fasting peak plasma levels occur in 2 to 3 hr; the drug undergoes first-pass metabolism and only about 50 percent is bioavailable by the oral route. Its half-life is approximately 2 hr; 65 percent of the dose is eliminated in the urine while 35 percent is found in the bile, largely as conjugates of both the unchanged drug and its metabolites. Some of the metabolites may have pharmacological activity. The drug is 99 percent bound to plasma albumin.

Toxicity

The most common adverse reactions are gastrointestinal disturbances and headache. A reversible elevation of serum transaminases occurs in 15 percent of patients. Diclofenac does increase platelet aggregation time, but other effects on clotting measurements are not clinically significant. Agranulocytosis, with an incidence approximately that for phenylbutazone, has been associated with diclofenac administration.

Preparation

Diclofenac sodium (*Voltaren*) is available as 25-, 50-, or 75-mg enteric-coated tablets.

Flurbiprofen

Flurbiprofen is indicated for the treatment of rheumatoid and osteoarthritis.

Fate

It is well absorbed orally; peak blood levels occur 0.5 to 4.0 hr after administration. The elimination half-life averages 5.7 hr. No accumulation of the drug occurs; up to 98 percent is excreted within 24 hr after the last dose. It is extensively metabolized, and excreted primarily in the urine: 20 percent as free drug and about 50 percent as hydroxylated metabolites. Typical of drugs of this class, it is highly bound (99%) to plasma proteins.

Toxicity

The most common adverse effects of flurbiprofen are similar to those of the other acidic NSAIDs.

Preparation

Flurbiprofen (*Ansaid*) is supplied as 50- and 100-mg tablets.

Etodolac (Lodine)

This acidic nonsteroidal antiinflammatory drug is indicated for the treatment of osteoarthritis only.

Fate

The systemic availability is at least 80 percent by the oral route, and significant first-pass metabolism does not occur. Peak blood levels are reached in about 80 min with a terminal half-life of about 7 hr. Intersubject variability in plasma levels is substantial. The drug is extensively biotransformed in the liver and excreted largely in the urine, primarily as metabolites.

Toxicity

The adverse effects are similar to those of other acidic NSAIDs.

Nabumetone (Relafen)

This agent, a weak inhibitor of cyclooxygenase, is metabolized to 6-methoxy-2-naphthylacetic acid (6-MNA), which is a strong inhibitor of the enzyme. Nabumetone is approved for both rheumatoid and osteoarthritis, and the drug is recommended to be given once a day.

Fate

Nabumetone is absorbed in the duodenum and is metabolized in the liver to 6-MNA, which has a terminal half-life of about 24 hr. Concentrations of the metabolite peak in about 2.5 hr on multiple dosing. The inactive metabolites of 6-MNA are excreted largely in urine and bile. Plasma concentrations of 6-MNA may increase in the elderly and in severe renal dysfunction.

Toxicity

As with most NSAIDs, gastrointestinal side effects are those most commonly reported. Since nabumetone is a nonacidic prodrug, less locally mediated gastric irritation

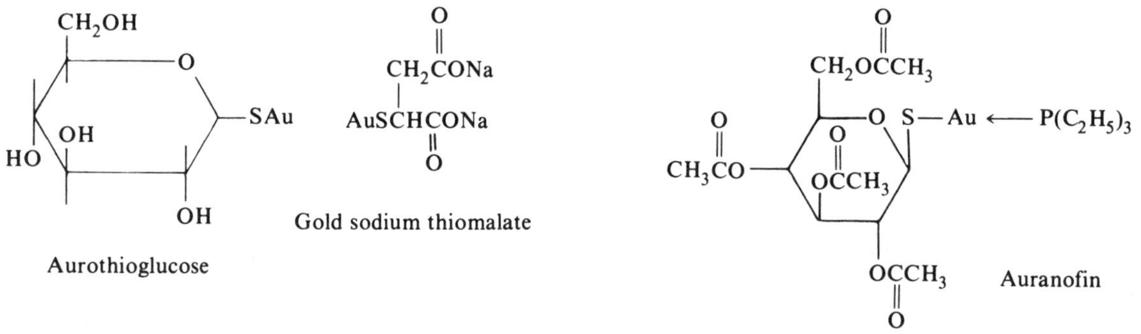

Figure 43-3. Commonly used gold preparations.

should be seen than with other NSAIDs. However, local irritation is not the sole cause of the adverse gastrointestinal effects of these drugs; knowledge as to whether reduced local irritation will significantly affect the incidence of peptic ulceration and gastrointestinal bleeding with nabumetone will require more experience.

Gold Preparations

The use of gold in treating rheumatoid arthritis was based originally on the substance's known antimicrobial activity and the belief that an infectious agent was responsible for the disease.

Chemistry

The gold preparations in use today contain gold in the monovalent state, although all valence states of gold have been evaluated for clinical effectiveness. Gold is quite inert chemically, and the ionic species tend to decompose to the elemental state. Advantage is taken of the strong affinity of aurous gold for sulfur to prepare relatively stable aurous gold for therapeutic use.

Although these complexes have been termed "gold salts," such a designation is not consistent with the nature of the Au-S bond, which is at least partly covalent in character. For this reason, and in order not to minimize the contribution of the ligand portion of the complex to the toxicological and pharmacological effects of the compounds, the designation of these complexes as "gold preparations" or "gold compounds" is observed in this chapter. Most of the therapeutic preparations in use are water soluble and contain hydrophilic groups in addition to the aurothio group. The structures of gold preparations available in the United States are shown in Fig. 43-3.

Mechanism of Action

The mechanism by which gold produces its antiarthritic effect is not known. The effects of gold on immune mechanisms are inconsistent and unimpressive. Since gold therapy can suppress the increased phagocytic activity of macrophages and polymorphonuclear leukocytes that occurs in patients with rheumatoid arthritis, it has been suggested that the antirheumatic activity of gold preparations might involve either the inhibition of the processing of antigens by macrophages or the inhibition of destructive lysosomal enzyme release in the joint. Gold preparations also are capable of directly inhibiting certain lysosomal enzymes that are contained in polymorphonuclear leukocytes and macrophages. These effects of gold on two important cell types involved in the inflammatory process may relate to its effectiveness in treating rheumatoid arthritis.

Absorption, Metabolism, and Excretion

With the exception of auranofin, all currently available gold preparations are poorly and erratically absorbed after oral administration and must be administered either intramuscularly (preferred route) or intravenously. The nature of the gold complex influences the rate of absorption as well as the distribution and excretion of the compound. The water-soluble preparations (aurothioglucose, gold sodium thiomalate, gold sodium thiosulfate), when administered intramuscularly as aqueous solutions, are rapidly absorbed, and maximal plasma levels are reached within a few hours. Peak plasma concentrations of gold are roughly proportional to the dosage administered. If the water-soluble preparations are suspended in oil and injected intramuscularly, somewhat lower peak plasma concentrations of gold are obtained. The lowest plasma concentrations of gold are obtained after the injection of oil suspensions of the water-insoluble preparations (e.g., aurothioglycanide).

Auranofin (*Ridaura*) is the first orally effective gold preparation to be approved in the United States. Only about 25 percent of an orally administered dose is absorbed, but this appears to be constant from day to day. Intact auranofin has not been detected in blood.

After absorption, the water-soluble gold preparations

are extensively bound to plasma protein, primarily serum albumin and α_1-globulin, and only insignificant amounts are associated with erythrocytes. After administration of the water-soluble gold preparations, the highest concentrations of gold occur in the kidney, with appreciable amounts also in liver and spleen. Colloidal suspensions of gold, on the other hand, are phagocytized by cells of the reticuloendothelial system and consequently higher levels are observed in the liver and spleen than in the kidneys. Long-term therapy with gold results in significant retention of the compound in other tissues, such as the lymph nodes and adrenal cortex. There is evidence that inflamed joints accumulate approximately twice as much gold as symptom-free joints.

Not much is known concerning the metabolic transformation of the gold preparations. The metal apparently remains complexed with ligands. Although the excretion of gold preparations is primarily through the kidneys, fecal excretion may be a major route of elimination in certain patients. In general, the most rapidly absorbed preparations are the most rapidly excreted. After a single IM injection of 50 mg of a water-soluble gold compound, approximately 85 percent of the gold is still present in the body after 7 days, and gold can still be detected in the urine of patients 15 months after discontinuance of administration.

Clinical Uses

Patients with active, progressive, erosive, and seropositive rheumatoid arthritis who have failed to respond adequately to more conservative measures are candidates for gold therapy (*chrysotherapy*). A clinical response to gold, if it occurs, is usually delayed in onset and therefore *treatment must be continued for at least a few months*. For those patients who are able to tolerate therapy, some benefit will be obtained in about 80 percent, and complete remission will be induced in perhaps 20 percent of cases. Remissions are maintained for varying periods of time after discontinuing therapy. The relapse rate has been reported in some instances to be as high as 80 percent. However, the relapse has been less severe than the original disease in the majority of patients and a second course of gold therapy in such patients usually produces beneficial effects.

Adverse Reactions

Toxic manifestations of gold therapy may occur at any time during treatment, but they are more common after a certain minimal total amount of gold has been administered (200–300 mg). Serious reactions necessitating discontinuance of therapy or antidotal therapy are encountered in perhaps 5 percent of the patients. The most frequent adverse reactions to auranofin are diarrhea, abdominal pain, nausea, and anorexia.

Dermatitis, which is almost invariably preceded and accompanied by pruritus, is the most frequent side effect observed with gold therapy. The skin reactions induced by gold may occur in a variety of forms, but the most serious is a generalized exfoliative dermatitis. This reaction generally occurs only after early warning symptoms (itching) have been ignored and gold therapy has been continued. Stomatitis may accompany dermatitis, which may be preceded by a metallic taste in the mouth of the patient.

Fatalities due to gold therapy have been reported, and are usually a consequence of a blood dyscrasia. The most common hematological abnormality is eosinophilia. Fortunately, serious blood dyscrasias, such as thrombocytopenia, agranulocytosis, and hypoplastic or aplastic anemia, are rare. Such reactions usually necessitate antidotal and supportive therapeutic measures.

A mild proteinuria is not uncommon in humans receiving gold therapy and does not always require discontinuance of therapy. A more severe proteinuria may indicate a toxic nephritis, and the nephrotic syndrome has been reported to occur in some patients. The proteinuria is usually reversible when gold administration is stopped.

To complement steroidal and other measures used in treating gold toxicity, it may be necessary to hasten the elimination of gold from the body. This action is accomplished by the use of chelating agents such as dimercaprol (British antilewisite, BAL), or penicillamine. The proper administration of either of these agents has been shown to markedly increase the excretion of gold and to alleviate the signs and symptoms of gold toxicity. Both BAL and penicillamine can produce toxic effects, some of which are dangerous, and caution is advised when one is using these agents.

Preparations and Dosage

The available gold preparations are listed in Table 43-5. Colloidal preparations of gold are usable in certain countries, but they are not recommended because they are rapidly phagocytized by cells of the reticuloendothelial system. The water-soluble preparations are preferred over water-insoluble preparations because of the slow absorption of the latter. There appears to be no difference in the therapeutic effect that is achieved between the two most commonly used preparations, aurothioglucose and gold sodium thiomalate.

Dosage schedules vary, but in general increasing doses given at weekly intervals are the rule.

Steroidal Antiinflammatory Agents

A more detailed discussion of the corticosteroids and their role in therapeutics can be found in Chap. 66. Certain aspects of their use as antiinflammatory agents are presented below.

Table 43-5. Gold Preparations

Compound	Trade name	Percent gold	Dosage form
Gold sodium thiomalate*	Myochrysine	50	Aqueous solution
Aurothioglucose*	Solganal	50	Suspension in oil
Gold sodium thiosulfate	Sanochrysine, Crisalbine, Sanocrysin	37	Aqueous solution
Aurothioglycanide	Lauron	54	Suspension in oil
Auranofin*	Ridaura	29	Capsules, 3 mg

*Available in the United States.

Chemistry

The antiinflammatory and glucocorticoid activities of steroids have never been separated despite intense efforts by synthetic chemists. The term *glucocorticoid* refers to the ability of the compounds to increase hepatic glucose output. This is a result of stimulating hepatic gluconeogenesis while inhibiting peripheral tissue protein synthesis. The mineralocorticoid and glucocorticoid activities of the adrenal corticosteroids have been successfully separated by molecular modification.

The basic steroidal structure required for antiinflammatory activity is that of hydrocortisone. Structural modifications of the hydrocortisone molecule have resulted in the development of a number of compounds with enhanced systemic antiinflammatory (and glucocorticoid) activity. These modified compounds include prednisone and prednisolone as well as the fluorinated steroids such as dexamethasone and triamcinolone. Prednisolone is about five times, and dexamethasone 30 times, as potent as hydrocortisone as an antiinflammatory agent. Other modifications of the hydrocortisone structure have been made, especially in those compounds primarily intended for dermatological use (Chap. 46).

Antiinflammatory Effects

The glucocorticosteroids can be shown experimentally to inhibit all phases of the inflammatory response. These phases are (1) the *vascular phase* (hyperemia and edema), (2) the *cellular phase* (infiltration of blood leukocytes), and (3) the *connective tissue phase* (repair phase). The vascular and cellular phases of inflammation appear to be mediated by factors elaborated or released (or both) by cells in the injured area. Some of these factors are histamine, kinins, prostaglandins, leukotrienes, lymphokines, complement, and products of lysosomal enzyme-catalyzed reactions. The connective tissue phase includes synthesis of new tissue and repair of the damaged area.

Steroids inhibit the accumulation of leukocytes in the inflamed area. This may be a consequence of inhibiting their response to chemotactic factors elaborated at the site of inflammation. The steroids, like the gold preparations, also have been shown to suppress the increased phagocytic activity of macrophages and polymorphonuclear leukocytes that occurs in patients with rheumatoid arthritis.

Their ability to prevent the conversion of membrane phospholipid to arachidonic acid may be the most relevant effect associated with the antiinflammatory action of the glucocorticoids. Arachidonic acid is the precursor of the prostaglandins and leukotrienes, which appear to be important mediators of the inflammatory response (see Chap. 42).

Finally, the effects of the glucocorticosteroids on the connective tissue phase of inflammation are well known. These compounds inhibit the proliferation of fibroblasts and prevent deposition of both the ground substance and collagen of connective tissue (see also Chap. 66).

Clinical Uses

Corticosteroids are never the treatment of choice and should never be the sole treatment for rheumatoid arthritis. The goal of corticosteroid therapy is to achieve adequate control of the arthritis, but not to ameliorate the condition totally. Total suppression of the inflammatory response does not appear to be possible with relatively "safe" doses of corticosteroids. Although corticosteroids do not arrest the progress of rheumatoid arthritis, they are capable of dramatically improving the well-being of the patient, at least temporarily.

Corticosteroid therapy is indicated in moderate to severe rheumatoid arthritis that is uncontrollable by more conservative measures, such as rest and administration of salicylates or other NSAIDs. Corticosteroids also are required when certain dangerous nonarticular manifestations such as vasculitis, hemolytic anemia, or iritis are present. In certain situations, such as life-threatening involvement of the heart or kidney in systemic lupus erythematosus, large doses of corticosteroids may be required to prevent death. There may also be socioeconomic reasons for instituting corticosteroid therapy in arthritics, for example, when the patient cannot be hospitalized for intensive, more conservative therapy because of obligations to job or family.

Adverse Reactions

The hazards of long-term therapy with corticosteroids are discussed in Chap. 66.

Preparations and Dosage

The glucocorticosteroids that are available for systemic use, and their equivalent doses, are given in Table 43-6. None of the more potent steroids offers any advantage over the less expensive prednisone and prednisolone, and these two are probably the most widely prescribed for inflammatory diseases. The dosage of prednisolone or prednisone for chronic palliative therapy generally is 2 to 10 mg/day. Any dose over 10 mg of prednisone, or its equivalent, is considered to be a high dose and carries with it an increasing risk of serious side effects.

In an attempt to minimize adrenal suppression, some physicians prefer to administer the dose of steroid in the morning, when adrenocorticotropic hormone (ACTH) levels are at their lowest. Alternate-day steroid therapy may not be appropriate for treating rheumatoid arthritis, since the disease does not appear to be controlled adequately under these conditions.

4-Aminoquinoline Antimalarials

Although the place of the 4-aminoquinolines as drugs for treatment of rheumatoid disease has not been agreed on, the weight of evidence suggests that they can be classified as compounds with definite, mild, long-term antirheumatic effects. A detailed discussion of the chemistry and pharmacology of the 4-aminoquinolines and their use as antimalarial compounds is presented in Chap. 57. The following discussion is limited to certain aspects of their use as antirheumatic agents.

Mechanism of Action

In animals, chloroquine can be shown to inhibit edema, the proliferation of connective tissue, contraction of smooth muscle, the tuberculin reaction, various enzymes, the aggregation of platelets, labilization of membranes, denaturation of proteins, and the migration, phagocytosis, and chemotaxis of leukocytes. Although any one of these properties might account for the clinical antirheumatic effect, the doses required for inhibition in most cases have been excessive, and none of these properties appears sufficient to explain the clinical effectiveness of chloroquine.

The interaction of the 4-aminoquinoline antimalarial drugs with biological macromolecules has been demonstrated many times. The aminoquinolines have been shown to form complexes with DNA, resulting in an inhibition of reactions in which the nucleic acid participates (e.g., DNA-dependent DNA and RNA polymerization, DNA hydrolysis). Chloroquine accumulates in tissues that are rich in nucleic acids, such as liver, spleen, kidney, lung, leukocytes, and parasitized erythrocytes. The ability to alter the properties of DNA and inhibit its replication may account for the antiplasmodial and antibacterial properties of the compounds, but the relationship, if any, of this interaction to their antirheumatic activity is obscure.

The effects of the aminoquinolines on polymorphonuclear leukocyte function may well be important to the antiinflammatory activity of these compounds. The demonstration of lysosomal membrane "stabilization" would suggest that the release of destructive enzymes in the joints by these cells would be hindered by the 4-aminoquinoline derivatives.

Clinical Uses

Therapy with the aminoquinolines is sometimes recommended for arthritic patients in whom LE cells* can be demonstrated. If a beneficial effect is obtained with aminoquinolines, it is usually delayed (weeks), and in this respect their therapeutic effects are similar to those of gold. Uncontrolled studies have suggested that 65 to 90 percent of arthritic patients receiving one of the antimalarial drugs respond favorably. The type of response has ranged from a mild amelioration of symptoms to remission of the disease.

Table 43-6. Glucocorticosteroids for Systemic Use

Steroid (trade name)	Approximate equivalent dose (mg)
Cortisone acetate	25
Hydrocortisone	20
Prednisone (Deltasone, Meticorten, Paracort)	5
Prednisolone (Delta-Cortef)	5
Triamcinolone (Aristocort, Kenacort)	4
Meprednisone (Betapar)	4
Methylprednisolone (Medrol)	4
Paramethasone acetate (Haldrone, Stemex)	2
Fluprednisolone (Alphadrol)	2
Dexamethasone (Decadron, Gammacorten)	0.75
Betamethasone (Celestone)	0.75

*Leukocytes characteristically found in patients with systemic lupus erythematosus that contain phagocytized nuclear-antinuclear antibody complexes.

Adverse Reactions

Serious toxic reactions observed in some patients receiving the aminoquinolines for connective tissue diseases are the result of the administration of high doses for prolonged periods. The dose of chloroquine required for the suppressive therapy of malaria is only about 500 mg/week; that used in the treatment of arthritis is 200 to 700 mg/day. The incidence of the most serious toxic reaction, irreversible retinopathy with resultant blindness, is dose related, and in recent years the daily dose of chloroquine (and other aminoquinolines) has been adjusted downward in the treatment of connective tissue disease.

Reversible side effects observed during high-dose, long-term therapy with the aminoquinolines include lichenoid skin lesions, leukopenia, neuromyopathy, hair loss, sensitivity to sunburn, and changes in the electrocardiogram.

Contraindications

Because the aminoquinolines accumulate in lung, kidney, and liver, any preexisting pathology in these tissues contraindicates their use. Similarly, any ocular pathology precludes their use. Psoriasis is frequently exacerbated by the administration of the aminoquinolines. Gold and an aminoquinoline probably should not be administered concurrently because of the propensity of each to produce dermatitis. Children should not receive the drugs.

Preparations

Hydroxychloroquine sulfate (*Plaquenil Sulfate*), is the most commonly used aminoquinoline for the treatment of connective tissue disease. It appears to be somewhat less toxic than, but equally effective as, chloroquine phosphate (*Aralen Phosphate*). Both drugs are taken orally in tablet form, either before or after meals.

Cytostatic-Cytotoxic and Antimetabolite Drugs

Two cytostatic-cytotoxic drugs used in the United States for the treatment of connective tissue diseases are azathioprine and cyclophosphamide. The pharmacology of these agents and their use in cancer chemotherapy are discussed in Chap. 62.

Cyclophosphamide and azathioprine, when given in sufficient quantity, reduce arthritic signs and symptoms in a significant proportion of patients who are able to tolerate the therapy. Fewer new erosions of the joint cartilage were present in patients receiving cyclophosphamide,

suggesting that the treatment actually arrested the disease process rather than just ameliorating symptoms. Furthermore, concomitant steroid therapy in these patients could be reduced without sacrificing adequate control of the disease.

The side effects associated with the cytostatic-cytotoxic drugs are well known (Chap. 62) and severely limit the use of such drugs. They are not considered to be a first or even a second choice in the treatment of rheumatoid arthritis. *Their use should be restricted to patients with severe active disease that has failed to respond to other forms of treatment.*

Methotrexate

This antimetabolite drug, when administered in low doses orally, intramuscularly, or intravenously, is effective in the treatment of rheumatoid arthritis. Its use, in a low-dose regimen, is reserved for patients inadequately controlled by other therapy.

When given in high doses, methotrexate exerts potent suppressing action on cellular and humoral immunity (see Chap. 63). When used in low doses to treat rheumatoid arthritis, evidence of immunosuppressive effects is lacking. At low doses methotrexate appears to be acting more as an antiinflammatory agent than as an antimetabolite. Its effects have been likened to those of a slow-acting steroid.

The absorption, metabolism, and excretion of methotrexate are fully described in Chap. 62.

Methotrexate is currently recommended for adults with severe active rheumatoid arthritis who have demonstrated an insufficient response to, or have an intolerance of, full-dose NSAIDs and have usually had a trial of at least one disease-modifying antirheumatic drug, such as penicillamine, hydroxychloroquine, or gold compounds. Its therapeutic effects are usually evident within 3 to 6 weeks.

Toxicity to methotrexate appears to be a function of the duration of exposure at a critical or threshold concentration rather than simply a function of peak blood level achieved. The threshold for toxicity varies from organ to organ, with bone marrow and gastrointestinal epithelium appearing most susceptible. When methotrexate is used in the low-dose regimen for rheumatoid arthritis, most immediate side effects are mild and can be managed by temporarily stopping the drug or reducing the dose. The most common symptoms are nausea, mucositis, gastrointestinal discomfort, rash, diarrhea, and headaches. Severe toxicity is also possible and may be a function of drug accumulation. These effects include hepatotoxicity progressing to cirrhosis, pneumonitis, and bone marrow depression with anemia, leukopenia, and thrombocytopenia.

Methotrexate is contraindicated in pregnancy, lactation, alcoholism or alcoholic liver disease, chronic liver disease, preexisting blood dyscrasias, and immunodeficiency syndrome, and in those individuals who are hypersensitive to the drug.

Methotrexate (*Rheumatrex*) is furnished as 2.5-mg tablets.

Penicillamine

Penicillamine (β,β-dimethylcysteine) is an effective agent in acute, severe rheumatoid arthritis in a large proportion of patients who are capable of tolerating the drug. Reductions in joint pain, edema, and stiffness all occur.

Mechanism of Action

Although a number of mechanisms have been proposed to explain the effectiveness of penicillamine in rheumatoid arthritis, none has gained wide acceptance. There is no evidence to suggest that penicillamine exhibits antiinflammatory activity. There are some indications that it exerts immunoregulatory actions (both immunosuppressive and immunostimulatory activities have been reported), but this has not been proved. Since *penicillamine is a metal chelator* (e.g., copper, mercury, zinc, and lead), a modification of trace metal metabolism may contribute to its efficacy in rheumatoid arthritis. The effect of the drug on macromolecules (macroglobulin dissociation, inhibition of collagen cross-linking) also could be involved in its mechanism of action, as could its antiviral activity. A better understanding of the apparent antiarthritic action of penicillamine is needed.

Clinical Uses

If a therapeutic effect is achieved in rheumatoid arthritis, it is usually delayed (4–12 weeks) in onset, and thus the drug is similar to the gold preparations in this respect. Drug-induced remissions of rheumatoid arthritis lasting several months after withdrawal of penicillamine have been reported. Penicillamine is not a first-choice treatment for rheumatoid arthritis but is becoming accepted in some centers as an alternative to gold, chloroquine, and the cytostatic agents.

Because of penicillamine's ability to chelate copper and promote its excretion, it is the drug of choice for Wilson's disease (hepatolenticular degeneration). It also has been used in other heavy metal (mercury, lead) intoxications. It has a dissociative effect on rheumatoid factor (anti–immunoglobulin G antibody) in vitro, and this observation formed the basis for the trial of the drug in patients with rheumatoid arthritis.

Adverse Reactions

Side effects necessitate discontinuance of penicillamine therapy in perhaps one-third of the patients taking the drug. The most common side effects are a maculopapular pruritic dermatitis, gastrointestinal upset, a loss of taste sensation, a mild to occasionally severe thrombocytopenia and leukopenia, and a mild proteinuria, which at times may progress to the nephrotic syndrome. The renal and blood complications are obviously the most serious, and monitoring of these areas in patients receiving penicillamine is necessary. Discontinuance of therapy usually results in a rapid disappearance of side effects.

Preparations and Dosage

Penicillamine (*Cuprimine*) is marketed as capsules and as tablets (*Depen*). It is readily absorbed from the gastrointestinal tract and is rapidly excreted in the urine, largely as the intact molecule. It is important to gradually increase the dose administered in order to minimize side effects.

New Approaches to the Treatment of Rheumatoid Arthritis

There is abundant evidence that both humoral and cell-mediated immunological phenomena are expressed in patients with rheumatoid arthritis. Their importance, if any, to the etiology of the disease remains obscure. The fact that these phenomena are present, however, provides the basis for the semiempirical treatment of rheumatoid arthritis with immunoregulatory agents.

Immunosuppressive therapy with cytostatic-cytotoxic agents, such as azathioprine, methotrexate, and cyclophosphamide, is obscured by the intrinsic antiinflammatory activity of these drugs. Thus, any amelioration of the disease after administration of these drugs may be due to antiinflammatory, rather than immunosuppressive, activity. However, results obtained in certain patients after administration of these immunosuppressive agents are qualitatively and quantitatively different from those obtained with therapeutic doses of "pure" antiinflammatory drugs; this suggests that additional mechanisms may be operative. Such observations justify continued investigation of the therapeutic usefulness of immunosuppressive agents.

The rationale for *immunopotentiation therapy* of rheumatoid arthritis is based on the following beliefs: (1) rheumatoid arthritis is an immune-deficiency disease in the sense that suppressor T lymphocytes are not functioning normally, thus allowing an unchecked autoimmune response to manifest itself, and (2) the underlying cause of rheumatoid arthritis is a persistent infection.

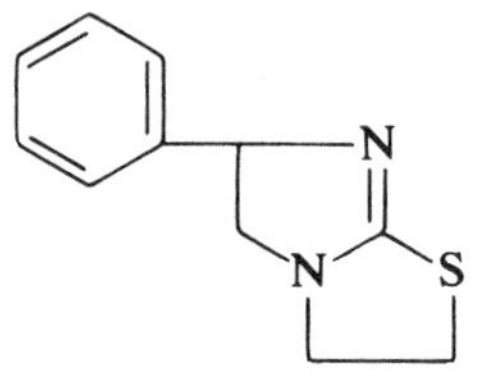

Figure 43-4. Levamisole.

The anthelmintic drug *levamisole* (Fig. 43-4) has received the most attention as an example of an immunopotentiating agent. Levamisole has been reported to produce significant improvement but with unacceptable toxicity in patients with rheumatoid arthritis. Investigation into the usefulness of immunopotentiating agents, such as levamisole, for the treatment of rheumatoid arthritis is being pursued.

Supplemental Reading

Brooks, P.M. (ed). *Slow Acting Anti-rheumatic Drugs and Immunosuppressives. Bailliere's Clinical Rheumatology, International Practice and Research,* Vol. 4, No. 3. Kent: Harcourt Brace Jovanovich, 1990.

Brooks, P.M., and Day, R.O. Nonsteroidal anti-inflammatory drugs—differences and similarities. *N. Engl. J. Med.* 324:1716, 1991.

Brooks, P.M., Keam, W., and Buchanan, W. *The Clinical Pharmacology of Antiinflammatory Agents.* Philadelphia: Taylor and Francis, 1986.

Buchanan, W.W. Implications of NSAID therapy in elderly patients. *J. Rheumatol.* 17 (Suppl. 20): 29, 1990.

Gabriel, S.E., and Bombardier, C. NSAID induced ulcers: An emerging epidemic? *J. Rheumatol.* 17:1, 1990.

Greene, J.M., and Winickoff, R.N. Cost-conscious prescribing of nonsteroidal antiinflammatory drugs for adults with arthritis. *Arch. Intern. Med.* 152:1995, 1992.

McCarty, D.J., and Koopman, W.J. *Arthritis and Allied Conditions: A Textbook of Rheumatology* (12th ed.). Baltimore: Lea & Febiger, 1992.

Ramos-Remus, C., Sibley, J., and Russell, A.S. Steroids in rheumatoid arthritis: The honeymoon revisited. *J. Rheumatol.* 19:667, 1992.

Stewart, C.F., and Evans, W.E. Drug-drug interactions with anti-rheumatic agents: Review of selected clinically important interactions. *J. Rheumatol.* 17 (Suppl. 22):16, 1990.

Vane, J., and Botting, R. Inflammation and the mechanism of action of anti-inflammatory drugs. *FASEB J.* 1:89, 1987.

Velo, G.P., and Milanino, R. Nongastrointestinal adverse reactions to NSAID. *J. Rheumatol.* 17 (Suppl. 20):42, 1990.

Weinblatt, M.E., and Maier, A.L. Longterm experience with low dose weekly methotrexate in rheumatoid arthritis. *J. Rheumatol.* 17 (Suppl. 22):33, 1990.

Weissmann, G. Aspirin. *Sci. Am.* 264:84, 1991.

44

Drugs Used in Gout

Knox Van Dyke

Gout is a disease or condition that is characterized biochemically as a disorder of uric acid metabolism and clinically by hyperuricemia and recurrent attacks of acute arthritis. Gouty arthritis is most frequently seen as an acute inflammation primarily in the large toe, instep, ankle, or heel. Less often, the initial symptoms appear in the knee or elbow; occasionally, they are seen in the wrist. If the condition remains untreated over a period of years, deposition of sodium urate crystals may occur in the subcutaneous tissue, joints, renal parenchyma, and renal pelvis. Uric acid stones may form in the lumen of the urinary tract, and a progressive renal failure often occurs in the later stages of untreated gout. Additionally, microcrystalline deposits of sodium urate frequently result in inflammatory bulges or bumps, termed *tophi,* appearing in the subcutaneous tissue of the ear lobes, elbows, and hands, and at the base of the large toe.

The elevated blood uric acid concentration in gout is an easily identified and readily treated abnormality. However, it is essential to identify the condition and institute therapy early to avoid the complications that result from a prolonged elevated uricemia. Complications include arthritis, tophi, urinary calculi, and a gouty nephropathy.

Although all forms of gout have the common trait of hyperuricemia, the causes of this condition can be manifold. *Primary, or genetic, gout results from either an increased synthesis of uric acid or a decreased renal excretion of the substance.* Some gout patients have an unusual shunt mechanism, which converts glycine directly into uric acid rather than into its normal metabolic products.

Secondary gout may result from either an overproduction or impaired elimination of uric acid. Overproduction is usually secondary to some other disorder, most frequently of hematological origin. For instance, in leukemia, myeloid metaplasia, lymphoma, polycythemia vera, and rapid weight loss (dieting), breakdown of cellular nucleoprotein is increased, which leads to an eventual excess formation of uric acid.

In secondary gout, diminished elimination of uric acid can be due to lead nephropathy, glycogen storage disease, and sickle cell anemia. In addition, several drugs, including salicylates, pyrazinamide, alcohol, ethambutol, nicotinic acid, cyclosporine, fructose, cytotoxic agents, and certain diuretics (e.g., thiazides, furosemide, bumetanide) will impair the renal elimination of uric acid. These drugs competitively inhibit the active secretion of uric acid (see Chap. 5) into the urine, with resulting hyperuricemia.

Chemistry of Uric Acid

Humans excrete approximately 0.7 gm uric acid daily. Most of this is derived from the metabolic breakdown of the purine bases adenine and guanine. The structure of uric acid is given in Fig. 44-1. Uric acid is the most highly oxidized of the endogenous purine compounds. It has a pK_a of 5.6 and is 50 percent ionized at that pH. It is less ionized and less water soluble at more acidic pHs. It exists mostly as the monovalent salt, *sodium urate.* However, uric acid itself, which is much less water soluble than is sodium urate, may be the predominant form found in an acid urine. Because the urine becomes more acidified as it moves through the renal tubular system, filtered urate is increasingly converted to uric acid. The relatively limited solubility of urate at a urinary pH of 5.0 is obviously clinically significant in patients with gout because of the possibility of the formation of uric acid stones.

The solubility of urate in plasma is higher than in aqueous solution, presumably owing to the presence of urate-binding plasma proteins. However, in vivo, the binding of uric acid to plasma proteins is relatively small and probably does not have great physiological significance. However, even this limited binding may be affected by administration of drugs, such as salicylates, phenylbutazone, probenecid, and sulfinpyrazone. These drugs probably affect urate protein binding only secondarily, that is, their principal action is to interfere with renal transport of uric

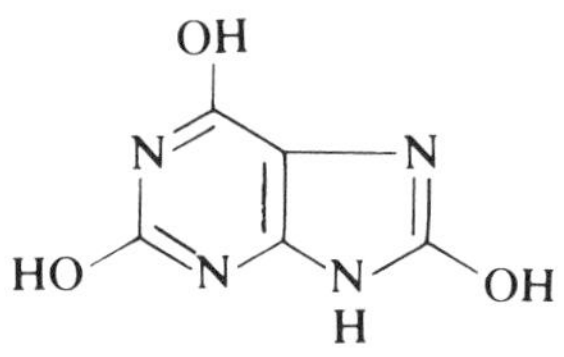

Figure 44-1. Uric acid.

acid, which, in turn, leads to alterations in plasma urate binding.

Renal Urate Homeostasis

The renal mechanisms involved in the handling of uric acid are extraordinarily complex. The processes involved include filtration, reabsorption, secretion, and possibly postsecretory reabsorption.

The proximal tubule is the principal site of both carrier-mediated reabsorption and secretion of urate. Urate is believed to be transported from the ultrafiltrate to the intracellular space by an anion exchange mechanism that is located in the *luminal membrane*. This active transport system can be inhibited by drugs, such as probenecid, sulfinpyrazone, and salicylate. The cellularly accumulated urate then moves passively across the basolateral membrane and into the peritubular fluid down its electrochemical gradient. Conversely, active tubular secretion of urate occurs as a consequence of carrier-mediated transport across the *basolateral membrane* of the proximal tubule. The cellularly accumulated urate then moves passively across the luminal membrane into the ultrafiltrate along its concentration gradient. The carrier-mediated secretion of urate can be inhibited by a variety of organic anions including the thiazide and loop diuretics.

The proximal tubule intracellular concentration of urate will ultimately be determined by the balance of influx and efflux. When the transport of urate from the peritubular fluid is high, there is a net elimination of urate across the luminal membrane. Under conditions in which transport of urate from luminal fluid is high, there is a net reabsorption across the basolateral membrane. Urate excretion in humans generally varies between 5 and 20 percent of that which is filtered at the glomerulus.

As discussed in the following sections, urate excretion is subject to modification by a variety of organic anions including uricosuric agents, phenylbutazone, diuretics, x-ray contrast agents, and certain anticancer compounds. A further complicating feature is that drug effects may be biphasic; that is, small amounts may depress urate excretion, while high dosages have uricosuric effects.

Relationship of Uric Acid Levels to Gout

The degree of risk of acquiring gouty arthritis is related primarily to the extent and duration of hyperuricemia. The risk is essentially zero at serum urate concentration below 7 mg/dl, whereas at concentrations of 10 to 11 mg/dl, the likelihood of having the disorder is very high. Gouty arthritis due to impaired renal excretion of uric acid may be diagnosed through a quantification of the patient's uric acid excretion. If a patient on a purine-restricted diet for 1 week excretes more than 600 mg uric acid per 24 hr, the individual is probably an overproducer. If, however, less than 350 mg uric acid is eliminated in 24 hr, impaired renal function can be suspected.

Since gout may have either a primary or secondary origin, it is essential to determine the nature of the gouty syndrome. In cases of primary gout, a reasonably accurate measure of the rate of urate synthesis may be obtained by using the low-purine diet procedure just described. A determination of renal function is also important. If the acute gouty arthritis is a secondary phenomenon, the precipitating cause must be determined. It may be secondary to a hematological disorder, chronic alcoholism, the drinking of "moonshine liquor" resulting in kidney disease (*lead, or saturnine, gout*), or possibly to the administration of drugs that can compete for the active renal secretory mechanisms involved in uric acid elimination.

Role of Phagocytosis in Acute Gouty Arthritis

The mere presence of urate crystals in the joint cannot be correlated with the appearance of acute gouty arthritic symptoms. Individuals who have never had any gouty arthritic problems have, nonetheless, still been found to have uric acid deposited on their articular cartilage. Acute attacks are generally the result of granulocytic phagocytosis of the urate crystals. This engulfing of the crystals is accompanied by a cellular release of chemotactic lipids, lysosomal enzymes, and acidic substances into the synovial tissues. The lipids appear to trigger further phagocytosis, whereas the acidic compounds decrease local pH to the point that increased urate crystal formation is favored.

In addition to the phagocytic activity of the leukocytes, there is an accumulation in the joint space of small peptide substances, such as the kinins, which are thought to be partially responsible for the local inflammatory response in gouty arthritis. The inflammation is associated with local vasodilation, increased vascular permeability, and pain. Recent studies point to activation of phagocytic cell membrane phospholipase H_2, and its activating protein (PLAP), by sodium urate crystals as being a key to inflammation in gout.

In summary, the two main components of acute gouty arthritis, hyperuricemia and local inflammation, are separable processes. One may or may not be accompanied by the other. Thus, treatment can be directed at either or both of these aspects of the disorder; however, drugs that control one process usually will alter the other as well.

General Principles of Gout Management

Initial treatment of gout and hyperuricemia must involve therapy directed toward terminating the painful inflammatory process that is a prominent feature of acute gouty arthritis. A variety of nonsteroidal antiinflammatory compounds (e.g., indomethacin, oxyphenbutazone, ibuprofen, naproxen, sulindac) can be administered either alone or in combination with *colchicine,* a relatively specific agent for use in acute gouty attacks. Glucocorticosteroids such as prednisone can be given as a tapered dose over 10 days to replace colchicine. These steroids cause fewer side effects than does colchicine. If the diagnosis is uncertain, then colchicine should be used, since a response to this drug is generally taken as establishing the presence of acute gouty arthritis.

Although the treatment of the hyperuricemia of gout revolves around the lowering of blood uric acid levels, most physicians caution against employing drugs such as *allopurinol, probenecid,* or *sulfinpyrazone* during an acute attack, since the therapy itself, at least during the initial stages, may actually exacerbate the condition. Once the acute symptoms are under control and the patient enters an asymptomatic period, appropriate treatment should include not only drug therapy but also management of body weight and control of dietary purine intake. Long-term treatment is directed toward decreasing uric acid production, increasing excretion, or both.

Uric acid production is more easily controlled by drug therapy than by dietary restriction because only a small portion of blood uric acid is derived from the dietary intake of purines. Most of the uric acid comes from the breakdown of purines that have been synthesized endogenously (i.e., through catabolism of nucleoproteins).

Excretion of uric acid may be increased by increasing the rate of urine flow or by using uricosuric agents. Since uric acid is filtered at the glomerulus, actively secreted by the proximal tubule cells, and actively reabsorbed from the ultrafiltrate, both approaches are effective.

Since overproducers are already excreting large quantities of uric acid in their urine, drugs that further increase the rate of excretion (i.e., uricosuric compounds) increase the likelihood of renal stone formation. In these patients, the use of a compound that inhibits uric acid synthesis (e.g., allopurinol) would be the preferable approach to gout control. Although, at first glance, the use of a combination of drugs—a drug that reduces production along with one that is uricosuric—would seem to be a rational therapeutic approach, in practice this has not worked well. Apparently, the effectiveness of a drug such as allopurinol is diminished by uricosuric agents (e.g., probenecid) and therefore the combination has less value than each drug used separately. Furthermore, side effects appear to occur more frequently during combination drug therapy.

Pharmacological Agents

Colchicine

Chemistry

Colchicine (Fig. 44-2), an alkaloid obtained from the autumn crocus, has long been used in the treatment of acute gouty arthritis.

Mechanism of Action

As was pointed out earlier, gouty inflammation of the tissues or joints is associated with the local accumulation of urate microcrystals by the phagocytic neutrophils. After sufficient amounts of these crystals have been taken up into the phagolysosomes of the neutrophil, these organelles disrupt and release their degradative enzymes, accumulated microcrystals (which may be rephagocytized), and chemotactic factors. It is these released substances that are responsible for much of the local inflammation and pain associated with acute attacks of gout.

Unlike many of the more recently developed agents for use in gout, *colchicine has minimal effects on uric acid synthesis and excretion;* it decreases inflammation associated with this disorder. It is thought that colchicine, in some way,

Figure 44-2. Colchicine.

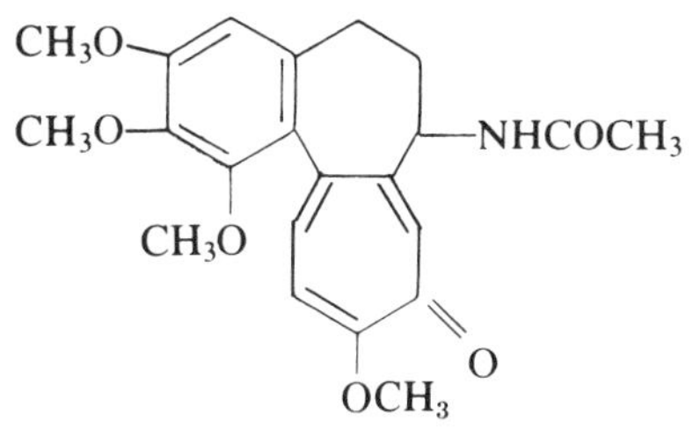

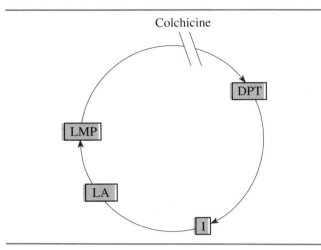

Figure 44-3. Illustration of probable mechanism by which colchicine breaks the cycle of inflammation in acute gouty arthritis. See text for more detail. LMP = leukocytic microcrystal phagocytosis; DPR = degradative product release; I = inflammation; LA = leukocytic attraction.

prevents the release of the chemotactic factors from the neutrophils, and this, in turn, decreases the attraction of more neutrophils into the affected area. The ability of colchicine to bind to leukocyte microtubules in a reversible covalent complex and cause their depolymerization also may be involved in decreasing the attraction of the motile leukocytes into the inflamed area. By these mechanisms, the cycle of inflammation is disrupted.

Absorption, Metabolism, and Excretion

Colchicine is rapidly absorbed after oral administration and tends to concentrate in the spleen, kidney, liver, and gastrointestinal tract. Leukocytes also avidly accumulate and store colchicine even after a single intravenous injection. Since colchicine can accumulate in cells against a concentration gradient, it is postulated that an active transport process may be involved in its cellular uptake. The drug is metabolized, primarily in the liver, by deacetylation. Fecal excretion plays a major role in the elimination of colchicine from the body, since it and its metabolites are readily secreted into the bile. Only about 15 to 30 percent of the drug is eliminated in the urine, except in patients with liver disease; urinary excretion becomes more important in these individuals.

Clinical Uses

The major use of colchicine is as an antiinflammatory agent in the treatment of acute gouty arthritis. *It is not effective in reducing inflammation in other disorders.* It also can be used prophylactically to prevent future attacks. Since colchicine is so rapidly effective in relieving the acute

symptoms of gout (substantial improvement is achieved within hours), it has been used as a diagnostic aid in this disorder.

Therapy with colchicine is usually begun at the first sign of an attack and is continued until symptoms subside, or adverse gastrointestinal reactions appear, or until a maximum dosage of 6 to 7 mg has been reached. The drug can be given intravenously as well as orally, but care must be exercised since extravasated drug may result in localized sloughing of skin and subcutaneous tissues. Relief of pain and inflammation usually occurs within 48 hr. Small doses of colchicine can be used during asymptomatic periods to minimize the reappearance or severity of acute attacks.

Adverse Reactions

Diarrhea, nausea, vomiting, and abdominal pain are the major limiting side effects that ultimately determine the tolerated dosage. These symptoms occur in approximately 80 percent of patients who take colchicine, especially in those taking high dosages. These symptoms may be controlled with appropriate drug therapy, but it must be remembered that gastrointestinal distress is often an early warning sign of colchicine intolerance or toxicity. The hepatobiliary recycling of colchicine and colchicine's antimitotic effect on cells that are rapidly turning over, such as those of the intestinal epithelium, account for its gastrointestinal toxicity. Gastrointestinal symptoms generally intervene before the appearance of more serious toxicity and thereby provide a margin of safety in drug administration.

Ingestion of large doses of colchicine may be followed by a burning sensation in the throat, bloody diarrhea, shock, hematuria, oliguria, and central nervous system (CNS) depression.

Preparations and Dosage

Colchicine is available as 0.5- and 0.6-mg tablets and sterile injectable solutions (0.5 mg/ml). The recommended dosage is 0.5 or 0.6 mg every hour for five doses, followed by 0.5 or 0.6 mg every 2 hr until gastrointestinal symptoms begin or relief is achieved. Most individuals cannot tolerate more than 6 or 7 mg orally.

Uricosuric Agents

The uricosuric drugs (or urate diuretics) are anions that are somewhat similar to urate in structure; therefore, they can compete with uric acid for transport sites. The rates of both active reabsorption and secretion of uric acid can be altered by appropriate drug therapy. Small dosages of uricosuric agents will actually decrease the total excretion of urate by inhibiting its active tubular secretion. The quantitative importance of the secretory mechanism is of relatively minor importance, however, and at high dosages these same drugs increase uric acid elimination by inhibiting its more important proximal tubular reabsorption. Thus, uricosuric drugs have a seemingly paradoxical effect on both serum and urinary uric acid levels: At low dosages, they increase serum levels while decreasing the urinary levels; they have the opposite effect on these two levels at high dosages.

The two uricosuric drugs that are most important clinically, probenecid and sulfinpyrazone, are organic acids. Since they are organic acids, their individual rates of renal clearance, and therefore their inhibitory potency, are affected by local pH. If the blood pH rises, more of the drug will be in its ionized, anionic form (i.e., the form necessary for the drug to be actively secreted into the proximal tubule). Alkalinization of the urine also will increase the amount of uricosuric agent found in this fluid, since increasing urinary pH impairs the passive back-diffusion of the drug.

The initial phase of therapy with uricosuric drugs is the most potentially dangerous period. Until uricosuric drug levels build up sufficiently to fully inhibit uric acid reabsorption as well as secretion, there may be a temporary increase in uric acid blood levels that significantly increases the risk of an acute gouty attack. Therefore, it is wise to begin with the administration of small dosages of colchicine before adding a uricosuric drug to the therapeutic regimen. In addition, the initial rise in urinary uric acid concentrations during uricosuric drug therapy may also result in renal stone formation. Such a complication can be obviated by increasing urinary output and mildly alkalinizing (above pH 6) the urine during this period of gout therapy.

Probenecid

Pharmacokinetics
Probenecid (Fig. 44-4) is a lipid-soluble compound that is rapidly absorbed after oral administration, with peak plasma levels usually achieved in 2 to 4 hr. Although the drug is extensively bound to plasma proteins, it does not have a very long body half-life (6–12 hr), because it and its metabolites are actively secreted by the proximal tubule anionic secretory system. Its urinary excretion increases with increasing urinary pH. Probenecid is rapidly metabolized, with less than 5 percent of an administered dose being eliminated in a 24-hr period. The major metabolite is an acylmonoglucuronide.

Mechanism of Action
When probenecid is given in sufficient amounts, *it will block the active reabsorption of uric acid that occurs in the proximal tubules,* thereby increasing the amount of urate eliminated. Paradoxically, if small dosages are administered,

Figure 44-4. Probenecid.

probenecid may actually decrease uric acid excretion and raise blood levels. Low dosages of probenecid appear to compete preferentially with plasma uric acid for the proximal tubule anionic transport system and block its access to this active secretory system. The uricosuric action of probenecid, however, is accounted for by the drug's ability to inhibit the active reabsorption of *filtered* urate.

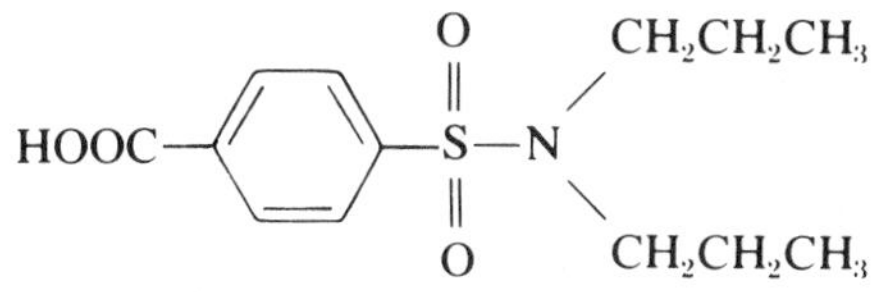

Clinical Uses
Probenecid is an effective and relatively safe agent for controlling hyperuricemia and preventing tophi deposition in tissues. Chronic administration will decrease the incidence of acute gouty attacks as well as diminish the complications usually associated with hyperuricemia, such as renal damage and tophi deposition. It is not useful in treating acute attacks of gouty arthritis or in cases of renal insufficiency when glomerular filtration rates have been reduced below 30 ml/min.

Proper use of probenecid requires that the patient be hydrated (3 liters H_2O/day) before and during the initial phases of drug administration. If the total amount of uric acid excreted is greater than 800 mg/day, the urine should be alkalinized with sodium bicarbonate or potassium citrate to increase the aqueous solubility of uric acid (i.e., convert it to the more soluble urate form). In addition to preventing kidney stone formation, alkalinization of the urine also serves to promote uric acid elimination by decreasing its rate of passive reabsorption.

Probenecid also is still used by some physicians to maintain high blood levels of penicillin, cephalosporin, acyclovir, and cyclosporine.

Adverse Reactions
Adverse reactions associated with probenecid therapy include occasional rashes, allergic dermatitis, upper gastrointestinal tract irritation, and drowsiness. The drug is contraindicated in patients with a history of renal calculi.

Drug Interactions
Probenecid can impair the renal active secretion of a variety of acidic compounds, including sulfinpyrazone, sulfonylureas, indomethacin, penicillin, sulfonamides, and 17-ketosteroids. If these agents are to be given concomitantly with probenecid, their dosage should be modified appropriately. For example, salicylates, including aspirin,

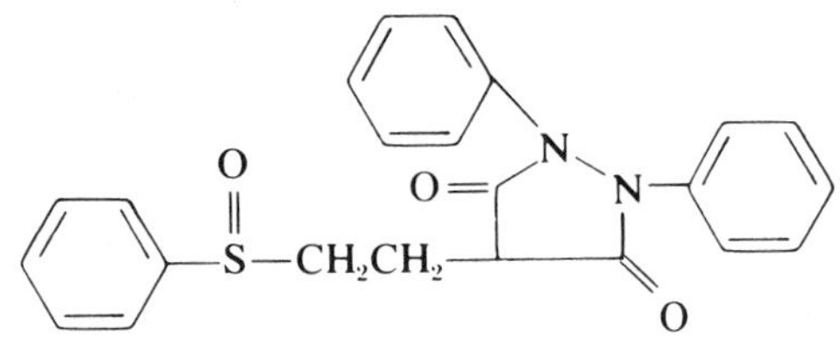

Figure 44-5. Sulfinpyrazone.

can almost completely block the uricosuric effect of probenecid. In addition, uricosuric agents can influence renal excretion, volume of distribution, and hepatic metabolism of a number of drugs.

Preparations and Dosage

Probenecid (*Benemid*) is marketed as 500-mg tablets. A combination of probenecid (500 mg) and colchicine (0.5 mg) is commercially available (*ColBENEMID*) and is suggested for use as maintenance therapy.

Sulfinpyrazone

Sulfinpyrazone (Fig. 44-5) is chemically related to the antiinflammatory and uricosuric compound phenylbutazone. However, it lacks the antiinflammatory, analgesic, and sodium-retaining properties of phenylbutazone.

Pharmacokinetics

Sulfinpyrazone is readily absorbed after oral administration, with peak blood levels being achieved 1 to 2 hr after ingestion. Sulfinpyrazone is more highly bound to plasma protein (98–99%) than is probenecid (84–94%), and it is a more potent uricosuric agent.

Most of the drug (90%) is eliminated through active proximal tubular secretion of the intact parent compound. Sulfinpyrazone also undergoes *p*-hydroxylation to form an active metabolite that is also uricosuric. The formation of such a metabolite undoubtedly contributes to the drug's prolonged activity (about 10 hr) and potency relative to probenecid. In contrast to probenecid, the rate of excretion of sulfinpyrazone is not enhanced by alkalinization of the urine, since at all urinary pHs the drug is largely ionized and therefore not a candidate for passive back-diffusion.

Mechanism of Action

The mechanism of sulfinpyrazone's uricosuric activity is similar to that described for probenecid. It also shares most of probenecid's undesirable side effects and precautions to be observed in clinical use. These two uricosuric drugs can be used in combination since they have an ad-

ditive effect. *Salicylates interfere with the clinical effects of both drugs and should be avoided in patients treated with uricosuric agents.*

Clinical Uses

Sulfinpyrazone, although less effective than allopurinol in reducing serum uric acid levels, remains useful for the prevention or reduction of the joint changes and tophi that would otherwise occur in chronic gout. It has no antiinflammatory properties. During the initial period of sulfinpyrazone use, acute attacks of gout may increase in frequency and severity. It is recommended, therefore, that either colchicine or a nonsteroidal antiinflammatory agent be coadministered during early sulfinpyrazone therapy.

A recent observation indicates that sulfinpyrazone inhibits platelet aggregation. The drug is now being investigated for use in the prophylactic treatment of myocardial infarction, since its administration may diminish the appearance of blood clots in coronary vessels.

Adverse Reactions

Abdominal pain, nausea, and possible reactivation of peptic ulcer have been reported. The drug should be used with caution in patients with compromised renal function. Adequate fluid intake should always accompany sulfinpyrazone administration in order to minimize the possibility of renal calculi formation.

Preparations and Dosage

Sulfinpyrazone (*Anturane*) is marketed as 200-mg capsules and 100-mg tablets.

Allopurinol

Allopurinol is the drug of choice in the treatment of chronic tophaceous gout, and is especially useful in those patients whose treatment is complicated by the presence of renal insufficiency.

Mechanism of Action

Allopurinol (Fig. 44-6), in contrast to the uricosuric drugs, *reduces serum urate levels through a competitive inhibition of uric acid synthesis* rather than by impairing renal urate reabsorption. This action is accomplished by inhibiting *xanthine oxidase,* the enzyme involved in the metabolism of hypoxanthine and xanthine to uric acid. After enzyme inhibition, the urinary concentration of uric acid is greatly reduced and a simultaneous increase in the excretion of the more soluble compounds xanthine and hypoxanthine occurs.

Allopurinol itself is metabolized by xanthine oxidase to

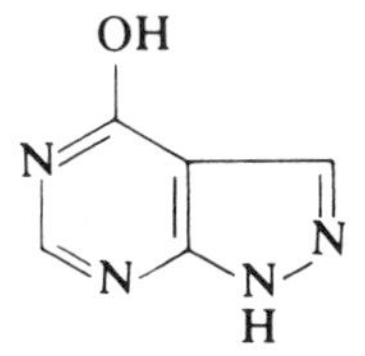

OH

Figure 44-6. Allopurinol.

form the active metabolite oxypurinol. The latter compound tends to accumulate after chronic administration of the parent drug, a phenomenon that contributes to the therapeutic effectiveness of allopurinol in long-term use. Most investigators believe that oxypurinol is primarily responsible for the antigout effects of allopurinol. Once produced, oxypurinol inhibits xanthine oxidase by forming a reversible complex with it. Although oxypurinol seems to be the principal inhibitor of the enzyme, oxypurinol itself is not administered because it is not absorbed orally as well as is allopurinol. Reabsorption of oxypurinol occurs at the same renal tubular site as the reabsorption of urate. This active reabsorption of oxypurinol greatly prolongs its biological half-life.

Absorption, Metabolism, and Excretion

Allopurinol is completely absorbed after oral ingestion, reaching peak blood levels in about 4 hr. In contrast to the uricosuric drugs, allopurinol is not appreciably bound to plasma proteins and is only a minor substrate for renal secretory mechanisms. Allopurinol is a substrate for xanthine oxidase and is metabolized by this enzyme to form oxypurinol, an active metabolite that also inhibits xanthine oxidase. The formation of this active metabolic product and the finding that oxypurinol is, in part, actively reabsorbed in the proximal tubule, accounts for the longer half-life of the metabolite (18–20 hr) compared with that of the parent drug (2–3 hr). This long half-life permits once-a-day drug administration.

Clinical Uses

Allopurinol is especially indicated in the treatment of chronic tophaceous gout, since patients receiving the drug show a pronounced decrease in their serum *and* urinary uric acid levels.

Because it does not depend on renal mechanisms for its efficacy, allopurinol is of particular benefit in patients who already have developed renal obstructions due to uric acid stones, patients with excessively high urate excretion (e.g., above 1,200 mg/24 hr), patients with a variety of blood disorders (e.g., leukemia, polycythemia vera), pa-

tients with excessive tophi deposition, or patients who fail to respond well to the uricosuric drugs. The actions of allopurinol are not antagonized by the coadministration of salicylates.

Allopurinol also is effective in inhibiting the appearance of reperfusion injury. This injury occurs when organs that either have been transplanted or have had their usual blood perfusion blocked for a period of time are reperfused with blood or an appropriate buffer solution. The cause of this injury involves the local formation of free radicals, such as the superoxide anion ($\cdot O_2^-$), hydroxyl free radical ($\cdot OH$), or peroxynitrite (OONO). These substances are strong oxidants and quite damaging to tissues. The toxic free radicals are produced by the action of the enzyme xanthine oxidase on tissue purine bases such as xanthine and hypoxanthine. The formation of free radicals can be inhibited by the administration of allopurinol, either directly to the patient or administered in the medium applied to the removed organ. Such a procedure has been shown to reduce the major cause of reperfusion injury. For example, kidneys ready for transplantation remain vital two to three times longer in the presence of allopurinol.

Adverse Reactions

The most common toxicities include a variety of skin rashes of differing severities, gastrointestinal upset, hepatotoxicity, and fever. These reactions are often sufficiently severe to dictate termination of drug therapy. It is advised that therapy not be initiated during an acute attack of gouty arthritis. As with the uricosuric drugs, therapy with allopurinol should be accompanied both by a sufficient increase in fluid intake to ensure a water diuresis and by alkalinization of the urine. These procedures help diminish the incidence of acute gout attacks that might otherwise accompany the initiation of drug therapy. Prophylactic use of colchicine also helps to prevent acute attacks of gout that may be brought on during the initial period of allopurinol ingestion.

A note of caution: The long-term risks involved in the chronic inhibition of purine and pyrimidine biosynthesis have not been established and it is therefore important to maintain careful surveillance of patients receiving prolonged allopurinol therapy.

Drug Interactions

Allopurinol has some inhibitory effects on hepatic microsomal drug-metabolizing enzymes. Thus, coadministration of drugs metabolized by this system should be done with caution. Because allopurinol can very effectively inhibit the oxidation of mercaptopurine and azathioprine, their administered dosage must be decreased by as much as 75 percent when they are given together with allopurinol. Allopurinol may also increase the toxicity of other cytotoxic drugs (e.g., vidarabine). Due to a complex interaction when probenecid and allopurinol are coadministered (e.g., chronic tophaceous gout), it is usually necessary to decrease the dosage of probenecid and increase the dosage of allopurinol.

Preparations and Dosage

Allopurinol (*Zyloprim*) is available as 100- and 300-mg tablets and is usually given in divided doses, up to 400 mg daily in mild cases of gout.

Other Drugs

A number of drugs other than those discussed in detail have been used to control the symptoms of acute gouty arthritis. Since the principal aspects of the pharmacology of these agents have been described elsewhere, they are mentioned only briefly here.

Indomethacin (see Chap. 43) exerts antiinflammatory, antipyretic, and analgesic properties. These qualities make it useful for the short-term management of the symptoms of acute gouty arthritis, although it has little effect on serum uric acid levels. Its antiinflammatory activity has been attributed to inhibition of prostaglandin synthesis, phosphodiesterase inhibition, inhibition of leukocytic phagocytosis, or a combination of these. The last-named action would be particularly valuable in treating the early stages of gout, because a decrease in the leukocytic phagocytosis of urate crystals should result in a stabilization of leukocyte lysosomes and hence decrease the amount of peptides, prostaglandins, and other substances released from these organelles. Acute attacks of gout are generally treated with 50 mg indomethacin (*Indocin*) three times a day for about 5 days.

Phenylbutazone (see Chap. 43) is a pyrazoline derivative that also displays antipyretic, analgesic, and antiin-flammatory activity. In addition, it possesses some uricosuric potency. It is most widely used for the treatment of acute attacks of gouty arthritis, in which it is about equal to colchicine in effectiveness. Although the drug does promote the renal excretion of uric acid, its usefulness is generally attributed to its antiinflammatory actions. Phenylbutazone (*Butazolidin, Azolid*) is available as 100-mg tablets and is generally administered for up to 7 days at a dosage of 200 mg three or four times on the first day, followed by diminishing daily dosages.

Oxyphenbutazone (*Oxalid, Tandearil*) is the principal uricosuric metabolite of phenylbutazone. It has the same indications and toxicities as phenylbutazone and can be given in approximately the same doses. It is marketed as 100-mg tablets.

Adrenal corticosteroids and corticotropin (adrenocorticotropic hormone) are also used to treat acute attacks of gouty arthritis. They are administered for brief periods (up to 3 days) and are generally reserved for severe cases. Additional details of their pharmacology can be found in Chaps. 65 and 66.

Supplemental Reading

Abramson, S., Hoffstein, S.T., and Weissman, G. Superoxide anion generation by human neutrophils exposed to monosodium urate. *Arthritis Rheum.* 25:174,1982.

Boss, G.R., and Seegmiller, J.E. Hyperuricemia and gout: Classification, complications and management. *N. Engl. J. Med.* 300:1459,1979.

Moller, J.V., and Sheikh, M.I. Renal organic ion transport system: Pharmacological, physiological, and biochemical aspects. *Pharmacol. Rev.* 34:315,1982.

Roberts, W.N., Liang, M.H., and Stern, S.H. Colchicine in acute gout: Reassessment of risks and benefits. *J.A.M.A.* 257:1920,1987.

Wedeen, R.P. Hyperuricemia and gouty nephropathy: Persisting controversy. *Drug Ther. Bull.* 11:45,1981.

Wyngaarden, J.B., and Kelley, W.N. *Gout and Hyperuricemia.* New York: Grune & Stratton, 1976.

45

Drugs Used in Asthma

Theodore J. Torphy and *Douglas W. P. Hay*

The word *asthma* is derived from a Greek word meaning difficulty in breathing. The clinical manifestations of asthma, wheezing and shortness of breath, are produced by a reversible narrowing of the airway. This results in an increased resistance to airflow and, consequently, a reduction in the efficiency with which air is carried to and from the alveoli. In addition to airway obstruction, cardinal features of asthma include airway inflammation and airway hyperreactivity. In contrast to *chronic obstructive pulmonary disease* (emphysema and chronic bronchitis), the airway obstruction associated with asthma is generally considered to be reversible. However, changes in the architecture of the airway occur in patients with severe long-standing asthma. These changes, including airway smooth muscle hypertrophy and bronchofibrosis, can result in an irreversible decrement in pulmonary function.

The clinical expression of asthma may vary from a mild intermittent wheeze or cough to severe chronic obstruction that is capable of restricting normal ambulatory activity. *Status asthmaticus* is a life-threatening exacerbation of the disease that must be treated aggressively.

An aberrant immune response associated with allergy appears to underlie asthma in most children over the age of 3 years and in most young adults; allergy-induced asthma is also known as *extrinsic asthma*. In contrast, a large number of patients, and especially those who acquire asthma as older adults, have no discernible immunological basis for their condition, although airway inflammation remains a characteristic of the disease; this type of asthma has been termed *intrinsic asthma*. In other patients, both allergic and nonallergic forms of asthma may coexist.

Three factors contribute to airway obstruction in asthma: (1) contraction of the smooth muscle that surrounds the airways; (2) excessive secretion of mucus and, in some, secretion of a thick, tenacious mucus that adheres to the walls of the airways; and (3) edema of the respiratory mucosa. Spasm of the bronchial smooth muscle can occur rapidly in response to a provocative stimulus and

likewise can be reversed rapidly by drug therapy. In contrast, respiratory mucus accumulation and edema formation are likely to require more time to develop and are only slowly reversible.

The recognition that asthma is a disease of *airway inflammation* (Fig. 45-1) has fundamentally changed the manner in which the disease is treated. Thus, it is useful to discuss the involvement of various mediators and inflammatory cells in antigen-induced asthma, an extensively studied, albeit simplistic model of the disease. In this model, antigens, such as ragweed pollen, sensitize individuals by eliciting the production of cytotrophic antibodies of the immunoglobulin E (IgE) type. Those antibodies attach themselves to the surface of *mast cells* and *basophils*. If the individual is reexposed to the same antigen days to months later, the resulting antigen-antibody reaction on lung mast cells will trigger the release of *histamine* and the *peptidoleukotrienes,* agents that produce bronchoconstriction, mucus secretion, and pulmonary edema. Mast cells also release a variety of chemotactic mediators such as *leukotriene B$_4$, platelet-activating factor,* and *cytokines.* These agents recruit and activate additional inflammatory cells, especially eosinophils. Eosinophils are major contributors to airway inflammation in chronic asthma; these cells release peptidoleukotrienes as well as a number of *cytotoxic peptides* that damage the airway epithelium. Alveolar macrophages are also activated and serve as yet another source for leukotrienes and cytokines. Ultimately, repeated antigen exposure establishes a chronic inflammatory state in the asthmatic airway.

Chronic airway inflammation is thought to produce a hyperreactivity of the asthmatic airway to a variety of stimuli. In addition to antigen(s), exposure to cold air, exercise, emotional stress, and chemical irritants can provoke an acute asthmatic episode, and it is probable that these stimuli, either directly or indirectly, bring about the release of mediators or contractile neurotransmitters. One specific cause of the excessive airway reactivity of asth-

Morphology of the Normal and Asthmatic Airway

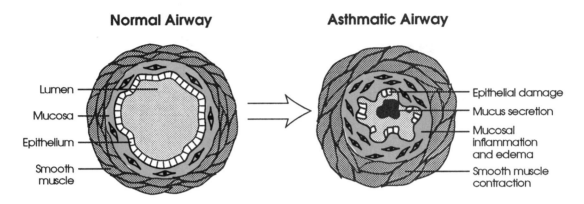

Mediators of Bronchial Asthma

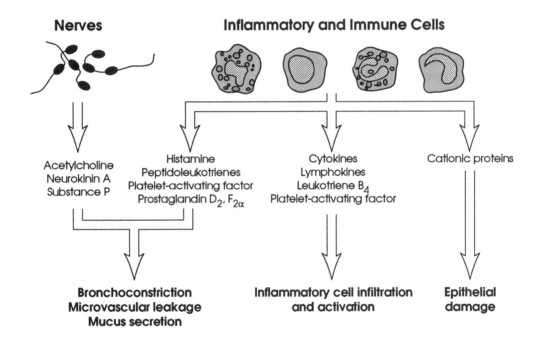

Figure 45-1. Pathophysiology of asthma.

matics to noxious stimuli is that airway sensory receptors are made more irritable or more accessible by eosinophil-induced damage to the airway epithelium.

Treatment Strategy

Clinical symptoms alone cannot be used as an accurate assessment of the severity of physiological impairment in the asthmatic patient, because a substantial degree of impairment may persist even after symptoms are relieved by treatment. Consequently, the overall objective of antiasthma therapy is to return lung function to as near normal as possible and, at the same time, prevent acute exacerbations of the disease. Bronchodilators are used both in maintenance therapy and on an as-needed basis to reverse acute attacks. Based on the underlying pathophysiology of the disease, antiinflammatory therapy is strongly recommended in all but the mildest asthmatics. In addition, all treatment regimens should include patient education

Airway Status	Symptoms	Lung Function*	Drug Therapy

Chronic Mild Asthma

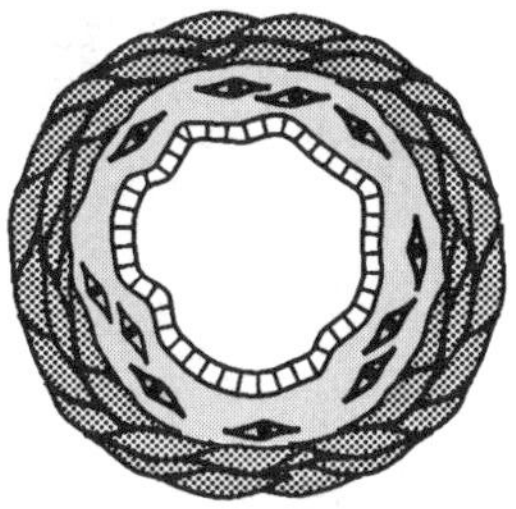

- Intermittent, brief (<1hr) dyspnea 2 times weekly
- Brief wheezing with activity or cold air
- Asymptomatic between exacerbations

Asymptomatic ≥ 80% baseline ➡ **Inhaled β₂-agonist** or **cromolyn** prn before exposure to allergen or other stimuli

Symptomatic varies 20% or more ➡ **Inhaled β₂-agonist** q 4 hours for duration of episode

Chronic Moderate Asthma

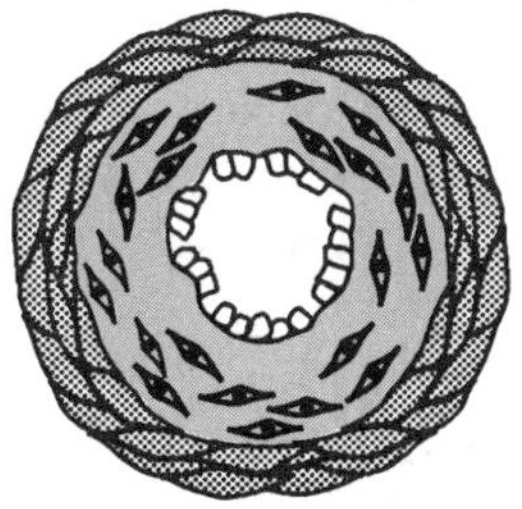

- Symptoms > 1-2 times weekly
- Exacerbations affect activity and may last several days
- Occasional emergency care

60-80% of baseline and varies 20-30% ➡ **Inhaled β₂-agonist** prn to qid and **Anti-inflammatory agents**
- Inhaled steroids *or*
- Cromolyn
If symptoms persist:
Additional therapy
- Increase inhaled steroids *and/or*
- Add theophylline *and/or*
- Add oral β₂-agonist

- Severe exacerbations

As above but varies > 30% ➡ Short course of **oral steroids**

Chronic Severe Asthma

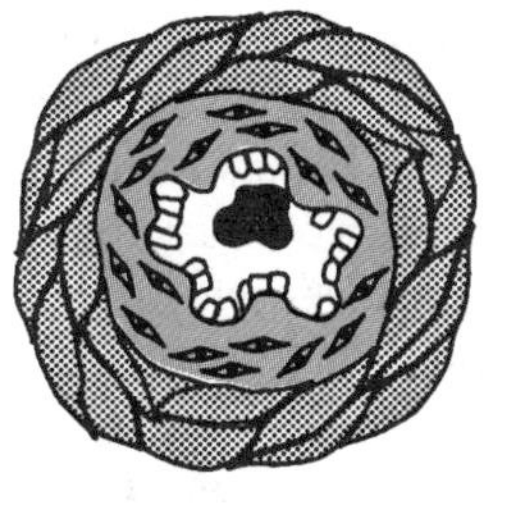

- Continuous symptoms
- Limited physical activity
- Frequent exacerbations
- Occasional hospitalization and emergency care

< 60% of baseline and highly variable ➡ **Inhaled β₂-agonist** qid & **Anti-inflammatory agents**
- Inhaled steroids *with or without*
- Cromolyn *with or without*
Theophylline
Oral β₂-agonist *and*
Oral steroids
- Short-term for active symptoms *consider*
- Daily or alternate day use

* Lung function expressed as a % of predicted standardized norms obtained from pulmonary function tests.

Figure 45-2. Guidelines for the treatment of asthma. (From National Asthma Education Program, *Guidelines for the Diagnosis and Treatment of Asthma.* PHS Publication No. 91-3042. Bethesda, Md.: Department of Health and Human Services, 1991.)

regarding the appropriate use of medications to control symptoms (e.g., proper technique for use of metered-dose inhalers) and signs of a deteriorating disease status (e.g., a progressive increase in the use of bronchodilators), as well as approaches toward prevention (e.g., avoidance of antigenic material, such as pollen, animal dander, and house mite dust).

The primary drugs used to treat asthma are *bronchodilators* and *antiinflammatory agents*. Bronchodilators include theophylline, a variety of *adrenomimetic amines,* and ipratropium bromide. Antiinflammatory therapy consists of the *corticosteroids.* A third class of drugs typified by *cromolyn sodium* normalize airway reactivity in an ill-defined manner.

Recommendations for the stepwise treatment of adult asthma are shown in Fig. 45-2. Recommendations for children are similar to those made for adults, except that corticosteroids are used more conservatively.

Table 45-1. Examples of Theophylline Preparations

Formulation	Trade names	Route	Dosage and frequency[a]
Conventional	—	IV[b]	0.6 mg/kg/hr[c]
	—	po	3 mg/kg/hr
Controlled release	Theo-Dur, Slo-bid, Uniphyl, Theo-24	po	7 mg/kg q12h
		po	13 mg/kg q24h

[a]Dosages are approximate since theophylline must be titrated in each patient to achieve therapeutic plasma concentrations.
[b]Only aminophylline is given IV.
[c]Loading dose of 6 mg/kg is given to patients not previously receiving theophylline.

Bronchodilators

When administered in sufficient quantities by an appropriate route, bronchodilators usually will reduce the work of breathing, relieve symptoms of asthma, and improve ventilation. By relaxing bronchial smooth muscle, bronchodilators can produce a substantial increase in pulmonary function by dilating the airways. Commonly used bronchodilators are listed in Tables 45-1 and 45-2.

Theophylline

Until recently theophylline and its more soluble ethylenediamine salt, aminophylline, were the bronchodilators of choice in the United States for the management of asthma. Although this primary role has now been taken by the β_2-adrenoceptor agonists, theophylline continues to have an important place in the therapy of asthma. Theophylline is also useful in treating the reversible component of the airway obstruction associated with emphysema and chronic bronchitis.

Chemistry

Theophylline is a methylated xanthine, which is chemically and pharmacologically related to caffeine and theobromine. Theophylline, caffeine, and theobromine are alkaloids that occur in varying proportions in coffee beans, tea leaves, cocoa seeds, and cola nuts.

Mechanism of Action

The mechanism by which theophylline relaxes bronchial smooth muscle is unknown. Increases in the intracellular concentration of adenosine 3'5'-cyclic phosphate (cAMP) are associated with relaxation of airway smooth muscle. Phosphodiesterase, the enzyme that inactivates cAMP, is inhibited by theophylline. Until recently, it has been accepted that inhibition of phosphodiesterase by the-ophylline results in an intracellular accumulation of cAMP and a subsequent relaxation of bronchial smooth muscle. However, phosphodiesterase is only slightly inhibited by concentrations of theophylline that are considered to be within the therapeutic range. Other mechanisms that may contribute to the action of theophylline in asthma include antagonism of adenosine, inhibition of mediator release, increased sympathetic activity, alteration in immune cell function, and reduction in respiratory muscle fatigue.

Pharmacological Actions

Smooth muscle relaxation, central nervous system (CNS) excitation, and cardiac stimulation are the principal pharmacological effects observed in patients treated with theophylline. The action of theophylline on the respiratory system is easily seen in the asthmatic by the resolution of obstruction and improvement in pulmonary function. Historically, the ability of theophylline to improve pulmonary function was attributed solely to its bronchodilator activity. Recently, however, it has been recognized that theophylline also may exert an antiinflammatory effect.

Plasma concentrations of theophylline between 10 and 20 μg/ml are generally considered to be optimal, although concentrations as low as 5 μg/ml have been clinically effective.

In addition to having an antiasthmatic effect, theophylline increases cardiac output and lowers venous pressure.

Absorption, Metabolism, and Excretion

The plasma concentration of theophylline cannot be predicted reliably from the dose administered. In one study, the oral dosage of theophylline required to produce plasma levels between 10 and 20 μg/ml varied between 400 and 3,200 mg/day. Heterogeneity among individuals in the rate at which they metabolize theophylline appears to be the principal factor responsible for the variability in plasma levels.

The average half-life of theophylline in the adult asth-

Table 45-2. Examples of Adrenomimetics and Anticholinergics Used as Bronchodilators

Class	Agent	Trade name(s)	Route	Dosage and frequency[a]
α/β-Adrenoceptor agonists	Epinephrine	—	SC	0.01 mg/kg
		Primatene	Inhalation	0.44 mg q4h
β-Adrenoceptor agonists	Isoproterenol	Isuprel Mistometer	Inhalation	0.25 mg q4h
	Metaproterenol	Alupent	po	20 mg q6–8h
			Inhalation	1.3 mg[b]
Selective β_2-adrenoceptor agonists	Albuterol	Proventil, Ventolin	po	2–4 mg q6h
	Bitolterol	Tornalate	Inhalation	0.75 mg q8h
	Pirbuterol	Maxair	Inhalation	0.4 mg q4–6h
	Terbutaline	Brethine	SC	0.25 mg
		Brethine	po	5 mg q6h
		Brethaire	Inhalation	0.4 mg q4–6h
Anticholinergics	Ipratropium bromide	Atrovent	Inhalation	0.07 mg q6h

[a]Dosages for inhalation represent the amount of compound delivered by two actuations (inhalations) of the individual metered-dose inhaler listed.
[b]Because of its short duration of action, inhaled metaproterenol is not used in maintenance therapy.

matic is 5.2 hr, although a range from 3.0 to 9.5 hr has been seen. The average half-life of theophylline in children 5 to 15 years of age is somewhat shorter at 3.6 hr. In smokers, the average half-life is 4.3 hr and in nonsmokers, 7.0 hr.

Theophylline is metabolized in the liver and eliminated in the urine as 1,3-dimethyl uric acid and 3-methyl xanthine. Less than 10 percent is excreted in the urine unchanged. Such conditions as heart failure, liver disease, and severe respiratory obstruction will slow the metabolism of theophylline.

Clinical Uses

The principal use of theophylline is in the management of asthma. It is also used to relieve dyspnea associated with pulmonary edema that develops from congestive heart failure.

Adverse Reactions

The most frequent complaints of patients taking theophylline are nausea and vomiting, which occur most frequently in patients receiving theophylline for the first time and when the plasma level approaches 20 μg/ml, but rarely occur at plasma concentrations <15 μg/ml. The fact that patients who receive the drug intravenously also have the same complaint suggests that the nausea and vomiting result from an action in the CNS.

When serum concentrations exceed 40 μg/ml, there is a high probability of seizures. Nausea will not always be a premonitory sign of impending toxicity. For instance, in children, restlessness, agitation, diuresis, or fever can occur even when nausea does not. A rapid intravenous injection of theophylline can cause arrhythmias, hypoten-

sion, and cardiac arrest. Thus, extreme caution should be used when giving the drug by this route. Since *it is not possible to predict blood levels on the basis of dosage,* toxicity is not uncommon by any route of administration. Consequently, it is recommended that plasma concentrations of theophylline be determined when a patient begins therapy and then at regular intervals of 6 to 12 months thereafter.

Cautions and Contraindications

Theophylline should be used with caution in patients with myocardial disease, liver disease, and acute myocardial infarction. The half-life of theophylline is prolonged in patients with congestive heart failure. Because of its narrow margin of safety, extreme caution is warranted when coadministering drugs, such as cimetidine, that may interfere with the metabolism of theophylline. It is also prudent to be careful when using theophylline in patients with a history of seizures.

Preparations and Dosage

Theophylline is available commercially in a large variety of forms (see Table 45-1). Aminophylline (theophylline ethylenediamine) can be given by slow intravenous injection and is used in the treatment of status asthmaticus. Because of the relatively short plasma half-life of theophylline, conventional oral formulations must be given four to six times a day to maintain therapeutic plasma concentrations. Sustained-release oral preparations that can be administered once or twice a day also are available (see Table 45-1). Oral dosages of theophylline vary depending on the formulation, but in general the total daily dose is approximately 13 mg/kg.

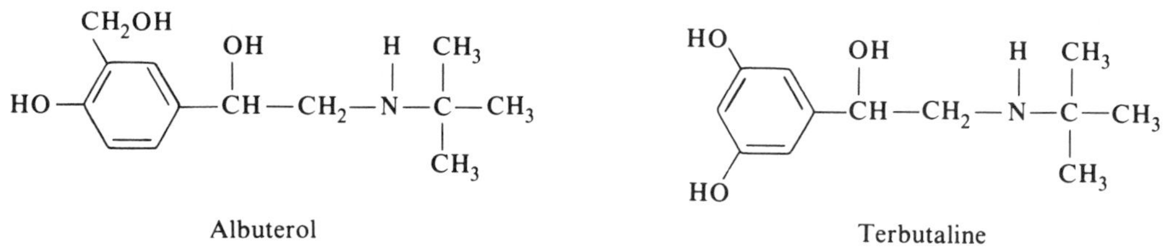

Figure 45-3. Structures of albuterol and terbutaline.

Adrenomimetic Amines

Adrenergic drugs that are currently used for the management of acute and chronic asthma are epinephrine, isoproterenol, and a group of adrenoceptor agonists including albuterol and terbutaline that are relatively selective for β_2-adrenoceptors (see Chap. 12). This latter class of agents has become the mainstay of modern bronchodilator therapy. These agents are used both on an as-needed basis to reverse acute episodes of bronchospasm and prophylactically to maintain airway patency over the long term.

Chemistry

Epinephrine and isoproterenol are catechols. The hydroxyl groups are located at positions 3 and 4 on the ring, and consequently both are substrates of catechol-O-methyltransferase and have very short plasma half-lives. *Albuterol* (Fig. 45-3), known as salbutamol outside of the United States, has ring substituents at positions 3 and 4, but only one of these is a hydroxyl group. The other is a hydroxymethyl group and therefore the molecule is not a substrate for catechol-O-methyltransferase (COMT). *Terbutaline* (see Fig. 45-3) also is not a substrate for COMT, since its hydroxyl groups are located at positions 3 and 5.

Epinephrine activates both α- and β-adrenoceptors, whereas isoproterenol is selective for β-adrenoceptors. The tertiary butyl derivatives, albuterol and terbutaline, represent an improvement over isoproterenol in targeting adrenomimetics to the airway in that these compounds have a higher affinity for β_2-adrenoceptors, the predominant subtype in the airway, than for β_1-adrenoceptors. Other β_2-selective adrenomimetics used as bronchodilators are bitolterol and pirbuterol. Metaproterenol, another

β-adrenomimetic used as a bronchodilator, is less selective for β_2-adrenoceptors than albuterol or terbutaline.

Mechanism of Action

The effects of the adrenomimetics are thought to be mediated by cAMP. Adrenomimetics enhance the production of cAMP by activating adenylyl cyclase, the enzyme that converts adenosine triphosphate (ATP) to cAMP. *The action of adrenomimetic bronchodilators in the lung is the result of relaxation of bronchial smooth muscle, an effect that is initiated by the combination of an agonist with β_2-adrenoceptors.*

Pharmacological Actions

The general pharmacological actions of adrenomimetics are described in detail in Chap. 12. The principal pharmacological effects that may be observed in humans treated for bronchospasm are bronchodilation, tachycardia, anxiety, and tremor. All of these actions are produced either directly or indirectly by stimulating β_2-adrenoceptors.

Epinephrine administered subcutaneously is used to manage severe acute episodes of bronchospasm and status asthmaticus. In addition to its bronchodilator activity through β-adrenoceptor stimulation, a portion of the therapeutic utility of epinephrine in these acute settings may be due to a reduction in pulmonary edema as a result of pulmonary vasoconstriction. The effects on pulmonary function are quite rapid, with peak effects occurring within 5 to 15 min. Measurable improvement in pulmonary function is maintained for up to 4 hr. The characteristic cardiovascular effects observed with doses of 0.3 to 0.5 mg, administered SC to normal or asthmatic subjects, are increased heart rate, increased cardiac output, increased stroke volume, an elevation of systolic pressure and decrease in diastolic pressure, and a decrease in systemic vascular resistance. The cardiovascular response to epinephrine represents the algebraic sum of both α- and β-adrenoceptor stimulation. A decrease in diastolic blood pressure and a decrease in systemic vascular resistance are reflections of vasodilation, a β_2-adrenoceptor response. The increase in heart rate and systolic pressure is the result of either a direct effect of epinephrine on the myocardium, primarily a β_1 effect, or a reflex action provoked by a decrease in peripheral resistance, mean arterial pressure, or both. Overt α-adrenoceptor effects, such as systemic vasoconstriction, are not obvious unless high dosages are used.

Isoproterenol is administered almost exclusively by inhalation from metered-dose inhalers or from nebulizers. The response to inhaled isoproterenol and other inhaled adrenomimetics is almost instantaneous. The duration of action of isoproterenol is generally considered to be brief, although an objective measurement of pulmonary function has shown an effective duration of up to 3 hr. When administered by inhalation, the cardiac effects of isoproterenol are relatively mild, although in some cases a substantial increase in heart rate occurs.

Isoproterenol has *equal* affinity for β_1- and β_2-adrenoceptors and therefore has equal capacity to produce bronchodilation and cardiac stimulation. Terbutaline and albuterol are *relatively selective* for β_2-adrenoceptors, and theoretically are capable of producing bronchodilation with minimal cardiac stimulation. It should be remembered, however, that the term β_2 *selectivity* is a pharmacological classification based primarily on the relative potency of an individual adrenomimetic to stimulate the pulmonary or the cardiovascular system.

Figure 45-4 represents the results of a study in which asthmatic patients were given intravenous infusions of isoproterenol on one occasion and a β_2-stimulant (albuterol) on another. A sufficient portion of the dose-response curves for pulmonary function and heart rate was described so comparisons could be made. The dose-response curves of isoproterenol on pulmonary function and heart rate are essentially superimposable, thus showing no selectivity of pulmonary over cardiovascular actions. A dose of isoproterenol that produced a 50 percent increase in FEV_1 produced an 80 percent increase in heart rate.

Albuterol, on the other hand, increased FEV_1 50 percent while producing only a 25 percent increase in heart rate. These results are consistent with albuterol being selective for β_2-receptors. A similar separation of cardiac and pulmonary effects has been demonstrated for terbutaline. It is important to recognize that separation of cardiac and pulmonary effects is relative and that β_2-agonists will produce tachycardia at higher dosages, either by activating sympathetic reflex pathways as a consequence of systemic vasodilation or by directly stimulating cardiac β_1-adreno-

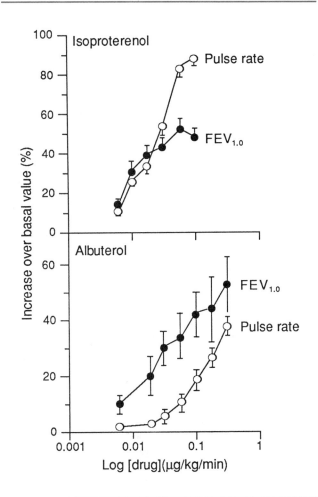

Figure 45-4. Effects of IV infusion of isoproterenol and albuterol on FEV_1 and heart rate of 10 asthmatic subjects. (From N. Svedmyr and G. Thiringer, Effects of Salbutamol and isoprenaline on β-receptors in patients with chronic obstructive lung disease. *Postgrad. Med. J.* 47 [Suppl.]:44, 1971.)

ceptors. In addition, a significant number of β_2-adrenoceptors are present in the human heart and stimulation of these receptors may contribute to the cardiac effects of β_2-adrenoceptor agonists.

Absorption, Metabolism, and Excretion

Epinephrine and isoproterenol are essentially ineffective when given orally because they are rapidly metabolized in the intestine and liver. When administered by inhalation or by injection, the first-pass effect (see Chap. 4) is avoided and the pattern of metabolism is different. Isoproterenol that is administered orally is inactivated by enzymes in the intestinal wall and liver, with 85 percent of the dose appearing in the urine as the sulfate conjugate.

When the drug is given intravenously, very little appears in the urine as the sulfate conjugate, most of the dose being recovered in the urine as unchanged isoproterenol. The metabolic pattern observed following inhalation from a metered-dose inhaler is very similar to that seen after oral administration. However, if isoproterenol is instilled directly into the bronchial tree, the metabolic pattern will resemble that seen after intravenous administration.

The similarity of the patterns following ingested and inhaled isoproterenol suggests that *most of the dose delivered by a metered-dose inhaler is swallowed* and inactivated in the gastrointestinal tract and that only a small fraction (about 10%) of the dose gets directly into the lungs. Therefore, the pharmacological effect of 200 μg inhaled isoproterenol is produced by the 20 μg or less that actually gets to the lung.

Terbutaline and albuterol are effective when administered orally or by inhalation. Terbutaline is not completely absorbed from the gastrointestinal tract. Peak plasma levels of terbutaline following oral administration are reached within 2 to 3 hr and its elimination half-life is 3 to 4 hr. Albuterol is well absorbed from the gastrointestinal tract. After oral administration peak plasma concentrations are reached within 2 to 3 hr and the elimination half-life is 5 to 6 hr.

The principal product of terbutaline metabolism is the sulfate conjugate; the quantity of the metabolite formed, however, depends on the route of administration. Terbutaline is eliminated in the urine as the sulfate conjugate and in the feces as the unchanged parent compound. Albuterol is eliminated in the urine, both as a metabolite and as the unchanged drug.

Clinical Uses

Epinephrine is used in a variety of clinical situations, and although concern has been expressed about the use of epinephrine in asthma, the drug is still used extensively for the management of acute attacks.

Isoproterenol is used principally by inhalation for the management of bronchospasm. It is also used intravenously for asthma and as a stimulant in cardiac arrest.

Terbutaline, albuterol, and other β₂-adrenoceptor agonists are used primarily in the management of asthma. In addition, terbutaline is used extensively to control premature labor, since contractions of uterine smooth muscle are abolished by adrenomimetics.

Adverse Reactions

Patients treated with recommended dosages of epinephrine will complain of feeling nervous or anxious. Some will experience tremor of the hand or upper extremity and many will complain of palpitations. Epinephrine is dangerous if recommended dosages are exceeded or if the drug is used in patients with coronary artery disease, arrhythmias, or hypertension. The inappropriate use of epinephrine has resulted in extreme hypertension and cerebrovascular accidents, pulmonary edema, angina, and ventricular arrhythmias including ventricular fibrillation.

At recommended dosages, adverse effects from inhaled isoproterenol are infrequent and not serious. When excessive dosages are used, tachycardia, dizziness, and nervousness may occur, and some patients may experience arrhythmias.

The limiting side effect associated with orally administered β₂-adrenoceptor agonists is *muscle tremor,* which results from a direct stimulation of β₂-adrenoceptors in skeletal muscle. This side effect is most notable on the initiation of therapy and gradually improves on continued use. β₂-Agonists also cause tachycardia and palpitations in some patients. When used by intravenous infusion for premature labor, β₂-agonists have been reported to produce tachycardia and pulmonary edema in the mother and hypoglycemia in the newborn. When administered by inhalation, the β₂-agonists produce only minor side effects.

Recent epidemiological studies suggest that the overuse of β-adrenoceptor agonists is associated with an overall deterioration in disease control and a slight increase in asthma mortality. This apparent trend could be caused by several factors, the most likely of which is that patients rely too heavily on bronchodilator therapy to control acute symptoms at the expense of antiinflammatory therapy to control the underlying disease process.

Preparations

A variety of β-adrenomimetics are used as bronchodilators and are available in a number of dosage forms (see Table 45-2).

Epinephrine is available in multidose vials in concentrations of 1:1,000. Epinephrine bitartrate is also available for inhalation from a metered-dose inhaler (*Medihaler-Epi*). Solutions of epinephrine are available for use in nebulizers.

Isoproterenol hydrochloride and isoproterenol sulfate are available in metered-dose inhalers (*Isuprel Mistometer* and *Medihaler-Iso,* respectively) and as solutions for inhalation from power-driven nebulizers.

In the United States, terbutaline sulfate (*Bricanyl, Brethaire*) is available in tablets as well as a metered-dose inhaler. An injectable solution also is available.

Albuterol (*Ventolin Inhaler, Proventil*) is available as tablets and as a metered-dose inhaler. Albuterol also is available as a dry powder formulation for inhalation (*Ventolin Rotocaps*). Drug contained within the capsule is delivered to the airway by a specially designed reusable device (*Rotahaler*) that is breath actuated. Unlike conventional metered-dose inhalers, this device does not rely on chlorofluorocarbons as propellants. Instead, the Rotahaler mechanically opens the capsule and disperses the drug into the airstream created as the patient inhales through the mouthpiece.

An obvious disadvantage of the currently available β_2-adrenoceptor agonists is that when used for prophylactic therapy, these agents must be taken three to four times a day. Formoterol and salmeterol are longer-acting inhaled β_2-adrenoceptor agonists with bronchodilator activity that lasts 12 to 18 hr. These agents are used in several countries but have not yet been approved for use in the United States.

Anticholinergics

The main neuronal control in human airways is exerted by the parasympathetic cholinergic pathway emanating from the vagus nerve. The cholinergic efferent nerves synapse in ganglia within the airways and from there short postganglionic fibers emerge to innervate the end organs, including the airway smooth muscle and mucous glands. Stimulation of these nerve fibers, and the resultant release of acetylcholine and activation of muscarinic cholinoceptors, elicits bronchoconstriction, mucous secretion, and bronchial vasodilatation. Thus, the cholinergic pathways play a key role in the maintenance of the caliber of the airways and contribute to the airway obstruction in both asthma and chronic obstructive pulmonary disease. The airway effects of released acetylcholine are mediated via activation of three distinct muscarinic receptor subtypes: M_1, located in parasympathetic ganglia and mucous glands; autoinhibitory M_2, found in parasympathetic nerve terminals, and M_3, located in airway smooth muscle and mucous glands.

Anticholinergic compounds have been utilized for the treatment of respiratory disorders, including asthma, for centuries. For example, preparations of the plants *Atropa belladonna* and *Datura stramonium,* which contain the classical muscarinic receptor antagonist atropine, were used in the treatment of asthma in the 17th century. However, although atropine and related compounds possessed bronchodilator activity, their use was associated with the typical spectrum of anticholinergic side effects (see Chap. 15). Since the introduction of the β_2-adrenoceptor agonists, which possess superior efficacy and an improved side-effect profile, atropine has no longer been used in the treatment of asthma.

To improve the clinical utility of anticholinergics, quaternary amine derivatives of atropine have been developed, which, by virtue of their positive charge, are absorbed poorly across mucosal surfaces and thus produce fewer side effects than atropine. This is particularly true when these agents are given by the inhaled route.

Ipratropium bromide (*Atrovent*) is an archetypical example of this class of quaternary amine derivatives. It is an isopropyl congener of atropine that is used in the treatment of chronic obstructive pulmonary disease and, to a lesser extent, asthma. This compound is available only for inhalation. Compared with β_2-adrenoceptor agonists, ipratropium is generally at least as effective in chronic obstructive pulmonary disease but less effective in asthma. In the latter disease ipratropium is not normally administered alone but is often given in conjunction with a β_2-adrenoceptor agonist. The combination of these agents is more effective and has a longer duration of action than either agent alone. Ipratropium has greater effectiveness than β_2-adrenoceptor agonists in two settings: in psychogenic asthma and in patients taking β_2-adrenoceptor antagonists.

The typical dose of ipratropium is two inhalations of 36 μg each four times a day. Ipratropium has a slower onset of action (1–2 hr for peak activity) than β_2-adrenoceptor agonists and, thus, may be more suitable for prophylactic use. Ipratropium is virtually devoid of the CNS side effects associated with atropine. The most prevalent peripheral side effects are dry mouth, headache, nervousness, dizziness, nausea, and cough. Unlike atropine, ipratropium does not inhibit mucociliary clearance and thus does not promote the accumulation of secretions in the lower airways.

Corticosteroids

The use of systemically administered corticosteroids in the treatment of asthma was pioneered nearly 40 years ago. Although they proved to be very effective in the management of this disease, their usefulness was counterbalanced by an array of significant side effects. A major breakthrough was the introduction in the 1970s of *aerosol corticosteroids,* which maintained much of the impressive therapeutic efficacy of parenteral and oral corticosteroids, but, by virtue of their local administration and markedly reduced systemic absorption, were associated with a greatly reduced incidence and severity of side effects. The success of inhaled steroids has led to a substantial reduction in the use of systemic corticosteroids. *Inhaled corticosteroids are now increasingly utilized as front-line therapy in asthma.*

Chemistry

The corticosteroids utilized in asthma possess a heterocyclic carbon nucleus and compounds for inhalation are analogues of hydrocortisone.

Mechanism of Action

The corticosteroids all have the same general mechanism of action as do the mineralocorticoids and sex hormones; that is, they pass through cell membranes and bind to specific cytoplasmic receptors. The steroid receptor complexes translocate to the cell nucleus, where they attach to nuclear binding sites and initiate synthesis of messenger ribonucleic acid (mRNA). The novel proteins that are formed may then exert a variety of effects on cellular functions. The precise mechanism(s) whereby the corticosteroids exert their therapeutic benefit in asthma remains unclear, although it is likely to be due to several rather than one specific action and is almost certainly related to their ability to inhibit inflammatory processes.

Pharmacological Actions

The corticosteroids have an array of actions in several systems that may be relevant to their effectiveness in asthma. These include inhibition of mediator release, attenuation of mucous secretion, up-regulation of β-adrenoceptor number, inhibition of IgE synthesis, attenuation of eicosanoid generation, vasoconstriction, and suppression of inflammatory cell influx and inflammatory processes. The effects of the steroids take several hours to days to develop and thus they cannot be used to quickly relieve acute episodes of bronchospasm.

Absorption, Metabolism, and Excretion

Corticosteroids can be given via parenteral, oral, and local routes of administration. Prednisone and prednisolone are absorbed rapidly when given orally, with peak plasma concentrations reached within 1 to 2 hr.

There are significant differences in the absorption of different corticosteroids when administered by the inhaled route. Inhaled betamethasone and dexamethasone are absorbed relatively well and produce systemic effects. In contrast, triamcinolone acetonide, beclomethasone dipropionate, and flunisolide are either poorly absorbed or, following absorption, are rapidly metabolized and inactivated. Accordingly, by virtue of their rapid inactivation by first-pass metabolism in the liver and poor absorption in the gastrointestinal tract, corticosteroids such as beclomethasone have greatly diminished systemic effects relative to hydrocortisone and dexamethasone when administered via inhalation. Cortisone and prednisone need to be hydroxylated to become active, whereas most other corticosteroids do not require biotransformation.

The corticosteroids can be categorized into three groups based on their biological and plasma half-lives. Hydrocortisone is short-acting; prednisone, prednisolone,

and methylprednisolone are intermediate-acting; and dexamethasone, triamcinolone, and betamethasone are long-acting.

Clinical Uses

The corticosteroids are effective in most children and adults with asthma. They are beneficial for the treatment of both acute and chronic aspects of the disease. However, *inhaled corticosteroids are not effective or utilized in the relief of acute episodes of severe bronchospasm.* Systemic corticosteroids are used for the treatment of asthma that does not respond to theophylline, β_2-adrenoceptor agonists, or aerosol corticosteroids and, along with other treatments, in the control of status asthmaticus.

Adverse Reactions

The side effects of corticosteroids range from minor to severe and life threatening. The nature and severity of side effects depend on the route, dose, and frequency of administration, as well as the specific agent used.

Side effects are much more prevalent with systemic administration than with inhalant administration. The potential consequences of systemic administration of the corticosteroids include adrenal suppression, cushingoid changes, growth retardation, cataracts, osteoporosis, CNS effects and behavioral disturbances, and increased susceptibility to infection. The severity of all of these side effects can be reduced markedly by alternate-day therapy.

Inhaled corticosteroids are generally well tolerated. However, the first compounds to be administered by inhalation, hydrocortisone and dexamethasone, produced significant systemic side effects. Adverse reactions following inhalant administration include thrush (*Candida albicans*) and dysphonia. These side effects can be reduced by rinsing the mouth after dosage or by using spacer devices that aid in delivering a higher proportion of the administered dose to the distal airways rather than oropharynx. Rare instances of immediate and delayed hypersensitivity reactions, including urticaria, angioedema, rash, and bronchospasm, have been reported with inhaled corticosteroids.

Contraindications and Cautions

Systemic administration of the corticosteroids causes suppression of the hypothalamus-pituitary-adrenal axis. Care should be taken in transferring patients from systemic to aerosol corticosteroids, as deaths due to adrenal insufficiency have been reported. In addition, allergic conditions, such as rhinitis, conjunctivitis, and eczema, pre-

Table 45-3. Examples of Oral and Aerosol Corticosteroids

Class	Agent	Trade name(s)	Route	Dosage and frequency[a]
Oral corticosteroids	Prednisone	Deltasone	po	5–60 mg/day
	Methylprednisolone	Medrol	po	2–60 mg/day
		Solu-Medrol	IV	60–80 mg IV bolus q6–8h
		Depo-Medrol	Parenteral	1 single injection/day equivalent to total daily oral dose
	Hydrocortisone	Hydrocortone	IV	2 mg/kg bolus q4h or 2 mg/kg bolus, then 0.5 mg/kg/hr IV infusion
Aerosol corticosteroids[b]	Triamcinolone acetonide	Azmacort	Inhalation	0.2–0.4 mg q6–12h
	Beclomethasone dipropionate	Beclovent	Inhalation	0.084 mg q6–8hr
		Vanceril		or 0.168 mg q12h
	Flunisolide	AeroBid	Inhalation	0.5–1 mg q12h

[a]Dosage and frequency depend on the severity of the disease.
[b]Doses for inhalation represent the amount of compound delivered by two to four actuations (inhalations) of the individual metered-dose inhaler listed.

viously controlled by systemic corticosteroids, may be unmasked when asthmatic patients are switched from systemic to inhaled corticosteroids. Care should be exercised when taking the corticosteroids during pregnancy as glucocorticoids are teratogenic. Systemic corticosteroids are contraindicated in patients with systemic fungal infections.

Preparation and Dosage

Dosing regimens for inhaled and systemically administered corticosteroids are shown in Table 45-3. The three aerosol corticosteroids that are widely used in the United States are beclomethasone dipropionate (*Beclovent, Vanceril*), triamcinolone acetonide (*Azmacort*), and flunisolide (*AeroBid*). Generally, dosing twice or three times a day (two inhalations) is sufficient for mild to moderate asthma, although dosing four times a day may be required for the control of severe conditions.

The dosage for orally administered prednisone is 5 to 60 mg/day, and in the treatment of severe acute asthma the dosage of hydrocortisone is 2 mg/kg intravenously every 4 to 6 hr. Beclomethasone in a dose of 400 μg/day has been shown to be as effective as 7.5 to 15.0 mg prednisone.

Cromolyn Sodium

Chemistry

Cromolyn sodium (*Intal, Aarane*), a bischromone, was developed from a research effort aimed at improving on the bronchodilator activity of the naturally occurring smooth muscle relaxant, khellin, which is a furanochro-

mone derived from the Mediterranean plant *Ammi visnaga* (*Umbelliferae*). Cromolyn sodium is a white, hydrated, hygroscopic powder that is hydrophilic, highly polar, and acidic with a pK_a of 2 (Fig. 45-5).

Mechanism of Action

Controversy persists as to the mechanism of action of cromolyn sodium. Unlike khellin, it does not directly relax smooth muscle. Thus, it does not antagonize the contractile activity of released mediators. However, it does antagonize antigen-induced bronchospasm and was proposed to act by "stabilizing" mast cells, thereby preventing the release of mediators. However, several other compounds exhibit greater potency than cromolyn sodium for "stabilization" of mast cells yet possess no clinical efficacy in asthma. This would suggest that the therapeutic activity of cromolyn sodium in asthma is related to another pharmacological mechanism(s). Postulates include inhibitory effects on irritant receptors, nerves, plasma exudation, and inflammatory cells in general.

Pharmacological Actions

Cromolyn sodium attenuates bronchospasm induced by various stimuli including antigen, exercise, cold dry air, and sulfur dioxide. It also suppresses inflammatory cell influx and chemotactic activity, as well as antigen-induced bronchial hyperreactivity. Cromolyn sodium inhibits the release of mediators from mast cells induced by specific antigen and also nonspecific stimuli, perhaps by inhibiting Ca^{2+} influx across mast cell membranes. Cromolyn sodium has been shown to inhibit C fiber sensory nerve activation in animal models and thus has been proposed to inhibit reflex-induced bronchospasm.

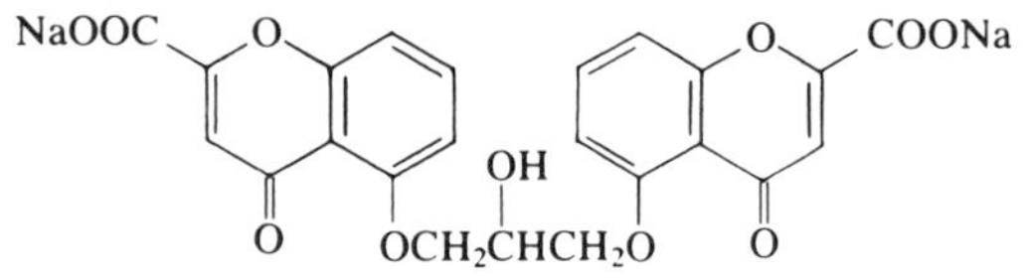

Figure 45-5. Cromolyn sodium.

Absorption, Metabolism, and Excretion

Less than 1 percent of cromolyn sodium is absorbed after oral administration and thus, it is only effective when given via inhalation. The amount of drug absorbed after inhalation depends on the dose and the delivery system. After inhalation peak plasma concentrations of cromolyn sodium are achieved within 15 min. The biological half-life of the compound is 45 to 100 min. A maximum of only 10 percent of cromolyn sodium is absorbed systemically after inhalation. Drug that is absorbed is excreted unchanged in bile and urine in equal proportions.

Clinical Uses

Cromolyn sodium is used almost exclusively for the prophylactic treatment of mild to moderate asthma and should not be used for the control of acute bronchospasm. Cromolyn sodium is effective in about 60 to 70 percent of children and adolescents with asthma. Unfortunately, there is no reliable means to predict which patients will be responsive. It is less effective in older patients and in patients with severe asthma. It may take up to 4 to 6 weeks of treatment for cromolyn sodium to be effective in chronic asthma, but it is effective acutely in exercise-induced asthma.

One of the major advantages of cromolyn sodium is its safety. It appears to be as effective as theophylline in chronic asthma, but it has fewer side effects. In some studies the combination of the two therapies has been shown to be more effective than other agents alone. There is some evidence that treatment with cromolyn sodium will permit a decrease in steroid use in some patients.

Adverse Reactions

Cromolyn sodium is the least toxic of presently available therapies for asthma. Adverse reactions are rare and generally minor. Those occurring in fewer than 1 in 10,000 patients include transient bronchospasm, cough or wheezing, dryness of throat, laryngeal edema, swollen parotid gland, angiodema, joint swelling and pain, dizziness, dysuria, nausea, headache, nasal congestion, rash, and urticaria. A few cases of anaphylaxis, gastroenteritis, myositis, and granulomas in the lung in addition to very severe bronchospasm have been reported.

Contraindications and Cautions

Cromolyn sodium is contraindicated in patients who exhibit hypersensitivity to the drug or other components in the administration devices. In view of the excretion of cromolyn sodium in bile and urine, caution should be observed in patients with renal or hepatic dysfunction.

Preparations and Dosages

Cromolyn sodium is available as a metered-dose inhaler (recommended dosage is two inhalations of 800 μg four times a day), dry powder inhaler (*Spinhaler,* drug encapsulated with lactose; one capsule of 20 mg four times a day), and nebulized solution (one ampule of 10 mg/ml four times a day).

Nedocromil Sodium

Nedocromil sodium (*Tilade*) is a newer drug, which shares many of the chemical and biological properties of cromolyn sodium. It is structurally similar to cromolyn and inhibits activation and mediator release from a variety of inflammatory cells, including mast cells, eosinophils, neutrophils, and macrophages. Like cromolyn sodium, it has been proposed that a component of its therapeutic activity in asthma is due to inhibition of neural reflexes. Although it has not been comprehensively studied, the information to date would suggest that from an efficacy standpoint nedocromil sodium will offer little advantage over cromolyn sodium.

Like cromolyn sodium, nedocromil sodium is recommended for prophylactic use in chronic asthma and not for relief from acute attacks. The recommended dosage is 4 mg twice a day, in contrast to cromolyn sodium, which must be taken four times a day. The frequency of administration of nedocromil sodium can be increased to four times a day if required. The bioavailability of nedocromil sodium after inhalation is less than 10 percent, with 2.5 percent due to absorption from the gastrointestinal tract. Nedocromil sodium is not metabolized and is well tolerated. The side effects are usually minor and transient, with the most common ones being distinctive taste, headache, nausea, vomiting, and dizziness.

Steroid-Sparing Drugs

Several studies using experimental drugs have demonstrated their ability to decrease the use of systemic steroids in corticosteroid-dependent asthmatics. The compounds shown to be effective include parenteral gold salts, used as antiinflammatory drugs for rheumatic diseases; troleandomycin (*Tao*), a macrolide antibiotic; and methotrexate, the immunosuppressant used in cancer chemotherapy. Each of these drugs produces significant side effects. These include chemical hepatitis and steroid-enhancing effects (troleandomycin), as well as nausea, vomiting, abdominal pain, and hematologic, hepatic, teratogenic, and pulmonary effects (methotrexate). Consequently, these agents should only be considered in patients with severe asthma in which systemically administered corticosteroids are producing unacceptable side effects.

Supplemental Reading

Barnes, P.J. Biochemistry of asthma. *Trends Biochem. Sci.* 16:365, 1991.

Barnes, P.J., and Fan Chung, K. Questions about inhaled β_2-adrenoceptor agonists in asthma. *Trends Pharmacol. Sci.* 13:20, 1992.

Barnes, P.J., Fan Chung, K., and Page, C.P. Inflammatory mediators and asthma. *Pharmacol. Rev.* 40:49, 1988.

Check, W.A., and Kaliner, M.A. Pharmacology and pharmacokinetics of topical corticosteroid derivatives used for asthma therapy. *Am. Rev. Respir. Dis.* 141:S44, 1990.

Cochrane, G.M. Bronchodilator treatment. *Practitioner* 230:555, 1986.

Djukanovic, R., et al. Mucosal inflammation in asthma. *Am. Rev. Respir. Dis.* 142:434, 1990.

Doods, H.N. Selective muscarinic antagonists as bronchodilators. *Drug News Perspec.* 5:345, 1992.

Holgate, S.T. Inflammatory cells and their mediators in the pathogenesis of asthma. *Postgrad. Med. J.* 64 (Suppl. 4):89, 1988.

Larsen, G.L. Asthma in children. *N. Engl. J. Med.* 326:1540, 1992.

Murphy, S., and Kelly, H.W. Cromolyn sodium: A review of mechanisms and clinical use in asthma. *Drug Intell. Clin. Pharm.* 21:22, 1987.

National Asthma Education Program. *Guidelines for the Diagnosis and Management of Asthma.* PHS Publication No. 91–3042. Bethesda, Md.: Department of Health and Human Services, 1991.

Persson, C.G.A. Overview of effects of theophylline. *J. Allergy Clin. Immunol.* 78:780, 1986.

Tattersfield, A.E., and Barnes, P.J. β_2-Agonists and corticosteroids: New developments and controversies. *Am. Rev. Respir. Dis.* 146:1637, 1992.

Weinberger, M. Treatment of chronic asthma with theophylline. *ISI Atlas Sci.* 3:53, 1988.

46

Drugs Used in Dermatological Disorders

Mary-Margaret Chren and *David R. Bickers*

Dermatological pharmacotherapy is unique because disease response to therapy by either the topical or systemic routes can be monitored visually. Furthermore, the skin itself serves not only as a route of administration of drugs but also as a drug reservoir and a site of drug metabolism.

Skin Structure

Knowledge of skin structure is important for understanding both dermatological disease and principles of topical application of medications. The skin consists of *epidermis,* a stratified squamous epithelium, overlying *dermis,* which contains connective tissue (Fig. 46-1). The epidermis has multiple layers of *keratinocytes,* which originate in the basal layer along the basement membrane. The most superficial layer of the epidermis, the *stratum corneum,* consists of enucleated keratinocytes full of keratin and an interfilamentous matrix; this layer is primarily responsible for the excellent barrier function of the skin. The differentiation of keratinocytes from the proliferative, undifferentiated cells found along the basement membrane to the highly differentiated, nondividing cells in the stratum corneum is a coordinated process that is regulated by a variety of intrinsic and extrinsic factors. The major protein component of keratinocytes is *α-keratin* (a hydrophilic structural protein). The resulting membrane is an effective barrier to many topically applied agents. The dermis contains blood and lymphatic vessels as well as fibroblasts; the latter cells make intercellular structural proteins such as collagen and elastin.

Percutaneous Absorption

The rate of diffusion of a chemical across the skin is related to, among other features:

Its concentration when applied
The surface area to which it is applied
Its mobility through the epidermis (the *diffusion constant*)
The relative tenacity with which it binds to its vehicle compared to epidermis (the *partition coefficient*)
The thickness of the stratum corneum

The amount of drug absorbed can be enhanced by increasing its applied concentration, increasing the size of the area to which it is applied, decreasing the barrier to its mobility through the layers (generally by hydrating the skin), and increasing its affinity for the skin (usually by increasing its hydrophobic component). Drug absorption is also greater in regions in which the skin is thinner.

Practical Considerations in Topical Drug Therapy

It is important to understand the principles of transmembrane transport as well as the structure of the skin, in designing effective topical drug therapy. One must remain aware of six factors (Table 46-1):

- *Dosage/surface area relationships:* In general, about 2 gm of a topical product is required to cover the head, face, or hand; 3 gm to cover an arm; 4 gm to cover a leg; and 30 to 60 gm to cover the entire body.
- *Hydration of the stratum corneum:* Hydration enhances the drug's solubility in and mobility through the skin (and its absorption) as much as tenfold. Hydration is usually achieved by using an occlusive vehicle or covering the treated skin with impermeable plastic film.
- *Type of vehicle:* In addition to their importance

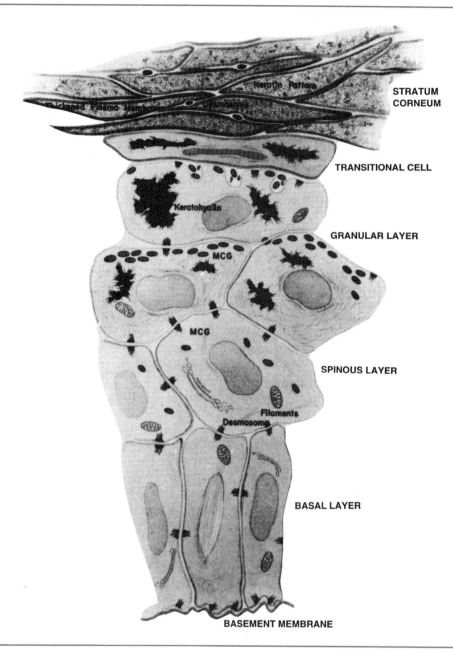

STRATUM
CORNEUM

TRANSITIONAL CELL

GRANULAR LAYER

SPINOUS LAYER

BASAL LAYER

BASEMENT MEMBRANE

Figure 46-1. Schematic diagram showing the layers of the epidermis. (Adapted from W. Montagna and P.F. Parakkal, *The Structure and Function of Skin* [3rd ed.]. New York: Academic, 1974.)

for hydration of the skin, vehicles vary in their partition coefficients (i.e., oil/water solubility ratio) for a given drug with respect to the stratum corneum. For example, a lipophilic drug moves more readily into the epidermis if it is in an aqueous vehicle (to which it is less tightly bound). Also, certain vehicles are more soothing in different types of skin eruptions; dry, chronic inflammation often improves more with drugs administered in lipophilic vehicles, whereas moist acute inflammation is best treated with aqueous preparations. Chemical constituents of vehicles can occasionally cause irritation or allergic sensitization that in turn may enhance penetration of drugs.

- *Variation in penetration at different anatomic sites:* Drug penetration is inversely related to stratum corneum thickness. Thus, permeability (and

Table 46-1. Factors to Consider in Topical Drug Therapy

Feature	Effect	
Dosage/surface relationships	*Treated area*	*Dose (approx)*
	Head, face, or hand	2 gm
	Arm	3 gm
	Leg	4 gm
	Entire body	30–60 gm
Hydration of stratum corneum	Enhances drug's mobility through skin	
Vehicle	Enhances drug's penetration into skin	
	Can function as irritant or allergen	
	Ointments more soothing in drier areas	
Site	Permeability greater where skin is thinner (face, groin)	
Inflammation	Permeability greater if skin is inflamed	
Age of patient	Children have increased risk of systemic toxicity	

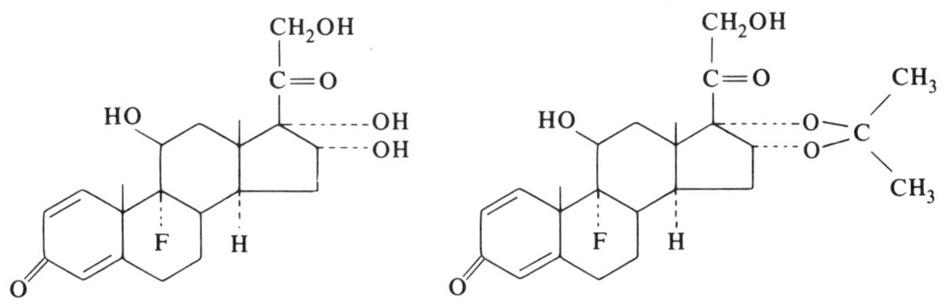

Figure 46-2. Triamcinolone and triamcinolone acetonide.

often toxicity) is greater in thinner areas such as the face or chafed regions.

- *Presence of inflammation:* Permeability to most drugs is greater in inflamed skin.
- *Age:* Systemic toxicity from topically applied drugs is more likely in infants and small children because of their higher surface area to body weight ratio.

Topical Corticosteroids

Corticosteroids have been a mainstay of dermatological therapy since the introduction of hydrocortisone in the 1950s. Since then, structural modifications have yielded a plethora of preparations that vary in potency and cost. The chemical modification most useful for increasing the potency of topically applied corticosteroids is enhance-

ment of their lipid solubility, which increases their movement from the vehicle into the skin. An example is triamcinolone acetonide, in which an acetonide replaces hydroxyl groups (Fig. 46-2), markedly increasing the drug's antiinflammatory potency.

Like systemic corticosteroids, topical corticosteroids bind to cytoplasmic receptors that transport the drug to the nucleus, where the steroid-receptor complex binds to DNA and alters protein synthesis. Such receptors have been identified in both epidermis and dermis. The drugs have myriad pharmacological effects, especially antiinflammatory (hence their usefulness in eczematous dermatitis) and catabolic (hence the toxicity of dermal atrophy). Given the complex pathophysiology of many steroid-responsive skin diseases such as psoriasis, however, the exact mechanism of drug action is unclear.

Topical corticosteroids are most useful in inflammatory dermatoses such as eczematous dermatitis and psoriasis; they may also be helpful in other skin diseases that have a prominent inflammatory component, such as autoimmune diseases (e.g., bullous pemphigoid and pemphigus vulgaris) and lupus erythematosus.

Factors that predispose to both systemic and local toxicity are the use of high-potency preparations (or even lower-potency drugs in children), application of the drug to larger areas, presence of inflamed areas, drug use for prolonged periods of time, and the use of occlusive dressings. Systemic toxicity from topical corticosteroids does occur, particularly from the more potent agents (Table 46-2). While Cushing's syndrome has been reported, it is rare. Milder suppression of the hypothalamic-pituitary-adrenal axis is more common, although the patient is usually asymptomatic and signs of suppression only can be detected through the use of clinical laboratory tests.

Local toxicity is relatively frequent and may not be reversible. Dermal atrophy, appearing as striae and telangiectasias, is especially likely in intertriginous (chafed) areas, where occlusion occurs naturally and the skin is often thinner. So-called "steroid purpura" is also related to the catabolic drug effects. Glaucoma and cataracts have been reported following chronic application around the eye. Less commonly, steroid-induced acneiform eruptions, rosacea, and perioral dermatitis can occur. Finally, the normal inflammatory response to local infections may be masked by corticosteroids, complicating diagnosis and therapy.

Hundreds of topical corticosteroid preparations are now available; therapeutic differences among them are often not obvious. Furthermore, many compounds are available in both proprietary and generic forms, and their bioequivalence has proved difficult to document. Nonetheless, the Food and Drug Administration (FDA) presently uses the vasoconstrictor assay to compare potencies, and these drugs can be classified into seven categories. (See Table 46-3 for the classification of a selected number of preparations.)

Frequent application of topical corticosteroids may not be necessary given the fact that the skin can function as a reservoir of drug. Tachyphylaxis to certain preparations is well recognized but poorly understood; change to an al-

ternate drug may be necessary. Also, discontinuation of therapy in many dermatoses is best accomplished by tapering to less potent preparations, since many skin diseases flare if therapy is stopped abruptly.

Finally, the vehicle in which the drug is compounded is important not only for its effects on penetration noted above but also for patient compliance. For example, eruptions on the scalp are best treated with nongreasy solutions, whereas ointments are most soothing in areas such as the palms and soles.

Table 46-3. Selected Topical Corticosteroid Preparations

Potency class*	Drug
1	Betamethasone dipropionate cream, ointment 0.05%
	Clobetasol propionate cream, ointment 0.05%
	Diflorasone diacetate 0.05%
2	Amcinonide ointment 0.1%
	Desoximetasone cream or ointment 0.25%, gel 0.05%
	Fluocinonide cream, ointment, gel 0.05%
	Halcinonide cream 0.1%
3	Betamethasone valerate ointment 0.1%
	Diflorasone diacetate cream 0.05%
	Triamcinolone acetonide ointment 0.1%, cream 0.5%
4	Amcinonide cream 0.1%
	Desoximetasone cream 0.05%
	Fluocinolone acetonide cream 0.2%
	Fluocinonide acetonide ointment 0.025%
	Hydrocortisone valerate ointment 0.2%
5	Betamethasone dipropionate lotion 0.05%
	Betamethasone valerate cream, lotion 0.1%
	Fluocinolone acetonide cream 0.025%
	Hydrocortisone valerate cream 0.2%
	Triamcinolone acetonide cream, lotion 0.1%
	Triamcinolone acetonide cream 0.025%
6	Aclometasone dipropionate cream 0.05%
	Desonide cream 0.05%
7	Hydrocortisone 0.5%, 1.0%, 2.5%

*Using the vasoconstrictor bioassay (see text), class 1 is most potent; class 7 is least potent.
Source: Adapted from K. A. Arndt, *Manual of Dermatologic Therapeutics.* Boston: Little, Brown, 1989.

Table 46-2. Toxicities of Topical Corticosteroids

Systemic
Cushing's syndrome
Milder suppression of hypothalamic-pituitary-adrenal axis

Local
Atrophy—including striae, telangiectasias, and purpura
Glaucoma/cataracts
Acne vulgaris
Acne rosacea
Persistence of untreated local infection

Retinoids

Retinoids are a family of both naturally occurring and synthetic analogues of vitamin A. The skin of subjects deficient in vitamin A becomes hyperplastic and keratotic (phrynoderma, or toad skin). The vitamin itself is employed in pharmacological doses in a wide variety of skin diseases, such as acne vulgaris, psoriasis, and the ichthyoses, but its therapeutic index generally precludes signifi-

Table 46-4. Available Synthetic Retinoids

Drug	Trade name	Route of administration	Major indication
Isotretinoin	Accutane	Oral	Acne vulgaris
Etretinate	Tegison	Oral	Psoriasis vulgaris
Tretinoin	Retin-A	Topical	Acne vulgaris

cant clinical benefit in these disorders. Synthetic retinoids, however, are more effective; Table 46-4 describes the three preparations available in the United States.

The usefulness of the retinoids in cutaneous disease is related to their ability to affect epidermal differentiation and keratinization, diminish sebum production, and reduce the induction of neoplasms by ultraviolet radiation (especially in patients with xeroderma pigmentosum, in whom large numbers of such lesions occur on sun-exposed skin). Their most important toxic biological effect is their profound teratogenicity when administered to pregnant women.

Isotretinoin

Isotretinoin is most useful for the treatment of severe nodulocystic acne vulgaris. It is rapidly absorbed orally, with peak blood concentrations occurring 3 hr after ingestion. It is not stored in tissue, and the elimination half-life is 10 to 20 hr both after a single dose or during chronic therapy.

Blockage of sebaceous follicles by keratin, and subsequent cyst formation, is believed to be important in the pathogenesis of acne vulgaris; isotretinoin alters keratinization in the follicular epithelium and also decreases the size of sebaceous glands. Furthermore, its antiinflammatory efficacy may be related to its ability to inhibit arachidonic acid release in macrophages, which is a component in the inflammatory response (see Chap. 42). The drug may also be helpful in other disorders of keratinization, such as the ichthyoses or Darier's disease, but it is not useful for psoriasis. Isotretinoin is helpful in preventing or reducing the frequency of induction of cutaneous malignancies in patients at increased risk, such as those with xeroderma pigmentosum, in whom intrinsic repair of DNA damage is impaired.

The most serious toxicity of isotretinoin is its *teratogenicity,* particularly in the first trimester. Pregnant women should not receive the drug, and women should not conceive for at least one month after its discontinuation. Counseling regarding this toxicity and the importance of avoiding pregnancy while on the drug, written informed consent, and a negative serum pregnancy test should be obtained before isotretinoin is prescribed to a woman of

childbearing age. The drug should be begun only on the second day of the menstrual period.

Other toxicities from isotretinoin are common, including

> *Skin complaints,* including xerosis, conjunctivitis, and cheilitis
> *Headache,* which in some cases may be attributable to pseudotumor cerebri
> *Hypertriglyceridemia* in about a quarter of patients (therapy should be discontinued if triglyceride levels exceed 500 mg/dl because of the risk of pancreatitis)
> *Arthralgias,* including skeletal changes, such as hyperostoses, tendinous calcifications, premature epiphysial closure, and pathological fractures
> *Elevation of liver function tests,* which is reversible

The usual dose of isotretinoin is 1 to 3 mg/kg/day. Doses as low as 0.1 mg/kg/day may be effective but generally induce shorter remissions. The usual course is 15 to 20 weeks; a second course is sometimes necessary. Remissions following therapy may persist for months to years. Isotretinoin (*Accutane*) is marketed as 10-, 20-, and 40-mg soft gelatin capsules.

Etretinate

Etretinate is most useful for the treatment of severe psoriasis that is refractory to other types of treatment. It is absorbed in the small intestine; peak blood concentrations are detectable 2 to 4 hr later. The drug accumulates in fat and liver; the elimination half-life after chronic administration is 80 to 100 days, and the drug is detectable in serum for at least 12 months after its discontinuation. A metabolite of etretinate, acitretin, has a shorter biological half-life and retains antipsoriatic activity, but is not available in the United States.

Etretinate does not significantly suppress sebum production and therefore is of little use in acne vulgaris. On the other hand, it is much more useful in psoriasis than is isotretinoin, perhaps because of its different effects on epidermal differentiation and inflammation. The drug is particularly effective for the pustular and erythrodermic variants of psoriasis; it is less helpful in plaque-type disease. Psoriatic nail changes and arthritis may also respond. Combining the drug with psoralen–ultraviolet A photochemotherapy (Re-PUVA) permits the use of lower doses of both etretinate and ultraviolet radiation. Other conditions in which the drug may be useful include palmoplantar hyperkeratoses and the ichthyoses.

Toxicities from etretinate are similar to those of isotretinoin: teratogenesis, cutaneous irritation and inflammation, hyperlipidemia, abnormal liver function tests, and tendinous and ligamentous calcifications. Given its long elimination half-life, etretinate should not be prescribed for women of childbearing age unless no acceptable alternative is available and the patient is fully informed of the risks.

Therapy with etretinate begins with 0.75 to 1.00 mg/kg/day in divided doses, tapering to 0.5 mg/kg/day as the disease responds. Repeat courses of the drug may be necessary with subsequent flares of the disease; ichthyotic and keratinizing disorders may require chronic therapy.

Tretinoin

Tretinoin is helpful in the therapy of comedogenic and papulopustular acne vulgaris. It is applied topically. Tretinoin, like isotretinoin, alters keratinization in the acroinfundibulum, which probably accounts for its usefulness in comedogenic acne. In addition, it causes a mild exfoliation and hence is sometimes useful in molluscum contagiosum, flat warts, and some ichthyotic disorders. It has been used for actinic keratoses, which are premalignant lesions on sun-exposed skin. The drug reverses some of the histological changes associated with ultraviolet radiation, and it has been used to lessen the clinical signs of "photoaging" (wrinkling and hyperpigmented macules), although the results of preliminary studies of this effect require confirmation, and the safety of its long-term use is unclear.

The major toxic effect of tretinoin is local erythema and irritation of the skin (which often improves with continued therapy) and photosensitivity.

Tretinoin preparations vary from a 0.025% cream (least irritating) to a 0.1% lotion (most irritating). It is usually applied once a day.

β-Carotene

β-Carotene is a naturally occurring retinoid, a dimer of vitamin A, that has been used in patients with erythropoietic protoporphyria. Its usefulness in this disorder may be related to its ability to inhibit free radical formation induced by porphyrins and light. Its major toxicity is yellow-orange discoloration of skin. The usual dose is 90 to 180 mg/day. β-Carotene (*Solatene*) is available as 30-mg capsules.

Photochemotherapy

Radiant energy can be used to treat the skin if it is first absorbed by a *chromophore* or photosensitizing chemical (the light must be in the chromophore's absorption spectrum); this absorption changes or excites the chromophore, which then mediates chemical reactions and their biological effects. Photochemotherapy refers to treatment in which the patient is exposed to light of an appropriate wavelength after the application or ingestion of a photosensitizing drug. The most common photosensitizing drugs used in dermatology are synthetic psoralens (which also occur naturally in many plants such as citrus fruits and celery), a therapy called *PUVA* (psoralen and ultraviolet A therapy).

Psoralen and Ultraviolet A Therapy

When exposed to light of the appropriate wavelength, psoralens form covalent linkages with pyrimidine bases in DNA and also, if oxygen is present, form reactive oxygen species that then may mediate other reactions. Although inhibition of DNA replication may account for much of the beneficial effect of psoralen therapy in psoriasis (in which epidermal hyperproliferation exists), PUVA has other important biological effects. The therapy suppresses contact hypersensitivity and may cause other immunological changes by affecting T lymphocytes and epidermal Langerhans cells. It increases melanin pigmentation in the skin and alters mast cell release, which may explain its usefulness in vitiligo and cutaneous mast cell disease.

Oral psoralens are rapidly absorbed (maximum photosensitivity for the most common preparation, 8-methoxypsoralen, is 1–1.5 hr); although their elimination half-life is 2.2 hr, the skin remains photosensitive for 8 to 12 hr. It is primarily excreted by the kidneys, and it does not accumulate. These drugs are systemically absorbed even if applied topically; after application to the entire body, therapeutic plasma levels can be detected.

PUVA is most useful for the treatment of severe psoriasis; most patients show marked improvement after an average of 20 treatments. Early-stage cutaneous T-cell lymphoma (CTCL) also responds to standard PUVA therapy, and the disease is also being treated with a newer regimen called *extracorporeal photopheresis*. Blood from a patient with CTCL who has taken psoralen is exposed to UVA light and returned to the patient. Lymphocytes are altered or destroyed by the treatment, and theoretically the return of these abnormal cells triggers an immune response directed against certain lymphocyte surface antigens. Although early results suggest that the majority of patients improve with this therapy, long-term results are not available.

Both topical and systemic PUVA are useful in some patients with vitiligo, although repigmentation is rarely complete. Other skin diseases for which PUVA may be helpful include atopic dermatitis, alopecia areata, dyshidrotic eczema, and polymorphous light eruption.

Nausea is the most common acute side effect (3–17%

of patients). Thirty-six to 48 hr after therapy, erythema and blistering can occur, especially if the UVA dose was too high or the patient had not avoided other sources of UVA (such as sunlight). Long-term toxicities include *hyperpigmentation* and the development of discrete dark macules called PUVA lentigines; *cataracts,* which have been demonstrated in animals given suprapharmacological doses; *nonmelanoma skin cancer* (basal cell and squamous cell carcinoma), for which the risk is increased tenfold; and *hepatotoxicity* (rarely).

The most commonly used oral preparation is a solution of 8-methoxypsoralen in soft gelatin capsules; it is usually taken one hour before UVA exposure. A topical lotion of 1% 8-methoxypsoralen is also available. Another psoralen, trioxsalen, is available in tablets and is usually taken 2 to 4 hr before UV exposure.

Coal Tar

Another photosensitizing agent used to treat skin disease is topical coal tar, a mixture of organic compounds produced by the distillation of coal. The active ingredient(s) and mechanism of action are unknown. The agent is active both in the dark and after exposure to ultraviolet radiation; presumably, reactive species in the coal tar bind to crucial cellular macromolecules, especially after photoexcitation. Little is known about the pharmacology of coal tar beyond the fact that it undergoes intraepidermal metabolism and urinary excretion.

Coal tar is a central component of a standard therapy for psoriasis, the *Goeckerman regimen,* which consists of ultraviolet B radiation therapy to psoriatic lesions to which coal tar has previously been applied. The contribution of coal tar to the treatment's effectiveness is controversial, however.

The major acute toxicity of coal tar is an acute phototoxic skin reaction called "tar smarts." Coal tar contains many known carcinogens, such as polyaromatic hydrocarbons, and occupational exposure to coal tar products in industrial workers is clearly associated with an increased incidence of squamous cell carcinoma of the skin. Population-based studies of patients with psoriasis have also demonstrated an increased incidence of skin cancer in patients who have received the Goeckerman regimen.

Coal tar is available in concentrations varying from 0.3 to 48.5% for topical use, primarily as a shampoo.

Photodynamic Therapy and Hematoporphyrins

Porphyrins are potent photosensitizing intermediates in heme synthesis and are thought to accumulate in malignant cells. This feature is used in photodynamic therapy, in which a synthetic porphyrin or porphyrin derivative (*Photofrin* I, or PF-I) is administered, followed by exposure of tissue to visible light. Malignant cells then fluoresce, which is helpful in early diagnosis and in targeting the cells for subsequent treatment. The regimen, while still experimental, may have some value in the therapy of skin cancers, although a limiting toxicity has been that patients remain extremely photosensitive for weeks after treatment because of the long elimination half-life of the drugs.

Dapsone

Although dapsone is most often used as an antibiotic, it has important antiinflammatory properties in many noninfectious skin diseases. Its pharmacology and toxicities are discussed in Chap. 53.

The mechanism of action of dapsone in skin disease is not clear. Most of the cutaneous diseases in which it is effective are characterized by an infiltration of neutrophils; the drug's antiinflammatory effect may be related either to its inhibition of intracellular neutrophil reactions, mediated by myeloperoxidase and hydrogen peroxide, or to its ability to scavenge reactive oxygen species, thus inhibiting inflammation.

Dapsone is approved for the treatment of an autoimmune blistering skin disease, dermatitis herpetiformis. This intensely pruritic eruption, characterized histologically by dense infiltration of the upper dermis and subepidermal vesicles by neutrophils, is usually associated with gluten-sensitive enteropathy (which may not be clinically significant). The response to dapsone in patients with this disease is rapid. Other skin diseases in which dapsone is helpful are linear immunoglobulin A (IgA) dermatosis, subcorneal pustular dermatosis, leukocytoclastic vasculitis, and a variety of rarer eruptions in which neutrophils predominate, including some forms of cutaneous lupus erythematosus.

Dapsone (*Alvosulfon*) is available as 25- and 50-mg tablets. The usual starting dose is 50 mg orally once a day, with gradual increase in dose (with close hematological monitoring) to 100 to 200 mg/day. Response occurs in about a week, and lower maintenance doses may be possible (especially in dermatitis herpetiformis, in which a gluten-free diet may also be therapeutic).

Antimalarial Drugs

Like dapsone, the antimalarial drugs chloroquine, hydroxychloroquine, and quinacrine are useful in some noninfectious skin diseases, although the mechanism of their therapeutic effect is unknown. Their pharmacology is discussed in Chap. 57.

Antimalarial drugs have myriad effects on cellular physiology, including an ability to impair or alter lysosomal phagosomal activity, inhibit iodination in and locomotion of neutrophils, and diminish macrophage and T-cell responsiveness in vitro. Chloroquine and hydroxychloroquine also form complexes with hepatic porphyrins, enhancing their urinary excretion. Both drugs also have an affinity for melanin, which may at least partially explain their ophthalmological toxicities.

Hydroxychloroquine is helpful for the treatment of both rheumatological and cutaneous lupus erythematosus; a majority of patients with chronic cutaneous (discoid) disease will respond. Both chloroquine and quinacrine are also effective in this skin disease. Low-dose chloroquine is used for therapy of porphyria cutanea tarda in patients in whom phlebotomy has failed or is contraindicated. Other skin diseases in which the drugs are useful (after sunscreens and avoidance of sun exposure) include polymorphous light eruption and solar urticaria.

The duration of treatment for skin disease is longer than for antimalarial therapy, and therefore dose-related toxicities are important to remember. (The toxicities of these drugs when used as antimalarial agents are discussed in Chap. 57.) The most serious toxicity of these drugs is ophthalmological. Reversible changes include ciliary body dysfunction and corneal changes with edema and deposits. Irreversible retinopathy also occurs but is much less common with quinacrine than with the other two drugs. Toxicity appears to involve actual drug deposition in the retina, and the earliest symptoms are night blindness, scotomas, or tunnel vision. Retinal examination reveals mottling of pigment at the macula, leading eventually to rings around the macula ("bull's eye"). The exact incidence of retinopathy is unclear, as is whether the toxicity appears to be daily dose–related or total dose (and duration of therapy)–related. Nonetheless, baseline and twice-yearly ophthalmological examinations should be performed, and the minimum effective dose of the drug should be employed.

In patients with porphyria cutanea tarda treated with chloroquine, a "chloroquine reaction" may occur—fever, nausea, abdominal pain, abnormal hepatocellular function, and massive uroporphyrinuria as a result of drug-porphyrin complex formation. Accordingly, low-dose regimens (twice weekly) are recommended for this disease.

Hydroxychloroquine is approximately twice as potent as chloroquine and four times as potent as quinacrine.

Systemic Antibiotics

Antibiotics are used in dermatology for both infectious and noninfectious skin eruptions. For infections of the skin such as impetigo or folliculitis, systemic antibiotics have been preferred because of concern that topical preparations do not penetrate skin sufficiently to eradicate infection. This preference may change, however, with the advent of more potent, proven topical preparations such as mupirocin (see below). Because most skin infections in the community are caused by *Streptococcus pyogenes* or *Staphylococcus aureus,* penicillin, erythromycin, or cephalosporins have been the drugs of choice.

Noninfectious skin eruptions such as acne vulgaris and acne rosacea are often treated with systemic antibiotics. The mechanism of action is not clear. Tetracycline is known to inhibit lipases derived from resident flora in the sebaceous follicle (*Streptococcus epidermidis, Propionibacterium acnes*). These lipases cleave irritating fatty acids from triglycerides in sebum, presumably contributing to inflammation in acne vulgaris.

The pharmacology and toxicities of the systemic antibiotics are discussed in Part VII. In general, the chronic therapy used in dermatology is tolerated well. Minocycline can cause slate-gray hyperpigmentation of the skin and teeth. Concern has also been raised about the theoretical risk of an interaction between oral contraceptives and long-term oral antibiotics; despite suggestive animal data, there is little experimental evidence to verify this interaction in humans.

Topical Antibiotics

Topical antibiotics are helpful in acne vulgaris, acne rosacea, and probably in reducing the frequency of infections related to intravenous catheters. One drug, mupirocin, applied as a 2% ointment, is the only topical antibiotic proved effective for impetigo contagiosa in controlled studies. Mupirocin is produced by *Pseudomonas fluorescens;* it binds to bacterial isoleucyl–transfer RNA synthetase and prevents the incorporation of isoleucine into protein sequences. It is most effective against gram-positive bacteria. Toxicity is uncommon.

Other selected topical antibiotics are described in Table 46-5.

Drugs for Cutaneous Fungal Infections

Two types of fungi infect the skin: dermatophytes (which digest keratin) and yeasts (most commonly *Candida* species). Antifungal agents are active against either one or both of these categories, and the choice of drug is guided by which category of organism is most likely to be causing the infection. Improvement in cutaneous fungal disease necessitates that therapy be continued until new,

Table 46-5. Selected Topical Antibiotics

Drug	Major use	Toxicity	Forms
Clindamycin	Acne vulgaris	Pseudomembranous colitis (rare)	1% solution, gel
Erythromycin	Acne vulgaris	Uncommon	1.5–2% solution, ointment, gel
Metronidazole	Acne rosacea	Uncommon	0.75% gel
Bacitracin	Superficial infection (gram-positive bacteria)	Uncommon	Single and combination preparations
Polymixin B	Superficial infection (gram-negative bacteria)	Uncommon	Combination preparations
Neomycin	Superficial infection (mainly gram-negative bacteria)	Allergic contact dermatitis	Single and combination preparations

Table 46-6. Selected Older Topical Agents for Cutaneous Fungal Disease

Drug	Active agent	Action	Use	Adverse effect
Selenium sulfide 2.5%	Same	Antibacterial, antifungal	Tinea versicolor	Uncommon
Hydroxyquinolines (iodoquinol, cloquinol)	Same	Antifungal, antibacterial	Dermatophyte infections, intertrigo	Yellow staining of skin, clothes
Castellani's paint	Basic fuchsin, phenol, resorcinol, acetone, alcohol	Fungicidal, bactericidal, mildly anesthetic	Moist, macerated areas	Red discoloration
Whitfield's ointment	Benzoic acid, salicylic acid	Fungistatic, keratolytic	Palms, soles	Irritation, salicylism (rare)
Gentian violet	Hexamethyl-pararosaniline	Against yeast	Mucosal infections	Purple discoloration

noninfected tissue is generated. For infections on non-hairy skin, the course is usually a minimum of 4 weeks; for hair infections, 4 to 6 weeks; and for nail infections (which usually begin in the nail matrix), 6 to 12 months for fingernails and 12 to 24 months for toenails. Except for toenail disease, in which up to a third of infections are unresponsive, most fungal infections of skin respond to therapy. Reinfection, however, is common, suggesting as yet undefined susceptibility factors.

Like bacterial infections of skin, cutaneous fungal infections are treated with either topical or systemic agents. The pharmacology and use of these agents are described in Chap. 59. In general, scalp and nail disease respond poorly to topical therapy alone. Table 46-6 describes selected older topical agents, many of which enhance sloughing of infected tissue in addition to inhibiting fungal growth. They are being prescribed less frequently since the development of newer topical agents.

Griseofulvin is active against the dermatophytes but not yeasts such as *Candida;* it remains the most useful drug for scalp and nail dermatophyte infections. It is generally well tolerated, even in the long-term courses necessary for nail disease.

Ketoconazole is active against both dermatophytes and yeasts such as *Candida.* It is helpful for treating fungal infections (especially of the nails) that are unresponsive to griseofulvin, or in patients who are unable to tolerate that drug. The long-term therapy that may be necessary, however, necessitates careful consideration of the risks (primarily hepatic) and the expense of the drug.

Fluconazole may be better absorbed and possibly less hepatotoxic than is ketoconazole, but it is considerably more expensive, an important consideration given the required length of therapy for most cutaneous fungal diseases.

Itraconazole is used for cutaneous deep fungal infections, but its usefulness in superficial mycosis is not yet established. It is intermediate in cost between ketoconazole and fluconazole.

Potassium iodide is used to treat the cutaneous lymphatic form of sporotrichosis, although newer agents are also effective in this disorder and may be better tolerated. It is also used in erythema nodosum and nodular vasculitis.

Terbinafine is a topically and orally administered allyl-amine that is currently available only for investigational use in the United States. It is highly concentrated in keratinous tissue, and is unique in that it is fungicidal. Its usefulness compared to drugs currently available is not established.

Drugs for Cutaneous Viral Infections

The specific antiviral agents used to treat cutaneous infections caused by herpes simplex and varicella-zoster viruses are discussed in Chap. 54.

Intralesional **interferons** α-2b and α-n3 have been shown to be effective for *condyloma acuminata* (genital warts). Interferons have both intrinsic antiviral effects and antiproliferative and immunomodulatory actions. Toxicities include flu-like symptoms, depression of the white blood cell count, mild diminution in hematocrit, and mild transient elevations of liver function tests.

Podophyllotoxin (*Podofilox*) is available alone (as a 0.5% solution) and as the main cytotoxic ingredient in *podophyllin* (25% podophyllum resin), a mixture of toxic chemicals derived from May apple plants. Both are used to treat genital warts; Podofilox is used by the patient, and podophyllin is administered by the physician. The mechanism of action is cytotoxic; the drug binds to microtubules in metaphase and prevents development of the mitotic spindle. Podofilox 0.5% is applied by the patient to the warts twice a day for 3 days, followed by a 4-day drug-free period; this cycle can be repeated up to four times. Podophyllin is applied by the physician every 7 to 10 days. The most common toxic effect is skin ulceration. Systemic absorption of podophyllin can occur (especially if applied to large, inflamed areas or mucosal surfaces), with subsequent gastrointestinal, hematological, renal, and hepatotoxic effects. In addition, seizures and peripheral neuropathy have been reported.

Cantharidin is a caustic chemical that causes intraepidermal vesiculation, which theoretically does not leave a residual scar on healing, although a pronounced inflammatory response after treatment can scar. It is available alone and in combination with podophyllin and salicylic acid.

Drugs for Scabies and Lice

Pyrethrins are naturally occurring pesticides derived from chrysanthemum plants. They are active against many insects and mites. Over-the-counter liquid and gel preparations of pyrethrins that also contain piperonyl butoxide are available for the treatment of pediculosis; piperonyl butoxide inhibits the hydrolytic enzymes that metabolize the pyrethrins in the arthropod. A synthetic pyrethroid, permethrin, is available in a 5% preparation by prescription and is probably superior to lindane for scabies. Toxicity from the pyrethrins and permethrin is uncommon.

Lindane is an effective pesticide most often used for scabies. Available as a cream, lotion, or shampoo, it is applied to the entire body from the neck down and washed off in 8 to 12 hr. Up to 10 percent of an applied dose is absorbed; alternative therapies such as permethrin are recommended in children and pregnant women due to the potential of lindane to cause central nervous system (CNS) toxicity following its topical absorption. The drug is also useful for pediculosis therapy, although it is probably not as effective as the pyrethrins.

Cytotoxic and Immunosuppressive Agents

Cytotoxic and immunosuppressive agents, which inhibit the synthesis or action of crucial cellular macromolecules such as nucleic acids, are used in three broad categories of skin disease: hyperproliferative disorders such as psoriasis, immunological disorders such as autoimmune bullous diseases, and skin neoplasias. The pharmacology of these drugs is discussed in Chap. 63; this section focuses on unique features of their use in skin disease, which are summarized in Table 46-7.

Methotrexate is approved for use in severe disabling psoriasis that is recalcitrant to other less toxic treatments;

Table 46-7. Selected Cytotoxic and Immunosuppressive Agents Used for Skin Disease

Drug	Major use	Special features
Oral use		
Methotrexate	Psoriasis	Cirrhosis, pancytopenia
Azathioprine	Autoimmune blistering diseases	"Steroid-sparing"*
Cyclophosphamide	Autoimmune blistering diseases, advanced CTCL	"Steroid-sparing"*
Cyclosporine	Psoriasis	
Colchicine	Leukocytoclastic vasculitis	Neutrophil inhibition
Topical use		
5-Fluorouracil	Actinic keratoses	
Nitrogen mustard	Early CTCL	
Intralesional use		
Vinblastine	Kaposi's sarcoma	
Bleomycin	Verruca vulgaris	Sclerodermoid skin changes

Key: CTCL = cutaneous T-cell lymphoma.
*Patients receiving these drugs often require lower doses of systemic corticosteroids to control their disease.

about 60 to 75 percent of patients will achieve 75 percent clearing of disease. The standard regimen is similar to low-dose therapy used for the treatment of rheumatoid arthritis (see Chap. 43): either a weekly single dose or three divided doses over a 36-hr period weekly. The usual dose is 7.5 to 30.0 mg/week. Although toxicities are similar to those described in the treatment of other diseases, hepatic cirrhosis and unexpected pancytopenia are of special concern given the long-term use of methotrexate in psoriasis. Cirrhosis, which appears to be related to the total cumulative dose, is probably not detectable by noninvasive tests, and liver biopsy is recommended either before or early in the treatment course and after cumulative methotrexate doses of 1.0 to 1.5 gm. Pancytopenia with low-dose methotrexate is probably multifactorial in etiology; monthly hematological monitoring is recommended.

Azathioprine is used in autoimmune blistering diseases such as bullous pemphigoid, either alone or in combination with corticosteroids.

Cyclophosphamide is approved for the treatment of advanced CTCL and is also used as a steroid-sparing agent for many immune system–mediated diseases, such as systemic lupus erythematosus and the autoimmune blistering diseases.

Cyclosporine is a potent immunosuppressive drug that has been used orally with some success in resistant psoriasis. There are other reports of its value in treating alopecia areata, pyoderma gangrenosum, and atopic dermatitis.

Colchicine, like the vinca alkaloids, podophyllin, and griseofulvin, arrests cellular mitosis in metaphase. In dermatology, it is used primarily for its inhibitory effects on neutrophil chemotaxis or action (for example, in leukocytoclastic vasculitis).

5-Fluorouracil, administered topically, is used for the treatment of actinic keratoses, which are premalignant lesions on sun-exposed skin. It is available in concentrations varying from 1 to 5%; the 5% strength is also approved for the treatment of superficial basal cell carcinomas if conventional therapies are impractical. The drug is usually applied once or twice a day; a brisk inflammatory reaction ensues. Therapy is continued until erosions develop (usually 2–6 weeks). The inflammation is aggravated by exposure to ultraviolet light. The major toxicities are local, with inflammation and postinflammatory changes.

Mechlorethamine is most often used in dermatology for the treatment of early CTCL; it is a potent contact sensitizer, an action that may contribute to the etiology of its effectiveness. The drug is dissolved in water or petrolatum at concentrations of 10 to 20 mg% and immediately applied to affected and unaffected skin for 8 to 12 hr. In addition to local inflammation, the drug is associated with an increased incidence of skin cancer.

Vincristine and vinblastine (both vinca alkaloids) are used intralesionally for localized Kaposi's sarcoma. Vinblastine is also approved for the treatment of advanced stages of CTCL.

Although not approved for dermatologic use except for palliative treatment of squamous cell carcinoma, bleomycin is also used intralesionally for resistant verruca vulgaris. Because skin and lung lack the inactivation enzyme bleomycin hydrolase, the drug is especially toxic to these tissues, and ulceration, atrophy, and sclerodermoid changes can occur.

Miscellaneous Topical Agents

Anthralin is a potent reducing agent whose mechanism of action is unknown. It is approved for the treatment of psoriasis and may also be helpful in alopecia areata. The major toxicities are discoloration of skin, hair, and nails, and irritant dermatitis. It is available as an ointment in concentrations from 0.1 to 1%.

Minoxidil is used for the treatment of androgenic alopecia of the scalp in both men and women. The drug appears to have a direct effect on the hair follicles. Response rates are low, however, and moderate or dense regrowth develops in only a minority of patients. It is available as a 2% solution, applied twice a day. Toxicity is uncommon.

Pramoxine is a local anesthetic used topically for pruritus. Adverse effects are uncommon. It is available in a variety of vehicles at 1% concentration, applied three to four times a day.

Capsaicin is a topical agent approved for the relief of pain following herpes-zoster infections (postherpetic neuralgia). The drug depletes neurons of substance P, an endogenous neuropeptide that may mediate cutaneous pain. It is available as a 0.025% cream applied to affected skin after open lesions have healed; local irritation may occur.

Masoprocol is newly approved for the topical treatment of actinic keratoses. The etiology of its action is unclear, but the drug is a potent 5-lipoxygenase inhibitor and has both antiinitiating and antipromoting activity in vitro. The major toxicity is allergic contact dermatitis. It is available as 10% cream and is applied to affected areas for 28 days.

Benzoyl peroxide is a potent oxidizing agent that has both antimicrobial and comedolytic properties; its primary use is in the therapy of acne vulgaris. It is converted in the skin to benzoic acid. Clearance of absorbed drug is rapid, and no systemic toxicity has been observed. The major toxicity is irritation and contact allergy in 10 percent of patients.

Salicylic acid is keratolytic and thus is effective in softening hyperkeratotic areas in psoriasis and warts.

Sunscreens

Sunscreens absorb ultraviolet radiation before it can be absorbed in the skin. They are recommended to protect the skin from the major toxicities of sun exposure: sunburn and skin cancer. Most available agents primarily absorb UVB, although newer preparations probably also give some protection against UVA. Sunblocks (which are generally opaque, like zinc oxide) block all ultraviolet radiation.

The frequency of application of sunscreen is guided by the sun protection factor (SPF) of the preparation. This derived value is the ratio of the time of ultraviolet exposure that causes erythema with the sunscreen to the time that causes erythema without the sunscreen. The higher the SPF, the less frequent the application of sunscreen. SPFs of available preparations vary from 2 to 50.

Supplemental Reading

Arndt, K.A. *Manual of Dermatologic Therapeutics.* Boston: Little, Brown, 1989.

Bickers, D.R., Hazen, P.G., and Lynch, W.S. *Clinical Pharmacology of Skin Disease.* New York: Churchill Livingstone, 1984.

Chren, M.M., and Bickers, D.R. Dermatological Pharmacology. In *Goodman and Gilman's The Pharmacological Basis of Therapeutics.* New York: Pergamon, 1990.

Elewski, B.E. (ed.). *Cutaneous Fungal Infections.* New York: Igaku-Shoin, 1992.

Harber, L.C., and Bickers, D.R. *Photosensitivity Diseases. Principles of Diagnosis and Treatment.* Toronto: B.C. Decker, 1989.

Mukhtar, H. (ed.). *Pharmacology of the Skin.* Boca Raton, Fla.: CRC, 1991.

Wolverton, S.E., and Wilkin, J.K. (eds.). *Systemic Drugs for Skin Diseases.* Philadelphia: Saunders, 1991.

VI

Chemotherapy

47

Introduction to Chemotherapy

Irvin S. Snyder and *Roger G. Finch*

Antimicrobial agents fall into two general classes: (1) synthetic chemicals, such as the sulfonamides, isonicotinic acid hydrazide, and the quinolones; and (2) antibiotics, such as penicillin, tetracycline, and chloramphenicol. *Antibiotics* are those compounds produced by microorganisms that, at high dilutions, are inhibitory to other microorganisms. Two groups of microorganisms, the bacteria and fungi, produce antibiotics, although many are now produced semisynthetically by chemical modifications of the naturally occurring compound. Some antibiotics, such as chloramphenicol, are now completely synthesized.

This ability to chemically modify compounds produced by bacteria and fungi has led to congeners with greater stability, improved pharmacokinetic properties, and an extended spectrum of antimicrobial activity. Table 47-1 is a compilation of antibiotics showing the susceptibility of microorganisms to commonly used natural and synthetic antimicrobial agents.

A large number of synthetic and natural chemicals inhibit growth of microbes in vitro, but few are useful as chemotherapeutic agents. To be useful in chemotherapy, the chemical should inhibit microbial growth in vivo and be harmless to the host. Thus, the ideal chemotherapeutic agent is *selectively* toxic. However, a number of antimicrobial agents capable of producing toxic effects in humans are used as chemotherapeutic agents because they have a favorable therapeutic index.

Antibiotics are often referred to as either *narrow-, broad-,* or *extended-spectrum* agents. Penicillin G is primarily active against gram-positive bacteria and is classified as a narrow-spectrum antibiotic. Tetracycline and chloramphenicol are examples of broad-spectrum antibiotics; that is, they are active against both gram-positive and gram-negative bacteria. Modification of the parent compound can extend the range of a narrow-spectrum antibiotic and is evident if one compares amoxicillin and ampicillin,

both congeners of penicillin G, to penicillin G (see Table 47-1).

Mode of Action: Static and Cidal Effects

Antimicrobial agents are frequently classified according to their effect on the microbe as either *static* (inhibitory) or *cidal* (lethal) agents. Antimicrobials affect microbial cells by interfering with one or more of the following processes: (1) protein synthesis, (2) maintenance of cell membrane integrity, (3) cell wall synthesis, (4) nucleic acid structure and function, or (5) production of folic acid (or some other key metabolite). Interference with some processes inhibits growth and replication, whereas inhibition of others results in bacterial cell death (Table 47-2).

The ability of an antimicrobial agent to chemically alter the organism's cell wall or membrane can result in cell death and a *cidal effect* on the microbe. Cell lysis may ensue because of the bacteria's high internal osmotic pressure or its destruction by autolytic enzymes. Similarly, drug-induced effects on replication and transcription of DNA can cause death of the bacterial cell. *Bacteriostatic effects* are obtained when antimicrobial therapy results in *reversible* changes in the microorganism. For example, inhibition of folic acid synthesis by the sulfonamides can be reversed by removal of the drug, by increasing the synthesis of the affected enzymes, or by providing the metabolic intermediates that occur at a point beyond the inhibited step.

In reality, bactericidal or bacteriostatic activity is determined not only by the mode of action of the compound but also by its concentration since low concentrations of an antimicrobial may be bacteriostatic and higher concentrations bactericidal.

Table 47-1. Sensitivity of Selected Bacteria to Common Antibacterial Agents

Agent	Staphylococcus aureus (penicillin-sensitive)	Staphylococcus aureus (penicillin-resistant)	Streptococcus pyogenes and Strep. pneumoniae	Enterococcus	Clostridium perfringens	Neisseria gonorrhoeae	Neisseria meningitidis	Haemophilus influenzae	Escherichia coli	Klebsiella
Pencillin V, G	+	R	+	R	+	+*	+	±	R	R
Methicillin, oxacillin, cloxacillin, dicloxacillin, nafcillin	+	+*	+	R	(+)	(±)	(±)	R	R	R
Ampicillin, amoxicillin	+	R	+	+	+	+	+	±	±	R
Carbenicillin, ticarcillin	(+)	R	(+)	R	+	(+)	(+)	(+)	±	±
Cefazolin	+	+*	+	R	(±)	(+)	(+)	±	+	±
Erythromycin	+	+	+	R	±	+	(+)	±	R	R
Clindamycin	+	+	+	R	+*	R	R	R	R	R*
Tetracyclines	+	+*	±	R	+	+	(+)	+	+	±
Chloramphenicol	+	+	+	+	+	+	+	+	+	±
Gentamicin, tobramycin, amikacin	+	+	R	R	R	R	R	+	+*	+
Sulfonamides	+	+	+	±	±	+	+	+	±	±
Trimethoprim-sulfamethoxazole	+	+	+	+	R	+	+	+	+	+
Ciprofloxacin	+	+	+	±	R	+	+	+	+	+

Key: + = sensitive; R = resistant; ± = some strains resistant; ( ) = not appropriate therapy; * = rare strains resistant.

Drug Combinations

The mode of action of a particular antimicrobial agent is important clinically where use of more than one agent is necessary. Combining antimicrobial agents with differing sites of action may result in inhibition (*antagonism*), enhancement (*synergy*), or no alteration (indifference) of antimicrobial activity. For example, the tetracyclines inhibit protein synthesis and are bacteriostatic. Penicillin affects cell wall synthesis and requires that bacteria be actively multiplying in order to be bactericidal. When penicillin and tetracycline are combined, the production of the enzymes needed for cell synthesis and growth is inhibited by tetracycline, so the bactericidal effect of penicillin is not expressed.

Synergism, or the enhancement of the action of one drug by another, can be demonstrated by the use of trimethoprim in combination with the sulfonamide sulfamethoxazole. Both these antimicrobials inhibit production of folic acid by acting sequentially in the folic acid biosynthetic pathway, thereby producing synergistic inhibition of bacterial growth. Another example of synergy is the combined use of penicillin and an aminoglycosidic aminocyclitol antibiotic (such as gentamicin) on the enterococcus. In this example, inhibition of cell wall synthesis by penicillin permits better penetration of the cell wall by the aminocyclitol and more effective inhibition of protein synthesis.

Antibiotics may interact with other drugs to modify their metabolism or excretion, thereby enhancing their toxicity. For example, chloramphenicol is known to impair the metabolism of anticoagulants and anticonvulsants. Ototoxicity, an adverse reaction common to the aminoglycosidic aminocyclitols, can be potentiated by the coadministration of diuretics, such as furosemide and ethacrynic acid.

Combining drugs in vitro may alter the physicochemical state of an agent and modify its antimicrobial activity. For example, inactivation or drug precipitation occurs if solutions of carbenicillin and gentamicin are mixed. Also, drugs such as heparin and hydrocortisone may be incompatible in solution with antibiotics. The pH stability of the drug in solution also must be considered. Benzylpenicillin is stable for 12 hr at a pH of 5.5 to 6.5, but unstable below pH 5.5 or above pH 7.5.

Proteus spp. (indole-negative)	Proteus spp. (indole-positive)	Serratia	Salmonella	Shigella	Pseudonomas	Bacteroides fragilis	Other Bacteroides spp.	Chlamydia	Mycoplasma pneumoniae	Rickettsia
R	R	R	R	R	R	R	+	R	R	R
R	R	R	R	R	R	R	(±)	R	R	R
+	R	R	+	±	R	R	+	R	R	R
+	±	±	(+)	(+)	+*	±	±	R	R	R
+	R	R	(+)	(+)	R	R	±	R	R	R
R	R	R	R	R	R	+	+	+	+	R
R	R	R	R	R	R	+	+	R	R	R
±	R	R	(+)	(±)	R	±	±	+	+	+
+	±	+	+	+	R	+	+	+	+	+
+	+	+*	(+)	(+)	+*	R	R	R	R	R
+	±	R	±	+	R	R	R	+	R	R
+	+	R	+	+	R	R	R	+	R	R
+	+	+	+	+	+	R	R	±	R	R

Pharmacological Principles

To be useful in vivo, an antimicrobial should penetrate body tissues and be maintained in concentrations sufficient to inhibit microbial growth. Obtaining an adequate drug concentration in tissue is dependent on factors including the rate and degree of drug absorption from the gut or site of injection, the drug concentration in blood, molecular size, ionic charge, rate of metabolism and excretion (half-life), lipid solubility, degree of protein and tissue binding, and the presence or absence of inflammation.

Not all antibiotics can be given orally. Some are destroyed by gastric acidity whereas others, because of poor lipid solubility, are not absorbed from the gastrointestinal tract. However, in treating an infection of the intestinal mucosa, a nonabsorbable antimicrobial may be ideal. Some poorly absorbed agents are given parenterally to achieve rapidly effective serum and tissue levels and are especially useful in treating serious infections.

Tissue penetration depends on factors that determine the passage of any chemical across biological membranes (e.g., diffusion coefficient, lipid solubility, and charge).

Diffusibility is determined by molecular size and pK_a, whereas lipid solubility depends on the degree of ionization and the partition coefficient of the drug and is therefore dependent on local pH. The intracellular pH will, in part, determine whether the drug becomes trapped inside the cell or escapes back into the blood. Once the antimicrobial agent enters the membrane, it crosses from the extracellular to the intracellular side, primarily by diffusion. Compounds such as the aminocyclitols, which are poorly soluble in lipids, are found in highest concentrations in the extracellular fluid. In contrast, drugs such as erythromycin and the quinolones achieve high intracellular concentrations.

Protein binding may be an important factor in determining an antimicrobial agent's clinical efficacy. Tissue distribution is affected by plasma protein binding, since protein-bound drug cannot cross tissue barriers. Protein binding also interferes with glomerular filtration and therefore reduces drug elimination. Although a protein-bound antimicrobial is not biologically active, binding is a dynamic, reversible process. The protein-bound drug serves as a temporary store of the antimicrobial and helps prevent large changes in the concentration of free drug.

Table 47-2. Action of Antibacterial Chemotherapeutic Agents

Mode of action	Specific effect	Static or cidal effect	Drug
Inhibits cell wall synthesis	Prevents cross-linking of linear peptidoglycan strands by inhibiting transpeptidase	Cidal	β-Lactam antibiotic
	Inhibits peptidoglycan synthetase and polymerization of linear peptide	Cidal	Glycopeptide antibiotics
	Inhibits regeneration of lipid carrier by preventing dephosphorylation of lipid pyrophosphate to lipid phosphate	Cidal	Bacitracin
	Prevents formation of uridine diphosphate (UDP) N-acetylmuramyl pentapeptide (by inhibiting D-alanyl-D-alanine synthetase and racemase)	Cidal	Cycloserine
Inhibits protein synthesis or structure	Interferes with initiation complex; causes misreading of messenger RNA (mRNA)	Cidal	Aminoglycosides
	Prevents translocation	Static	Spectinomycin
	Inhibits peptidyl transferase and peptide band formation	Static	Chloramphenicol
	Releases nascent oligopeptidyl transfer RNA (tRNA) and inhibits translocation	Static	Macrolides, lincosamides
	Inhibits binding of aminoacyl tRNA to ribosome	Static	Tetracylines
	Inhibits translation of mRNA specific for inducible enzymes	Static	Nitrofurans
	Alkylates proteins	Cidal	Methenamine
Interferes with cell membrane function	Cationic detergent	Cidal	Polymyxin B, colistin
Interferes with DNA/RNA synthesis	Inhibits DNA-dependent RNA polymerase	Cidal	Rifampin
	Interferes with supercoiling of DNA by action on DNA gyrase	Cidal	Nalidixic acid, other 4-quinolones
Inhibits metabolism	Inhibits lipid synthesis	Cidal or static	Isoniazid Ethambutol
	Prevents synthesis of folic acid	Static	Sulfonamide, sulfones, p-aminosalicylic acid, trimethoprim
	Produces reactive 5-nitro anion, superoxide, and other free radicals	Static	Nitrofurans

(For a further discussion of the factors that affect drug absorption, distribution, metabolism, and excretion, see Chaps. 3, 4, and 5.)

Microbial Factors

Even if adequate drug concentrations can be achieved at the site of infection, failure of drug therapy is still possible unless the antimicrobial agent is delivered to a sensitive site in the bacterial cell at a concentration sufficient to cause a bacteriostatic or bactericidal effect.

Some organisms are naturally resistant to certain antimicrobials. Microorganisms also can become resistant either by mutation, adaptation, or gene transfer. The mechanisms accounting for innate or acquired resistance are essentially the same. Spontaneous mutations in bacterial cells occur at a frequency of about 1 in 10^6 cells and may confer resistance to the antimicrobial agent. The occurrence of spontaneous mutations is not of major concern unless the use of the antimicrobial results in selection and subsequent population of the host with these resistant mutants.

Resistance to an antimicrobial can be the result of one or more mechanisms. Alterations in the lipopolysaccharide structure of gram-negative cells can affect the uptake of lipophilic drugs. Similarly, changes in porins can affect uptake of hydrophilic drugs. Once the drug enters the cell, it may be enzymatically inactivated. Recently, active efflux systems that remove antimicrobials from the bacterial cell have been described. The efflux system prevents the antimicrobial from reaching a critical concentration in the cell. If the antimicrobial does persist in the cell, it may not affect the cell because the target site (e.g., penicillin-binding proteins [PBPs], DNA gyrase, or ribosomal proteins) may be insensitive due to mutation and change.

Multiple resistance, whereby the bacterium becomes resistant to several antimicrobials, may occur. In recent years, drug resistance has been recognized as a major problem in controlling bacterial infections and may be either chromosomally or plasmid mediated. *Plasmids* (extrachromosomal genetic elements), which code for enzymes that inactivate antimicrobials, can be transferred by conjugation and transduction from resistant bacteria to previously sensitive bacteria. Enzymes coded by plasmids (e.g., penicillinase, cephalosporinase, and acetylases) that are specific for a given antimicrobial inactivate the drug either by the removal or addition of a chemical group from the molecule or by breaking a chemical bond. *Transposons* are segments of genetic material with insertion sequences at each end of the gene. These sequences allow genes from one organism to be easily inserted into the genetic material of another organism. Some of these transposons code for antibiotic resistance.

Adverse Effects

The adverse effects associated with the use of antimicrobial agents include (1) allergic reactions, (2) toxic reactions resulting from high doses or drug interactions, (3) idiosyncratic reactions, and (4) reactions related to alterations in normal body flora.

Allergic responses are probably the most frequently observed reactions, and range in intensity from mild skin rashes to fatal anaphylaxis. Most antimicrobials are safe when employed at appropriate dosage for recommended periods of time. However, high concentrations of certain antimicrobial agents can result in such toxic effects as neuropathy, ototoxicity, hepatotoxicity, nephrotoxicity, or electrolyte imbalance. Since the kidney is the major excretory pathway for many antimicrobials, impaired renal function may result in prolonged and elevated drug levels and toxicity.

Some adverse reactions are unrelated to either an immune response or to a known pharmacological property of the antimicrobial and are described as *idiosyncratic.* For instance, sulfonamides may precipitate acute hemolysis in people who are genetically deficient in the enzyme glucose 6-phosphate dehydrogenase. Another example is the development of a peripheral neuropathy following isoniazid therapy in those who are genetically slow acetylators of isoniazid (see Chap. 4).

Many antibiotics alter the microbial flora of the body. Sensitive bacteria are suppressed or killed, thereby removing their inhibitory effects on other organisms. Overgrowth or repopulation with resistant organisms, in turn, may result in infection (*superinfection*). Several variables

appear to influence the development of superinfection. It is more often seen in the young, in the elderly, and in patients with severe underlying disease, such as those found in critical care units. The length of antimicrobial treatment is also important, since the incidence of superinfection is uncommon when a drug is given for less than a week. Finally, the microbiological activity of the antimicrobial is important since broad-spectrum agents, such as ampicillin and the cephalosporins, cause a greater suppression of normal flora and thereby increase the risk of superinfection.

Laboratory Aspects of Antimicrobial Therapy

Sensitivity Tests

Laboratory tests of in vitro sensitivity of a microorganism to specific antimicrobial agents are used to predict in vivo efficacy. Two methods are generally used. The more common method uses an agar-filled Petri dish that is streaked with the organism. A small filter-paper disc containing a known amount of the antimicrobial agent is placed on the agar surface and allowed to diffuse into the medium over an 18- to 24-hr incubation period. After incubation, a zone of growth inhibition of the microorganism will occur if it is sensitive to the drug. For a given antimicrobial, the diameter of the zone of inhibition (no growth) correlates with the sensitivity of the organism to clinically achievable levels of the drug; the larger the zone, the more sensitive the organism is to that agent. The use of tables that correlate the zone size with the minimal inhibitory concentration in vitro permits the organism to be described as *sensitive, resistant,* or *of intermediate sensitivity* to the drug.

An alternative method of measuring microbial drug sensitivity incorporates dilutions of a known concentration of the antimicrobial agent in a broth or agar medium. The medium is then inoculated with the organism. After incubation, the concentration that inhibits growth is determined; it is known as the *minimum inhibitory concentration (MIC).*

MICs can also be done using commercial tests. One of these employs microdilutions of antibiotic and an automated system for reading and recording the presence or absence of growth, that is, the sensitivity or resistance of an organism. A second test is a modification of the disc diffusion test. It employs a plastic strip containing a gradient of antibiotic.

Some organisms, for example, *Staphylococcus aureus, Neisseria gonorrhoeae,* and *Haemophilus influenzae,* may produce β-lactamase and be resistant to penicillin and its congeners. Testing for β-lactamase production by isolates enables early decision on the use of penicillin and congeners in treatment of the disease. The use of a chromogenic cephalosporin substrate allows detection of the β-lactamase in a few minutes.

In Vivo Measurements

The concentrations of antimicrobial agent in blood, cerebrospinal fluid (CSF), or urine can be measured to determine whether sufficient levels are present to inhibit bacterial growth or whether drug levels toxic to the host have been reached. Assays can be performed using either chemical or biological techniques.

In certain situations (e.g., bacterial endocarditis) it may be necessary to determine if the patient's blood contains antimicrobial activity sufficient to kill the infecting organism. Dilutions of the patient's serum are incubated with the organism isolated from the patient and the MBC determined as described. Generally, the physician hopes to obtain a trough serum level of antibiotic in the patient that will still inhibit bacterial growth at a dilution of 1:8 to 1:32.

Immunoassays and high-performance liquid chromatographic assays have been developed for measurement of antibiotic levels in tissue.

Use and Selection of Antimicrobial Agents

Antimicrobial agents are among the most widely used and safest agents available to the clinician. However, physicians must first consider the etiological agent responsible for the disease, to choose the most effective drug. Although sensitivity testing is usually required, it is unnecessary for certain infections, such as those caused by *Streptococcus pneumoniae* and *Streptococcus pyogenes,* since these organisms are usually sensitive to penicillin.

Whenever possible, specimens suitable for laboratory diagnosis should be obtained before initiating treatment. Once the etiological agent is identified, the physician should decide whether modification of the initial choice of drug is appropriate.

Antimicrobials are, regrettably, frequently prescribed in the absence of either laboratory or clinical evidence of a definite, or even a probable, bacterial infection. Surveys have indicated that up to 60 percent of the antimicrobials prescribed for hospitalized patients may be inappropriate. For example, *antibiotics are frequently, but inappropriately, given for an upper respiratory tract infection of viral origin.*

Selection of an antimicrobial agent requires consideration of the route of administration, dosage, duration of treatment, cost of the drug regimen, and awareness of the possible adverse reactions that may occur. The route of administration depends on many factors. For example, gastrointestinal problems, such as surgical resection or malabsorptive states, can seriously impair the absorption of orally administered drugs. There is also impaired absorption of oral tetracycline and quinolones when given simultaneously with aluminum- or magnesium-containing antacids. Some drugs, such as methicillin, are inactivated if given by mouth, whereas others, such as neomycin, are too toxic for systemic use. Thus, despite laboratory information indicating an organism's susceptibility to a particular antimicrobial, the final choice of agent and route of administration depends on the site of infection, the physiological status of the host, and the pharmacokinetics and toxicity of the drug.

Dosage selection should be related to the site of infection. Drugs used in the treatment of bladder bacteriuria appear in the urine in very high concentrations. However, the same drug dosage regimen may be inadequate for the treatment of renal parenchymal infections, for which higher dosages and parenteral administration frequently become necessary. Since many drugs are excreted by the kidney, dosage modification is essential in renal insufficiency if toxicity is to be avoided. The aminoglycosidic aminocyclitols are prime examples of compounds whose half-lives and toxicity are increased significantly in patients with renal failure. In these patients, the dosage either must be reduced, or the intervals between doses increased. On the other hand, nitrofurantoin, a drug used in the treatment of urinary tract infections, is present in the urine in suboptimal amounts when renal function is impaired.

Combination Therapy

Most infections can be treated with a single antimicrobial agent. If a single agent is known to be effective, then the simultaneous use of more than one antimicrobial should be avoided to reduce both the risk of adverse reactions and the cost of medication. Nevertheless, some situations exist in which it is advantageous to use combination therapy. For example, in the treatment of endocarditis, penicillin and gentamicin have a synergistic effect on enterococci; that is, the combined use of these two drugs is superior to the effects produced by either agent alone.

Combined therapy for the prevention of drug resistance is well illustrated by the use of two or three agents for the treatment of *Mycobacterium tuberculosis* infections (see Chap. 53). Occasionally, combined therapy is indicated for a true mixed infection, although it is more commonly used as initial therapy in the treatment of serious infections in which the pathogen is unknown. In the latter instance, however, the regimen should be modified once laboratory investigations identify both the pathogenic organism and its sensitivity to antimicrobial drugs.

The use of fixed-dose combinations is rarely justified. One exception is the combination of trimethoprim-sulfamethoxazole (see Chap. 48), which is commonly used to treat urinary tract as well as other infections.

Prophylactic Use

The use of antimicrobials prophylactically to prevent infection is appropriate only under certain circumstances. For example, the purpose of surgical chemoprophylaxis is to prevent postoperative sepsis by inhibiting the growth of bacteria that may gain entry into the tissues at the time of surgery. Proper chemoprophylaxis demands a knowledge of the likely pathogen and a careful selection of a reasonably safe and effective agent, which is administered immediately before operation and for a maximum of 24 to 48 hr postoperatively, thereby providing bactericidal tissue levels during the perioperative period. The small total dose involved rarely produces adverse reactions.

Patient Compliance

Patients must be made aware of the importance of taking the antibiotic as prescribed. As pointed out previously, the presence of certain foods or divalent cations will impair absorption of some antimicrobials. Also, patients frequently discontinue antibiotic therapy when they feel better. Unfortunately, these individuals may then self-prescribe the remaining antibiotic for themselves or for others at some later date.

Antibiotics and Host Resistance

Perhaps the most important effect of antibiotics on host resistance is their effect on normal flora. Antibiotic therapy may remove inhibitory effects exerted by drug-sensitive normal flora, thereby permitting the establishment of exogenously derived organisms or overgrowth of endogenous organisms. This occurrence can have a devastating

effect on the host. As an example, *Clostridium difficile,* which is found in small numbers in the intestine and which is resistant to clindamycin, as well as to some other antibiotics, can grow and produce toxins in antibiotic-treated patients and cause pseudomembranous colitis.

A further risk of antibiotic treatment is the selection of resistant organisms, which can spread to susceptible hosts. A prime example is the recurrent problem of staphylococcal infection caused by antibiotic-resistant staphylococci carried on the skin and in the nose of patients and staff. In recent years, gram-negative bacilli, such as *Klebsiella, Enterobacter, Serratia,* and *Pseudomonas aeruginosa,* have become serious hospital pathogens by virtue of their resistance to many commonly prescribed antibiotics. In other cases, treatment does not shorten the duration of the disease but it prolongs excretion and enhances spread of infectious organisms.

To be most effective, antimicrobials require a host with a functional immune system. However, antimicrobials can act as immunomodulators. For example, they can suppress antibody production (e.g., chloramphenicol) and alter leukocyte chemotaxis and complement activation (e.g., tetracycline). In humans, rifampin decreases the number of T lymphocytes and depresses cutaneous hypersensitivity. Treatment of certain infections impairs antibody production because growth of the organism and consequent antigenic stimulation are prevented. Some antibiotics, such as chloramphenicol and the sulfonamides, may cause a granulocytopenia and bone marrow aplasia. These effects are not well understood but emphasize the importance of judicious use of those important agents.

Although the results have been somewhat variable, certain antibiotics release IL-1α, IL-6, and TNF from human monocytes and IL-4 and IFN-γ from lymphocytes in vitro. These cytokines are important in inflammatory and immunological responses and could, in some cases, contribute to the severity of disease or, in other situations, act as immunomodulators and enhance antimicrobial activity.

Supplemental Reading

Finch, R.G. Antibacterial chemotherapy. *Med. International* 104:4374, 1992.

Kucers, A., and Bennent, N. McK. *The Use of Antibiotics* (4th ed.). London: William Heinemann, 1990.

Leff, R.D., and Roberts, R.J. Host factors influencing the response to antimicrobial agents. *Pediatr. Clin. North Am.* 30:93, 1983.

Levy, S.B. Active efflux mechanisms for antimicrobial resistance. *Antimicrob. Agents Chemother.* 36:695, 1992.

Levy, S.B., Burke, J.P., and Wallace, C.K. Antibiotic use and antibiotic resistance world-wide. *Rev. Infect. Dis.* 3:745, 1987.

Marr, J.J., Moffet, H.L., and Kunin, C.M. Guidelines for improving the use of antimicrobial agents in hospital: A statement by the Infectious Diseases Society of America. *J. Infect. Dis.* 157:869, 1988.

Milatovic, D. Effects of Antibiotics on Phagocytic Cell Functions. In P.K. Peterson and J. Verhoef (eds.), *The Antimicrobial Agents Annual 1.* Amsterdam: Elsevier, 1986. P. 446.

Rosenblatt, J.E. Laboratory tests used to guide antimicrobial therapy. *Mayo Clin. Proc.* 66:942, 1991.

Sanders, C.C. β-Lactamases of gram negative bacteria: New challenges for new drugs. *Clin. Infect. Dis.* 14:1089, 1992.

Tufano, M.A., et al. Antimicrobial agents induce monocytes to release IL-1 α, IL-6, and TNF, and induce lymphocytes to release IL-4 and IFNγ. *Immunopharmacol. Immunotoxicol.* 14:769, 1992.

48

Synthetic Organic Antimicrobials (Sulfonamides, Trimethoprim, Nitrofurans, Quinolones, Methenamine)

Roger G. Finch and *Irvin S. Snyder*

Antimicrobial chemotherapy began in 1935, when Domagk showed that Prontosil, a dye, prevented streptococcal infections in mice. Prontosil was subsequently shown to be metabolized in vivo to the active antibacterial compound sulfanilamide (Fig. 48-1), an observation that provided a basis for the synthesis of many other chemicals with antibacterial potency. The synthetic chemotherapeutic agents available for clinical use include the sulfonamides, sulfones, quinolones, *p*-aminosalicylic acid (PAS), trimethoprim, pyrimethamine, nitrofurantoin, isoniazid, pyrazinamide, and methenamine.

Sulfonamides

Chemistry

The sulfonamides comprise a large group of compounds that are structural analogues of *p*-aminobenzoic acid (PABA) (Fig. 48-1). They differ primarily in the substituents on either the sulfonamide or the amino group (Fig. 48-2). Substitutions on the sulfonamide group modify the drug's solubility characteristics, thus resulting in congeners with different rates of absorption and excretion. Some sulfonamides, such as sulfacetamide and mafenide, are designed for topical use, whereas phthalylsulfathiazole, because it is poorly absorbed from the intestinal tract, has been used against intestinal organisms.

Mechanism of Action

The sulfonamides interfere with microbial growth by *competitively inhibiting incorporation of PABA into folic acid* and thereby preventing the synthesis of folic acid, a compound *essential to bacterial growth*. In its reduced form, folic acid functions as a coenzyme in the transport of one-carbon units from one molecule to another. These one-carbon transfers are necessary for the synthesis of thymidine, purines, and some amino acids. *Humans cannot synthesize folic acid* and must acquire it through their diet; thus, the sulfonamides selectively inhibit microbial growth.

Resistance to the sulfonamides can be the result of decreased bacterial permeability to the drug, an increased production of PABA, or production of an altered dihydropteroate synthetase (the enzyme required for synthesis of dihydropteroic acid). The inhibitory effect of the sulfonamides also can be reversed by the presence of pus, tissue fluids, and drugs that contain PABA.

Antibacterial Spectrum

The sulfonamides are *broad-spectrum* antimicrobials that are effective against gram-positive organisms, some gram-negative organisms, and *Chlamydia*. They also are used in treating infections caused by *Toxoplasma gondii* and, occasionally, by chloroquine-resistant *Plasmodium falciparum*. In combination with trimethoprim, they are the drugs of choice for the treatment of *Pneumocystis carinii* infections.

Pharmacokinetic Properties

Absorption

Sulfonamides are usually given orally, although the soluble sodium salts can be given parenterally. The sulfonamides are rapidly absorbed from the intestinal tract

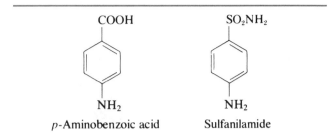

Figure 48-1. Structural comparison of *p*-aminobenzoic acid and sulfanilamide.

and usually can be found in serum within 30 min after ingestion. Peak serum levels are obtained in 2 to 3 hr.

Distribution

The systemic sulfonamides readily distribute throughout body fluids. They pass the placental barrier and enter the cerebrospinal fluid (CSF) even in the absence of inflammation. The degree of protein binding, the half-life, and the drug's solubility in urine will vary considerably from one sulfonamide to another (Table 48-1).

Metabolism and Excretion

The sulfonamides are degraded in the liver by acetylation and oxidation. Both parent compound and metabolites are excreted in the urine, primarily by glomerular filtration; some tubular reabsorption does occur.

Clinical Use

Sulfonamides have a long record of successful use in the treatment of a wide range of both gram-positive and gram-negative bacterial infections. However, the current indications for their use are more limited because of the availability of better and safer agents.

Acute uncomplicated urinary tract infections caused by *Escherichia coli* and other pathogens generally respond promptly to one of the short-acting sulfonamides. Recurrent urinary tract infections are often related to some structural abnormality in the tract and are frequently caused by sulfonamide-resistant bacteria.

Sulfonamides have been widely used for the treatment of meningococcal meningitis and shigellosis. Because resistant bacteria are frequently encountered, sulfonamides should not be used in these conditions without laboratory evidence of susceptibility.

Sulfadiazine and sulfisoxazole still play a useful role in the prophylaxis of streptococcal infections in patients with rheumatic fever who are hypersensitive to penicillin.

Trisulfapyrimidine (a combination of sulfadiazine, sulfamerazine, and sulfamethazine), trimethoprim-sulfamethoxazole, or sulfisoxazole is used as an alternative drug for the treatment of melioidosis caused by *Pseudomonas pseudomallei* and for infections produced by *Nocardia*.

A number of infections caused by *Chlamydia trachomatis*, such as trachoma, inclusion conjunctivitis, pneumonia, and urethritis, can be treated with topical or systemic sulfonamides, although tetracycline or erythromycin is preferred.

Sulfonamides, such as trisulfapyrimidine, in combination with pyrimethamine, are helpful in the treatment of symptomatic toxoplasmosis. Some regimens have included a sulfonamide (sulfadoxine) in combination with pyrimethamine (*Fansidar*) for the treatment of chloroquine-resistant malaria caused by *Plasmodium falciparum*.

Topically active sulfonamides are useful in preventing infections in burn patients. Mafenide acetate (*Sulfamylon Cream*) is the most widely used compound and is effective against *Pseudomonas aeruginosa,* an organism that frequently colonizes burns. It is less effective against staphylococci, another organism that colonizes burns. Local absorption of the acetate preparation, which is acidic, can result in respiratory alkalosis. Silver sulfadiazine in a 1% cream can be used as an alternative to mafenide and has good activity against gram-negative bacteria.

Haemophilus (*Gardnerella*) *vaginalis* infections are treated intravaginally with a triple sulfa preparation consisting of sulfathiazole, sulfacetamide, and sulfabenzamide.

Sulfacetamide is used topically for treatment of ocular infections.

Adverse Reactions

The sulfonamides are relatively safe agents, but hypersensitivity reactions (e.g., rashes, eosinophilia, and drug fever) occur in a small number of patients. Other rare allergic reactions include vasculitis, photosensitivity, agranulocytosis, and thrombocytopenia. The Stevens-Johnson syndrome is also associated with sulfonamide use; it is characterized by fever, malaise, erythema multiforme, and ulceration of the mucous membranes of the mouth and genitalia. A hemolytic anemia may develop in persons with a genetic deficiency of red blood cell glucose 6-phosphate dehydrogenase.

Sulfonamides compete for sites on plasma proteins that are responsible for the binding of bilirubin. As a result, less bilirubin is bound and, in the newborn, the unbound bilirubin can be deposited in the basal ganglia and subthalamic nuclei, causing *kernicterus,* a toxic encephalopathy.

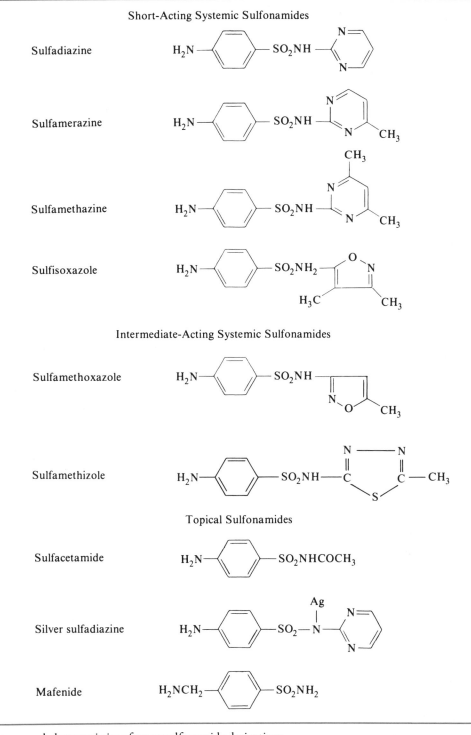

Figure 48-2. Structures and characteristics of some sulfonamide derivatives.

Table 48-1. Characteristics of the Systemic Sulfonamides

Compound	Serum half-life (hr)	Protein binding (%)	Solubility (urine)
Sulfadiazine	17	20–60	1+
Sulfamethazine	7	60–80	3+
Sulfisoxazole	6	90	3+
Sulfamethoxazole	11	85–90	1+
Sulfacetamide	12	20	3+
Sulfamethizole	2.5	90	3+

For this reason, *sulfonamides should not be administered to newborns or to women during the last 2 months of pregnancy.*

If the concentration of the sulfonamide is sufficiently high and its aqueous solubility is sufficiently low, the free drug or its metabolites may form crystals and cause bleeding or complete obstruction of the kidneys. This adverse effect is extremely uncommon with the more soluble sulfonamides currently in use.

Preparations and Dosage

Short-Acting Sulfonamides

Individual short-acting, intermediate-acting, and topical sulfonamides are shown in Fig. 48-2. Many preparations consisting of several sulfonamides, as well as combinations of a sulfonamide and another antibacterial agent, are available.

Trimethoprim

Chemistry and Mechanism of Action

Trimethoprim (Fig. 48-3) is a structural analogue of dihydrofolic acid that can inhibit the synthesis of folic acid. However, trimethoprim differs from the sulfonamides in that it acts at a second step in the folic acid synthetic pathway; that is, it competitively inhibits dihydrofolate reductase, the enzyme that catalyzes the reduction of dihydrofolic acid to tetrahydrofolic acid. Dihydrofolate reductase is present in both mammalian tissue and bacteria, but 20,000 to 60,000 times more drug is required to inhibit the mammalian enzyme; this accounts for its *selective toxicity* against bacteria.

Antibacterial Spectrum

Trimethoprim exhibits broad-spectrum activity. It is most commonly used in combination with sulfamethoxazole and is active against most aerobic and facultative

gram-positive and gram-negative organisms. However, *Pseudomonas aeruginosa* is resistant and there is little activity against anaerobic bacteria.

Resistance can develop from alterations in dihydrofolate reductase, impermeability to the drug, and by overproduction of the dihydrofolate reductase. The most important mechanism of bacterial resistance to the drug clinically is production of plasmid-encoded trimethoprim-resistant forms of dihydrofolate reductase.

Because trimethoprim and sulfamethoxazole each have their effects at different points in the folic acid synthetic pathway, a synergistic effect results when the two are administered together. Because the combination affects different steps in folic acid synthesis, the incidence of bacterial resistance to the combination is less than that observed when the drugs are used individually.

Absorption, Metabolism, and Excretion

Trimethoprim is well absorbed from the gastrointestinal tract, and peak blood levels are achieved in about 2 hr. Tissue levels often exceed those of plasma, and the urine concentration of trimethoprim may be 100 times that of the plasma. Trimethoprim readily enters the CSF if inflammation is present. The half-life of the drug is approximately 11 hr. Sulfamethoxazole is frequently coadministered with trimethoprim in a dose ratio of 5:1 (sulfamethoxazole:trimethoprim). Peak drug levels in plasma are achieved in 2 to 4 hr. At this time, the sulfamethoxazole-trimethoprim plasma ratio is 20:1, which is the ratio most effective for producing a synergistic effect against most susceptible pathogens. Both drugs bind to plasma protein and both are metabolized in the liver. Both parent drugs and their metabolites are excreted by the kidney.

Clinical Use of Trimethoprim-Sulfamethoxazole

Trimethoprim-sulfamethoxazole is used in the treatment of urinary, intestinal, and lower respiratory tract infections, otitis media, and prostatitis caused by susceptible bacteria. *Escherichia coli,* enterococci, *Proteus mirabilis,* and

Figure 48-3. Trimethoprim.

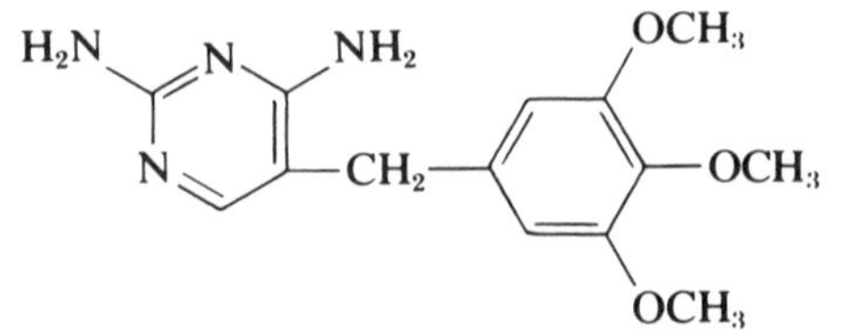

Klebsiella pneumoniae are usually sensitive to this combination therapy. In some patients with recurrent urinary tract infections, most notably women of childbearing age, the long-term use of one tablet taken at night is an effective form of chemoprophylaxis.

Trimethoprim is a weak base and is present in vaginal secretions in high enough levels to be active against many of the organisms responsible for recurrent urinary tract infections. Trimethoprim-sulfamethoxazole is also used in the treatment of infection caused by ampicillin-resistant *Shigella* and for antibiotic-resistant *Salmonella*.

Because trimethoprim accumulates in the prostate, trimethoprim-sulfamethoxazole is used to treat prostatitis caused by sensitive organisms. Therapy may have to be prolonged (4–6 weeks) and repeat courses of therapy may be necessary. Trimethoprim alone is used in the initial treatment of uncomplicated urinary tract infections.

Purulent exacerbations of chronic bronchitis respond well to the trimethoprim-sulfamethoxazole combination, since it is active against both *Streptococcus pneumoniae* and *Haemophilus influenzae*, the bacteria most frequently associated with such a condition. Gonorrhea, typhoid fever, and brucellosis have been treated with trimethoprim-sulfamethoxazole with cure rates comparable to those attained by standard therapy. The combination also has been used in the treatment of nocardial infections.

The combination is effective in both the treatment and prevention of infections caused by *Pneumocystis carinii*, a protozoan that causes a serious pneumonitis in patients with hematological malignancies and acquired immuno-deficiency syndrome (AIDS). In those with AIDS, treatment is more prolonged and relapse is common. Hence, long-term low-dose chemoprophylaxis with trimethoprim-sulfamethoxazole is widely used.

Adverse Reactions

Trimethoprim-sulfamethoxazole can cause the same adverse effects as those associated with sulfonamide administration, including skin rashes, central nervous system (CNS) disturbances, and blood dyscrasias. Skin rashes are particularly common in patients with AIDS. Most of the adverse effects of this combination are due to the sulfamethoxazole component. Trimethoprim may increase the hematological toxicity of sulfamethoxazole. Long-term use of trimethoprim in persons with borderline folic acid deficiency, such as alcoholics and the malnourished, may result in megaloblastic anemia, thrombocytopenia, and granulocytopenia.

The use of trimethoprim is contraindicated in patients with blood dyscrasias, hepatic damage, and renal impairment, although infections such as those caused by *P. carinii* frequently occur in patients with such problems and require careful dosaging and monitoring.

Preparations and Dosage

Trimethoprim-sulfamethoxazole (*Septra, Bactrim, Sulfatrim*) is available as an oral suspension (each 5 ml containing 40 mg trimethoprim and 200 mg sulfamethoxazole), in tablet form (80:400 mg, 160:800 mg), and for intravenous administration (5 ml containing 80 mg trimethoprim and 400 mg sulfamethoxazole).

Trimethoprim (*Trimpex, Proloprim*) is available as 100-mg tablets.

Nitrofurans

Structure and Mechanism of Action

A number of 5-nitro-2-furaldehyde derivatives (Fig. 48-4), called *nitrofurans*, are used in the treatment of microbial infections.

The mechanism for the antimicrobial activity of the 5-nitrofurans is still not clear, but recent evidence suggests that reduction of the 5-nitro group to the nitro anion results in bacterial toxicity. Evidence also indicates that the nitro anion undergoes recycling with the production of superoxide and other toxic oxygen compounds. It is presumed that the nitrofurans are selectively toxic to microbial cells because, in the human, high serum concentrations are not reached and these drugs are readily inactivated in the liver.

Figure 48-4. Nitrofurantoin and nitrofurazone.

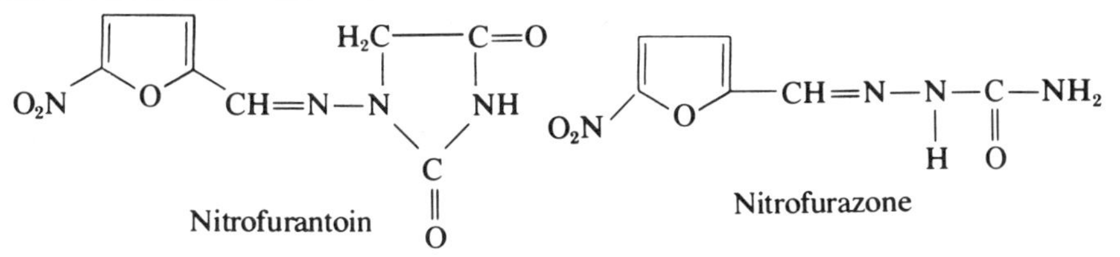

Antibacterial Spectrum

The nitrofurans are *broad-spectrum* compounds that are active against gram-positive and gram-negative bacteria. They inhibit *E. coli, Klebsiella, Enterobacter, Salmonella, Shigella,* and *Vibrio cholerae* as well as staphylococci and enterococci. Most *Proteus* species and *Pseudomonas aeruginosa* are resistant.

Absorption, Metabolism, and Excretion

Nitrofurantoin is administered orally and is rapidly and almost completely absorbed from the small intestine; however, only low levels of activity are achieved in serum because the drug is rapidly metabolized. Nitrofurantoin is rapidly excreted by glomerular filtration and tubular secretion, and this results in a serum half-life of only about 20 min. About 40 percent of the drug is excreted in the active form. Although serum drug concentrations are low, high concentrations are found in renal interstitial fluids and in urine. Alkalinization of the urine increases urinary concentrations of the drug but decreases its antibacterial efficacy.

Nitrofurazone is used topically and is not readily absorbed from the skin.

Clinical Use

The only indication for nitrofurantoin is in the treatment and prophylaxis of urinary tract infections caused by susceptible bacteria. These bacteria usually include *E. coli,* enterococci, indole-positive *Proteus* and *Klebsiella. Pseudomonas aeruginosa* is usually resistant and *Proteus mirabilis* is variable in its susceptibility.

Since inadequate urinary levels are achieved in renal insufficiency, the use of nitrofurantoin is contraindicated under these circumstances. Inadequate serum levels prohibit its use for treating episodes of septicemia that may complicate urinary tract infections. A macrocrystalline formulation of nitrofurantoin is more slowly absorbed, thereby delaying peak serum and urinary levels; it is better tolerated than the parent form, but is more expensive and no more effective.

Nitrofurazone, a topical antibiotic, is occasionally used in the treatment of burns or skin grafts, in which bacterial contamination may cause rejection.

Adverse Reactions

Nausea and vomiting are the most commonly observed adverse effects. Allergic reactions to the nitrofurans include rashes, urticaria, angioneurotic edema, eosinophilia, and drug-induced fevers. Two types of pulmonary reactions have been described: an acute and probably allergic reaction characterized by fever, cough, myalgia, dyspnea, pulmonary infiltrates (especially at the base of the lung), and pleural effusion that disappears with cessation of treatment, and a second type of pneumonic complication, characterized as interstitial fibrosis.

Nitrofurantoin also has been associated with a sensorimotor peripheral neuropathy, most notably in association with impaired renal function. Megaloblastic anemia and cholestasis have been reported. Hemolysis can occur in patients with erythrocytic enzyme deficiencies (e.g., glucose 6-phosphate dehydrogenase). Hepatotoxicity is rare and is usually reversible.

Nitrofurazone is a relatively safe topical agent. Skin sensitization has been reported.

Preparations and Dosage

Nitrofurantoin (*Furadantin, Macrodantin*) is available as tablets, capsules, and a suspension.

Nitrofurazone (*Furacin*) comes as a cream (0.2%), powder (0.2%), soluble dressing (0.2%), and a solution (0.2%).

Nalidixic Acid and Other 4-Quinolone Agents

Mechanism of Action

Nalidixic acid, a 4-quinolone, and several chemically related compounds, for example, fluoroquinolones (Fig. 48-5), are antimicrobial agents that inhibit DNA synthesis. This is accomplished through a specific action on *DNA gyrase,* the enzyme that is responsible for the unwinding and supercoiling of bacterial DNA within the bacterium before its replication. Resistance is related to changes in the DNA gyrase and to alterations in porins resulting in decreased uptake of the drug. Recently, an active efflux system for transport of the drug out of the cell has been described. Plasmid-mediated resistance does not occur. Cross-resistance between the 4-quinolones can occur.

Antibacterial Spectrum

Nalidixic acid inhibits gram-negative organisms and is used to treat urinary tract infections produced by *E. coli, Klebsiella,* and *Proteus.* The chemically related compounds cinoxacin and oxolinic acid possess a similar spectrum and degree of activity as nalidixic acid. Some of the newer agents have the additional advantage of possessing high

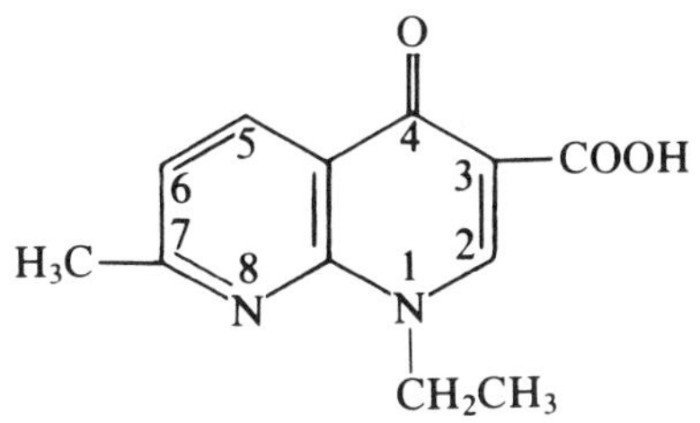

Figure 48-5. Antibacterial 4-quinolones.

activity against *Neisseria gonorrhoeae;* some also affect *Chlamydia trachomatis* and *Ureaplasma urealyticum.* Several other 4-quinolones, such as enoxacin, norfloxacin, ofloxacin, lomefloxacin, and ciprofloxacin, are even more potent against common gram-negative bacteria and are also active against staphylococci and *Pseudomonas aeruginosa.* The antipseudomonal activity of ciprofloxacin, norfloxacin, ofloxacin, and lomefloxacin is due to the piperazine moiety.

Absorption, Metabolism, and Excretion

Nalidixic acid is administered orally and is rapidly and almost completely absorbed from the intestinal tract. Concentrations in plasma of 20 to 40 μg/ml are achieved 1 to 2 hr after administration of a 1-gm dose; about 95 percent of the drug is bound to serum protein. The plasma half-life is approximately 90 min, but it may be extended in patients with renal failure. In the liver, nalidixic acid is converted to hydroxynalidixic acid, a biologically active metabolite, and to an inactive glucuronide. Nalidixic acid and its metabolites are eliminated through the kidney, and urine concentrations (150–200 μg/ml) are severalfold greater than those of serum. About 80 percent of the administered nalidixic acid is eliminated as the active hydroxynalidixic acid.

Oxolinic acid is moderately well absorbed although its absorption can be somewhat delayed by the presence of food in the gastrointestinal tract. The drug is widely distributed in the tissues although plasma concentrations tend to be low. It is extensively metabolized and only some 5 percent of the drug appears in the urine in the active form, the remainder being present largely as the glucuronide.

Cinoxacin is well absorbed, with peak serum concentrations of 15 μg/ml being reached 1 to 2 hr after a 500-mg dose. The serum half-life is 1.5 hr, with most of the dose excreted in 24 hr, about 60 percent in the unaltered active form.

Norfloxacin, after a dose of 200 or 400 μg, gives peak serum levels of 0.8 to 1.5 μg/ml in 1 hr. It has a half-life of 3 to 4 hr. About 1 to 15 percent is protein bound.

Ciprofloxacin, at an oral dose of 250 mg, gives maximum blood levels of 1.2 μg/ml in 1 to 2 hr after treatment. Intravenous infusion of 250 mg has resulted in peak serum concentrations of 2.1 μg/ml. The plasma half-life is from 4 to 6 hr. High tissue concentrations are achieved. About 50 percent of the drug is excreted unchanged in urine with 20 to 40 percent protein bound.

Ofloxacin is rapidly absorbed after oral administration with 98 percent of the drug bioavailable. After a dose of 200 mg, peak plasma levels of 1.5 μg/ml are obtained. Intravenous administration of 200 mg has resulted in peak plasma concentrations of 2.7 μg/ml. Ofloxacin distributes widely in tissue at high concentrations. Approximately 32 percent of this quinolone is protein bound. Excretion is largely renal, with some biliary excretion. The half-life is 5 to 7 hr.

Lomefloxacin, like ofloxacin, is rapidly absorbed with most of the drug bioavailable. Peak plasma concentration after administration of 200 mg reaches 1.4 μg/ml. The drug distributes widely in tissue. Approximately 10 percent is protein bound. Lomefloxacin is excreted in urine, with about 65 percent of the administered drug excreted unchanged. The half-life is 8 hr.

Enoxacin is rapidly absorbed from the intestinal tract with peak serum levels reached in about 2 hr. The drug's half-life is 3.3 to 6.2 hr and it has a 32 to 43 percent serum protein binding. It is excreted in urine with about 60 to 72 percent of the drug unchanged.

Clinical Uses

With the exception of *Pseudomonas aeruginosa,* nalidixic acid is active against most gram-negative bacteria associated with urinary tract infections. It is an effective urinary tract antiseptic, and this remains its main indication. In patients with renal insufficiency, the metabolites accumulate but are nontoxic, and the urinary concentrations of the active drug remain adequate. Other agents, however, are preferred in renal insufficiency.

Bacteria can become resistant to the drug, particularly if it is used for lengthy periods, and therefore it is not recommended for long-term chemoprophylaxis of urinary tract infections.

Both oxolinic acid and cinoxacin are promoted for the treatment of urinary tract infections. They appear to offer little advantage over nalidixic acid and have been less extensively evaluated. Drug resistance can emerge on treatment, especially with oxolinic acid.

Among the new quinolones most experience has been gained with ciprofloxacin. Its potent activity against gram-negative enteric bacteria including *P. aeruginosa* has resulted in extensive clinical use. It has proved effective in the treatment of urinary tract infection including those unresponsive to existing agents and especially where structural abnormalities impede the chemotherapeutic response. Intraabdominal and biliary infections have also been treated satisfactorily although the drug lacks activity against anaerobic bacteria. Ciprofloxacin, given orally, is useful in the treatment of osteomyelitis due to gram-negative enteric organisms. In addition, patients suffering from cystic fibrosis complicated by *P. aeruginosa* infections of the lung have also responded satisfactorily although drug resistance has occasionally occurred. Oral administration is a major advantage over existing treatment for pseudomonad infections. All forms of gonorrhea are extremely susceptible to ciprofloxacin. Its activity against bacterial bowel pathogens, such as *Shigella, Salmonella,* and *Campylobacter,* suggests a possible future role in their treatment and in the prevention of traveler's diarrhea.

Ofloxacin use is similar to that of ciprofloxacin. High blood and tissue levels are obtained that balance its slightly lower in vitro activity. It is not considered suitable for treating *P. aeruginosa* infections.

Norfloxacin is used in the treatment of uncomplicated urinary tract infections including those caused by gram-negative rods and gram-positive cocci.

Enoxacin is used in treatment of gonorrhea, urinary tract infections, and chronic bronchitis.

Adverse Reactions

The most frequently reported side effect for the quinolones is nausea, but vomiting, diarrhea, and abdominal pain also may result. Allergic reactions (e.g., rashes, urticaria, and eosinophilia) have been observed. Central nervous system (CNS) effects, such as drowsiness, weakness, headache, dizziness and, in severe cases, convulsions and toxic psychosis, have been reported. These drugs have on some occasions been associated with cholestatic jaundice, blood dyscrasias, hemolytic anemia, hypoglycemia, and nephrotoxicity.

The variety of adverse reactions experienced with the more recently introduced quinolones, including ciprofloxacin, is similar to those seen with nalidixic acid.

Preparations and Dosage

Nalidixic acid (*NegGram*) is available as 250-mg, 500-mg, and 1-gm tablets and as a suspension containing 250 mg/5 ml.

Cinoxacin (*Cinobac*) is available as 250- and 500-mg capsules.

Enoxacin (*Penetrex*) is available as 200- and 400-mg tablets.

Norfloxacin (*Noroxin*) is available as 400-mg tablets and as an ophthalmic solution (*Chibroxin*).

Ciprofloxacin (*Cipro*) is supplied as 250-, 500-, and 750-mg tablets. Solutions containing 200 and 400 mg (*Cipro IV*) are available for IV use. An ophthalmic preparation (*Ciloxan*) is also available.

Ofloxacin (*Floxin*) is available as tablets containing 200, 300, and 400 mg for oral use and as solutions containing 20 and 40 mg/ml.

Lomefloxacin hydrochloride (*Maxaquin*) is available as 400-mg tablets.

Methenamine

Chemistry and Mode of Action

Methenamine (hexamethylenetetramine) is an aromatic acid that is hydrolyzed at an acid pH to liberate ammonia and the alkylating agent formaldehyde (Fig. 48-6). The formaldehyde that is released denatures protein and is bactericidal. Methenamine is usually administered as a salt of mandelic, ascorbic, or hippuric acid. The acids not only acidify the urine, which is necessary for degradation of methenamine, but the low urine pH also is bacteriostatic for some organisms.

Antibacterial Spectrum

Methenamine is active against gram-negative bacteria, particularly *E. coli,* a major cause of urinary tract infections. Bacterial resistance to formaldehyde does not develop.

Absorption, Distribution, and Excretion

Methenamine is administered orally and is well absorbed from the intestinal tract. However, 10 to 30 percent decomposes in the stomach unless the tablets are protected by an enteric coating. The inactive form (methenamine) is distributed throughout the body, but since formaldehyde is generated only at an acid pH, the antimicrobial effect of methenamine is expressed only in acidic urine. Acidifying agents can be coadministered to lower urinary pH and thereby potentiate the action of methenamine.

Clinical Uses

The hydrolysis of methenamine in an acid environment of pH 5.5 or less has made it useful for the treatment

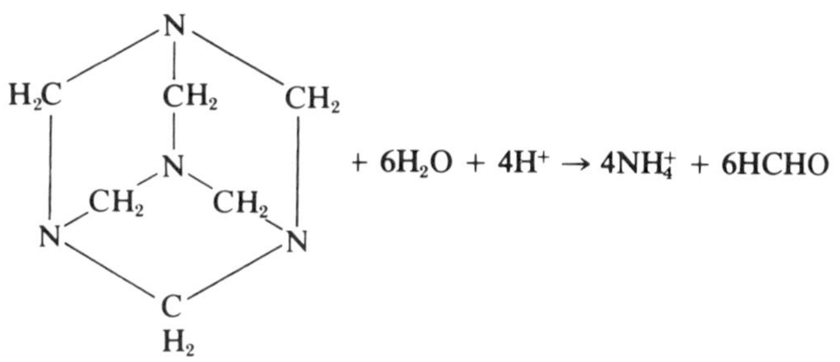

$$+ 6H_2O + 4H^+ \rightarrow 4NH_4^+ + 6HCHO$$

Figure 48-6. Methenamine, showing its hydrolysis at an acid pH.

and prevention of urinary tract infections. Some bacteria, notably *Proteus* species, produce ammonia from urea and thereby prevent the normal urinary acidification necessary for the hydrolysis of methenamine. A number of methenamine preparations, therefore, include mandelic or hippuric acid to acidify the urine. Alternatively, acidifying agents, such as ascorbic acid or methionine, can be taken separately. *The importance of checking the urine pH and maintaining it below pH 5.5 is vital for the effective use of methenamine.*

The availability of alternative well-tolerated antimicrobial agents has substantially reduced the use of methenamine in the management of urinary tract infections.

Adverse Reactions

Methenamine is usually well tolerated, although gastric distress and allergic reactions are occasionally reported. Bladder irritation (e.g., dysuria, polyuria, hematuria, and urgency) may occur. The mandelic salt can crystallize in urine if there is inadequate urine flow and should not be given to patients with renal failure.

Preparations and Dosage

Methenamine is commercially available as the hippurate salt (*Hiprex, Urex*) and as the mandelate salt (*Mandelamine*).

Supplemental Reading

Bergan, T. Pharmacokinetics of ciprofloxacin with reference to other fluorinated quinolones. *J. Chemotherapy* 1:10, 1989.

Brogden, R.N., et al. Trimethoprim: A review of its antibacterial activity, pharmacokinetics and therapeutic use in urinary tract infections. *Drugs* 23:405, 1982.

Campoli-Richards, D.M., et al. Ciprofloxacin. A review of its antibacterial activity, pharmacokinetic properties and therapeutic use. *Drugs* 35:373, 1988.

CuNa, B.A. Nitrofurantoin—current concepts. *Urology* 32:67, 1988.

Foltzer, M.A., and Reese, R.E. Trimethoprim-sulfamethoxazole and other sulphonamides. *Med. Clin. North Am.* 71:1177, 1987.

Gleckman, R., et al. Drug therapy reviews: Nalidixic acid. *Am. J. Hosp. Pharm.* 36:1071, 1979.

Gonzalez, J.P., and Henwood, J.M. Pefloxacin: A review of its antibacterial activity, pharmacokinetic properties and therapeutic use. *Drugs* 37:628, 1989.

Holmberg, L., et al. Adverse reactions to nitrofurantoin. Analysis of 921 reports. *Am. J. Med.* 69:733, 1980.

Huovinen, P. Trimethoprim resistance. *Antimicrob. Agents Chemother.* 31:1451, 1987.

Rowen, R.C., Michel, D.J., and Thompson, J.C. Norfloxacin: Clinical pharmacology and clinical use. *Pharmacotherapy* 7:92, 1987.

Scavone, J.M., Gleckman, R.A., and Fraser, D.G. Cinoxacin: Mechanism of action, spectrum of activity, pharmacokinetics, adverse reactions, and therapeutic indications. *Pharmacotherapy* 2:266, 1982.

Symposium. Focus on ofloxacin—a new 4-quinolone antimicrobial agent. *J. Antimicrob. Chemother.* 22 (Suppl. C): 1, 1988.

Vree, T.B., and Hekster, Y.A. Renal excretion of sulphonamide. *Antibiot. Chemother.* 34:66, 1985.

49

β-Lactam Antibiotics

Irvin S. Snyder and Roger G. Finch

The discovery of penicillin by Sir Alexander Fleming in 1928 resulted from the contamination of laboratory cultures by the mold *Penicillium notatum*. Fleming noted a zone of inhibition of bacterial growth around the mold; he subsequently demonstrated antimicrobial activity in culture filtrates of the mold. Sir Howard Florey and others later isolated and purified the active antimicrobial component. These findings eventually led to the discovery of several different penicillins and to their subsequent chemical modification to form a number of useful antibiotics.

Since the discovery of penicillin, antibiotics produced by fungi of the genus *Cephalosporium* have been identified. These antibiotics are called cephalosporins and contain, in common with the penicillins, a β-lactam ring.

In addition to the numerous penicillins and cephalosporins currently in use, three other classes of β-lactam antibiotics are now clinically available. These are the carbapenems, the carbacephems, and the monobactams.

Penicillins

Chemistry

The penicillins represent a large group of compounds with the same basic chemical nucleus. In all but one, the basic chemical structure is 6-aminopenicillanic acid (Fig. 49-1). The exception is amdinocillin, which has a 6-amidinopenicillanic acid (Table 49-1) group at its core. The essential constituents of the penicillin nucleus are a β-lactam ring and a thiazolidine nucleus.

The antimicrobial activity of penicillin resides in the β-lactam ring. The splitting of this ring by either acid or specific bacterial enzymes (*β-lactamases*) results in the formation of penicilloic acid, an inactive product. Addition of a side chain (R) results in the formation of a class of compounds having the same mechanism of action as penicillin G, but with differing chemical and biological properties.

For example, the analogues may be resistant to acid hydrolysis or unaffected by β-lactamase, have broad- or extended-spectrum activity, or be better absorbed from the intestinal tract (see Table 49-1).

The penicillins can be divided into three groups: *naturally occurring* penicillins (penicillin G, phenoxymethyl, and phenoxymethyl penicillins), *penicillinase-resistant* penicillins (methicillin, nafcillin, oxacillin, cloxacillin, and dicloxacillin), and *broad- or extended-spectrum* penicillins. The broad- or extended-spectrum penicillins are those with activity against gram-negative organisms, including the enterics and *Pseudomonas*. The latter group consists of several subgroups based on chemical structure and includes the aminopenicillins (ampicillin, hetacillin, and amoxicillin), the carboxypenicillins (carbenicillin and ticarcillin), and the acylureidopenicillins (mezlocillin, azlocillin, and piperacillin). A newer penicillin, amdinocillin, lacks the common 6-β-amino group that links the R group to the β-lactam nucleus. The 6-β-amino group is replaced by a 6-β-amidino group in amdinocillin.

Mechanisms of Action

Both the penicillins and the cephalosporins have the same mechanism of action; that is, they *prevent bacterial cell wall synthesis* and, in doing so, are bactericidal.

The final reaction in cell wall synthesis is a cross-linking of adjacent peptidoglycan strands by a transpeptidation reaction (Fig. 49-2). This reaction involves cleavage of the terminal alanine from the pentapeptide attached to D-alanine on one linear peptide and L-lysine on another linear peptide, thus completing the cross-linking of adjacent peptidoglycan polymers.

The penicillins, and also the cephalosporins, are structurally similar to the terminal D-alanyl-D-alanine portion and therefore can compete for and bind to proteins (enzymes) that catalyze transpeptidation and cross-linking. These proteins are called *penicillin-binding proteins (PBP)*

555

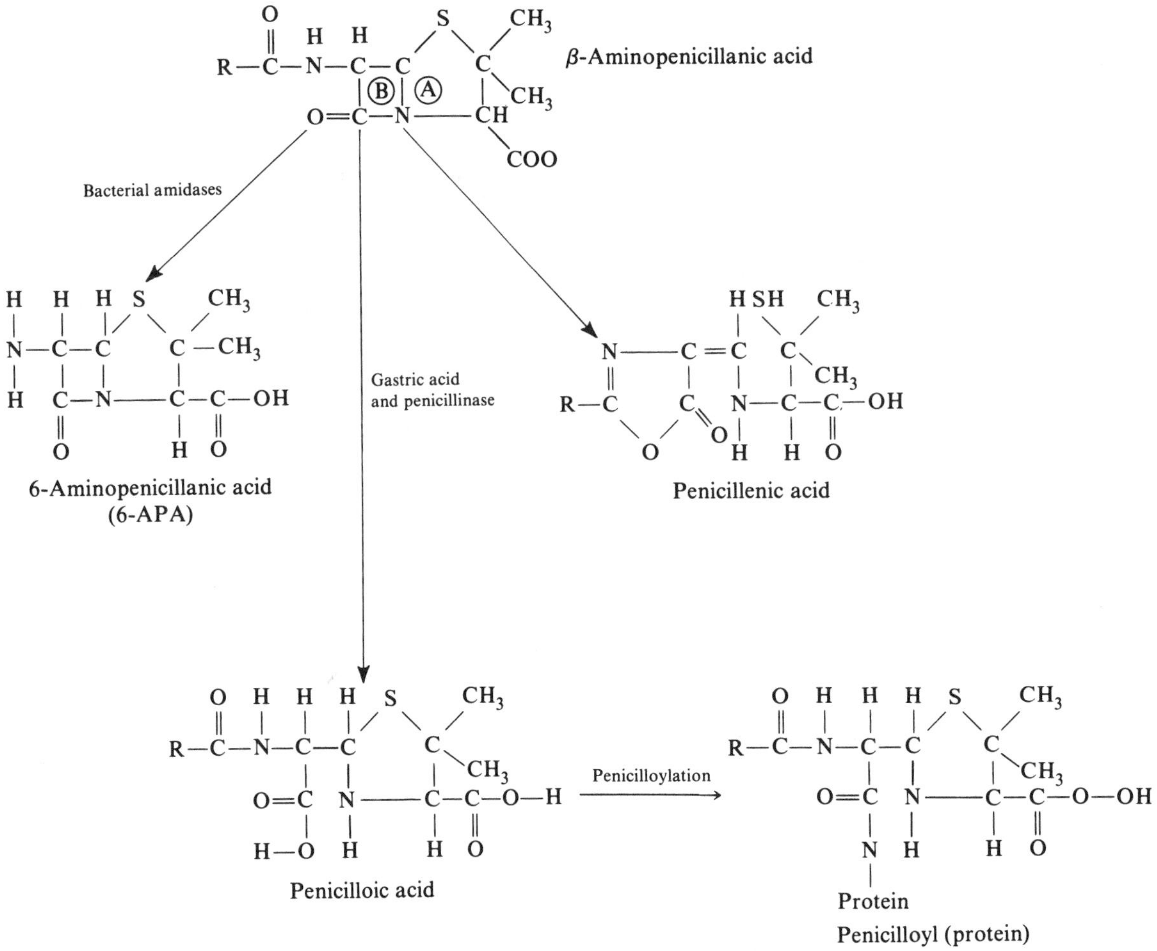

Figure 49-1. The basic chemical structure of penicillin. The actions of bacterial amidases result in formation of 6-aminopenicillanic acid, whereas the actions of gastric acid or β-lactamase (penicillinase) result in the formation of penicilloic acid. These penicilloyl derivatives may combine with protein carriers to form the major determinant of penicillin allergy (see text). Penicillenic acid is an additional breakdown product of benzylpenicillin, which can also appear in vitro. (A) = thiazolidine nucleus; (B) = β-lactam ring.

and consist of transpeptidases, transglycosylases, and D-alanine carboxykinases. The transpeptidases have different functions in the cell, and selective inactivation of each transpeptidase and carboxykinase results in a different effect on the bacterial cells (e.g., cell lysis, production of spherical cells or elongated cells). *Interference with the PBPs responsible for the cross-linking of the peptidoglycan polymers results in the formation of a structurally weakened cell wall, aberrant morphological forms, and, ultimately, cell death.* Lysis is due to the action of cell wall autolytic enzymes.

Alterations in the binding of penicillins or cephalosporins to PBPs can also result in resistance to the antibiotics. Resistance is also expressed by organisms that produce β-

lactamases, enzymes that cleave the N-C bond in the β-lactam ring.

β-Lactamase Inhibitors

The inactivation of many β-lactam antibiotics by β-lactamase-producing organisms limits the effectiveness of these compounds in treating infections. A novel approach that extends the usefulness of these antibiotics has been to incorporate a β-lactamase inhibitor into the antibiotic formulation. Clavulanic acid and sulbactam are β-lactams with only weak antibacterial properties. However, they not only inactivate extracellular β-lactamases, but they

Table 49-1. Pharmacology and Pharmacokinetics of Penicillins

Agent	Route of administration	Oral absorption	$t_{1/2}$ (hr)	Protein bound (%)	Penicillinase resistance	Acid stable	Spectrum of activities
Natural penicillins							
Penicillin G	o, IM, IV	15–30	0.7	60	No	No	Narrow
Penicillin V	o	60	0.8	80	No	No	Narrow
Penicillin resistant							
Methicillin	IM, IV	Minimal	0.45	40	Yes	No	Narrow
Nafcillin	o, IM, IV	Low	0.5–1.0	90	Yes	Yes	Narrow
Oxacillin	o, IM, IV	33	0.4–0.7	94	Yes	Yes	Narrow
Cloxacillin	o	49	0.5	95	Yes	Yes	Narrow
Dicloxacillin	o	37	0.8	98	Yes	Yes	Narrow
Extended spectrum							
Ampicillin	o, IM, IV	30–50	1.0–1.3	20	No	Yes	Broad
Amoxicillin	o	74–80	1.0–1.3	20	Yes	Yes	Broad
Carbenicillin	IM, IV	Minimal	1.1	50	No	No	Broad
Ticarcillin	IM, IV	None	1.2	45	No	No	Broad
Piperacillin	IM, IV	None	1.0	16	No	No	Extended

Key: $t_{1/2}$ = half-life; o = oral; IM = intramuscular; IV = intravenous.

penetrate cell walls and inactivate bound enzyme. These inhibitors of β-lactamase are called "suicide inhibitors" because, when they bind to β-lactamase, products are formed that covalently bind to the enzyme and permanently inactivate it.

Clavulanate potassium, the potassium salt of clavulanic acid, is presently available in combination with amoxicillin (*Augmentin*) and ticarcillin disodium (*Timentin*). Unlike the β-lactam antibiotics, clavulanic acid is excreted by glomerular filtration and therefore probenecid does not affect its serum levels. However, probenecid does extend the half-life of sulbactam.

Antibacterial Spectrum

The *natural penicillins* (penicillins G and V) are narrow-spectrum antibiotics and are only active against facultative gram-positive cocci and rods and gram-negative cocci (see Table 49-1). Several anaerobic gram-negative rods are sensitive to penicillin, with the notable exception of *Bacteroides fragilis*.

The *penicillinase-resistant penicillins* (methicillin, nafcillin, oxacillin, cloxacillin, and dicloxacillin) are active primarily against gram-positive cocci and *Staphylococcus aureus*. Both *Staph. aureus* and *Staphylococcus epidermidis* are sensitive to the penicillinase-resistant penicillins.

The *broad-spectrum penicillins* (ampicillin, carbenicillin, and ticarcillin) differ from the natural and semisynthetic penicillinase-resistant congeners in that they have activity against a number of aerobic gram-negative rods. For example, *Escherichia coli* and *Proteus mirabilis* are sensitive to ampicillin whereas *Enterobacter* and *Pseudomonas aeruginosa* are sensitive to carbenicillin and ticarcillin. Amdinocillin

is an unusual penicillin in that it has poor activity against gram-positive cocci but is extremely active against gram-negative bacteria. It is not effective against *P. aeruginosa* or anaerobic bacteria.

The *ureidopenicillins* (mezlocillin and piperacillin) are broad (extended)-spectrum agents, but unlike methicillin they are not active against penicillin-resistant *Staph. aureus*. In addition, both piperacillin and azlocillin have excellent in vitro activity against *P. aeruginosa*.

Pharmacokinetic Properties

Table 49-1 lists some of the pharmacological and pharmacokinetic characteristics of the penicillins and should be referred to for information on specific compounds.

Absorption

The oral absorption of most penicillins, with the exception of penicillin V and amoxicillin, is poor and is impaired by the presence of food; it is recommended that they be taken 30 to 60 min before eating. In general, peak serum concentrations are obtained 1 to 2 hr after drug ingestion.

Slight chemical modifications of some of the congeners result in marked changes in the compound's pharmacological properties. The addition of a bulky group to the basic penicillin molecule (methicillin, nafcillin, and oxacillin) protects the β-lactam nucleus against penicillinase. Cloxacillin differs structurally from oxacillin by a single chlorine atom, a difference that results in better absorption and higher blood levels. Addition of a second chlorine atom produces dicloxacillin, which has an extended half-

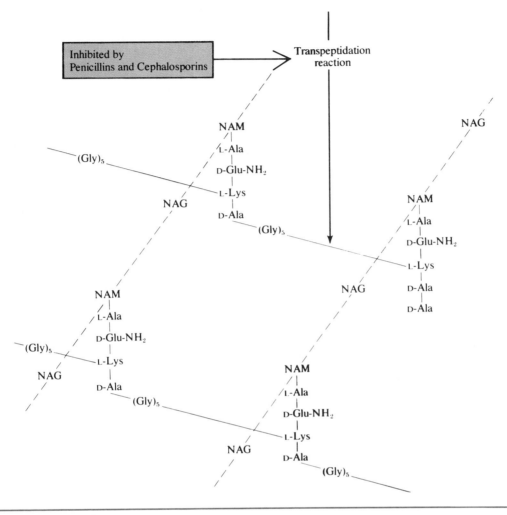

Figure 49-2. Mode of action of penicillins and cephalosporins. Both antibiotics interfere with cross-linking of adjacent peptidoglycan polymers. Absence of cross-linking results in a weakened cell wall. Action is noted only on cells that are growing, and therefore synthesizing, cell wall materials. NAG = *N*-acetylglucosamine; NAM = *N*-acetylmuramic acid; L-Ala = L-alanine; D-Glu-NH₂-D = glutamate; L-Lys = L-lysine; D-ala =D-alanine; (Gly)₅ = polyglycine. (Adapted from R. F. Boyd and J. J. Marr, *Medical Microbiology.* Boston: Little, Brown, 1980.)

life and gives even higher blood levels. Amoxicillin, which differs from ampicillin by the presence of a hydroxyl group, is better absorbed orally than is ampicillin.

Another approach aimed at increasing gastrointestinal absorption is the formation of an ester to produce a *prodrug* (proampicillin). Bacampicillin and hetacillin are two proampicillins that are inactive until they are absorbed and hydrolyzed. Bacampicillin is a biologically inactive ethoxycarbonyloxyethyl ester of ampicillin. The ester is stable in gastric fluids but is rapidly hydrolyzed to ampicillin in blood and tissue by nonspecific esterases. Bacampicillin is more rapidly absorbed than is ampicillin, and its

administration results in higher blood levels. Indanyl carbenicillin is another example of a prodrug. Carbenicillin is not absorbed from the intestinal tract but indanyl carbenicillin is. Hydrolysis of the ester results in the availability of the active form, carbenicillin.

The amount of drug bound to plasma proteins differs widely among the various penicillinase-resistant penicillins. Ampicillin is about 20 percent bound, whereas nafcillin, oxacillin, cloxacillin, and dicloxacillin are greater than 90 percent bound. These differences in protein binding do not appear to affect significantly the efficacy of the drug.

Penicillin G, methicillin, carbenicillin, and ticarcillin are *acid labile,* and biological activity is lost when they are given orally. However, they all are absorbed rapidly after an intramuscular injection, and peak blood levels are achieved in about 1 hr. *Repository* forms of penicillin G, such as procaine penicillin G and benzathine penicillin G, are absorbed slowly from intramuscular sites, and this results in low, but sustained, levels of penicillin for 24 hr and 4 weeks, respectively. The ureidopenicillins (mezlocillin, azlocillin, and piperacillin) are not acid stable and must be given parenterally.

Distribution

The penicillins are relatively insoluble in lipid and therefore penetrate cells and the blood-brain barrier poorly. In the presence of inflammation, however, increased permeability permits entry of these antibiotics into the cerebrospinal fluid (CSF). The penicillins are readily distributed into interstitial fluids, synovial fluid, bone, and serosal cavities; the penicillins will cross the placenta.

Metabolism and Excretion

Most of the penicillins are rapidly excreted in the urine as the active drug. Approximately 10 percent of the drug undergoes glomerular filtration, while elimination of most of the remainder is accounted for by *tubular secretion.* Blocking tubular secretion using *probenecid* results in higher penicillin blood levels. The penicillins also may be excreted into bile in high concentration.

The half-life of penicillin in serum ranges from 0.4 to 1.3 hr in the normal individual to as long as 20 hr in the anuric patient. Serum levels vary with the congener employed and generally reflect the different pharmacokinetic properties of each agent. The serum levels of nafcillin, oxacillin, cloxacillin, and dicloxacillin do not markedly increase in anuric patients because resultant increases in drug metabolism and biliary excretion compensate for the diminished urinary elimination.

The ureidopenicillins are given in large dosages and achieve high serum concentrations with half-lives varying between 0.8 and 1.3 hr. In the anuric state, drug accumulation occurs but to a lesser degree than with carbenicillin.

Clinical Uses

Penicillin G is the most active of the penicillins on a weight-for-weight basis. Therefore, whenever a penicillin is indicated (for prophylaxis or treatment), penicillin G or one of its longer-acting derivatives should be given primary consideration.

Streptococcal Infections

Serogroups A, B, C, and G streptococci and *Streptococcus pneumoniae* are extremely sensitive to the penicillins. During the 40 years that penicillin has been available, clinically significant resistance to this antimicrobial by the *β*-hemolytic streptococci has not developed. Recently, however, there have been reports, especially from Europe, of an increasing number of strains of *Strep. pneumoniae* that are penicillin resistant.

Pneumococcal pneumonia responds rapidly to penicillin G; oral penicillin V also has been used, but it is not recommended for initial therapy.

Pneumococcal meningitis is an extremely serious condition for which high dosages of penicillin G are used. Ampicillin or amoxicillin is often prescribed for infections, such as otitis media and chronic bronchitis, where *Haemophilus influenzae* frequently accompanies *Strep. pneumoniae.*

Streptococcus pyogenes is a frequent cause of acute tonsillitis and responds rapidly to oral penicillin V, although severe attacks may require parenteral therapy. Ten days of therapy are necessary to eradicate *Strep. pyogenes* from the throat and reduce the risk of poststreptococcal rheumatic fever and recurrent infection. In contrast, the occurrence of poststreptococcal glomerulonephritis is little influenced by penicillin therapy.

Bacterial endocarditis is most frequently caused by the viridans group of streptococci. Benzylpenicillin, given intravenously, is usually sufficient. Alternatively, 2 weeks of intravenously administered penicillin G followed by large oral doses of penicillin V or amoxicillin for a further 2 weeks is also satisfactory.

Enterococci are less susceptible to penicillin. When they cause endocarditis, a combination of penicillin G or ampicillin along with an aminoglycoside, such as gentamicin or streptomycin, given intravenously for a minimum of 4 weeks, is often used. This is one of the few situations in which a combination of antibiotics is used to obtain a synergistic bactericidal effect. Laboratory determination of the minimum inhibitory and minimum bactericidal concentration of antibiotic is a great help in the management of these serious diseases.

Resistance of *Staph. aureus* to penicillin develops because of *penicillinase production* by the organism. These strains make up approximately 90 percent of the isolates found in hospitals and are frequent causes of serious hospital-acquired infections. Even in the community, penicillinase-resistant staphylococci are in the majority. Some strains of *Staph. aureus* are resistant both to penicillin and the penicillinase-resistant penicillins.

Since *Staph. aureus* is frequently associated with local abscess formation, surgical incision and drainage of the lesion represent a most important part of the clinical management. Antibiotics are indicated for bacteremia as well as tissue infections, such as cellulitis, osteomyelitis, and pneumonia. Since endocarditis may complicate bacteremia, 4 weeks of high-dose antistaphylococcal penicillin therapy is often recommended.

Penicillin has been the drug of choice for all forms of gonorrhea for many years, despite the steady increase in resistance to penicillin that has developed. This situation has been compounded by the more recent occurrence of β-lactamase–producing isolates that are totally resistant to penicillin. Therapeutic regimens for uncomplicated gonococcal infection include amoxicillin (3 gm) or ampicillin (3.5 gm) by mouth, or aqueous procaine penicillin G (4.8 million units) divided and administered IM to two sites, together with 1 gm probenecid by mouth 0.5 hr before the penicillin injection. However, ceftriaxone or spectinomycin is the preferred agent. If the organisms are susceptible, crystalline penicillin G followed by amoxicillin or ampicillin can be used for gonococcal arthritis, disseminated gonococcal infection, or gonococcal infections complicated by salpingitis, prostatitis, or epididymitis. Likewise, gonococcal ophthalmia neonatorum can be treated with either aqueous crystalline penicillin G, plus frequent topical application of penicillin eye drops, or alternatively with ampicillin or amoxicillin and probenecid if the organisms are sensitive to the antibiotic.

Penicillin G is the most effective agent for the treatment of either meningococcal bacteremia or meningitis. However, it is unreliable for eradicating pharyngeal infections by *Neisseria meningitidis;* sulfonamides are usually effective in this condition, but where sulfonamide resistance is a problem, rifampin or minocycline is recommended.

Syphilis

Penicillin is the mainstay of syphilis therapy, irrespective of the stage of the disease. For early forms of syphilis (primary, secondary, and latent infection of less than 1 year's duration) either a single IM injection of 2.4 million units of benzathine penicillin G or 600,000 units of aqueous procaine penicillin G daily for 8 days is recommended. For infections of more than 1 year's duration (latent syphilis of unknown origin, cardiovascular, late benign, and neurosyphilis), either three IM injections of 2.4 million units of benzathine penicillin G at weekly intervals or aqueous procaine penicillin G, 600,000 units daily for 15 days, is recommended. In neurosyphilis, it is recommended that penicillin G, 2 to 4 megaunits IV every 4 hr for between 8 and 10 days be given or, alternatively, procaine penicillin G, 2 to 4 megaunits daily IM plus 0.5 gm probenecid daily by mouth for a total of 10 days. It is important to continue to monitor the progress of the treatment to determine clinical and serologic cure.

In over half the patients with early forms of syphilis, the *Jarisch-Herxheimer reaction* develops within hours of receiving penicillin therapy. This reaction consists of fever, chills, muscle aches, arthralgia, headaches, and a greater prominence of syphilitic skin lesions. The reaction is self-limiting and requires only symptomatic treatment. Recent evidence suggests that this reaction is caused by the release of endotoxin from the treponemes.

Anaerobic Infections

Penicillin G is highly active against a wide range of anaerobic and microaerophilic bacteria. It has been used effectively for treating anaerobic brain and lung abscesses and remains the drug of choice for actinomycosis. Clostridial infections, such as tetanus and gas gangrene, also are treated with penicillin G, although antibiotics play a secondary role to the use of antitoxin and surgical debridement, respectively, in these life-threatening conditions. *Bacteroides fragilis,* which is frequently isolated from abdominal infections, is generally resistant to penicillin. Its presence should be considered when treating infections suspected to be caused by anaerobic organisms. Trench mouth, which is associated with fusobacterial infections, responds rapidly to penicillin G.

Haemophilus influenzae Infections

Ampicillin was the drug of choice in the treatment of meningitis, osteomyelitis, epiglottitis, pneumonia, and septic arthritis. β-Lactamase-producing strains that are resistant to ampicillin now make up approximately a quarter of isolates and have resulted in a preference for the highly active cephalosporins, such as cefotaxime, ceftriaxone, or ceftizoxime. In infants and young children, otitis media and sinusitis caused by *H. influenzae* can be treated with oral ampicillin or amoxicillin. However, because of β-lactamase–producing strains, amoxicillin-clavolanate or an oral cephalosporin is being used increasingly often.

Typhoid Fever

High-dose ampicillin is an effective alternative to chloramphenicol for the treatment of infections caused by *Salmonella typhi* and *Salmonella paratyphi*. It is also occasionally useful in eliminating the carrier state in patients in whom the biliary or renal tract remains infected. High levels of ampicillin are obtained in the biliary tract if the gallbladder is normal and its ability to contract is preserved. The rate of appearance of drug-resistant strains is increasing, and an alternative choice for treatment is ciprofloxacin.

Urinary Tract Infections

Ampicillin and amdinocillin achieve high levels in urine and are effective against *E. coli, P. mirabilis,* and the enterococci, which are frequent causes of urinary tract infection. Drug resistance among uropathogens has increased, so that the penicillins have become second-line agents. The indanyl ester of carbenicillin is occasionally useful for the oral treatment of urinary tract infections caused by *P. aeruginosa* and indole-positive *Proteus* species.

Mezlocillin and piperacillin are highly active against many gram-negative enteric bacteria responsible for a wide range of serious infections of the urinary, respiratory, and biliary tracts as well as intraabdominal sepsis. Azlocillin is less active against gram-negative enteric bacteria but is more active against *P. aeruginosa,* for which it is widely prescribed in combination with an aminoglycoside. In many ways, piperacillin combines the spectrum, indications, and efficacy of mezlocillin and azlocillin. Pending the results of laboratory investigation, piperacillin is used in the empirical treatment of serious infections, often in combination with an aminoglycoside.

Other Infections

Other conditions in which penicillin G is the agent of choice include leptospirosis, *Pasteurella multocida* infections, and rat-bite fever. Ampicillin is the drug of choice for treatment of *Listeria monocytogenes* infections.

Rheumatic Fever

Penicillin has been used prophylactically to prevent recurrent attacks of acute rheumatic fever. Benzathine penicillin G, 1.2 million units IM every 4 weeks, will provide serum levels above the minimal inhibitory concentration for *Strep. pyogenes.* Alternatively, either 200,000 units of penicillin G or 250 mg of penicillin V, twice daily by mouth, can be used. It is not infrequent for this regimen to be given for life, although it is unusual for an adult to have a further attack of acute rheumatic fever once a 5-year attack-free period has elapsed.

Bacterial Endocarditis

Penicillins are used prophylactically to prevent bacterial endocarditis of either prosthetic or damaged heart valves in patients with congenital or acquired disease. The principle behind the treatment is to provide high blood levels at the time of a surgical procedure and for a subsequent period of 24 hr, thereby eliminating any transient bacteremia that may result. The penicillins, either alone or in combination with an aminoglycoside, such as streptomycin or gentamicin, provide an effective regimen. The serious consequences of an infection to a prosthetic heart valve also warrant the prophylactic use of antimicrobial agents.

Most dental procedures and upper respiratory tract procedures such as bronchoscopy, adenoidectomy, and ton-

sillectomy carry the risk of inducing bacteremia with the viridans streptococci; hence prophylaxis is directed toward these organisms. On the other hand, gastrointestinal surgery and surgery or instrumentation of the genitourinary tract can induce an enterococcal bacteremia; prophylaxis requires modification for this potential pathogen. Recommendations have been made by the American Heart Association and should be consulted for appropriate treatment. Prosthetic heart valves are occasionally infected at the time of surgery by *Staph. aureus* or *epidermidis.* A semisynthetic penicillin (such as methicillin or oxacillin) or cephalothin and, less often, vancomycin is frequently used to prevent infection introduced at the time of valve insertion.

Adverse Reactions

The penicillins are among the most widely used and least toxic antibiotics available. However, adverse reactions may range from the trivial to the life threatening and include both hypersensitivity reactions and direct toxic effects. Direct toxicity to benzylpenicillin is rare and tends to be related to prolonged high dosage. Neurotoxicity resulting in convulsions has followed intrathecal injections of penicillin, although this method of administration is rarely indicated.

Glossitis and stomatitis occur infrequently, but superinfection by *Candida albicans,* notably with ampicillin, can be troublesome. Diarrhea is frequently observed in patients receiving ampicillin and on occasion with amoxicillin and indanyl carbenicillin.

Large doses of the sodium or potassium salt of penicillin G can result in excessive blood levels of these cations. This effect may also occur with carbenicillin and ticarcillin, but it is less likely to result from the ureidopenicillins. Individuals particularly at risk are those with renal insufficiency.

Other side effects occasionally seen include a granulocytopenia associated with methicillin and cloxacillin. Oxacillin can cause an elevation of hepatic transaminase levels. Both carbenicillin and ticarcillin may interfere with platelet aggregation and, occasionally, cause bleeding problems. This is less frequently seen with the use of the ureidopenicillins.

No serious side effects are associated with clavulanic acid or sulbactam preparations apart from occasional nausea, vomiting, and diarrhea.

Hypersensitivity

The amount of drug required to produce a hypersensitivity reaction may be quite small, or the reaction may follow prolonged high-dose therapy. The overall incidence of hypersensitivity reactions to penicillins is 0.004

to 8.0 percent, according to the type of reaction and agent used. Several factors are important in determining whether a response will occur. One is the type of penicillin preparation; *procaine penicillin G gives the highest reaction rate* (about 5%), whereas both oral penicillins and benzathine penicillin G have the lowest (0.3%).

The route of administration and immune status of the patient also are relevant. The importance of questioning the patient carefully about previous drug reactions is obvious for the prevention of a hypersensitivity reaction. However, it is equally important not to accept a patient's statement concerning "allergic" reactions without careful questioning. To do so would deny the use of this most useful group of antibiotics and, in turn, may result in the use of more toxic and less effective agents.

Allergic reactions to the penicillins can be classified as immediate, accelerated, and late.

Immediate Reactions

These reactions usually occur within 20 min and most frequently follow parenteral, rather than oral, administration of penicillin. The incidence is estimated as 0.004 to 0.4 percent and, although a previous history of penicillin allergy is usual, it is not inevitable. *Anaphylaxis* is the extreme form of an immediate reaction and is characterized by apprehension, pruritus, paresthesia, wheezing, choking, fever, generalized urticaria, and edema, which may then lead to hypotension, shock, and loss of consciousness. Death can occur within a few minutes. In the United States, an estimated 300 deaths per year result from acute anaphylaxis. Other immediate reactions include angioedema, urticaria, rhinitis, wheezing, flushing, and diffuse pruritus.

Accelerated Reactions

These reactions occur from 1 to 72 hr after drug administration and are almost always manifested by urticaria; more rarely, laryngeal or angioneurotic edema is seen. Mortality is exceedingly rare.

Late Reactions

These reactions occur from 72 hr to several weeks after therapy begins and are characterized by skin rashes, which are usually maculopapular and itchy, but can be vesicular, bullous, urticarial, and rarely exfoliative. In addition, Coombs-positive hemolytic anemia, and, occasionally, serum sickness syndrome of fever, arthralgia, myalgia, lymphadenopathy, and splenomegaly can occur.

Skin rashes are most frequently associated with the semisynthetic penicillins. For instance, ampicillin carries a 9 percent risk of producing skin rashes. Furthermore, if ampicillin is administered to patients with infectious mononucleosis, the incidence of a skin eruption is as high as 90 percent; however, it appears to be a toxic reaction

rather than a hypersensitivity phenomenon. Ampicillin-related drugs, such as amoxicillin and proampicillins, produce a similar reaction.

Other hypersensitivity phenomena include eosinophilia, bronchospasm, fever (either alone or with accompanying rash), and arthralgia. Interstitial nephritis resulting in hematuria, albuminuria, pyuria, renal casts, and, occasionally, oliguric renal failure accompanied by a generalized allergic vasculitis, have been reported with some penicillins, notably methicillin. A contact dermatitis is occasionally seen in pharmacists, nurses, and physicians who prepare the drug for parenteral administration.

Mechanisms of Hypersensitivity Reactions

Penicillin is degraded in vivo to produce a number of antigenic breakdown products (see Fig. 49-1). The penicilloyl derivatives act as a hapten and combine with protein carriers to form the *major determinant* of penicillin allergy. Additionally, penicillic acid, which also can react with tissues, accumulates in aqueous solutions of benzylpenicillin stored at room temperature or at a low pH. Other breakdown products can act as haptens and are known as the *minor determinants;* they include benzylpenicillin itself and sodium benzylpenicilloate.

Penicillin antibodies are widely distributed in the population. They are either immunoglobulin M or G (IgM or IgG) antibodies and are largely directed against the benzylpenicilloyl derivative. These can be present in individuals who have never received penicillin therapeutically and probably result from exposure to small quantities of penicillin in milk and other foodstuffs.

Immediate reactions, including anaphylaxis, appear to be mediated by IgE antibodies to the minor determinants, whereas accelerated and late urticarial reactions are usually mediated by antibodies to the major determinants. The reactions terminate as blocking antibodies develop.

Two types of skin test preparations have been used to predict reactions in patients with a possible history of penicillin hypersensitivity. First, penicilloyl-polylysine (PPL) is commercially available and is used to determine sensitivity to the major determinant. PPL-positive tests indicate a high risk of accelerated urticarial reactions. To determine sensitivity to minor determinants, aqueous penicillin G is first given by a scratch test before intradermal administration. A positive skin test indicates a significant risk of anaphylaxis if systemic penicillin therapy is used. If penicillin therapy is clinically indicated and alternative agents are inappropriate, pretreatment with corticosteroids and antihistamines can reduce the severity of reactions. In addition to a history of a previous penicillin reaction, a strongly positive personal or family history of atopic allergy may be associated with an increased risk of hypersensitivity.

Management of Penicillin Hypersensitivity

Immediate reactions require the prompt administration of epinephrine (SC or IM); antihistamines, such as diphenhydramine; oxygen; and volume expanders and vasopressors if persistent hypotension develops. If airway obstruction occurs due to laryngeal edema, tracheostomy may be necessary.

Preparations

Penicillins are available in many dosage forms: tablets, capsules, oral suspensions, and intravenous and intramuscular injectables. Table 49-2 lists commercially available preparations.

Table 49-2. Commercially Available Penicillins

Generic name	Trade name(s)
Penicillin G sodium,	Pentids, Pfizerpen, SK-
Penicillin G potassium	Penicillin G
Penicillin V potassium	Pen-Vee, V-Cillin
	V-Cillin K, Ledercillin VK, Penapar VK, Uticillin VK, Veetids, Beepen, Betapen VK, Pen-Vee K, Robicillin VK
Aqueous penicillin procaine G	Pfizerpen-AS, Duracillin, Crysticillin, Wycillin
Amoxicillin	Amoxil, Polymox, Trimox, Utimox, Wymox, Larotid
Amoxicillin-clavulanate potassium[a]	Augmentin
Ampicillin	Omnipen, Polycillin Principen, Totacillin, Amcil
Ampicillin sodium with sulbactam sodium[b]	Unasyn
Penicillin G benzathine	Bicillin L-A, Permapen
Carbenicillin disodium	Geopen, Pyopen
Carbenicillin indanyl sodium	Geocillin
Cloxacillin sodium	Tegopen, Cloxapen
Dicloxacillin sodium	Dynapen, Pathocil, Dycil
Methicillin sodium	Staphcillin
Nafcillin sodium	Nafcil, Unipen, Nallpen
Oxacillin sodium	Bactocill, Prostaphlin
Ticarcillin disodium	Ticar
Ticarcillin disodium—clavulanate potassium[a]	Timentin
Bacampicillin hydrochloride	Spectrobid
Hetacillin	Versapen
Amdinocillin	Coactin
Azlocillin	Azlin
Mezlocillin	Mezlin
Piperacillin sodium	Pipracil

[a]The addition of clavulanic acid extends the agent's antibacterial range to β-lactamase–producing organisms.
[b]The addition of sulbactam extends ampicillin's antibacterial range to β-lactamase–producing organisms.

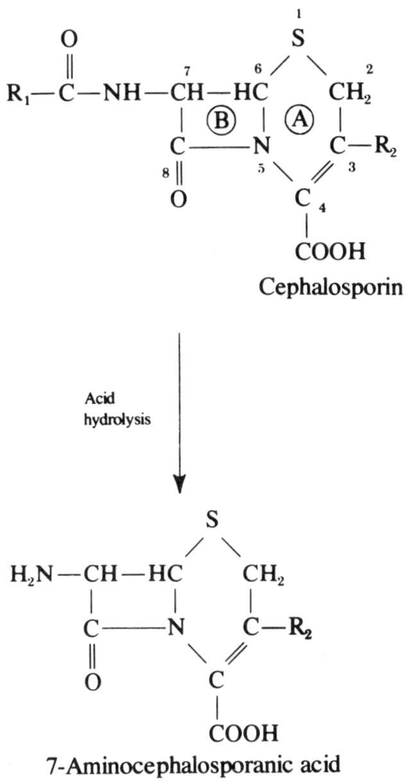

Figure 49-3. Cephalosporins. (A) = dihydrothiazine nucleus; (B) = β-lactam ring; R_1 and R_2 are sites for substitution.

Cephalosporins

Chemistry

The cephalosporins are produced by the mold *Cephalosporium acremonium* and have a structure similar to that of penicillin. The basic nucleus is a 7-aminocephalosporanic acid that is composed of a dihydrothiazine nucleus and a β-lactam ring identical to that of the penicillins (Fig. 49-3, Table 49-3). As with the penicillins, the β-lactam ring is the chemical group associated with antibacterial activity. The differing pharmacological and pharmacokinetic properties of the individual cephalosporins result from substitution of the various R_1 and R_2 groups. In general, substitution of the 7-acyl group (R_1) and C7 (β-lactam nucleus) determines the degree of antibacterial activity displayed by a congener, whereas substitution at position 3 (R_2) affects the compound's pharmacokinetic properties (see Fig. 49-3).

β-lactamases (penicillinases) inactivate some cephalosporins, but are much less efficient than *cephalosporinases* (β-lactamases specific for the cephalosporins). Resistance to cephalosporins also can result from a modification of

Table 49-3. Pharmacology and Pharmacokinetics of Selected Cephalosporins

Compound	Route of administration	$t_{1/2}$ (hr)	Protein bound (%)	Percent metabolized	Relative resistance to β-lactamase	
					Gram positive	Gram negative
First generation						
Cephalothin	IM, IV	0.5–0.7	65	33	3+	—
Cefazolin	IM, IV	2.0	74–86	Minimal	3+	—
Cephalexin	o	1.0	10–15	Minimal	3+	+
Cefadroxil	o	1.2–2.5	20	Minimal	3+	+
Second generation						
Cefoxitin	IM, IV	0.8	65–79	Minimal	3+	3+
Cefuroxime	IM, IV	1–2	50	Minimal	3+	3+
Cefaclor	o	0.6–0.9	25	30	3+	3+
Third generation						
Cefotaxime	IM, IV	1.0	40	*	3+	3+
Ceftriaxone	IM, IV	7–8	83–96	Minimal	3+	3+
Ceftazidime	IM, IV	1.8	17	Minimal	3+	3+
Cefotetan	IM, IV	3.0–4.6	88	Minimal	3+	3+
Cefpodoxine (prodrug)	o	1.9–3.7	18–23	Minimal	3+	3+
Cefixime	o	3.0	70	Minimal	3+	3+

Key: o = oral; IM = intramuscular; IV = intravenous.
*50% metabolized to desacetyl derivative.

the microbial penicillin-binding proteins. Large numbers of cephalosporins are currently available and several others are undergoing clinical trial. These differ in acid stability and susceptibility to inactivation by β-lactamases.

Antibacterial Spectrum

The cephalosporins have been classified into *generations,* which indicate improvements in their antibacterial spectrum, stability to β-lactamase, and potency. Table 49-3 shows the pharmacological characteristics of some of the cephalosporins currently available.

The *first-generation* cephalosporins have a range of activity similar to that of the broad-spectrum penicillins, but are more resistant to the effects of some β-lactamases. In contrast to the penicillins, they are relatively ineffective against *Bacteroides* species, enterococci, and most indole-positive *Proteus* species.

The *second-generation* cephalosporins have greater stability against β-lactamase inactivation and possess a broader spectrum of activity to include gram-negative rods and anaerobic organisms. Cefoxitin is highly active against the majority of clinically significant anaerobic pathogens including *Bacteroides* as well as some *Serratia* species. On the other hand, cefamandole and especially cefuroxime have good activity against indole-positive *Proteus* strains, *Enterobacter* species, and also *H. influenzae,* including β-lactamase-producing strains.

The extended spectrum, or *third-generation,* cephalo-

sporins possess a high degree of in vitro potency, β-lactamase stability, and a broader spectrum of action against many common gram-negative enteric bacteria and anaerobes while retaining good activity against streptococci. They are less active against staphylococci than the earlier cephalosporins. This class of agents is ineffective in the treatment of enterococcal infections. They are highly active against *Neisseria* and *H. influenzae,* including β-lactamase-producing strains.

Pharmacokinetic Properties

Absorption

Some of the pharmacological properties of this large group of antibiotics are presented in Table 49-3. Cephradine, cephalexin, cefaclor, and cefadroxil are acid-stable cephalosporins, which are well absorbed from the intestinal tract and thus can be taken orally. Absorption of cephalexin is impaired by food.

Of the parenterally effective first-generation cephalosporins, cefazolin has the longest half-life (approximately 2 hr), and its administration results in the highest serum levels. Administration twice daily is sufficient to maintain high levels, although more frequent dosing can be given for serious infections. Cephradine also can be given parenterally to produce high blood levels.

With the exception of cefuroxime axetil (prodrug of cefuroxime), cefixime, and cefpodoxime proxetil, the *sec-*

ond- and *third-generation cephalosporins* must be given by the parenteral route. These parenteral preparations give higher serum levels than the first-generation cephalosporins. Cefixime and cefpodoxime proxetil have longer half-lives than the orally administered first- and second-generation cephalosporins.

Distribution

The cephalosporins readily pass into pleural, pericardial, and joint fluids and reach high concentrations in skin, muscles, heart, stomach wall, liver, spleen, and kidney. Low concentrations are found in brain and bone. As with the penicillins, the cephalosporins are largely lipid insoluble and do not readily penetrate cells or the blood-brain barrier. The concentrations of the first-generation cephalosporins achieved in CSF in the absence of inflammation are not predictable. This is, in part, related to the metabolic instability of the first-generation parenteral cephalosporins. Inflammation increases the penetration of these drugs through the meninges, but they are not recommended for the treatment of meningeal infections. There is considerable variation among the first-generation cephalosporins in degree of protein binding (see Table 49-3). With the exception of cephradine (10% binding), the rest vary from 40 to 80 percent.

The second- and third-generation cephalosporins are also widely distributed throughout most body fluids and tissues; their degree of CSF penetration is increased by the presence of inflammation. Several of these compounds, including cefotaxime, ceftizoxime, ceftazidime, and ceftriaxone, have been used to treat meningitis. Cefotaxime is metabolized to desacetyl cefotaxime, which remains microbiologically active and is also detectable in the CSF. Ceftriaxone has an extremely long half-life permitting once- or twice-daily dosing for the treatment of meningitis and other serious infections. Cefuroxime, although a member of the second-generation cephalosporins, has also proved effective in the treatment of common bacterial meningitides, although it is less effective than the third-generation agents in treating *H. influenzae* infections. Serum protein binding of the second- and third-generation cephalosporins is also variable.

Metabolism and Excretion

Most cephalosporins, like the penicillins, are excreted into the urine in high concentration and in active form. Since they are *eliminated largely by tubular secretion,* serum levels can be increased through the use of probenecid. Depending on the congener employed, from 75 to 100 percent of the drug is excreted in the urine. Two of the first-generation cephalosporins, cephalothin and cephapirin, are deacetylated in the liver and excreted in urine. Most of the third-generation cephalosporins are also excreted in urine. Cefoperazone is deacetylated in the liver and excreted in bile.

Clinical Uses

Although cephalosporins have a spectrum of activity similar to that of the broad-spectrum penicillins, until recently there have been few primary indications for their use.

The oral cephalosporins have proved to be useful for the treatment of urinary tract and both upper and lower respiratory tract infections in patients who are hypersensitive to other compounds. However, the first-generation cephalosporins have variable degrees of activity against one of the major respiratory tract pathogens, *H. influenzae.* The increased activity of cefaclor, and to a greater extent cefixime and cefuroxime axetil, against *H. influenzae* gives them some advantage over other oral cephalosporins.

The second-generation parenteral cephalosporins are highly active against many gram-negative bacilli, including most strains of *H. influenzae.* As a result they have been used widely in the treatment of many common infections, including those of the skin and respiratory, biliary, and urinary tracts, and in intraabdominal sepsis. The use of second-generation cephalosporins has diminished somewhat since the advent of the third-generation compounds. Cefoxitin and cefotetan are both cephalosporins with good anaerobic activity and are widely used in the treatment and prophylaxis of intraabdominal and gynecological sepsis.

The third-generation compounds are used extensively in the treatment and prophylaxis of infections in hospitalized patients. Their broad-spectrum and high intrinsic activity, combined with their relative safety, has led to their widespread use in the treatment of many serious infections, including those caused by gram-negative enteric bacteria. In addition, their excellent activity against both streptococci and *H. influenzae* has made them truly broad-spectrum compounds. As such, they have been used extensively in the treatment of lower respiratory tract, urinary, and bile tract infections and the many causes of intraabdominal sepsis. Ceftazidime is particularly useful in managing *Pseudomonas* infections.

The third-generation cephalosporins are also highly effective in the treatment of penicillin-resistant gonorrhea, where ceftriaxone, 250 mg as a single IM dose, is recommended for uncomplicated gonorrhea. The cephalosporins are now widely used in the treatment of meningitis, where their activity against gram-negative bacilli as well as the more common causes of bacterial meningitis, such as pneumococcal, meningococcal, and *H. influenzae* infections, have proved to be extremely valuable. In the case of gram-negative bacillary infections, the third-generation cephalosporins are now a useful alternative to the aminoglycosides. Ceftriaxone is useful in the treatment of Lyme disease.

Adverse Reactions

The cephalosporins are relatively nontoxic. Local adverse effects include thrombophlebitis and pain at the site of an intramuscular injection. This reaction appears less commonly with cefazolin and cefamandole than with cephalothin. Allergic reactions, such as rash, urticaria, fever, serum sickness, hemolytic anemia, and eosinophilia, have been reported in 3 to 5 percent of patients taking these drugs.

Because of the similarities in structure between the cephalosporins and penicillins, it is not surprising that *patients who are hypersensitive to penicillin occasionally exhibit similar sensitivity when treated with a cephalosporin.* Therefore, it is important to inquire about both penicillin and cephalosporin hypersensitivity, especially the immediate variety, before administering any of these agents. Cephalosporin-associated nephrotoxicity is potentiated by the simultaneous use of diuretics (e.g., furosemide) or nephrotoxic agents, such as gentamicin.

Superinfections with *Pseudomonas, Klebsiella, Enterobacter, E. coli, Proteus, Serratia,* and *Candida* have been reported.

The use of the third-generation cephalosporins has resulted in two additional problems of superinfection. Overgrowth and infection caused by enterococci have been recognized and reflect the poor activity of this class of antibiotics against this organism. Reports of superinfection caused by *Enterobacter* species that are resistant to these cephalosporins have been noted and reflect the varying ability of these potent antibiotics to induce β-lactamase activity. Although relatively infrequent, these new problems are a cause for some concern.

A further complication of the use of selected extended-spectrum cephalosporins has been the development of coagulation disorders, which, on occasion, have resulted in overt bleeding. This problem has been recognized with a number of agents, including cefoperazone, cefamandole, and cefmenoxime.

A disulfiram-like reaction has also been noted with some of these agents, such as cefoperazone.

Preparations and Dosage

Preparations of the cephalosporins and their dosages are indicated in Table 49-4.

Table 49-4. Commercially Available Cephalosporins

Generic name	Trade name(s)
First generation	
Cephalothin sodium	Keflin, Seffin
Cefazolin sodium	Ancef, Kefzol
Cephapirin sodium	Cefadyl
Cephalexin	Keflex, Keflet, Keftab, Biocef, Cetanex, Zartan
Cephradine	Velosef, Anspor
Cefadroxil	Duricef, Ultracef
Second generation	
Cefamandole nafate	Mandol
Cefoxitin	Mefoxin
Cefuroxime sodium	Zinacef, Kefurox
Cefuroxime axetil	Ceftin
Cefonicid monosodium	Monocid
Ceforanide	Precef
Cefaclor	Ceclor
Third generation	
Cefotaxime sodium	Claforan
Ceftizoxime sodium	Cefizox
Ceftazidime	Fortaz, Tazidime, Ceptaz, Tazicef
Cefoperazone sodium	Cefobid
Cefotetan disodium	Cefotan
Ceftriaxone sodium	Rocephin
Cefixime	Suprax
Cefpodoxime proxetil	Vantin

Cephems and Penems

Two new classes of β-lactam antibiotics are currently in use. These new antibiotics contain a methylene group in place of the sulfur atom in the five-membered thiazolidine ring of penicillin (carbapenem) and in the six-membered dihydrothiazine ring of cephalosporin (carbacephem). The mode of action is the same as described for other β-lactam antibiotics, that is, inhibition of cell wall synthesis by interference with function of penicillin-binding proteins.

Imipenem

Imipenem is an analogue of thienamycin, a carbapenem produced by *Streptomyces cattleya* (Fig. 49-4). The addition of an *N*-formimidoyl side chain to thienamycin increases its chemical stability. The hydroxyethyl side chain on the β-lactam ring results in resistance to β-lactamase and the low molecular weight allows it to readily enter the cell through porins. The ease of penetration and resistance to β-lactamase imparts a broad spectrum of antimicrobial activity against most aerobic and anaerobic bacteria with the exception of *Xanthomonas maltophila,*

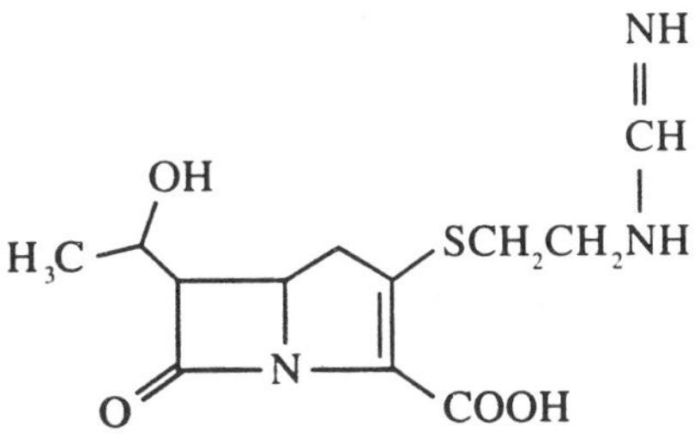

Imipenem

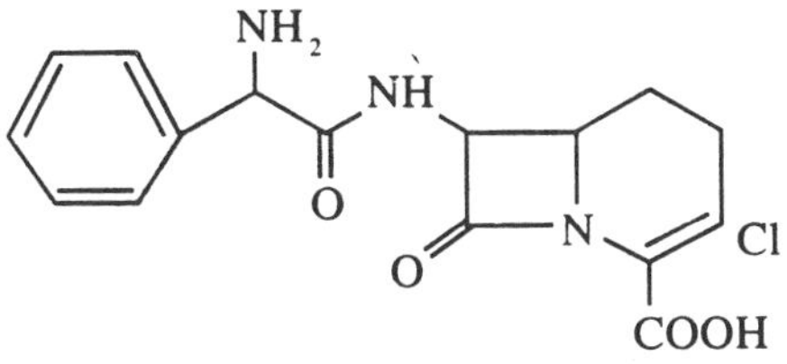

Loracarbef

Figure 49-4. Structure of imipenem (a carbapenem) and loracarbef (a carbacephem).

occasional *Pseudomonas* strains, and some *Staph. epidermidis.*

Imipenem is administered either intramuscularly or intravenously, and is generally well tolerated. It is hydrolyzed and inactivated in vivo by renal dipeptidase. This problem has been cleverly solved by the coadministration of cilastin, an inhibitor of renal dipeptidase activity, along with the carbapenem. Imipenem is administered with cilastin in a 1:1 ratio. Its half-life is approximately 1 hr. Binding to serum proteins is about 20 percent. Imipenem-cilastin (*Primaxin*) is available for IM or IV administration.

Loracarbef

Loracarbef is a synthetic β-lactam antibiotic of the carbacephem class (Fig. 49-4). It is an analogue of cefaclor but has a higher degree of stability. It is well absorbed (90%) after oral administration, although food interferes with absorption and results in lower peak plasma levels and a delay in reaching peak levels. Its half-life is one hour. Approximately 25 percent is bound to serum proteins. Loracarbef is not metabolized and is excreted by the kidneys.

In vitro this carbacephem is active against gram-positive and gram-negative aerobes and anaerobes, including

β-lactamase-producing *Staph. aureus, H. influenzae,* and *Moraxella catarrhalis.* Adverse reactions are essentially those expected with other oral β-lactam antibiotics. Loracarbef (*Lorabid*) is available in pulvules and an oral suspension.

Monobactams

Another interesting and potentially valuable group of compounds produced by several bacterial genera are the monocyclic β-lactams (*monobactams*). The natural monobactams have little, if any, antimicrobial activity. However, they are simple compounds that can be readily synthesized and modified. A synthetic derivative, aztreonam, is unique in that it has excellent activity against facultative gram-negative organisms and *P. aeruginosa;* it has no significant activity against gram-positive bacteria or anaerobes. The specific activity against facultative gram-negative organisms is related to the aminothiazole oxime moiety on the acyl side chain. The addition of two methyl groups and a carboxylic acid group on the oxime side chain enhances activity against *P. aeruginosa.* Aztreonam is stable to most β-lactamases (chromosomal and plasmid) and does not induce β-lactamases; this effect is related to the 1-sulfone side group and the 4-α-methyl group. The pharmacokinetic properties of aztreonam are similar to those of the penicillins and cephalosporins. The serum half-life is 1.7 hr. About 56 percent of the drug is bound to serum with about two thirds of an administered dose excreted into the urine. Of interest is the low potential of aztreonam to produce hypersensitivity reactions, even in patients with known β-lactam allergy. Most of the adverse reactions reported have been at the site of injection. Other effects, for example, hematological effects, nephrotoxicity, and pseudomembranous colitis, have been infrequently reported.

Aztreonam represents the first of a unique series of antibiotics that has been engineered to have activity directed against specific groups of organisms.

Aztreonam (*Azactam*) is available as 500-mg, 1-gm, and 2-gm powders for intravenous and intramuscular administration.

Supplemental Reading

Allan, J.D., Eliopoulos, G.M., and Moellering, R.C., Jr. The expanding spectrum of β-lactam antibiotics. *Adv. Intern. Med.* 31:119, 1986.

Balant, L., Dayer, P., and Auckenthaler, R. Clinical pharmacokinetics of the third generation cephalosporins. *Clin. Pharmacokinet.* 10:101, 1985.

Barriere, S.L., and Flaherty, J.F. Third-generation cephalosporins: A critical evaluation. *Clin. Pharm.* 3:351, 1984.

Barza, M. Imipenem: First of a new class of β-lactam antibiotics. *Ann. Intern. Med.* 103:552, 1985.

Blanca, M., et al. Cross-reactivity between penicillins and cephalosporins: Clinical and immunologic studies. *J. Allergy Clin. Immunol.* 83:381, 1989.

Brogden, R.N., and Campoli-Richards, D.M. Cefixime. A review of its antibacterial activity, pharmacokinetic properties and therapeutic potential. *Drugs* 38:524, 1989.

Brogden, R.N., and Heel, R.C. Aztreonam: A review of its antibacterial activity, pharmacokinetic properties and therapeutic use. *Drugs* 31:96, 1986.

Bush, K. Characterization of β-lactamases. *Antimicrob. Agents Chemother.* 33:259, 1989.

Carmine, A.A., et al. Cefotaxime. A review of its antibacterial activity, pharmacological properties and therapeutic use. *Drugs* 25:223, 1983.

Conference. Clavulanate/β-lactam antibiotics: Further experience. *J. Antimicrob. Chemother.* 24 (Suppl. B):1, 1989.

Emmerson, A.M. Cefuroxime axetil. *J. Antimicrob. Chemother.* 22:101, 1988.

Frampton, J.E., et al. Cefpodoxime proxetil. A review of its antibacterial action, pharmacokinetic properties and therapeutic potential. *Drugs* 44:889, 1992.

Nahata, M.C., and Barson, W.H. Ceftriaxone: A third generation cephalosporin. *Drug Intell. Clin. Pharm.* 19:900, 1985.

Omura, S. (ed.). *Macrolide Antibiotics. Chemistry, Biology, and Practice.* Orlando, Fla.: Academic, 1984.

Rolinson, G.N. β-Lactam antibiotics. *Antimicrob. Chemother.* 17:5, 1986.

Rolinson, G.N. β-Lactamase induction and resistance to lactam antibiotics. *Antimicrob. Chemother.* 23:1, 1989.

Waxman, D.J., and Strominger, J.L. Penicillin-binding proteins and the mechanism of action of β-lactam antibiotics. *Annu. Rev. Biochem.* 52:825, 1983.

Williams, J.D. The cephalosporin antibiotics. *Drugs* 34 (Suppl. 2):1, 1987.

Aminoglycoside-Aminocyclitol Antibiotics

Roger G. Finch and *Irvin S. Snyder*

Streptomycin and Related Aminoglycosidic Aminocyclitols

Chemistry

The aminocyclitol antibiotics include streptomycin, neomycin, paromomycin, kanamycin, gentamicin, tobramycin, netilmicin, amikacin, and spectinomycin. Except for gentamicin and netilmicin, the aminocyclitols are produced by members of the genus *Streptomyces;* gentamicin and netilmicin are produced by the mold *Micromonospora* species.

Structurally, all the aminocyclitols are similar (see Fig. 50-1 for a representative structure). With one exception, they all have an aminocyclitol moiety linked glycosidically to an amino sugar; they are referred to as *aminoglycosides* or *aminoglycosidic aminocyclitols*. The exception is spectinomycin, an aminocyclitol linked to a neutral sugar through a glycosidic bond (Fig. 50-2). Spectinomycin is an aminocyclitol but not an aminoglycoside. It is discussed separately at the end of this chapter. Paromomycin is used in the treatment of intestinal protozoa infections and is discussed in Chap. 56.

Mechanism of Action

All of the aminoglycosides are bactericidal and affect the bacterial cell by similar mechanisms. The aminoglycosides are cationic and bind to anionic sites on the outer membrane by displacing Mg^{2+}. This results in increasing permeability of the outer surface and permits enhanced uptake of additional drug. This loss of membrane integrity can, at least in part, account for the cidal effect of the antibiotic. Translocation of aminoglycoside across the cell membrane is energy dependent. The effect on the cell membrane may also interfere with ori C binding and DNA replication.

Inside the cell, the aminoglycosides have been shown to inhibit protein synthesis. Though they bind to the 30S ribosome, each has different binding sites. As one might expect, binding of streptomycin to ribosomes is not prevented by other aminoglycosides. Irrespective of differences in binding sites and some differences in mechanism of action, all the aminoglycosides affect protein synthesis, either by direct synthesis inhibition or by decreasing fidelity in reading the genetic code.

Streptomycin causes premature release of ribosomes from messenger RNA (mRNA) and stimulates polysome breakdown to monosomes. The monosomes resulting from polysome breakdown bind to mRNA but are inactive.

The errors in protein synthesis induced by the aminoglycosides have been related to a mispairing between codon and the aminoacyl transfer RNA (tRNA) and to faulty proofreading.

Resistance

Resistance to the aminoglycosides results either from reduced accumulation of the drug in the bacterial cell (decreased membrane transport), alteration of the ribosomal binding sites, or enzymatic inactivation. Mutational resistance of the ribosomal subunit is responsible for the high level of resistance to streptomycin that is sometimes encountered. Enzymatic inactivation is controlled by resistance (R) factors and is an example of transmissible resistance. This last mechanism is the most important in the development of resistance to all aminoglycosides except amikacin. Since amikacin is resistant to the adenylating,

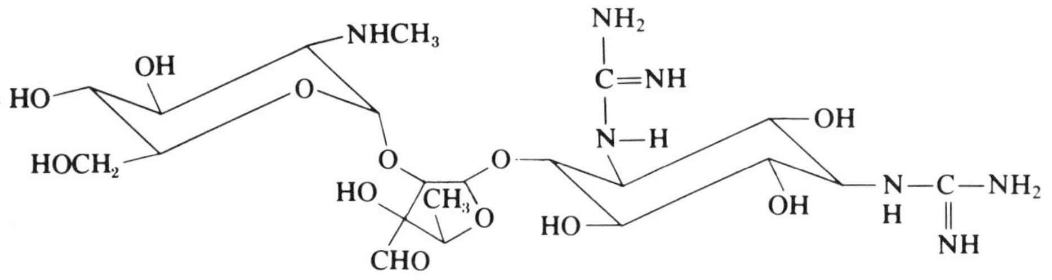

Figure 50-1. Structural formula of Streptomycin, an aminoglycosidic aminocyclitol antibiotic.

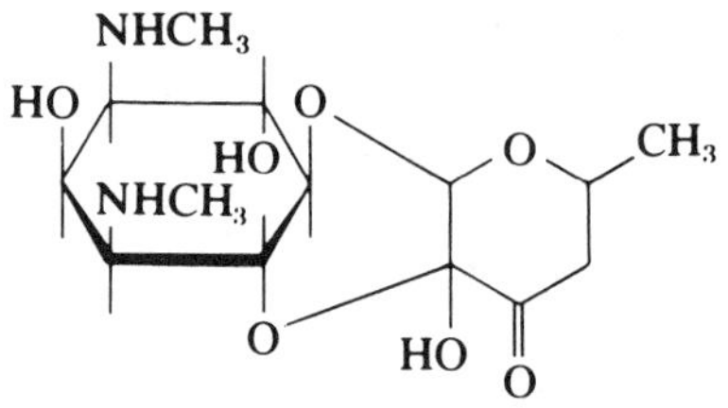

Figure 50-2. Spectinomycin.

phosphorylating, and acetylating enzymes that inactivate other aminoglycosides, resistance to amikacin is usually related to permeability changes.

Antimicrobial Spectrum

All aminoglycosides have a similar spectrum of antimicrobial action. They are most active against gram-negative enteric bacteria and some gram-positive bacteria, in particular *Staphylococcus aureus*. Anaerobic bacteria are generally resistant. *Mycobacterium tuberculosis* is susceptible to streptomycin, kanamycin, amikacin, and gentamicin.

Pharmacokinetic Properties

Absorption

The aminoglycosides are poorly absorbed from the gastrointestinal tract. Because of this limited absorption, neomycin, and paromomycin are occasionally given orally to reduce intestinal flora or control intestinal disease. Because of its toxicity, neomycin is not administered parenterally but is applied topically, since absorption through the skin and mucosa is poor.

Distribution

The aminoglycosides are highly polar molecules and therefore are generally insoluble in lipids. Consequently, they do not penetrate most cells, fatty tissue, or organs, such as the eye and central nervous system (CNS). They have a volume of distribution approximately equivalent to that of the extracellular fluid, which is about 30 percent of lean body weight and amounts to about 20 liters (L) in the average adult. Their binding to plasma proteins is minimal. Peak serum concentrations range from 4 to 10 μg/ml for gentamicin, tobramycin, and netilmicin and up to 25 μg/ml for amikacin, kanamycin, and streptomycin. To raise the level of aminoglycosides in the cerebrospinal fluid (CSF), intrathecal or, occasionally, intraventricular administration may be necessary. These antibiotics have a marked affinity for renal cortical tissue, where they are concentrated 10 to 50 times higher than in serum.

Metabolism and Excretion

The aminoglycosides are eliminated in unchanged form by glomerular filtration, with about 50 to 90 percent of an administered dose excreted in the urine within 24 hr. There is little, if any, biotransformation of the drugs. The half-life of the aminoglycosides is approximately 2 hr in patients with normal kidneys, but it is greatly extended in patients with impaired glomerular filtration (Table 50-1) when accumulation to toxic levels will occur unless the dosage is modified.

Clinical Uses

Streptomycin

Streptomycin was the first aminoglycoside to become available for clinical use. With the advent of more potent aminoglycosides, such as gentamicin, amikacin, netilmicin, and tobramycin, indications for its use have diminished.

Table 50-1. Characteristics of the Aminoglycosides

Drug	Half-life (hr)	Therapeutic serum level (μg/ml)	Toxic serum levels (μg/ml)
Streptomycin	2–3	25	50
Neomycin	3	5–10	10
Kanamycin	2.0–2.5	8–16	35
Gentamicin	1.2–5.0	4–10	12
Tobramycin	2.0–3.0	4–8	12
Amikacin	0.8–2.8	8–16	35
Netilmicin	2.0–2.5	0.5–10	16

Source: Adapted from *Drug Facts and Comparisons.* St. Louis: Lippincott, 1985. P. 1372.

Worldwide, one of the more important uses of streptomycin has been in the treatment of tuberculosis (see Chap. 53). It has been part of the standard triple-drug regimen for many years. However, its low degree of activity, greater potential for toxicity, the necessity for intramuscular administration, and the availability of other highly effective tuberculocidal agents have led to a reappraisal of the need for streptomycin in antituberculosis therapy.

The synergistic effect of penicillin G or ampicillin, in combination with streptomycin or gentamicin, makes the combination important in the treatment of confirmed enterococcal endocarditis and as prophylaxis in persons with known valvular disease undergoing surgery or instrumentation of the gastrointestinal or urogenital tracts.

Other indications for streptomycin include the treatment of plague (*Yersinia pestis*), tularemia (*Francisella tularensis*), and infections with *Brucella* species. In the last, a combination of streptomycin and tetracycline has been shown to be effective.

Kanamycin

Kanamycin is effective in the treatment of facultative gram-negative bacterial infections, with the notable exception of *Pseudomonas aeruginosa*. It has been used parenterally for the management of septicemia, meningitis, and urinary tract infections. However, it is now uncommonly prescribed because of the introduction of more active and less toxic drugs. Kanamycin is used in the treatment of tuberculosis when resistance or intolerance to standard drugs exists.

Neomycin

Serious toxicities associated with the systemic use of neomycin have restricted its use to oral and topical application. Its spectrum of activity is similar to that of kanamycin.

Orally administered neomycin has been used to reduce the facultative flora of the gut in hepatic coma, thereby reducing the load on the liver from endogenously produced amino acids. Neomycin, in combination with erythromycin, has significant activity on the anaerobic bowel flora and is used prophylactically in the preoperative preparation of patients undergoing large bowel surgery.

Neomycin is included in a wide variety of topical preparations, often in combination with other antibiotics and adrenal corticosteroids. By combining it with other antibiotics, such as polymyxin B and bacitracin, the antibacterial spectrum is increased, and the risk of drug resistance is reduced. However, prolonged skin application can result in sensitization and allergic reactions.

One of the hazards of neomycin use is its possible absorption either from the skin or gut mucosa. Skin absorption can occur much more readily if the epithelium is ulcerated. Although in normal individuals only 1 to 3 percent of an orally administered dose is excreted in the urine, this can be increased greatly by mucosal ulceration or prolonged gastrointestinal transit time. Ototoxicity has followed the topical use of neomycin while renal insufficiency also may increase the probability of neomycin toxicity.

Gentamicin, Tobramycin, Netilmicin, and Amikacin

These four aminoglycosides are essentially similar in their range of activity and clinical indications. They are all highly active against facultative gram-negative bacilli, including *P. aeruginosa* as well as *Staph. aureus*. They are indicated for the treatment of infections caused by *Escherichia coli*, *Klebsiella pneumoniae*, *Proteus* species, *Serratia*, *Acinetobacter*, *Citrobacter*, and *Enterobacter* species. In the treatment of *P. aeruginosa* infections, they are either used alone or in combination with carbenicillin, ticarcillin, azlocillin, or an antipseudomonal cephalosporin. Such a combination is particularly valuable in the treatment of septicemia and pneumonia caused by *P. aeruginosa* in the granulocyte-depleted patient undergoing treatment for hematologic malignancies, since synergistic inhibition can be demonstrated against about half the strains.

The activity of these aminoglycosides against other facultative gram-negative organisms makes them useful in treating a wide range of infections, such as septicemia, meningitis, urinary tract infections, pneumonia, endocarditis, and bone and joint infections. They also are used in the initial therapy of sepsis, before the causative pathogen has been identified and its sensitivities known. A combination of penicillin (or ampicillin) and gentamicin or streptomycin is useful in the treatment of enterococcal endocarditis.

The choice of a particular aminoglycoside is determined by microbial susceptibility testing, but where all appear to be equally effective, toxic manifestations also need to be considered. Gentamicin has been in clinical use for many years and, at present, remains the most widely used drug against sensitive bacteria. However, tobramycin and netilmicin are somewhat less nephrotoxic and probably less ototoxic than either gentamicin or amikacin.

A variety of dosage regimens are in use, but most employ a loading dose based on the weight and age of the patient. Since toxicity is related to drug accumulation, it is advisable to monitor serum creatinine and plasma antibiotic levels in all patients and especially in those with renal insufficiency immediately before giving the next dose. The toxic serum levels are given in Table 50-1.

Experimental and limited clinical data suggest that aminoglycosides may also be effective when administered as a single daily dose. This produces high peaks and prolonged serum levels and also makes use of the prolonged postantibiotic effect of the aminoglycosides. The postantibiotic effect is the ability of a drug to interfere with multiplication after exposure to subinhibitory concentrations.

In patients with renal insufficiency, the dosage should be reduced in proportion to the serum creatinine levels. This can be achieved either by reducing individual doses and maintaining the same dosage interval or by keeping the individual doses constant and lengthening the dosage interval. Nomograms that take age, sex, weight, and renal function into consideration are available for determining the appropriate dosages of several of these agents. Gentamicin is sometimes administered directly into the CSF by the lumbar route or directly into the ventricular system. These routes are chosen in order to achieve therapeutic concentrations of antimicrobial in the CSF for the treatment of gram-negative bacillary meningitis.

Eye infections have been treated successfully with subconjunctival injections of gentamicin. Therapeutic levels are produced in the aqueous humor within 2 hr.

In some countries and in certain institutions in the United States, the incidence of gentamicin-resistant bacteria has increased to very high levels. In part, this has followed its topical use in the treatment of burns and other superficial infections and as part of a bowel decontaminating regimen in granulocytopenic states. Topical use of such a valuable drug is not encouraged.

Adverse Reactions

The margin of safety that exists between toxic and therapeutic concentrations of the aminoglycosides is narrow. The most frequently reported adverse reactions are nephrotoxicity and ototoxicity; the latter may be either cochleotoxic or vestibulotoxic. Ototoxicity follows the selective destruction of the outer hair cells in the organ of Corti with degeneration of the auditory nerve fibers. The aminoglycosides concentrate and persist for long periods within the endolymph and perilymph of the inner ear. Symptoms of ototoxicity may include tinnitus, deafness, vertigo, or unsteadiness of gait. High-frequency hearing loss is relatively common but is often undetected unless it progresses to a more severe hearing loss. Cochleotoxic injury is often irreversible. Streptomycin and gentamicin mainly affect vestibular function; kanamycin, amikacin, netilmicin, and neomycin mainly affect hearing. Tobramycin affects auditory and vestibular function equally.

The risk of drug toxicity increases with advancing age, underlying renal disease, preexisting hearing loss, or prior administration of aminoglycosides and diuretics. Nephrotoxicity is related to the rapid uptake of the drug by the proximal tubular cells and subsequent active concentration of the drug within the renal cortex to some 5 to 50 times serum levels. Streptomycin is the least nephrotoxic of the aminoglycosides.

Aminoglycoside-induced neuromuscular blockade may result in weakness of skeletal muscles and respiratory depression. These reactions rarely occur in the absence of predisposing factors, such as myasthenia gravis, severe hypocalcemia, or the concurrent administration of neuromuscular blocking agents. The mechanism of neuromuscular blockade involves both the inhibition of the presynaptic release of acetylcholine and the blockade of the postsynaptic nicotinic receptor sites for this transmitter. The blockade can be reversed by the administration of calcium salts.

Other toxic reactions are uncommon, but they include skin rashes and fever. Malabsorption also has occasionally been observed following the oral administration of neomycin, kanamycin, and paromomycin.

Drug Combinations

The aminoglycosides are often combined with other antibiotics. However, certain drug incompatibilities must be kept in mind when this is done. For instance, gentamicin is inactivated if premixed with carbenicillin or cephalothin. Aminoglycoside activity is decreased in acid conditions, and acidifying agents should not be used with these antibiotics. Heparin precipitates aminoglycosides.

Preparations

Amikacin sulfate (*Amikin*) is a water-soluble aminocyclitol synthesized by the acylation of kanamycin A. It is available only for parenteral use.

Gentamicin sulfate (*Garamycin, Jenamicin*) is available for topical (ophthalmic ointment and solution) and parenteral use. A preparation for intrathecal use is available.

Kanamycin sulfate (*Kantrex, Klebcil*) is available as parenteral formulations.

Neomycin sulfate (*Mycifradin Sulfate, Neobiotic*) is marketed for oral and topical use. Although a sterile powder for injection is available, neomycin is not recommended for parenteral administration.

Netilmicin sulfate (*Netromycin*) is a semisynthetic water-soluble antibiotic of the aminoglycoside group. It is available for injection.

Streptomycin sulfate (available in generic form) is given parenterally.

Tobramycin sulfate (*Nebcin*) is a water-soluble compound administered intramuscularly or intravenously.

Spectinomycin

Structure and Mode of Action

Spectinomycin is an aminocyclitol that is structurally different from streptomycin and related compounds (see Fig. 50-2). It is not an aminoglycoside, because it contains an aminocyclitol linked glycosidically to a *neutral sugar* rather than to an amino sugar. Unlike the aminoglycosides, which are bactericidal, spectinomycin is *bacteriostatic*. This antibiotic inhibits protein synthesis by binding to the 30S ribosomal subunit. It binds to a specific site and inhibits translocation.

Antibacterial Spectrum

Spectinomycin is used only in the treatment of infections caused by *Neisseria gonorrhoeae*, where penicillin is contraindicated. Although spectinomycin shows moderate activity in vitro against a wide range of gram-positive and gram-negative bacteria, including some anaerobes, other drugs demonstrate superior activity and clinical efficacy. The fairly rapid development of resistance by some *Staph. aureus* is a problem with spectinomycin therapy.

Absorption, Distribution, and Excretion

Spectinomycin is not absorbed orally and is administered by IM injection. Peak serum concentrations of about 100 μg/ml are found about 1 hr after the injection of a single 2-gm dose. Spectinomycin does not penetrate the CNS and is not found in aqueous humor. It is excreted by glomerular filtration in its active form and produces high urinary concentrations. The total amount of a single injection appears in the urine within 48 hr.

Clinical Use

The indications for use of spectinomycin are in the treatment of infections caused by *N. gonorrhoeae* in the penicillin-hypersensitive individual and in the treatment of infections caused by penicillin-resistant strains of *N. gonorrhoeae*. Resistance to spectinomycin is rare in these organisms, but when it occurs, the bacteria generally remain sensitive to penicillin. Spectinomycin is less effective than penicillin in the treatment of gonococcal pharyngeal infections, and, unlike penicillin, it cannot be relied on to abort incubating syphilis. Serologic and clinical follow-up, therefore, are essential in such patients.

Adverse Effects

Few side effects are associated with spectinomycin therapy. Those effects reported include pain at the site of injection, rash, headache, dizziness, vomiting, and nervousness. Alterations in vestibular function are not found with this antibiotic.

Preparation

Spectinomycin hydrochloride (*Trobicin*) is available as a powder to be prepared for solution.

Supplemental Reading

Collatz, F., Carbon, C., and Humbert, G. Aminoglycosides (Aminocyclitols). In P.K. Peterson and J. Verhoef (eds.), *The Antimicrobial Agents Annual 2.* New York: Elsevier, 1987. P. 1.

Craig, W.A., Gudmundsson, S., and Reich, R.M. Netilmicin sulfate: A comparative evaluation of antimicrobial activity, pharmacokinetics, adverse reaction and clinical efficacy. *Pharmacotherapy* 3:305, 1983.

Holloway, W.J. Spectinomycin. *Med. Clin. North Am.* 66:169, 1982.

Hostetler, K.Y., and Hall, L.B. Inhibition of kidney lysosomal phospholipases A and C by aminoglycoside antibiotics. Possible mechanism of aminoglycoside toxicity. *Proc. Natl. Acad. Sci. U.S.A.* 79:1663, 1982.

Mattie, H., Craig, W.A., and Pechere, J.C. Determinants of efficacy and toxicity of aminoglycosides. *J. Antimicrob. Chemother.* 24:281, 1989.

Mitscher, L.A., and Martin, F.G. Nonlactam Antibiotics. In M. Verderame (ed.), *Handbook of Chemotherapeutic Agents.* Vol. 1. Boca Raton, Fla: CRC, 1986. P. 99.

Moore, R.D., et al. Risk factors for nephrotoxicity in patients treated with aminoglycosides. *Ann. Intern. Med.* 100:352, 1984.

Nordstrom, L., et al. Does administration of an aminoglycoside in a single daily dose affect its efficacy and toxicity? *J. Antimicrob. Chemother.* 25:159, 1990.

Ristuccia, A.M., and Cunha, B.A. The aminoglycosides. *Med. Clin. North Am.* 66:303, 1982.

Ristuccia, A.M., and Cunha, B.A. An overview of amikacin. *Ther. Drug Monit.* 7:12, 1985.

Spyker, D.A., and Guerrant, R.L. Dosage nomograms for aminoglycoside antibiotics. *Hosp. Formulary* 16:132, 1981.

Walby, A.P., and Kerr, A.G. Streptomycin sulphate and deafness: A review of the literature. *Clin. Otolaryngol.* 7:63, 1982.

Winstanley, T.G., and Hastings, J.G.M. Synergy between penicillin and gentamicin against enterococci. *J. Antimicrob. Chemother.* 25:551, 1990.

Tetracyclines, Chloramphenicol, Macrolides, and Lincosamides

Irvin S. Snyder and *Roger G. Finch*

All the antibiotics discussed in this chapter inhibit bacterial protein synthesis by an effect either on the 30S or 50S ribosomal unit. They are broad-spectrum antibiotics in that they inhibit the growth of both gram-positive and gram-negative facultative and anaerobic organisms. Although they have similar modes of action, they have different chemical structures and are produced by different species of *Streptomyces*. Structural analogues of these compounds have been synthesized to improve pharmacokinetic properties and antimicrobial activity.

Tetracyclines

Structure and Mechanism of Action

The tetracyclines have a common polycyclic structure (Table 51-1). Although several biological processes in the bacterial cell are modified by the tetracyclines, their *primary mode of action is through inhibition of protein synthesis.* Tetracyclines bind to the 30S ribosome and thereby prevent the binding of aminoacyl transfer RNA (tRNA) to the A site (acceptor site) on the 50S ribosomal unit. The tetracyclines affect both eukaryotic and prokaryotic cells but are selectively toxic for bacteria, because they readily penetrate microbial membranes and accumulate in the cytoplasm through an energy-dependent transport system for tetracycline that is absent from mammalian cells.

Resistance is related largely to changes in cell permeability and a resultant decreased accumulation of drug due to increased efflux from the cell by an energy-dependent mechanism. Other mechanisms, such as production of a protein that alters the interaction of tetracycline with the ribosome and enzymatic inactivation of the drug, have been reported.

Antibacterial Spectrum

The tetracyclines display broad-spectrum activity and are effective against both gram-positive and gram-negative bacteria, including *Rickettsia, Coxiella, Mycoplasma,* and *Chlamydia.* Tetracycline resistance has increased among pneumococci and gonococci, thus limiting their use in the treatment of infections caused by these organisms.

Although several congeners of the tetracyclines are available, they all have a similar spectrum of in vitro activity. Minocycline, however, is somewhat more active and oxytetracycline and tetracycline are somewhat less active than other members of this group.

Pharmacokinetic Properties

Absorption

These antibiotics are partially absorbed from the stomach and upper-gastrointestinal tract. *Food impairs absorption* of all tetracyclines except doxycycline and minocycline. Absorption of doxycycline and minocycline is improved with food. Since *they form insoluble chelates with calcium, magnesium, and other metal ions,* their simultaneous administration with milk (calcium), magnesium hydroxide, aluminum hydroxide, or iron will interfere with absorption. Because some of the tetracyclines are not completely absorbed, any drug remaining in the intestine may inhibit sensitive intestinal microorganisms and alter the normal intestinal flora.

Distribution

The tetracyclines are distributed throughout body tissues and fluids in concentrations that reflect the lipid sol-

575

Table 51-1. Structures and Some Properties of Tetracycline and its Congeners

Drug (trade name)	R_1	R_2	R_3	R_4	Route	Serum half-life (hr)	Serum protein binding (%)
Tetracycline hydrochloride (*Achromycin, Panamycin Hydrochloride*)	H	CH_3	OH	H	Oral, IV	8	25–60
Chlortetracycline hydrochloride (*Aureomycin*)	Cl	CH_3	OH	H	Oral, IV	6	40–70
Oxytetracycline hydrochloride (*Terramycin Hydrochloride*)	H	CH_3	OH	OH	Oral, IV	9	20–35
Demeclocycline hydrochloride (*Declomycin*)	Cl	H	OH	H	Oral	12	40–90
Methacycline hydrochloride (*Rondomycin*)	H	CH_2	—	OH	Oral	13	75–90
Doxycycline (*Vibramycin*)	H	CH_3	H	OH	Oral, IV	18	25–90
Minocycline hydrochloride (*Minocin, Vectrin*)	N | $(CH_3)_2$	H	H	H	Oral, IV	16	70–75

ubility of each individual agent. Minocycline and doxy-cycline are the most lipid soluble, while oxytetracycline is the least lipid soluble. The tetracyclines penetrate (but somewhat unpredictably) the uninflamed meninges and cross the placental barrier. Peak serum levels of 3 to 5 μg/ml are reached approximately 2 hr after oral administration. Peak serum levels achieved after the intravenous injection of tetracycline, doxycycline, or minocycline are 15 to 30 μg/ml; cerebrospinal fluid (CSF) levels are only one-fourth those of plasma.

The various congeners differ in their half-lives and their protein binding ability (see Table 51-1). The significant differences in serum half-life allows the grouping of the tetracyclines into subclasses: *short-acting* (tetracycline, chlortetracycline, and oxytetracycline); *intermediate-acting* (demeclocycline and methacycline), and *long-acting* (minocycline and doxycycline).

Metabolism and Excretion

The tetracyclines are metabolized in the liver and are concentrated in the bile. Bile concentrations can be up to five times those of the plasma. Doxycycline, minocycline, and chlortetracycline are excreted primarily in the feces. The other tetracyclines are eliminated primarily in the urine by glomerular filtration. Obviously, these tetracyclines have greater urinary antibacterial activity than those (e.g., doxycycline) that are excreted by nonrenal mechanisms.

Clinical Uses

Since their introduction, the tetracyclines, because of their broad spectrum of activity, have been used extensively to treat a wide range of infectious diseases.

There is little difference in clinical response among the various tetracyclines. The selection of an agent, therefore, is based on tolerance, ease of administration, and cost. The restriction of their use in pregnancy and in patients under the age of 8 years applies to all preparations.

Two tetracyclines have sufficiently distinctive features to warrant separate mention. Doxycycline, with its longer half-life and lack of nephrotoxicity, is a popular choice for patients with preexisting renal disease or those who are at risk of developing renal insufficiency. The lack of nephrotoxicity is related mainly to biliary excretion, which is the primary route of doxycycline elimination. Doxycycline is the preferred parenteral tetracycline. Minocycline is an effective alternative to rifampin for the eradication of meningococci, including sulfonamide-resistant strains, from the nasopharynx. However, the high incidence of dose-related vestibular side effects renders it less acceptable. Although minocycline has good in vitro activity against *Nocardia* species, further studies are necessary to confirm its clinical efficacy.

The tetracyclines are still the *drugs of choice* for the treatment of cholera, diseases caused by *Rickettsia* and *Coxiella*, granuloma inguinale, relapsing fever, the chlamydial diseases (trachoma, lymphogranuloma venereum, and psittacosis), and nonspecific urethritis. They are also effective in the treatment of brucellosis and tularemia and infections caused by *Pasteurella* and *Mycoplasma*, although other agents may be equally effective. For many other infections, tetracyclines are a second choice. These diseases include syphilis, chancroid, gonorrhea, actinomycosis, anthrax, and shigellosis.

Tetracyclines are clinically effective in acne (in which long-term, low-dose therapy is popular), Whipple's disease, tropical sprue, exacerbations of chronic bronchitis, and certain urinary tract infections. Mild to moderate attacks of pelvic inflammatory disease often respond to tetracycline, probably as a result of the drug's action on anaerobic bacteria.

Tetracyclines no longer can be entirely relied on in the treatment of streptococcal infections; up to 40 percent of *Streptococcus pyogenes* and 10 percent of *Streptococcus pneumoniae* are resistant.

Adverse Reactions

A wide range of side effects is associated with the administration of the tetracyclines. Oral administration can cause nausea, vomiting, epigastric burning, stomatitis, and glossitis, whereas intravenous injection can cause phlebitis. Given over long periods of time, use of these agents can result in a negative nitrogen balance, which may lead to an elevated blood urea nitrogen. Hepatotoxicity occurs infrequently but is of particular severity during pregnancy, when the combination of uremia and increasing jaundice can be fatal. In addition, these antibiotics are occasionally nephrotoxic and should not be administered with other potentially nephrotoxic drugs. Staining of both the deciduous and permanent teeth, as well as retardation of bone growth, can occur if tetracyclines are administered after the fourth month of gestation or if they are given to children less than 8 years of age; this is a further reason for avoiding their use during pregnancy.

Photosensitivity, observed as abnormal sunburn reaction, is particularly associated with demeclocycline and doxycycline administration. Superinfection may result in oral, anogenital, and intestinal *Candida albicans* infections, whereas *Staphylococcus aureus* or *Clostridium difficile* overgrowth may cause an enterocolitis. Minocycline can produce vertigo.

Preparations

Demeclocycline and demeclocycline hydrochloride (*Declomycin*) are available for oral administration as pediatric drops, syrup, capsules, and tablets.

Doxycycline (*Vibramycin Doxy*), doxycycline calcium (*Vibramycin Calcium*), doxycycline hyclate (*Vibramycin Hyclate, Vivox, Doxychel, DOXY-CAPS, Doryx, Ramycin*), and doxycycline monohydrate (*Vibramycin Monohydrate*) are analogues of oxytetracycline. The calcium salt is marketed as a syrup, the hyclate as capsules and powder, and the monohydrate as a powder for suspension.

Methacycline hydrochloride (*Rondomycin*) is a semisynthetic derivative of oxytetracycline and is available in capsules.

Minocycline hydrochloride (*Minocin*) is a semisynthetic derivative of tetracycline available for both oral and parenteral use.

Oxytetracycline hydrochloride (*Terramycin Hydrochloride, E.P. Mycin*), oxytetracycline (*Oxymycin*), and oxytetracycline calcium (*Uritet*): The hydrochloride salt is marketed as tablets and as solutions for intramuscular injection, the calcium salt as pediatric drops and syrup.

Tetracycline hydrochloride (*Achromycin, Tetracyn, Cyclinex, Sumycin, Panmycin Hydrochloride, Cyclopar, Robitet, Nor-tet, Retet, Tetralan, Tetram*): The hydrochloride salt penetrates tissues well and is marketed in a variety of oral, topical, and parenteral forms and dosages.

Chloramphenicol

Structure and Mode of Action

Chloramphenicol is a nitrobenzene derivative (Fig. 51-1). There are no other congeners of this broad-spectrum antibiotic available in the United States, although thiamphenicol is available elsewhere. Chloramphenicol affects protein synthesis by binding to the 50S ribosomal subunit and preventing peptide bond formation. It prevents the attachment of the amino acid end of aminoacyl-tRNA to the A site and the subsequent association of peptidyltransferase with the amino acid substrate. Resistance is due to changes in the ribosome-binding site, resulting in a de-

Figure 51-1. Chloramphenicol.

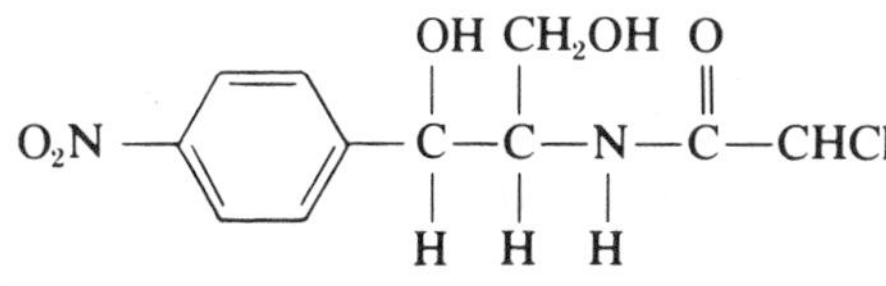

$$O_2N - \bigcirc - \underset{\underset{H}{|}}{\overset{\overset{OH}{|}}{C}} - \underset{\underset{H}{|}}{\overset{\overset{CH_2OH}{|}}{C}} - \underset{\underset{H}{|}}{\overset{}{N}} - \overset{\overset{O}{||}}{C} - CHCl_2$$

creased affinity for the drug, decreased permeability, and plasmids that code for enzymes that degrade the antibiotic.

The drug-induced inhibition of mitochondrial protein synthesis is probably responsible for the associated toxicity.

Antibacterial Spectrum

Chloramphenicol is a broad-spectrum antibiotic. As with tetracyclines, it is effective against gram-positive and gram-negative bacteria, including *Rickettsia, Mycoplasma,* and *Chlamydia.* Chloramphenicol is also effective against most anaerobic bacteria, including *Bacteroides fragilis.*

Pharmacokinetic Properties

Absorption

Chloramphenicol, a low-molecular-weight antibiotic, is rapidly and completely absorbed from the gastrointestinal tract. Unlike many antibiotics, chloramphenicol absorption is not affected by food ingestion or metal ions. Since absorption is rapid and complete after oral administration, parenteral administration is generally reserved for situations in which oral therapy is contraindicated, as in the treatment of meningitis and septicemia or where vomiting prohibits oral administration.

Distribution

Chloramphenicol penetrates body fluids and tissues well. Serum levels of 15 to 20 μg/ml are found 1 to 2 hr after oral administration and almost immediately after the IV administration of 1 gm. The biological half-life of chloramphenicol is 1.5 to 3.5 hr. Up to 60 percent of the drug is bound to serum albumin. The drug penetrates the brain and CSF and crosses the placental barrier.

Metabolism and Excretion

Chloramphenicol is inactivated in the liver by glucuronyltransferase and is rapidly excreted (80–90% of dose) in the urine. About 5 to 10 percent of the administered drug is excreted unchanged. Renal elimination is by tubular secretion and glomerular filtration.

Clinical Uses

The serious and potentially fatal nature of chloramphenicol-induced bone marrow suppression restricts its use to a few life-threatening infections in which the ben-

efits outweigh the risks. *There is no justification for its use in treating minor infections.* By restricting the daily dosage and also the total dosage, toxic manifestations can be limited, although the idiosyncratic aplastic anemia can still occur (see Adverse Reactions).

There are few absolute indications for the use of chloramphenicol since, in most instances, effective alternative drugs are available. Since effective CSF levels are obtained, it is a good choice for the treatment of pyogenic meningitis, particularly that caused by *Haemophilus influenzae.* It is also effective in treating other invasive infections caused by *H. influenzae,* such as meningitis, arthritis, osteomyelitis, and epiglottitis. The appearance of ampicillin-resistant strains of *H. influenzae* has increased the use of chloramphenicol in these situations, although the third-generation cephalosporins are preferred. If the patient is hypersensitive to β-lactams, chloramphenicol administration constitutes appropriate therapy for meningitis caused by *Neisseria meningitidis* and *Strep. pneumoniae.*

A major use of chloramphenicol is in the treatment of typhoid and paratyphoid fever, although ampicillin and trimethoprim-sulfamethoxazole are also effective. However, the clinical response to these agents is often slower. Plasmid-mediated drug resistance is an increasing problem in *Salmonella* species and therefore the final selection of an antibiotic will depend on laboratory testing. Other *Salmonella* infections, such as osteomyelitis, meningitis, and septicemia, are also indications for the use of chloramphenicol. However, nontyphoidal *Salmonella* enteritis is not helped by treatment with chloramphenicol or other antibiotics. In fact, it is unusual for antibiotics to shorten the period of infection; antibiotics commonly prolong the period of fecal excretion of *Salmonella.*

Chloramphenicol also is widely used for the topical treatment of both ear and eye infections. It is a very effective agent because of its extremely broad spectrum of activity and its ability to penetrate ocular tissue.

Chloramphenicol is an alternative to tetracycline for rickettsial diseases. Another indication for chloramphenicol is in the treatment of serious anaerobic infections caused by penicillin-resistant bacteria, such as *B. fragilis.* Clindamycin and metronidazole are other effective agents and are now preferred. Chloramphenicol, in combination with surgical drainage, is useful in treating cerebral abscesses caused by anaerobic bacteria, particularly those that are resistant to penicillin.

Adverse Reactions

Newborn infants, especially those born prematurely, are unable to adequately conjugate chloramphenicol to form the glucuronide; they also have depressed rates of glomerular and tubular secretion. Because of these metabolic deficiencies, high levels of free chloramphenicol may accumulate and cause a potentially fatal toxic reaction, the *gray baby syndrome*. This syndrome is characterized by abdominal distention, vomiting, progressive cyanosis, irregular respiration, hypothermia, and vasomotor collapse. The mortality is high. The syndrome also has been observed in older children and is associated with high serum levels of chloramphenicol, probably also arising from a defect in glucuronidation.

The most publicized adverse effects are those involving the hematopoietic system; they are manifested by toxic bone marrow depression or idiosyncratic aplastic anemia. The bone marrow depression is dose related and is seen most frequently when daily dosages exceed 4 gm and plasma concentrations exceed 25 μg/ml. It is recognized as anemia, sometimes with leukopenia or thrombocytopenia, but it is reversible on discontinuation of the chloramphenicol.

Aplastic anemia occurs in only about 1 in 24,000 to 40,000 cases of treatment. It is not a dose-related response and can occur either while the patient is taking chloramphenicol or days to months after completion of drug therapy. The aplastic or hypoplastic response involves all cellular elements of the marrow and is usually fatal. The mechanism is not known, but it occurs more frequently with oral administration. Thiamphenicol is apparently devoid of this idiosyncratic effect but may produce dose-related marrow toxicity.

Preparations

Chloramphenicol (*Chloromycetin*), chloramphenicol palmitate (*Chloromycetin Palmitate*), and chloramphenicol sodium succinate (*Chloromycetin Sodium Succinate*): The base is available for oral, topical (ophthalmic, skin, and otic preparations), and parenteral use. The palmitate salt is provided only as an oral suspension, while the succinate salt is available only in powder form.

Macrolide Antibiotics

Structure

The *macrolide antibiotics* are those that consist of a large lactone ring to which sugars are attached. Antibiotics in this group include erythromycin, clarithromycin, azithromycin, and oleandomycin. Erythromycin (Fig. 51-2) is produced by *Streptomyces erythraeus*, while *Streptomyces antibioticus* is the source of oleandomycin. Clarithromycin differs from erythromycin by an O-methyl substitution in the lactone ring. Azithromycin, chemically an azalide, is similar to erythromycin except that a methyl-substituted nitrogen is inserted into the lactone ring. Erythromycin

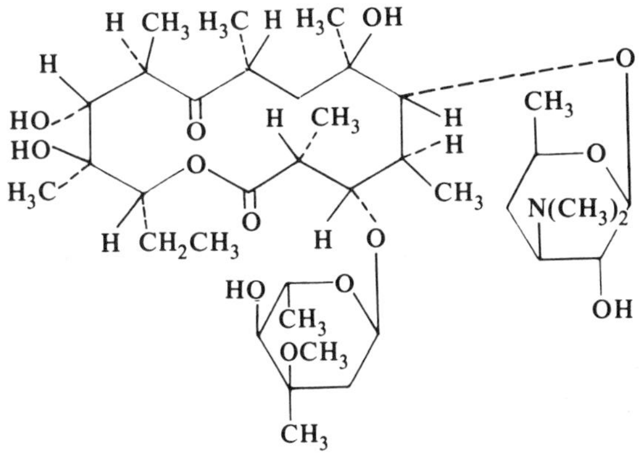

Figure 51-2. Erythromycin.

and its derivatives (clarithromycin, azithromycin) are the only macrolides in common use, although the acetylated derivative of oleandomycin (troleandomycin) is available for oral use.

Mode of Action

Macrolides bind to the 50S ribosomal subunit of bacteria, but not to the 80S mammalian ribosome; this accounts for its selective toxicity. Binding to the ribosome occurs at a site near peptidyltransferase, with a resultant inhibition of translocation, peptide bond formation, and release of oligopeptidyl tRNA. However, unlike chloramphenicol, the macrolides do not inhibit protein synthesis by intact mitochondria, and this suggests that the mitochondrial membrane is not permeable to erythromycin.

Antibacterial Spectrum

The macrolides are effective against a number of organisms, including *Mycoplasma* species, *H. influenzae*, *Streptococcus* species (including *Strep. pyogenes* and *Strep. pneumoniae*), staphylococci, gonococci, *Legionella pneumophila*, and other *Legionella* species. Staphylococci resistant to erythromycin are resistant to all macrolides. The hemolytic streptococci also exhibit varying degrees of cross-resistance to the macrolides and to lincomycin and clindamycin, although the macrolides are chemically unrelated to the last two agents. There are only minor variations in the antibacterial spectrum of the newer macrolides. Clarithromycin is very active against *H. influenzae* and *Legionella*, whereas azithromycin is superior against *Branhamella*, *Neisseria*, and *H. influenzae*.

Pharmacokinetic Properties

Absorption

The macrolides are absorbed from the intestinal tract. Food interferes with absorption and part of the dose is destroyed because of the relative acid lability of these antimicrobials. To minimize destruction and enhance absorption, erythromycin is administered as a stearate or oleate salt or is enteric coated. Because erythromycin stearate and estolate are not acid labile, these formulations result in higher blood levels. The O-methyl substitution of erythromycin that results in clarithromycin allows acid stability and better absorption with food.

Distribution

The macrolides diffuse readily into tissues and cross placental membranes. With the stearate and estolate formulations, serum levels of 5 to 15 $\mu g/ml$ can be achieved 1 to 4 hr after oral administration of 500 mg. CSF levels are about 20 percent of plasma levels, while biliary concentrations are about 10 times plasma levels. The serum levels of clarithromycin and azithromycin are low. However, these antibiotics concentrate in tissue and reach high levels.

Metabolism and Excretion

Erythromycin and azithromycin are excreted primarily in active form in bile with only low levels found in urine. Clarithromycin is metabolized to the biologically active 14-OH metabolite and is eliminated largely by the kidney. The half-life of erythromycin is approximately 1.4 hr, whereas the half-life of clarithromycin is 3 to 7 hr. For azithromycin, it is prolonged and approaches 68 hr. Partial deactivation occurs by demethylation in the liver.

Clinical Uses

Although erythromycin is a well-established antibiotic, there are relatively few primary indications for its use. These indications include the treatment of *Mycoplasma pneumoniae* infections, eradication of *Corynebacterium diphtheriae* from pharyngeal carriers, the early preparoxysmal stage of pertusses, chlamydial infections, and, more recently, the treatment of legionnaires' disease and *Campylobacter* enteritis.

Erythromycin is effective in the treatment and prevention of *Strep. pyogenes* and *Strep. pneumoniae* infections, but not those caused by the more resistant fecal streptococci. Staphylococci are generally susceptible to erythromycin and therefore this antibiotic is a suitable alternative drug for the penicillin-hypersensitive individual. It is a second-line drug for the treatment of gonorrhea and syphilis. Erythromycin is popular among pediatricians for the treatment of middle ear and sinus infections, since the causative agents, *H. influenzae* and *Strep. pneumoniae*, are usually sensitive.

The new macrolides have similar indications for use as erythromycin but with some additional areas of potential value. Clarithromycin has activity against *Toxoplasma gondii* and *Mycobacterium intracellulare*, and it is undergoing assessment in infections caused by these organisms. Azithromycin has been shown to be effective in pelvic infections and urethritis/cervicitis caused by chlamydia and gonococci.

Adverse Reactions

The incidence of side effects associated with erythromycin therapy is very low. Mild gastrointestinal upset with nausea, diarrhea, and abdominal pain is reported to occur more commonly when the propionate and estolate salts are used. Rashes are seen infrequently, but may be a part of a generalized hypersensitivity reaction that includes fever and eosinophilia. Thrombophlebitis may follow intravenous administration as may transient impairment of hearing.

Cholestatic hepatitis may occur when drug therapy lasts longer than 10 days or repeated courses are prescribed. The hepatitis is characterized by fever, enlarged tender liver, hyperbilirubinemia, dark urine, eosinophilia, elevated serum bilirubin, and elevated transaminase levels. Hepatitis has been associated with the estolate salt of erythromycin, but not with other formulations. Although the hepatitis usually occurs 10 to 20 days after the initiation of therapy, it can occur within hours in a patient who previously has had such a reaction. The hepatitis is believed to be the result of both a hepatotoxic effect and a hypersensitivity reaction; this latter effect is reversible on withdrawal of the drug. Erythromycin and derivatives induce hepatic microsomal enzymes and interfere with various drugs including theophylline and carbamazepine.

Preparations

Erythromycin (*Ilotycin, E-Mycin, Ery-Tab, Robimycin, ERYC*) is available as erythromycin estolate (*Ilosone*), erythromycin ethylsuccinate (*Erythrocin Ethyl Succinate, Pediamycin, EryPed, E-Mycin E, Wyamycin E*), erythromycin glucepate (*Ilotycin Glucepate*), erythromycin lactobionate (*Erythrocin Lactobionate-IV*), and erythromycin stearate (*Erythrocin Stearate, Wyamycin S, Ethril, Eramycin, Erypar*) salts. All the erythromycin forms have the same spectrum of activity. Erythromycin is marketed in a variety of oral, topical, rectal, and parenteral forms and dosages.

Clarithromycin (*Biaxin*) is available as tablets while azithromycin (*Zithromax*) is supplied as capsules of 250 mg.

Troleandomycin (*Tao*) is not widely used because of its toxicity and relatively limited effectiveness. It is available for oral use as capsules (250 mg).

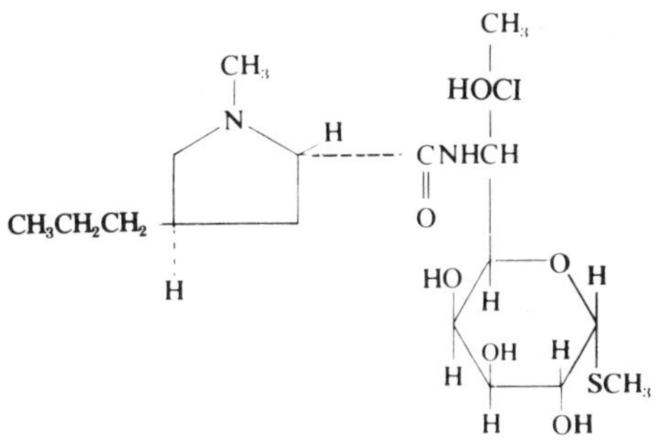

Lincosamides

Structure and Mode of Action

The lincosamide family of antibiotics includes lincomycin and clindamycin. Lincomycin is produced by *Streptomyces lincolnensis*. Clindamycin is the 7-chloro derivative of lincomycin (Fig. 51-3). They are both inhibitors of protein synthesis. They bind to the 50S ribosomal subunit at a binding site close to, or overlapping, the binding sites for chloramphenicol and erythromycin. They block peptide bond formation by interference at either the A or P site on the ribosome.

The antibacterial spectrum of clindamycin is similar to that of lincomycin but it has increased antibacterial activity and rate of gastrointestinal absorption. For these reasons, clindamycin has rendered lincomycin obsolete.

Antibacterial Spectrum

Lincomycin and clindamycin are active against staphylococci, streptococci (excluding enterococci), and most anaerobic bacteria.

Pharmacokinetic Properties

Absorption

Food in the stomach does not interfere with the absorption of clindamycin or lincomycin. Peak serum levels of 10 to 45 μg/ml can be obtained 1 hr after the IV administration of 600 mg of clindamycin. Approximately 90 percent of the antibiotic is protein bound.

Distribution

Lincomycin and clindamycin penetrate most tissues well, including bone. Therefore, bone and joint infections caused by susceptible organisms respond well to treatment with clindamycin. These drugs also concentrate within phagocytic cells, which may offer a therapeutic advantage. Lincomycin and clindamycin do not readily pene-

Figure 51-3. Clindamycin.

trate the normal or inflamed meninges. They do, however, pass readily through the placental barrier. Their half-lives are 2.0 to 2.5 hr.

Metabolism and Excretion

Both clindamycin and lincomycin are metabolized by the liver, and 90 percent of the inactivated drug is excreted in the urine. If renal function is impaired, the amount of drug excreted in the feces will be increased.

Clinical Uses

Clindamycin is highly active against staphylococci and streptococci other than enterococci. However, the adverse reaction of pseudomembranous colitis has limited its use to those individuals who are unable to tolerate other antibiotics and to the treatment of penicillin-resistant anaerobic bacterial infections.

Both clindamycin and chloramphenicol have excellent activity against anaerobic bacteria but have potentially life-threatening adverse reactions and should not be used without good justification.

Adverse Reactions

The major adverse reactions reported are hypersensitivity rashes and diarrhea. The rash is usually itchy, morbilliform, and generalized. Gastrointestinal intolerance with abdominal pain, nausea, and vomiting occurs infrequently. Diarrhea is fairly common but is rarely incapacitating. Hepatotoxicity and bone marrow suppression have been noted.

It is important to differentiate between gastrointestinal irritation and pseudomembranous colitis. In its most extreme form, the colitis results in mucosal ulceration and bleeding, and infrequently may necessitate colectomy. On rare occasions, it has proved to be fatal. The majority of patients in whom colitis develops have had recent surgery. Milder forms of the colitis are frequently reversible on discontinuation of clindamycin administration. Pseudomembranous colitis is caused by the overgrowth and production of toxins by strains of *Clostridium difficile* that are resistant to clindamycin; *C. difficile* is sensitive to vancomycin, which is given orally and is the drug of choice for treatment of this complication.

Preparations

Clindamycin hydrochloride (*Cleocin Hydrochloride*), clindamycin palmitate hydrochloride (component of *Cleocin Pediatric*), and clindamycin phosphate (*Cleocin Phosphate*) are semisynthetic derivatives of lincomycin that are available as capsules, as granules for suspension, and for parenteral use. Clindamycin is also available as a topical solution and as a gel.

Lincomycin hydrochloride (*Lincocin Hydrochloride*) is marketed in both oral and injectable formulations.

Supplemental Reading

Bartlett, J.G. Chloramphenicol. *Med. Clin. North Am.* 66:19, 1982.

Congress. Azithromycin (CP-62, 993): The first azalide antimicrobial agent. *J. Antimicrob. Chemother.* 25 (Suppl. A):1, 1990.

Cunha, B.A., Sibley, C.M., and Ristuccia, A.M. Review. Doxycycline. *Ther. Drug Monit.* 4:115, 1982.

Derrick, C.W., Jr., and Reilly, K.M. Erythromycin, lincomycin and clindamycin. *Pediatr. Clin. North Am.* 30:63, 1983.

Dhawan, V.K., and Thadepalli, H. Clindamycin: A review of fifteen years of experience. *Rev. Infect. Dis.* 4:1133, 1982.

Finch, R.G., and Mandragos, C. In *Antibiotics and Chemotherapy* (6th ed.). Edinburgh: Churchill Livingstone, 1992. P. 277.

Hardy, D.J., et al. Comparative in vitro activities of new 14-, 15-, and 16-membered macrolides. *Antimicrob. Agents Chemother.* 32:1710, 1988.

Kirst, H.A., and Sides, G.D. New directions for macrolide antibiotics. *Antimicrob. Agents Chemother.* 33:1413, 1419, 1989.

Klainer, A.S. Clindamycin. *Med. Clin. North Am.* 71:1169, 1987.

Kucers, A. Chloramphenicol, erythromycin, vancomycin, tetracyclines. *Lancet* 2:425, 1982.

Malmborg, A.S. The renaissance of erythromycin. *J. of Antimicrob. Chemother.* 18:293, 1986.

Mitscher, L.A., and Martin, F.G. Nonlactam Antibiotics. In M. Verderame (ed.), *Handbook of Chemotherapeutic Agents.* Boca Raton, Fla.: CRC, 1986. P. 99.

Nahata, M.C. Serum concentrations and adverse effects of chloramphenicol in pediatric patients. *Chemotherapy* 33:322, 1987.

Peters, D.H., and Clissold, S.P. Clarithromycin. A review of its antimicrobial activity, pharmacokinetic properties and therapeutic potential. *Drugs* 44:117, 1992.

Speer, B.S., Shoemaker, M.B., and Salyers, A.A. Bacterial resistance to tetracycline: Mechanism, transfer, and clinical significance. *Clin. Microbiol. Rev.* 5:387, 1992.

Symposium. Macrolides-lincosamides-streptogramins. *J. Antimicrob. Chemother.* 16(Suppl.A):1, 1985.

Wright, A.L., and Colver, G.B. Tetracyclines—how safe are they? *Clin. Exp. Dermatol.* 13:57, 1988.

52

Bacitracin, Glycopeptide Antibiotics, and the Polymyxins

Roger G. Finch and *Irvin S. Snyder*

Bacitracin and the polymyxins are polypeptide antibiotics. They are relatively toxic drugs and have only limited use in chemotherapy. Vancomycin, a glycopeptide, although not without side effects, is widely used. Teichoplanin is a new glycopeptide antibiotic that is available in other countries. Approval for use in the United States is expected. The modes of action of this group differ: Bacitracin and the glycopeptides affect cell wall synthesis, whereas the polymyxins affect the cell membrane. Bacitracin and the glycopeptides are used for the treatment of infections caused by gram-positive bacteria; the polymyxins are used for treating gram-negative infections and are active against *Pseudomonas aeruginosa*.

Bacitracin

Structure and Mechanism of Action

Bacitracin is a mixture of polypeptide antibiotics produced by *Bacillus subtilis*. As with penicillin, it contains a thiazolidine nucleus attached through L-leucine to a peptide composed of both D- and L-amino acids. However, it does not contain a β-lactam ring (Fig. 52-1). Bacitracin prevents cell wall synthesis by binding to a lipid pyrophosphate carrier that transports cell wall precursors to the growing cell wall. Bacitracin inhibits the dephosphorylation of this lipid carrier, a step essential to the carrier molecule's ability to accept cell wall constituents for transport.

Antimicrobial Spectrum

Bacitracin inhibits gram-positive cocci, including *Staphylococcus aureus* and streptococci, and a few gram-negative organisms.

Absorption, Distribution, and Excretion

Bacitracin is a *topical* antibiotic. Previously, it was administered intramuscularly, but the toxicity associated with its parenteral administration has precluded systemic use. The bacitracins are not absorbed from the gastrointestinal tract following oral administration.

Clinical Uses

Bacitracin is highly active against staphylococci and *Streptococcus pyogenes*. The high degree of activity against the group A streptococci is used in the laboratory as a means of differentiating between the Lancefield group A streptococci and other streptococci.

Bacitracin is well tolerated topically and is frequently used in combination with other agents (notably polymyxin B and neomycin) in the form of creams, ointments, and aerosol preparations. Hydrocortisone has been added to the combination for its antiinflammatory effects.

Bacitracin preparations are effective in the treatment of impetigo and other superficial skin infections. However, poststreptococcal nephritis has followed the topical treatment of impetigo and therefore oral penicillin therapy is preferred.

Adverse Effects

Because of the risk of serious nephrotoxicity, the *parenteral use of bacitracin is not justified*.

Preparations

Bacitracin and a variety of generic preparations are available in both regular and ophthalmic ointment forms.

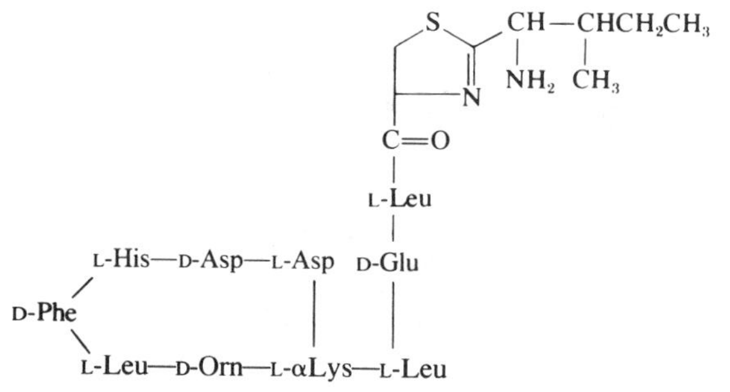

Figure 52-1. Bacitracin A, one of the bacitracin polypeptides. Bacitracin contains a thiazolidine ring, but not the β-lactam ring as does penicillin.

When bacitracin is used as one component of a mixture (see Clinical Uses), the zinc salt is commonly employed. It is also available as a powder for injection.

Glycopeptides: Vancomycin and Teicoplanin

Structure and Mechanism of Action

Vancomycin is a tricyclic glycopeptide antibiotic produced by *Streptomyces orientalis*. It has a complex structure and consists of a disaccharide (vancosamine and glucose), three substituted phenylglycines, two β-hydroxychlorotyrosines, *N*-methylleucine, and an aspartic acid residue. It is not related to the aminocyclitol antibiotics produced by other *Streptomyces* species.

Teicoplanin is derived from *Actinoplanes* (*Actinomyces*) *teichomyceticus*. It has two major components: a phosphoglycolipid (A₁) and five chlorine-containing glycopeptides (A₂).

The glycopeptides are inhibitors of cell wall synthesis. They bind to the terminal carboxyl group on the D-alanyl-D-alanine terminus of the *N*-acetylglucosamine-*N*-acetylmuramic acid peptide and *prevent polymerization* of the linear peptidoglycan by peptidoglycan synthase. They are bactericidal in vitro.

Antimicrobial Spectrum

The glycopeptides are narrow-spectrum agents that are active against staphylococci and streptococci. Like vancomycin, teicoplanin is bacteriostatic against *Streptococcus faecalis* in vivo. Gram-positive rods, such as *Bacillus anthracis*, *Corynebacterium diphtheriae*, *Clostridium tetani*, and *Clostridium perfringens*, are sensitive to the glycopeptides,

as are some isolates of *Neisseria*. The glycopeptides are not effective against gram-negative rods, mycobacteria, or fungi.

Absorption, Distribution, and Excretion

Vancomycin is poorly absorbed from the gastrointestinal tract, resulting in high concentrations in the feces. Except for the treatment of staphylococcal enterocolitis and pseudomembranous colitis, it is administered intravenously. Serum levels of 25 µg/ml are achieved 2 hr after the IV administration of 1 gm and about 55 percent is bound to serum protein. In normal adults the serum half-life is 5 to 11 hr. With impaired renal function, the half-life is 7 to 9 days.

After intravenous administration, vancomycin diffuses into serous cavities and across inflamed, but not normal, meninges. It is rarely used in the treatment of meningitis, although it has been administered by direct intrathecal injection. It is also given via ventriculoatrial or ventriculoperitoneal shunts when these become infected.

Renal excretion is predominant, with 80 to 90 percent of an administered dose eliminated in 24 hr. Only small amounts appear in the stool and bile after intravenous administration.

Teicoplanin, like vancomycin, is not absorbed from the intestinal tract. Peak plasma concentrations of 45 mg per liter (L) are obtained 30 min after an intravenous bolus of 400 mg. Peak plasma levels after intramuscular injection are achieved about 2 hr after administration. The drug distributes widely in tissues. Plasma protein binding is about 90 percent. The half-life approximates 50 hr, which is considerably longer than that of vancomycin. The long half-life allows once-daily administration. Like vancomycin, teicoplanin is excreted via the renal route.

Clinical Uses

Vancomycin and teicoplanin display excellent activity against staphylococci and streptococci, but because of the wide availability of equally effective and less toxic drugs, they are *second-line drugs in the treatment of most infections*. They have attained much wider use in recent years as a consequence of the reemergence of methicillin-resistant *Staphylococcus aureus* infections and, in particular, the growing importance of *Staphylococcus epidermidis* infections associated with the use of intravascular catheters and in patients with peritonitis who are on continuous ambulatory peritoneal dialysis.

Vancomycin is also an effective alternative therapy for the treatment of staphylococcal enterocolitis and endocarditis. The combination of vancomycin and either streptomycin or gentamicin acts synergistically against enterococci and is used effectively for the treatment or prevention of enterococcal endocarditis. Teicoplanin demonstrates similar synergy and is under evaluation for the treatment of endocarditis.

Staphylococcal vascular shunt infections in persons undergoing renal dialysis have been successfully treated with vancomycin. Two factors, the drug's prolonged half-life in patients with renal failure and the relatively small amount of drug that passes across dialysis membranes, combine to produce therapeutic drug levels for days after a single 0.5- to 1.0-gm dose.

Teicoplanin has the advantage of once-daily administration. It has also been used to treat peritonitis complicating peritoneal dialysis.

Vancomycin is also the drug of choice in patients in whom a *Clostridium difficile* colitis has developed.

Adverse Reactions

The earlier preparations of vancomycin were associated with significant toxicity. Purification of this antibiotic has led to a very useful product with little toxicity.

The major adverse effect associated with vancomycin therapy is ototoxicity, which may result in tinnitus, high-tone hearing loss, and deafness in extreme instances. Ototoxicity generally occurs when serum levels exceed 30 $\mu g/ml$ so that dosage modification is essential in the presence of renal failure. More commonly, the intravenous infusion of vancomycin can result in the occurrence of chills, fever, and a maculopapular skin rash often involving the head and upper thorax ("red man syndrome"). The red man syndrome is associated with increased levels of serum histamine. Vancomycin is rarely nephrotoxic.

Teicoplanin has advantages over vancomycin in that it rarely causes red man syndrome. Evidence for nephrotoxicity is lacking.

Preparations and Dosage

Vancomycin hydrochloride (*Vancocin Hydrochloride*) is available in powder form, both for oral (1 and 10 gm) and parenteral (500-mg ampule) use. Solutions prepared for oral use are stable for 2 weeks when stored at room temperature.

Teicoplanin (*Targocid*) is not yet available in the United States.

The Polymyxins

The polymyxins comprise a group of antibiotics produced by *Bacillus polymyxa,* two of which, polymyxin B

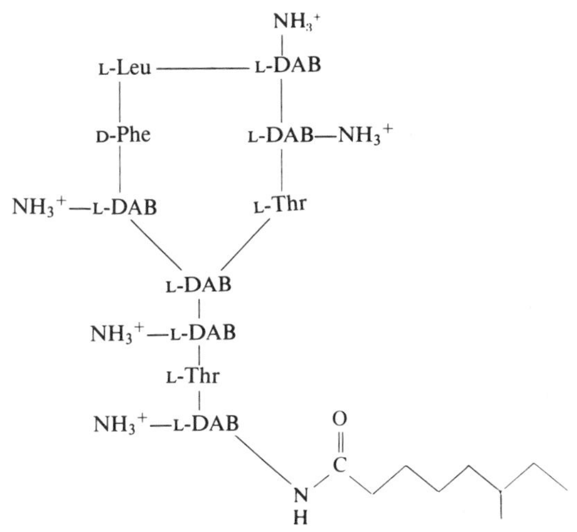

Figure 52-2. Polymyxin B. The terminal diamino-butyric acid (DAB) is acetylated by 6-methyloctanoic acid.

and colistin (polymyxin E), are used in the treatment of bacterial diseases.

Structure and Mechanism of Action

The polymyxins are polypeptide antibiotics (Fig. 52-2) that contain both hydrophilic and lipophilic regions. These antibiotics accumulate in the cell membrane and probably interact with membrane phospholipids. Most likely, the fatty acid portion of the antibiotic penetrates into the hydrophobic portion of the membrane phospholipid, while the polypeptide ring binds to the exposed phosphate groups of the membrane. Such an interaction would result in a distortion of the membrane, a loss of its selective permeability, leakage of metabolites, and inhibition of cellular processes.

These antibiotics also are toxic to mammalian cells, probably by a mechanism that is similar, if not identical, to that described for their antimicrobial activity.

Antimicrobial Spectrum

The polymyxins are active against facultative gram-negative bacteria, and *P. aeruginosa* in particular.

Absorption, Metabolism, and Excretion

Because polymyxin B and colistin are not well absorbed from the gastrointestinal tract they have been used for treating bacterial diarrhea. An intramuscular injection of the polymyxins results in high drug concentrations in the liver and kidneys, but the antibiotic does not enter the cerebrospinal fluid (CSF), even in the presence of inflammation.

The polymyxins are slowly excreted by glomerular filtration; the slow elimination rate is due to binding in tissues. Elimination is decreased in patients with renal disease, and drug accumulation can lead to toxicity. Sodium colistimethate, the parenteral preparation, binds less to tissue and is excreted faster than the free base.

Clinical Uses

With the advent of potent broad-spectrum antibiotics, such as the aminocyclitols and third-generation cephalosporins, the indications for the use of the polymyxins, with their serious potential for toxicity, are few.

In combination with neomycin, polymyxin B has achieved some popularity as a bladder irrigant to reduce the risk of catheter-associated infections. This use remains controversial. Polymyxin B also is applied topically in combination with other antibiotics in a variety of formulations, but this use also is not universally accepted since it has not proved to be efficacious.

Adverse Reactions

Colistin and polymyxin B cause similar toxicities, the most frequent of which is renal tubular necrosis. A preexisting renal insufficiency will potentiate the nephrotoxicity caused by these antibiotics.

Neurotoxicity is a rare adverse reaction recognized by perioral paresthesia, numbness, weakness, ataxia, and blurred vision. These drugs may precipitate respiratory arrest both in patients given muscle relaxants during anesthesia and in persons suffering from myasthenia gravis.

Preparations and Dosage

Colistimethate sodium (*Coly-Mycin M*) is a derivative of colistin that has been used in the treatment of urinary tract diseases, especially when infections do not respond to less toxic antimicrobial agents. It is administered parenterally.

Colistin sulfate (*Coly-Mycin*) is a water-soluble form of colistin for suspension; it is given IV or IM. A powder for oral suspension is also available.

Polymyxin B sulfate (*Aerosporin*) has been administered parenterally (e.g., IM, IV, intrathecally) by inhalation, and topically (ophthalmic ointment). The use of polymyxin B by inhalation to treat *Pseudomonas* infections is quite controversial. It is marketed as a powder for injection and in combination with other antibiotics, such as bacitracin and neomycin, in a variety of creams and ointments (e.g., *Neosporin*).

Supplemental Reading

Bailie, G.R., and Neal, D. Vancomycin ototoxicity and nephrotoxicity. A review. *Medical Toxicology and Adverse Drug Experience* 3:376, 1988.

Barna, J.C., and Williams, D.H. The structure and mode of action of glycopeptide antibiotics of the vancomycin group. *Annu. Rev. Microbiol.* 38:339, 1984.

Cheung, R.P., and Dipiro, J.T. Vancomycin: An update. *Pharmacotherapy* 6:153, 1986.

Healy, D.P., et al. Vancomycin-induced histamine release and "red man syndrome": Comparison of 1- and 2-hour infusion. *Antimicrob. Agents Chemother.* 34:550, 1990.

Johnson, A.P., et al. Resistance to vancomycin and teicoplanin: An emerging clinical problem. *Clin. Microbiol. Rev.* 3:280, 1990.

Katz, B.E., and Fisher, A.A. Bacitracin: A unique topical antibiotic sensitizer. *J. Am. Acad. Dermatol.* 17:1016, 1987.

Lagast, H., Dodion, P., and Klasterky, J. Comparison of pharmacokinetics and bactericidal activity of teicoplanin and vancomycin. *J. Antimicrob. Chemother.* 18:513, 1986.

McHenry, M.C., and Gavan, T.L. Vancomycin. *Pediatr. Clin. North Am.* 30:31, 1983.

Polk, R.E., et al. Vancomycin and the red-man syndrome: Pharmacodynamics of histamine release. *J. Infect. Dis.* 157:502, 1988.

Williams, A.H., and Gruneberg, R.N. Teicoplanin revisited. *J. Antimicrob. Chemother.* 22:397, 1988.

53

Drugs Used in Tuberculosis and Leprosy

Irvin S. Snyder and *Roger G. Finch*

A number of *Mycobacterium* species produce infections in humans that clinically resemble tuberculosis. However, only one organism, *M. leprae,* causes leprosy.

The incidence of tuberculosis has increased markedly since 1984, in part because of the number of human immunodeficiency virus (HIV)-infected persons, who are susceptible not only to *Mycobacterium tuberculosis* infection but also to infection with other *Mycobacteria* species. In addition, spread of the disease to persons in institutional settings, such as correctional facilities, shelters for the homeless, nursing homes, and hospitals, has increased.

Along with the increase in cases of tuberculosis has come an increase in multidrug-resistant (MDR) tuberculosis. Some of the MDR isolates are resistant to as many as seven of the commonly employed and useful antimycobacterial drugs. Clearly, this presents a major problem in treatment and control of this important disease.

Control of this epidemic will require a number of initiatives, including revitalization of tuberculosis control programs, improved and rapid methods for growth and antimicrobial sensitivity testing, the development of new antimycobacterial drugs, and increased suspicion on the part of clinicians and health care workers.

Treatment of Tuberculosis

Because of the slow growth rate of mycobacteria and their intracellular location, drug administration must be used for a longer period of time than is usual in other infectious diseases. The risks of adverse reactions, therefore, must be a major consideration in drug selection. Furthermore, to prevent the emergence of resistant strains which occur naturally at very low frequencies *it is vital to employ combined therapy with at least two agents to which the organism is susceptible.* For instance, resistance to isoniazid occurs in approximately 1 to 10^5 bacilli, whereas streptomycin resistance appears in approximately 1 in 10^6 bacilli. Thus, one can expect only 1

in 10^{11} bacilli to be resistant to both drugs. Since it is uncommon for there to be as many as 10^{11} bacilli in an individual with active tuberculosis, the risk of drug failure from bacterial resistance is quite small when combined drug therapy is employed. In addition to use of combined therapy, successful treatment and avoidance of selection of resistant organisms require patient compliance in taking the chemotherapy.

Antituberculous drugs are categorized into *first-line* and *second-line drugs* on the basis of their efficacy, activity, and risk of adverse reactions. The drugs and their common adverse reactions are summarized in Table 53-1.

Second-line drugs are indicated only when the *Mycobacterium tuberculosis* organisms are resistant to the first-line agents. In general, second-line drugs are more toxic, and in some cases less effective, than first-line drugs. The choice of a second-line drug is usually dictated by the results of susceptibility testing. Two, and preferably three, drugs to which the organism is sensitive are used against organisms resistant to first-line antimicrobial agents. Therapy with second-line agents may have to be prolonged beyond the standard period of treatment, depending on clinical, radiographic, and microbiological responses to therapy.

In general, drugs with similar toxicities should not be used together. For example, streptomycin, kanamycin, capreomycin, and viomycin are all potentially ototoxic and nephrotoxic. Some of these antimycobacterial agents have been described in earlier chapters and, except for their use in the treatment of tuberculosis, are not discussed further here.

The current recommended treatment for pulmonary tuberculosis caused by *M. tuberculosis* is a 6-month regimen of isoniazid, rifampin, and pyrazinamide for 2 months followed by isoniazid and rifampin for 4 months. Where isoniazid resistance is suspected, ethambutol should be added. A 9-month regimen of isoniazid and rifampin following an initial 2-week period of added ethambutol is also effective. In the case in which the organ-

Table 53-1. Drugs Used in the Treatment of Tuberculosis

Drug	Common adverse reactions
First-line drugs	
Ethambutol	Optic neuritis (rare with 15 mg/kg), rash
Isoniazid	Hepatitis, peripheral neuropathy, hypersensitivity
Rifampin	Hepatitis, fever, thrombocytopenia
Pyrazinamide	Hepatotoxicity, hyperuricemia
Second-line drugs	
Aminosalicylic acid	Gastrointestinal intolerance, hypersensitivity, hepatotoxicity, sodium overload
Capreomycin	Ototoxicity, nephrotoxicity
Cycloserine	Personality alterations, psychoses, seizures, rash
Ethionamide	Gastrointestinal intolerance, hepatotoxicity, hypersensitivity
Kanamycin	Ototoxicity, nephrotoxicity
Streptomycin	Ototoxicity, nephrotoxicity
Viomycin	Ototoxicity, nephrotoxicity

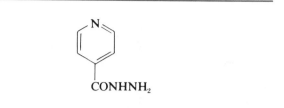

Figure 53-1. Isoniazid.

ism is resistant to isoniazid, rifampin and ethambutol with pyrazinamide should be given initially for at least 12 months. This regimen is also effective in extrapulmonary tuberculosis.

Isoniazid

Structure and Mechanism of Action

Isoniazid (isonicotinic acid hydrazide) (Fig. 53-1) may affect mycobacteria by inhibiting the synthesis of mycolic acids and inhibiting a desaturase enzyme. The double bonds produced by the desaturase are methylated to produce cyclopropane ring structures that are critical for the cell envelope. The mycolic acids are constituents of the bacterial cell envelope and their loss affects the integrity of the cell envelope and hence cell stability. Alternatively, isoniazid may be hydrolyzed to isonicotinic acid, which accumulates and competes with nicotinic acid in the synthesis of nicotinamide adenine dinucleotide (NAD). In vitro, isoniazid is bacteriostatic against resting organisms and bactericidal for dividing organisms. Resistance to isoniazid occurs and is due to the failure of the drug to enter the bacterial cell.

Pharmacokinetic Properties

Absorption

Isoniazid is water soluble and can be administered orally or parenterally. It is readily absorbed from the gastrointestinal tract, yielding peak serum levels in 1 to 2 hr. Absorption is reduced if antacids are administered concurrently.

Distribution

Isoniazid does not bind to serum proteins and readily distributes in tissue fluids. Therapeutic levels are found in pleural fluid, ascitic fluid, saliva, skin, muscle, and cerebrospinal fluid (CSF), both in the presence and absence of inflammation. An important attribute of the drug is that it penetrates caseous tuberculous lesions.

Metabolism and Excretion

Isoniazid is acetylated to acetylisoniazid by *N*-acetyltransferase, an enzyme present in liver, bowel mucosa, and kidney. The acetylated derivative and a small amount of unaltered isoniazid are excreted by the kidneys, with 75 to 90 percent of the drug being metabolized and excreted in 24 hr. The ratio of acetylisoniazid to free isoniazid is determined by the rate of acetylation.

Genetically rapid acetylators (see Chap. 4) will have a higher ratio of acetylisoniazid to isoniazid than will slow acetylators. Since acetylisoniazid is more rapidly excreted by the kidney than the parent compound, the overall rate of drug excretion will depend on whether the patient is a fast or slow acetylator. The blood levels of isoniazid also will depend on the rate of acetylation.

Clinical Uses

Isoniazid is among the safest and most active of the mycobactericidal agents. The high levels achieved in all body fluids, including CSF, make it an appropriate choice for all types of tuberculous infections. It is included in the *first-line* drug combinations and is also the drug of choice when single-agent therapy is employed as chemoprophylaxis in persons who show a positive purified protein derivative (PPD) skin reaction but have no radiographic or other clinical evidence to suggest tuberculosis.

The genetically determined rapid or slow inactivation of isoniazid is rarely important clinically although slow inactivators tend to develop a peripheral neuropathy more readily. If an individual has a severe preexisting renal insufficiency and is a slow acetylator, dose reduction is indicated to prevent toxicity. A single daily adult dosage of 300 mg for 6 to 9 months is usually sufficient when isoniazid is combined with one or more of the other antituberculous drugs. The rare occurrence of an isoniazid-induced pyridoxine-deficient peripheral neuropathy can be prevented by administration of 50 mg of pyridoxine daily.

Patients who convert from a negative to a positive tuberculin skin test should be considered for chemoprophylaxis. The risk of developing tuberculosis is greatest among recent skin test converters, particularly in the first year or so after conversion, when there is a 5 percent chance of developing active tuberculosis. This risk applies particularly to children below 6 years of age. Members of the same household and close associates of a patient with a recently diagnosed case should be skin tested at 3-month intervals even if their skin test is initially negative. Children, and some adults, may merit chemoprophylaxis even if the initial skin test is negative. Drug administration is stopped after 3 months if the skin test remains negative. *In HIV-infected persons, the risk of tuberculosis is high.* Chemoprophylaxis is recommended for those with skin test evidence of mycobacterial infection.

Since the risk of an isoniazid-induced hepatitis increases with age, chemoprophylaxis is not recommended in individuals over 35 unless some additional risk factor is present. These predisposing factors include long-term therapy with adrenocorticosteroids or immunosuppressant drugs and preexisting conditions, such as leukemia, lymphoma, diabetes mellitus, and gastrectomy.

Infections by *Mycobacterium kansasii* are usually sensitive to the standard multiple drug regimen, which includes isoniazid. *Mycobacterium avium-intracellulare* infections, however, frequently show in vitro resistance to many of the antituberculous drugs and generally are managed through the use of a combination of four or more drugs, including isoniazid, quinolone, or macrolide regimens. Surgery may be necessary if drug therapy fails.

Adverse Reactions

Neurotoxicity, hepatotoxicity, and allergic reactions have been associated with the use of isoniazid; the most significant of these is hepatotoxicity. Evidence of liver dysfunction (e.g., increased serum glutamic-oxaloacetic transaminase [SGOT]) is reported in 10 to 20 percent of patients receiving isoniazid therapy. Advancing age and underlying liver disease are predisposing factors. Although hepatotoxicity is reversible in most patients, even with continued isoniazid administration, some individuals will develop overt hepatitis. Rapid acetylators have a higher incidence of liver damage; this may be related to the appearance of *acetylhydrazine,* a product of acetylisoniazid metabolism, which in experimental animals has been shown to bind to liver cells and produce liver necrosis.

Neurotoxicity, primarily a peripheral neuritis, may occur in patients who are malnourished, chronic alcoholics, or slow acetylators. The symptoms include a numbness and tingling in the lower extremities and, occasion-

ally, paresthesias in the hands and fingers. Central nervous system (CNS) effects, notably excitability, also have been described. Pyridoxine administration prevents the neurotoxic effects of isoniazid, but it does not alter its bactericidal action. Rash, urticaria, fever, and other allergic reactions also may occur during isoniazid therapy.

Preparations

Isoniazid (*INH, Laniazid, Teebaconin, Nydrazid*) is available for both oral and parenteral use.

Rifampin

Structure and Mechanism of Action

Rifampin is a semisynthetic antimicrobial agent derived from rifamycin B, one of the rifamycins produced by *Streptomyces mediterranei.* It is a large, lipid-soluble molecule (Fig. 53-2). Its mode of action involves *inhibition of RNA synthesis* through the formation of a stable complex with DNA-dependent RNA polymerase, thereby preventing the action of the enzyme. The receptor for rifampin is the β subunit of the enzyme. The polymerase in rifampin-resistant strains does not bind rifampin. Mammalian enzymes are not affected by the drug.

Antibacterial Spectrum

In addition to being a potent antituberculous drug, rifampin has broad activity against other bacteria, notably staphylococci, as well as chlamydiae and certain viruses.

Pharmacokinetic Properties

Absorption

Rifampin is administered orally and is well absorbed from the gastrointestinal tract, with peak blood levels achieved after 2 to 4 hr. Drug absorption is impaired if rifampin is taken immediately after a meal.

Figure 53-2. Rifampin.

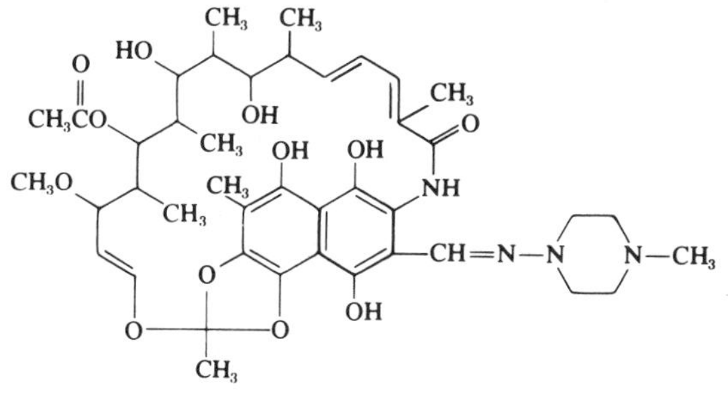

Although rifampin's half-life is approximately 3 to 5 hr after an initial dose of 600 mg, this can be reduced to 2 hr after 1 or 2 weeks of daily administration. This is probably due to an induction of drug-metabolizing enzymes. About 85 percent of the drug is bound to protein.

Distribution

Rifampin penetrates tissues well and therapeutic levels are achieved in lung, bronchial secretions, CSF, pleural fluid, liver, bile, urine, and the tuberculous cavity. It penetrates macrophages and is effective against extracellular as well as intracellular organisms.

Metabolism and Excretion

Rifampin is deacetylated in the liver and excreted primarily in the bile, with a smaller amount appearing in the urine. Unlike many other antimicrobial agents, in rifampin the deacetylated drug is active. Rifampin administration can result in the induction of liver enzymes and enhancement of drug metabolism. The effectiveness of concomitantly administered drugs that are also substrates for microsomal enzymes may be decreased if induction occurs.

Clinical Uses

Rifampin is a *first-line* antituberculous drug. The cost of rifampin, however, is a major obstacle to its use in developing countries. It is highly bactericidal and has permitted shorter courses of therapy than in the past.

The drug is well tolerated but, on occasions, it can be hepatotoxic. As in all antituberculous regimens, the necessity for regular and continuous rifampin dosage cannot be stressed too highly. Patient noncompliance is a well-known cause of relapse. Intermittent or irregular therapy frequently results in the appearance of an immune-mediated syndrome of fever, malaise, and influenza-like symptoms. Bacterial resistance emerges rapidly if rifampin is taken alone.

The multiple-drug approach to the treatment of mycobacterial infections reduces the very real risk of emergence of resistant strains. Rifampin also is indicated in the eradication of pharyngeal carriage of sulfonamide-resistant *Neisseria meningitidis* or in those instances when the patient is unable to tolerate minocycline. More recently, rifampin, in combination with other antibiotics, has been used in the treatment of methicillin-resistant *Staphylococcus aureus* and *Staphylococcus epidermidis* infections.

Adverse Reactions

The adverse effects associated with rifampin administration are many and varied. The most commonly observed side effects involve gastrointestinal disturbances and nervous system complaints, such as headache, drows-iness, ataxia, dizziness, and fatigue. The most serious problem is liver damage, expressed as jaundice. The incidence of liver damage appears to be higher in patients who also are slow inactivators of isoniazid or who have a prior history of liver disease. The combined use of isoniazid and rifampin may increase the risk of hepatotoxicity. Rifampin and its metabolites can color the urine, feces, saliva, sweat, and tears red-orange, which may cause patient anxiety.

Intermittent therapy is associated with the highest incidence of adverse reactions, many of which are suspected as having an immunological basis. These reactions, which include anemia, thrombocytopenia, acute renal failure, chills, fever, myalgia, arthralgia, vomiting, and diarrhea, emphasize the importance of advising patients not to skip doses of rifampin.

Preparations and Dosage

Rifampin (*Rifadin, Rimactane*) is available as capsules and for injection. *Rifamate* contains 300 mg rifampin and 150 mg isoniazid in a capsule.

Aminoglycosidic Aminocyclitols

Both the aminoglycosidic aminocyclitols, streptomycin and kanamycin, have been used in the treatment of tuberculosis. Their structures, mode of action, and pharmacology have been described in Chap. 50.

Clinical Uses

Streptomycin is no longer a first-line drug in the treatment of tuberculosis. When used it is administered by intramuscular injections and, very occasionally, by the intrathecal route. It has the potential to cause both ototoxicity and nephrotoxicity. Side effects have limited its usefulness in inpatient chemotherapy when first-line agents are contraindicated.

Mycobacterium tuberculosis strains that are resistant to streptomycin are usually sensitive to kanamycin. Its potential for causing nephrotoxicity and ototoxicity demands careful patient monitoring. Kanamycin is preferred to viomycin by some physicians because of its lower toxicity. However, should kanamycin-resistant organisms emerge, they usually are sensitive to viomycin.

Aminosalicylic Acid

Structure and Mode of Action

Aminosalicylic acid (*p*-aminosalicylic acid, PAS) (Fig. 53-3), like the sulfonamides (see Chap. 48), is a structural analogue of *p*-aminobenzoic acid (PABA). *It inhibits folic*

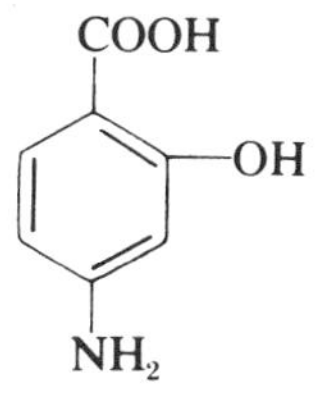

COOH

—OH

NH₂

Figure 53-3. Aminosalicylic acid.

acid synthesis, and consequently interferes with the transfer of one-carbon units. Aminosalicylic acid, however, inhibits only certain mycobacteria. This specificity may be due either to differences in bacterial permeability to PAS or to a greater drug sensitivity of the mycobacterial enzyme that incorporates PABA into folate. Aminosalicylic acid is a bacteriostatic drug.

Absorption, Metabolism, and Excretion

Aminosalicylic acid is readily absorbed from the intestinal tract and is widely distributed throughout body tissues, including the tuberculous lesion. Peak blood levels of about 7.5 μg/ml are reached within 1 to 2 hr of the administration of a 4-gm dose. The drug has a half-life of about 1 hr, and plasma concentrations are quite low, 4 to 5 hr after a single dose. Aminosalicylic acid is primarily metabolized in the liver by acetylation; both the acetylated and the unaltered drug are excreted rapidly.

Clinical Uses

Before the widespread use of rifampin and ethambutol, aminosalicylic acid (in combination with streptomycin and isoniazid) was included in the first-line regimen for the treatment of tuberculosis. Aminosalicylic acid, although only bacteriostatic, delays the emergence of mycobacterial resistance to streptomycin and isoniazid and increases the concentration of free isoniazid in the blood when the two drugs are coadministered; it serves as an alternative substrate for the hepatic enzymes involved in isoniazid acetylation.

The use of aminosalicylic acid remains popular in developing countries because it is inexpensive and relatively nontoxic. Intermittent administration (i.e., 2 or 3 times weekly) appears no less effective than daily dosing and offers certain advantages for outpatient treatment.

Adverse Reactions

Aminosalicylic acid is a relatively safe drug. Gastrointestinal irritation is common, however, and bleeding may be produced; caution is required when treating patients with peptic ulcers. Liver damage and decreased iodine uptake by the thyroid also have been reported.

Hypersensitivity reactions, including fever, rash, pruritus, and hepatotoxicity, can result, especially within the first few weeks of treatment. These symptoms will disappear if drug treatment is terminated.

Because aminosalicylic acid is most commonly employed as part of a three-drug regimen, it may be necessary to stop all drug administration and then cautiously reintroduce each drug singly in low test doses to identify the offending agent. Corticosteroids may be necessary to suppress severe hypersensitivity reactions.

The administration of large doses of the sodium salt of aminosalicylic acid may cause a sodium overload and result in fluid retention. This occurrence is a particular problem for tuberculous patients who also may suffer from renal or cardiac failure. The calcium salt of aminosalicylic acid can be used in this situation.

Preparations and Dosage

Aminosalicylate sodium (*P.A.S. Sodium, Teebacin*) is available as 0.5- and 1.0-gm tablets and as a bulk powder.

Ethambutol

Structure and Mechanism of Action

Ethambutol (Fig. 53-4) is a synthetic antituberculosis agent. It is bacteriostatic and its mechanism of action is presently uncertain, although recent studies indicate that synthesis and function of polyamines are inhibited.

Antibacterial Spectrum

Most strains of *M. tuberculosis* and *M. marinum* are sensitive to ethambutol. The sensitivity of other mycobacteria is variable, with about 50 percent of *M. kansasii* being sensitive. *M. avium-intracellulare* organisms are usually resistant.

Pharmacokinetic Properties

Absorption
Ethambutol is administered orally and approximately 80 percent of a given oral dose is absorbed from the gastrointestinal tract. Peak serum concentrations of 2 to 5 μg/ml are obtained 2 to 4 hr after an oral dose of 25 mg/kg body weight. Its half-life is 3.3 hr. Absorption is not affected by food.

Distribution
Ethambutol is found in most body tissues and fluids, including erythrocytes, kidneys, lungs, and saliva. Ethambutol enters the CSF even in the absence of inflammation.

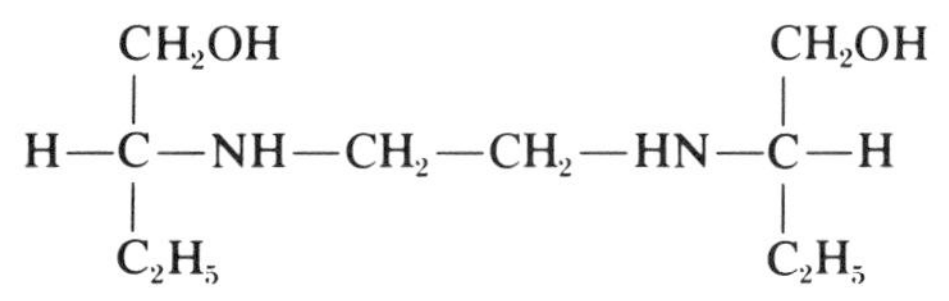

$$CH_2OH \qquad\qquad CH_2OH$$
$$H-\underset{\underset{C_2H_5}{|}}{\overset{\overset{|}{}}{C}}-NH-CH_2-CH_2-HN-\underset{\underset{C_2H_5}{|}}{\overset{\overset{|}{}}{C}}-H$$

Figure 53-4. Ethambutol.

Metabolism and Excretion

Ethambutol is partially metabolized in the liver. About 50 percent of the nonmetabolized drug and 8 to 15 percent of the metabolized drug (as aldehyde and dicarboxylic acid derivatives) are excreted in the urine. Twenty percent of the unchanged drug is found in the feces. Ethambutol is rapidly excreted and is virtually undetectable 24 hr after the last dose.

Clinical Uses

Ethambutol has replaced aminosalicylic acid as a first-line drug for use in combination with isoniazid and rifampin. It is much better tolerated than aminosalicylic acid, and the risk of causing serious toxicity is lower. Therapy usually begins with the administration of 25 mg/kg/day for 4 to 6 weeks, after which the dosage is reduced to 15 mg/kg/day. Before treatment is initiated, it is recommended that the patient undergo an ophthalmological examination and be questioned carefully concerning any impairment of visual acuity or inability to distinguish green from red.

Adverse Reactions

Ethambutol is well tolerated. The major side effect associated with its use is an optic neuritis that affects the central fibers of the optic nerve, resulting in loss of central vision and an impaired red-green discrimination. These effects may be unilateral or bilateral and are usually reversible on stopping the drug. The optic neuritis occurs in approximately 3 percent of individuals taking the standard dosage for some months. This is almost totally avoidable by using a maintenance dosage of 15 mg/kg/day. A second, but less common, type of neuritis affects the peripheral fibers of the optic nerve, resulting in constriction of peripheral vision, but with no loss of visual acuity.

Mild gastrointestinal upset, allergic reactions, fever, headache, malaise, mental confusion, and dizziness have been reported. Serum levels of uric acid may increase and can result in gout. This last effect is the result of an ethambutol-induced impaired renal clearance of urate. The drug-induced hyperuricemia responds to probenecid, sulfinpyrazone, or allopurinol.

Preparations

Ethambutol hydrochloride (*Myambutol*) is marketed as oral tablets.

Ethionamide

Structure and Mechanism of Action

Ethionamide is a thioamide analogue of isonicotinic acid (Fig. 53-5) and thus bears some structural similarity to isoniazid. It has only about one-tenth the activity of isoniazid. Its mechanism of action is not known, although there are indications that it may function as an antimetabolite or it may inhibit synthesis of mycolic acid. It is bacteriostatic. Although resistance to ethionamide develops rapidly when it is given alone, resistance can be delayed when ethionamide is administered with other antituberculous drugs.

Absorption, Metabolism, and Excretion

Ethionamide is absorbed after oral administration and doses of 1 gm can yield plasma levels of about 20 μg/ml within 3 hr after administration. The drug is distributed to all body tissues and fluids, including the CSF. As with aminosalicylic acid, ethionamide can function as an alternative substrate and thereby block hepatic acetylation of isoniazid. Metabolism of ethionamide is extensive (resulting largely in dihydropyridine metabolites), and less than 1 percent of an administered dose is eliminated in the urine as active parent drug. Ethionamide has a shorter half-life than does the closely related compound isoniazid.

Clinical Uses

Ethionamide is more active against M. tuberculosis in vitro than is streptomycin, but it is inferior to isoniazid. Ethionamide is administered orally, although serious toxicity severely limits its use. With the increased use of ethambutol and rifampin, the indications for ethionamide

Figure 53-5. Ethionamide.

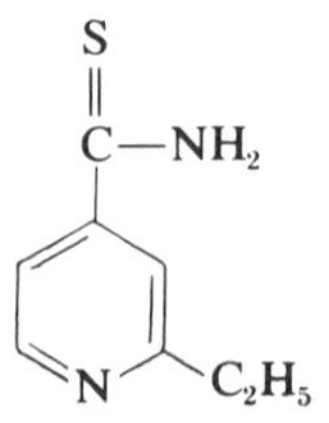

therapy have diminished. As with other *second-line* compounds, it is essential to combine it with at least one other drug.

Adverse Reactions

Gastrointestinal intolerance is frequent, resulting in nausea, vomiting, pain, and diarrhea. Hepatitis, allergic reactions, impotence, and gynecomastia also have been reported.

Preparations and Dosage

Ethionamide (*Trecator-SC*) is provided solely for oral use as 250-mg tablets.

Pyrazinamide

Structure and Mode of Action

Pyrazinamide (Fig. 53-6) is a synthetic tuberculocidal analogue of nicotinamide. Its mode of action is unknown, although it may affect electron transport. Pyrazinamide is effective against intracellular mycobacteria. Resistance to pyrazinamide develops, but this can be delayed by coadministering it with other antituberculous drugs.

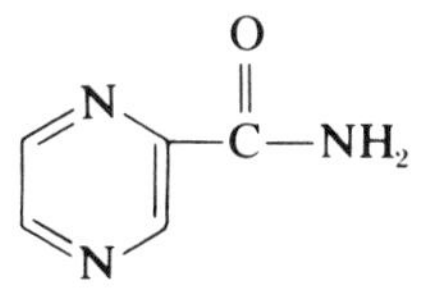

Absorption, Metabolism, and Excretion

Pyrazinamide is absorbed from the intestinal tract after oral administration. A dose of 1 gm results in plasma levels of 40 to 50 μg/ml in 2 hr. The drug distributes widely in tissues and penetrates macrophages and tuberculous cavities. It is active only in a slightly acidic environment and is therefore active against the intracellular mycobacteria. Pyrazinamide is deaminated by the microsomal drug-metabolizing enzyme pyrazinamide deaminase to form pyrazinoic acid. The hyperuricemic effect of pyrazinamide appears to be due to this metabolite. The principal metabolite found in the urine is 5-hydroxypyrazinoic acid. The half-life is 9 to 10 hr. Renal glomerular filtration serves as the major excretory pathway for pyrazinamide and its metabolites.

Clinical Uses

Pyrazinamide, in combination with isoniazid, is effective against resistant strains of *M. tuberculosis.* Previously this drug was used infrequently in Western Europe and North America except as a *second-line* drug, although it was used widely in developing countries, notably Africa. However, its potent tuberculocidal activity has led to a reappraisal of its value as shorter regimens for treatment of

Figure 53-6. Pyrazinamide.

tuberculosis have become recommended. Its advantages are that it can be totally synthesized and is therefore relatively inexpensive.

It is now used in combination with drugs such as isoniazid, rifampin, and ethambutol for the abbreviated (i.e., 6–9 months) treatment of tuberculosis. Pyrazinamide also can be given on an intermittent basis, once or twice a week, and still produce acceptable cure rates.

Adverse Reactions

Hepatotoxicity occurs with some regularity, and its development is related to the dosage and duration of treatment. Hyperuricemia has been reported in *all* patients receiving pyrazinamide and clinical gout has occurred in some. Pyrazinamide-induced gout *does not respond* to uricosuric therapy with probenecid. Acetylsalicylic acid (2.4 gm/day), which also may produce uric acid retention, reverses the hyperuricemic effect of pyrazinamide; the mechanism is unknown. Aminosalicylic acid also has been reported to prevent or delay the appearance of hyperuricemia.

Preparations and Dosage

Pyrazinamide is available in 500-mg tablets for oral use.

Cycloserine

Structure and Mechanism of Action

Cycloserine, an antibiotic produced by *Streptomyces orchidaceus,* is a structural analogue of D-alanine (Fig. 53-7). It is a competitive inhibitor of D-alanyl-D-alanine synthetase and alanine racemase; both enzymes are required for bacterial cell wall synthesis. Alanine racemase converts L-alanine to D-alanine, whereas the synthetase is necessary for the subsequent production of the dipeptide D-alanyl-D-alanine. The terminal D-alanyl-D-alanine is required for cross-linking of the linear peptidoglycan. Inhibition of dipeptide formation prevents formation of the uridine diphosphate (UDP)-acetylmuramyl pentapeptide, a precursor required for cell wall synthesis.

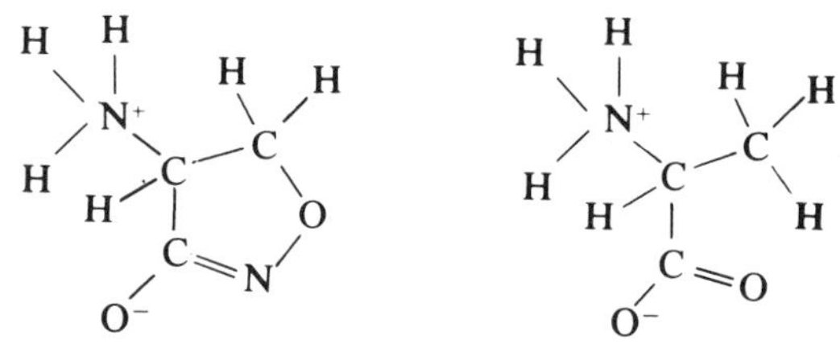

Figure 53-7. D-Cycloserine and D-alanine (zwitterion forms). Note similarity in conformation.

Antibacterial Spectrum

Cycloserine is a *second-line* drug that inhibits growth of *M. tuberculosis.* It also inhibits the growth of other facultative gram-positive and gram-negative bacteria.

Absorption, Metabolism, and Excretion

Cycloserine is administered orally; blood levels of 15 to 35 μg/ml can be obtained 3 to 4 hr after a single dose. It penetrates most tissues and fluids, including macrophages and CSF; tissue levels approximate plasma levels. Cycloserine is only partially metabolized, and 60 to 80 percent is excreted by glomerular filtration as the unchanged parent molecule. The drug reaches high concentrations in urine and is quite useful in treating renal tuberculosis. Cycloserine is most active at acid pH.

Clinical Uses

Although cycloserine has relatively low activity against *M. tuberculosis,* resistance to it emerges slowly. The development of resistance can be prevented by combining cycloserine with other antituberculous drugs. Cycloserine is rarely used for the treatment of tuberculosis.

Adverse Reactions

Cycloserine can cause headache, tremors, seizures, agitation, confusion, hallucinations, and psychoses. Some of these side effects may be related to the low levels of magnesium in the CSF, which often accompany cycloserine administration. Patients with epilepsy or mental depression should not be given cycloserine. On occasion, hepatic damage, peripheral neuropathy, and malabsorption also can occur.

Preparations and Dosage

Cycloserine (*Seromycin*) is administered only orally and is available as 250-mg capsules.

Viomycin and Capreomycin

Viomycin and capreomycin are antibiotics that are infrequently used in the treatment of tuberculosis. They have properties similar to those of the aminoglycosidic aminocyclitols.

Viomycin has a clinical spectrum of activity that is similar to that of streptomycin, although its toxicity is greater and its antibacterial activity is lower. It is given by injection daily or on an alternate-day regimen to avoid toxicity. Viomycin-resistant strains usually are also resistant to streptomycin and kanamycin, but fortunately the reverse is not so. Viomycin is rarely used in children. Capreomycin is a useful second-line drug against strains of *M. tuberculosis* and atypical mycobacteria.

Capreomycin and viomycin can cause both ototoxicity and nephrotoxicity, adverse reactions that are potentiated by preexisting renal insufficiency. Urinalysis may show proteinuria, red and white blood cells, and casts. However, a cautious continuation of treatment is still possible even under these circumstances. Elevation of the blood urea nitrogen (BUN) and serum creatinine cannot be ignored and, when this occurs, the drug administration should be stopped.

Preparations and Dosage

Capreomycin sulfate (*Capastat Sulfate*) is a polypeptide antibiotic derived from *Streptomyces capreolus* and is available only for parenteral (IM) administration.

Viomycin sulfate (*Viocin Sulfate*) is an antibiotic derived from an actinomycete whose chemistry and pharmacology are quite similar to those of capreomycin. It is used clinically in a similar manner to that described for capreomycin.

Treatment of Leprosy

The treatment of leprosy is a specialized area. Host defenses are crucial in determining the patient's response to the disease and, consequently, the clinical presentation and the bacillary load. These factors dictate the length of therapy and the risk of adverse reactions to medication. Drug sensitivity to *Mycobacterium leprae* cannot be tested for in vitro.

Tuberculoid leprosy is characterized by intact cell-mediated immunity, a positive skin-test reaction to lepromin, granuloma formation, and a relative paucity of bacilli. At the other extreme, *lepromatous leprosy* produces no granulomas and numerous bacilli are present in a palisade arrangement within the tissues; there is markedly depressed cell-mediated immunity and the skin-test reaction to lep-

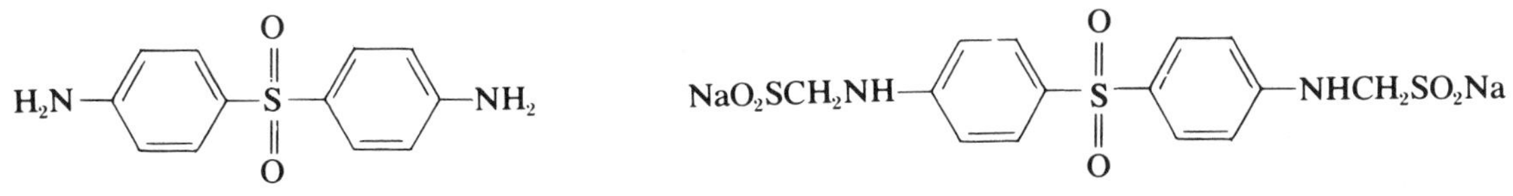

Figure 53-8. Dapsone (diaminodiphenylsulfone) and sulfoxone sodium.

romin is negative. Within these two extremes are patients with features that place them in an intermediate or borderline category. Early in the disease, an indeterminate or mixed form of leprosy occurs that displays few clinical features. In this form, a variable reaction to lepromin occurs and biopsy material usually shows only a few bacilli. The disease may then progress to either tuberculoid or lepromatous leprosy.

The aim of drug therapy is to kill all viable bacilli. Within 3 to 6 months of drug administration, viable bacilli are eliminated from the blood and nasal secretions. Following this, a period of prolonged chemotherapy is necessary to prevent relapse. The length of therapy is dependent on clinical response. For example, patients with tuberculoid leprosy are frequently treated for 1 to 2 years after the resolution of their lesions. Patients with lepromatous leprosy are treated for at least 5 years, owing to a higher incidence of relapse. Lifelong therapy is not unusual, particularly for patients with lepromatous leprosy who fail to recover lepromin reactivity.

Drug therapy is only one aspect of the management of this physically, psychologically, and socially crippling disease. Surgery, physical therapy, education, and rehabilitation are integral parts in the total approach to the treatment of leprosy.

Sulfones

The sulfones have been widely used to treat all forms of leprosy. The most widely used agent has been *dapsone* (diaminodiphenylsulfone). An increasing worldwide problem of drug resistance has led to alternative regimens, which include rifampin, clofazimine, amithiozone (thiacetazone), ethionamide, and prothionamide.

Structure and Mechanism of Action

The sulfones (Fig. 53-8) are structural analogues of PABA and are competitive inhibitors of folic acid synthesis (Chap. 48). *The sulfones are bacteriostatic and are used only in the treatment of leprosy.* Although the sulfones are highly active against most strains of *M. leprae,* a small number of organisms are less susceptible and can persist for many years, resulting in a relapse of infection, notably in lepromatous leprosy.

Absorption, Metabolism, and Excretion

The sulfones are slowly, but completely, absorbed from the intestinal tract and are widely distributed in tissues and body fluids. Peak plasma concentrations are reached in 1 to 3 hr, and about 50 percent of the drugs are bound to serum protein. The sulfones tend to be retained in skin, muscle, liver, and kidney. The concentration in inflamed skin is 10 to 15 times that found in normal skin. The sulfones are excreted in the bile and then reabsorbed by the intestine, thereby prolonging blood levels for up to 12 days. With repeated doses, these drug levels persist for up to 35 days. The sulfones are metabolized in the liver, where they undergo acetylation and glucuronide formation.

Adverse Reactions

The sulfones can produce a nonhemolytic anemia, methemoglobinemia, and sometimes an acute hemolytic anemia in persons deficient in the enzyme glucose 6-phosphate dehydrogenase. Treatment of leprosy with sulfones can cause an acute exacerbation of skin lesions and may result in permanent paralysis of muscles served by the involved nerves. Erythema nodosum skin rashes, including Stevens-Johnson syndrome ("dapsone dermatitis"), and hepatotoxicity are also seen.

Preparations and Dosage

Dapsone (*Alvosulfon*) is included in all regimens used in the treatment of all types of leprosy. The drug is administered orally and is available as 25- and 100-mg tablets.

Sulfoxone sodium (*Diasone Sodium*) is available as enteric-coated tablets containing 165 mg.

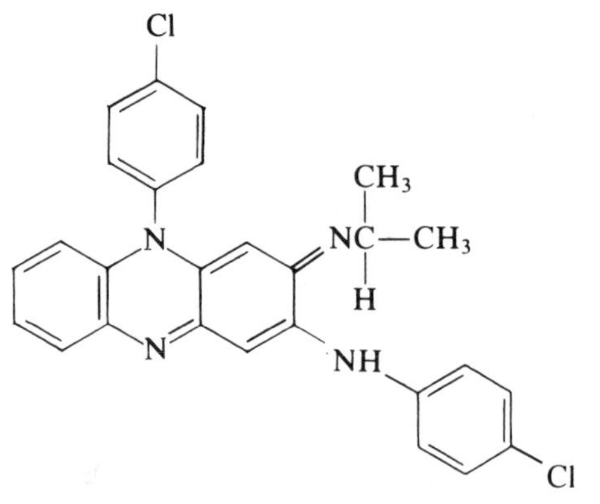

Figure 53-9. Clofazimine.

Other Antilepromatous Drugs

Clofazimine

Clofazimine (B663, *Lamprene*) is a phenazine dye (Fig. 53-9). It is bactericidal, probably through binding of the drug to DNA. Although clofazimine is administered orally, its degree of gastrointestinal absorption is quite variable. The drug is well tolerated in dosages of 100 mg per day. Low serum concentrations (0.4–3.0 μg/ml) are obtained with a half-life of approximately 2 months. The drug is lipophilic and widely distributed in tissues, including phagocytic cells, and significant amounts of drug can accumulate. Clofazimine is excreted primarily in bile with only small amounts excreted in urine.

The major adverse reaction associated with its administration is a reddish-brown pigmentation of the skin that occurs particularly in light-skinned persons. This reaction is frequently unacceptable to the patient and can seriously limit the usefulness of the drug. Gastrointestinal intolerance occurs occasionally.

An advantage of clofazimine over and above its antilepromatous action is its antiinflammatory properties. The appearance of erythema nodosum leprosum, which can interrupt treatment with dapsone, appears to be inhibited by clofazimine. *Mycobacterium ulcerans,* which is responsible for Buruli ulcer, also responds to clofazimine.

Rifampin

Rifampin is the most active antilepromatous drug available. Its structure, mode of action, and pharmacological properties were discussed earlier in this chapter. A dosage of 600 mg per day will kill the majority of bacilli in the host within a few days. Its cost seriously limits its wider appli-

cation in developing countries, where it is used more commonly in combination drug therapy on an intermittent basis.

Clinical Use of Antilepromatous Drugs

The treatment of leprosy has become more complicated as a result of drug resistance to dapsone. The current recommendations by the World Health Organization (WHO) suggest that *all forms of leprosy should be treated with a combination of drugs* rather than reliance on therapy with dapsone alone.

Treatment of multibacillary leprosy, which includes borderline lepromatous and lepromatous leprosy, is with a triple regimen of dapsone, 50 to 100 mg per day, together with clofazimine, 50 mg per day, and an additional 300-mg dose once a month, plus rifampin, 600 mg once a month. All drugs are given by mouth. This regimen is given for a minimum of 2 years, but it should be prolonged until skin biopsies and scrapings become negative for acid-fast bacilli. The risk of adverse reactions with intermittent rifampin therapy has led to a preference for the daily use of this drug by some experts. This occurrence substantially increases the cost of treatment.

For the treatment of paucibacillary leprosy, which includes tuberculoid and smear-negative borderline tuberculoid leprosy, WHO suggests a regimen of rifampin, 600 mg once a month for a 6-month period, together with 100 mg dapsone daily for 6 months. Again, both drugs are given orally. Follow-up for a 2-year period is advisable to detect relapse. The smaller number of bacilli in tuberculoid forms of the disease allow for this shorter course of treatment. Drug combination therapy has the added advantage of minimizing the emergence of drug-resistant strains. Some physicians prefer to use rifampin on a daily basis for 6 months and extend the use of dapsone for 2 to 5 years.

Other agents, such as ethionamide and prothionamide, are second-line agents where drug resistance is a problem or when first-line drugs are poorly tolerated. These compounds are used only occasionally in the treatment of lepromatous leprosy.

Supplemental Reading

Acocella, G., et al. Pharmacokinetic studies on antituberculosis regimens in humans. *Am. Rev. Respir. Dis.* 132:510, 1985.

American Thoracic Society. Treatment of tuberculosis and tuberculosis infection in adults and children. *Am. Rev. Respir. Dis.* 134:355, 1986.

Baciewicz, A.M., and Self, T.H. Isoniazid interactions. *South. Med. J.* 78:714, 1985.

British Thoracic Society. Control and prevention of tuberculosis in Britain: An updated code of practice. *Br. Med. J.* 300:995, 1990.

Bullock, W.E. Rifampin in the treatment of leprosy. *Rev. Infect. Dis.* 5 (Suppl.3):606, 1983.

Chaisson, R.E., and Slutkin, G. Tuberculosis and human immunodeficiency virus infection. *J. Infect. Dis.* 159:96, 1989.

Citron, K.M. Ocular toxicity from ethambutol. *Thorax* 41:737, 1986.

Dutt, A.K., Moers, D., and Stead, W.W. Short course chemo-therapy for extrapulmonary tuberculosis. *Ann. Intern. Med.* 104:7, 1986.

Ellard, G.A. Chemotherapy of leprosy. *Br. Med. Bull.* 44:775, 1988.

Girling, D.J., et al. Extrapulmonary tuberculosis. *Br. Med. Bull.* 44:738, 1988.

Sensi, P. Antimycobacterial Agents. In M. Verderame (ed.), *Handbook of Chemotherapeutic Agents.* Vol. 1. Boca Raton, Fla.: CRC, 1986. P. 195.

Wheate, H.W. Management of leprosy. *Br. Med. Bull.* 44:791, 1988.

54

Antiviral Drugs

Knox Van Dyke

The least exploited area of chemotherapy is that of selective chemical attack on viruses. According to data from the Centers for Disease Control, approximately 4,800 unnecessary deaths occur each year during the influenza season. Childhood diseases, such as viral pneumonia, may cause 10,000 deaths a year. Approximately one third of all office visits to practicing physicians are concerned with influenza or upper-respiratory virus infections. Herpes simplex virus type 1, the virus responsible for cold-sore infections of the lip, is present in one third to one half of the human population. Simplex type 2 infection of the genitals is a venereal disease that is currently widely transmitted. Acquired immunodeficiency syndrome (AIDS) has spread at an amazing pace, with more than 100,000 deaths in the United States in 1992.

Viruses are among the simplest living organisms. They are composed of one or more strands of a linear or helical nucleic acid core, consisting of either DNA or RNA, but not both. The particular type of nucleic acid present will determine the initial classification of the virus. Further subdivision is usually based on some morphological characteristic, cellular site of viral multiplication, and so forth. Many viruses possess an outer protein or lipoprotein envelope.

The viruses must enter living cells to maintain their growth and to reproduce. Thus, they are essentially intracellular parasites that utilize many of the biochemical mechanisms and products of the host cell to sustain their viability. This fact makes it particularly difficult to find a drug that is selective for the virus and that does not interfere with host cell function. A mature virus (called a *virion*) can exist outside a host cell and still retain its infective properties. However, to reproduce, the virus must enter the host cell, take over the host cell's mechanisms for nucleic acid and protein synthesis, and direct the host cell to make new viral particles. Many different viruses have been isolated from both animal and plant sources.

Recent increased knowledge of viral function suggests that some structures, enzymes, and replicative mechanisms are unique to the virus. This recognition is permitting the development of drugs that have a greater antiviral specificity than has been heretofore possible. The realization that the host cell possesses surface receptors to which viruses can attach is leading to the development of a new class of antiviral drugs.

Three basic approaches are used to control viral diseases. The first and foremost of these has been through immunological control. In addition, both chemotherapy and the stimulation of natural resistance mechanisms in the host (which could also be a form of chemotherapy) have been attempted.

Vaccination has been used successfully to prevent measles, rubella, mumps, poliomyelitis, yellow fever, smallpox, and hepatitis B. Unfortunately, the usefulness of vaccines appears to be limited when many serotypes are involved (e.g., rhinoviruses). Furthermore, vaccines have little or no use once the infection has been established, since they cannot prevent the spread of active infections within the host. Passive immunization as an aid in assisting the body's own defense mechanisms is also commonly employed. Human immune globulin, equine antiserum, or antiserum from vaccinated humans has been used in this regard.

The main problem in the chemotherapy of viruses is in finding a drug that will be selectively toxic to the virus without producing major toxic reactions in the host. The drug should distribute to the site of viral activity, that is, the particular host cells that are supporting viral replication. In addition, the drug should not be metabolized so quickly by the host that it becomes inactivated before adequate tissue concentrations are reached. For instance, adenine arabinoside (ara-A) and cytosine arabinoside (ara-C) are so rapidly deaminated that they must be either continuously infused or their metabolism somehow blocked to be most effective. Sometimes, the antiviral activity of a compound can be increased if the drug is suitably dissolved in a solvent that increases drug membrane penetration (e.g., ara-C dissolved in dimethyl sulfoxide).

There are several important stages at which viral invasion may be impaired. They are listed in the following section.

Steps in Viral Infection and Replication

Phase 1: Attachment and Penetration

The virus attaches to the host cell membrane. Specific receptor sites on the host cell are recognized by corresponding areas on the specific virus. The virus penetrates the host membrane by a phagocytosis-like mechanism and is then encapsulated by the host cell cytoplasm, forming a vacuole.

Phase 2: Uncoating

The protein coat of the virus is dissolved by viral enzymes liberating free viral DNA or RNA, depending on the given type of virus (i.e., the viral genome).

Phase 3: Synthesis of Viral Components

The genome of the virus is duplicated and viral proteins are synthesized in the appropriate sequence. At this time, host synthesis of nucleic acids or protein, or both, is inhibited.

Phase 4: Assembly of the Virus Particle

In phase 4, the viral components are assembled to form the mature virus particle. The viral genome is encapsulated by viral protein or, in some cases, not encapsulated, for example, adenovirus or poliovirus. Sometimes, as in poxviruses, the viral DNA becomes surrounded by multiple membranes.

Phase 5: Release of the Virus

Release of the virus from the host cell may be rapid and is accompanied by host cell lysis and cell death. Other viruses are released more slowly by means of a budding-like process, and the host cell may survive.

The chemotherapy of virus infections, theoretically, could involve interference with any or all of the above steps. In practice, however, antiviral drugs generally inhibit only one of the phases. Of course, all steps subsequent to the particular one inhibited also will be affected, although not by direct drug action.

Immune Globulin (Gamma Globulin)

Chemistry

Immune globulin, or, more commonly, gamma globulin (IgG), is a fraction obtained from the plasma of normal individuals and is rich in most of the antibodies found in whole blood. Although it is not really a drug in the classic sense, gamma globulin contains a variety of antibodies against specific viral antigens.

Mechanism of Action

Our understanding of gamma globulin's mode of action as an antiviral drug is somewhat unclear, but it is assumed to block penetration of the virus particle into the host cell (*phase 1 inhibitor*).

Clinical Uses

Gamma globulin is not effective orally and must be administered by parenteral means. Intramuscular injections given during the early infectious stage can partially alleviate the progression of hepatitis, measles, rabies, poliomyelitis, and probably other viral disorders. Protection lasts for 2 to 3 weeks after a single injection, although for prolonged infections, injections can be repeated every 2 to 3 weeks. This procedure confers a *passive immunity* to the virus. Gamma globulin also can be used as an adjunctive form of therapy with other therapeutic approaches.

Adverse Reactions

Side effects associated with gamma globulin administration are rare. However, since immune globulin does have some tendency to form large polymers, these aggregates may be the cause of an occasional anaphylactoid reaction.

Preparations and Dosage

Immune globulin (human) (*Gamastan*) is available for IM administration. Formulations of immune globulin intravenous (*Gamminume, Sandoglobulin*) are available for use in patients who require an immediate increase in immunoglobulin levels. The usual dosage is 100 mg/kg once a month.

Amantadine Hydrochloride

Chemistry and Mechanism of Action

Amantadine (Fig. 54-1) is a synthetic antiviral compound whose structure differs considerably from all other antimicrobial agents. It is a *phase 1 inhibitor* and acts by somehow impairing the ability of the virus to uncoat its RNA in host cells. A derivative, rimantadine, has similar activities toward influenza A viruses. Rimantadine hydrochloride has been approved in Europe but not in the U.S.

Absorption, Metabolism, and Excretion

Amantadine is rapidly and completely absorbed from the gastrointestinal tract after oral administration, and peak blood levels are achieved in 2 to 4 hr. The serum half-life of amantadine is about 20 hr. It does not undergo significant hepatic metabolism. Most of the drug (90%) is excreted in the urine as the unchanged compound. Because the drug may accumulate in patients with renal disease, the dosage should be modified in these patients.

Clinical Uses

Amantadine appears to be especially useful in the prevention and treatment of diseases caused by the type A_2 (Asian) influenza virus. It protects approximately 70 to 90 percent of patients receiving it prophylactically from infection by influenza A_2 viruses. It is particularly valuable for high-risk patients, such as the elderly or those with other underlying disease. It is not effective, however, against influenza B or myxoviruses. Its use in the treatment of an already established influenza A_2 infection remains somewhat controversial. Amantadine is also employed in the therapy of parkinsonism (see discussion in Chap. 38).

Adverse Reactions

Side effects of amantadine are most prominent at increased dosages and include depression, congestive heart failure, orthostatic hypotension, psychosis, and urinary retention. Dizziness, insomnia, nervousness, and skin rash also have been reported.

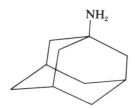

Figure 54-1. Amantadine.

Contraindications and Warnings

Amantadine is used with caution in patients with impaired liver and kidney function, epilepsy, or psychosis, or during pregnancy. The drug should not be used in children under 15 years of age who have been exposed to rubella or in the treatment of patients with already established influenza or other respiratory infections not caused by influenza virus A. Increased amantadine toxicity has been reported following concomitant use with anticholinergic drugs, phenelzine, and thiazide-triamterene diuretics.

Preparations and Dosage

Amantadine hydrochloride (*Symmetrel*) is available for oral administration in the form of capsules (100 mg) and syrup (50 mg/5 ml). Patients more than 65 years of age should take no more than 100 mg once a day. Therapy is usually maintained for at least 10 days following a known exposure or throughout the risk period (6–8 weeks).

Vidarabine (Adenine Arabinoside)

Chemistry and Mechanism of Action

Vidarabine (adenine arabinoside) is a purine nucleoside obtained from cultures of *Streptomyces antibioticus*. The drug is a *phase 3 inhibitor* and impairs the early steps in viral DNA synthesis, presumably by inhibiting virus-specific DNA polymerase. Vidarabine is phosphorylated in vivo, and while the phosphorylated nucleoside can inhibit both viral and cellular DNA polymerase, the viral enzyme is inhibited to a much greater extent.

Antiviral Spectrum

Vidarabine has particular activity against DNA viruses related to herpes simplex types 1 and 2, cytomegalovirus, varicella-zoster, and vaccinia viruses. Vidarabine has only limited effects on most RNA and nonherpes DNA viruses, such as adenovirus.

Absorption, Metabolism, and Excretion

Vidarabine is only administered topically as an ophthalmic ointment or intravenously as an infusion; therefore, absorption from the gastrointestinal tract is not a consideration. The drug has relatively limited solubility and is not absorbed after ophthalmic application. After intravenous administration, vidarabine is rapidly deaminated to its principal metabolite, arabinosylhypoxanthine, which retains some degree of antiviral activity. The drug is widely distributed in body tissues, including cerebrospinal fluid (CSF). The primary route of elimination is by renal excretion of the metabolite. The plasma half-life of the metabolite is about 4 hr.

Clinical Uses

The principal use of vidarabine is in the treatment of infections caused by herpes simplex viruses. Encephalitis, keratoconjunctivitis, and recurrent epithelial keratitis are particularly responsive. Systemic administration has not yet proved to be effective in the management of encephalitis caused by varicella-zoster or vaccinia virus, although it does appear to have some efficacy in the treatment of localized herpes zoster and chickenpox infections in immunocompromised adults and children, respectively. It is *ineffective* against bacterial, fungal, and adenovirus infections.

Adverse Reactions

Anorexia, nausea, vomiting, and diarrhea are the most commonly observed side effects of vidarabine infusion. Central nervous system (CNS) symptoms, including dizziness, hallucinations, psychosis, and ataxia, also have been reported. Pain at the site of injection is not infrequent. The most commonly observed side effects associated with the ophthalmic product are lacrimation, burning, irritation, pain, and photophobia.

Contraindications and Cautions

The drug should not be administered intramuscularly or subcutaneously. Systemic vidarabine is contraindicated if patients show signs of hypersensitivity reaction. In addition, since animal studies have shown vidarabine to have oncogenic and mutagenic potential, the use of the compound in pregnant patients should be reserved for life-threatening illnesses. Patients with impaired renal function may require dose adjustment. Liver function and hematological tests are recommended, since alterations in serum glutamic oxaloacetic transaminase (SGOT), bilirubin, hematocrit, and white blood cell count have occasionally been associated with vidarabine therapy.

Preparations and Dosage

Vidarabine (adenine arabinoside, ara-A, *Vira-A*) is available as an IV infusion (200 mg/ml) and as a 3% ophthalmic ointment. The parenteral preparation is given as a slow infusion to achieve a blood level of 3 to 6 μg/ml (adenine arabinoside) or 0.2 to 0.4 μg/ml (arabinosylhypoxanthine).

Zidovudine (Azidothymidine, AZT)

Zidovudine is a synthetic pyrimidine deoxynucleoside with an N_3 (azide) group attached to the deoxyribose at the 3' position. It is commonly referred to by its code designation, AZT.

Zidovudine is indicated for the management of patients with symptomatic human immunodeficiency virus (HIV) infections, that is, AIDS and advanced AIDS-related complex. See Chap. 55 for a complete discussion of this compound.

Ribavirin

Chemistry and Mechanism of Action

Ribavirin is a synthetic nucleoside that possesses broad antiviral inhibitory activity against respiratory syncytial, herpes simplex, and influenza viruses. Its exact mechanism of action is unknown, but its antiviral activity can be inhibited by the coadministration of either guanosine or xanthosine. This observation suggests that ribavirin has antimetabolite activity and therefore probably functions as a *phase 3 inhibitor*. It may interfere with the formation of viral messenger RNA (mRNA) and viral polymerase, resulting in a decrease in ribonucleic protein synthesis.

Absorption, Metabolism, and Excretion

Ribavirin is administered as an aerosol using a small-particle aerosol generator. When administered by this route, the drug has only minimal systemic absorption yielding a plasma concentration of approximately 0.76 μM. The drug concentration in respiratory tract secretions may be 100-fold higher than that found in plasma. The plasma half-life is 9.5 hr when ribavirin is administered for 2.5 hr/day for 3 days, while the half-life of the drug in erythrocytes is 40 days. Ribavirin is metabolized to at least one major metabolite. About 50 percent of the drug or metabolites appear in the urine within 72 hr.

Clinical Use

Ribavirin aerosol is indicated in the treatment of selected hospitalized infants and young children with severe lower respiratory tract infections due to respiratory syncytial virus. Resistance to ribavirin has not been reported.

Ribavirin aerosol begun within 24 hr of the appearance of symptoms associated with various influenza A and B infections may reduce fever and systemic symptoms. High-dose intravenous ribavirin therapy may be lifesaving in Lassa fever.

Adverse Reactions

Pulmonary function may decline if the drug is used in adults who have chronic respiratory disease. In addition, the drug should be used with caution in asthmatics. Dyspnea and chest soreness have been seen in patients with compromised lung function. Rash, conjunctivitis, and anemia also have been reported.

Contraindications

Ribavirin is teratogenic and should not be used in pregnant patients.

Preparations and Dosage

Ribavirin (*Virazole*) is supplied in 100-ml glass vials containing 6 gm of sterile, lyophilized drug to be reconstituted and administered using a small-particle aerosol generator in an oxygen tent or mask. The average aerosol concentration for a 12-hr period is 190 μg per liter (L) of air. The reconstituted solutions are stable only for 24 hr.

Cytarabine (Cytosine Arabinoside)

As with adenine arabinoside, cytarabine (cytosine arabinoside, ara-C, *Cytosar-U*) also displays activity against herpesviruses. However, this is not a Food and Drug Ad-

ministration (FDA)-approved use of the drug. Its sole use at present is in cancer chemotherapy (see Chap. 62).

Idoxuridine

Chemistry and Mechanism of Action

Idoxuridine is a water-soluble iodinated derivative of deoxyuridine that is thought to be a *phase 3 viral inhibitor*. It is considered to exert toxicity primarily through its introduction into viral DNA, which results in the formation of less stable DNA and in aberrant viral protein synthesis. Effects on pyrimidine formation and nucleotide interconversions also have been demonstrated. The active form of the drug is the triphosphorylated derivative, which can inhibit both viral and cellular DNA synthesis. Unfortunately, the drug has host cytotoxicity and cannot be used to treat systemic viral infections.

Antiviral Spectrum

Idoxuridine is active against herpes virus, varicella, vaccinia, polyoma virus, and several others. Its actions are directed particularly against DNA viruses. The development of drug resistance is common.

Absorption, Metabolism, and Excretion

The drug is marketed strictly for topical ophthalmic use and therefore systemic pharmacokinetics need not be seriously considered. However, studies of individuals who have accidentally ingested idoxuridine have shown that the drug is rapidly metabolized and excreted, and tends not to accumulate in body tissues.

Clinical Uses

The only approved use of idoxuridine is in the treatment of herpes simplex infections of the eyelid, conjunctiva, and cornea. It is most effective against surface infections, since it has little ability to penetrate the tissues of the eye.

Adverse Reactions

Idoxuridine may cause local irritation, mild edema, itching, and photophobia. Corneal clouding and small punctate defects in the corneal epithelium have been reported. Allergic reactions are rare.

Preparations

Idoxuridine (*Herplex Liquifilm, Stoxil*) is marketed as a 0.1% ophthalmic solution and as a 0.5% ophthalmic ointment.

Acyclovir

Acyclovir is a guanine analogue that has an acyclic side chain instead of ribose at position 9 (Fig. 54-2). Acyclovir has potent antiviral activity against most herpes viruses and is particularly effective against the herpes simplex virus.

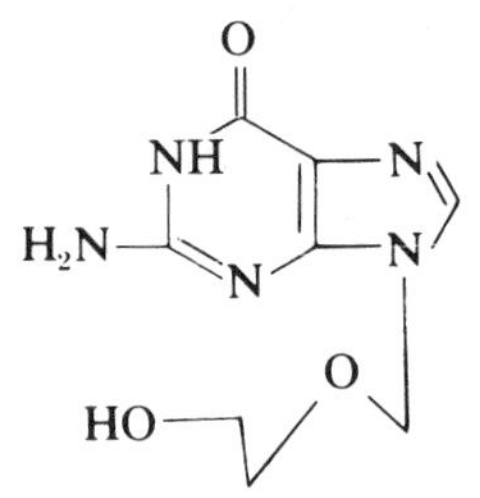

Mechanism of Action

In order to be effective as an antiviral agent, acyclovir must be converted to a phosphorylated derivative. Viral thymidine kinase readily acts on acyclovir to form acyclovir monophosphate. The monophosphate is then converted to the diphosphate and triphosphate by host cellular enzymes. *Acyclovir triphosphate* is the active antiviral agent that selectively inhibits the herpesvirus DNA polymerase. Acyclovir inhibits herpesvirus DNA replication in two ways. First, it inhibits the incorporation of deoxynucleotide triphosphate into the viral DNA. Second, any acyclovir that is incorporated into a viral DNA chain will terminate further replication, since no other nucleotides can be added; acyclovir lacks the 3′-hydroxy group necessary for further chain elongation. Much higher concentrations of acyclovir are required to inhibit host cell growth.

Antiviral Spectrum

Acyclovir is primarily effective against herpes simplex virus, but it has some activity against varicella-zoster virus, cytomegalovirus, and Epstein-Barr virus.

Absorption, Metabolism, and Excretion

Absorption is variable and incomplete following oral administration, with about 15 percent of the dose appearing in the urine as unchanged acyclovir. A small portion is excreted as an oxidized inactive metabolite. Acyclovir is distributed throughout body tissues and is only about 20 percent bound to plasma protein. Acyclovir is both filtered at the glomeruli and actively secreted. A dosage adjustment is necessary in patients with impaired renal function. The plasma half-life of acyclovir in patients with normal renal function is 3–4 hr.

Figure 54-2. Acyclovir.

Clinical Uses

Acyclovir can be administered topically, orally, and parenterally for a variety of herpes infections.

In the treatment of initial episodes of genital herpes, acyclovir has been found to (1) reduce viral shedding, (2) increase the spread of healing of lesions, and (3) decrease the duration of pain and new lesion formation. Acyclovir appears to be less effective in the treatment of recurrent herpes genitalis, although its administration does result in a somewhat decreased rate of recurrences, a reduction in the duration of viral shedding, and a slight reduction in the time necessary for healing. Acyclovir is not able to eradicate the nonreplicating virus, but there is evidence that if therapy is initiated early enough after the primary infection, it may be possible to prevent the secondary infection. For the treatment of genital herpes, acyclovir is usually given orally or as an ointment applied topically to the lesion.

The application of acyclovir as a topical ointment is an effective treatment for herpes keratoconjunctivitis. Acyclovir, given intravenously, shows promise in the treatment of herpes simplex encephalitis and appears to be superior to vidarabine. Acyclovir also accelerates healing in patients with herpes zoster (shingles), but it does not affect postherpetic neuralgia.

Patients receiving immunosuppressive drugs for the treatment of leukemia or those who have received organ transplants have a high incidence of severe reactivated herpes simplex infections. In these patients, acyclovir has been shown to be effective for the prophylaxis and therapy of herpes simplex virus infections and for the therapy of herpes zoster. AIDS patients often are infected with the herpes simplex virus and may require treatment with acyclovir.

Adverse Reactions

Acyclovir toxicity to date has been minimal and consists largely of headache, nausea, and vomiting. Less frequently observed are skin rash, fatigue, fever, increased hair loss, and depression. Rarely, a reversible renal dysfunction has been reported. There are reports of the occurrence of viral resistance to acyclovir, but the extent and significance of this finding are not known.

The potential for drug interactions, particularly with other drugs that are actively secreted by the proximal tubules, should be considered. Probenecid has been shown to inhibit the renal clearance of acyclovir.

Preparations and Dosage

Acyclovir (*Zovirax*) is available for oral administration as 200-mg capsules. For the initial treatment of genital herpes infections the dosage is 1 gm every day for 10 days. For the treatment of recurrent herpes, the same dosage is given for 5 days.

Zovirax Ointment 5% is available as a formulation for topical application.

Interferons

The enhanced production of the antiviral proteins called *interferons* is one of the body's earliest responses to a viral infection. It is thought that the interferons help contain viral infections until the immune system can be fully activated (Fig. 54-3). All cells appear to have the capacity to produce these substances; exposure to an appropriate stimulus (e.g., virus, double-stranded RNA, a protozoal parasite, lipopolysaccharide, or an antibiotic such as kanamycin) is all that is needed to increase a cell's rate of interferon synthesis.

A number of distinct interferon molecules have been identified in human cells. The principal interferon synthesized by white blood cells (interferon-α) differs both from that produced by connective tissue fibroblasts (interferon-β) and that formed by the T lymphocytes (interferon-γ) of the immune system. After their intracellular formation, the interferon molecules diffuse from their site of origin to adjacent cells, where they attach to surface receptors. This attachment in some way initiates the production of additional antiviral proteins.

Interferons can be detected in the blood soon after the introduction of a virus infection, with peak plasma concentrations occurring within approximately 24 hr; interferon levels begin to decline after about 4 days. All the interferons isolated to date are glycoproteins with molecular weights of 18,000 to 20,000; each contains approximately 150 amino acids.

Although it is known that *interferons can prevent viruses from reproducing,* their mode of action is not entirely clear. It has been suggested that once the interferons are released from virus-infected cells, they appear to induce the synthesis of specific proteins in other, noninfected cells.

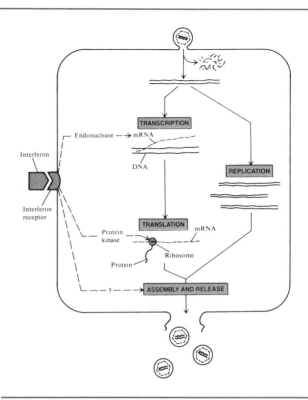

Figure 54-3. Interferons bind to receptor molecules on the surface membrane of an infected cell (left) and may then exert their antiviral effect at several junctures in the viral replication cycle. One is the transcription of the viral DNA: the process by which viral genetic information is copied into messenger RNA (mRNA). Interferons can initiate biochemical events that activate an endonuclease, an enzyme that breaks down the viral mRNA. Another possible target of interferons is translation: the production of proteins from the mRNA template, which occurs on organelles known as ribosomes. Interferons can stimulate the cells to make a protein kinase that inactivates a factor taking part in translation. A third target may be the final step in viral replication: the assembly of new virus particles from viral proteins and replicated genetic material and the release of the particles. The mechanism by which interferons may block virus assembly and release is not known. (From M. S. Hirsch and J. C. Kaplan, Antiviral therapy. April, p. 83. Copyright © 1987 by *Scientific American,* Inc. All rights reserved.)

These proteins probably impair the translation of viral mRNA and thereby prevent further viral multiplication. In addition, the interferons, particularly interferon-γ, stimulate macrophages to greatly increase their oxidative metabolism.

The interferons, in addition to being used to treat viral infections, are being extensively investigated for use in AIDS and cancer therapy. Human cancers showing some responsiveness to interferon administration include osteogenic sarcoma, multiple myeloma, melanoma, breast cancer, and certain leukemias and lymphomas. These substances show particular promise in the treatment and prevention of viral infections in patients whose immune systems have been compromised either by previous drug therapy or by cancer. The possible use of interferons before organ transplantation in patients whose immune systems have been suppressed is also being evaluated.

Interferon research and clinical application have been hampered by the limited availability of these substances. Now exogenous interferons have been produced using recombinant DNA techniques. Interferons-α, -β, and -γ have been produced, and two derivatives of interferon-α (α-2a and -2b) have been approved by the FDA for use against hairy cell leukemia.

Interferon-α is available in three different preparations that have essentially similar activity: α-2a (*Roferon-A*), α-2b (*Intron A*), and α-n3 (*Alferon N*). These agents differ with respect to single amino acid constituents. Interferon-α is effective for condylomata acuminata (papillomavirus infection) and chronic hepatitis B virus (HBV) infection. Parenteral injection of α-2b has resulted in loss of HBV DNA and clinical improvement in 40 percent of patients. A 50 percent response to interferon α-2b has been seen in patients with chronic hepatitis C. It has been suggested that interferon α-2b may prevent chronic liver toxicity. However, chronic hepatitis of autoimmune origin may be worsened by treatment with interferon. Interferon-α also can be used to treat hairy cell leukemia.

Injection of interferon-α can cause "flu-like" symptoms during the first week of therapy. High-dose or chronic therapy has caused bone marrow suppression and neurotoxicity. The following have also been seen: fatigue, depression, muscle weakness, weight and appetite loss,

change in thyroid function, autoantibody formation, and possibly cardiotoxicity.

Interferon-γ has been used to reverse chronic granulomatous disease. Patients treated with interferon-γ experience arthritic side effects. However, the use of this interferon can prevent chronic and life-threatening bacterial infections.

Supplemental Reading

DeClercq, E., and Walker, R.T. (eds.). *Antiviral Drug Development.* New York: Plenum, 1988.

DeMaeyer, E., and DeMaeyer-Guignard, J. *Interferons and Other Regulatory Cytokines.* New York: Wiley, 1988.

Dolin, R. Antiviral chemotherapy and chemoprophylaxis. *Science* 227:1296, 1985.

Evans, A.S. (ed.). *Viral Infections of Humans.* New York: Plenum, 1989.

Field, H.J. *Antiviral Agents: The Development and Assessment of Antiviral Chemotherapy.* Boca Raton, Fla.: CRC, 1988.

Jaffe, H.S., Bucalo, L.R., and Sherwin, S.A. (eds.). *Anti-Infective Applications of Interferon-Gamma.* New York: Marcel Dekker, 1992.

Oxford, J.S., Field, H.J., and Reeves, D.S. (eds.). *Drug Resistance in Viruses, Other Microbes, and Eukaryotes.* New York: Academic, 1986.

Stuart-Harris, C.H., and Oxford, J. (eds.). *Problems of Antiviral Therapy.* Orlando, Fla.: Academic, 1984.

Taylor-Papadimitrious, J. (ed.). *Interferons: Their Impact in Biology and Medicine.* New York: Oxford, 1985.

55

Drugs Used in Acquired Immunodeficiency Syndrome

Knox Van Dyke

Acquired immunodeficiency syndrome (AIDS) is one of the most significant infections to appear in the last decade. This epidemic is not confined to a single segment of the population and its spread is not blocked by natural barriers or international boundaries. Millions have died in Africa and many more individuals are infected worldwide. In the United States more than 100,000 people have died and at least 1 million more are presently infected with the virus. This pandemic shows no signs of abating.

AIDS was first diagnosed in male homosexuals who exhibited a variety of infections of fungal (*Candida albicans*), protozoal (*Pneumocystis carinii, Toxoplasma gondii*), and viral (*Herpes zoster*) origin. Many of these individuals also had an increased incidence of Kaposi's sarcoma and lymphoma. They had a depressed T helper/T suppressor cell ratio and an absence of delayed hypersensitivity responses. Collectively, these observations suggested a deficiency in cell-mediated immunity.

The causative agent in AIDS is an RNA retrovirus called the *human immunodeficiency virus*(HIV I or HIV II) (Fig. 55-1). Currently, there is no known cure for AIDS. However, some progress has been made in understanding and treating this infection. A number of drugs and biological therapies are available that can prolong survival and minimize symptoms. Additionally, it is recognized that the disease is largely preventable by practicing safe sex, carefully controlling the blood supply, and adequately sterilizing instruments used in the health care industry (e.g., needles, syringes, etc.). Current approaches to treatment generally involve immunotherapy (e.g., vaccines against whole killed HIV and a variety of HIV surface glycoproteins) directed at the HIV as well as pharmacological intervention in the HIV infectious process.

The first drug licensed for use in HIV treatment became available in 1987; it was zidovudine (AZT). In the early 1990s, dideoxyinosine (DDI) and dideoxycytidine (DDC) were approved by the Food and Drug Administration (FDA). AZT and DDI were approved for monotherapy while DDC is most likely to be useful in combination with one of the other drugs.

The HIV Infection Process

Human immunodeficiency virus is a retrovirus that possesses an envelope glycoprotein (gp120) that has a high affinity for the CD4 receptor on T helper cells. The infectious process begins when the virus penetrates the body (e.g., through use of an infected needle, sexual transmission, etc.) and enters the bloodstream. The surface glycoprotein (gp120) of the virus binds to the T helper cell CD4 receptor of the host (Fig. 55-2). The virus then fuses with the lymphocyte surface membrane, loses its coat, and releases its RNA core and reverse transcriptase enzyme into the host cell cytoplasm (Fig. 55-3).

The HIV reverse transcriptase (also called DNA polymerase) enzyme copies the RNA message, producing first a single-stranded, and then a double-stranded, DNA (circular complementary DNA). This newly formed double-stranded DNA becomes incorporated into the host chromosomal DNA once it enters the host cell nucleus. This incorporated viral DNA may remain dormant or, on activation, will produce viral messenger RNA (mRNA). The viral mRNA codes for proteins that are important in viral replication. Glycoprotein will then envelop the RNA genome resulting in the production of infectious viral particles; completed viral particles are then released to infect other host cells.

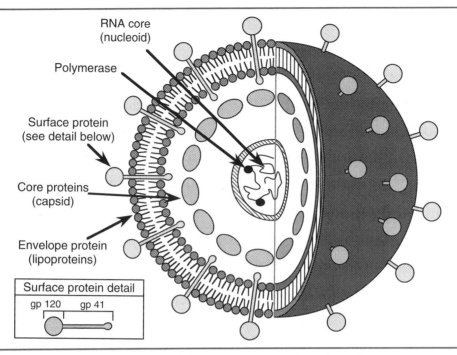

RNA core
(nucleoid)

Polymerase

Surface protein
(see detail below)

Core proteins
(capsid)

Envelope protein
(lipoproteins)

Surface protein detail

gp 120   gp 41

Figure 55-1. Exploded view of the human immunodeficiency virus. It is an RNA (retrovirus) virus that contains surface proteins composed of a knob-like glycoprotein (gp120) linked to a transmembrane stalk (gp41). These surface proteins are the infective mechanism that allows the virus to bind to CD4 proteins of cells, such as T4 lymphocytes and monocytes.

Approved Drugs for AIDS Treatment

In theory any of the steps of viral replication or release could be points of attack against the virus. However, in reality, the most important procedure is the prevention of the initiation of the viral infectious process, that is, prevention of undue exposure to the virus. Once the virus enters the body and begins the uncoating process, a fatal outcome is almost inevitable. The AIDS virus markedly impairs the host immune system and leads to the subsequent appearance of several opportunistic infections and, possibly, cancer.

The major chemotherapeutic attack by available drugs is at the level of inhibition of viral reverse transcriptase (Fig. 55-4). *None of the nucleoside anti-AIDS drugs can cure the HIV infection.* The drugs can delay the onset of symptoms in the early stages of the disease, however. As the disease progresses, the use of AZT can decrease the frequency and severity of AIDS-related infections. AIDS-related neurological symptoms often are improved but patient survival time may not be extended.

Zidovudine

Zidovudine (azidothymidine, AZT) is a 3'-azido derivative of thymidine (Fig. 55-5). The presence of the azido

group on the sugar prevents the formation of the phosphate linkage needed by the virus to complete the DNA polymer. AZT is converted by host kinases to azidothymidine triphosphate, which then competes with host thymidine triphosphate and is incorporated into the growing viral DNA during reverse transcription of the viral RNA. Since this compound is missing the 3'-hydroxyl group, no additional nucleosides can be added to the DNA strand; this results in early termination of viral DNA chain elongation.

Pharmacokinetics

AZT is readily available after oral drug administration and demonstrates good penetration into the central nervous system, probably as a result of its favorable lipid solubility. The serum half-life is approximately one hour. The majority of the drug is metabolized by glucuronidation in the liver, although approximately 25 percent of unchanged AZT may be eliminated by renal mechanisms.

Clinical Effects

AZT is used for the management of patients diagnosed with HIV disease including AIDS and AIDS-related complex (ARC). These patients generally have *P. carinii* pneumonia (PCP) or show an excessively low CD4 (T4

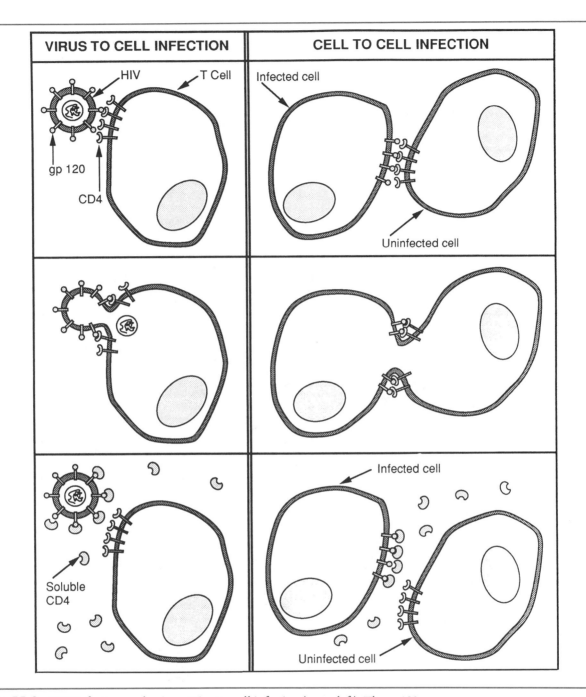

Figure 55-2. HIV infective mechanisms. Virus to cell infection (upper left). The gp120 knob-like surface protein contacts the CD4 receptor on T lymphocytes or other cells (lower left). The virus fuses with the cell and RNA is uncoated (middle left). If soluble CD4 molecules are present, they can bind to the gp120 projections on the HIV virus and prevent infection of the host cell. Once a cell is infected, it can infect noninfected cells by fusion of processed surface gp120 with CD4 receptors of the uninfected cells (upper right). By fusion of infected and multiple noninfected cells, a multinucleated giant cell can be produced (middle right). If soluble CD4 proteins exist, cell-to-cell fusion could be prevented (lower right).

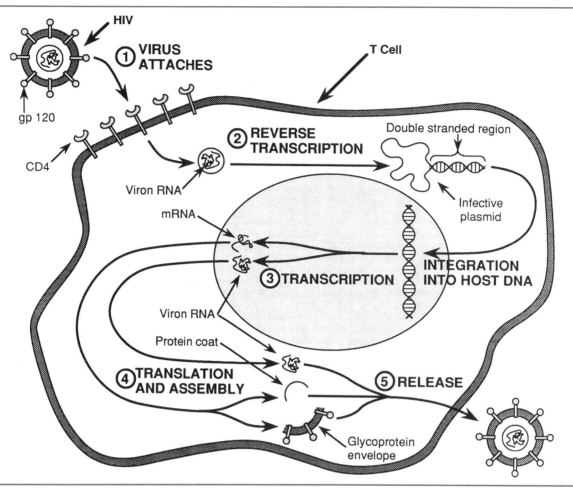

Figure 55-3. Steps that occur in infection and viral replication. Step 1: HIV retrovirus infection of T cell. The gp120 viral knob attaches to a CD4 lymphocyte receptor. Step 2: HIV viral RNA produces a DNA copy using reverse transcriptase. The linear DNA has long terminal repeats at each end that are complementary, and can participate in the formation of a partly double-stranded DNA plasmid. This infective plasmid migrates into the nucleus of the host cell and integrates into its DNA. At some point host DNA, RNA, and protein synthesis is shut off and viral RNA and protein synthesis is turned on, resulting in transcription of RNA. Step 3: Transcription. Step 4: Translation. Translation into protein and assembly of viral particles surrounded by an envelope glycoprotein now occur. Step 5: Release of the completed virus.

helper/inducer) lymphocyte count in the peripheral blood. AZT (500 mg/day) can significantly slow the progression of the infection. In addition, AZT treatment can increase CD4 lymphocyte counts while decreasing serum P24 viral antigen levels. When the drug is given early in the infection, it can decrease opportunistic infections, cause regression of some Kaposi's sarcoma lesions, and improve delayed hypersensitivity reactions.

Patients with HIV disease often have dementia. This condition appears to respond to higher doses of AZT (approaching 1,500 mg/day). At this dose, improved cognition, motor skills, memory, attention span, and general mental speed usually result.

Resistance to AZT

During treatment with AZT, the CD4 lymphocyte count initially rises and then, eventually, falls in part due to drug resistance. Five different mutations have been shown to occur in the viral reverse transcriptase. These mutation sites are involved with nucleotide binding. Data indicate that the degree of resistance correlates with the number of viral mutations present.

Adverse Effects

AZT should be used with caution in patients with bone marrow suppression since both anemia and granulocyto-

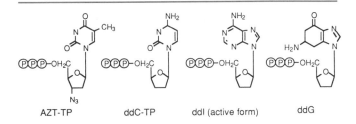

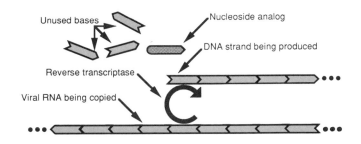

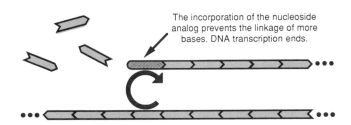

Figure 55-4. Mechanism of inhibition of HIV reverse transcriptase by deoxynucleoside triphosphate analogues. AZT and other pyrimidine and purine deoxynucleoside triphosphates incorporate into the DNA strand by splitting off inorganic pyrophosphate (PPI) and linking to previous DNA nucleotides by a 3',5' linkage. Since the 3' linkage on AZT, DDC, DDI, and DDG is absent, the DNA polymerase is chemically stopped and DNA transcription ends.

plasia can result (Table 55-1). The anemia and granulocytopenia can be helped by administration of recombinant erythropoietin (*Epogen*) and granulocyte-stimulating hormone (G-CSF; *Neupogen*), respectively. The cost of these drugs, however, is often a limiting factor. AZT therapy may result in nausea, myalgias, and insomnia as well as headache and fatigue. Myopathy may appear after several years of treatment.

Preparations and Dosage

Zidovudine or AZT (*Retrovir*) is available as 100-mg capsules, as a 50-mg/teaspoon syrup, and as a 10-mg/ml injection. It is often given every 4 hr in 200-mg doses during the first month of treatment. Careful monitoring of hematological indices is generally required.

Figure 55-5. 3-Azidothymidine (AZT, zidovudine).

Didanosine (Dideoxyinosine)

The second drug approved for use in the treatment of AIDS was didanosine (DDI) (Fig. 55-6). The deoxyribose of DDI has no hydroxyl at either positions 2' or 3'. In the cell DDI is converted to dideoxyadenosine and is then phosphorylated to dideoxyadenosine triphosphate by appropriate kinase enzymes. ddATP is the compound that inhibits viral reverse transcriptase and acts as a chain terminator in a manner similar to that of AZT. Because of the lack of OH group on the 3' position of the deoxysugar, the DNA polymer is terminated and RNA does not produce a proper DNA copy from the viral RNA message.

Pharmacokinetics

DDI is well absorbed after oral administration. Although its plasma half-life is only 1.4 hr, compared to 1.1 for AZT, its active metabolite, ddATP, has a half-life of 8 to 24 hr. Therefore, twice-daily dosing can be used, compared to the five to six times in 24 hr required for AZT. The concentration of DDI in cerebrospinal fluid is only 20 to 50 percent of plasma levels taken concurrently. DDI is taken with antacids or buffer because it is degraded in gastric acid or at a low pH.

Clinical Uses

DDI is used in patients with AIDS or AIDS-related complex. CD4 lymphocyte counts are increased 30 percent over baseline after 8 weeks of drug therapy. After 16 weeks, CD4 levels drop 20 percent below baseline. Response is greatest in patients with higher CD4 counts who have higher steady-state plasma levels of DDI. In addition, viral P24 antigen levels are decreased, indicating that

Table 55-1. Toxic Side Effects of the Nucleoside Analogues

System affected	Observed toxicity	AZT	DDI	DDC
Gastrointestinal	Elevated transaminase	+ +	+	+ +
	Pancreatitis	−	+ + +	+
	Nausea	+ +	+	+
	Diarrhea	+	+ +	+
	Stomatitis	−	−	+ + +
	Abdominal pain	−	+ +	−
	Anorexia	+	−	−
Constitutional	Fatigue/malaise	+ +	+	+
	Headache	+ +	+	+
	Fever	−	−	+
Hematologic	Neutropenia	+ +	+	+
	Granulocytopenia	+	+	+
	Anemia	+ + +	−	−
	Thrombocytopenia	−	+	+
	Macrocytosis	+ +	−	−
Musculoskeletal	Myalgias	+ +	+	−
	Myositis	+ + +	−	−
	Arthralgias	−	−	+
Neurologic	Peripheral neuropathy	−	+ +	+ + +
	Restlessness/agitation	+	+ +	+
	Insomnia	+	−	−
	Seizures	−	−	+
Metabolic	Hyperamylasemia	−	+ +	+
	Hypertriglyceridemia	−	+	−
	Hyperuricemia	−	+ +	−
Dermatologic	Rash	−	−	+ +

Key: The number of plus signs indicates the relative frequency of occurrence.

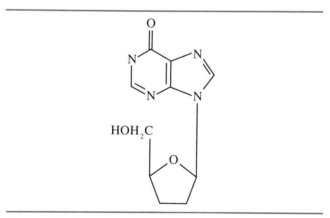

Figure 55-6. Didanosine (dideoxyinosine). This drug is metabolized to dideoxyadenosine and eventually to its active triphosphate form.

viral load was lowered. DDI is indicated for patients who are intolerant to AZT or who become resistant to this drug.

Viral Resistance to DDI

Resistance to DDI has been documented in patients treated initially with AZT and then given DDI. Some patients show clear improvement when switched from AZT to DDI. Eventually, these patients become more sensitive to AZT and sensitivity to DDI decreases.

Adverse Effects

DDI has not been in clinical trial long enough to have a clear picture of all toxicities associated with its use. Pancreatitis is the most serious side effect noted thus far (Table 55-1). Since this can cause death, immediate withdrawal is necessary once pancreatitis is diagnosed. Pancreatitis occurs in fewer than 10 percent of patients. It appears to occur more often in patients whose previous history includes alcoholism. Pancreatitis usually causes nausea, vomiting, abdominal pain, and increased serum amylase. A serum amylase three times normal is found in a number of these patients.

DDI can cause a *peripheral neuropathy*, especially at doses higher than 9 mg/kg/day. *Hyperuricemia* is also associated with higher doses of DDI. Since the drug is a purine, higher doses could increase purine salvage load, precipitating gout. *Hypercalcemia* has been seen in some patients. Hematologic abnormalities are rare.

Zalcitabine (Dideoxycytidine)

In 1992, zalcitabine (DDC) (Fig. 55-7) was approved in combination therapy for infection by HIV. This com-

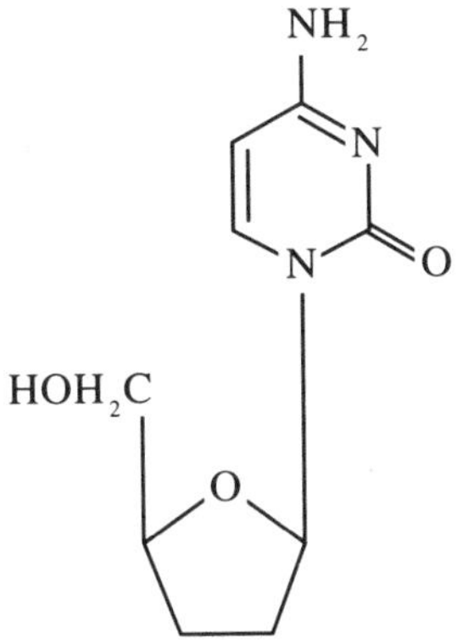

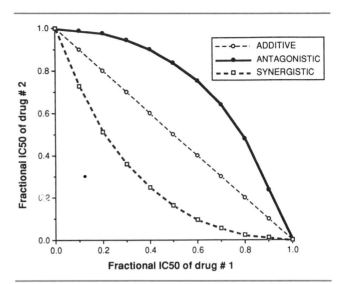

Figure 55-7. Zalcitabine (dideoxycytidine).

pound is a pyrimidine nucleoside that enters cells and is converted by kinases to dideoxycytidine triphosphate (ddTP). ddTP inhibits viral reverse transcriptase and terminates the DNA chain. Thus, DNA cannot be synthesized from the viral RNA primer.

Pharmacokinetics

DDC is a potent orally effective drug. It is well absorbed orally and reaches maximal activity in 1 to 2 hr. It penetrates into cerebrospinal fluid and reaches 20 percent of blood concentrations assayed simultaneously. DDC also decreases P24 antigen levels from the HIV virus and transiently decreases CD4 lymphocyte counts. In some studies DDC seemed to be superior to AZT. However, this is not yet clear.

Clinical Uses

DDC was approved for use with AZT to treat patients with severe HIV infection. Currently, it is not to be used as monotherapy. Resistance to DDC has been observed to develop.

Adverse Effects

Few clinical trials with DDC have been published. In general, adverse reactions are similar to those of DDI, although some differences do exist (Table 55-1). Peripheral neuropathy, stomatitis, and rash occur less often with DDI than with DDC, pancreatitis is seldom seen with DDC. Skin rashes are observed in 8 to 10 percent of patients while fatigue and gastrointestinal effects occur less often than with AZT. Anemia and decreased platelets occur in fewer than 4 percent of patients, but decreased granulocytes or neutrophils are seen in 8 to 10 percent of patients, which indicates that peripheral blood counts need to be monitored.

Figure 55-8. Drug isobologram. An isobologram results when fractions of the 50 percent inhibitory concentration (IC$_{50}$) of one drug are plotted against corresponding values for a second drug. If the actions of two drugs, when used together, are additive, a linear relationship will exist in such a plot. If the drugs act synergistically, the resulting curve is concave, reflective of the need for lower doses of each drug. If the two drugs are mutually antagonistic, the curve is convex showing that higher doses of each of the combined drugs are needed.

Possible Application of Sequential Blockade and Synergism to AIDS Treatment

When two points of a sequential metabolic pathway are inhibited, smaller amounts of drug can be utilized at both points compared to the amount of drug necessary to inhibit a single point of the pathway. Not only is this method of treatment often more effective, but it is also more difficult for an organism to mutate against two points of attack compared to one.

This may prove to be the case with AIDS therapy. Combination therapy, therefore, may be much more effective than monotherapy. Usually, such combinations display synergism; that is, the combination is more effective than the additive effects of either drug alone. This can be illustrated with an isobologram; that is, a graph of the fraction at 50 percent inhibitory concentrations of drugs plotted against each other (Fig. 55-8).

DNA is composed of four different bases: adenine, thymidine, guanine, and cytidine. Therefore, when the RNA of the AIDS virus is copied to produce a DNA copy, each base could be a point of attack by competitive drugs such as the dideoxy derivative of each base. Instead of using mono- or ditherapy, it would appear to be logical to use all four base antagonists (tetratherapy) simultaneously. This would put maximum stress against the replication of DNA from RNA and make it maximally difficult for the virus to mutate against four points of attack simultaneously. In addition, less of each competitor could be used because of the existence of synergism between the competitors. Rather than causing more toxicity to the host, it could be expected that because of the inherent synergism between the drugs less toxicity might be expected.

Treatment of AIDS-Related Diseases

Pneumocystis carinii *Pneumonia*

The most common infection in advanced AIDS is PCP. Recently, this disease was found to be a fungal infection rather than a parasitic or bacterial disease. Previously, pneumonia developed in 80 percent of AIDS patients at least once. It is often the actual cause of death from AIDS infection.

Current therapies for PCP use cotrimoxazole and parenteral pentamidine. Either therapy is effective but side effects limit their effectiveness in 30 to 60 percent of patients. An alternative drug therapy is the combined use of dapsone and trimethoprim. A combination of oral primaquine and clindamycin is 90 percent effective for prophylaxis and treatment of PCP. Another combination useful for *Pneumocystis* is cotrimazole, dapsone, and trimethoprim.

Aerosolized pentamidine has been used to decrease parenteral toxicity and should be administered in mild to moderate disease. Pentamidine delivered by jet nebulizer once a month (300 mg) decreases PCP recurrence 80 percent among patients with AIDS. Two cotrimoxazole tablets are more effective prophylactically than is aerosol pentamidine. Dapsone also can be used for prophylaxis. Prednisone, 40 mg twice a day for 5 days, in addition to the standard PCP therapy, is used to inhibit AIDS-related pulmonary inflammation.

Fungal Infections

Fungal infections (e.g., coccidioidomycosis) often complicate advanced AIDS infections and even cause death. In dry regions such as the Southwest, coccidioidomycosis is the third highest ancillary infection in AIDS. AIDS patients with deep-seated mycosis respond well to amphotericin B, but after a year 90 percent need retreatment, compared to 10 to 20 percent in patients who do not have AIDS. Ketoconazole has been used, but the failure rate is 50 percent in patients with AIDS.

Candidiasis in oral or vaginal cavities, or both, occurs early and in many patients. The more invasive fungal infections usually are seen later in severe AIDS.

In the Midwest, histoplasmosis is an endemic infection in a large proportion of the population. This disease is seen in 5 to 10 percent of AIDS patients there. Itraconazole has been used effectively in patients with AIDS to treat primary or secondary infections.

Cryptococcosis occurs in 2 to 13 percent of patients with AIDS as meningitis, pneumonitis, or disseminated diseases. Standard therapy with amphotericin B alone or with flucytosine is effective in patients with AIDS, but relapse occurs often. Fluconazole taken orally has been approved for cryptococcosis.

Reactivation of histoplasmosis associated with AIDS usually affects the brain. Since the standard therapy of pyrimethamine and sulfadiazine is more toxic in AIDS patients, clindamycin and pyrimethamine are used. Cotrimoxazole is also effective against both diseases.

Viral Infections

Herpes viral infection is often seen with AIDS infections and, therefore, acyclovir is used continuously. Resistance often occurs via alterations in the viral thymidine kinase necessary for drug activation. Alternatively, vidarabine (ara-A) or phosphonoformate trisodium could be used. When topical therapy is needed, trifluridine has been used effectively.

Cytomegalovirus (CMV) contributes to illness and death in patients with AIDS. Often, autopsy reveals CMV infections of eye, lungs, liver, gut, and central nervous system. AIDS retinitis is a major problem with a 20 percent incidence and the virus can cause irreversible necrosis of the retina. Both ganciclovir and foscarnet have been approved for CMV retinitis. Both are effective, but foscarnet is more toxic. These drugs are 80 to 100 percent effective initially, but drug resistance often occurs later.

Mycobacterial Infections

Infections with mycobacteria can become very aggressive in an immunocompromised host. In patients with AIDS, tuberculosis can develop when CD4 lymphocyte counts fall. If an AIDS patient is infected with a drug-sensitive strain of tuberculosis, it can be readily treated. However, drug-resistant isolates have been found in New York and Miami, and these require aggressive therapy with all four antituberculosis drugs (see Chap. 53).

AIDS-Associated Cancers

Suppression of the immune system either by drugs or by AIDS carries the risk of inducing Kaposi's sarcoma or

Hodgkin's lymphoma. The mucocutaneous form of Kaposi's sarcoma has been treated with irradiation and/or administration with interferon-α, etoposide (VP-16), vincristine, vinblastine, or possibly taxol. Disseminated Kaposi's sarcoma can be much more severe and must be treated aggressively.

Non-Hodgkin's lymphoma (NHL) occurs in transplant recipients as well as in AIDS patients at fairly high rates (~15%). NHL tends to follow bone marrow suppression. Central nervous system lymphoma is becoming more prevalent in AIDS.

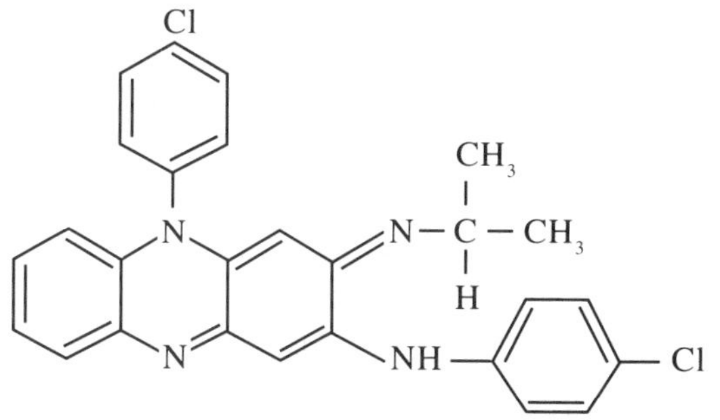

Drugs for Treatment of AIDS-Related Diseases

Clofazimine

Clofazimine is used to treat individuals with *Mycobacterium avium–intracellulare, M. leprae,* or possibly *M. tuberculosis*. Clofazimine is a phenazine dye (Fig. 55-9) with antimycobacterial and antiinflammatory activity. It binds preferentially to mycobacterial DNA by a nonintercalative mechanism. It seems to have a predilection for guanine-cytosine base pairs in DNA.

Clofazimine is a highly lipophilic compound that is only partially orally absorbed (45–50%). It is not metabolized and distributes in fatty tissues, but does not enter the central nervous system. Its half-life is 8 days. It is excreted in the feces.

It can cause discoloration of the conjunctiva of the eye and gastrointestinal side effects including abdominal pain, nausea, and vomiting.

Pentamidine

Pentamidine isoethionate is primarily an antifungal or antiprotozoal drug. It is a secondary drug for both the treatment of PCP infection and leishmaniasis or African sleeping sickness. It is less toxic given by the inhalational route in PCP infections. Since many AIDS patients cannot tolerate sulfisoxazole/trimethoprim, inhalational pentamidine is often used.

Pentamidine binds to DNA and inhibits replication of susceptible organisms that cause PCP, leishmaniasis, and trypanosomiasis.

Pentamidine is not well absorbed orally and is either inhaled or given intravenously or intramuscularly. Tissue binding is extensive, with detectable drug levels found in plasma 6 to 8 weeks after dosing. It is excreted essentially unmetabolized.

When pentamidine is given by the IM or IV route, adverse reactions occur frequently. Infusion must be done

Figure 55-9. Clofazimine.

slowly to prevent ventricular arrhythmias, tachycardia, vomiting, shortness of breath, headache, and hypotension. Diabetic patients should have blood sugar monitored frequently. Renal function and the appearance of blood dyscrasias also need to be monitored. Upon cessation of therapy, side effects generally subside. Inhalational drug is much better tolerated by AIDS patients.

Drug interactions have been reported to occur with aminoglycosides, gentamicin, acyclovir, amphotericin B, bumetanide, carmustine, cisplatin, cyclosporine, ethacrynic acid, furosemide, plicamycin, and streptozocin.

Foscarnet

Foscarnet is a secondary drug used for AIDS retinitis caused by cytomegalovirus infection. It inhibits the synthesis of cytomegalovirus DNA.

Foscarnet is not well absorbed after oral administration, and is usually given intravenously. Its half-life is about 3 hr; the drug is not metabolized and is excreted unchanged. Foscarnet is deposited in bone.

Nephrotoxicity and anemia are the main toxicities associated with the use of foscarnet. The drug causes tremor, headache, fatigue, nausea, and vomiting. Foscarnet has been reported to have interactions with aminoglycosides (amikacin, etc.), amphotericin B, edetate disodium, and pentamidine.

Ganciclovir

Ganciclovir is used to treat CMV infections, which are prevalent in immunocompromised and AIDS patients. It is given intravenously because of its poor absorption via the oral route. More than 90 percent of ganciclovir is excreted unchanged by the kidneys.

The common adverse reactions associated with the use of ganciclovir are granulo- and thrombocytopenia. Anemia, fever, rash, and abnormal liver function tests have been reported in some patients.

Probenicid competes with the renal tubular secretion of ganciclovir. Nephrotoxic agents, for example, imipenem/cilastatin and AZT, increase the risk of renal dysfunction.

Supplemental Reading

Hersh, E.M. Current status of immunotherapy of patients with HIV infection. *Int. J. Immunopharmacol.* 13:9, 1991.

White, D.A., and Gold, J.W. Medical management of AIDS patients. *Med. Clin. North Am.* 76:1–287, 1992.

Yarchoan, R., et al. Treatment of Acquired Immunodeficiency Syndrome. In H.M. Pinedo, B.A. Chabner, and D.L. Longo (eds.), *Cancer Chemotherapy and Biological Response Modifiers Annual II.* Elsevier: New York, 1990.

Youle, M., et al. *AIDS—Therapeutics in HIV Disease.* Edinburgh: Churchill Livingstone, 1988.

56

Antiprotozoal Drugs

Roger G. Finch and *Irvin S. Snyder*

Protozoal and helminthic infections are a major cause of disease in many parts of the world. Although some of these diseases are endemic to the United States, or can be found in migrant workers or individuals returning from an endemic area, many other such infections are rarely seen in the United States. However, physicians should be aware of these diseases and seek advice from those experienced in their diagnosis and treatment.

A number of compounds are available for the treatment of infections caused by protozoa. Drugs used in the treatment of malaria are discussed in Chap. 57. While most antiprotozoal agents are products of laboratory synthesis, a few antibiotics are available for the treatment of amebiasis and one variety of leishmaniasis. Although the mode of action of many antiprotozoals is not well understood, Table 56-1 summarizes the assumed or known modes of action of a number of the agents.

Protozoal Diseases

Amebiasis and Balantidial Dysentery

The protozoan *Entamoeba histolytica* causes amebiasis, an infection that is endemic in parts of the United States. The parasite can be present in the host either as an encysted or trophozoite form. Initial ingestion of the cyst may result either in no symptoms or in a severe amebic dysentery characterized by the frequent passage of blood-stained stools. The latter symptom occurs after invasion of the intestinal mucosa by the actively motile and phagocytic trophozoite form of the protozoan.

Trophozoites may spread to the liver through the portal vein and produce an acute amebic hepatitis or, more rarely, the trophozoites may encyst and produce an amebic liver abscess many years later. On rare occasions, amebic abscesses are found in other organs, such as the lungs or the brain.

Many patients continue to excrete cysts for several years after recovery from the acute disease and, therefore, are a hazard to themselves and other persons; the public health risk is greatest when persons employed as food handlers are affected. More recently, it has been recognized that infection can be transmitted by homosexual activities.

The pharmacological management of diseases caused by *E. histolytica* is shown in Table 56-2.

Balantidium coli is the largest of the protozoans that infect humans. The trophozoite form is covered with cilia, which impart mobility. Infection is acquired through the ingestion of cyst-contaminated soil, food, or water. The trophozoite causes a superficial necrosis or deep ulceration in the mucosa and submucosa of the large intestine. Otherwise healthy persons commonly exhibit symptoms of nausea, vomiting, abdominal pain, and diarrhea, whereas debilitated or nutritionally stressed patients may develop severe dysentery.

Trichomoniasis and Giardiasis

Trichomoniasis is a genital infection produced by the protozoan *Trichomonas vaginalis*. Infections frequently are asymptomatic in the male, whereas in the female a vaginitis characterized by a frothy pale-yellow discharge is common. Relapses occur if the infected person's sexual partner is not treated simultaneously.

Giardiasis is caused by the protozoan *Giardia lamblia* and is characterized by gastrointestinal symptoms ranging from an acute self-limiting diarrhea to a chronic condition associated with episodic diarrhea and occasional instances of malabsorption. The parasite is similar to *E. histolytica* in that it exists in two forms, an actively motile trophozoite

Table 56-1. Chemotherapeutic Agents Used in Treatment of Protozoal Disease

Drug	Specific effects	Mode of action
Arsenicals (melarsoprol, tryparsamide), antimonials	Binds with SH groups and selectively inhibits pyruvate kinase	Affects protein structure, function and synthesis
Emetine and dehydroemetine	Interferes with elongation of polypeptide by inhibiting translocation	
Paromomycin	Interferes with initiation complex; causes misreading of mRNA	
Diamidines (pentamidine)	Binds to kinetoplast DNA	Affects synthesis or structure of nucleic acids
Metronidazole	Inhibits DNA replication	
Nifurtimox	Generation of toxic oxygen radicals	Unknown
Suramin	Binds to intestinal epithelium; inhibits glucose utilization	Unknown
Iodoquinol, diloxanide furoate	Unknown	Unknown
Eflornithine	Inhibits ornithine decarboxylase and biosynthesis of polyamines	Affects cell division and differentiation

Key: SH = sulfhydryl; mRNA = messenger RNA.

Table 56-2. Drug Treatment of Amebiasis

State of disease	Drug of choice	Alternate drug
Asymptomatic	Iodoquinol or paromomycin	Diloxanide furoate
Intestinal disease (dysenteric or nondysenteric)	Metronidazole followed by iodoquinol or paromomycin	Dehydroemetine + iodoquinol
Hepatic abscess	Metronidazole followed by iodoquinol or paromomycin	Dehydroemetine followed by chloroquine phosphate + iodoquinol

(usually confined to the upper small bowel) and a cyst (commonly excreted in the feces).

Leishmaniasis and Trypanosomiasis

The flagellate leishmania is transmitted to humans by the bite of the female sandfly of the genus *Phlebotomus*. Three principal diseases result from infection with leishmania. *Leishmania donovani* causes visceral leishmaniasis (kala-azar), *L. tropica* and *L. major* produce cutaneous leishmaniasis, and *L. braziliensis* causes South American mucocutaneous leishmaniasis. In visceral leishmaniasis, the protozoan parasitizes the reticuloendothelial cells, and this results in an enlargement of the lymph nodes, liver, and spleen; the spleen can become massive. Cutaneous leishmaniasis remains localized at the site of inoculation, where it forms a raised ulcerative and disfiguring lesion. South American leishmaniasis is variable in its presentation. It is characterized by ulceration of the mucous mem-

branes of the nose, mouth, and pharynx; there also may be some disfiguring skin involvement.

African trypanosomiasis follows the bite of a tsetse fly infected with the protozoan *Trypanosoma brucei*. The ensuing illness (*sleeping sickness*) is initially characterized by fever, headache, and lymph node enlargement. These symptoms are followed by wasting, mental disturbances, and drowsiness as nervous system involvement progresses. There are geographical variations of the disease. *Rhodesian sleeping sickness* is a much more acute and rapidly progressive disease than *Gambian sleeping sickness,* in which the incubation period can be more prolonged and the disease more protracted.

Chagas' disease is the South American variety of trypanosomiasis and is caused by *Trypanosoma cruzi*. It is quite different from African trypanosomiasis in its clinical and pathological presentation and in its failure to respond to agents effective in that disease. It has both an acute and chronic phase. The latter frequently results in gastrointestinal and myocardial disease that ultimately ends in death.

Antiprotozoal Drugs

Metronidazole

Structure and Mechanism of Action

Metronidazole (Fig. 56-1) is a 5-nitroimidazole that exerts activity against most anaerobic bacteria and several protozoa. The drug freely penetrates protozoal and bacterial cells, but not mammalian cells. It has a redox potential lower than that of the electron transfer protein ferredoxin, which is found in anaerobic or microaerophilic

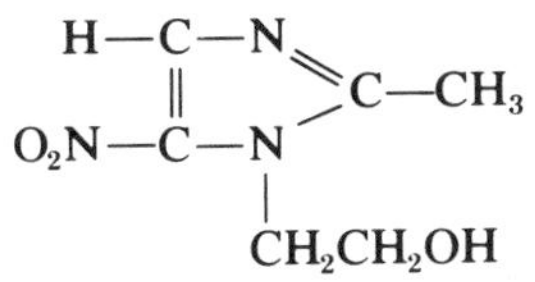

H—C—N
‖   ⧵
         C—CH₃
O₂N—C—N
        |
      CH₂CH₂OH

Figure 56-1. Metronidazole.

organisms. As a result, metronidazole can function as an electron sink, and because it does so, its 5-nitro group is reduced. Nitroreductase, found only in anaerobic organisms, reduces metronidazole and thereby activates the drug. The unstable nitro anion radical and hydroxylamine derivative are the proposed toxic intermediates. Reduced metronidazole incubated with DNA causes multiple single-strand breaks, disrupts replication and transcription, and inhibits DNA repair.

Antimicrobial Spectrum

Metronidazole is inhibitory to *E. histolytica, G. lamblia, T. vaginalis, Blastocystis hominis,* and *Balantidium coli,* and to the helminth *Dracunculus medinensis.* It is also bactericidal for obligate anaerobic gram-positive and gram-negative bacteria, with the exception of *Actinomyces* species. It is not active against aerobes or facultative anaerobes. Drug resistance is rare.

Absorption, Metabolism, and Excretion

Absorption from the intestinal tract is usually good. Food delays but does not reduce absorption. The drug is distributed in body fluids and has a half-life of about 8 hr. High levels are found in plasma and cerebrospinal fluid (CSF). Less than 20 percent binds to plasma proteins. Metronidazole is metabolized by oxidation and glucuronide formation in the liver and is primarily excreted by the kidneys, although small amounts can be found in saliva and breast milk. Dose reduction is generally unnecessary in renal failure.

Clinical Uses

Metronidazole is the most effective agent available for the treatment of all forms of amebiasis with, perhaps, the exception of the person who is asymptomatic but continues to excrete cysts. In that situation, diiodohydroxyquin is the most effective intraluminal amebicide. Metronidazole is active against intestinal and extraintestinal cysts and trophozoites. However, the dose required varies according to the situation.

Metronidazole was used originally in the treatment of trichomoniasis. A 7-day course of metronidazole is highly effective in treating this form of vaginitis. The sexual partner of the infected person should be treated simultaneously to prevent reinfection.

Although quinacrine hydrochloride (see Chap. 57) remains the drug of choice for the treatment of giardiasis, many physicians prefer metronidazole for its greater efficacy. Furazolidone is an alternate choice.

Metronidazole is highly active against the majority of anaerobic bacteria pathogenic to humans. It is currently the drug of choice for treating anaerobic bacterial infections in Europe, although concern about possible carcinogenicity has led to some caution in its use in the United States.

Adverse Reactions

The most frequently observed adverse reactions include nausea, vomiting, cramps, diarrhea, and a metallic taste. The urine is often dark or red-brown. Less frequently, unsteadiness, vertigo, ataxia, paresthesias, peripheral neuropathy, encephalopathy, and neutropenia have been reported. In most instances these adverse reactions are reversed by stopping treatment. Alcohol should be avoided during treatment with metronidazole, since a disulfiram-like reaction can occur, as can psychotic reactions.

Although metronidazole has been used in adults for many years with no apparent fetal toxicity, some concern remains. Animal toxicity studies have shown an association between high-dose metronidazole administration and lung cancer in rats. Bacteria exposed to metronidazole have an increased mutation rate, which suggests that there may be a risk of teratogenicity for humans. For these reasons, the drug is not recommended for use during pregnancy, although evidence of human toxicity is lacking.

Preparations and Dosage

Metronidazole (*Flagyl, Metrogel, Protostat*) is provided as 250-mg tablets. It is also available for intravenous use.

Emetine and Dehydroemetine

Structure and Mode of Action

Emetine (Fig. 56-2) and its derivative dehydroemetine are synthesized from ipecac alkaloids. They inhibit protein synthesis in eukaryotic cells by preventing translocation of peptidyl-transfer RNA (tRNA) from the acceptor site to the donor site on the ribosome. Why these drugs fail to inhibit protein synthesis in mammalian cells is not known.

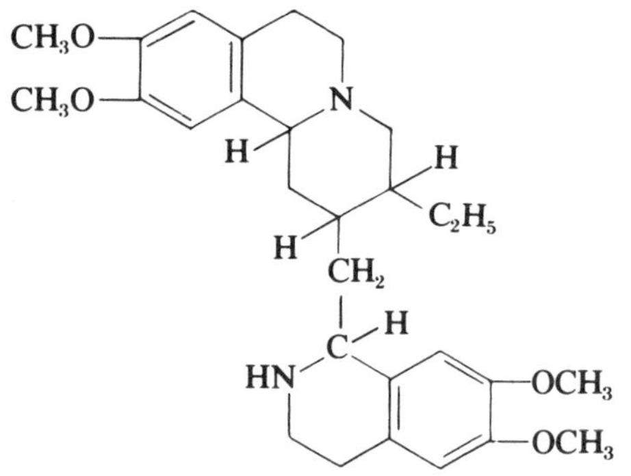

Figure 56-2. Emetine.

Antimicrobial Spectrum

Emetine and dehydroemetine kill the trophozoite stage of E. histolytica, but only when it is in tissues. They have no effect on either the cyst or trophozoite forms present in the intestinal lumen.

Absorption, Distribution, and Excretion

Emetine and dehydroemetine are rapidly absorbed from the injection site and are concentrated and stored in several tissues, including the liver, lungs, spleen, and kidney. The principal route of excretion in humans is assumed to be the kidneys, but some animal studies have shown most of the drug to be present in the feces. Excretion of emetine is slow and the drug can readily accumulate; therefore, the dosage administered must be monitored carefully. Dehydroemetine is excreted more rapidly than emetine, which probably accounts for its lower toxicity.

Clinical Uses

Emetine and dehydroemetine are not widely used. They are given in combination with other drugs in alternative regimens for the treatment of severe intestinal amebiasis and hepatic abscess caused by E. histolytica.

Adverse Reactions

Emetine and dehydroemetine produce local and systemic reactions. Both drugs are irritants and their administration frequently produces pain, tenderness, and muscular weakness at the site of injection.

Gastrointestinal toxicity due to a direct stimulation of the smooth muscle in the gut is common and is manifested by diarrhea, cramps, and vomiting. These side effects should not be confused with similar symptoms seen in amebic dysentery. If the side effects are very severe, drug treatment must be stopped.

Muscular aches, tenderness, stiffness, and weakness can occur and may be indicative of more serious toxic effects on the cardiovascular system. Hypotension, tachycardia, shortness of breath, precordial chest pain, and electrocardiographic (ECG) effects are the most serious. Mild ECG changes (e.g., prolongation of the P–R and Q–T intervals and flattening of the T waves) occur in 25 to 50 percent of patients; rhythm changes are rare. Careful monitoring of the patient is essential to prevent lasting myocardial damage, and undue exercise should be prohibited. Preexisting cardiac disease is a contraindication to the use of emetine and dehydroemetine unless the amebic infection is life threatening.

Dehydroemetine is claimed to have a similar therapeutic efficacy and fewer and less severe toxic manifestations than emetine. However, these claims are not universally accepted.

Preparations

Emetine hydrochloride is available only for parenteral use. It is usually administered by IM or SC injection.

Dehydroemetine dihydrochloride can be obtained from the Parasitic Diseases Division, Centers for Disease Control, Atlanta, Ga. 30333.

Iodoquinol

Structure and Mode of Action

Iodoquinol (diiodohydroxyquin) is a halogenated 8-hydroxyquinoline derivative (Fig. 56-3). The precise mechanism of action is not known, although it can inhibit several parasite enzymes.

Antimicrobial Spectrum

Iodoquinol kills the trophozoite forms of E. histolytica, B. coli, B. hominis, and Dientamoeba fragilis.

Absorption, Metabolism, and Excretion

Iodoquinol is absorbed from the gastrointestinal tract and excreted in the urine as glucuronide and sulfate conjugates. Most of an orally administered dose is excreted in the feces. Iodoquinol has a plasma half-life of about 12 hr. A single oral dose of 250 mg results in serum levels of 5 μg within 4 to 8 hr.

Clinical Use

Iodoquinol is the drug of choice in the treatment of asymptomatic amebiasis and D. fragilis infections. It is also

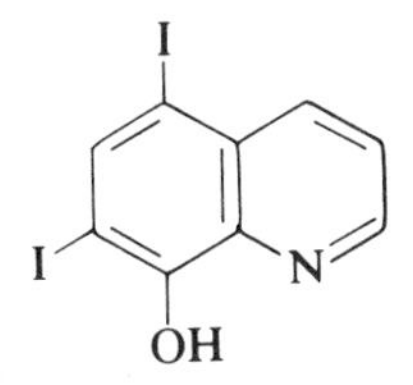

Figure 56-3. Iodoquinol.

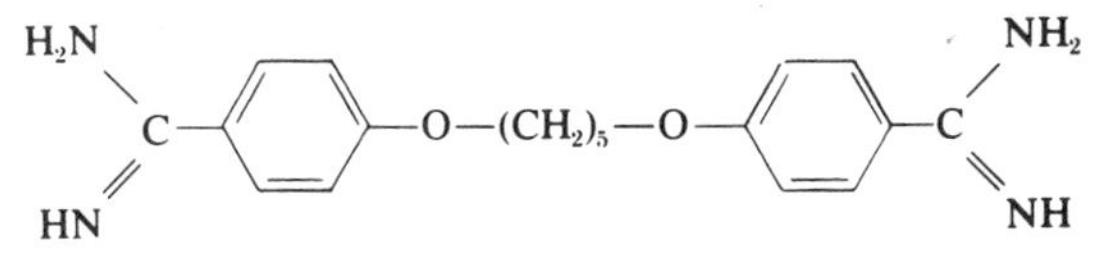

Figure 56-4. Pentamidine.

used in combination with other drugs in the treatment of other forms of amebiasis and as an alternative to tetracycline in the treatment of balantidiasis. The use of iodoquinol in the treatment of "traveler's diarrhea" is no longer recommended, since this disease is of short duration and the use of trimethroprim, trimethoprim-sulfamethoxazole, or a 4-quinolone is preferred.

Adverse Reactions

Adverse reactions are related to the iodine content of the drug; the toxicity is often expressed as skin reactions, thyroid enlargement, and interference with thyroid function studies. Headache and diarrhea also occur.

Preparations and Dosage

Iodoquinol (*Yodoxin, Moebiquin*) is marketed as 210- and 650-mg tablets and as a 25-gm powder.

Pentamidine

Structure and Mechanism of Action

Pentamidine is an aromatic diamidine (Fig. 56-4). The drug binds to DNA and may inhibit DNA replication. An effect on organism respiration, especially at high doses, also may play a role.

Antimicrobial Spectrum

Pentamidine is active against *Pneumocystis carinii* and trypanosomes.

Absorption, Distribution, and Excretion

Pentamidine is not well absorbed from the intestinal tract after oral administration and generally is given by intramuscular injection. The drug binds to tissues, particularly the kidney, and is slowly excreted, mostly as the unmodified drug. It does not enter the central nervous system (CNS). Its sequestration in tissues accounts for its prophylactic use in trypanosomiasis.

Clinical Use

Pentamidine is an alternative agent for the treatment of *P. carinii* pneumonia. Although it is more toxic than trimethoprim-sulfamethoxazole, it has been widely used in patients with acquired immunodeficiency syndrome (AIDS), in whom *P. carinii* infection is common (see Chap. 55), and often associated with hypersensitivity reactions to trimethoprim-sulfamethoxazole.

Clinical Use

Pentamidine is an alternative drug for visceral leishmaniasis, especially in those situations in which sodium stibogluconate has failed or is contraindicated. Pentamidine is also a reserve agent for the treatment of trypanosomiasis before the CNS is invaded. This characteristic largely restricts its use to Gambian trypanosomiasis.

Adverse Reactions

Since adverse reactions occur frequently with pentamidine, considerable caution is necessary when it is used. Pain at the site of injection is not unusual; although the drug was previously given by intramuscular injection, the intravenous route is now preferred. Rapid infusion may produce tachycardia, vomiting, shortness of breath, headache, and a fall in blood pressure. Changes in blood sugar (hypoglycemia or hyperglycemia) necessitate caution in its use, particularly in patients with diabetes mellitus. Renal function should be monitored and blood counts checked for dyscrasias. Fortunately, the majority of the above adverse reactions are reversible.

Preparations

Pentamidine isethionate (*Pentam 300*) is marketed in the United States only for treatment and prevention of *P. carinii* pneumonia in those with HIV infection.

Suramin

Structure and Mechanism of Action

Suramin is a derivative of a nonmetallic dye (Fig. 56-5). Its antiparasitic mechanism of action is not clear. Sur-

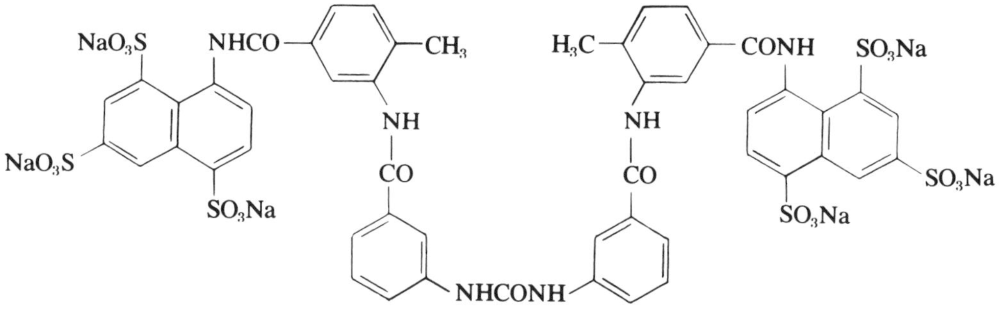

Figure 56-5. Suramin.

amin has been shown to inhibit glucose metabolism of trypanosomes. However, glucose utilization does not appear to be altered in treated helminths. In worms, suramin apparently binds to intestinal epithelium after ingestion and causes alterations in the structure and function of the epithelium. In *Onchocerca volvulus,* it inhibits dihydrofolate reductase. Whether the effect on the worm is due to this alteration, however, is not clear. Because it is a large, negatively charged molecule, it may bind to cationic sites on protein. Suramin does not readily penetrate mammalian cells; this may account for its selective toxicity.

Absorption, Distribution, and Excretion

Suramin is not absorbed from the intestinal tract and is administered intravenously. Although the initial high plasma levels drop rapidly, suramin binds tightly to, and is slowly released from, plasma proteins, and so persists in the host for up to 3 months. Suramin neither penetrates cells nor enters the CNS. It is excreted by glomerular filtration, largely as the intact molecule.

Clinical Uses

Suramin is used primarily to treat African trypanosomiasis, for which it is the drug of choice. It is effective in treating disease caused by *Trypanosoma gambiense* and *T. rhodesiense,* but not *T. cruzi* (i.e., Chagas' disease). It can be used alone prophylactically or during the initial stages of the disease. Later stages of the disease, particularly those involving the CNS, are more commonly treated with a combination of suramin and the arsenical tryparsamide.

The drug used for treatment of sleeping sickness is determined by the presence or absence of CNS involvement. Suramin is the most effective agent in the early stages of the disease and for prophylaxis. When CNS involvement occurs, the poor penetration of suramin and pentamidine into the CSF requires alternative forms of chemotherapy,

such as melarsoprol or tryparsamide in combination with suramin. In treating *O. volvulus* infections, suramin is an alternative to ivemectin. Suramin is used after initial treatment with diethylcarbamazine.

Adverse Reactions

It is important to test for drug sensitivity by administering a small (200 mg) dose by slow IV injection before giving the full amount of suramin. Since adverse reactions occur with greater frequency and severity among the malnourished, greater caution is necessary for patients with advanced trypanosomiasis. An acute reaction in sensitive individuals results in nausea, vomiting, colic, hypotension, urticaria, and even unconsciousness; fortunately, this reaction is rare. Rashes, photophobia, paresthesias, and hyperesthesia may occur later; these symptoms may presage a peripheral neuropathy. Mild albuminuria is not uncommon, but hematuria with casts suggests nephrotoxicity and the need to stop treatment.

Preparations

Suramin sodium (*Germanin*) is usually administered IV as a 10% solution in water for injection. It is available from the Parasitic Diseases Division, Centers for Disease Control.

Eflornithine

Eflornithine (difluoromethylornithine) is a unique antiprotozoal agent in that its mode of action is by inhibition of a specific enzyme, ornithine decarboxylase. In eukaryotes, decarboxylation of ornithine is required for biosynthesis of polyamines, which are important in cell division and differentiation.

Eflornithine is given intravenously. About 80 percent

of the drug is excreted in urine within 24 hr. It does not bind significantly to plasma proteins and has a terminal plasma half-life of about 3 hr. It crosses the blood-brain barrier and is one of the drugs of choice for treating the hemolymphatic and meningoencephalitic stage of *Trypanosoma brucei gambiense.* The most significant side effects are anemia and leukopenia. Diarrhea, thrombocytopenia, and seizures are occasionally reported.

Eflornithine (*Ornidyl*) is available in 100-ml vials with a concentration of 200 mg/ml.

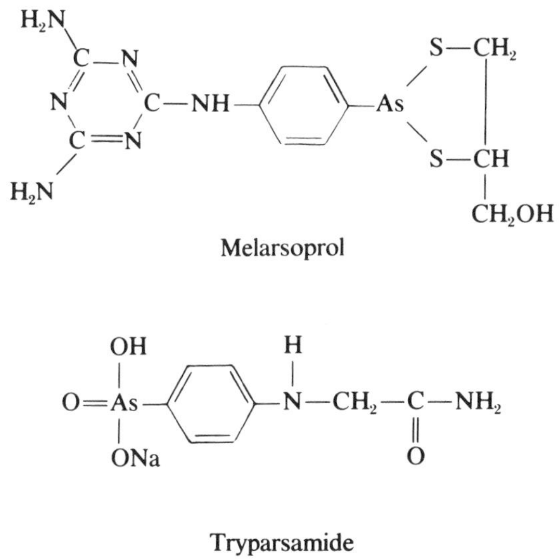

Arsenicals

Structure and Mechanism of Action

Melarsoprol (trivalent) and tryparsamide (pentavalent) (Fig. 56-6) are organic compounds containing arsenic. Arsenicals bind to sulfhydryl (SH) groups in proteins, thereby affecting cellular structure and function. The action of arsenic is nonspecific and any selective toxicity achieved is related to differences in drug permeability and SH content of the affected structure or enzyme. Melarsoprol shows some selectivity for trypanosome enzymes. This may be due to the greater sensitivity of the trypanosomal pyruvate kinase compared to the corresponding mammalian enzyme. Resistance has started to emerge among trypanosomes responsible for African trypanosomiasis.

Absorption, Distribution, and Excretion

These drugs are administered intravenously. Their value lies in their ability to penetrate the CNS, and hence they are useful in treating meningoencephalitis caused by trypanosomes. The CNS concentration ranges from 2 to 20 percent of the plasma concentration. The drugs are eliminated rapidly.

Clinical Uses

The arsenicals are trypanocidal. Melarsoprol is highly active against all stages of trypanosomiasis, but its toxicity restricts its application to the meningoencephalitic phase of the disease. Tryparsamide, the pentavalent arsenical, is more toxic than melarsoprol and is used as an alternative drug along with suramin in treating CNS disease.

Adverse Reactions

Vomiting and abdominal cramping occur, but may be minimized by slow injection in the supine fasting patient. Great care should be taken to prevent painful drug extravasation into the tissue. The most frequently observed adverse reaction is an encephalopathy, which develops on or

Figure 56-6. Trivalent (melarsoprol) and pentavalent (tryparsamide) arsenicals.

about the third day of therapy. It can be fatal despite the use of corticosteroids or the chelating agent dimercaprol. Other side effects include fever, rashes, proteinuria, peripheral neuropathy, and, rarely, agranulocytosis. Since the overall incidence of side effects to tryparsamide is quite high, it largely has been replaced by melarsoprol in the treatment of trypanosome infestation.

Preparations and Dosage

Melarsoprol is available as a 3.6% solution for injection. It is provided through the Parasitic Diseases Division, Centers for Disease Control.

Nifurtimox

Structure and Mechanism of Action

Nifurtimox (Fig. 56-7) is a nitrofuran derivative. The likely mechanism of action for killing of trypanosomes is through production of activated forms of oxygen. Nifurtimox is reduced to the nitro anion radical in the presence of pyridine nucleotides. The anion then reacts with oxygen to produce superoxide and regeneration of nifurtimox. This recycling and production of activated oxygen results in toxicity to cells.

Absorption, Metabolism, and Excretion

The drug is given orally and is well absorbed from the gastrointestinal tract. It is rapidly metabolized and only

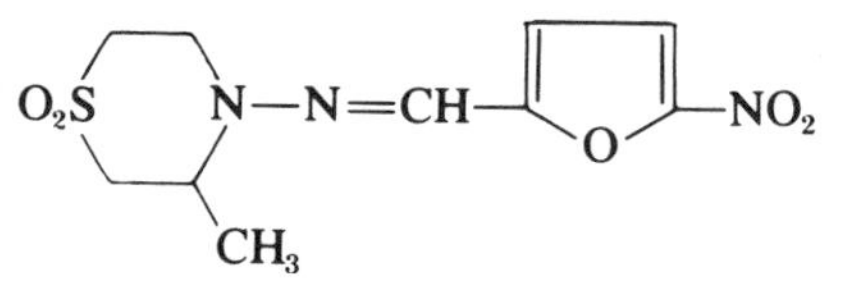

Figure 56-7. Nifurtimox.

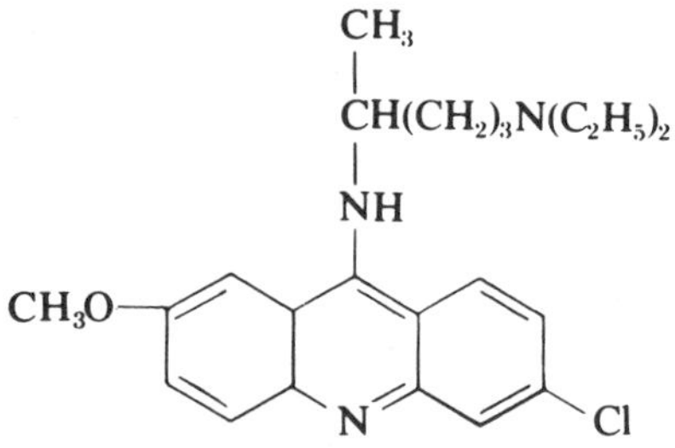

Figure 56-8. Quinacrine.

low levels are found in blood and tissues. The drug is excreted in the urine, primarily in the form of metabolites.

Clinical Uses

Nifurtimox is trypanocidal and exerts an effect on the trypomastigote and amastigote forms of *T. cruzi*. It is effective in the treatment of the acute form of Chagas' disease but is less effective once the disease becomes chronic. The drug is moderately well tolerated. Treatment lasts 3 to 4 months. Cure rates of 80 to 90 percent have been reported. Since much of the tissue damage caused by the disease is irreversible, early diagnosis and treatment are important.

Adverse Reactions

Although side effects occur in approximately half the patients treated with nifurtimox, it is necessary to discontinue treatment in only a minority. Nausea, vomiting, abdominal pain, skin rashes, headache, insomnia, convulsions, and myalgia all have been reported. It is generally recommended that nifurtimox be administered only to hospitalized patients where close supervision and supportive measures are readily available. However, since Chagas' disease is so serious, the drug has been used on an outpatient basis when hospitalization is not practical.

Preparations and Dosage

Nifurtimox (*Lampit*) is provided by the Parasitic Diseases Division, Centers for Disease Control, as 100-mg tablets.

Quinacrine

Structure and Mechanism of Action

Quinacrine (Fig. 56-8) is an acridine derivative that binds to DNA through an intercalation mechanism, thereby blocking the activity of DNA and RNA polymerase and preventing the synthesis of nucleic acids. Whether this is the ultimate mechanism for its antiparasitic effect is unknown.

Absorption, Metabolism, and Excretion

Quinacrine is administered by the oral route and is readily absorbed from the intestinal tract. It is distributed widely in tissues, where it tends to accumulate. Because it is slowly excreted, it may be detected in urine for up to 2 months after drug administration is discontinued.

Clinical Use

Quinacrine is still considered the drug of choice in the treatment of infections caused by *G. lamblia,* although metronidazole is preferred by many. Patients should be given only a liquid diet the day before treatment with quinacrine and should fast on the day of treatment. Its former use as an antimalarial drug is discussed in Chap. 57.

Adverse Effects

The most frequent side effects associated with quinacrine use are headache, dizziness, and vomiting. Occasionally, drug therapy may lead to a yellow staining of the skin and sclera and a deposition of a blue and black pigment in the nail beds. Exfoliative dermatitis, urticaria, blood dyscrasias, and toxic psychosis also have been reported. Aplastic anemia and acute hepatic necrosis are rare complications.

Preparations and Dosage

Quinacrine hydrochloride (*Atabrine Hydrochloride*) is marketed as 100-mg tablets.

Antimonials

Structure and Mechanism of Action

Sodium stibogluconate (Fig. 56-9), a pentavalent antimonial, binds to SH groups on proteins and forms thioantimonites. Whether thioantimonites are formed in vivo with the pentavalent form is not known; some evidence

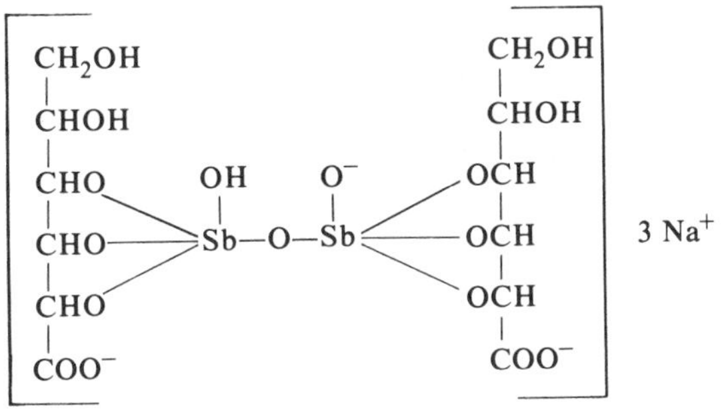

Figure 56-9. Sodium stibogluconate, a pentavalent antimonial drug.

suggests that the pentavalent form may be reduced in vivo to the trivalent antimonial before binding.

Trivalent antimonials inhibit phosphofructokinase, a rate-limiting enzyme in glycolysis, and organisms whose growth is dependent on the anaerobic metabolism of glucose are unable to survive without the active enzyme. Whether this is the mechanism by which pentavalent antimonials inhibit protozoa is unclear.

Absorption, Distribution, and Excretion

Antimonials are irritating to the intestinal mucosa and thus are administered by intramuscular or slow intravenous injection. They bind to cells, including erythrocytes, and are found in high concentrations in the liver and spleen. As compared with the trivalent antimonials, which are no longer used, the pentavalent antimonials bind to tissue less strongly. This results in higher blood levels, more rapid excretion, and lowered toxicity. Pentavalent antimonials are rapidly excreted in the urine, with up to one-half of the administered dose excreted in 24 hr.

Clinical Use

The pentavalent antimony compound *sodium stibogluconate is the drug of choice for all three forms of leishmaniasis.* It can be given by the intravenous or intramuscular route. In addition, local infiltration of the lesion in cutaneous leishmaniasis is highly effective.

Adverse Effects

As indicated above, the pentavalent antimonials are less toxic than trivalent antimonials. Adverse reactions particularly associated with the trivalent antimonials are coughing, occasional vomiting, myalgia, arthralgia, and changes in the ECG. The antimonial derivatives occasionally cause rashes, pruritus, abdominal pain, diarrhea, and

anaphylactoid collapse. Liver damage with jaundice is a rare side effect. Toxic reactions are more common with repeated courses of treatment.

Preparations and Dosage

Sodium stibogluconate (*Pentostam, Triostam*) is available for parenteral administration as a sterile aqueous solution containing 330 mg/ml. It is provided by the Parasitic Diseases Division, Centers for Disease Control.

Diloxanide Furoate

Diloxanide furoate (*Furamide*) (Fig. 56-10) is an amebicide that is effective against trophozoites in the intestinal tract. It is not effective against extraintestinal parasites but is a useful alternative drug for the treatment of an asymptomatic carrier. The drug is only administered orally (500-mg tablets) and is rapidly absorbed from the gastrointestinal tract following hydrolysis of the ester group. Diloxanide is excreted in the urine, largely as the glucuronide. It is available from the Parasitic Diseases Division, Centers for Disease Control.

Antibiotics

Several antibiotics have been used to treat intestinal protozoal infections. Erythromycin and tetracycline do not have a direct effect on the protozoa, but act by altering intestinal bacterial flora and preventing secondary infection. Tetracycline also reduces the normal gastrointestinal bacterial flora on which the amebas depend for growth. It has also been used in the management of intestinal amebiasis with mucosal involvement.

The aminoglycoside paromomycin has a mode of action identical to that of the other aminocyclitols (see Chap. 50) and is directly amebicidal. It is not absorbed from the intestinal tract and thus has its primary effect on bacteria, some amebas (e.g., *E. histolytica*), *T. vaginalis,* and some helminths found in the lumen of the intestinal tract. Its use is now limited to that of an alternative agent in the treatment of intestinal amebiasis.

Paromomycin sulfate (*Humatin*) is marketed for oral

Figure 56-10. Diloxanide furoate.

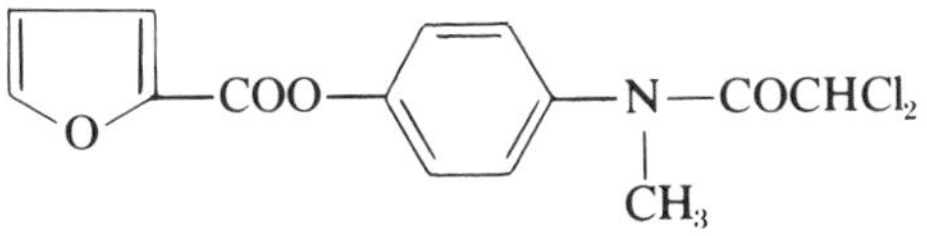

administration as 250-mg capsules and as a syrup (125 mg/5 ml).

Amphotericin B is a polyene and is discussed more fully in Chap. 52. It has produced healing of the mucocutaneous lesions of American leishmaniasis, but its potential for nephrotoxicity makes it a drug of second choice.

Supplemental Reading

Barrett-Connor, E. Drugs for the treatment of parasitic infection. *Med. Clin. North Am.* 66:245, 1982.

Docampo, R., and Moreno, S.N.J. Free-radical Intermediates in the Antiparasitic Action of Drugs and Parasitic Cells. In W.A. Pryor (ed.), *Free Radicals in Biology.* Vol. 6. New York: Academic, 1984. P. 243.

Drugs for parasitic infections. *Med. Lett. Drugs Ther.* 34:17, 1992.

Goldman, P. Metronidazole. *N. Engl. J. Med.* 303:1212, 1980.

Gustafsson, L.L., Beermann, B., and Abdi, Y.A. (eds.). *Handbook of Drugs for Tropical Parasitic Infections.* New York: Taylor & Francis, 1987.

Hastings, R.C., and Franzblau, S.G. Chemotherapy of Leprosy. *Annu. Rev. Pharmacol. Toxicol.* 28:231, 1988.

Hooper, M. (ed). *Chemotherapy of Tropical Diseases.* New York: Wiley, 1987.

Lerman, S.J., and Walker, R.A. Treatment of giardiasis. Literature review and recommendation. *Clin. Pediatr.* 21:409, 1982.

Lossick, J.G. Treatment of *Trichomonas vaginalis* infection. *Rev. Infect. Dis.* 4 (Suppl.):S801, 1982.

Voogd, T., et al. Recent research on the biological activity of suramin. *Pharmacol. Rev.* 45:147, 1993.

57

Antimalarial Drugs

Knox Van Dyke and *Zuguang Ye*

Malaria is a parasitic disease endemic in those parts of the world where moisture and warmth permit the disease vector, mosquitoes of the genus *Anopheles,* to exist and multiply. Extensive programs for the eradication of malaria undertaken shortly after World War II were only partially successful. The disease again became a major problem when local mosquito eradication programs were gradually eliminated after a decrease in the incidence of reported cases of malaria. Furthermore, many of the programs still functioning operate at less than peak efficiency because of administrative, organizational, and financial difficulties. The emergence of both drug-resistant strains of malarial parasites and insecticide-resistant strains of *Anopheles* also has contributed significantly to the extensive reappearance of this infection. The annual global incidence of malaria is estimated to be approximately 200 million cases, and in tropical Africa alone, malaria is responsible for the deaths of more than 1 million children under the age of 14 every year.

Although malaria was once endemic in the United States, the disease has been virtually eliminated through the use of pesticides, such as DDT. However, when travelers go from a nonendemic area (e.g., North America) to an endemic one (e.g., Africa or Asia), they are generally more susceptible to the disease because of their lack of antibodies against the parasite. Most cases of malaria in the United States result from individuals who have contracted the disease before their entry into this country. It is also possible to contract malaria during a blood transfusion if the transfused blood has been taken from a malaria-infected individual. Additionally, hypodermic needles previously contaminated by blood containing malarial parasites can be the source of an infection; this has occurred when needles are shared among drug addicts.

While vaccines have proved useful in animal models, they have been ineffective in human studies. Since antigens of the parasite constantly change and recombine, as in trypanosomes, it seems unlikely that an effective vaccine will be forthcoming.

New approaches to drug therapy are being actively investigated. One of the plasmodial species, *Plasmodium falciparum,* can now be grown in culture in human red cells continuously. The development of this culture system is making it possible to learn considerably more about parasite biochemistry and to pinpoint those pathways that are most susceptible to pharmacological intervention.

Effective treatment of malaria is dependent on early diagnosis. Since the patient's symptoms are often relatively nonspecific, it is crucial to examine stained blood smears for the presence of the parasite. Even this procedure may be inconclusive during the early stages of the infection, since the levels of parasitemia can be quite low. Thus, it is important to repeat the blood smear examination several times if malaria is suspected.

Once the presence of malarial parasites has been confirmed, it is vital to identify the particular plasmodial strain involved, since appropriate use of chemotherapy depends on the particular species responsible for the acute attack. Unfortunately, mixed infections, that is, simultaneous infections with more than one species of plasmodia, are often observed. If more than a single species is involved, treatment appropriate for the elimination of all strains must be instituted to avoid delayed attacks or misinterpretations.

Life Cycle of the Malarial Parasite

The malarial parasite is a single-cell protozoan (plasmodium). Although more than 50 different species of plasmodia have been identified, only four are capable of infecting humans (*P. malariae, P. ovale, P. vivax,* and *P. falciparum*); the rest attack a variety of animal hosts. *Plasmodium falciparum* and *P. vivax* malaria are the two most common forms.

Plasmodium vivax malaria is the most prevalent type of infection and is characterized by periodic acute attacks involving chills and fever, profuse sweating, enlarged spleen and liver, anemia, abdominal pain, headaches, and lethargy. A hyperactivity of the reticuloendothelial system is the principal cause of the enlarged spleen and liver; these effects often result in anemia, leukopenia, thrombocytopenia, and hyperbilirubinemia. The cyclical nature of the acute attacks (48 hr for *P. vivax* and *P. falciparum*) is characteristic of malaria and reflects the relatively synchronous passage of the parasites from one red blood cell stage in their life cycle to another. If *P. vivax* malaria is not treated, the symptoms may subside for several weeks or months and then recur. These "relapses" are due to a latent liver form of the parasite (see the following section), which is not present in *P. falciparum* strains. Although the fatality rate of *P. vivax* malaria is low, it is an exhausting infection and renders the patient more susceptible to other diseases.

Unchecked *P. falciparum* malaria is the most serious and most lethal form of the disease. It is responsible for 90 percent of the deaths from malaria. The parasitemia achieved can be quite high and will be associated with an increased incidence of serious complications (e.g., hemolytic anemia, encephalopathy). *Plasmodium falciparum* malaria produces all the symptoms listed for *P. vivax* malaria and, in addition, can cause renal failure and pulmonary and brain edema. The tissue anoxia occurring in *P. falciparum* infections results from the unique sequestering of infected erythroytes deep in the capillaries during the last three fourths of the intraerythrocytic cycle.

Members of the genus *Plasmodium* have a complex life cycle (Fig. 57-1). A sexual stage occurs in the *Anopheles* mosquito, while asexual stages take place in an animal host, for example, human. Malaria is actually transmitted from one human to another through the insect vector. Initially, a female mosquito is infected by biting a human with the disease whose blood contains male and female *gamete* forms of the parasite. Fertilization takes place in the mosquito gut and, after differentiation and multiplication, the mature *sporozoite* forms migrate to the insect's salivary glands. At the mosquito's next feeding, the sporozoites are injected into the bloodstream of another human to begin the asexual stages. After a relatively brief residence (less than 1 hr) in the systemic circulation, the sporozoites invade liver parenchymal cells, where they divide and develop asexually into multinucleated *schizonts*. These are the primary exoerythrocytic tissue forms of the parasite. When this primary stage of development is completed (6–12 days), the schizonts will rupture, releasing *merozoites* into the blood. These latter forms invade host erythrocytes, where they again grow and divide asexually (*erythrocytic schizogony*) and become red cell schizonts. Some of the parasites differentiate into sexual (male and female) forms, or *gametocytes*. If the diseased human is bitten by a mosquito at this time, the gametes will be taken up into the gut to reinitiate the sexual cycle. The gametocytes and

the exoerythrocytic liver forms of the *Plasmodium* are not associated with the appearance of clinical symptoms of malaria.

The asexual intraerythrocytic parasites, that is, those that do not differentiate into gametocytes, also multiply and grow until they rupture the cells in which they are located; these new merozoites are released into the bloodstream. This occurrence not only sets up the subsequent cyclical red blood cell stages of the plasmodium cycle, but also gives rise to the symptoms associated with malarial infections. The recurrent chills and fever are thought to be related to the lysis of erythrocytes and the accompanying release of lytic material and parasite toxins into the bloodstream. Although the appearance of a cyclic fever is useful for diagnosis, this symptom may not occur during the early stages of the infection.

In individuals infected with either *P. vivax* or *P. ovale*, the exoerythrocytic tissue (e.g., liver) forms can persist after a latent period and give rise to relapses. In *P. falciparum* and *P. malariae* malaria, however, there do not appear to be any secondary liver forms that persist. Thus, in both of these forms of malaria, the physician must contend only with the asexual erythrocytic forms and the gametes, and not with the latent liver forms found in *P. vivax* and *P. ovale* (and possibly *P. malariae*).

Patients who have blood transfusion malaria are infected with the asexual erythrocytic parasites only; exoerythrocytic tissue forms apparently do not develop. *Plasmodium malariae* has been known to produce an infection after transfusion, even when the blood was obtained from a person whose only contact with malaria was 40 years previous to the donation of blood.

Therapeutic Considerations

The main objective in the clinical management of patients suffering from an *acute* malaria attack is the prompt elimination of the parasite form responsible for the symptoms, that is, the asexual erythrocytic form. Drugs that are particularly effective in this regard are called *schizontocidal*, or *suppressive*, agents. They include such compounds as amodiaquine, chloroguanide, chloroquine, hydroxychloroquine, pyrimethamine, quinine, and tetracycline. These drugs have the potential for effecting a *clinical cure*; that is, they can reduce the parasitemia to zero. The term *radical cure* also has been used and it, in contrast to clinical cure, implies the total elimination of all parasite forms from the body. A radical cure of malaria infections produced by all four species of *Plasmodium* is possible, although infections with *P. malariae* are known to last for many years.

Once the primary therapeutic objective has been achieved, attention can be focused on such additional con-

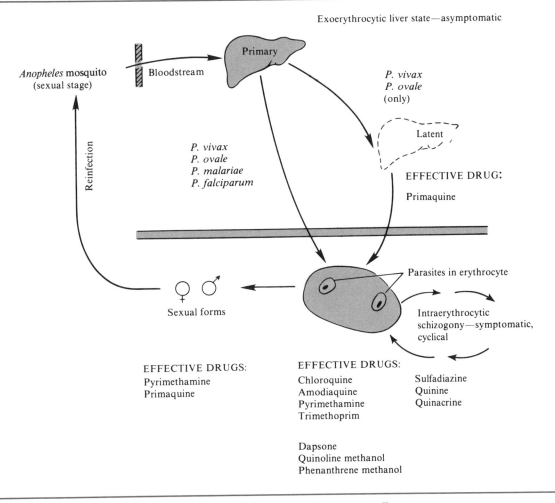

Exoerythrocytic liver state—asymptomatic

Figure 57-1. Life cycle of malaria parasites and locations where specific drugs are effective. Note that the life cycles are not identical for every species.

siderations as elimination of the gametocytes and the tissue forms of the parasite. Success in these areas would help to ensure that relapses do not occur. Since no latent liver forms are associated with mosquito-induced, drug-sensitive *P. falciparum* malaria, administration of chloroquine for up to 3 months after the patient leaves a malarious area will usually bring about a complete or radical cure, *unless* the organism is resistant to chloroquine.

The emergence of parasites resistant to chloroquine is an increasingly important problem. Several strains of chloroquine-resistant *P. falciparum* have been identified. The strains are not, however, equally resistant. It is also possible that parasite drug resistance may increase even during chloroquine administration. This resistance would lead to the reappearance of overt symptoms of *P. falciparum* malaria.

Plasmodium falciparum malaria may be accompanied by an infection caused by one of the other three plasmodial forms (*mixed infection*). As long as all the parasites are

drug-sensitive, the parasitemia can be eliminated. However, it must be remembered that even though *P. falciparum* malaria may be ameliorated or eliminated, relapses due to *P. vivax* and *P. ovale* still can occur. In these cases, patients probably should be given primaquine after therapy with chloroquine has been completed.

Broad guidelines or recommendations for drug regimens in particular clinical situations can be found at the end of this chapter.

Antimalarial Drugs

Chloroquine

Chemistry and Mechanism of Action

Chloroquine (Fig. 57-2) is one of several 4-aminoquinoline derivatives that display antimalarial activity.

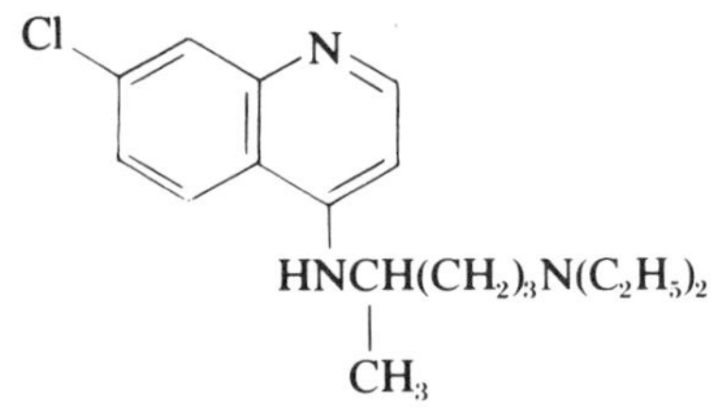

Figure 57-2. Chloroquine.

The addition of a chlorine atom to the quinoline portion of the molecule markedly increases the antimalarial activity of this series of compounds. Chloroquine is particularly effective against intraerythrocytic forms because it is concentrated within the parasitized erythrocyte. This preferential drug accumulation appears to occur as a result of specific uptake mechanisms that are present in the parasite. Chloroquine appears possibly to poison the feeding mechanism of the parasite by interfering with the digestion of endocytotic vesicles of hemoglobin that are delivered to the parasite's food vacuole.

Antimalarial Spectrum

The drug is effective against all four types of malaria with the exception of chloroquine-resistant *P. falciparum.* Chloroquine destroys the blood stages of the infection and therefore ameliorates the clinical symptoms seen in *P. vivax, P. ovale,* and sensitive *P. falciparum* forms of malaria. The disease will return in *P. vivax* and *P. ovale* malaria, however, unless the liver stages are sequentially treated, first with chloroquine and then with primaquine. Chloroquine also can be used prophylactically.

Absorption, Metabolism, and Excretion

The absorption of chloroquine from the gastrointestinal tract is rapid and complete. The drug is distributed widely and is extensively bound to body tissues, with the liver containing 500 times the blood concentration. The primary pathway involved in the hepatic metabolism of chloroquine is de-ethylation; desethylchloroquine is the major metabolite. Both the parent compound and its metabolites are slowly eliminated by renal excretion. The half-life of the drug is 6 to 7 days.

Clinical Uses

In addition to its use as an effective antimalarial compound, chloroquine, because it possesses antiinflammatory properties, is used in the treatment of rheumatoid arthritis and lupus erythematosus (see Chap. 43). Chloroquine also has been found useful in treating extraintes-

tinal amebiasis, especially that caused by *Entamoeba histolytica* (see Chap. 56), and in treating photoallergic reactions and *Clonorchis sinensis* infection (Chap. 58).

Adverse Reactions

The toxicity of chloroquine is related to dosage and duration of treatment. In low dosages (which are suppressive to the parasite), there is little major toxicity, although dizziness, headache, itching, skin rash, vomiting, and blurring of vision may occur. In higher dosages these symptoms are more common and exacerbation or unmasking of lupus erythematosus or discoid lupus as well as toxic effects in skin, blood, and eyes can occur. Since the drug concentrates in melanin-containing structures, prolonged administration of high doses can result in corneal deposits and lead to blindness. Children are especially sensitive to the toxic effects of chloroquine.

Contraindications

Chloroquine should not be used in the presence of retinal or visual field changes.

Preparations and Dosage

Chloroquine phosphate (*Aralen Phosphate*) is marketed as plain and enteric-coated tablets containing 500 mg. Chloroquine hydrochloride (*Aralen Hydrochloride*) is available only in injectable form.

Hydroxychloroquine

Hydroxychloroquine (Fig. 57-3), like chloroquine, is a 4-aminoquinoline derivative. As with chloroquine, it is used for the suppressive and acute treatment of malaria caused by *P. vivax, P. malariae, P. ovale,* and susceptible strains of *P. falciparum.* It also has been used for rheumatoid arthritis and discoid and systemic lupus erythematosus. Hydroxychloroquine has not been proved to be more effective than chloroquine. Adverse reactions associated with its use are similar to those described for chloroquine.

Figure 57-3. Hydroxychloroquine.

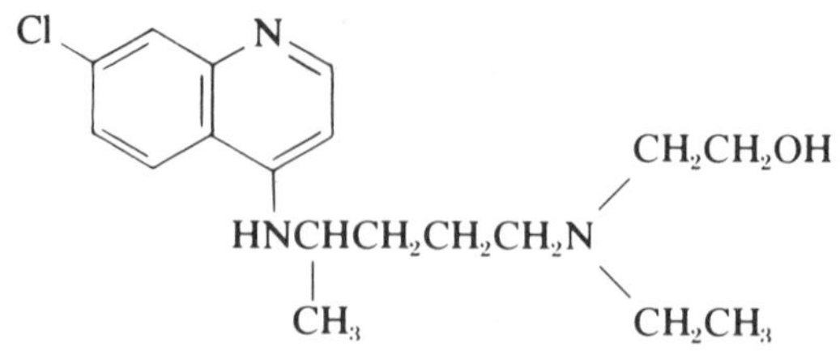

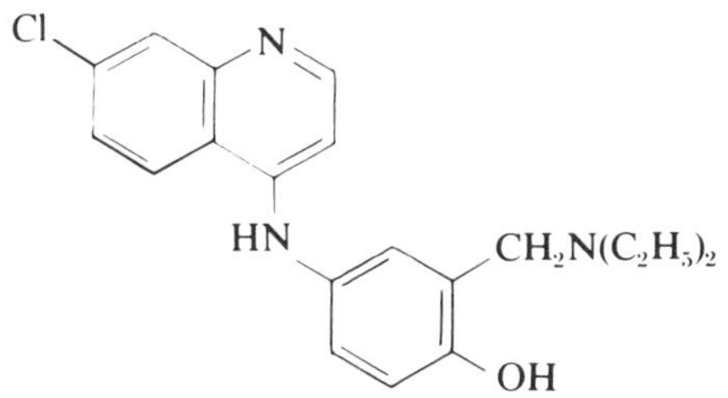

Figure 57-4. Amodiaquine.

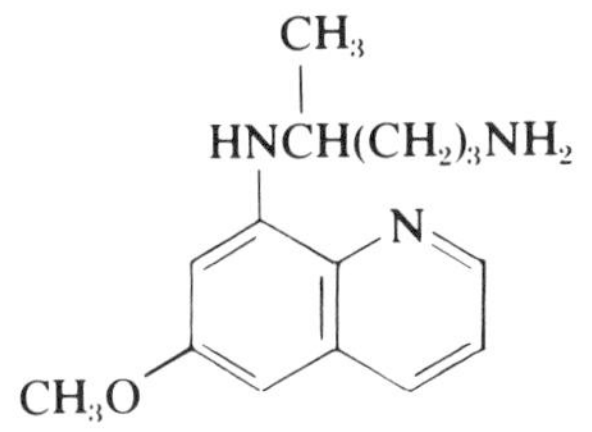

Figure 57-5. Primaquine.

The drug should not be used in patients with psoriasis or porphyria, since it may exacerbate these conditions. Hydroxychloroquine sulfate (*Plaquenil Sulfate*) is available as oral tablets (200 mg). The dosage regimens employed are similar to those for chloroquine.

Amodiaquine

Amodiaquine (Fig. 57-4) is another 4-aminoquinoline derivative whose antimalarial spectrum and adverse reactions are similar to those of chloroquine. Prolonged treatment may result in pigmentation of the palate, nail beds, and skin. Amodiaquine hydrochloride (*Camoquin Hydrochloride*) is marketed as oral tablets (200 mg).

Primaquine

Chemistry and Mechanism of Action

Primaquine (Fig. 57-5) is the least toxic and most effective of the 8-aminoquinoline antimalarial compounds. The degree of toxicity these derivatives possess appears to be directly related to the extent of substitution on the terminal amino group: The primary amine has the lowest toxicity. The mechanism by which 8-aminoquinolines exert their antimalarial effects is unknown.

Antimalarial Spectrum

There is some disagreement concerning the best use of primaquine in the treatment of malaria, especially when its utility in prophylaxis is discussed. There is little disagreement that the drug has a prophylactic effect, but its relatively short duration of action has led some physicians to conclude that this effect does not have practical value. However, the drug is still used widely for prophylaxis.

Primaquine is an important antimalarial because it is essentially the only drug effective against the liver (*exoerythrocytic*) forms of the malarial parasite. The drug also kills the gametocytes, and patients recovering from *P. falciparum* malaria can be given primaquine for its gametocyticidal properties. It should be noted, however, that primaquine is relatively ineffective against the asexual erythrocyte forms. The drug finds its greatest use in providing a radical cure for *P. vivax* malaria.

Absorption, Metabolism, and Excretion

Primaquine is readily absorbed from the gastrointestinal tract and, in contrast to chloroquine, is not bound extensively by tissues. It is rapidly metabolized, and the metabolites are reported to be as active as the parent drug itself. Peak plasma levels are reached in 4 to 6 hr after an oral dose, with almost total drug elimination occurring by 24 hr. The drug is best given 12 hr before a probable exposure to the parasite. The half-life is short and daily administration is usually required.

Adverse Reactions

Although primaquine has a good therapeutic index, a number of important side effects are associated with its administration. In individuals with a genetically determined glucose 6-phosphate dehydrogenase deficiency, primaquine can cause a lethal hemolysis of red cells. This genetic deficiency occurs in 5 to 10 percent of black males, in Asians, and in some Mediterranean peoples. With higher dosages or prolonged drug use, gastrointestinal distress, nausea, headache, pruritus, and leukopenia can occur. Occasionally, agranulocytosis also has been observed. Many soldiers engaged in the Vietnam conflict found that continuous use of the primaquine-chloroquine combination made them ill, and therefore patient compliance was low.

Preparations and Dosage

Primaquine phosphate is available as oral tablets (15 mg). The drug is commonly administered with a 4-aminoquinoline derivative (e.g., chloroquine, amodiaquine), especially for the prevention of relapses.

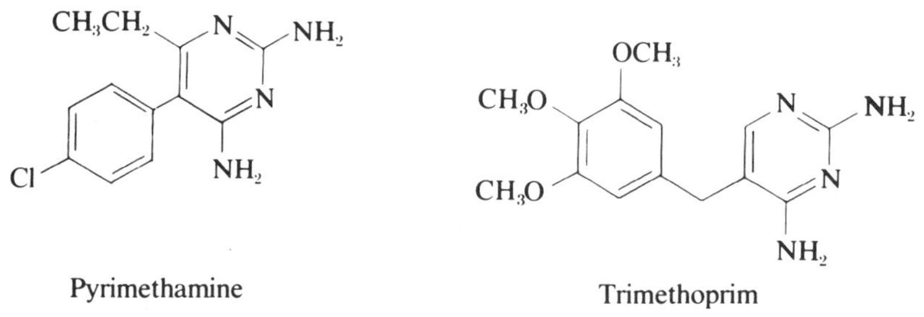

Figure 57-6. Pyrimethamine and trimethoprim.

Pyrimethamine

Chemistry

Pyrimethamine (Fig. 57-6) is the best of a number of 2,4-diaminopyrimidines that were synthesized as potential antimalarial and antibacterial compounds. Trimethoprim (see Fig. 57-6) is a closely related compound.

Mechanism of Action

The only antimalarial drugs whose mechanisms of action are reasonably well understood are the drugs that inhibit the parasite's ability to synthesize folic acid. Parasites cannot use preformed folic acid and therefore must synthesize this compound from the following precursors obtained from their host: p-aminobenzoic acid (PABA), pteridine, and glutamic acid. The dihydrofolic acid formed from these precursors must then be hydrogenated to form tetrahydrofolic acid. The latter compound is the coenzyme that acts as an acceptor of a variety of one-carbon units. The transfer of one-carbon units is important in the synthesis of the pyrimidines and purines, which are essential in nucleic acid synthesis.

Whereas the sulfonamides and sulfones inhibit the initial step whereby PABA and the pteridine moiety combine to form dihydropteroic acid (see Chap. 48), pyrimethamine and trimethoprim inhibit the conversion of dihydrofolic acid to tetrahydrofolic acid, a reaction catalyzed by the enzyme dihydrofolate reductase. The basis of pyrimethamine's selective toxicity resides in the *preferential binding* of the drug to the parasite's reductase enzyme.

The combined use of sulfonamides or sulfones with dihydrofolate reductase inhibitors such as trimethoprim (*Bactrim, Septra*) or pyrimethamine (*Fansidar*) is a good example of the synergistic possibilities that exist in multiple-drug chemotherapy. This type of impairment of the parasite's metabolism is termed *sequential blockade.* Using drugs that inhibit at two different points in the same biochemical pathway produces parasite lethality at lower drug concentrations than are possible when either drug is used alone (see Fig. 57-1).

Antimalarial Spectrum

Pyrimethamine is recommended for prophylactic use against all susceptible strains of plasmodia. It should not be used as the sole therapeutic agent for treating acute malarial attacks. As mentioned previously, *sulfonamides should always be coadministered with pyrimethamine (or trimethoprim)*, since the combined antimalarial activity of the two drugs is significantly greater than when either drug is used alone. Resistance also develops more slowly to the combination.

Clinical Uses

In addition to its antimalarial effects, pyrimethamine is indicated (in combination with a sulfonamide) for the treatment of toxoplasmosis. The dosage required, however, is 10 to 20 times higher than that employed in malarial infections.

Absorption, Metabolism, and Excretion

Pyrimethamine is well absorbed after oral administration, with peak plasma levels occurring within 3 to 7 hr. An initial loading dose to saturate nonspecific binding sites is not required, as it is with chloroquine. However, the drug binds to tissues and therefore its rate of renal excretion is slow. Pyrimethamine has a half-life of about 4 days. Although the drug does undergo some metabolic alterations, the metabolites formed have not been totally identified.

Adverse Reactions

There are relatively few side effects associated with the usual antimalarial dosages. However, signs of toxicity are evident at higher dosages, particularly those used in the management of toxoplasmosis. Many of these reactions reflect the interference of pyrimethamine with host folic acid metabolism, especially that occurring in rapidly dividing cells. Toxic symptoms include anorexia, vomiting, anemia, leukopenia, thrombocytopenia, and atrophic glossitis. Central nervous system (CNS) stimulation, including convulsions, may follow an acute overdosage. The side effects associated with the pyrimethamine-sulfadoxine combination include those associated with the sulfonamide and pyrimethamine alone. In addition, there is some evidence of a greater incidence of allergic reactions, particularly Stevens-Johnson syndrome, with the combination.

Preparations and Dosage

Pyrimethamine (*Daraprim*) is used in tablet form (25 mg) for the prophylaxis of malaria. *Fansidar* is a combination of sulfadoxine (500 mg) and pyrimethamine (25 mg) and is most widely used prophylactically for the prevention of malaria caused by chloroquine-resistant strains of *P. falciparum.*

Chloroguanide

Chloroguanide also interferes with parasite folic acid synthesis. It is a dihydrofolate reductase inhibitor that is used for the prophylaxis of malaria caused by all susceptible strains of plasmodia. The side effects and spectrum of antimalarial activity for chloroguanide hydrochloride (*Paludrine Hydrochloride*) are quite similar to those described for pyrimethamine.

Quinine

Chemistry

Historically, quinine (Fig. 57-7) was a very important antimalarial compound. It is one of several alkaloids derived from the bark of the cinchona tree.

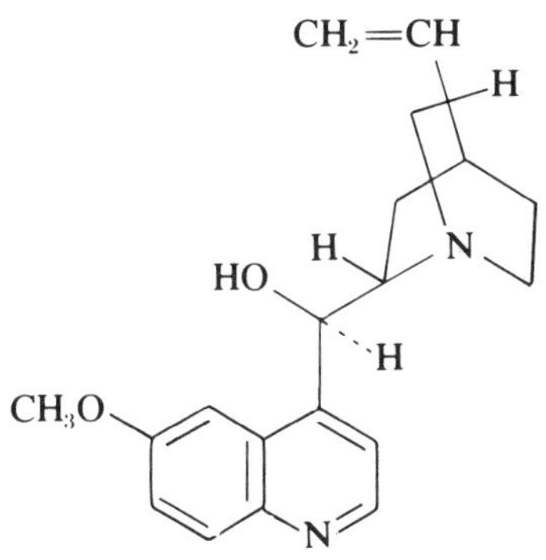

Mechanism of Action

The mechanism by which quinine exerts its antimalarial activity is not known. It does not bind to DNA at dosages that are antimalarial. Its effects may relate to a poisoning of the parasite's feeding mechanism. The drug has been termed a general protoplasmic poison, since many organisms are affected by it.

Antimalarial Spectrum

The primary present-day indication for quinine is in the treatment of chloroquine-resistant malaria caused by *P. falciparum.*

Absorption, Metabolism, and Excretion

Quinine is rapidly absorbed following oral ingestion, with peak blood levels achieved in 1 to 4 hr. About 70 per-

Figure 57-7. Quinine.

cent of the drug is bound to plasma proteins. Quinine is extensively metabolized, with only about 5 percent of the parent compound eliminated in the urine.

Clinical Uses

Aside from its use as an antimalarial compound, quinine is used for the prevention and treatment of nocturnal leg muscle cramps, especially those resulting from arthritis, diabetes, thrombophlebitis, arteriosclerosis, and varicose veins.

Adverse Reactions

Cinchonism is the term used to describe the toxic state induced by quinine when the plasma levels exceed 10 to 12 $\mu g/ml$. Symptoms include sweating, ringing in the ears, impaired hearing, blurred vision, nausea, vomiting, and diarrhea. Quinine has an irritant effect on the gastrointestinal mucosa. Also, a variety of relatively rare hematological changes occur, including leukopenia and agranulocytosis. Quinine is potentially neurotoxic in high dosages and a variety of CNS effects may occur. Severe hypotension may occur following intravenous administration.

Preparations and Dosage

Quinine sulfate is marketed as 130-, 200-, and 325-mg tablets and capsules. Quinine dihydrochloride is available in powder form for intravenous administration.

Quinacrine

Quinacrine is no longer used extensively as an antimalarial drug. It has been largely replaced by the 4-aminoquinolines. It exerts some inhibitory activity against the blood stages of the malarial parasite. Quinacrine binds strongly to nucleic acids and presumably acts by a mechanism referred to as *intercalation;* that is, the drug inserts itself edgewise between the base pairs of the DNA helix, thereby blocking DNA polymerization. Concentrations of quinacrine needed to intercalate DNA are roughly the same as those needed to affect the malarial parasite. This is the only clear-cut example of an antimalarial drug working by this mechanism. Quinacrine is the drug of choice for the treatment of giardiasis (see Chap. 56).

Dapsone

Dapsone (see Chap. 53, Fig. 53-8) is a sulfone used in the clinical management of leprosy, and most of its pharmacology has been described in Chap. 53. Although it was once used in the treatment and prophylaxis of chloroquine-resistant falciparum malaria, the toxicities associated with its administration (e.g., agranulocytosis, hemolytic anemia) have severely reduced its use. Occasionally, dapsone (25 mg daily) has been added to the usual chloroquine therapeutic regimen for the prophylaxis of chloroquine-resistant *P. falciparum* malaria.

Mefloquine

Mefloquine is a 4-quinolinemethanol derivative that shows promise against resistant *P. falciparum* malaria. Only one form of the racemic mixture is antimalarial. The drug is being used both prophylactically and acutely. It is ineffective against the liver stage of vivax malaria.

While its detailed mechanism of action is unknown, it is an effective blood schizonticide; that is, it acts against the mature form of the parasite. Orally administered mefloquine is well absorbed and has an absorption half-life of about 2 hr; the elimination half-life is 2 to 3 weeks. Among its side effects are vertigo, visual alterations, vomiting, and such CNS disturbances as psychosis, hallucinations, confusion, anxiety, and depression.

Mefloquine hydrochloride (*Lariam*) is available as 250-mg tablets.

Drugs in Development

Chinese scientists have isolated several compounds with antimalarial activity from species of *Artemisia.* These include artemisinin (*Qinghaosu*), artesunate, and artemether. These sesquiterpene peroxides are potent and rapidly acting antimalarial drugs that show relatively low human toxicity. They are active against blood stages and cerebral malaria, especially against chloroquine-resistant malarial infections. They possess activity against the erythrocytic stages of human malaria and have no effect on the liver or exoerythrocytic stage of the parasite; their gameticidal activity is not clear. They are most useful in treating life-threatening cerebral edema.

These drugs are rapidly absorbed and metabolized resulting in compounds with short half-lives. The peroxide is rapidly split in the blood, thereby inactivating the compounds. Their use is associated with a transient reticulocytopenia and a relatively high return of the malarial infection, possibly because of their short half-life. Animal experiments have shown some embryotoxic effects. Presently, artemisinin, artesunate, and artemether are available outside the United States in either suppository or parenteral forms.

Selection of Drugs

The particular agent employed in the treatment of acute malarial infections will depend on the severity of the infection, the strain of the infecting plasmodium, and the degree to which the organism is drug resistant. In addition, *chemoprophylaxis* is considered a valid indication for the use of antimalarial drugs when individuals are traveling in areas where malaria is endemic. The following paragraphs may provide useful guidelines in the therapeutic management and prevention of malarial infections.

Prophylactic Measures While in Endemic Areas

Drugs useful for malaria prophylaxis are summarized in Table 57-1. *Chloroquine is the drug of choice* even in areas of chloroquine-resistant *P. falciparum.* It is combined with chloroguanide for the treatment of highly chloroquine-resistant strains. Drugs should be continued for 6 to 8 weeks after leaving the endemic areas.

Treatment of an Acute Uncomplicated Attack

Chloroquine phosphate, administered orally, is again the drug of choice unless one suspects the presence of a chloroquine-resistant organism. Amodiaquine hydrochloride is a suitable alternative drug. For severe infections, chloroquine hydrochloride, intramuscularly, is indicated.

Mechanism of Chloroquine Resistance

Recent studies point to the cause of the development of chloroquine resistance in the malarial parasite. A particular protein (P_{170} glycoprotein) has been identified in the resistant parasite that appears to function as a drug-transporting pump mechanism. This resistance mechanism is

Table 57-1. Drugs Used in the Prophylaxis and Presumptive Treatment of Malaria Acquired in Areas with Chloroquine-Resistant *Plasmodium falciparum* (CRPF)

Drug (trade name)	Routine prophylaxis		Presumptive treatment	
	Adult dose	Pediatric dose	Adult dose	Pediatric dose
Chloroquine phosphate (*Aralen Phosphate*)	300 mg base (500 mg salt) orally, once/wk	5 mg/kg base (8.3 mg/kg salt) orally, once/wk, up to maximum adult dose of 300 mg base	Chloroquine is not recommended for the presumptive treatment of malaria acquired in areas of known chloroquine resistance	
Amodiaquine hydrochloride (*Camoquin Hydrochloride, Flavoquine*)[a]	400 mg base (520 mg salt) orally, once/wk	7 mg/kg base (9 mg/kg salt) orally, once/wk, up to maximum adult dose of 400 mg base	Amodiaquine is not recommended for the presumptive treatment of malaria acquired in areas of known chloroquine resistance	
Pyrimethamine-sulfadoxine (*Fansidar*)[b]	1 tablet (25 mg pyrimethamine and 500 mg sulfadoxine) orally, once/wk	2–11 mo: ⅛ tablet/wk, 1–3 yr: ¼ tablet/wk, 4–8 yr: ½ tablet/wk, 9–14 yr: ¾ tablet/wk, >14 yr: 1 tablet/wk	3 tablets (75 mg pyrimethamine and 1,500 mg sulfadoxine), orally, as a single dose	2–11 mo: ¼ tablet 1–3 yr: ½ tablet 4–8 yr: 1 tablet 9–14 yr: 2 tablets >14 yr: 3 tablets as a single dose
Doxycycline[c]	100 mg orally, once/day	>8 yr: 2 mg/kg body weight, orally/day up to adult dose of 100 mg/day	Tetracyclines are not recommended for the presumptive treatment of malaria	

[a]Unavailable in the United States but widely available overseas.
[b]The use of *Fansidar* is contraindicated in persons with histories of sulfonamide or pyrimethamine intolerance, in pregnancy at term, and in infants under 2 months of age. Physicians who prescribe the drug to be used as presumptive treatment in the event of a febrile illness when professional medical care is not readily available should ensure that such prescriptions are clearly labeled with instructions to be followed in the event of a febrile illness. If the drug is used as weekly prophylaxis, travelers should be advised to discontinue its use immediately in the event of a possible adverse effect, especially if any mucocutaneous signs or symptoms develop.
[c]The use of doxycycline is contraindicated in pregnancy and in children under 8 years of age. The FDA considers the use of tetracyclines as antimalarials to be investigational. Physicians who prescribe doxycycline as malaria chemoprophylaxis should advise their patients to limit direct exposure to the sun to minimize the possibility of a photosensitivity reaction.
Source: From *M.M.W.R.* 34:185, 1985.

similar to the multidrug resistance system in cancer. A variety of lipophilic drugs inhibit this chloroquine exit pump. Thus, when drug enters the organism it is rapidly removed before it can exert its toxicity. This protein is present only in small amounts in chloroquine-sensitive malarial parasites. Drug therapy directed at inhibiting this pump mechanism may be able to reverse this drug resistance. In laboratory studies, the calcium channel blocking drugs, such as verapamil, in combination with chloroquine did appear to reverse resistance. This is a potentially important new approach to the chemotherapy of malaria.

Prevention of Relapse from P. Vivax and P. Ovale

Primaquine phosphate is recommended at an adult dosage of 26.3 mg (15 mg base) per day for 14 days. The pediatric dosage is 0.3 mg base/kg/day for 14 days.

Treatment of Chloroquine-Resistant P. Falciparum Infection

If a patient has traveled to an area where resistant *P. falciparum* occurs, or if the patient does not show a prompt response to chloroquine, a chloroquine-resistant species should be suspected. As a prophylactic measure in areas where chloroquine-resistant *P. falciparum* is common, pyrimethamine (50 mg) plus sulfadiazine (1,000 mg) once every week is indicated for adults. For infants one-fourth tablet (6.25 mg) of pyrimethamine is recommended. For children 1 to 3 years old, one-half tablet; 4 to 8 years old, one tablet; and 9 to 14 years old, one and one-half tablets. A combination of pyrimethamine-sulfadoxine may, however, be the treatment of choice. An acute attack of malaria caused by chloroquine-resistant *P. falciparum* may be terminated with quinine sulfate alone or with quinine plus pyrimethamine or sulfadiazine, or both. Mefloquine has been used in place of chloroquine in chloroquine resistance, but serious CNS side effects (e.g., flashbacks) are frequently seen with its use.

Mixed Infections

Every patient with malaria should be examined for the possible presence of a simultaneous infection with more than one species of *Plasmodium*. Infections with both *P. falciparum* and *P. vivax* are among the most commonly encountered mixed infections. In patients with falciparum malaria, attacks of *P. vivax* malaria may later develop; it is important not to misinterpret this delayed *P. vivax* form as a possible relapse of *P. falciparum* infection. If a mixed infection is identified, a combination of 4-aminoquinoline and primaquine should be administered. The combination helps to eliminate any persisting tissue forms of *P. vivax*.

Supplemental Reading

Klayman, D.L. *Qinghaosu* (artemisinin): An antimalarial drug from China. *Science* 228:1049, 1985.

Mefloquine for malaria. *Med. Lett. Drugs Ther.* 31:13, 1990.

Miller, L.H., et al. *Science* 234:1349, 1986.

Peters, W. *Chemotherapy and Drug Resistance in Malaria* (2nd ed.). New York: Academic, 1987.

Peters, W., and Richards, W.H.G. (eds.). *Antimalarial Drugs: Biological Background, Experimental Methods, and Drug Resistance.* New York: Springer-Verlag, 1984.

Randall, G., and Seidel, J.S. Malaria. *Pediatr. Clin. North Am.* 32:893, 1985.

Ye, Z., and Van Dyke, K. Reversal of chloroquine resistance in falciparum malaria independent of calcium channels. *Biochem. Biophys. Res. Commun.* 155:476, 1988.

58

Anthelmintic Drugs

Irvin S. Snyder and *Roger G. Finch*

Infection by *helminths* (worms) may be limited solely to the intestinal lumen or may involve a complex process, with migration of the adult or immature worm through the body before localization in a particular tissue. Complicating our understanding of the host-parasite relationship and the role of chemotherapy in helminth-induced infections is the complex life cycle of many of these organisms. Whereas some helminths may have a simple cycle of egg deposition and development of the egg to produce a mature worm, others must progress through one or more hosts and one or more morphological stages before emerging as an adult. Furthermore, an infective form may be either an adult worm or an immature worm. Not uncommonly, treatment is further complicated by infection with more than one genus of helminth. Helminths can be divided into three groups: *cestodes* (flatworm), *nematodes* (roundworm), and *trematodes* (flukes). The following discussion of anthelmintics takes advantage of this grouping.

The complex life cycle and host-parasite relationship means that treatment is sometimes difficult and may need to be protracted. Table 58-1 lists the diseases, causative organisms, and recommended drugs. Other drugs are available but, because of toxicity or the availability of superior agents, they are neither included in the table nor discussed in this chapter.

The mode of action of most drugs used in the treatment of helminthic infections is only partially understood; it is discussed separately for each drug and is also summarized in Table 58-2. Some of the drugs used in the treatment of diseases caused by helminths also are used in the treatment of some protozoal diseases.

Treatment for Infections Caused by Cestodes

Cestodes, commonly referred to as tapeworms, are flattened dorsoventrally and are segmented. The tapeworm has a head with round suckers or a sucking groove. In some cases, there is a projection (*rostellum*) that bears hooks. This head, or *scolex* (also referred to as the holdfast organ), is used by the worm to attach to tissues. Drugs that affect the scolex permit expulsion of the organisms from the intestine. Attached to the head is the neck region, which is the region of growth. The rest of the worm consists of a number of segments, called *proglottids,* each of which contains both male and female reproductive units. These segments, after filling with fertilized eggs, are released from the worm and discharged into the environment.

Cestodes that parasitize humans have complex life cycles that usually require development in a second or intermediate host. Following their ingestion, the infected larvae develop into adults in the small intestine. Although a majority of patients remain symptom-free, some experience a vague abdominal discomfort, hunger pains, indigestion, and anorexia, and may develop a vitamin B deficiency. In some cestode infections, eggs containing larvae are ingested; the larvae invade the intestinal wall, enter a blood vessel, and lodge in such tissues as muscle, liver, and eye. Symptoms are associated with the particular organ affected.

Niclosamide

Chemistry and Mechanism of Action

Niclosamide (Fig. 58-1) is an insoluble chlorosalicylamide derivative that inhibits the uptake of glucose and the production of energy derived from anaerobic metabolism. Inhibition of anaerobic incorporation of inorganic phosphate into adenosine triphosphate (ATP) is detrimental to the parasite. Niclosamide can uncouple oxidative phosphorylation in mammalian mitochondria, but this action requires dosages that are higher than those commonly used in treating worm infections. Niclosamide also exerts an effect on the worm that is spastic, paralytic, or both.

Table 58-1. Drugs for the Treatment of Helminthic Disease

Organism	Drug(s) of choice	Alternative drugs
Cestodes		
Diphyllobothrium latum	Niclosamide or praziquantel	None
Hymenolepis nana	Praziquantel	Niclosamide
Taenia saginata	Niclosamide or praziquantel	None
Taenia solium	Niclosamide or praziquantel	None
F. buski	Niclosamide or praziquantel	None
Nematodes		
Ancylostoma duodenale	Mebendazole or pyrantel pamoate	None
Ascaris lumbricoides	Mebendazole or pyrantel pamoate	Piperazine citrate
Dracunculus medinensis	Metronidazole	Thiabendazole
Enterobius vermicularis	Mebendazole or pyrantel pamoate	None
Filariasis (Brugia malayi, Dipetalonema perstans, Loa loa, Wuchereria bancrofti)	Diethylcarbamazine	None
Onchocerca volvulus	Ivermectin	Diethylcarbamazine followed by suramin
Necator americanus	Mebendazole or pyrantel pamoate	None
Strongyloides stercoralis	Thiabendazole	None
Trichuris trichiura	Mebendazole	None
Trichostrongylus spp.	Thiabendazole	Pyrantel pamoate
Trichinella spiralis	Thiabendazole	Mebendazole
Trematodes		
Schistosoma haematobium	Praziquantel	None
Schistosoma japonicum	Praziquantel	None
Schistosoma mansoni	Praziquantel	Oxamniquine
Fasciola hepatica	Bithionol	Praziquantel
Paragonimus westermani	Praziquantel	Bithionol
Clonorchis sinensis	Praziquantel	None

Table 58-2. Mode of Action of Drugs Employed in the Chemotherapy of Helminthic Diseases

Drug	Mode of action	Specific effect
Paromomycin	Inhibits protein synthesis	Interferes with initiation complex; causes misreading of messenger RNA (mRNA)
Piperazine	Paralyzes helminth muscle	Blocks myoneural junction and causes hyperpolarization and flaccid paralysis
Ivermectin	Paralyzes helminth muscle	Blocks γ-aminobutyric acid (GABA)-mediated transmission of nerve signals
Pyrantel	Paralyzes helminth muscle	Depolarization and spastic paralysis
Niclosamide, mebendazole	Inhibits production of energy	Inhibits uptake of glucose with resultant loss of glycogen and decreased adenosine triphosphate (ATP) synthesis
Mebendazole	Inhibits protein function	Binds to tubulin
Diethylcarbamazine	Enhances phagocytosis and killing	Uncertain
Praziquantel	Paralyzes helminth muscle	Causes increase in membrane permeability, increased uptake of calcium
Thiabendazole	Inhibits energy production	Inhibits fumarate reductase and ATP synthesis
Bithionol	Inhibits energy production	Uncouples oxidative phosphorylation

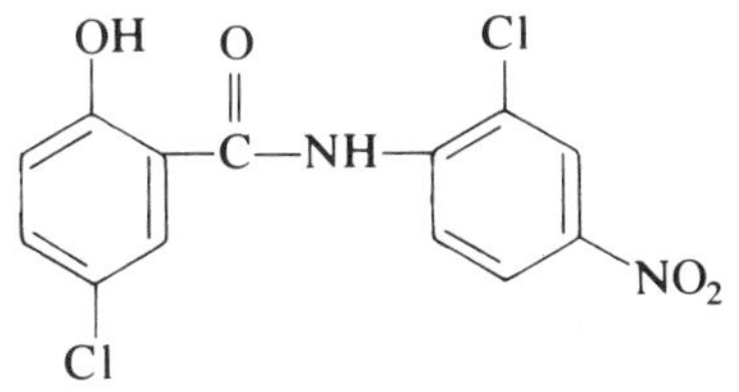

Figure 58-1. Niclosamide.

The drug affects the scolex and proximal segments of the cestodes, resulting in a detachment of the scolex from the intestinal wall and eventual evacuation of the cestodes from the intestine by the normal peristaltic action of the host's bowel. Niclosamide is insoluble in aqueous media and, because it is not absorbed from the intestinal tract, high concentrations can be achieved in the intestinal lumen, the environment of the parasite. The drug is not ovicidal.

Anthelmintic Spectrum

Niclosamide has been used extensively in the treatment of tapeworm infections caused by *Taenia saginata*, *Taenia solium*, *Diphyllobothrium latum*, *Fasciolopsis buski*, and *Hymenolepis nana*.

Clinical Uses

The broad range of activity of niclosamide against cestodes and the absence of significant side effects associated with its use have made it valuable in the treatment of *T. saginata* (beef tapeworm), *H. nana* (dwarf tapeworm), *D. latum* (fish tapeworm), *T. solium* (pork tapeworm), and *F. buski* (intestinal fluke) infestations. It is administered by mouth after the patient has fasted overnight and is followed by purging to encourage complete expulsion of the cestode, although this is not always considered necessary. With *T. solium* there is a risk of cysticercosis from ova released into the lumen of the bowel by the dead worm; purgation is usually necessary to reduce this risk. More recently, praziquantel, a broad-spectrum anthelmintic agent, has been extremely effective in treating many of the above infections (see the following discussion).

Adverse Reactions

No serious side effects are associated with niclosamide, although some patients may report abdominal discomfort and loose stools.

Preparation and Dosage

Niclosamide (*Niclocide*) is only available as oral tablets (500 mg).

Treatment for Infections Caused by Nematodes

Nematodes are elongated, cylindrical, nonsegmented worms that are tapered at both ends. Because of their shape, they are commonly referred to as roundworms. Some intestinal nematodes contain a mouth with three lips and, in some, the mouth has been modified and contains cutting plates. Infection occurs after ingestion of embryonated eggs or tissues of another host that contain larval forms of the nematodes.

Some of the nematodes (filarial worms and guinea worms) live in blood, lymphatics, and other tissues and are referred to as blood-and-tissue nematodes. Others are found primarily in the intestinal tract. One group, hookworms, undergoes a developmental cycle in soil. The larvae penetrate the skin of humans, enter the venules, and are carried to the lungs, where they enter the alveoli, sometimes causing pneumonitis. The larvae then migrate up the trachea and are swallowed. In the intestine, they attach to the mucosa and, using the cutting plates and a muscular esophagus, feed on host blood and tissue fluid. This occurrence may result in vague abdominal pains, diarrhea, and, if many worms are present, anemia.

Other intestinal nematodes are acquired by ingestion of eggs from soil. These groups lack cutting plates and may not cause anemia. Still other nematodes, such as pinworms, migrate from the anus to lay eggs, which are transmitted by fingers or through the air. The eggs are ingested and the adult worm develops in the intestinal tract. In some cases, the appendix may be invaded, resulting in symptoms of appendicitis. In most cases, the symptoms are perianal pruritus and a restlessness associated with the migration of the female worm through the anus to the perianal skin. Other nematodes, such as *Ascaris*, are ingested in egg form, but have a migration similar to that of the hookworm.

The filarial worms differ from other nematodes in that they are threadlike and are found in blood and tissue. The infective larvae enter following the bite of an infected arthropod (fly or mosquito). They then enter the lymphatics and lymph nodes. Fever, lymphangitis, and lymphadenitis are associated with the early stage of the disease. Chronic infections may be characterized by elephantiasis as a result of lymphatic obstruction. Some species of filarial worms migrate in the subcutaneous tissues and produce nodules and blindness (onchocerciasis).

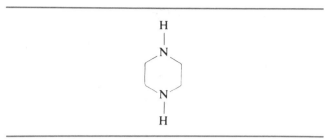

Figure 58-2. Piperazine.

Piperazine

Mechanism of Action

Piperazine (Fig. 58-2) acts on the musculature of the helminths, causing a flaccid paralysis and expulsion of the worm by the normal peristaltic action of the host's intestine. Since piperazine increases the resting potential of the helminth muscle, a pacemaker that is presumably present in the muscle membrane is suppressed. It has been suggested that piperazine is an analogue of an inhibitory transmitter present in helminths. This suggestion, which proposes different control mechanisms for helminth and mammalian tissue, would account for the lack of piperazine toxicity in mammalian nervous tissue. Piperazine has been shown to block the response of *Ascaris lumbricoides* muscle to acetylcholine.

Anthelmintic Spectrum

Piperazine has been used to treat *A. lumbricoides* and *Enterobius vermicularis* infections, although mebendazole is now the agent of choice.

Absorption and Excretion

Piperazine is administered orally and is readily absorbed from the intestinal tract. Most of the drug is excreted in the urine within 24 hr.

Clinical Uses

Piperazine is an appropriate alternative to mebendazole for the treatment of ascariasis; cure rates of greater than 80 percent are obtained following a 2-day regimen.

Adverse Reactions

Piperazine salts are well tolerated. Side effects occasionally include gastrointestinal distress, urticaria, and dizziness. Neurologic symptoms of ataxia, hypotonia, visual disturbances, and exacerbations of epilepsy can occur in patients with preexisting renal insufficiency.

Preparations

Piperazine citrate (*Vermizine*) is available as oral tablets and as a syrup.

Diethylcarbamazine

Mechanism of Action

Diethylcarbamazine citrate (Fig. 58-3) is a piperazine derivative. Although piperazine itself is inactive in the treatment of filarial infections, diethylcarbamazine (a substituted piperazine) is active against several microfilaria and adult filarial worms. The drug causes an increase in muscle tone, particularly of the organ of attachment. More important, the drug may cause the release of enzymes from eosinophils, which then alter the surface of the worms, making them susceptible to phagocytosis. The drug is not filaricidal in vitro.

Anthelmintic Spectrum

Diethylcarbamazine is highly effective in eliminating the microfilariae of *Loa loa, Wuchereria bancrofti,* and *Brugia malayi* that circulate in the bloodstream. It also kills the adult worm of *L. loa* and *B. malayi,* but it has little effect on the adult worm of *W. bancrofti.* Although in onchocerciasis the microfilariae disappear from the skin, the drug affects neither the adult worm nor the microfilariae present in the lymph nodes. Ivermectin is now the preferred agent for onchocercosis. Diethylcarbamazine also is inactive against both adult filariae and microfilariae of *Dipetalonema perstans.*

Absorption, Metabolism, and Excretion

Diethylcarbamazine is absorbed from the gastrointestinal tract, and peak blood levels are obtained in 4 hr; the drug disappears from the blood within 48 hr. The intact drug and its metabolites are excreted in the urine.

Clinical Uses

Since diethylcarbamazine is not universally active against filarial infections, a specific diagnosis based on blood smears, biopsy samples, and a geographic history is important. The drug's rapid action against susceptible microfilariae can result in severe systemic effects if the parasite load is heavy (see Adverse Reactions).

Adverse Reactions

Caution is necessary when using this agent, particularly when treating onchocerciasis. The sudden death of the microfilariae can produce mild to severe reactions

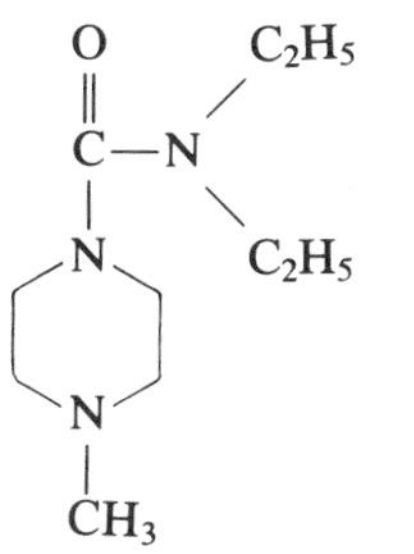

O
‖
C—N
C₂H₅

C₂H₅

N

N

CH₃

Figure 58-3. Diethylcarbamazine.

within hours of drug administration. These are manifested by fever, lymphadenopathy, cutaneous swelling, leukocytosis, and intensification of any preexisting eosinophilia, edema, rashes, tachycardia, and headache. Corticosteroids may be necessary for severe reactions. Other side effects are relatively mild and range from malaise, headache, and arthralgias to gastrointestinal symptoms.

An encephalopathy is occasionally seen in patients treated for *L. loa* with diethylcarbamazine.

Preparations and Dosage

Diethylcarbamazine citrate (*Hetrazan*): Oral tablets (50 mg each) are administered in gradually increasing doses (to a maximum dose of 2 mg/kg) three times a day for the treatment of wuchereriasis (14–21 days of treatment) and loiasis (14–21 days of treatment). In onchocerciasis, diethylcarbamazine followed by a course of suramin (see Chap. 56) is an alternative to ivermectin.

Ivermectin

Structure and Mechanisms of Action

Ivermectin is a semisynthetic macrocyclic lactone. It is a derivative of a naturally occurring compound produced by *Streptomyces avermitilis*. It acts by increasing the release and binding of γ-aminobutyric acid (GABA), thereby producing paralysis. Ivermectin does not cross the mammalian blood-brain barrier.

Anthelmintic Spectrum

Ivermectin has broad-spectrum activity in that it can affect nematodes, insects, and acarine parasites. It is active against the microfilariae of *Onchocerca volvulus*.

Absorption, Metabolism, and Excretion

Ivermectin is administered by the oral and subcutaneous route. It is rapidly absorbed. Most of the drug is excreted in the feces as unaltered drug. The half-life is approximately 12 hr.

Clinical Use

Ivermectin has been widely used in veterinary medicine. It is used in treating humans infected with *O. volvulus*. It appears to be better tolerated and more effective than diethylcarbamazine.

Adverse Effects

The side effects are minimal, with pruritus, fever, and tender lymph nodes occasionally seen. The side effects are considerably less than those seen after diethylcarbamazine administration.

Preparation

Ivermectin (*Mectizan*) is available from the manufacturer.

Pyrantel Pamoate

Structure and Mechanism of Action

Pyrantel pamoate (Fig. 58-4) is an insoluble pyrimidine derivative that causes both the depolarization of helminth muscle and an inhibition of cholinesterase. This activity results in a spastic paralysis and loss of muscle activity.

The drug is selectively toxic primarily because the neuromuscular junction of helminth muscle is more sensitive to the drug than is mammalian muscle. Pyrantel and piperazine have opposing mechanisms of action.

Anthelmintic Spectrum

Pyrantel pamoate is active against several roundworms: *A. lumbricoides*, *Ancylostoma duodenale*, *Necator americanus*, and *E. vermicularis*.

Absorption, Metabolism, and Excretion

This drug is administered orally and, because very little is absorbed, high levels are achieved in the intestinal tract. Less than 15 percent of the drug and its metabolites are excreted in urine.

Clinical Use

Pyrantel is an alternative drug of choice in treating infections with *A. lumbricoides*, *E. vermicularis* (pinworms), and hookworms (*N. americanus* and *A. duodenale*). It is not recommended for pregnant patients or for children under the age of 1 year.

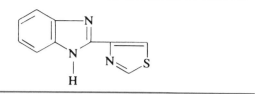

Figure 58-4. Pyrantel.   **Figure 58-5.** Thiabendazole.

Adverse Reactions

Although most of the drug remains in the intestinal lumen, enough can be absorbed systemically to cause headache, dizziness, and drowsiness. In addition, gastrointestinal symptoms may occur.

Preparation and Dosage

Pyrantel pamoate (*Antiminth*) is marketed as a 250-mg/5 ml suspension.

Benzimidazoles

Several benzimidazoles are currently in use for the treatment of helminthic infections. Two of these, mebendazole and thiabendazole, are described in this section.

Thiabendazole

Chemistry and Mechanism of Action

Thiabendazole is a benzimidazole derivative (Fig. 58-5) that inhibits fumarate reductase and electron transport-associated phosphorylation in helminths. Interference with ATP generation decreases glucose uptake and glycogen synthesis, and affects the energy available for metabolism. In helminths, but not in mammals, fumarate is the terminal electron acceptor in anaerobic metabolism.

Anthelmintic Spectrum

Thiabendazole shows a broad spectrum of activity against the following nematodes: *A. lumbricoides, N. americanus, A. duodenale, E. vermicularis, Strongyloides stercoralis,* and *Trichuris trichiura* (whipworm). Thiabendazole affects adult worms, is larvicidal, and prevents the development of eggs.

Absorption, Metabolism, and Excretion

Thiabendazole is administered orally and is rapidly absorbed from the intestinal tract, with peak plasma levels achieved in about 1 hr. The drug is metabolized in the liver and excreted in urine within 24 to 48 hr as glucuronide and sulfate esters. Approximately 10 percent is found in feces.

Clinical Uses

At present, thiabendazole is the drug of choice for the treatment of cutaneous larva migrans (creeping eruption), strongyloidiasis, and trichostrongyliasis and trichinosis. When used to treat severe trichinosis, it is used in conjunction with steroids. Severe forms of visceral larva migrans also can be treated with the drug. Mild forms are usually self-limiting.

Adverse Reactions

Side effects are fairly frequent with the standard dosage of 25 mg/kg/day for 2 days. However, these reactions may be alleviated by taking the drug after a meal. Anorexia, nausea, vomiting, drowsiness, and vertigo occur in up to one-third of the patients. Diarrhea, pruritus, rash, hallucinations, crystalluria, and leukopenia are less common; shock, hyperglycemia, lymphadenopathy, and the Stevens-Johnson syndrome are rare. Some patients report that their urine smells like asparagus. This reaction is related to the excretion of a metabolite.

Preparations

Thiabendazole (*Mintezol*) is available both as chewable tablets and as an oral suspension.

Mebendazole

Chemistry and Mechanism of Action

Mebendazole, also a benzimidazole derivative, inhibits glucose uptake. Unlike thiabendazole, it does not inhibit fumarate reductase. Mebendazole also binds to both mammalian and nematode tubulin. The difference in binding affinities may explain the selective action of the drug. Mebendazole accumulates in the parasite but, unlike its metabolism in mammalian cells, the nematodes do not metabolize the drug rapidly. Mebendazole is toxic to both adults and eggs.

Anthelmintic Spectrum

The drug is used for the treatment of infections caused by *A. lumbricoides, E. vermicularis, T. trichiura, N. americanus,* and *A. duodenale.* A large number of nematodes and cestodes are susceptible to mebendazole (e.g., *O. volvulus*).

Absorption, Metabolism, and Excretion

Mebendazole is given orally. It is poorly soluble and very little is absorbed from the intestinal tract. Peak plasma levels approach only 0.3 percent of the total administered dose. About 5 to 10 percent, principally the decarboxylated derivatives, is recovered in the urine; most of the orally administered drug is found in the feces within 24 hr.

Clinical Uses

Mebendazole is used primarily for the treatment of *A. lumbricoides, T. trichiura, E. vermicularis,* and hookworm infections, in which it produces high cure rates. It is an alternative agent in the treatment of trichinosis. Owing to its broad-spectrum anthelmintic effect, mixed infections (ascariasis, hookworm infestation, or enterobiasis, in association with trichuriasis) frequently respond to therapy.

Adverse Reactions

The drug is well tolerated, although it is poorly absorbed. Abdominal discomfort and diarrhea may occur when the worm load is heavy. Embryonic defects and teratogenic effects have been demonstrated in rats; therefore, its use is contraindicated during pregnancy.

Preparation

Mebendazole (*Vermox*) is available as chewable tablets.

Treatment for Infections Caused by Trematodes

Trematodes (flukes) are nonsegmented flattened helminths that are often leaflike in shape. Most have two suckers, one found around the mouth (oral sucker) and the other located ventrally. They are usually hermaphroditic. The eggs, which are passed out of the host in sputum, urine, or feces, undergo several stages of maturation in other hosts before the larvae enter humans. The larvae are acquired either through food (aquatic vegetation, fish, crayfish) or by direct penetration of the skin. After ingestion, most trematodes mature in the intestinal tract (intestinal flukes); others will migrate and mature in the liver and bile duct (liver flukes), whereas still others penetrate the intestinal wall and migrate through the abdominal cavity to the lung (lung flukes). Diarrhea, abdominal pain, and anorexia are common symptoms associated with trematode infestation. Liver flukes may cause bile duct blockage, liver enlargement, upper right quadrant pain, and diarrhea. Liver function tests are usually altered. Lung flukes produce pulmonary symptoms such as cough, hemoptysis, and chest pain.

The *schistosomes* (blood flukes) represent a distinct group of trematodes. These helminths are cylindrical at the anterior end and flattened at the posterior end. The sexes are separate. The larvae penetrate skin that is in contact with contaminated water and then migrate through the lymphatics and blood vessels to the liver. After maturing, schistosomes migrate into the mesenteric or vesicular vein, where the adults mate and release eggs. The eggs secrete enzymes that enable them to pass through the wall of the intestine (*Schistosoma mansoni* and *Schistosoma japonicum*) or bladder (*Schistosoma haematobium*). In addition, some eggs may be carried to the liver or the lung by the circulation. Penetration of the skin is associated with petechial hemorrhage, some edema, and a pruritus that disappears after about 4 days. Approximately 3 weeks after trematode penetration, patients complain of malaise, fever, and vague intestinal symptoms. With the laying of eggs, acute symptoms of generalized malaise, fever, urticaria, abdominal pain, and liver tenderness are reported. Diarrhea or dysentery is associated with infestations by *S. mansoni* and *S. japonicum,* whereas hematuria and dysuria are commonly caused by *S. haematobium.* In the chronic form of the disease, fibrosis and hyperplasia can occur in those tissues in which the eggs are located.

Praziquantel

Structure and Mechanism of Action

Praziquantel (Fig. 58-6) is one of a number of stereoisomers of prazinoisoquinolines. It causes changes in membrane permeability and produces tetanic-like contractions within the muscle system of the fluke, possibly by altering the influx of calcium ions. Vacuolization and disintegration of the schistosome integument also occur.

Anthelmintic Activity

Praziquantel is the most effective of the drugs used in the treatment of schistosomiasis. Unlike other agents, it is active against all three major species (*S. haematobium, S. mansoni,* and *S. japonicum*). In addition, it has activity against other flukes such as *Clonorchis sinensis, Fasciola hepatica, Paragonimus westermani, Opisthorcis viverrini,* and the

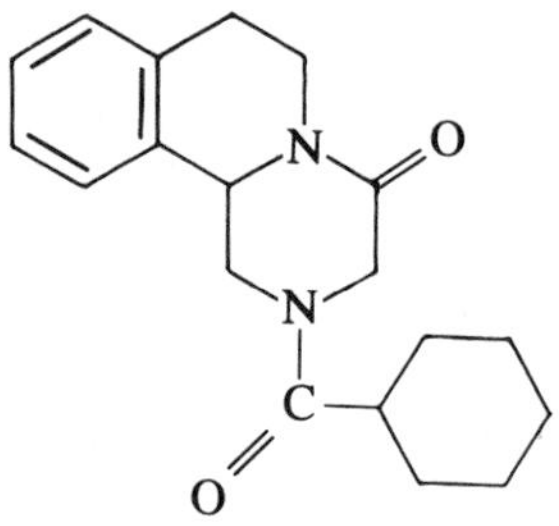

Figure 58-6. Praziquantel.

tapeworms (*D. latum, H. nana, T. saginata,* and *T. solium*). It is the drug of choice to treat neurocysticercosis.

Absorption, Metabolism, and Excretion

Praziquantel is readily (80% in 24 hr) absorbed after oral administration. Serum concentrations are maximal in 1 to 3 hr; the drug has a half-life of 0.8 to 1.5 hr. Praziquantel is excreted by the kidneys.

Clinical Uses

Praziquantel is an extremely active, broad-spectrum anthelmintic that is well tolerated and has become the drug of choice for the treatment of schistosomiasis. It is also used effectively in the treatment of clonorchiasis and paragonimiasis. The drug is also an effective alternative agent to niclosamide in the treatment of tapeworm infestations.

Adverse Reactions

Adverse reactions tend to occur within a few hours of administration and include gastrointestinal intolerance with nausea, vomiting, and abdominal discomfort.

Preparation and Dosage

Praziquantel (*Biltricide*) is available for oral administration as a lacquered tablet containing 600 mg of drug.

Oxamniquine

Oxamniquine is a tetrahydroquinolone that stimulates parasite muscular activity at low concentrations but causes paralysis at higher concentrations. It is given orally and is readily absorbed from the intestinal tract. Peak concentrations in plasma are obtained in about 3 hr. The drug is excreted in urine mostly as a 6-carboxyl derivative. Oxamniquine has a restricted range of efficacy, being active only

against *S. mansoni* infections. It is an alternative drug for these infections. The drug is reasonably well tolerated and has been used both for the treatment of individuals as well as for community use in control programs. Side effects include central nervous system (CNS) toxicity with unsteadiness and, occasionally, seizures. The drug is given as a single dose of 15 mg/kg, although it appears that African strains of *S. mansoni* are less susceptible and require higher doses.

Oxamniquine (*Vansil*) is available in capsules of 250 mg.

Bithionol

Chemistry and Mechanism of Action

Bithionol (Fig. 58-7) is a phenolic derivative. Its mode of action is related to uncoupling of oxidative phosphorylation.

Anthelmintic Spectrum

Bithionol is active against flukes, including *F. hepatica* (sheep liver fluke) and *P. westermani* (lung fluke).

Absorption, Metabolism, and Excretion

The drug is administered orally and is absorbed from the intestinal tract. Peak blood levels are achieved in 4 to 8 hr. Excretion is mainly by the kidneys.

Clinical Uses

Trematode infections of livestock are of major economic importance. Most of the drugs available for the treatment of animals are too toxic for human use. Bithionol is one exception. It is used in treatment of *F. hepatica* infections and as an alternative to praziquantel in the treatment of infestation by *P. westermani*. It is highly active against the adult worm but exerts no action against the migratory stages. Careful postdrug monitoring of the patient is essential to determine clinical cure.

Figure 58-7. Bithionol.

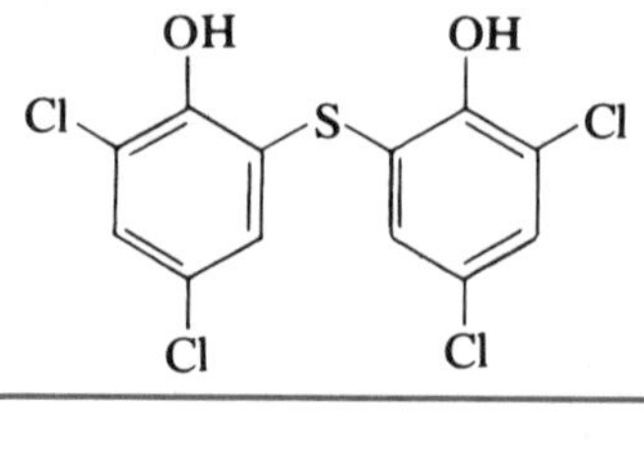

Adverse Reactions

Side effects are generally mild and transient and include nausea, vomiting, diarrhea, headache, dizziness, urticaria, and other skin rashes.

Preparation and Dosage

Bithionol (*Actamer*) is administered orally at a dose of 40 to 50 mg/kg every other day for up to 15 doses. The drug is available from the Parasitic Diseases Division, Centers for Disease Control, Atlanta, Ga. 30333.

Supplemental Reading

Andrew, P. Praziquantel: Mechanisms of anti-schistosomal activity. *Pharmacol. Ther.* 29:129, 1985.

Bruce, J.I. Anthelmintics. *Int. J. Parasitol.* 17:131, 1987.

Campbell, W., and Rew, R.S. (eds.). *Chemotherapy of Parasitic Diseases.* New York: Plenum, 1986.

Cook, J.A. Schistosome infection in humans: Perspectives and recent findings. *Ann. Intern. Med.* 97:740, 1982.

Davis, A., and Wegner, D.H.G. Multicentre trials of praziquantel in human schistosomiasis: Design and techniques. *Bull. WHO* 57:767, 1979.

Drugs for parasitic infections. *Med. Lett. Drugs Ther.* 34:17, 1992.

Kilpatrick, M.E., et al. Treatment of *Schistosomiasis mansoni* with oxamniquine—5 years' experience. *Am. J. Trop. Med. Hyg.* 30:1219, 1981.

Pearson, R.D., and Guerrant, R.L. Praziquantel: A major advance in anthelmintic therapy. *Ann. Intern. Med.* 99:195, 1983.

Van den Bossche, H., Thienpont, D., and Janssen, P.G. (eds.). *Chemotherapy of Gastrointestinal Helminths.* New York: Springer-Verlag, 1985.

Verderame, M. and MacKiewicz, J. Antihelmintics. In M. Verderame (ed.), *Handbook of Chemotherapeutic Agents.* Vol. 2. Boca Raton, Fla.: CRC, 1986.

59

Antifungal Drugs

Roger G. Finch and Irvin S. Snyder

Treatment of fungal infections is considerably more difficult than treatment of bacterial infections. Many fungal infections occur in poorly vascularized tissues or avascular structures such as the superficial layer of the skin, nails, and hair. Treatment of these infections presents a problem in distribution and retention of adequate amounts of chemotherapeutic agents owing to the poor solubility of some of these drugs. Deep-seated mycoses, such as those caused by *Blastomyces dermatitidis, Histoplasma capsulatum,* and others, are particularly difficult to treat. This reflects the slow-growing nature of these organisms, the eukaryotic structure of the cell, and the granulomatous tissue response, which may interfere with drug penetration.

Amphotericin B (a polyene), flucytosine (5-fluorocytosine, a fluorinated pyrimidine), miconazole, ketoconazole (imidazoles), and fluconazole (triazole) are the most useful agents for treating systemic fungal infections. Topical infections are susceptible to a wider range of drugs than are systemic infections. Table 59-1 summarizes the mechanisms of action of presently available antifungal agents.

Amphotericin B

Chemistry and Mechanism of Action

Amphotericin B, which is produced by *Streptomyces nodosus,* is characterized by a large ring structure, part of which is hydroxylated and hydrophilic, and part of which contains conjugated double bonds and is lipophilic (Fig. 59-1).

The polyenes inhibit fungi through an interaction with ergosterol, a fungal membrane sterol. This effect results in the loss of both membrane selective permeability and intracellular components. In addition, amino acid uptake is impaired. These antibiotics are selective for fungi and do not affect bacteria because, with the exception of

Mycoplasma, sterols are not found in bacterial membranes. Mammalian cell membranes also contain sterols, which account for the host toxicity associated with these antibiotics. However, the polyenes bind more effectively to ergosterol, the principal sterol in fungal membranes, than to other sterols; this, in fact, may account for their relatively selective toxicity. Depending on the concentration employed, the polyenes have either a fungistatic or fungicidal effect.

Antifungal Spectrum

Amphotericin B is used to treat systemic infections caused by *Cryptococcus neoformans, Histoplasma capsulatum, Coccidioides immitis, Blastomyces dermatitidis,* and *Sporothrix schenckii.* The *Aspergillus* species and the phycomycetes are variable in their sensitivity.

Absorption, Distribution, and Metabolism

Amphotericin B is poorly absorbed from the intestinal tract. Consequently, it is usually administered either intravenously or topically. After intravenous injection, the drug is rapidly sequestered in tissues and then is slowly released. The initial half-life of the injected drug is about 24 hr; however, there is a second elimination phase with a half-life of 15 days. The initial phase represents elimination from both a central intravascular and a rapidly equilibrating extravascular compartment, whereas the second, more prolonged, phase represents elimination from storage sites in a slowly equilibrating extravascular compartment. The drug concentrations achievable in cerebrospinal fluid (CSF) and aqueous humor are lower than those found in the blood.

Amphotericin B is slowly excreted by the kidney, with about 5 percent excreted daily as the active drug. The drug can be detected in urine for at least 7 weeks after therapy

Table 59-1. Mechanism of Action of Antifungal Chemotherapeutic Agents

Agent (or class)	Mechanism of action	Cidal or static
Polyene antibiotics: amphotericin B; nystatin	Bind to fungal membrane sterols and alter selective permeability of fungal membrane	Cidal
Griseofulvin	Binds to fungal microtubules; prevents cell division	Static
Flucytosine	Inhibits synthesis of fungal pyrimidines and RNA	Static
Azoles	Inhibit cytochrome P-450, demethylation of lanosterol and ergosterol synthesis	Static
Ciclopirox olamine	Transport of precursors for macromolecular synthesis	Cidal
Tolnaftate	Unknown	Static
Allylamines	Inhibit squalene epoxidase	Cidal

is stopped. Compromised renal function does not affect serum levels. The major route of excretion is extrarenal. Amphotericin B is 90 percent bound to serum proteins; the drug is not removed by hemodialysis.

Clinical Uses

Amphotericin B is a *broad-spectrum* antifungal agent that is active against yeast and yeastlike fungi as well as dimorphic and filamentous fungi. There has been varying success in the treatment of protozoal infections caused by the free-living amebae of the *Naegleria* and *Hartmannella* genera as well as in treating mucocutaneous lesions of American leishmaniasis.

Although the drug is toxic if given in sufficient quantities, the seriousness of the systemic mycoses justifies its use. In the United States, it remains the drug of choice for the treatment of localized and disseminated blastomycosis, coccidioidomycosis, and histoplasmosis. Disseminated infections with *Candida albicans*, *Torulopsis* species, and *Cryptococcus neoformans* as well as meningitis caused by the last-named microorganisms usually respond to treatment with amphotericin B. In the case of cryptococcal meningitis, amphotericin B is usually combined with 5-fluorocytosine, which often provides a synergistic combination and limits the total duration of therapy to 4 weeks. Treatment of these systemic mycoses is by no means universally successful. Host factors play an important role in determining prognosis. For example, human immunodeficiency virus (HIV)-infected patients with cryptococcal meningitis frequently relapse so that further treatment is necessary. In this situation, fluconazole has been shown to be effective therapeutically in combination with amphotericin B.

Many of the fungal infections, notably those caused by *Candida*, *Cryptococcus*, and *Torulopsis*, are opportunistic in nature and develop in patients whose immune system is suppressed either by disease (e.g., leukemias, lymphomas, disseminated malignancies, and acquired immunodeficiency syndrome [AIDS]) or by treatment with cytotoxic agents or corticosteroids. The length of treatment will vary with the severity of the disease and the patient's response to therapy, but it is seldom less than 4 weeks and requires a minimum total dose of approximately 1 gm.

Figure 59-1. Amphotericin B.

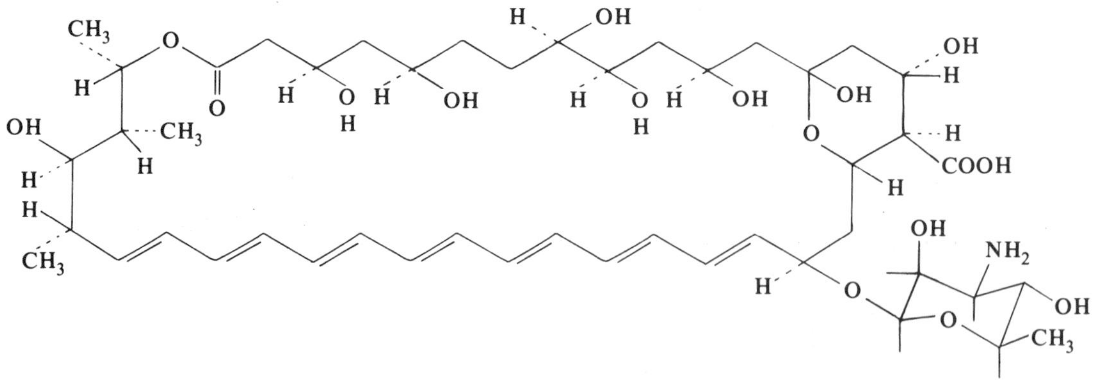

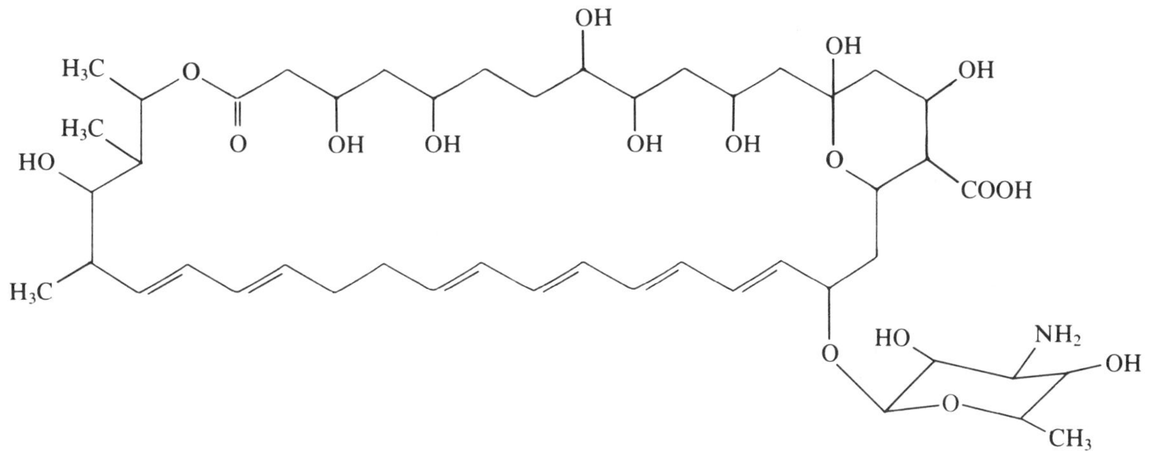

Figure 59-2. Nystatin.

Adverse Reactions

Amphotericin B is a toxic drug and its use demands great care. An acute hypersensitivity reaction is unusual but, occasionally, it may cause anaphylaxis, generalized pain, and seizures. Phlebitis at the site of injection is not uncommon but may be prevented by the addition of heparin to the infusion. Headache, anorexia, vomiting, fever, and chills also can occur. Aspirin or acetaminophen, diphenhydramine, or prochlorperazine and 25 to 50 mg hydrocortisone added to the infusion may decrease fever and chills. A reversible anemia of the normochromic and normocytic type also may develop.

The most serious and most common adverse effect is nephrotoxicity, an effect that can be made less severe by alternate-day therapy. Hypokalemia, hypomagnesemia, and tubular acidosis also are observed. A variety of histological changes can occur in the kidney; they include thickening of the glomerular basement membrane, tubular degeneration, nephrocalcinosis, and glomerular hyalinization. Renal function usually improves on discontinuation of treatment.

Fungal infections of the meninges have been treated by intrathecal injection of amphotericin B. Despite the small doses given, side effects are frequent and range from headache, paresthesias, and arachnoiditis to nerve palsy; problems with micturition also occur.

Preparations and Dosage

Amphotericin B (*Fungizone*) is marketed as a topical 3% cream, lotion, and ointment as well as a powder (50 mg) for injection.

Liposomal Amphotericin B

Liposomal encapsulation of drugs is a promising development in drug formulation that is especially suited for highly lipophilic drugs. Various liposomal amphotericin B formulations have been used in experimental infections. They are currently undergoing extensive clinical trials. The ability to increase therapeutic concentrations of drugs in organs such as the liver, lungs, and spleen is a particular advantage, especially in immunocompromised patients who are susceptible to fungal infections. It also holds the promise of reduced toxicity compared with the original formulation.

Nystatin

Chemistry and Mechanism of Action

Nystatin (Fig. 59-2) is a polyene antibiotic isolated from *Streptomyces noursei*. It is insoluble in water and plasma, and quickly decomposes in solution. Its mode of action is identical to that of amphotericin B; that is, it complexes with sterols and alters the permeability of the fungal membrane. Generally, resistance to this drug does not occur.

Antifungal Spectrum

Nystatin is used to treat superficial infections caused by *Candida albicans*. However, *C. neoformans, H. capsulatum,*

B. dermatitidis, and dermatophytes also are sensitive to the drug. It has both fungicidal and fungistatic activity. Cross-resistance with amphotericin B does occur.

Clinical Use

Nystatin is used topically or is administered orally in the treatment of mucocutaneous infections caused by *Candida albicans.* These infections may take the form of stomatitis (thrush), esophagitis, vaginitis, paronychia, or, rarely, intestinal candidiasis; they are seen more frequently in patients with leukemia or diabetes mellitus, and in those receiving corticosteroids, cytotoxic agents, or broad-spectrum antibiotics, such as the tetracyclines.

Preparations and Dosage

Nystatin (*Mycostatin, Nilstat, Nystex*) is available as oral (500,000 units) and vaginal (100,000 units) tablets as well as in ointment, cream, and powder formulations.

Griseofulvin

Chemistry and Mechanism of Action

Griseofulvin is an antibiotic (Fig. 59-3) produced by *Penicillium griseofulvin.* It affects fungi by binding to their microtubules (the protein structures found in eukaryotic cells that are responsible for the formation of mitotic spindles). Unlike other drugs that bind to microtubules and inhibit assembly, griseofulvin affects the function of the polymerized proteins. Destruction of microtubules alters the processing of new cell wall components needed for fungal growth.

Antifungal Spectrum

Griseofulvin is fungistatic and is used for treating infections caused by the dermatophytes: *Epidermophyton, Microsporum,* and *Trichophyton* species.

Absorption, Metabolism, and Excretion

Because of poor solubility, griseofulvin is not well absorbed from the intestinal tract; however, absorption may be improved if the drug is milled into fine, crystalline particles, thus increasing the surface area of the griseofulvin crystals. Unlike other antibiotics, the absorption of griseofulvin is enhanced when it is given with a fatty meal. Absorption occurs primarily from the small intestine,

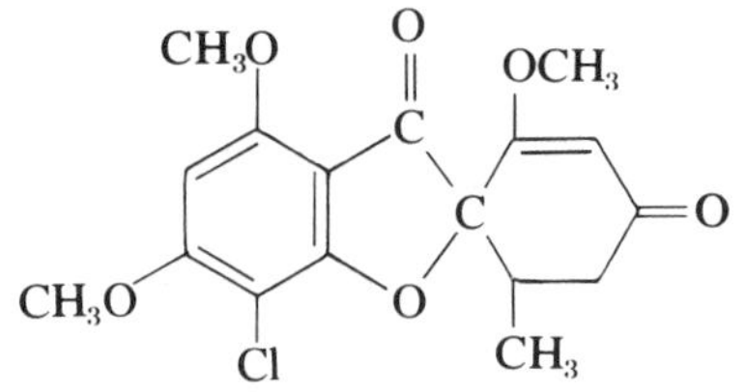

Figure 59-3. Griseofulvin.

with peak serum levels obtained 4 hr after drug administration.

Griseofulvin specifically binds to keratin, and high concentrations are found in the stratum corneum and outermost layer of the epidermis; it is also taken up by nails. Keratin binding can be demonstrated after either oral or topical use. The drug also binds to keratin precursor cells, making them resistant to fungal infection.

Griseofulvin is metabolized in the liver by demethylation and glucuronide formation. Less than 1 percent of the intact drug is excreted in the urine; the bulk of the drug is found unchanged in the feces.

Adverse Reactions

Griseofulvin is normally well tolerated. However, side effects include headache, lapses of memory, and impairment of judgment. Skin rashes, gastrointestinal distress, and a variety of skin reactions, including angioedema and photosensitivity reactions, also have been described. Hepatotoxicity and leukopenia can occur. Because griseofulvin can induce symptoms of porphyria, the drug should not be used in persons with porphyria or advanced liver disease.

Preparations

Griseofulvin (*Grifulvin V, Fulvicin-U/F, Grisactin*) is marketed as oral tablets or capsules and as an oral suspension. Ultramicrosize griseofulvin (*Fulvicin P/G*) tablets also are available.

Flucytosine (5-Fluorocytosine)

Chemistry and Mechanism of Action

Flucytosine (5-fluorocytosine) is a fluorinated pyrimidine (Fig. 59-4), which becomes toxic only after it enters the cell via cytosine permease. Inside the cell, it is deam-

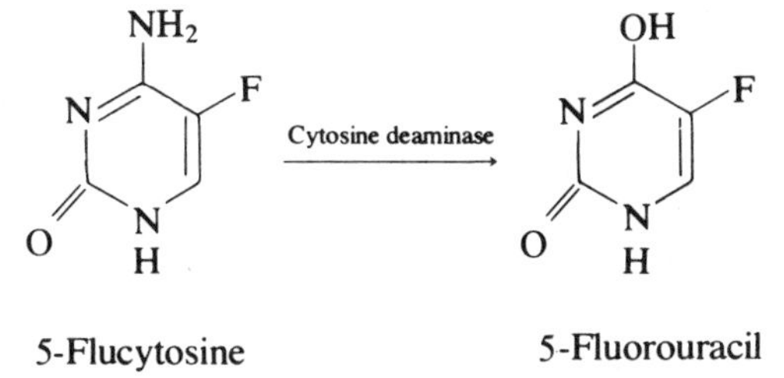

Figure 59-4. Flucytosine, showing its conversion to 5-fluorouracil.

inated by fungal cytosine deaminase to form the active metabolite 5-fluorouracil (5-FU). Thymidylate synthetase and DNA synthesis are inhibited by 5-fluoro-2'-deoxyuridylic acid, a metabolite of 5-fluorocytosine. Mammalian cells lack cytosine deaminase and are not affected by the drug. Flucytosine is a fungistatic agent. Incorporation of the metabolite into RNA results in defective RNA and altered protein synthesis.

Antifungal Spectrum

Cryptococcus neoformans, C. albicans, Torulopsis glabrata, and *S. schenckii,* as well as *Cladosporium* species, and *Phialophora* species, the fungi responsible for chromomycosis, are susceptible to flucytosine. There are marked differences in sensitivity among fungal isolates and resistance has been reported. Resistance may be a reflection of a deficiency in the enzymes involved in the transport of the drug into the cytoplasm, or it may be due to a compensatory ability of the organism to increase its rate of pyrimidine synthesis.

Absorption, Distribution, and Excretion

Flucytosine is well absorbed (about 90%) from the intestinal tract after oral administration and is detectable in serum after 30 min. Peak serum values of 25 to 100 μg/ml are obtained after 4 to 6 hr. Since serum protein binding is minimal, the drug can be removed by hemodialysis.

Flucytosine is widely distributed in body fluids and readily penetrates into the CSF, where it reaches concentrations that are 60 to 80 percent of the serum level. Its half-life is about 3 to 5 hr. Flucytosine also is found in the urine, aqueous humor, and in bronchial secretions. The drug is not metabolized in humans, and most (approximately 90%) of an administered dose can be detected unchanged in the urine. Since it is excreted primarily by glomerular filtration, dose reduction is necessary in renal failure.

Adverse Reactions

The adverse effects associated with flucytosine administration are few but include abdominal bloating and diarrhea. Leukopenia, thrombocytopenia, and elevated serum glutamic oxaloacetic transaminase (SGOT) and alkaline phosphatase also have been described, but these alterations have not been clearly ascribed to flucytosine. Marrow depressant effects are more likely to be seen in patients with abnormal renal function. Since flucytosine is excreted primarily in the urine, blood levels of the drug should be monitored in patients with renal insufficiency.

Preparations and Dosage

Flucytosine (*Ancobon*) is only available for oral administration in the form of 250- and 500-mg capsules.

Azoles

The azoles represent a large and emerging group of synthetic antifungal agents. The azoles contain a five-membered azole ring attached by an N-C bond to other chemical structures. The *imidazoles* comprise the largest group of these clinically useful drugs, with ketoconazole being the most important imidazole. The imidazole antifungal agents include the topical agents clotrimazole, econazole, tioconazole, oxiconazole, and terconazole. Ketoconazole and miconazole are used as both superficial and systemic agents. Two new azole antifungal agents, itraconazole and fluconazole, are systemically active; they are classified as *triazoles*. The imidazoles have two nitrogens in the azole ring, whereas the triazoles have three nitrogens in the azole nucleus (Fig. 59-5).

The azoles all have the same mechanism of action. They bind through either the N-3 (imidazoles) or N-4 (triazoles) to the heme iron of cytochrome P-450 and inhibit demethylation of 14-α-methylsterols to ergosterol. They may also have a direct effect on fungal membrane phospholipids. Selective toxicity is related to the differences in affinity of the drug for mammalian and fungal cytochrome P-450. In addition, humans use preformed exogenous sterols.

Imidazoles

Clotrimazole

Antifungal Spectrum

Clotrimazole has broad antifungal activity. It is primarily fungistatic and is active against dermatophytes as

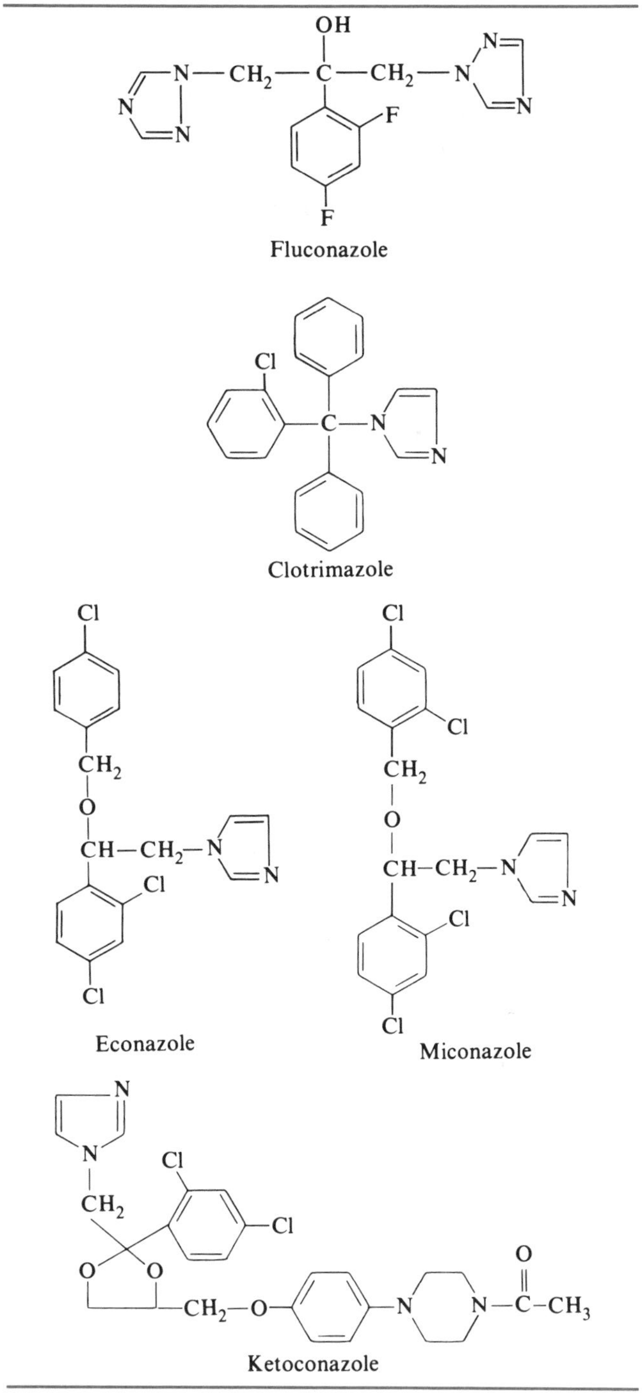

Figure 59-5. Representative azoles.

well as *C. albicans, C. neoformans, S. schenckii,* and *B. dermatitidis.*

Absorption, Metabolism, and Excretion

Topical use results in therapeutic concentrations of clotrimazole in the epidermis and in the mucosa. Negligible amounts are found in serum.

Clinical Uses

Use of clotrimazole is limited to the topical treatment of oral, skin, and vaginal infections caused by *Candida albicans.* It appears to be as effective as nystatin when given for genital candidiasis in the form of a vaginal tablet. Another indication is in the treatment of dermatophytic infections caused by *Epidermophyton, Microsporum,* and *Trichophyton* species.

Adverse Reactions

Topically applied clotrimazole is well tolerated. Adverse reactions are minor and primarily involve local irritation, although abdominal cramps and increased urination have been reported. An elevated SGOT level has been observed in some patients. However, liver enzyme values return to normal after discontinuation of therapy. The hepatic changes may be the result of a stimulation of microsomal enzymes.

Preparations and Dosage

Clotrimazole (*Lotrimin, Gyne-Lotrimin, Mycelex*) is available as a 1% cream or solution and as 100- and 500-mg vaginal tablets. *Mycelex* is available as a lozenge containing 10 mg clotrimazole.

Terconazole

Antifungal Spectrum

Terconazole is active against *Candida albicans,* other *Candida* species, and dermatophytes.

Absorption, Metabolism, and Excretion

A small amount of the drug is absorbed systemically following topical vaginal therapy. The drug is rapidly metabolized in the liver and excreted in urine and feces. The half-life is 6 to 12 hr.

Clinical Use

The use of terconazole is limited to topical vaginal therapy in the treatment of candidiases.

Adverse Reactions

The adverse reactions are similar to those of other imidazoles. Transient headache, fever, chills, and hypotension have been reported in some patients.

Preparations and Dosage

Terconazole (*Terazol*) is available in a 0.4% vaginal cream and as 80-mg vaginal suppositories.

Miconazole

Antifungal Spectrum

Miconazole, like clotrimazole, has broad-spectrum activity against fungi. In vitro, it is inhibitory to *Candida* species, *T. glabrata, C. neoformans, C. immitis,* and *Pseu-*

doallescheria boydii. Some species of *Aspergillus* also are susceptible.

Absorption, Metabolism, and Excretion

Miconazole can be given either topically, intravenously, or intrathecally. Only small amounts are absorbed through the skin or from vaginal mucous membranes. Peak blood levels of 7.5 µg/ml can be obtained after IV administration of 600 to 1,000 mg. Initially, the drug has a half-life of 20 to 30 min, but after continued drug administration the half-life is increased to about 24 hr. The drug is rapidly metabolized in the liver. About 15 percent of the drug is excreted, mostly as inactive metabolites. Excretion is primarily by a nonrenal pathway. The half-life is only minimally affected by renal insufficiency. Greater than 90 percent of the injected miconazole is bound to serum protein.

The drug penetrates well into inflamed joints, the vitreous fluid of the eye, and the peritoneal cavity. Penetration into the saliva, sputum, and central nervous system (CNS) is poor.

Clinical Uses

Vulvovaginitis caused by *Candida albicans* responds rapidly and reliably to 2% miconazole cream. Other topical uses for miconazole are in the treatment of dermatophyte infections caused by *Epidermophyton, Trichosporum, Trichophyton* species, and *C. albicans.* The injectable preparation has been used, with varying degrees of success, to treat coccidioidomycosis, paracoccidioidomycosis, cryptococcosis, systemic candidiasis, and mucocutaneous candidiasis. For the treatment of relatively resistant infections, direct intrathecal or intravesicular (bladder) administration is occasionally indicated. However, the systemic indications for the use of miconazole have been largely superseded by the availability of other less toxic azoles such as ketoconazole and fluconazole.

Adverse Reactions

The most commonly observed side effect after intravenous use is thrombophlebitis. This effect can be prevented by administering the drug through central venous catheters. Nausea may develop in some patients, but in most cases it will disappear within a few hours after therapy. Anaphylaxis and cardiotoxicity are rare adverse reactions.

Side effects after topical use are few and uncommon. Burning and skin maceration can occur following cutaneous use. Itching, burning, urticaria, headache, and cramps have been associated with the use of the vaginal preparation.

Preparations and Dosage

Miconazole nitrate (*Micatin, Monistat, Monistat-Derm*) is available as a 2% cream or lotion for either topical or vaginal use and as vaginal suppositories (100 and 200 mg).

Miconazole (*Monistat I.V.*) is available for IV use as a sterile solution containing 10 mg/ml miconazole.

Ketoconazole

Antifungal Spectrum

Ketoconazole is effective against a variety of fungi and yeasts, including *B. dermatitidis, Candida, C. immitis, H. capsulatum,* and dermatophytes.

Absorption, Distribution, and Excretion

Ketoconazole, unlike other imidazoles, is readily absorbed after oral administration. It is insoluble at neutral pH but in the acid pH of the stomach, it readily enters the vascular system. However, absorption is variable, with peak plasma levels of approximately 3.5 µg/ml achieved 1 to 2 hr after administration of 200 mg. The initial half-life in plasma is 2 hr. After 8 to 10 hr, the half-life increases to about 9 hr. Food does not interfere with absorption. The drug is metabolized in the liver and inactive metabolites are excreted in bile with a small amount in urine. Greater than 90 percent is bound to serum protein.

Clinical Uses

Ketoconazole is a broad-spectrum antifungal effective for a variety of dermatophyte, mucosal, and systemic fungal infections. It has been helpful in treating ringworm, although its expense suggests that it should be limited to those cases unresponsive to griseofulvin. In the treatment of mucocutaneous candidiasis, ketoconazole has proved to be highly effective, although treatment must be prolonged. Mucosal candidiases of the mouth, esophagus, and vagina also respond well to ketoconazole, although there is little evidence to suggest that oral thrush responds better to ketoconazole than to nystatin when this occurs in the granulocytopenic patient.

A broad range of systemic fungal diseases also have been treated with ketoconazole with encouraging results. This applies particularly to paracoccidioidomycosis, although coccidioidomycosis responds less well. Both blastomycosis and histoplasmosis also have been treated with ketoconazole with varying responses. Histoplasmosis involving the lungs and other body tissues has responded to ketoconazole, although treatment must be prolonged for many months. Blastomycosis responded much less favorably. In both these conditions, amphotericin B remains the agent of choice.

Other fungal diseases that have been treated with ketoconazole include cryptococcosis and systemic candidiasis; the results of treatment of the latter infection, however, have been variable. Amphotericin B remains the drug of choice although fluconazole is often effective in the nonimmunocompromised patient.

The antiandrogenic activity of ketoconazole has led to its use in the management of prostatic carcinoma on an investigational basis.

Adverse Reactions

The commonest adverse reactions are gastrointestinal intolerance with nausea and vomiting; these symptoms may be improved by coadministration with food. Hepatotoxicity is not uncommon but is generally asymptomatic with reversible elevation of serum transaminases. However, in approximately 1 in 10,000 courses, progressive hepatotoxicity has been reported and has occasionally proved to be fatal. Another adverse reaction related to the depressive effect that ketoconazole has on serum testosterone is gynecomastia. This effect is dose related and has been utilized in the management of prostatic cancer.

Preparations and Dosage

Ketoconazole (*Nizoral*) is available as a 2% cream, 200-mg tablets, and as an oral suspension containing 100 mg/5ml.

Econazole

Econazole is an imidazole that is used topically for the treatment of superficial fungal infections of skin. The drug binds to skin with high levels in the stratum corneum. Very small amounts are absorbed following topical application. Econazole is equivalent to clotrimazole and miconazole in safety and effectiveness.

Econazole nitrate (*Spectazole*) is available as a cream.

Tioconazole

Tioconazole is an imidazole that is used in the treatment of dermatophyte infection and candidiasis. It is a nonprescription drug.

Triazoles

Though *itraconazole* and *fluconazole* are both triazoles, they are chemically and pharmacologically quite different. Itraconazole is water insoluble and lipophilic, and requires a low pH to be ionized; it is highly protein bound and excreted in bile. Fluconazole is a water-soluble fluorine–substituted bis-triazole that does not require a low gastric pH for absorption; it is poorly bound to serum proteins and is eliminated by renal excretion. An important feature of fluconazole is that it reaches high concentrations in the normal and inflamed CNS.

Fluconazole

Antifungal Spectrum

Fluconazole has broad-spectrum activity and in animal models is active in the treatment of aspergillosis, blastomycosis, candidiasis, cyptococcosis, and histoplasmosis. It is given either orally or intravenously. After oral administration, fluconazole is rapidly absorbed (90% of administered dose) and high concentrations of the drug appear in plasma. The half-life in adults ranges between 27 and 37 hr. Binding to plasma proteins is low (11%) and the drug distributes widely in tissue. It penetrates inflamed and normal meninges, and reaches concentrations in the CSF that are 60 to 80 percent those of serum levels. Fluconazole is excreted largely through the kidney with approximately 80 percent unchanged.

Fluconazole is effective in the treatment of dermatomycoses and oropharyngeal, esophageal, and vaginal candidiasis; it also has been used successfully in systemic candidal infections and is proving valuable in the treatment and prophylaxis of cryptococcosis in patients with AIDS, in whom relapse is common and long-term prophylaxis with amphotericin B is impractical. It is well tolerated, with nausea, gastrointestinal upset, and asymptomatic elevation of hepatic enzymes occurring in fewer than 5 percent of the patients.

Fluconazole (*Diflucan*) is available for oral and intravenous use.

Itraconazole

Itraconazole has an antifungal spectrum similar to that of ketoconazole except that it is also active against *Aspergillus* species and *S. schenckii*. Itraconazole, like ketoconazole, requires a low gastric pH to be absorbed. Absorption, however, is variable, with peak plasma concentrations of 0.02 to 0.18 mg/liter obtained following a 100-mg dose. Food enhances absorption. In lipophilic tissues, the concentration of drug is 2 to 20 times higher than plasma concentrations. The plasma half-life following a single dose is 15 to 20 hr. After multiple doses the half-life extends to 30 to 35 hr. Greater than 99 percent of the drug is protein bound. It is metabolized by the liver; excretion is biliary. Hydroxyitraconazole, a metabolite, retains antifungal activity.

Itraconazole is effective in a broad range of dermatomycoses, pityriasis, and oral and vaginal candidiasis. It is also effective against a variety of systemic mycoses, including blastomycosis, histoplasmosis, coccidioidomycosis, and paracoccidioidomycosis. Experience in treating systemic candidiasis and *Aspergillus* infections, although encouraging, is unlikely to make this the agent of choice.

Generally, itraconazole is well tolerated. Gastrointestinal disturbances, headache, and dizziness have been noted.

Itraconazole (*Sporanox*) is available as 100-mg capsules.

Naftifine Hydrochloride

Naftifine hydrochloride (Fig. 59-6) is the first of a new class of antifungal agents. It is a synthetic allylamine that inhibits squalene epoxidase and decreases ergosterol syn-

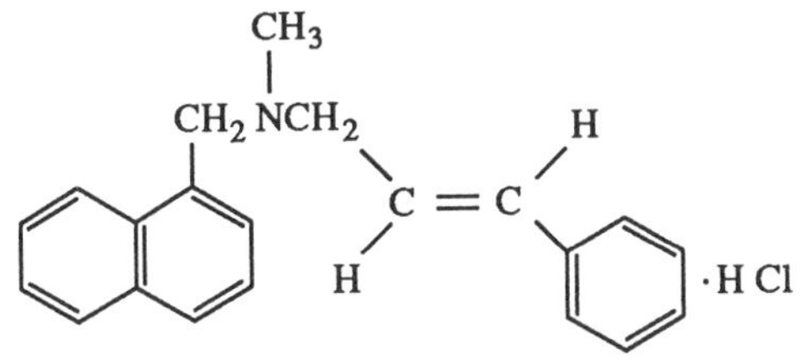

Figure 59-6. Naftifine hydrochloride.

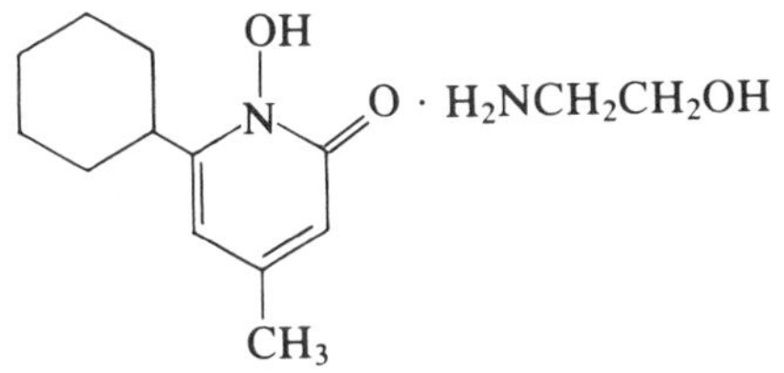

Figure 59-7. Ciclopirox olamine.

thesis. It has broad-spectrum fungicidal activity against dermatophytes and yeasts. Despite this broad-spectrum activity, it is approved only for topical use in treating dermatophyte infections. Its adverse effects are minimal, although an allergic dermatitis has occurred. Naftifine hydrochloride (*Naftin*) is available as a 1% cream.

Terbinafine is also an allylamine. It is the most active agent of this group. It is given orally, and distributes in skin, sebum, and nails. Its half-life is approximately 22 hr. It is fungicidal and effective in treating dermatophyte infections.

Ciclopirox Olamine

Ciclopirox olamine (Fig. 59-7) is a broad-spectrum fungicide with activity against dermatophytes. It inhibits growth, probably by interfering with the uptake of precursors needed for the synthesis of macromolecules, possibly through an effect on the fungal membrane. It is used topically for the treatment of dermal infections. Only small amounts (1%) are absorbed into the bloodstream. Levels in the dermis approach 10 to 15 times the minimum inhibitory concentration (MIC) for dermatophytes. Adverse reactions are few but may include pruritus and burning.

Ciclopirox olamine (*Loprox*) is available as a 1% cream for topical use.

Potassium Iodide

Potassium iodide (KI) is an inorganic, water-soluble salt. Its mode of action is unknown, but it may involve an iodination of proteins in the fungal cell wall and membrane. It is readily absorbed from the intestinal tract. It is given orally and is primarily distributed in extracellular fluids. Excretion is by the kidneys.

Potassium iodide is used only for the treatment of cutaneous forms of infections caused by *S. schenckii*. The dosage is slowly increased daily while the patient is mon-

itored for signs of toxicity. Extracutaneous sporotrichosis is treated with amphotericin B.

Iodides are well tolerated; however, iodism or chronic iodine toxicity is often encountered. The first symptoms are usually a metallic or unpleasant taste and coryza. Acneiform lesions may occur on skin areas prone to heavy sweating. Nausea, heartburn, diarrhea, and swelling of the parotid gland also may occur.

Potassium iodide is available as a saturated solution (1 mg/ml) for the oral treatment of cutaneous lymphatic sporotrichosis.

Tolnaftate

Tolnaftate (*Tinactin*) (Fig. 59-8) is a water-insoluble synthetic topical drug that has proved to be successful in treating a number of dermatophyte infections, including tinea versicolor, when applied twice a day for 7 to 21 days. It is not effective in treating fungal infections of the nails, or tinea capitis caused by *Microsporum audouini* or *Trichophyton tonsurans*. Cure rates for susceptible dermatophyte infections are comparable to those achieved by griseofulvin. Its mechanism of action is unknown. It is available for topical application as a cream, solution, and powder.

Whitfield's Ointment and Undecylenic Acid

Two traditional medications used in the treatment of tinea pedis are Whitfield's ointment and undecylenic acid

Figure 59-8. Tolnaftate.

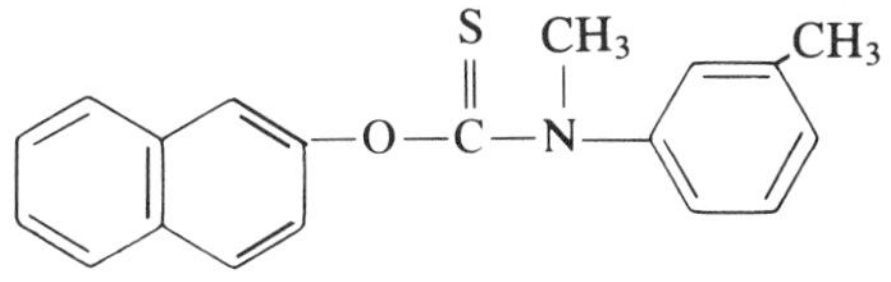

(*Desenex*). They are both fungistatic and require several weeks of application.

Whitfield's ointment contains benzoic acid, which is fungistatic, and salicylic acid, which acts as a keratolytic agent, in a ratio of 2:1. Undecylenic acid or its salt, zinc undecylenate, is available in a variety of concentrations for use both on the skin and mucous membranes. Relapse is common with both of these preparations, and hence their use is declining.

Supplemental Reading

Borgers, M. Mechanism of action of antifungal drugs, with special reference to the imidazole derivative. *Rev. Infect. Dis.* 2:520, 1980.

Daneshmend, T.K., and Warnock, D.W. Clinical pharmacokinetics of systemic antifungal drugs. *Clin. Pharmacokinet.* 8:17, 1983.

Fromtling, R.A. Overview of medically important antifungal azole derivatives. *Clin. Microbiol. Rev.* 1:187, 1988.

Gallis, H.A., Drew, R.H., and Packard, W.W. Amphotericin B: 30 years of clinical experience. *Rev. Infect. Dis.* 12:308, 1990.

Hay, R.J., Dupont, B., and Graybill, J.R. First International Symposium on Itraconazole. *Rev. Infect. Dis.* 9(Suppl. 1): 1987.

Kerridge, D. Mode of action of clinically important antifungal drugs. *Adv. Microb. Physiol.* 27:1, 1986.

Lyman, C.A., and Walsh, T.J. Systemically administered antifungal agents. A review of their clinical pharmacology and therapeutic applications. *Drugs* 44:9, 1992.

Saag, M.S., and Dismukes, W.E. Azole antifungal agents: Emphasis on new triazoles. *Antimicrob. Agents Chemother.* 32:1, 1988.

Walsh, T.J., and Pizzo, A. Treatment of systemic fungal infections: Recent progress and current problems. *Eur. J. Clin. Microb. Infect. Dis.* 7:460, 1988.

Antiseptics, Disinfectants, and Sterilization

Irvin S. Snyder and *Roger G. Finch*

General Principles

The proper use of antiseptics and disinfectants has received increasing attention in recent years. One reason is the recognition of the importance of *nosocomial,* or hospital-acquired, infections and the need to minimize the transfer of microorganisms to susceptible patients. Those individuals whose defense mechanisms have been compromised by preexisting disease or whose clinical management has resulted in suppression of normal immunity are particularly at risk. A second reason for understanding the use of antiseptics and disinfectants comes from the realization that some of the agents previously considered safe may produce toxic effects with prolonged use (e.g., hexachlorophene).

The most effective methods for reducing the number of microbes and for sterilization are heat and irradiation. However, since high temperatures, such as those obtained in an autoclave with pressurized steam (121°C), cannot be used for heat-labile materials, one must use other chemical or physical methods. Irradiation is an effective alternative to heat. Although ultraviolet radiation can be used to sterilize heat-labile materials, unfortunately it does not penetrate glass or liquids very well, and one has to monitor the light carefully to be sure that the appropriate wavelength and intensity are emitted. The use of ultraviolet light to reduce the bacterial load in air is being reemphasized because of the increase of tuberculosis among certain populations and the high risk of transmission in health care facilities and shelters for the homeless. Other types of radiation, such as β and γ emitters, are now used for sterilization of heat-sensitive plastics and other materials.

Removal of bacteria from heat-labile liquids is often done by passing the liquid through filters with pore sizes that screen out bacteria and fungi. Filtration of air through specially constructed filters, termed *high-efficiency particulate air (HEPA) filters,* is used to reduce the load of microorganisms in clean rooms and under hoods where sterile solutions are prepared. HEPA filters are often used to reduce the bacterial loads in selected areas in health care facilities.

Chemical agents, generally classified as antiseptics or disinfectants, are used to reduce the microbial content of surfaces, either living or inanimate. There are several modes of action by which chemical agents function. They may alter proteins by oxidation, alkylation, dehydration, or reaction with sulfhydryl groups; also, they may affect cell permeability through an interaction with bacterial membranes (Table 60-1).

Antiseptic is the term that is generally applied to chemical agents that are used on body surfaces to kill or inhibit growth of microorganisms and prevent infection (sepsis), whereas *disinfectant* refers to those materials that are employed, usually on inanimate objects, to kill pathogenic organisms. Disinfectants that are used to reduce microbial numbers to levels that are considered safe by public health standards are referred to as *sanitizers.* It must be emphasized that the use of an antiseptic or disinfectant does not imply that sterilization has been achieved.

From a practical standpoint, a chemical disinfectant or antiseptic must have several properties. It must be safe to use; that is, it must be selectively toxic. Since many chemical disinfectants and antiseptics are used repeatedly by physicians, nurses, and other medical personnel, the agents should not irritate tissues or cause hypersensitivity reactions with repeated use. These substances should be water soluble and have a low surface tension, so that they wet the surface, thereby allowing better contact with microorganisms. Compatibility with a detergent is desirable, because detergents improve surface wetting properties. Ideally, if the disinfectant is adsorbed, it will be maintained on the surface and provide a longer disinfecting action.

Some disinfectants and antiseptics are inactivated by the protein found in exudates and excreta. Therefore, the ideal agent is one that maintains activity or is minimally affected by the presence of organic materials. Staining of

Table 60-1. Characteristics of Selected Antiseptics and Disinfectants

Site of action	Mode of action	Chemical agents
Proteins	Alkylation	Ethylene oxide; glutaraldehyde; formaldehyde
	Dehydration	Alcohols
	Oxidation	Iodine; iodophors
	Bind to sulfhydryl groups	Silver- and mercury-containing compounds
Membranes	Affect permeability	Soaps, detergents (quaternary amines), chlorhexidine

materials and tissue is generally undesirable but may be of some value in skin antiseptics or disinfectants where one wants to define a "clean area."

Several factors must be considered in the use of chemical agents. First, the nature of the microorganisms to be treated is important. Bacterial spores, for example, are more resistant to killing than are vegetative bacteria. Various microorganisms, such as *Mycobacterium*, viruses, and fungi, will differ in their susceptibility to chemical agents. Thus, the ideal chemical agent would be one that displays activity against a wide spectrum of microorganisms, including bacterial spores. Table 60-2 compares the activities of some commonly used chemical disinfectants.

The time necessary to disinfect a surface will vary with the concentration of the organisms present, the relative susceptibility or resistance of the organism, and the concentration of the chemical employed. Since temperature affects the rate of biological and chemical reactions, the rate of reaction between the chemical agent and the microbe (and therefore the rate of killing) will be affected by ambient temperature. Local pH is important because it

may affect not only the degree of ionization of the chemical agent but also the biological process taking place in the microbial cell. It is obvious that a rapid effect that is lethal (cidal) rather than static is desirable.

The rate of germicidal action approaches first-order kinetics and is dependent on the concentration of drug, pH, and temperature. However, the kinetics can be more complex when the contributions of chemical diffusion, binding, and cellular penetration are considered. Also, many antiseptics and disinfectants contain more than one active component, and hence the total observed activity will be a reflection of the activity of all the components.

Organisms can become resistant to disinfectants and, in some cases, the disinfectant has become a source of infection for the susceptible person. For example, *Pseudomonas aeruginosa* can survive and grow in benzalkonium chloride as well as in iodophors; subsequent use of these contaminated disinfectants and antiseptics has been responsible for nosocomial infection.

The development and use of antiseptics, disinfectants, and sanitizers represent a complex problem that requires consideration of the chemical agents, the material to be treated, and the nature of the microorganism and its environment.

Evaluation of Disinfectants and Antiseptics

Chemical agents are rated by the *phenol coefficient test.* This is a standardized test in which the dilution of the chemical agent being evaluated that kills a standard number of bacteria in 10 min is compared to the dilution of phenol that accomplishes the same task. The coefficient is calculated as follows:

$$\text{Phenol coefficient} = \frac{\text{dilution of chemical agent}}{\text{dilution of phenol}}$$

Table 60-2. Microbial Spectrum of Selected Disinfectants and Antiseptics

Compound	Microbicidal activity				Virucidal	
	Gram-positive bacteria	Gram-negative bacteria	Bacterial spores	*Myobacterium tuberculosis*	Nonenveloped	Enveloped
Phenols	Good	Good	Poor	Fair	Poor	Good
Cationic detergents	Good	Fair	None	None	Poor	Good
Halogens						
Chlorine	Good	Good	Poor	Good	Good	Good
Iodine	Good	Good	Poor	Good	Good	Good
Alkaline glutaraldehyde	Good	Good	Good	Good	Good	Good
Chlorhexidine	Good	Fair	None	Poor	Uncertain	Uncertain
Alcohols (70–85%)	Good	Good	None	Good	Poor	Good
Ethylene oxide	Good	Good	Good	Good	Good	Good

If the coefficient is greater than 1, it is assumed that the substance is better than phenol in killing activity. The test has some faults in that the standard test organisms are *Salmonella typhi, P. aeruginosa,* and *Staphylococcus aureus,* and not the gram-negative bacteria that are usually associated with nosocomial infection. Also, good activity against standard test organisms may not reflect efficiency under conditions of everyday use. Consequently, many modifications of the standard phenol coefficient test have been developed.

Oxidizing Agents

Halogens

Only two of the halogens, *chlorine* and *iodine,* are used as disinfectants or antiseptics. The halogens are highly reactive elements and their mode of action, irrespective of the halogen employed or its formulation, is identical. They *oxidize sulfhydryl groups* to the S-S form and thereby affect protein structure and function. Formation of chloramines also may contribute to antimicrobial activity, but this is not the primary effect of the halogens.

Chlorine, chloramine-T, and *hypochlorite* generally are used to treat water and to surface-sanitize equipment; they are not used as antiseptics and are clinically useful for inactivating spillage of blood/secretions infected with hepatitis B or human immunodeficiency (HIV) viruses.

Iodine in ethanol (tincture) and the iodophors (iodine combined with a solubilizing agent or carrier) are bactericidal for a wide spectrum of microbes and also have sporicidal activity. Irrespective of the formulation, *the bactericidal activity is related to the free iodine generated.* The iodide ion and triiodide have little or no activity. Iodine is effective over a wide pH range. Iodophors have an advantage over iodine solutions in that they slowly liberate free iodine and thus have a longer-lasting antiseptic effect. They supposedly are less volatile and less irritating.

Iodophors, such as povidone-iodine preparations (*Betadine*), have achieved wide popularity as skin disinfectants, surgical scrubs, and disinfectants of some instruments. Repeated use for hand washing has a cumulative antimicrobial action because of the slow release of iodine. Skin sensitization is less frequent than with iodine solutions but still can be troublesome.

Iodine also is commonly used as a skin antiseptic and is safe if used in the concentrations that are commercially available. Hypersensitivity reactions are the most important adverse effect and can result in a wide variety of skin eruptions, varying from a mild eczematous reaction to an exfoliative dermatitis. Absorption of iodine can occur from denuded and mucosal surfaces, but this generally does not cause serious adverse effects. If swallowed, iodine is corrosive to the mucosa and produces reflex vomiting, abdominal pain, and diarrhea, which may result in fluid and electrolyte depletion.

Iodophors contaminated during preparation have been associated with nosocomial infections.

Hydrogen Peroxide

Hydrogen peroxide is an oxidizing agent that is highly unstable and, in the presence of tissue or blood catalase, rapidly breaks down to form water and oxygen. Hydrogen peroxide is bactericidal due to its ability to generate hydroxyl free radicals and their effect on membrane lipids and other cell components. The bubbling action of the released oxygen mechanically loosens infected material and particles and thereby contributes to the drug's cleansing action.

Acids

Benzoic acid, undecylenic acid, and other organic acids are often used to inhibit microbial growth. Their major use is as antifungal agents and as such are discussed in Chap. 59. Acetic acid is bactericidal to many organisms. It is particularly effective against *P. aeruginosa* and has been used in the treatment of infected burns and for the decontamination of ventilation equipment. Boric acid is a toxic compound that can cause acute poisoning if enough is absorbed from the gastrointestinal tract, serous cavities, and abraded or inflamed skin. Boric acid should be limited to use as an ophthalmic solution.

Dehydrating Agents

Alcohols

The agents most widely used as disinfectants or antiseptics are ethyl and isopropyl alcohol. Aliphatic alcohols are germicidal in proportion to their lipid solubility. The effects produced by alcohols are concentration dependent; alcohols are most effective when used at 70 to 90 percent concentration by weight. They cause a bactericidal effect through dehydration of protein, the subsequent change in the protein's secondary structure, and hence its function. Alcohols have little effect on spores.

Although the disinfecting effect of alcohol is modest, the mechanical removal of squamous cells effected by scrubbing is important in the disinfection of skin. In addition, the alcohols do not irritate tissues. Unfortunately, since ethanol does precipitate protein, it may coagulate the protein found in wounds and thus form a protective layer over the microorganisms.

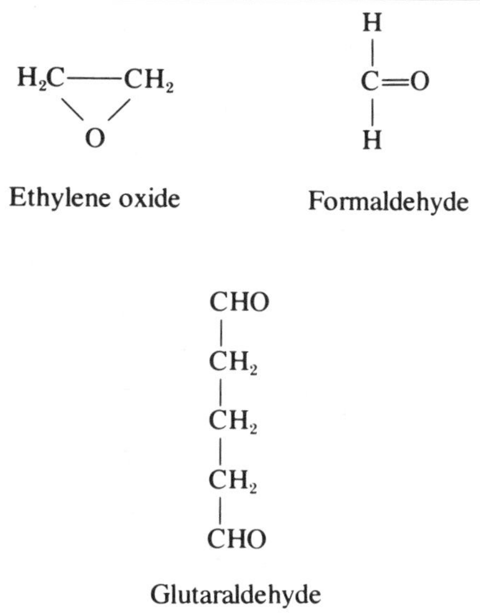

H₂C——CH₂ [Ethylene oxide structure]

Formaldehyde structure:
H
|
C=O
|
H

Ethylene oxide   **Formaldehyde**

Glutaraldehyde structure:
CHO
|
CH₂
|
CH₂
|
CH₂
|
CHO

Glutaraldehyde

Figure 60-1. Three alkylating agents.

Alkylating Agents

Several agents (Fig. 60-1) used for sterilization and disinfection are alkylating agents. Alkylating agents cause a replacement of the hydrogen atoms in amino, carboxyl, sulfhydryl, and hydroxyl groups with an alkyl group, thereby altering structure and function. Ethylene oxide, formaldehyde, and glutaraldehyde are alkylating agents that are used for sterilization of instruments and other materials, and are cidal for spores, bacteria, and viruses.

Ethylene oxide has its primary effect on nucleic acids, whereas formaldehyde affects both proteins and nucleic acids. Glutaraldehyde has its primary effect on proteins, principally with the amino acid lysine.

Ethylene Oxide

Ethylene oxide has good penetrating power. Disadvantages associated with ethylene oxide sterilization include the long time required for sterilization (4 hr) and the 10- to 12-hr period required for the dissipation of the gas from the sterilized materials. The gas is explosive at concentrations above 3 percent and must be used in an atmosphere of 30 to 40 percent humidity. Commercial equipment is available that can meet these conditions. The sterilization of instruments by this method must be followed by an adequate period of aeration. Trace amounts of ethylene oxide remaining on materials or instruments have caused burns, thrombophlebitis, and tracheitis. It is mutagenic,

carcinogenic, and irritating to eyes and mucous membranes. Inhalation of ethylene oxide gas in sufficient concentrations can produce nausea, vomiting, and neurological symptoms and can present a problem to personnel in sterilization units. The need for regular maintenance of sterilizing equipment cannot be emphasized too strongly.

Formaldehyde

Formaldehyde gas has an unpleasant odor. Because it leaves a film on surfaces and is corrosive, and because of its slow action, it is not widely used. It has high antimicrobial activity but poor penetrability and thus is useful only for surface sterilization.

Glutaraldehyde

Glutaraldehyde, as an alkaline solution and with the addition of a surfactant, has excellent antimicrobial activity. The activity of glutaraldehyde is due to its free aldehyde groups. It is bactericidal, virucidal, and sporicidal and has a short killing time. Glutaraldehyde is used to sterilize instruments, such as cystoscopes, hemostats, bronchoscopes, and respiratory equipment. It is also used for decontamination of dental instruments and surfaces contaminated with hepatitis B virus. It is much safer and more effective than formaldehyde, but is also irritating to skin and mucous membranes.

Sulfhydryl Combining Agents

Soluble salts of heavy metals, such as mercury and silver, combine with sulfhydryl, amino, and other groups and interfere with normal protein structure and function. The action of mercury salts is reversible if exogenous sulfhydryl groups are provided; their effect in tissue is primarily bacteriostatic. Silver salts precipitate protein and have a bactericidal effect.

Silver nitrate at a concentration of 1% (Credé's solution) is an example of a heavy metal that is used to control gonococcal ophthalmia. Silver nitrate placed in the eyes of newborns prevents infection with *Neisseria gonorrhoeae.* Silver nitrate was used in the past to prevent the infection of burns by *P. aeruginosa,* but because it can cause electrolyte disturbances, it largely has been replaced by mafenide (*Sulfamylon*) or silver sulfadiazine (see Chap. 48).

Several different formulations of mercury, for example, merbromin (*Mercurochrome*), thimerosal (*Merthiolate*), and nitromersol (*Metaphen*), have been used widely as antiseptics and skin disinfectants, but their use is diminishing with the availability of better agents. Furthermore, they are only bacteriostatic. Contaminated preparations have been responsible for nosocomial infections.

Zinc, as either a sulfate or an oxide, also is used as a topical antiseptic. Its effect is weak and is related primarily to its astringent property, that is, its ability to precipitate protein.

Agents Affecting Permeability

Anionic Detergents

Anionic detergents (soap) are, at best, weakly bactericidal. They are good emulsifiers of fats and oils and their major value is in the mechanical removal of microorganisms and dead epithelial cells. The anionic detergents are most active at an *acid* pH; they are relatively ineffective against gram-negative bacteria because of the lipopolysaccharide in the outer membrane of those organisms. Anionic agents can chemically neutralize cationic detergents and therefore these two should not be used together.

Cationic Detergents

The cationic detergents are used widely and are effective disinfectants and antiseptics. These detergents possess many of the properties of ideal disinfectants and antiseptics. For example, they exert a rapid effect and are nontoxic. They wet surfaces, penetrate skin, and have emulsifying, keratolytic, and detergent properties. They cause relatively little toxicity, although poisoning can occur if they are swallowed. Irritation of the skin and allergic reactions are rare.

The most important and effective of the cationic detergents are the quaternary ammonium compounds such as benzalkonium chloride (*Zephiran Chloride*), cetylpyridinium chloride (*Ceepryn*), and benzethonium chloride (*Phemerol Chloride*). This class of compounds has four carbon atoms linked to nitrogen through covalent bonds. The anion, usually chloride or bromide, is linked to the nitrogen atom by an electrovalent bond (Fig. 60-2); R_1, R_2, R_3, and R_4 are alkyl groups. Because of their net posi-

tive charge, the quaternary ammonium compounds react with the negatively charged phosphate groups on membrane phospholipids. Penetration of the hydrophobic interior of the cell membrane by the nonpolar portion of the quaternary ammonium molecule results in an increased cellular permeability.

Cationic detergents are most effective at an *alkaline* pH and act on a wide range of bacteria. They are more effective against gram-positive cells and do not affect spores. Some gram-negative organisms can survive and even multiply in benzalkonium chloride. The quaternary ammonium compounds are inactivated by soaps and other anionic detergents.

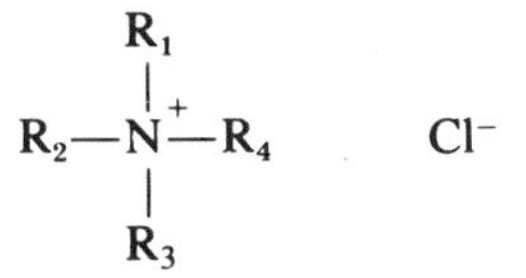

Nonionic Detergents

Nonoxynol-9, a nonionic detergent used as a spermicide, has been reported to be active against a wide variety of organisms. It is incorporated also into antimicrobial hand soap preparations.

Phenols

Phenol and a number of substituted phenols are commonly used as disinfectants. Although they have several effects on the microbial cell, their primary site of action is probably on the cell membrane. They also can lower surface tension and denature proteins. The activity of phenolic compounds is related to the free hydroxyl group. Unlike many disinfectants, the phenols are not significantly neutralized by organic material.

Phenol denatures protein and readily penetrates skin and mucosa; concentrated solutions will cause extensive tissue necrosis. If absorbed systemically, phenol has a marked antipyretic action and can produce depression of the central nervous system (CNS) as well as vasomotor collapse. The *cresols* (alkyl-substituted phenols) are used for the disinfection of exudates and equipment. The cresols are less toxic and more effective than phenols.

Figure 60-3. Hexachlorophene.

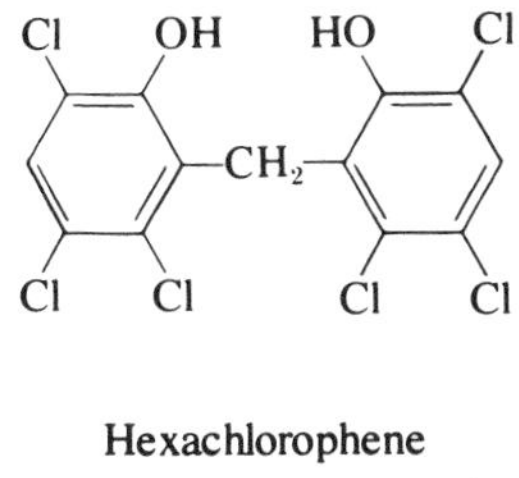

Hexachlorophene

Figure 60-2. Basic chemical structure of quaternary ammonium compounds.

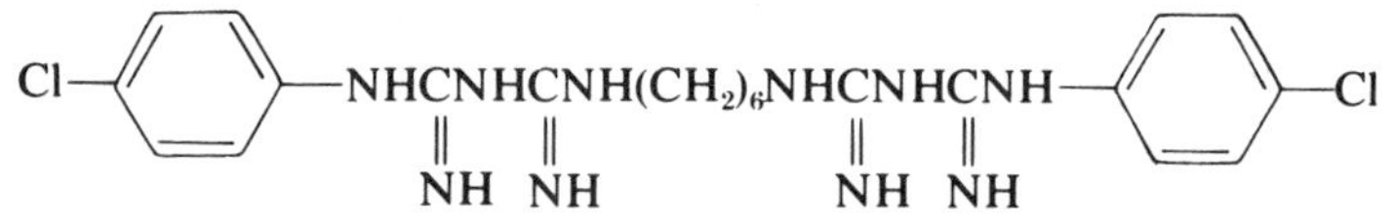

Cl—⬡—NHCNHCNH(CH₂)₆NHCNHCNH—⬡—Cl
        ‖ ‖   ‖ ‖
        NH NH   NH NH

Figure 60-4. Chlorhexidine.

Bisphenols contain two phenolic groups. The bisphenol most widely used to disinfect skin is *hexachlorophene* (Fig. 60-3). Organic matter prevents the rapid action of the bisphenols, but does not affect activity under conditions of long-term contact.

Hexachlorophene (*pHisoHex*) is less irritating to tissue than is phenol. Its action is primarily on gram-positive organisms and it is used to reduce the flora on the skin. Hexachlorophene has a range of toxic effects similar to those of phenol, although the degree of toxicity produced is much less. If swallowed, the agent causes nausea, vomiting, abdominal cramps, and CNS depression. Systemic toxicity and death have followed repeated application of hexachlorophene to the skin. This reaction has occurred most notably in newborn infants, particularly if premature, and where ulceration of the skin exists; this last condition promotes systemic absorption. Lethargy, twitching, respiratory depression, and convulsions may be produced and postmortem studies have shown a spongy degeneration of the brain. For these reasons, hexachlorophene is *no longer used routinely in nurseries* to prevent skin sepsis in newborns.

Chlorhexidine

Chlorhexidine gluconate (*Hibiclens*) (Fig. 60-4) is a cationic biguanide and has its primary effect on the bacterial cell membrane. At low concentrations, it causes cellular constituents to leak from the cell. At high concentrations, chlorhexidine results in a precipitation of cell membrane and cytoplasmic constituents. Concentrations of 10 μg/ml inhibit gram-positive organisms. Gram-negative organisms require up to 50 μg/ml for inhibition. The recommended concentration for use as a bactericidal agent is 200 μg/ml.

Chlorhexidine is precipitated by inorganic anions, such as those found in hard water. It is not significantly neutralized by soaps, body fluids, or other organic compounds and is active over a wide pH range (5–8). It is widely used, frequently as a surgical scrub and for hand washing, and has a prolonged bactericidal action that is cumulative with repeated use. It is well tolerated and rarely causes skin reactions such as dermatitis or photosensitivity.

Incorporation of chlorhexidine into an instant release matrix on the inner surface of latex gloves has been reported effective in killing bacterial and viral pathogens. This would be important given the concern about pathogens entering through puncture holes and through stressed surfaces. The levels of chlorhexidine gluconate released have not caused dermal irritation or sensitization.

Supplemental Reading

Block, S.S. *Disinfection, Sterilization and Preservation* (4th ed.) Philadelphia: Lea & Febiger, 1991.

Dineen, P. Hand-washing degerming: A comparison of povidone-iodine and chlorhexidine. *Clin. Pharmacol. Ther.* 23:63, 1978.

Kensit, J.G. Hexachlorophene: Toxicity and effectiveness in prevention of sepsis in neonatal units. *J. Antimicrob. Chemother.* 1:263, 1975.

Miner, N.A., et al. Antimicrobial and other properties of a new stabilized alkaline glutaraldehyde disinfectant/sterilizer. *Am. J. Hosp. Pharm.* 34:376, 1977.

Modak, S., et al. Rapid inactivation of infectious pathogens by chlorhexidine-coated gloves. *Infect. Control Hosp. Epidemiol.* 13:463, 1992.

Peterson, A.F., Rosenberg, A., and Alatary, S.D. Comparative evaluation of surgical scrub preparations. *Surg. Gynecol. Obstet.* 146:63, 1978.

61

The Rational Basis for Cancer Chemotherapy

Branimir I. Sikic

Modern cancer chemotherapy originated in the 1940s with the demonstration that nitrogen mustard possessed antitumor activity against human lymphomas and leukemias. During the next 40 years, steady progress has been made in the treatment of cancer with drugs. Some milestones in cancer chemotherapy are listed in Table 61-1. Presently, 10 types of human cancer are curable in the majority of cases with chemotherapy alone or chemotherapy plus surgery or radiation. Cure is defined for this purpose as the disappearance of any evidence of tumor for several years and a high actuarial probability of a normal life span.

Human cancers in which chemotherapy alone, or chemotherapy combined with other treatment modalities, has resulted in apparent cure in 40 to 80 percent of patients are listed in Table 61-2. Patients with other types of unresectable cancer also may benefit from chemotherapy, as evidenced by prolongation of life, shrinkage of tumor, and improvement in symptoms. Notable among these are ovarian epithelial and breast carcinomas, oat cell (small-cell undifferentiated) carcinoma of the lung, and acute myelocytic leukemia. Cancers that are, for the most part, resistant to currently used agents include melanoma, colorectal and renal carcinomas, and non–oat cell cancers of the lung.

Concepts in Tumor Cell Biology

The Normal Cell Cycle

The *normal cell cycle* consists of a definable sequence of events that characterize the growth and division of cells and can be observed by morphological and biochemical means. A schematic representation of the cell cycle is presented in Fig. 61-1. Two of the four phases of the cell cycle can be studied directly: the *M-phase,* or mitosis, is easily visible using light microscopy because of the processes of chromosomal condensation, spindle formation, and cell division taking place. The *S-phase* is the period of DNA synthesis and is observed by measuring the incorporation of tritiated thymidine into cell nuclei.

The *mitotic index* is the fraction or percentage of cells in mitosis within a given cell population. The *thymidine labeling index* is the fraction of cells incorporating radioactive thymidine. They represent cells in M-phase and S-phase and serve to define the proliferative characteristics of normal and tumor cells.

The Tumor Cell Cycle

The duration of the S-phase in human tumors is 10 to 20 hr. This period is followed by the G_2-*phase,* or period of preparation for mitosis, in which cells contain a tetraploid number of chromosomes. The G_2-phase lasts only 1 to 3 hr for most cell types, with mitosis itself lasting approximately 1 hr. The two daughter cells then enter the G_1-*phase,* whose duration varies from several hours to days. The G_1-phase also can give rise to a resting state, termed G_0, in which cells are relatively inactive metabolically and are resistant to most chemotherapeutic drugs.

The *generation time,* or T_c, is the time required to complete one cycle of cell growth and division. The T_c will vary depending on the duration of the G_1-phase. The factors that influence daughter cells to enter the G_0, or resting stage, are not well understood. The ability to cause such resting cells to reenter the cell cycle would be potentially quite useful, since proliferating cells generally are more sensitive to chemotherapy.

Table 61-1. Milestones in Cancer Chemotherapy

1946	Nitrogen mustard reported as first effective anti-cancer drug and alkylating agent
1948	Aminopterin (and later methotrexate) as first major antimetabolite
1950s	Analogues of alkylating agents and antimetabolites synthesized; cure of gestational choriocarcinoma with methotrexate or dactinomycin
1964	MOPP (mechlorethamine, vincristine, procarbazine, prednisone) for Hodgkin's disease
1975	CMF (cyclophosphamide, methotrexate, 5-fluorouracil) adjuvant chemotherapy for breast cancer
1977	PVB (cisplatin, vinblastine, bleomycin) chemotherapy for testicular carcinomas
1982	Monoclonal antibody-induced remission in B-cell lymphoma
1986	Multidrug resistance (MDR) gene cloned and proved to cause MDR
1991	Bone marrow colony stimulating factors introduced

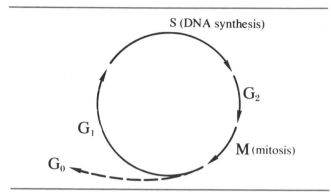

Figure 61-1. The cell cycle. S, G_1, G_2, and G_0 represent phases of the cell cycle (see text).

Table 61-2. Cancers with 40 to 80 Percent Cure Rates

Age	Type of cancer
Childhood	Acute lymphocytic leukemia
	Burkitt's sarcoma
	Ewing's sarcoma
	Retinoblastoma
	Rhabdomyosarcoma
	Wilms' tumor
Adult	Hodgkin's disease
	Non-Hodgkin's disease
	Trophoblastic choriocarcinoma
	Testicular and ovarian germ cell cancers

Drugs and the Cell Cycle

Various classification schemes have been proposed to describe the effects of drugs on the cell cycle. One such classification divides the anticancer drugs into three categories:

1. *Class 1 agents* (e.g., radiation, mechlorethamine, and carmustine) exert their cytotoxicity in a *nonspecific* (i.e., nonproliferation-dependent) manner. They kill both normal and malignant cells to the same extent.

2. *Class 2 agents* are phase-specific and reach a plateau in cell kill with increasing dosages. Only a certain *proportion* of cells are sensitive to the toxic effects of these drugs. For example, hydroxyurea and cytarabine are drugs that kill only cells that are in the S-phase. Similarly, bleomycin is most toxic to cells in G_2- and early M-phase. Because they affect only a small fraction of the cell population at any one time, it has been suggested that these

drugs should be given either by continuous infusion or in frequent small doses. Such a dosage regimen would increase the number of tumor cells exposed to the drug during the sensitive phase of their cell cycle.

3. *Class 3 agents* kill *proliferating* cells in preference to resting cells. It has been recommended that these proliferation-dependent, but non-phase-specific, agents be administered in single large doses to take advantage of their sparing effect on those normal cells that may be in G_0. Unfortunately, many human cancers have a large proportion of cells in the resting phase, and these cells are also resistant to the class 3 agents. These agents include cyclophosphamide, dactinomycin, and fluorouracil.

There are limitations inherent in this classification of anticancer drugs, however. For instance, it may be difficult to generalize about the phase specificity of a particular drug, since this may vary among different cell types. Several techniques are available that can synchronize cell populations in such a way that the great majority of cells will be in the same phase of the cell cycle. After synchronization, one can treat cells in each phase and determine their relative sensitivity to drugs throughout the cell cycle.

Although some drugs may exert their maximum cytotoxicity during the S-phase of the cycle, they also may prevent cells from progressing through the cell cycle to the S-phase; this is accomplished by a sublethal inhibition of RNA and protein synthesis. The antimetabolites methotrexate, fluorouracil, and mercaptopurine all can inhibit RNA synthesis in G_1- and G_2-phases as well as inhibit DNA synthesis during S-phase. This inhibition of cell cycle progression actually may result in reduced cytotoxicity, and such agents have been termed *S-phase-specific, but self-limited*.

Tumor Growth and Growth Fraction

The rate of growth of human and experimental cancers is initially quite rapid (exponential) and then slows until a plateau is reached. The decrease in growth rate with increasing tumor size is related both to a decrease in the proportion of cancer cells actively proliferating (termed the *growth fraction*) and to an increase in the rate of cell loss due to hypoxic necrosis, poor nutrient supply, immunological defense mechanisms, and other processes.

The rate of spontaneous cell death for some human tumors is thought to be a significant factor in limiting growth. However, the growth fraction, or percentage of cells in the cell cycle, is the most important determinant of overall tumor enlargement. The "doubling times" of human tumors have been estimated, by direct measurement of chest x-ray lesions or palpable masses, to be from 1 to 6 months.

The *growth fraction* represents dividing cells that are potentially sensitive to chemotherapy; thus, it is not surprising that tumors with high growth fractions are the ones most easily curable by drugs. Among human tumors, only Burkitt's lymphoma and trophoblastic choriocarcinoma are readily curable by single-agent chemotherapy; both these tumors have growth fractions close to 100 percent. As tumors grow larger, the growth fraction within the tumor decreases, and the greater the distance of cells from nutrient blood vessels, the more likely they are to be in the G_0-, or resting, phase. The growth fraction is less than 10 percent for slow-growing cancers of the colon or lung.

A number of factors must be considered before chemotherapy is instituted for a human cancer that has a low growth fraction. For instance, the larger the tumor, the more cells will be present in the nonproliferating, relatively resistant state. Therefore, the earlier chemotherapy is instituted, the greater the chance of a favorable response. A "debulking" of tumors by surgery or radiation therapy may be a means of stimulating the remaining cells into active proliferation. Small metastases may respond to drugs more dramatically than will large primary tumors or a larger metastasis in the same patient.

Several cycles of treatment may be necessary to achieve substantial reduction in tumor size. The chemotherapeutic regimen, especially when one is dealing with large solid tumors, probably should include agents that have cytotoxic activity against resting cells.

The Log-Cell Kill Hypothesis

Cytotoxic drugs act by *first-order kinetics,* that is, at a given dose, they kill a *constant fraction* of the tumor cells rather than a fixed number of cells. For example, a drug dose that would result in a three–log-cell kill (i.e., 99.9%)

cytotoxicity) would reduce the tumor burden of an animal that has 10^8 leukemic cells to 10^5 cells. This killing of a fraction of cells rather than an absolute number per dose is called the *log-cell kill hypothesis.*

The earliest detectable human cancers usually have a volume of at least 1 cc and contain 10^9 (1 billion) cells. This number reflects the result of at least 30 cycles of cell division, or cell doublings, and represents a kinetically advanced stage in the tumor's growth. Most patients actually have tumor burdens that are greater than 10^9. Since the major limiting factor in patient chemotherapy is cytotoxicity to normal tissues, only a limited log-cell kill can be expected with each individual treatment.

Even in the absence of tumor regrowth, several cycles of therapy would be required for eradication of the tumor, assuming it was sensitive to the drugs employed. When a tumor has decreased in size to around 10^8 cells, it is generally no longer detectable clinically and would be considered a "clinically complete remission." Regrowth of residual cells is the obvious cause of relapse in patients who have achieved clinically complete remissions.

Drug Resistance

Many patients undergoing chemotherapy fail to respond to treatment from the outset; their cancers are resistant to the currently available agents. Other patients may respond initially, only to relapse.

Cancers can be regarded as populations of cells undergoing spontaneous mutations. The population becomes increasingly heterogeneous as the tumor grows and increasing numbers of mutations occur. Tumors of the same type and size will vary in their responsiveness to therapy because of the chance occurrences of drug-resistant mutations during tumor growth.

Assuming the same initial drug sensitivity, smaller tumors are generally more curable than larger tumors because of the increased probability of drug-resistant mutations in the larger tumors. Therefore, therapy *earlier* in the course of tumor growth should increase the chance for cure. *Combination chemotherapy* (e.g., Table 61-3) is often more effective than treatment with single drugs. Those tumors that are resistant to drugs from the outset will always have a largely drug-resistant population and will be refractory to treatment.

Many different kinds of biochemical resistance to anticancer drugs have been described. The biochemical and genetic mechanisms of resistance to *methotrexate* are now known in some detail. Three major resistance pathways have been described: (1) decreased drug transport into cells; (2) an alteration in the structure of the target enzyme, dihydrofolate reductase (DHFR), resulting in reduced drug affinity; and (3) an increase in DHFR content of tumor cells. The increase in DHFR content has been

Table 61-3. The MOPP Regimen for Hodgkin's Disease

Drug	Dosage/sq m body surface	Schedule	Rest period
Mechlorethamine	6 mg, IV	Days 1 and 8	Days 15–28
Oncovin (vincristine sulfate)	1.4 mg, IV	Days 1 and 8	Days 15–28
Procarbazine	100 mg, po	Daily, days 1–14	Days 15–28
Prednisone	40 mg, po	Daily, days 1–14*	Days 15–28

*Only on cycles 1 and 4 out of six total cycles, repeated every 28 days.

shown to occur through a process of *gene amplification,* that is, a reduplication or increase in the number of copies per cell of the gene coding for DHFR. Amplification of various genes may be a relatively frequent event in tumor cell populations and an important genetic mechanism for generating resistance to drugs.

Tumor cells may become generally resistant to a variety of cytotoxic drugs on the basis of decreased uptake or retention of the drugs. This form of resistance is termed *pleiotropic, or multidrug, resistance,* and it is the major form of resistance to anthracyclines, vinca alkaloids, etoposide, paclitaxel, and dactinomycin. The gene that confers multidrug resistance (termed *mdr I*) has been cloned. It encodes a high-molecular-weight membrane protein called *P-glycoprotein,* which acts as a drug efflux pump in many tumors and normal tissues.

Possible biochemical mechanisms of resistance to *alkylating agents* include changes in cell DNA repair capability, increases in cell thiol content (which, in turn, can serve as alternate and benign targets of alkylation), decreases in cell permeability, and increased activity of glutathione transferases. Increased methallothionein content has been associated with tumor cell resistance to cisplatin.

Drugs that require metabolic activation for antitumor

activity, such as the *antimetabolites* 6-fluorouracil and 6-mercaptopurine, may be ineffective if a tumor is deficient in the required activating enzymes. Alternatively, a drug may be metabolically inactivated by resistant tumors, which is the case with cytarabine (pyrimidine nucleoside deaminase) and bleomycin (bleomycin hydrolase). Leukemias have been shown to develop resistance to L-asparaginase due to a drug-related induction of the enzyme asparagine synthetase.

Major mechanisms of cellular resistance to anticancer drugs are depicted in Fig. 61-2.

Cancer Therapy and the Immune System

Although manipulation of the host immune response in animal tumor models has at times yielded impressive therapeutic results, attempts to extend these results to human cancers generally have been disappointing.

Several proteins that stimulate subsets of lymphocytes involved in various aspects of the immune response are now produced by recombinant DNA techniques. The pharmacology of these "lymphokines" as potential anticancer agents is being investigated. *Interleukin-2 (IL-2),* originally described as a T-cell growth factor, induces the production of cytotoxic lymphocytes (lymphokine-activated killer cells, or LAK cells). IL-2 produces remissions in 10 to 20 percent of patients with melanoma or renal cell carcinoma when infused at high doses either alone or with lymphocytes that were previously harvested from the patient and incubated with IL-2 in vitro.

The ability of certain anticancer agents to suppress both humoral and cellular immunity has been exploited in the field of organ transplantation and in diseases thought to be caused by an abnormal or heightened immune response. In particular, the alkylating agents cyclophosphamide and chlorambucil have been used in this context, as have several of the antimetabolites, including methotrexate, mercaptopurine, azathioprine, and thioguanine. Daily treatment with these agents rather than high-dose intermittent therapy is the preferred schedule for immune suppression.

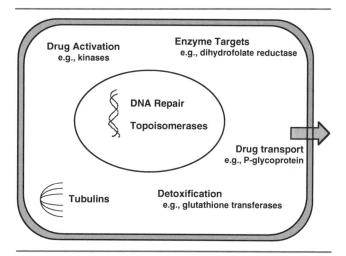

Figure 61-2. Mechanisms of cellular resistance to anticancer drugs.

Toxicological Properties of Anticancer Drugs

Most of the drugs used in cancer treatment have a therapeutic index that approaches unity, exerting toxic effects on both normal and tumor tissues even at optimal dosages. This *lack of selective toxicity* is the major limiting factor in the chemotherapy of cancer. Rapidly proliferating normal tissues, such as bone marrow, gastrointestinal tract, and hair follicles, are the major sites of acute toxicity of these agents. In addition, chronic and cumulative toxicities may occur. The most commonly encountered toxicities of antineoplastic agents are described in the following section; more detailed information on individual agents is presented in Chap. 62.

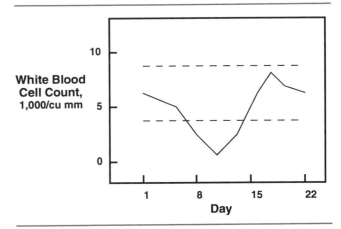

Figure 61-3. The typical course of white blood cell decrease and recovery after chemotherapy.

Bone Marrow Toxicity

Chemotherapy may result in the destruction of actively proliferating hematopoietic precursor cells. White blood cell and platelet counts may, in turn, be decreased, resulting in an increased incidence of life-threatening infections and hemorrhage. Maximum toxicity usually is observed 10 to 14 days after initiation of drug treatment, with recovery by 21 to 28 days. In contrast, the nitrosourea drugs exhibit a delayed hematological toxicity 4 to 6 weeks after beginning treatment.

The risk of serious infections has been shown to increase greatly when the peripheral blood granulocyte count falls below 1,000 cells/mm³. A chronic bone marrow toxicity or hypoplastic state may develop after long-term treatment with nitrosoureas, other alkylating agents, and mitomycin C. Thus, patients frequently will require progressive reduction in dosages of *myelosuppressive* drugs if undergoing long-term therapy, since such treatment may result in chronic pancytopenia. The time course of blood count decrease and recovery after chemotherapy is shown in Fig. 61-3.

The genes for several growth factors that stimulate cell production by the normal bone marrow have been cloned, and their protein products are useful in ameliorating the marrow toxicity of anticancer drugs. These "cytokines" include *granulocyte colony stimulating factor,* or G-CSF, the closely related *granulocyte-macrophage colony stimulating factor,* or GM-CSF, and *erythropoietin* (stimulates production of red blood cells).

Bone marrow transplantation offers the possibility of rescuing patients from very high dosages of myelosuppressive drugs, thus potentially increasing the cure rate of certain tumors. Compatible donors have been used for such marrow transplantation in acute leukemias, making possible treatment with otherwise lethal doses of drugs and radiation. For tumors that do not invade the bone marrow, the patient's own marrow can be harvested before high-dose therapy and then reinfused to hasten recovery of blood counts, a process termed *autologous bone marrow transplantation.*

Bleomycin, L-asparaginase, and the hormonal agents are notably without significant toxicity to the bone marrow.

Gastrointestinal Tract Toxicity

The nausea and vomiting frequently observed after anticancer drug administration are actually thought to be caused by a stimulation of the vomiting center or chemoreceptor trigger zone in the central nervous system (CNS) rather than by a direct gastrointestinal effect. These symptoms are ameliorated by treatment with phenothiazines and other centrally acting antiemetics. Great patient variability is seen in the degree of nausea produced by a given drug. In addition, some patients will begin vomiting before treatment or at the thought of visiting the hospital or oncology office, a conditioned behavioral response termed "anticipatory nausea." More commonly, nausea begins 4 to 6 hr after treatment and lasts 1 or 2 days. Although this symptom is distressing to patients, it is rarely severe enough to require cessation of therapy. Anorexia and alterations in taste perception also may be associated with chemotherapy.

A new antinausea drug, the serotonin antagonist ondansetron (*Zofran*), has proved very effective in the prevention of nausea and vomiting with chemotherapy.

Damage to the normally proliferating mucosa of the gastrointestinal tract may produce stomatitis, dysphagia, and diarrhea several days after treatment. Oral ulcerations, esophagitis, and proctitis may cause pain and bleeding.

Mucositis is more frequently observed when drugs, such as fluorouracil and bleomycin, are administered by continuous infusion for several days.

Hair Follicle Toxicity

Most anticancer drugs damage hair follicles and produce partial or complete alopecia. Patients should be advised of this symptom, especially if paclitaxel, cyclophosphamide, doxorubicin, vincristine, methotrexate, or dactinomycin is used. Hair usually regrows normally after completion of chemotherapy.

Local Toxicity

Several agents (e.g., anthracyclines, vinca alkaloids, mechlorethamine, dactinomycin, mithramycin, nitrosoureas, and mitomycin C) are potent irritants and may cause phlebitis or local tissue necrosis. They must not be injected subcutaneously or intramuscularly, and special care should be taken to avoid extravasation. An intravenous injection should be stopped immediately if pain is produced at the injection site.

Radiation Recall Reactions

Doxorubicin and dactinomycin have been reported to cause flare-ups of dermatitis or esophagitis in areas that were previously treated with radiation therapy. Radiation is known to produce long-standing arteriolar endothelial injury, which may be exacerbated by anticancer drugs. The exact mechanisms involved in producing such *recall* phenomena, however, are not well understood.

Metabolic Abnormalities

A rapid destruction of tumor cells by anticancer drugs results in an increased metabolism of the nucleic acids *released* from these cells. This, in turn, raises uric acid production to levels that may precipitate in renal tubules and cause nephrotoxicity. This complication can be prevented either by prior administration of allopurinol or by adequate hydration of the patient and the alkalinization of urine. Rarely, massive tumor lysis may result in the liberation of amounts of intracellular potassium and phosphate that are sufficient to cause severe hyperkalemia and hyperphosphatemia. Hyponatremia due to inappropriate secretion of antidiuretic hormone has been reported following administration of cyclophosphamide and vincristine.

Hepatic Toxicity

Hepatic fibrosis and even cirrhosis are reported to occur in about 20 percent of patients who receive chronic low doses of methotrexate. Transient increases in serum transaminase also are seen. It has been recommended that such patients be placed on an intermittent dosage schedule, be discouraged from alcohol intake, and have yearly liver biopsies to detect subclinical hepatic toxicity. Liver toxicity also may be caused by L-asparaginase, mercaptopurine, and azathioprine.

Urinary Tract Toxicity

Renal tubular damage is the major toxic symptom associated with cisplatin, streptozocin, and high-dose methotrexate therapy. Vigorous hydration during infusion appears to reduce cisplatin nephrotoxicity, and intravenous hydration and urine alkalinization are required to prevent the renal toxicity of high-dose methotrexate.

Acute hemorrhagic cystitis may complicate cyclophosphamide and ifosfamide therapy, especially when large intravenous doses are administered. Patients should be advised to maintain a large oral intake of fluids during therapy, and a urinalysis should be performed periodically to detect microscopic hematuria. Chronic cyclophosphamide therapy occasionally has been associated with bladder fibrosis and, rarely, with carcinoma of the bladder. To diminish the risk of cystitis, ifosfamide should be administered together with *mesna,* a thiol compound that inactivates the toxic metabolite acrolein.

Cardiac Toxicity

The anthracyclines, doxorubicin and daunorubicin, produce both acute and chronic cardiotoxicity (see Chap. 62). Cyclophosphamide in high intravenous dosages has been reported to cause subendocardial hemorrhage in rare instances.

Pulmonary Toxicity

Bleomycin is a potent pulmonary toxin in humans and is lethal in approximately 1 percent of the patients receiving the drug. Busulfan, like bleomycin, has been associated with a chronic pulmonary interstitial fibrosis, especially after long-term treatment. Acute and chronic lung injury also have been reported with several other *alkylating agents,* notably melphalan and carmustine, but they occur much less commonly than after treatment with bleomycin and busulfan. Methotrexate has caused a hypersensitivity pneumonitis, or allergic interstitial pneumonia, which is associated with fever and eosinophilia. If pulmonary toxicity is suspected subsequent to antineoplastic therapy, administration of that drug should be discontinued permanently.

Nervous System Toxicity

Vincristine is the only antineoplastic agent that has a dose-limiting neurotoxicity. Paresthesias of the hands and feet, loss of deep tendon reflexes, and weakness occur in almost all patients. These effects are usually, but not always, reversible and are more severe in older patients. Myalgias, paresthesias, and weakness severe enough to cause foot drop frequently require discontinuation of therapy. Seizures may occur rarely. Autonomic nervous system toxicity may result in chronic constipation, orthostatic hypotension, or bowel obstruction. Vinblastine also may produce these symptoms. Hexamethylmelamine and cisplatin occasionally produce peripheral neuropathies characterized by weakness and sensory impairment. Paclitaxel causes a sensory neuropathy with numbness and tingling of hands and feet, which is usually mild and resolves before the next cycle of therapy.

Procarbazine, L-asparaginase, and ifosfamide may cause disorientation, somnolence, and other CNS changes. These effects are reversible when drug administration is discontinued. Intrathecally administered methotrexate has produced headaches and delayed meningoencephalopathy in children with acute leukemia. Rarely, fluorouracil treatment has resulted in acute cerebellar dysfunction with ataxia.

Reproductive Function Toxicity

Menstrual irregularities and premature menopause may occur during long-term treatment with alkylating agents. Oligospermia and infertility occur in men, although testosterone production by the testis is not affected. Young patients with a good prognosis should be advised to consider sperm banking before beginning chemotherapy.

Most antineoplastic agents have been shown in animal studies to cause fetal abnormalities, and methotrexate, in particular, is a potent teratogen. Although there are many reports of women bearing normal children after receiving cytotoxic drugs during pregnancy, the long-term effects on these children of such intrauterine exposure is not known.

Carcinogenic Properties

Preclinical tests show that the alkylating agents, anthracyclines, and procarbazine are mutagenic and carci-

nogenic. There is evidence that patients treated with these compounds have an increased incidence of second malignancies. A combination of radiation therapy and chemotherapy with alkylating agents increases substantially the risk of acquiring acute myelocytic leukemia.

Pharmacokinetic Considerations in Cancer Chemotherapy

Pharmacokinetic Sanctuaries

The existence of the blood-brain barrier is an important consideration in the chemotherapy of neoplastic diseases of the brain or meninges. Poor drug penetration into the CNS has been a major cause of treatment failure in acute lymphocytic leukemia in children. Treatment programs for this disease now routinely employ craniospinal irradiation and intrathecally administered methotrexate as prophylactic measures for the prevention of relapses. The testes also are organs in which inadequate antitumor drug distribution can be a cause of relapse of an otherwise responsive tumor.

The multidrug transporter, P-glycoprotein, is expressed in the endothelial lining of the brain and testis, but not in other organs, and is thought to be a major component of the blood-brain and blood-testis drug barriers.

Schedules of Administration

Although the effects of various schedules are not always predictable, drugs that are rapidly metabolized, excreted, or both, especially if they are phase-specific and thus act on only one portion of the cell cycle (e.g., cytarabine), appear to be more effective when administered by continuous infusion or frequent dose fractionation than by high-dose intermittent therapy. On the other hand, intermittent high-dose treatment of Burkitt's lymphoma with cyclophosphamide is more effective than fractionated treatment, since cyclophosphamide acts on all phases of the cell cycle, and almost 100 percent of the tumor cells in that disease are actively proliferating.

The classic example of *schedule dependency* is cytarabine, a drug that specifically inhibits DNA synthesis and is cytotoxic only to cells in S-phase. Continuous infusion or frequent administration of cytarabine hydrochloride is superior to intermittent injection of the drug. Bleomycin is another drug for which continuous infusion may increase therapeutic efficacy.

Administration of some anticancer drugs by *continuous infusion* has been shown to improve their therapeutic index through selective reduction of toxicity with retained or enhanced antitumor efficacy. The cardiac toxicity of doxorubicin, the pulmonary toxicity of bleomycin, and the myelosuppression of fluorouracil are diminished by continuous infusion compared to bolus injection.

Routes of Administration

In addition to the usual intravenous or oral routes, some anticancer agents have been administered by regional intraarterial perfusion to increase drug delivery to the tumor itself and, at the same time, diminish systemic toxicity. Thus, patients with metastatic carcinomas of the liver and little or no disease elsewhere (a common occurrence in colorectal cancer) can be treated with a continuous infusion of fluorouracil or floxuridine through a catheter implanted in the hepatic artery.

Intracavitary administration of various agents has been used for patients with malignant pleural or peritoneal effusions. *Intraperitoneal instillations* of cisplatin, etoposide, bleomycin, 5-fluorouracil, and interferon are well tolerated and are being investigated in patients with ovarian carcinomas, in whom the tumor is frequently restricted to the peritoneal cavity.

Other routes of administration can be employed in certain situations. Methotrexate and cytarabine are given *intrathecally or intraventricularly* to prevent relapses in the meninges in acute lymphocytic leukemia and to treat carcinomatous meningitis. Thiotepa and bleomycin have been administered by intravesical instillation to treat early bladder cancers. Fluorouracil can be applied topically for certain skin cancers.

Drug Interactions

Antineoplastic drugs may be involved in several types of drug interactions. Methotrexate, for example, is highly bound to serum albumin and can be displaced by salicylates, sulfonamides, phenothiazines, phenytoin, and other organic acids. The induction of hepatic drug-metabolizing enzymes by phenobarbital may alter the metabolism of cyclophosphamide to both active and inactive metabolites. Mercaptopurine metabolism is blocked by allopurinol, an occurrence that may result in lethal toxicity if the dosage of mercaptopurine is not reduced to one-fourth the usual dosage. Methotrexate is secreted actively by the renal tubules, and its renal clearance may be delayed by salicylates.

Procarbazine exhibits an interesting interaction with ethanol, resulting in headaches, diaphoresis, and facial erythema; patients taking this drug should be forewarned to abstain from alcohol. Procarbazine is also a monoamine oxidase (MAO) inhibitor and may potentiate the effects of drugs that are substrates for this enzyme.

The biliary and renal excretion of some drugs (anthracyclines, vinca alkaloids, dactinomycin, etoposide) by the multidrug transporter P-glycoprotein can be inhibited by other drugs that are also transported by P-glycoprotein. These other drugs include verapamil, reserpine, phenothiazines, and cyclosporine. The reaction results in delayed excretion and may increase the toxicity of the anticancer agents.

Competitive inhibition of P-glycoprotein offers a possible avenue for therapy of drug-resistant cancers. The cancers for this mechanism of resistance that are thought to be important include acute leukemias, lymphomas, and several others, including breast and ovarian carcinomas and various malignancies in children. Several clinical trials are exploring this approach of reversal or "modulation" of multidrug resistance.

Combination Chemotherapy

The treatment of acute lymphocytic leukemia (ALL) with methotrexate in the 1940s produced remissions for the first time in a previously untreatable cancer. It soon became apparent that single-agent treatment produced only partial and brief remissions. After several years, when other drugs became available, the VAMP regimen (an acronym for the combination of *v*incristine, *a*methopterin [methotrexate], *m*ercaptopurine, and *p*rednisone) produced complete and durable remissions in ALL.

The value of combination chemotherapy has been proved in humans. The combined use of two or more drugs often is superior to single-agent treatment in many different cancers (Table 61-4), and certain principles have been used in designing such treatments:

1. Each drug used in the combination regimen should have some *individual* therapeutic activity against the particular tumor being treated. A drug that is not active against a tumor when used as a single agent is likely to increase toxicity without increasing the therapeutic efficacy of a combined drug regimen.

2. Drugs that *act by different mechanisms* may have additive or synergistic therapeutic effects. Tumors may contain heterogeneous clones of cells that differ in their susceptibility to drugs. Combination therapy will thus increase log-cell kill and diminish the probability of emergence of resistant clones of tumor cells.

3. To avoid cumulative damage to a single organ, drugs with *different dose-limiting toxicities* should be used.

Table 61-4. Response of Hodgkin's Disease to Chemotherapy with Single Agents

Drug	Partial and complete responses (%)
Mechlorethamine	61
Cyclophosphamide	59
Vinblastine	64
Vincristine	63
Procarbazine	75
Carmustine	47
Bleomycin	50
Prednisone	40
Adriamycin (doxorubicin hydrochloride)	33
Dacarbazine *(DTIC)*	56

Source: V. T. DeVita et al. The chemotherapy of Hodgkin's disease: Past experiences and future direction. *Cancer* 42:979, 1978.

Table 61-5. The ABVD Regimen for Advanced Hodgkin's Disease

Drug	Dosage/sq m body surface	Schedule
Adriamycin (doxorubicin hydrochloride)	25 mg, IV	Administer every 2 weeks if blood counts permit, or alternate monthly with MOPP regimen for 12 months
Bleomycin	15 units, IV	
Vinblastine	4 mg, IV	
Dacarbazine *(DTIC)*	350 mg, IV	

4. Intensive *intermittent schedules* of drug treatment should allow time for recovery from the acute toxic effects of antineoplastic agents, primarily bone marrow toxicity. The use of nonmyelosuppressive agents can be considered during the recovery period, especially when one is treating fast-growing cancers.

5. Several *cycles of treatment* should be given, since one or two cycles of therapy are rarely sufficient to eradicate a tumor. Most curable tumors require at least six to eight cycles of therapy.

The chemotherapy of advanced Hodgkin's disease is one of the best examples of successful combination chemotherapy. Combination therapy with the MOPP regimen (mechlorethamine, *Oncovin* [vincristine sulfate], procarbazine, prednisone), alternating with ABVD (*Adriamycin* [doxorubicin hydrochloride], bleomycin, vinblastine, dacarbazine), has resulted in cure rates of 50 to 60 percent. The treatment scheme for these two regimens is presented in Tables 61-3 and 61-5.

The treatment of Hodgkin's disease also illustrates the use of combined modalities, that is, radiation plus chemotherapy. The relative importance of these two modalities is still being defined for certain stages of Hodgkin's disease, but it appears that local treatment of large tumor masses by radiation may prevent the recurrences previously observed following chemotherapy alone. The combined modality approach to several childhood tumors (e.g., Ewing's sarcoma, Wilms' tumor, and rhabdomyosarcoma) has dramatically increased the cure rates for these diseases.

Adjuvant chemotherapy involves the use of antineoplastic drugs in those instances where surgery or radiation therapy has eradicated the primary tumor, but historical experience with similar patients indicates a high risk of subsequent relapse due to micrometastases. Adjuvant chemotherapy should employ drugs that are known to be effective in the treatment of advanced stages of the particular tumor being treated. Therapy generally is continued for 6 to 12 months. Because a large percentage of patients may survive for several years, drugs with minimal chronic toxicity should be used. For instance, since antimetabolites are less mutagenic, they should be employed in preference to alkylating agents where possible. Adjuvant chemotherapy has played a major role in the cure of several types of childhood cancers as well as breast cancer, colorectal cancer, and osteosarcoma in adults. Its role in many other malignancies is currently being studied.

Prospects for Future Treatment

Despite important successes in the past few years, cancer chemotherapy remains a challenging, if often frustrating, area. Continued progress in the understanding of drug action mechanisms may aid in the improvement of therapy and the reduction of toxicity. Better drugs are still needed for the treatment of solid tumors (e.g., colorectal, lung, renal, and melanoma) resistant to current therapy. Identification of drug resistance in tumor specimens by measurements of biochemical markers of resistance or by growth assays in vitro may improve the specificity of chemotherapy.

Immunotherapy, which thus far has been relatively ineffective, may eventually develop into an effective fourth modality of cancer treatment. In this regard, the advent of monoclonal antibodies for diagnosis and treatment of various cancers is especially exciting. Investigations of modulators of the immune system, such as the interferons and interleukin-2, are ongoing. Careful, controlled clinical research with the presently available drugs also may be expected to continue to improve the results of treatment for many of the neoplastic diseases.

The concept of "dose intensity," or increasing the amount of chemotherapy delivered per unit of time, is being tested in many different cancers. The technologies that contribute to the feasibility of this approach include the development of bone marrow growth stimulating factors and methods of harvesting and purifying bone marrow stem cells. Drugs such as granulocyte colony stimulating factor (G-CSF, filgrastim) accelerate the recovery of blood counts after chemotherapy. They can also be used to stimulate release of bone marrow stem cells into the peripheral blood circulation; it is from here that the stem cells are purified and reinfused into patients after high-dose chemotherapy. The latter method of peripheral stem cell harvesting is increasingly replacing bone marrow transplantation, which requires an operation with anesthesia. Some drugs are limited in their application to dose-intense regimens because of side effects other than blood counts, such as the cardiac toxicity of doxorubicin and the renal toxicity of cisplatin. Nevertheless, the ability to deliver higher doses of chemotherapy safely is likely to increase cure rates in many different cancers.

Supplemental Reading

Chabner, B.A., and Collins, J.M. (eds.). *Cancer Chemotherapy: Principles and Practice.* Philadelphia: Lippincott, 1990.

DeVita, V.T. The consequences of the chemotherapy of Hodgkin's disease: The 10th David A. Karnofsky Memorial Lecture. *Cancer* 47:1,1981.

DeVita, V.T., Hellman, S., and Rosenberg, S.A. (eds.). *Cancer: Principles and Practice of Oncology* (4th ed.). Philadelphia: Lippincott, 1993.

Goldie, J.H., Coldman, A.J., and Gudauskas, G.A. Rationale for the use of alternating, non–cross-resistant chemotherapy. *Cancer Treat. Rev.* 66:439, 1982.

Roninson, I.B. (ed.). *Molecular and Cellular Biology of Multidrug Resistance in Tumor Cells.* New York: Plenum, 1990.

Yahanda, A.M., et al. Phase I trial of etoposide with cyclosporine as a modulator of multidrug resistance. *J. Clin. Oncol.* 10:1624, 1992.

62

Antineoplastic Agents

Branimir I. Sikic

Alkylating Agents

The alkylating agents are the largest class of anticancer agents, comprising 12 commonly used drugs and 5 subgroups: nitrogen mustards, alkyl sulfonates, nitrosoureas, ethylenimines, and triazenes (Table 62-1). In addition, several other agents including procarbazine, hexamethylmelamine, dacarbazine, estramustine, and mitomycin C, are thought to act, at least in part, by alkylation.

By definition, *alkylating agents* are compounds that are capable of introducing alkyl groups into nucleophilic sites on other molecules through the formation of *covalent bonds*. These nucleophilic targets for alkylation include the sulfhydryl, amino, phosphate, hydroxyl, carboxyl, and imidazole groups that are present in macromolecules and low-molecular-weight compounds contained within cells. The reaction between the alkylating agent and the nucleophilic target generally involves one of two mechanisms: (1) a first-order nucleophilic substitution (Sn1) with the initial formation of a solvated, highly reactive, electrophilic carbonium ion, followed by a reaction with a nucleophile; or (2) a second-order nucleophilic substitution (Sn2) in which a transition complex is immediately formed between the drug and its target molecule.

Several macromolecular sites of alkylation damage have been identified, including DNA, RNA, and various enzymes. The inhibition of DNA synthesis occurs at drug concentrations that are lower than those required to inhibit RNA and protein synthesis, and *the degree of DNA alkylation correlates especially well with the cytotoxicity* of these drugs. This interaction also accounts for the mutagenic and carcinogenic properties of the alkylating agents. The reactions of various alkylating agents with DNA have been studied in detail, and the 7-nitrogen (N7) and 6-oxygen (O6) of guanine have been shown to be particularly susceptible to attack by electrophilic compounds. There are several possible consequences of N7 guanine alkylation:

1. *Cross-linkage.* Bifunctional alkylating agents, such as the nitrogen mustards, may form covalent bonds with each of two adjacent guanine residues, with the 2-chloroethyl groups functioning as a covalent bridge between strands of DNA. Such interstrand cross-linkages will *inhibit DNA replication and transcription*. Intrastrand cross-links also may be produced between DNA and a nearby protein.

2. *Mispairing of bases.* Alkylating at N7 changes the O6 of guanine to its enol tautomer, which can then form base pairs with thymine. This occurrence may lead to gene miscoding, with adenine-thymine pairs replacing guanine-cytosine. The result is the production of *defective proteins*.

3. *Depurination.* 7-Nitrogen alkylation may cause cleavage of the imidazole ring and excision of the guanine residue, thus leading to *DNA strand breakage*.

Although all alkylating agents are potentially capable of causing the kinds of genetic damage just discussed, individual drugs will differ from one another in their electrophilic reactivity, the structure of their reactive intermediates, and their pharmacokinetic properties. These differences will be reflected in the spectrum of their antitumor activities and in the toxicities they produce in normal tissues.

Nitrogen Mustards

Mechlorethamine

Mechlorethamine (nitrogen mustard), a derivative of the war gas sulfur mustard, is considered to be the first modern anticancer drug. In the early 1940s it was discovered to be effective in the treatment of human lymphomas. A major disadvantage of mechlorethamine is insta-

Table 62-1. Classification of the Anticancer Drugs*

I. Alkylating agents
  A. Nitrogen mustards
    1. Mechlorethamine hydrochloride (*Mustargen,* HN$_2$, nitrogen mustard)
    2. Cyclophosphamide (*Cytoxan*)
    3. Chlorambucil (*Leukeran*)
    4. Melphalan (*Alkeran, L-PAM,* L-phenylalanine mustard)
    5. Ifosfamide (*Ifex*)
  B. Alkyl sulfonates
    1. Busulfan (*Myleran*)
  C. Nitrosoureas
    1. Carmustine (BCNU, *BiCNU*)
    2. Lomustine (CCNU, *CeeNU*)
    3. Semustine (methyl-CCNU)
    4. Streptozocin (*Zanosar,* streptozotocin)
  D. Ethylenimines
    1. Thiotepa
  E. Triazenes
    1. Dacarbazine (*DTIC-Dome*)
II. Antimetabolites
  A. Folate antagonist
    1. Methotrexate (*Folex, Mexate*)
  B. Purine analogues
    1. Thioguanine (6-TG, 6-thioguanine)
    2. Mercaptopurine (6-MP, *Purinethol*)
    3. Fludarabine (*Fludara*)
    4. Pentostatin (deoxycoformycin, *Nipent*)
    5. Cladribine (2-chloro-deoxyadenosine, *Leustatin*)
  C. Pyrimidine analogues
    1. Cytarabine (cytosine arabinoside, *Cytosar-U,* ara-C)
    2. Fluorouracil (5-FU, 5-fluorouracil)
III. Antibiotics
  A. Anthracyclines
    1. Doxorubicin hydrochloride (*Adriamycin*)
    2. Daunorubicin (daunomycin, *Cerubidine*)
    3. Idarubicin (*Idamycin*)
  B. Bleomycins
    1. Bleomycin sulfate (*Blenoxane*)
  C. Mitomycin (mitomycin C, *Mutamycin*)
  D. Dactinomycin (actinomycin D, *Cosmegen*)
  E. Plicamycin (*Mithracin*)

IV. Plant-derived products
  A. Vinca alkaloids
    1. Vincristine (*Oncovin*)
    2. Vinblastine (*Velban*)
  B. Epipodophyllotoxins
    1. Etoposide (VP-16, *Vepesid*)
    2. Teniposide (VM-26, *Vumon*)
  C. Taxanes: paclitaxel (*Taxol*)
V. Enzymes
  A. L-Asparaginase (*Elspar*)
VI. Hormonal agents
  A. Glucocorticoids
  B. Estrogens/antiestrogens
    1. Tamoxifen citrate (*Nolvadex*)
    2. Estramustine phosphate sodium (*Emcyt*)
  C. Androgens/antiandrogens
    1. Flutamide (*Eulexin*)
  D. Progestins
  E. Luteinizing hormone–releasing hormone (LH-RH) antagonists
    1. Buserelin (*Suprefact*)
    2. Leuprolide (*Lupron*)
  F. Octreotide acetate (*Sandostatin*)
VII. Miscellaneous agents
  A. Hydroxyurea (*Hydrea*)
  B. Procarbazine (N-methylhydrazine, *Matulane, Natulan*)
  C. Mitotane (o,p'-DDD, *Lysodren*)
  D. Hexamethylmelamine (HMM)
  E. Cisplatin (*cis*-platinum II; *Platinol*)
  F. Carboplatin (*Paraplatin*)
  G. Mitoxantrone (*Novantrone*)
VIII. Monoclonal antibodies
IX. Immunomodulating agents
  A. Levamisole (*Ergamisol*)
  B. Interferons
    1. Interferon alfa-2a (*Roferon-A*)
    2. Interferon alfa-2b (*Intron A*)
  C. Interleukins: aldesleukin (interleukin-2, IL-2, *Proleukin*)
X. Cellular growth factors
  A. Filgrastim (G-CSF; *Neupogen*)
  B. Sargramostim (GM-CSF, *Leukine, Prokine*)

*Proprietary (*italics*) and other names are given in parentheses.

bility of the 2-chloroethyl groups, which readily react with water molecules and hydroxyl ions. Several mechlorethamine analogues have been synthesized that are less reactive and now largely supplant it in clinical use (Fig. 62-1).

Mechanism of Action

Mechlorethamine, when placed in aqueous solution, loses a chloride atom and forms a cyclic ethylenimonium ion. This carbonium ion interacts with nucleophilic groups, such as the N7 and O6 of guanine, and leads to an interstrand cross-linking of DNA.

Although there is great variability among normal and tumor tissues in their sensitivity to mechlorethamine, the drug is generally more toxic to proliferating cells than to resting or plateau cells.

Pharmacokinetics

Mechlorethamine has a chemical and biological half-life in plasma of less than 10 min after intravenous injection. There is little or no intact drug excreted in urine.

Clinical Uses

The major indication for mechlorethamine is Hodgkin's disease; the drug is given in the MOPP regimen (mechlorethamine, vincristine, procarbazine, prednisone;

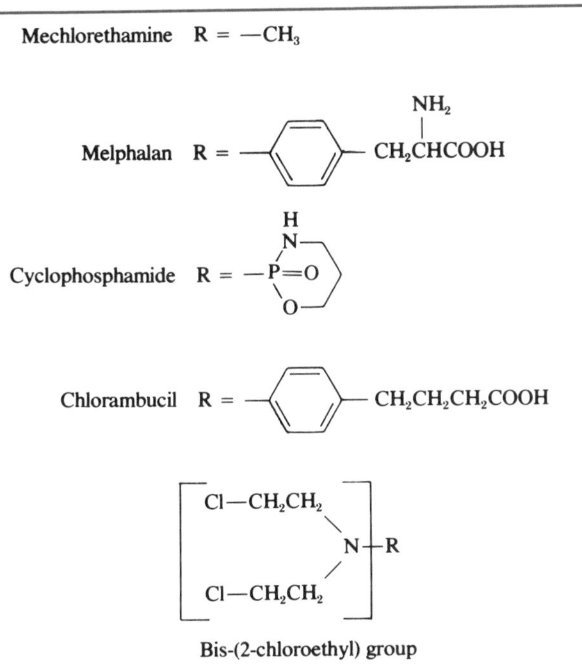

Mechlorethamine R = —CH₃

Melphalan R = [benzene ring]—CH₂CHCOOH (with NH₂ group)

Cyclophosphamide R = [ring structure with H, N, P=O, O]

Chlorambucil R = [benzene ring]—CH₂CH₂CH₂COOH

$$
\begin{bmatrix} Cl-CH_2CH_2 \\ Cl-CH_2CH_2 \end{bmatrix} N-R
$$

Bis-(2-chloroethyl) group

Figure 62-1. Nitrogen mustard alkylating agents.

see Chap. 61, Table 61-3). The other, less reactive, nitrogen mustards are now preferred for the treatment of non-Hodgkin's lymphomas, leukemias, and various solid tumors.

Adverse Reactions

The dose-limiting toxicity of mechlorethamine is *myelosuppression;* maximal leukopenia and thrombocytopenia occur 10 to 14 days after drug administration, and recovery is generally complete at 21 to 28 days. Lymphopenia and immunosuppression may lead to activation of latent herpes zoster infections, especially in patients with lymphomas. Mechlorethamine will affect rapidly proliferating normal tissues and cause alopecia, diarrhea, and oral ulcerations. *Nausea and vomiting* may occur 1 to 2 hr after injection and can last up to 24 hr. Since mechlorethamine is a potent vesicant, care should be taken to avoid extravasation into subcutaneous tissues or even spillage onto the skin. Areas of skin accidentally exposed to the drug should be washed immediately with 2% sodium thiosulfate, and 4% sodium thiosulfate should be infiltrated into areas of subcutaneous extravasation to provide nucleophilic reactants for the drug.

Reproductive toxicity includes amenorrhea and inhibition of oogenesis and spermatogenesis. About half the premenopausal women and almost all men treated for 6 months with MOPP (see Chap. 61) chemotherapy become permanently infertile. The drug is teratogenic and carcinogenic in experimental animals.

Preparation and Dosage

Mechlorethamine hydrochloride (*Mustargen*) is available in vials containing 10 mg of drug for IV use. The dosage in the MOPP regimen is 6 mg/sq m on days 1 and 8 of a 28-day drug administration cycle.

Cyclophosphamide

Cyclophosphamide is the most versatile and useful of the nitrogen mustards. In preclinical testing, it was shown to have a favorable therapeutic index and to possess the broadest spectrum of antitumor activity of all the alkylating agents. The parent drug is inactive and must be enzymatically converted to cytotoxic metabolites.

Mechanism of Action

As with the other nitrogen mustards, cyclophosphamide administration results in the formation of cross-links within DNA due to a reaction of the two chloroethyl moieties of cyclophosphamide with adjacent nucleotide bases. Cyclophosphamide must be activated metabolically by microsomal enzymes of the cytochrome P450 system before ionization of the chloride atoms and subsequent formation of the cyclic ethylenimonium ion can occur. The metabolites phosphoramide mustard and acrolein are thought to be the ultimate active cytotoxic moieties derived from cyclophosphamide.

Absorption, Metabolism, and Excretion

Cyclophosphamide can be given orally, intramuscularly, or intravenously. The plasma half-life of intact cyclophosphamide is 6.5 hr (range 4–8 hr) in patients receiving 6 to 80 mg/kg IV. Only 10 to 15 percent of the circulating parent drug is protein bound, whereas 50 percent of the alkylating metabolites are bound to plasma proteins. The liver is the site of formation of most of the initial active metabolite, 4-OH-cyclophosphamide. Peak blood levels of the alkylating metabolites occur 2 to 3 hr after parenteral administration. Cyclophosphamide does not cross the blood-brain barrier.

The major pathways involved in both activation and inactivation of cyclophosphamide are shown in Fig. 62-2.

In addition to the products depicted in this reaction, several other metabolites of cyclophosphamide have been identified, including the weak alkylating agent nornitrogen mustard.

Since cyclophosphamide and its metabolites are eliminated primarily by the kidneys, renal failure will greatly prolong their retention. Respiratory and fecal excretion are negligible. Small amounts of the drug or its metabolites are found in saliva, sweat, and milk.

Clinical Uses

Cyclophosphamide has a wide spectrum of antitumor activity. In lymphomas, it is frequently used in combina-

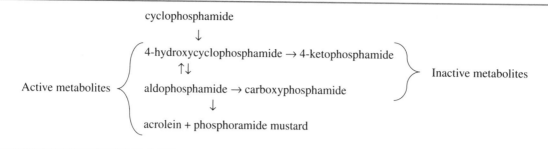

Figure 62-2. Pathways in the activation and inactivation of cyclophosphamide.

tion with vincristine and prednisone (CVP [or COP] regimen) or as a substitute for mechlorethamine in the MOPP regimen (C-MOPP). High dosages of intravenously administered cyclophosphamide are often curative in Burkitt's lymphoma, a childhood malignancy with a very fast growth rate. Oral daily dosages are useful for less aggressive tumors, such as nodular lymphomas, myeloma, and chronic leukemias.

Cyclophosphamide is a component of CMF (cyclophosphamide, methotrexate, 5-fluorouracil) and other drug combinations used in the treatment of breast cancer. Cyclophosphamide, in combination, may produce complete remissions in some patients with ovarian cancer and oat cell (small-cell) lung cancer. Other tumors in which beneficial results have been reported include non–oat cell lung cancers, various sarcomas, neuroblastoma, and carcinomas of the testes, cervix, and bladder.

Cyclophosphamide also can be employed as an alternative to azathioprine in suppressing immunologic rejection of transplant organs. Its immunosuppressive properties also are utilized in the treatment of Wegener's granulomatosis, childhood nephrosis, and severe rheumatoid arthritis. In these noncancerous but life-threatening conditions, the potential benefits of such therapy must be weighed against the drug's potential for producing serious toxicity to normal tissues.

Adverse Reactions

Bone marrow suppression that affects white blood cells more than platelets is the major dose-limiting toxicity. Maximal suppression of blood cell count occurs 10 to 14 days after drug administration; recovery is generally seen 21 to 28 days after injection. Nausea may occur a few hours after administration. *Alopecia* is more common than with other mustards, with loss of scalp hair a few weeks after treatment and regrowth after completion of therapy.

Cyclophosphamide reduces the number of circulating lymphocytes and impairs the function of both humoral and cellular (i.e., B and T cell) aspects of the immunologic system. Chronic therapy increases the risk of infections. These individuals should not be immunized with live vaccines.

A toxicity that is unique to cyclophosphamide and ifosfamide is cystitis, which can occur with both high-dose intravenous and low-dose oral administration. It is thought that the irritation of the bladder mucosa is caused by a metabolite, acrolein. Cystitis is relatively common, occurring in up to 20 percent of patients treated for several months. Dysuria and decreased urinary frequency are the most common symptoms; these symptoms subside within 2 to 3 days after discontinuation of therapy. Rarely, fibrosis and a permanently decreased bladder capacity may ensue. The risk of development of carcinoma of the bladder also is increased. Patients taking cyclophosphamide orally should be advised to take their medication in the morning and to drink liberal amounts of fluid during the day to reduce the urinary concentration of acrolein.

Large IV dosages (greater than 50 mg/kg) have resulted in impairment of renal water excretion, hyponatremia, and increased urine osmolarity. The mechanism for this effect is not clear but it may involve the presence of alkylating metabolites in the urine. Large dosages of cyclophosphamide also have been associated with hemorrhagic subendocardial necrosis, arrhythmias, and congestive heart failure. As is the case with several other alkylating agents, cyclophosphamide can occasionally produce interstitial pulmonary fibrosis after chronic treatment. Other effects of chronic drug treatment include infertility, amenorrhea, and possible mutagenesis and carcinogenesis.

Drug Interactions

Because enzymatic activation and inactivation are important determinants of cyclophosphamide effectiveness, drug interactions may occur. In humans, phenobarbital acts as a microsomal enzyme inducer to increase the rate of formation of both alkylating and inactive metabolites in such a way that peak levels are increased and plasma half-life is decreased. Allopurinol prolongs the plasma half-life of cyclophosphamide but does not alter the total amount of alkylating metabolites formed.

Preparations and Dosage

Cyclophosphamide (*Cytoxan*) is available as 25- and 50-mg tablets, and as vials for injection containing 100, 200, and 500 mg. The drug is stable in refrigerated solution for several days. The usual daily oral dosage for lymphoma, myeloma, or chronic immunosuppression is 2 to 3 mg/kg/day, or 50 to 100 mg/sq m daily. Dosage should be adjusted according to the white blood cell (WBC) count. In cyclical combination chemotherapy, IV dosages of 500 to 1,000 mg/sq m are employed every 3 to 4 weeks, or on days 1 and 8 of a 28-day cycle.

Ifosfamide

Ifosfamide (*Ifex*) is an analogue of cyclophosphamide in which one of the chloroethyl groups is present on the ring nitrogen atom. It requires activation by microsomal oxidation to 4-hydroxyifosfamide. In general, the metabolism, serum half-life, and excretion of ifosfamide are similar to those of cyclophosphamide, although the microsomal activation of ifosfamide proceeds at a slower rate and is saturable at high doses of the drug.

Ifosfamide is active against a broad spectrum of tumors, including germ cell cancers of the testis, lymphomas, sarcomas, and carcinomas of the lung, breast, and ovary. It is thought to be more active than cyclophosphamide in germ cell cancers and sarcomas.

Ifosfamide is less myelosuppressive than cyclophosphamide but is more toxic to the bladder. Ifosfamide can also produce other toxicities shared by alkylating agents including alopecia, nausea and vomiting, infertility, and the induction of second tumors, particularly acute leukemias. Neurological symptoms including confusion, somnolence, and hallucinations have also been reported as side effects of the drug. The high risk for hemorrhagic cystitis from its metabolite acrolein has resulted in the recommendation that ifosfamide be coadministered with the thiol compound mesna (*Mesnex*). A urinalysis should be obtained before each dose. The presence of microscopic hematuria is a contraindication to the use of ifosfamide.

Ifosfamide (*Ifex*) is available in vials for injection containing 1 gm. The usual dose in combination chemotherapy is 1.2 gm/sq m IV per day for 5 consecutive days, repeated every 3 to 4 weeks. As a single agent, doses of 1.5 to 1.8 gm/sq m IV for 5 days can be used. The drug should be given as an IV infusion over 30 to 45 min, with at least 2 liters (L) of oral or IV hydration per day.

The uroprotective agent mesna (sodium 2-mercaptoethanesulfonate; *Mesnex*) is available in ampules for IV injection containing 200 mg, 400 mg, and 1 gm mesna. It should be administered in divided doses of 20 percent of the ifosfamide dose IV immediately before ifosfamide, and then at 4 to 8 hr later.

Melphalan

Melphalan (L-phenylalanine mustard) is an amino acid derivative of mechlorethamine and was synthesized with the hope that some tumor cells might have specific transport systems for phenylalanine. Malignant melanoma cells utilize this amino acid as a precursor for melanin synthesis. Although melphalan has not proved to be effective against melanoma, it does possess the same general spectrum of antitumor activity as do the other nitrogen mustards.

Mechanism of Action

Melphalan acts similarly to mechlorethamine and does not require metabolic activation. However, the substituted phenyl ring greatly reduces the reactivity of the molecule in solution by slowing the rate of ionization of the chlorides and cyclization of the ethylimino groups.

Pharmacokinetics

The plasma half-life of oral melphalan is around 90 min. Alkylating activity has been detected in plasma for up to 6 hr after oral administration. However, the bioavailability of the oral preparation is quite variable (25–90%) from one patient to another. Poor systemic absorption should be suspected if blood count suppression does not occur after melphalan treatment.

Clinical Uses

The major indications for melphalan are in the palliative therapy of multiple myeloma and cancers of the breast or ovary. Because it does not produce alopecia, melphalan is occasionally substituted for cyclophosphamide in the CMF regimen for breast cancer.

Adverse Reactions

Melphalan produces less nausea and vomiting than does cyclophosphamide and does not cause alopecia. However, the bone marrow suppression of melphalan tends to be more prolonged and affects both white cells and platelets. Peak suppression of blood counts occurs 14 to 21 days after a 5-day course of drug therapy; recovery is generally complete within 3 to 5 weeks. Pulmonary fibrosis has been reported recently in a few patients undergoing chronic melphalan treatment. Atypical epithelial proliferation of alveolar lining cells has been observed in the lungs of these patients; it is similar to the pulmonary histopathology produced more commonly by bleomycin.

The carcinogenic potential of melphalan and other alkylating agents was analyzed in a large group of women

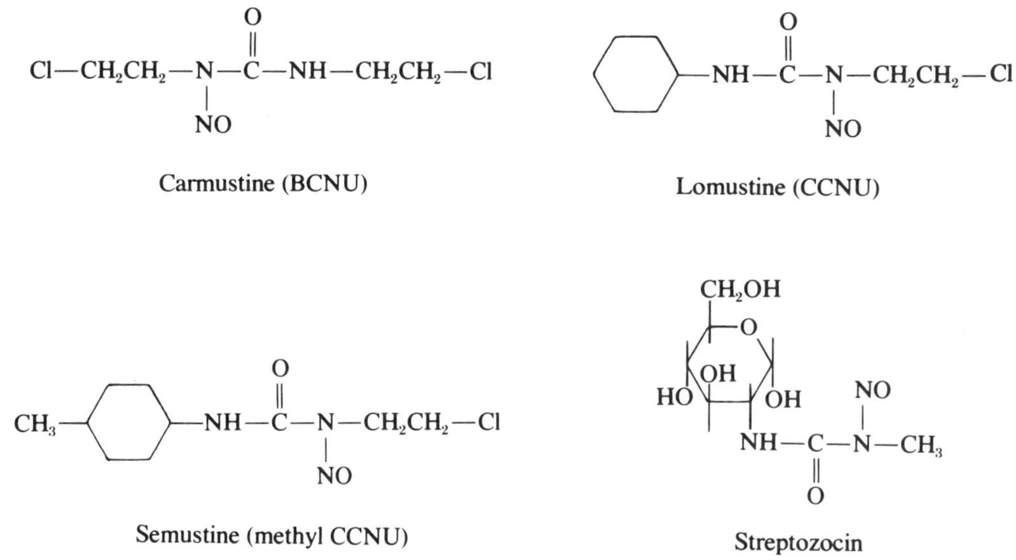

Figure 62-3. Nitrosoureas.

with ovarian cancer in whom second malignancies developed during or after treatment. An increased incidence of acute nonlymphocytic leukemia was found, with a risk over 2 years of 171 times that expected for patients who were not exposed to these drugs.

Preparations and Dosage

Melphalan (*Alkeran*) is marketed as 2-mg tablets. An IV formulation is available only for clinical investigation. The usual dosage is 0.1 to 0.2 mg/kg/day for 5 days; this is repeated every 4 to 6 weeks, depending on blood counts.

Chlorambucil

Chlorambucil is an aromatic nitrogen mustard intermediate in chemical reactivity between mechlorethamine and melphalan. Its mechanisms of action and range of antitumor activity are similar to theirs. It is well absorbed orally, but detailed information concerning its metabolic fate in humans is lacking.

Chlorambucil is used primarily as daily palliative therapy for chronic lymphocytic leukemia, Waldenström's macroglobulinemia, myeloma, and other lymphomas. In England, it is used frequently instead of cyclophosphamide for breast and ovarian cancer. Direct comparisons of the two drugs in patients have not been made.

Bone marrow toxicity is the major side effect of chlorambucil. Nausea is uncommon or mild, and hair loss does not occur. Chlorambucil shares the immunosuppressive, teratogenic, and carcinogenic properties of the nitrogen mustards.

Chlorambucil (*Leukeran*) is available as 2-mg tablets,

and the usual daily dosage is 0.1 to 0.2 mg/kg. It is not available for intravenous use.

Nitrosoureas

Carmustine, Lomustine, and Semustine

Chemistry. The nitrosoureas are alkylating agents with the general formula

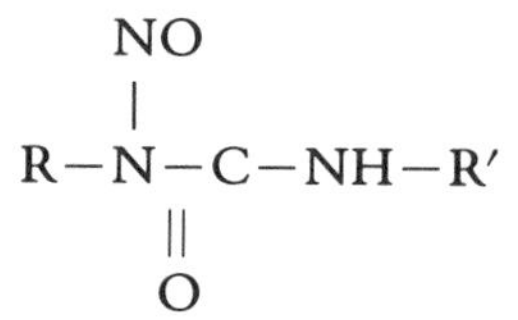

$$
\begin{array}{c}
NO \\
| \\
R-N-C-NH-R' \\
\| \\
O
\end{array}
$$

Three of these agents are highly lipid soluble and share similar pharmacological and clinical properties: carmustine (BCNU), lomustine (CCNU), and semustine (methyl-CCNU) (Fig. 62-3). A fourth nitrosourea, streptozocin, is a water-soluble natural product of a *Streptomyces* species and is considered separately.

Carmustine, lomustine, and semustine are chemically unstable, forming highly reactive decomposition products. The chemical half-life of these drugs in plasma is only 5 to 15 min. Their marked lipid solubility facilitates distribution into the brain and cerebrospinal fluid (CSF).

Mechanism of Action

The chloroethyl moiety of these nitrosoureas is capable of alkylating nucleic acids and proteins and producing single-strand breaks and interstrand cross-linkage of DNA. In addition, isocyanates of the general structure $R-N=C=O$ are formed during drug decomposition and can react by carbamoylating the lysine residues of proteins. Carbamoylation of proteins by the 2-chloroethyl isocyanate of carmustine has been shown to inhibit the repair of DNA strand breaks. *Both alkylation and carbamoylation* contribute to the therapeutic and toxic effects of the nitrosoureas. These agents can kill cells in *all* phases of the cell cycle, including resting, or G_0-phase cells.

Absorption, Metabolism, and Excretion

Oral absorption of lomustine and semustine is complete, but degradation and metabolism is so rapid that the parent drug cannot be detected after oral administration. Although the plasma half-lives of the parent drugs are only a few minutes, degradation products with antitumor activity may persist for longer periods. In addition to spontaneous decomposition, metabolism by microsomal oxygenases has been described for lomustine. After injection of the radiolabeled drugs in humans, radioactivity in the CSF reaches 15 to 30 percent of plasma levels.

Clinical Uses

Carmustine and lomustine can produce remissions that last from 3 to 6 months in 40 to 50 percent of patients with primary brain tumors. Both drugs also are used as secondary treatment of Hodgkin's disease and in experimental combination chemotherapy for various types of lung cancer. Other tumors in which remission rates of 10 to 30 percent have been obtained are non-Hodgkin's lymphomas, multiple myeloma, melanoma, renal cell carcinoma, and colorectal cancer.

Adverse Reactions

The nitrosoureas produce severe nausea and vomiting in most patients 4 to 6 hr after administration. The major site of dose-limiting toxicity is the bone marrow; leukopenia and thrombocytopenia occur after 4 to 5 weeks. This *delayed myelosuppression* is thought to be due to effects on bone marrow stem cells. The myelosuppression is cumulative, necessitating progressive dose reduction. Less frequent side effects include alopecia, stomatitis, and mild abnormalities of liver function. Pulmonary toxicity is becoming increasingly recognized as a complication of long-term nitrosourea treatment; it is manifested by cough, dyspnea, and interstitial fibrosis. As alkylating agents, these drugs are potentially mutagenic, teratogenic, and carcinogenic.

Preparations and Dosage

Carmustine (BCNU, *BiCNU*) is available in vials containing 100 mg of the drug. Because of poor aqueous solubility, the drug is first dissolved in 3 ml of ethanol, and then in 27 ml of sterile water, which can be further diluted with saline or dextrose. Under these conditions, the drug is stable for several hours. The ethanol in the solution frequently causes a pain or burning sensation at the injection site that can be ameliorated by infusing the drug over 1 to 2 hr. Extravasation should be avoided. The usual dosage as a single agent is 200 mg/sq m every 6 weeks.

Lomustine (CCNU *CeeNU*) and semustine (methyl-CCNU) are both administered orally. Lomustine is available as 10-, 40-, and 100-mg capsules. The recommended dosage as a single agent is 130 mg/sq m every 6 weeks. In combination chemotherapy regimens the lomustine dosage is 60 to 80 mg/sq m. The usual dosage of semustine is 200 mg/sq m every 6 weeks.

Streptozocin

Chemistry

Streptozocin is a water-soluble nitrosourea produced by the fungus *Streptomyces achromogenes*. It differs from the lipid-soluble nitrosoureas by a methyl group in place of chloroethyl and a glucosamine sugar at the other end of the molecule (see Fig. 62-3).

Mechanism of Action

Methylation of nucleic acids and proteins is thought to be the major cytotoxic mechanism involved in the action of streptozocin. In addition, it produces rapid and severe depletion of the pyridine nucleotides nicotinamide adenine dinucleotide (NAD) and its reduced form (NADH) in liver and pancreatic islets.

Absorption and Excretion

Streptozocin is not well absorbed from the gastrointestinal tract and must be administered intravenously or intraarterially. In preclinical studies, the plasma half-life was 5 to 10 min, with concentration of the drug in liver and kidney.

Clinical Uses

Streptozocin produces remission in 50 to 60 percent of patients with islet cell carcinomas of the pancreas. It is also useful in malignant carcinoid tumors.

Adverse Reactions

Almost all patients experience nausea and vomiting. The major toxicity is *renal tubular damage,* which may be severe in 5 to 10 percent of patients taking streptozocin. In the majority of patients, some sign of renal toxicity, including proteinuria, hypophosphatemia, aminoaciduria, and renal tubular acidosis, will develop. Treatment of metastatic insulinomas may result in release of insulin from the tumor; hypoglycemic coma may result within 24 hr of treatment. Less severe toxicities found in 10 to 30 percent of patients include diarrhea, anemia, and mild alterations in glucose tolerance or liver function tests. Of note is the virtual absence of toxicity to either white blood cells or platelets.

Preparation and Dosage

Streptozocin is available in vials containing 1.0 gm. The drug can be given by IV injection or infusion. For the treatment of liver metastases, 500 mg/sq m is administered daily for 5 days every 2 to 4 weeks, or 1.5 gm/sq m is given weekly.

Alkyl Sulfonates

Busulfan

Busulfan (Fig. 62-4) is a bifunctional methanesulfonic ester.

Mechanism of Action

Cleavage of the alkyl-oxygen bond produces an electrophilic butyl compound that forms intrastrand cross-linkages with DNA.

Absorption, Metabolism, and Excretion

The drug is well absorbed after oral administration, and has a plasma half-life of less than 5 min. Metabolites and degradation products are excreted primarily in the urine and include methanesulfonic acid and several unidentified alkyl species.

Clinical Use

Busulfan is used in the palliative treatment of chronic granulocytic leukemia. Daily oral therapy results in decreased peripheral WBCs and improved symptoms in almost all patients during the chronic phase of the disease. Excessive uric acid production from rapid tumor cell lysis should be avoided by coadministration of allopurinol. Busulfan is not useful for the treatment of "blast crisis" or transformation of chronic granulocytic leukemia into acute leukemia.

Adverse Reactions

At usual therapeutic dosages, busulfan is selectively toxic to granulocyte precursors rather than lymphocytes. Thrombocytopenia and anemia also may occur and, less commonly, nausea, alopecia, mucositis, and sterility. Unusual side effects of busulfan include gynecomastia, a generalized increase in skin pigmentation, and interstitial pulmonary fibrosis. The lung toxicity usually becomes manifest as a dry cough, dyspnea, and increased interstitial markings on the chest x-ray after 2 to 3 years of continuous treatment.

Preparation and Dosage

Busulfan (*Myleran*) is available as 2-mg tablets. The initial daily dosage is 4 to 8 mg, which can be reduced to a 1- to 3-mg maintenance dosage if needed.

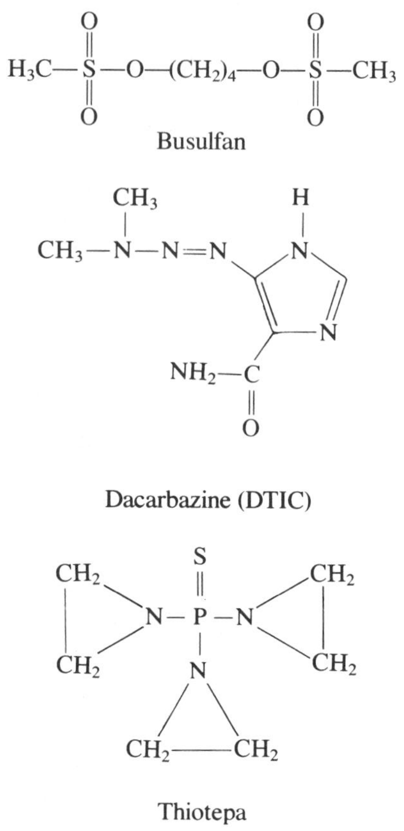

Figure 62-4. Alkylating agents.

Ethylenimines

Thiotepa

Thiotepa was developed as an anticancer drug because of its similarity to the ethylenimonium ions generated by the nitrogen mustards (Fig. 62-4). The sulfur atom of thiotepa confers stability to the cyclic ethylenimine groups.

Mechanism of Action

Although thiotepa is chemically less reactive than the nitrogen mustards, it is thought to act by similar mechanisms.

Absorption, Metabolism, and Excretion

Oral absorption of thiotepa is erratic. After intravenous injection, the plasma half-life is less than 2 hr. Urinary excretion accounts for 60 to 80 percent of injected radiolabeled drug in humans, but less than 1 percent of that is the parent compound.

Clinical Uses

Thiotepa has antitumor activity against ovarian and breast cancers and lymphomas. However, its use in these diseases has been largely supplanted by cyclophosphamide and other nitrogen mustards. It is also used by direct instillation into the bladder for multifocal, localized bladder carcinoma.

Adverse Reactions

Nausea and myelosuppression are the major toxicities of thiotepa. It is not a local vesicant and has been safely injected intramuscularly and even intrathecally.

Preparation and Dosage

The usual IV dosage of thiotepa is 0.2 mg/kg/day for 5 days, which is repeated every 4 weeks. For bladder instillation, 60 mg is usually given in 60 ml of sterile water and retained in the bladder for 2 hr once a week for 4 weeks, then every 4 to 6 weeks.

Triazenes

Dacarbazine

Dacarbazine (Fig. 62-4) was originally synthesized as a potential inhibitor of purine synthesis. Subsequent studies have indicated that alkylation is its primary mode of action.

Mechanism of Action

The parent drug is activated by photodecomposition and by enzymatic *N*-demethylation. Eventual formation of a methylcarbonium ion results in methylation of DNA and RNA and inhibition of nucleic acid and protein synthesis. *As with other alkylating agents, cells in all phases of the cell cycle are susceptible to dacarbazine.*

Distribution, Metabolism, and Excretion

The plasma half-life of dacarbazine in patients is biphasic, with a distribution phase of 19 min and an elimination phase of 5 hr. The drug is not appreciably protein bound, and it does not enter the central nervous system (CNS). Cumulative urinary excretion of unchanged drug is 40 percent in 6 hr and involves renal tubular secretion. Dacarbazine metabolism and decomposition is complex, with initial *N*-demethylation by microsomal mixed-function oxidases. Aminoimidazole-carboxamide is the major urinary metabolite.

Clinical Uses

Dacarbazine is the most active agent used in metastatic melanoma, producing a 20 percent remission rate. It is also combined with doxorubicin and other agents in the treatment of various sarcomas and Hodgkin's disease.

Adverse Reactions

Dacarbazine may cause severe nausea and vomiting. Leukopenia and thrombocytopenia occur 2 weeks after treatment, with recovery by 3 to 4 weeks. Less common is a flulike syndrome of fever, myalgias, and malaise. Alopecia and transient abnormalities in renal and hepatic function also have been reported.

Preparations and Dosage

Dacarbazine (*DTIC-Dome*) is available in 100-mg and 200-mg vials for injection. The drug can undergo photodecomposition and should be protected from light. Injection must be IV, since subcutaneous extravasation can cause severe tissue damage. The usual dosage is 250 mg/sq m IV daily for 5 days, which is repeated every 3 to 4 weeks.

Antimetabolites

Folate Antagonists

In general, antimetabolites used in cancer chemotherapy are drugs that are *structurally related to naturally occurring compounds,* such as vitamins, amino acids, or nucleotides. These drugs can compete for binding sites on enzymes or can themselves become incorporated into DNA or RNA and thus interfere with cell growth and proliferation. The antimetabolites in clinical use include the folic acid analogue methotrexate, the pyrimidines (fluorouracil and cytarabine), and the purines (thioguanine, mercaptopurine, fludarabine, pentostatin, and cladribine).

Methotrexate

In 1948, it was reported that antagonists of the vitamin folic acid, a substance that functions as a cofactor in the transfer of one-carbon units in several metabolic pathways, could produce remissions of acute leukemia in children. Some years later, methotrexate (Fig. 62-5) was found to produce long-term complete remissions of trophoblastic choriocarcinoma in women, the first demonstration of the curative potential of chemotherapy in human cancer.

Mechanism of Action

Methotrexate competitively inhibits the binding of folic acid to the enzyme dihydrofolate reductase. This enzyme catalyzes the formation of tetrahydrofolate, as follows:

$$\text{Folic acid} \xrightarrow{\text{dihydrofolate reductase}} \text{tetrahydrofolate}$$
$$(\text{FH}_2) \qquad\qquad\qquad (\text{FH}_4)$$

Tetrahydrofolate is, in turn, converted to N^5, N^{10}-methylenetetrahydrofolate, which is an essential cofactor for the synthesis of thymidylate, purines, methionine, and

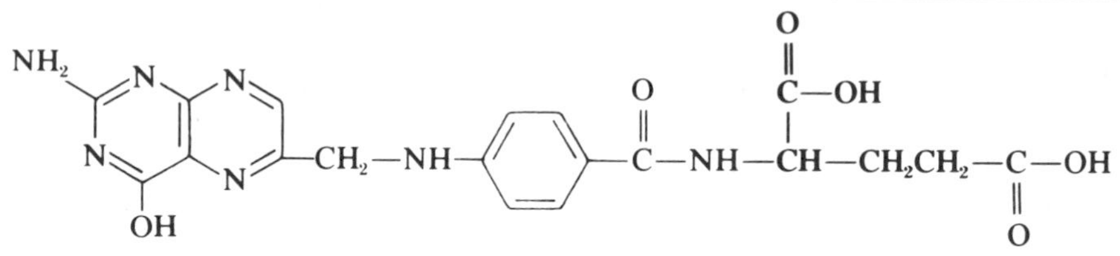

Figure 62-5. Folic acid and its analogue, methotrexate.

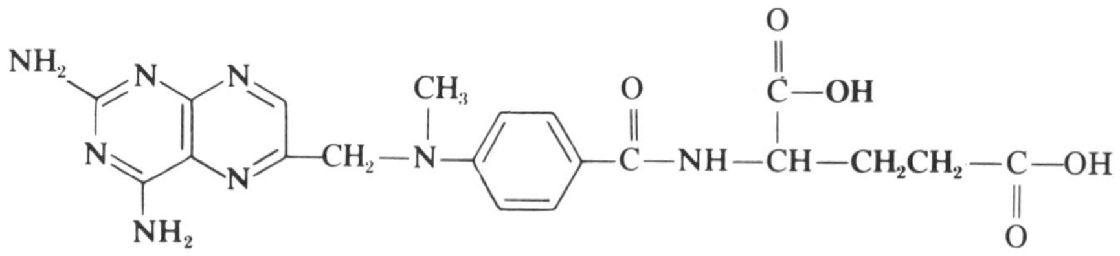

glycine. Binding by methotrexate to dihydrofolate reductase is noncovalent but extremely strong. The major mechanism by which methotrexate brings about cell death appears to involve inhibition of DNA synthesis through a blockage of the biosynthesis of thymidylate and purines.

Cells in S-phase are most sensitive to the cytotoxic effects of methotrexate. RNA and protein synthesis also may be inhibited to some extent and may delay progression through the cell cycle, particularly from G_1 to S.

Resistance

Several mechanisms of resistance to methotrexate are known in mammalian cells. These mechanisms include an increase in intracellular dihydrofolate reductase levels, appearance of altered forms of dihydrofolate reductase with decreased affinity for methotrexate, and a decrease in methotrexate transport into cells (see Chap. 61). The relative importance of each of these mechanisms of resistance in various human tumors is not known.

Cellular uptake of the drug is by carrier-mediated active transport. Drug resistance due to decreased transport can be overcome by greatly increasing extracellular methotrexate concentration, thus providing a rationale for "high-dose" methotrexate therapy. Since bone marrow and gastrointestinal cells do not have impaired folate-methotrexate transport, these normal cells can be selectively "rescued" with reduced folate, thus bypassing the block of dihydrofolate reductase. Leucovorin (citrovorum factor, folinic acid, 5-formyltetrahydrofolate) is the agent commonly used for rescue.

Absorption, Metabolism, and Excretion

Methotrexate is well absorbed orally up to a dosage of 30 mg/sq m, above which absorption is incomplete. At usual dosages the drug is 50 percent bound to plasma proteins. The plasma decay that follows an IV injection of 30 mg/sq m is triphasic, with a distribution phase of 0.7 hr, an initial elimination phase of 3.5 hr, and a prolonged elimination phase of 27.0 hr. The last phase is thought to reflect a slow release from tissues of methotrexate bound to dihydrofolate reductase.

The major route of excretion is renal, involving both glomerular filtration and active tubular secretion. After IV administration of 25 to 75 mg/sq m, about 80 percent of the dose is excreted in the urine within the first 24 hr, with more than 90 percent as unchanged parent drug. After 24 hr, or following oral administration, an increasing fraction of metabolites appears; these include 7-hydroxymethotrexate and 2,4-diamino-N-10-methylpteroic acid.

The formation of polyglutamic acid conjugates of methotrexate has been observed in tumor cells and in the liver and may be an important determinant of cytotoxicity. These methotrexate polyglutamates are retained intracellularly and are also potent inhibitors of dihydrofolate reductase.

Clinical Uses

Methotrexate is part of a curative combination chemotherapy for acute lymphoblastic leukemia, Burkitt's lymphoma, and trophoblastic choriocarcinoma. It is also useful in adjuvant therapy of breast carcinoma as well as in the palliation of metastatic breast, head and neck, cervical, and lung carcinomas and in mycosis fungoides.

High-dose methotrexate administration with leucovorin rescue has produced remissions in 30 percent of patients with metastatic osteogenic sarcoma.

Methotrexate is one of the few anticancer drugs that can be safely administered intrathecally for the treatment of meningeal metastases. Its routine use as prophylactic intrathecal chemotherapy in acute lymphoblastic leukemia has greatly reduced the incidence of recurrences in the CNS and has contributed to the cure rate in this disease. Daily oral doses of methotrexate are used for severe cases of the nonneoplastic skin disease psoriasis (see Chap. 46) and methotrexate has been used as an immunosuppressive agent in severe rheumatoid arthritis.

Adverse Reactions

The major dose-limiting toxicity associated with methotrexate therapy is myelosuppression, with leukopenia and thrombocytopenia appearing 7 to 14 days after treatment. Gastrointestinal toxicity may appear in the form of an ulcerative mucositis and diarrhea. Nausea, alopecia, and dermatitis are common with high-dose methotrexate. The greatest danger of high-dose therapy is renal toxicity due to precipitation of the drug in the renal tubules. The resulting prolonged high plasma levels may lead to lethal bone marrow and gastrointestinal toxicity unless adequate amounts of leucovorin are administered.

Intrathecal administration may produce neurological toxicity, ranging from mild arachnoiditis in 30 percent of patients shortly after treatment to a severe and progressive myelopathy or encephalopathy in about 10 percent of the individuals receiving methotrexate.

Chronic low-dose methotrexate therapy, as used for psoriasis, may result in cirrhosis of the liver. A more acute liver toxicity is commonly seen in a few days after high-dose methotrexate therapy, accompanied by transient increases in serum transaminases. This reaction does not preclude further treatment once the enzymes have returned to baseline levels.

Occasionally, methotrexate may produce an acute, potentially lethal lung toxicity, which is thought to be an allergic or hypersensitivity pneumonitis. An open lung biopsy demonstrating eosinophilic infiltration may be required to distinguish pulmonary toxicity from infection.

Methotrexate is a potent teratogen and abortifacient, but it has less long-term mutagenic and carcinogenic potential than do the alkylating agents.

High doses of methotrexate (50–250 mg/kg) have been associated with a number of deaths due to renal toxicity leading to delayed drug excretion. Vigorous intravenous hydration and alkalinization of the urine to increase drug solubility will reduce the risk of renal toxicity. Monitoring of plasma drug levels during high-dose therapy is useful in determining leucovorin dosage and duration or rescue. *Since methotrexate and leucovorin compete for*

intracellular uptake, prolonged treatment with high doses of leucovorin may be required if renal excretion is impaired.

Duration of exposure of cells to methotrexate is an important determinant of cytotoxicity. Thus, 48 hr of exposure to 10^{-8}M methotrexate is the minimum concentration and time threshold for bone marrow toxicity. Patients with malignant effusions may develop severe myelosuppression due to initial drug distribution into the ascites or pleural effusion; this site of drug accumulation acts as a reservoir for the slow release of methotrexate into the systemic circulation.

Intrathecal methotrexate therapy also results in a delayed distribution of the drug into the systemic circulation, and it may require low-dose leucovorin rescue to prevent bone marrow or gastrointestinal toxicity.

Contraindications

Because the major route of methotrexate elimination is urinary excretion, it should not be used in patients with renal impairment. Special precautions must be taken to avoid renal toxicity with high-dose therapy (50–250 mg/kg IV). Large volumes of intravenous fluid containing bicarbonate should be given, since maintenance of urine pH above 7.0 greatly increases methotrexate solubility. Renal function and plasma drug levels should be monitored. Leucovorin rescue is usually begun 24 hr after initiation of high-dose methotrexate infusion.

Drug Interactions

Salicylates, probenecid, and sulfonamides inhibit the renal tubular secretion of methotrexate and may displace it from plasma proteins. Asparaginase inhibits protein synthesis and may protect cells from methotrexate cytotoxicity by delaying progression from G_1-phase to S-phase. Methotrexate may either enhance or inhibit the action of fluorouracil, depending on its sequence of administration.

Preparations and Dosage

Methotrexate is supplied in vials containing 5 or 50 mg for IV or IM injection and as 2.5-mg tablets. Conventional dosages without leucovorin rescue are in a range of 2.5 mg/sq m daily (orally) for psoriasis to 75 mg/sq m (IV) weekly for solid tumors. The recommended dosage for intrathecal methotrexate is 6 to 12 mg/sq m weekly, with a maximum single dose of 12 mg.

Purine Analogues

Thioguanine (6-Thioguanine)

Chemistry

Thioguanine is an analogue of the natural purine guanine, in which a hydroxyl group has been replaced by a sulfhydryl group in the 6 position (Fig. 62-6).

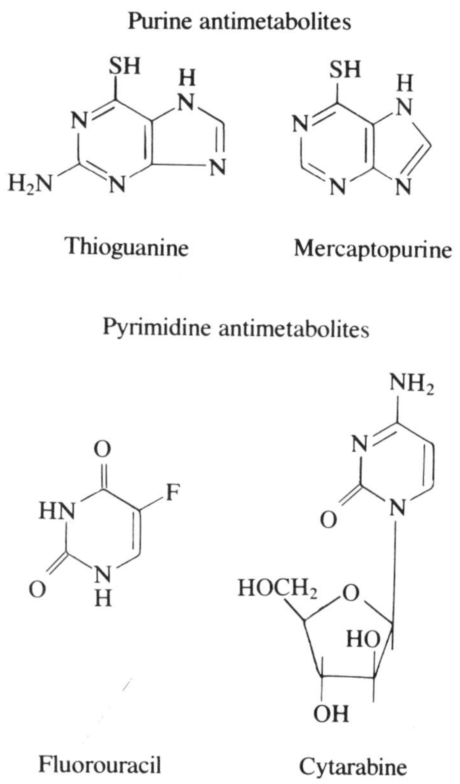

Figure 62-6. Purine and pyrimidine antimetabolites.

Mechanism of Action

Two major mechanisms of cytotoxicity have been proposed for 6-thioguanine: (1) incorporation of the thionucleotide analogue into DNA or RNA, and (2) feedback inhibition of purine nucleotide synthesis. Both these actions require initial activation of the drug by the enzyme hypoxanthine guanine-phosphoribosyltransferase (HGPRTase), as follows:

$$\text{6-Thioguanine} \xrightarrow{\text{HGPRTase}} \text{6-thioguanosine-5-mono-}$$
$$\text{(6-TG)} \qquad \text{phosphate (6-TGMP)}$$

The product of this reaction, 6-TGMP, can eventually be converted to deoxy-6-thioguanosine-triphosphate (dTGTP), which has been shown to be incorporated into DNA. This mechanism appears to be more important than feedback inhibition of purine synthesis in accounting for the antitumor effects of thioguanine.

Resistance of human leukemia cells to thioguanine has been correlated with decreased activity of HGPRTase as well as increased inactivation of the thionucleotides by alkaline phosphatase.

Absorption, Metabolism, and Excretion

Thioguanine is slowly absorbed after oral administration; parent drug levels are barely detectable and peak levels of metabolites (inorganic sulfate, 6-methylthioguanine, and 6-thiouric acid) occur only after 6 to 8 hr. Total urinary excretion of metabolites in the first 24 hr are 24 to 46 percent of the administered dose. Since the xanthine oxidase pathway is not a major route of metabolism of thioguanine, dosages do not need to be reduced for patients receiving allopurinol.

Clinical Uses

Thioguanine is used primarily as part of a combined induction of chemotherapy in acute myelogenous leukemia.

Adverse Reactions

Myelosuppression, with leukopenia and thrombocytopenia appearing 7 to 10 days after treatment, and mild nausea are the most common adverse effects. Liver toxicity with jaundice has been reported in some patients but appears to be less common than with mercaptopurine.

Preparation and Dosage

Thioguanine is available as 40-mg tablets. The usual dosage is 2 mg/kg orally, or 100 mg/sq m.

Mercaptopurine (6-Mercaptopurine)

Mercaptopurine is an analogue of hypoxanthine, in which the hydroxyl at the 6 position is replaced with a sulfhydryl group (see Fig. 62-6). The drug was one of the first agents shown to be active against acute leukemias and is now used as part of maintenance therapy in acute lymphoblastic leukemia.

Mechanism of Action

As with thioguanine, mercaptopurine must be activated to a nucleotide by the enzyme HGPRTase:

$$\text{6-Mercaptopurine} \xrightarrow{\text{HGPRTase}} \text{6-thio-inosine-5-mono-}$$
$$\text{phosphate (6-TIMP)}$$

This metabolite is capable of inhibiting the synthesis of the normal purines, adenine and guanine, at the initial aminotransferase step as well as inhibiting the conversion of inosinic acid to the nucleotides adenylate and guanylate at several steps. Some mercaptopurine is also incorporated into DNA in the form of thioguanine. The relative significance of these mechanisms to the antitumor action of mercaptopurine is not clear.

Resistance to mercaptopurine may occur as a result of a decreased drug activation by HGPRTase or an increased inactivation by alkaline phosphatase.

Absorption, Metabolism, and Excretion

The plasma half-life of an intravenous bolus injection of mercaptopurine is 21 min in children and 47 min in adults. After oral administration, peak plasma levels are attained within 2 hr. The drug is 20 percent bound to plasma proteins and does not enter the CSF.

A primary enzyme involved in the metabolic inactivation of mercaptopurine is xanthine oxidase; metabolism yields 6-thiouric acid. This pathway is blocked by allopurinol, which may result in an important drug interaction. To avoid possible lethal toxicity, patients receiving concurrent therapy with mercaptopurine and allopurinol should receive only 25 percent of the standard dosage of mercaptopurine.

Clinical Uses

Mercaptopurine is used in the maintenance therapy of acute lymphoblastic leukemia. It also displays activity against acute and chronic myelogenous leukemias.

Adverse Reactions

The major toxicities of mercaptopurine are myelosuppression, nausea and vomiting, and hepatic toxicity. Liver toxicity occurs in up to one third of patients and is manifested as a cholestatic jaundice. Death may result from hepatic failure if the drug is not discontinued.

Preparation and Dosage

Mercaptopurine (6-MP, *Purinethol*) is available as 50-mg tablets. The usual dosage is 2.5 mg/kg.

Fludarabine

Fludarabine is a fluorinated purine analogue of the antiviral agent vidarabine. The active metabolite, 2-fluoro-ara-adenosine triphosphate (ATP), inhibits various enzymes involved in DNA synthesis, including DNA polymerase alpha, ribonucleotide reductase, and DNA primase. Unlike most antimetabolites, it is toxic to nonproliferating as well as dividing cells, primarily lymphocytes and lymphoid cancer cells.

The drug is highly active in the treatment of chronic lymphocytic leukemia, with approximately 40 percent of patients achieving remissions after previously failing therapy with alkylating agents. Activity is also seen in the low-grade lymphomas. The major side effect is myelosuppression, which contributes to fevers and infections in as many as half the treated patients. The metabolic abnormalities of tumor lysis syndrome may occur within a few days of initial therapy. Nausea and vomiting are mild. Occasional neurotoxicity has been noted at higher doses, with agitation, confusion, and visual disturbances. Fludarabine (*Fludara*) is available in vials for IV injection containing 50 mg of drug. The usual dose is 25 mg/

m²/day for 5 consecutive days, administered as a 30-min infusion, and repeated every 4 weeks.

Pentostatin

Pentostatin (deoxycoformycin) is a purine isolated from fermentation cultures of the microbe *Streptomyces antibioticus*. Its mechanism of action is inhibition of the enzyme adenosine deaminase, which plays an important role in purine salvage pathways and DNA synthesis. The resulting accumulation of deoxy-ATP is highly toxic to lymphocytes (and is the underlying defect in the severe combined immunodeficiency syndrome, a genetic disease with low levels of adenosine deaminase).

Pentostatin is highly active in the therapy of hairy cell leukemia, producing remissions in 80 to 90 percent of patients and complete remissions in more than 50 percent. The major toxic effects of the drug include myelosuppression, nausea, and skin rashes. The drug is primarily excreted in the urine, and dose adjustments are necessary for patients with abnormal renal function.

Pentostatin (*Nipent*) is available in vials containing 10 mg of drug for IV injection. The recommended dose is 4 mg/m² every other week, with IV hydration of patients before and after the treatment.

Cladribine

Cladribine (2-chloro-deoxy-adenosine) is a synthetic purine nucleoside that is converted to an active cytotoxic metabolite by the enzyme deoxycytidine kinase. Like the other purine antimetabolites, it is relatively selective for both normal and malignant lymphoid cells, and kills resting as well as dividing cells by mechanisms that are not completely understood.

The drug is highly active against hairy cell leukemia, producing complete remissions in more than 60 percent of patients treated with a single 7-day course. Activity has also been noted in other low-grade lymphoid malignancies. The major side effect is myelosuppression, with associated fevers and infections.

Cladribine (*Leustatin*) is available in single-use vials containing 10 mg of drug. The recommended dose is 0.09 mg/kg/day by continuous IV infusion for 7 consecutive days. The drug is stable for 7 days in 0.9% normal saline (but not in 5% dextrose solution).

Pyrimidine Analogues

Cytarabine

Chemistry

Cytarabine (cytosine arabinoside, ara-C, 1-β-D-arabinofuranosylcytosine) is an analogue of the pyrimidine nucleosides cytidine and deoxycytidine, with an arabinose sugar moiety replacing ribose or deoxyribose (see Fig. 62-6). It is one of the most active agents available for the treatment of acute myelogenous leukemia.

Mechanism of Action

Cytarabine kills cells in the S-phase of the cycle by competitively inhibiting DNA polymerase. The drug must first be activated by pyrimidine nucleoside kinases to the triphosphate nucleotide, ara-cytosinetriphosphate (ara-CTP). The susceptibility of tumor cells to cytarabine is thought to be a reflection of their ability to activate the drug more rapidly (by kinases) than to inactivate it (by deaminases).

Metabolism and Excretion

Cytarabine is rapidly metabolized in the liver, kidney, intestinal mucosa, and red blood cells by cytidine deaminase. Its half-life in plasma is only 10 min after intravenous bolus injection. The major metabolite, uracil arabinoside (ara-U), can be detected in the blood shortly after cytarabine administration. About 80 percent of a given dose is excreted in the urine within 24 hr, with less than 10 percent appearing as cytarabine; the remainder is ara-U. When the drug is given by continuous infusion, cytarabine levels in CSF approach 40 percent of those in plasma. The half-life of cytarabine in CSF following intrathecal injection is 2 hr.

Clinical Uses

Cytarabine is used in the chemotherapy of acute myelogenous leukemia, usually in combination with an anthracycline agent or thioguanine, or both. It is less useful in acute lymphoblastic leukemia and the lymphomas and has no known activity against other tumors. It has been used intrathecally in the treatment of meningeal leukemias and lymphomas as an alternative to methotrexate.

Adverse Reactions

Myelosuppression is a major toxicity of cytarabine; the development of a severe bone marrow hypoplasia is a calculated risk of induction chemotherapy in acute leukemia. The drug is more toxic to granulocytes than to lymphocytes. Recovery of normal marrow after successful induction therapy may take 2 to 4 weeks. Nausea and mucositis also may occur.

Intrathecal administration occasionally produces arachnoiditis or more severe neurological toxicity. The relative risk of cytarabine administration compared to intrathecal methotrexate has not been assessed adequately.

Preparations and Dosage

Cytarabine (*Cytosar-U*) is available in vials containing 100 or 500 mg for IV, IM, or SC injection. Because the drug is cell cycle phase–specific and rapidly inactivated, continuous IV infusion is the preferred mode of adminis-

tration; the usual dosage is 100 mg/sq m daily for 7 to 10 days. The dosage for intrathecal administration is 25 to 50 mg/sq m once or twice a week.

Fluorouracil

Chemistry

Fluorouracil (5-fluorouracil, 5-FU) is a halogenated pyrimidine analogue, in which fluorine replaces hydrogen at the C5 position of uracil (see Fig. 62-6).

Mechanism of Action

5-FU must be activated metabolically, and it undergoes a series of intraconversions common to pyrimidines. The active metabolite that inhibits DNA synthesis is the deoxyribonucleotide 5-fluoro-2′deoxyuridine-5′-phosphate (FdUMP).

Generation of 5-FdUMP has been correlated with the antitumor effects of 5-FU. *5-Fluorouracil is selectively toxic to proliferating, rather than nonproliferating, cells and is active in both the G_1- and S-phases.* The target enzyme inhibited by 5-FU is thymidylate synthetase, which catalyzes the following reaction:

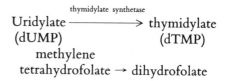

The carbon-donating cofactor for this reaction is N^5, N^{10}-methylenetetrahydrofolate, which is converted to dihydrofolate. The reduced folate cofactor occupies an allosteric site on thymidylate synthetase, which allows for the covalent binding of 5-FdUMP to the active site of the enzyme.

Another action proposed for 5-FU may involve the incorporation of the nucleotide 5-fluorouridine triphosphate (5-FUTP) into RNA. The cytotoxic role of these "fraudulent" 5-FU-containing RNAs is not well understood.

Drug Resistance

Several possible mechanisms of resistance to 5-FU have been identified. These mechanisms include an increased synthesis of the target enzyme, an altered affinity of thymidylate synthetase for FdUMP, deletion of enzymes (especially uridine kinase) that activate 5-FU to nucleotides, an increase in the pool of the normal metabolite deoxyuridylic acid (dUMP), and an increase in the rate of catabolism of 5-FU.

Absorption, Metabolism, and Excretion

The drug has been administered orally, but absorption by this route is erratic. The plasma half-life of 5-FU after intravenous injection of 15 mg/kg is 10 to 20 min. It readily enters CSF. Less than 20 percent of the parent compound is excreted into the urine, the rest being largely metabolized in the liver through the enzyme dihydrouracil dehydrogenase. Subsequent cleavage of the pyrimidine ring yields fluoro-β-alanine, urea, ammonia, and CO_2.

Clinical Uses

5-Fluorouracil is used in several combination regimens in the treatment of breast cancer. It also has palliative activity in gastrointestinal adenocarcinomas, including those originating in the stomach, pancreas, liver, colon, and rectum. Other tumors in which some antitumor effects have been reported include carcinomas of the ovary, cervix, oropharynx, bladder, and prostate.

Topical 5-FU cream has been useful in the treatment of premalignant keratoses of the skin and superficial basal cell carcinomas, but it should not be used in invasive skin cancer.

Hepatic arterial infusion of 5-FU has an increased therapeutic effect with a reduced systemic toxicity in the treatment of patients with hepatocellular carcinomas or liver metastases.

Adverse Reactions

The toxicities of 5-FU vary, depending on the schedule and mode of administration. Nausea is usually mild, if it occurs at all. Myelosuppression is most severe after intravenous bolus administration, with leukopenia and thrombocytopenia appearing 7 to 14 days after an injection; recovery takes place within a few days. Daily injection or continuous infusion is most likely to produce oral mucositis, pharyngitis, diarrhea, and alopecia, compared to weekly bolus injection. Skin rashes and nail discoloration have been reported, as have photosensitivity and increased skin pigmentation on sun exposure.

Neurological toxicity is manifested as an acute cerebellar ataxia in 1 to 2 percent of patients; it is thought to be due to the *metabolite* fluorocitrate. The ataxia may occur within a few days after treatment and may last 1 to 6 weeks.

Preparations and Dosage

Fluorouracil (*Efudex, Adrucil*) is supplied in ampules containing 500 mg for IV or intraarterial injection. Topical solutions of 2% and a 5% cream are also available.

The usual dosage for weekly IV injections is 12 to 15 mg/kg/day for 5 days, which is repeated every 4 weeks if necessary. Continuous infusion of 15 to 25 mg/kg/day can be given IV or intraarterially for 7 to 14 days. When one is using these schedules, the earliest detected sign of toxicity is usually gastrointestinal mucositis; the appearance of diarrhea or oral lesions is an indication for at least temporary discontinuance of infusion therapy.

Ftorafur and Floxuridine

Two analogues of 5-FU, ftorafur and floxuridine, have undergone extensive clinical testing. *Ftorafur* is a tetrahydrofuryl conjugate of 5-FU that is metabolized to, and functions as, a slow-release form of 5-FU. It is more lipid soluble than 5-FU and therefore is better absorbed orally. However, it produces a much higher incidence of neurological toxicity. *Floxuridine (FUDR)* is the nucleoside of 5-FU, which is readily converted into 5-FU in vivo. It has similar pharmacological effects, but is preferred over 5-FU for hepatic arterial infusions because it is more extensively metabolized in the liver than 5-FU, with lesser systemic toxicity.

Antibiotics

Anthracyclines

Doxorubicin and Daunorubicin

Chemistry

The anthracycline antibiotics are fermentation products of *Streptomyces peucetius*. Their chemical structures consist of a planar anthracycline ring system, which is attached by a glycosidic linkage to the sugar daunosamine (Fig. 62-7). Daunorubicin is used to treat acute leukemias, but its structural analogue doxorubicin is extensively employed against a broad spectrum of cancers. Although the two drugs have similar pharmacological and toxicological properties, doxorubicin is more potent against most animal and human tumors and will be discussed in greater detail.

Mechanism of Action

Doxorubicin binds tightly to DNA by its ability to *intercalate* between base pairs and, therefore, is preferentially concentrated in nuclear structures. Intercalation results in inhibition by steric hindrance of DNA synthesis and DNA-dependent RNA synthesis and the production of single-strand breaks in DNA. The enzyme topoisomerase II is thought to be involved in the generation of DNA strand breaks by the anthracyclines. *Cells in S-phase are most sensitive to doxorubicin*, although cytotoxicity also occurs in other phases of the cell cycle.

In addition to the intercalation mechanism described, the anthracycline ring of doxorubicin can undergo a one-electron reduction to form free radicals and participate in further electron transfer. These highly active substances can then react with tissue macromolecules. This type of interaction suggests an alternative mechanism of cytotoxicity for the anthracyclines. In particular, the cardiac toxicity of anthracyclines may result from the generation of

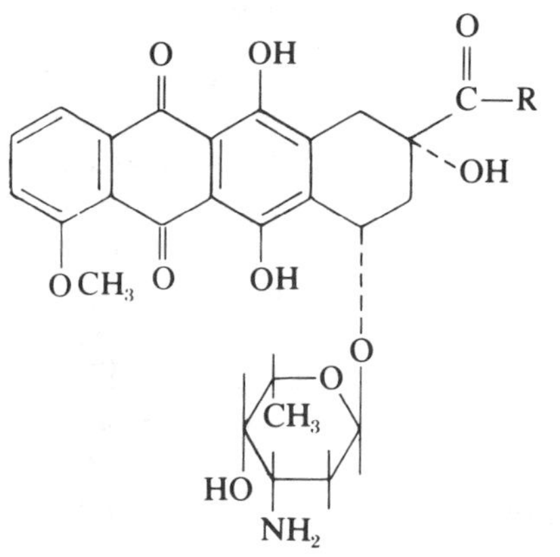

Doxorubicin (*Adriamycin*):   R = —CH₂OH

Daunorubicin: R = —CH₃

Figure 62-7. The anthracycline antibiotics, doxorubicin and daunorubicin.

free radicals of oxygen in the presence of the drug and NADPH-dependent reductases.

Drug Resistance

Resistance to the anthracyclines usually involves decreased drug accumulation due to *enhanced active efflux* of drug. This form of drug resistance is common among the large, heterocyclic, naturally derived anticancer agents. It is termed *multidrug resistance* because of the high degree of cross-resistance among the anthracyclines, vinca alkaloids, dactinomycin, and podophyllotoxins (see also Chap. 61).

Absorption, Metabolism, and Excretion

Doxorubicin is not absorbed orally, and because of its ability to cause tissue necrosis, must not be injected intramuscularly or subcutaneously. The plasma decay of doxorubicin is biphasic, with phase half-lives of around 1 and 17 hr in humans. Distribution studies indicate rapid uptake in all tissues except the CNS. Extensive tissue binding, primarily intranuclear, accounts for the prolonged elimination half-life. The drug is extensively metabolized in the liver to hydroxylated and conjugated metabolites and to aglycones that are primarily excreted in the bile.

Clinical Uses

Doxorubicin is one of the most effective agents used in the treatment of carcinomas of the breast, ovary, endometrium, bladder, thyroid, and oat cell cancer of the lung. It is included in several combination regimens for diffuse lymphomas and Hodgkin's disease. Doxorubicin can be used as an alternative to daunorubicin in acute leukemias and is useful in Ewing's sarcoma, osteogenic sarcoma,

soft-tissue sarcomas, and neuroblastoma. Some activity has been reported in non-oat cell lung cancer, multiple myeloma, and adenocarcinomas of the stomach, prostate, and testis.

Adverse Reactions

The most important toxicities caused by doxorubicin involve the heart and bone marrow. Acutely, doxorubicin may cause transient cardiac arrhythmias and depression of myocardial function. Chronic cardiotoxicity was reported to occur in 25 to 30 percent of patients who received total doses greater than 550 mg/sq m, but in only 1 percent of patients who received less than 550 mg/sq m.

The histopathological features of the cardiotoxicity include mitochondrial swelling and inclusions, myofibrillar degenerations, and focal necrosis of myocytes. Clinically undetectable cardiac damage seems to occur with each dose of doxorubicin. In the absence of overt toxicity, it is currently recommended that therapy be discontinued after a total dose of 550 mg/sq m has been administered. Radiation therapy to the mediastinum increases the risk of doxorubicin-induced cardiac toxicity, and such patients should receive no more than 450 mg/sq m total dose. Both concurrent cyclophosphamide therapy and uncontrolled hypertension exacerbate doxorubicin cardiotoxicity.

Therapy with doxorubicin should be discontinued at the earliest sign of congestive heart failure or if the total limb lead QRS voltage on the patient's electrocardiogram (ECG) decreases to less than 70 percent of the pretreatment value. Measurement of cardiac output by radionuclide ventriculography is also useful in assessing the degree of cardiac dysfunction. Congestive heart failure may occur at low total doses or several months after discontinuation of treatment and frequently responds poorly to the standard treatment of digitalization and diuresis.

The underlying biochemical mechanism of doxorubicin cardiac toxicity is not known, although free radical generation and lipid peroxidation have been implicated. Some structural analogues of doxorubicin are being investigated that appear to have decreased cardiac toxicity while retaining their antitumor efficacy.

The leukopenia and, to a lesser extent, thrombocytopenia that usually occur 10 to 14 days after doxorubicin injection generally subside by day 21. In almost all patients, a reversible alopecia develops. Nausea and vomiting occur 4 to 6 hr after treatment and may last for several hours. Stomatitis and esophagitis may occur 5 to 10 days after treatment.

Doxorubicin may cause "radiation recall" reactions, with flare-ups of dermatitis, stomatitis, or esophagitis that had been produced previously by radiation therapy. These reactions may be severe enough to limit further therapy with the drug. Other less severe toxicities include phlebitis and sclerosis of veins used for injection, hyperpigmentation of nail beds and skin creases, and conjunctivitis. Because of its intense red color, doxorubicin will impart a reddish color to the urine for 1 or 2 days after administration.

Since the liver is the major organ of metabolism and excretion of doxorubicin, impairment in hepatic function may lead to severe myelosuppressive toxicity with the usual therapeutic dosages. It is recommended, therefore, that only 50 percent of the usual dosage be administered if a patient's serum bilirubin level is between 1.2 and 3.0 mg/L, and only 25 percent of the usual dosage if the bilirubin is above 3.0 mg/L.

Preparations and Dosage

Doxorubicin hydrochloride (*Adriamycin*) is available in vials containing 10 or 50 mg of drug for IV injection. The usual IV dose is 60 to 75 mg/sq m every 3 weeks if it is used as a single agent, or 30 to 50 mg/sq m if used in combination regimens. A schedule of 20 mg/sq m of doxorubicin weekly has been reported to result in decreased cardiac toxicity, with no apparent loss of therapy activity. Continuous IV infusion of doxorubicin over 96 hr is also reported to decrease the risk of cardiac toxicity. If bolus administration is used, IV injection should be performed over a 10- to 15-min period rather than as a quick bolus, since acute cardiac arrhythmias and phlebitis have been associated with rapid injection. It is recommended that the drug be injected with a rapid-flowing IV infusion of normal saline or 5% dextrose. Special care must be taken to prevent extravasation of the drug since extravasated doxorubicin can cause extensive local tissue necrosis.

Daunorubicin hydrochloride (*Cerubidine*) is available in vials containing 20 mg of drug for IV injection. The usual IV dosage is 30 to 60 mg/sq m daily for 3 days. Similar precautions should be taken for daunorubicin as for doxorubicin.

Idarubicin

Idarubicin differs from its parent compound, daunorubicin, by the absence of the methoxy group in the anthracycline ring structure. Its mechanisms of action and resistance are similar to those of doxorubicin and daunorubicin. It is more lipophilic and more potent than these other anthracyclines. The drug undergoes extensive hepatic metabolism and biliary excretion. Some but not all comparative trials have shown that idarubicin is superior to daunorubicin in the primary therapy of acute myelocytic leukemia, with higher rates of complete remission and longer survivals. Preclinical studies show lower cardiac toxicity for idarubicin compared to daunorubicin, although this has not been demonstrated conclusively in clinical trials. The other adverse reactions of idarubicin are similar to those of its congeners: myelosuppression, alopecia, nausea and vomiting, and stomatitis.

Idarubicin (*Idamycin*) is available in vials containing 5 and 10 mg of the drug. The recommended dose for leukemia induction therapy is 12 mg/sq m IV daily for 3 days. The drug is a vesicant and will produce severe local inflammation and necrosis if it extravasates into subcutaneous tissues during intravenous infusion.

Bleomycins

Bleomycin

Chemistry

The bleomycins are a group of glycopeptides that are isolated from *Streptomyces verticillus*. The clinical preparation, bleomycin sulfate (*Blenoxane*), is a mixture of several components, primarily bleomycin A_2 (55–70%) and bleomycin B_2 (25–32%), which differ in their amine side chain (Fig. 62-8).

Mechanism of Action

Bleomycin binds to DNA, in part through an intercalation mechanism, without markedly altering the secondary structure of the nucleic acid. The drug produces both single- and double-strand scission and fragmentation of DNA. It is thought that the bleomycins, which are avid metal-chelating agents, form a bleomycin-Fe^{2+} complex, which can donate electrons to molecular oxygen, thus forming the superoxide and hydroxyl free radicals; it is these highly reactive intermediates that then attack DNA. These free radicals generated by bleomycin produce DNA strand breakage and maximum cytotoxicity in the late C_2- and early M-phases of the cell cycle.

Absorption, Metabolism, and Excretion

Bleomycin is poorly absorbed orally, but it can be given by various parenteral routes, including intravascular, intramuscular, intraarterial, and subcutaneous. The plasma half-life is not affected by renal dysfunction as long as creatinine clearance is greater than 35 ml/min. However, since the kidneys serve as the primary organ of drug excretion, use of bleomycin should be avoided or the dosage greatly reduced in patients with renal failure.

Bleomycin hydrolase, which inactivates bleomycin through deamination of an aminoalanine moiety, is an enzyme that is abundant in liver and kidney but virtually absent in lungs and skin; the latter two organs are the major targets of bleomycin toxicity. It is thought that bleomycin-induced dermal and pulmonary toxicities are related to the persistence of relatively high local concentrations of active drug.

Clinical Uses

Bleomycin, in combination with cisplatin or etoposide, is important as part of the potentially curative combina-

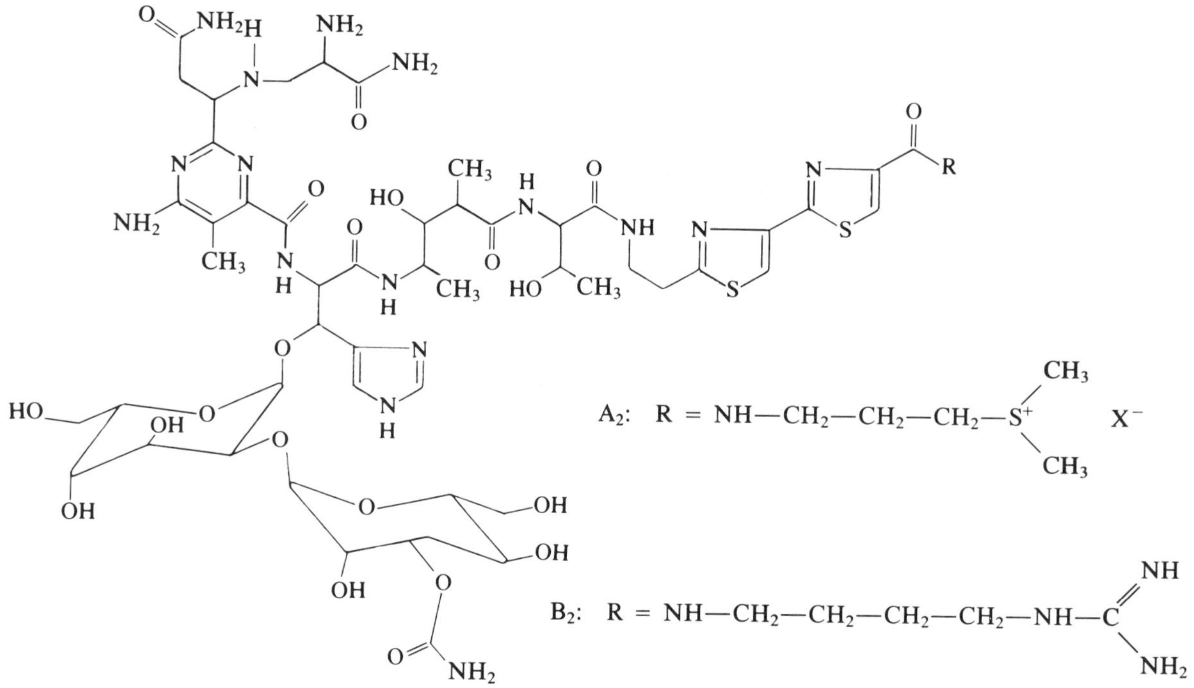

Figure 62-8. Bleomycins A$_2$ and B$_2$, the major constituents of bleomycin mixture.

tion chemotherapy of advanced testicular carcinomas. Bleomycin is used in some standard regimens for the treatment of Hodgkin's and non-Hodgkin's lymphomas, and it is useful against squamous cell carcinomas of the head and neck, cervix, and skin.

Adverse Reactions

A potentially fatal lung toxicity occurs in 10 to 20 percent of patients receiving bleomycin. Patients particularly at risk are those who are over 70 years of age and have had prior radiation therapy to the chest, and those who receive a total cumulative bleomycin dose above 400 units. Rarely, bleomycin also may cause an allergic pneumonitis, with peripheral eosinophilia. This condition, unlike the more common direct lung toxicity, frequently responds to treatment with glucocorticoids, and can be diagnosed by lung biopsy.

Bleomycin skin toxicity is manifested by hyperpigmentation, erythematous rashes, and thickening of the skin over the dorsum of the hands and at dermal pressure points, such as the elbows.

In many patients a low-grade, transient fever will develop within 24 hr of receiving bleomycin. Less common adverse effects include mucositis, alopecia, headache, nausea, and an arteritis of the distal extremities that is similar to Raynaud's disease. An acute, fulminating, anaphylactoid reaction has been reported in patients with lym-

phoma after the first or second dose. Although this reaction has been reported in only about 1 percent of lymphoma patients, it is the manufacturer's recommendation that a test dose of 2 units be administered to patients with lymphoma before treatment with standard dosages. Treatment for the anaphylactoid reaction should include epinephrine, an antihistamine, intravenous fluids, and glucocorticoids.

Preparation and Dosage

Bleomycin sulfate (*Blenoxane*) is supplied in vials containing 15 units of the drug. The drug is administered either by IV or IM injection, and the usual dosage is 10 to 20 units/sq m/week, or by continuous IV or intraarterial infusion of 10 to 15 units/sq m/day for 3 to 7 days. A continuous infusion of bleomycin appears to be superior to a bolus injection, since both increased antitumor efficacy and decreased pulmonary toxicity result when continuous infusion is used.

Mitomycin

Mitomycin (mitomycin C) is an antibiotic that is derived from a species of *Streptomyces* (Fig. 62-9). It is sometimes classified as an alkylating agent, because it can covalently bind to and cross-link DNA.

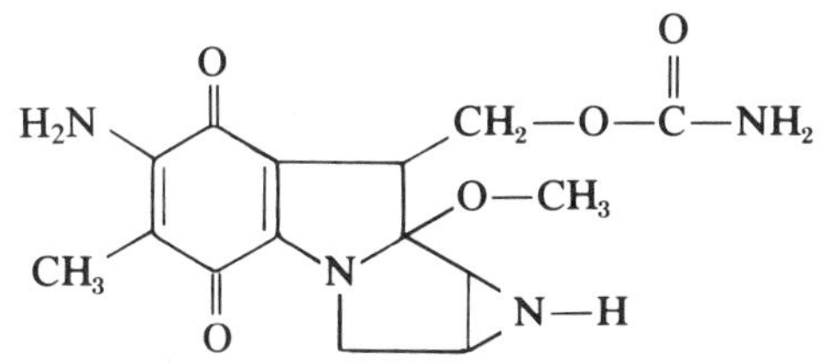

Figure 62-9. Mitomycin.

Mechanism of Action

Mitomycin is thought to inhibit DNA synthesis through its ability to alkylate double-strand DNA and bring about interstrand cross-linking. There is evidence that enzymatic reduction by an NADPH-dependent reductase is necessary to activate the drug and that a half-reduced semiquinone free radical may be the active intermediate. Oxygen-derived free radicals also may be formed by a chain reaction from activated mitomycin; single-strand cleavage of DNA may result.

Pharmacokinetics

The drug is rapidly cleared from serum after intravenous injection; it is not distributed to the brain. Metabolites have not been characterized.

Clinical Uses

Mitomycin has limited palliative effects in carcinomas of the stomach, pancreas, colon, breast, and cervix.

Adverse Reactions

The major toxicity associated with mitomycin therapy is an unpredictably long and cumulative myelosuppression, which affects both white blood cells and platelets. Since suppression is usually maximal 4 to 6 weeks after treatment, drug administration more often than every 6 to 8 weeks should be avoided. A syndrome of microangiopathic hemolytic anemia, thrombocytopenia, and renal failure has been described in 5 to 10 percent of patients receiving mitomycin C therapy. The underlying pathogenesis is not clear, but it appears that immune mechanisms are involved in this treatment-related toxicity. Renal toxicity with glomerular sclerosis may occur in about 2 percent of patients. Nausea after injection is usually mild. Hepatic toxicity has been reported but is uncommon. Pulmonary toxicity has been reported in patients in whom chest x-ray and histological findings have shown a diffuse interstitial fibrosis. The drug is teratogenic, carcinogenic, and a local vesicant.

Preparations and Dosage

Mitomycin (*Mitocin-C, Mutamycin*) is available in vials containing 5 mg, for IV injection. The drug is light-sen-sitive. Care should be taken to avoid subcutaneous extravasation. The usual dosage is 10 to 20 mg/sq m, IV, every 6 to 8 weeks.

Dactinomycin

Dactinomycin (actinomycin D) is one of a family of chromopeptides produced by *Streptomyces* (Fig. 62-10).

Mechanism of Action

Dactinomycin is known to bind noncovalently to double-strand DNA by partial intercalation, inhibiting DNA-directed RNA synthesis. The drug is more toxic to proliferating cells, but it is not specific for any one phase of the cell cycle. *Resistance* to dactinomycin is caused by a decreased ability of tumor cells to take up and retain the drug, and it is associated with cross-resistance to vinca alkaloids, the anthracyclines, and certain other agents (multidrug resistance).

Distribution, Metabolism, and Excretion

Dactinomycin is cleared rapidly from plasma, does not enter the brain, is not appreciably metabolized or protein bound, and is gradually excreted in both bile and urine. Studies in humans confirm prolonged drug retention, with only 30 percent of the dose recovered in urine and stool even after 1 week. The plasma elimination half-life is 36 hr. Less than 10 percent of the administered drug is metabolized, and virtually no drug is detected in CSF.

Clinical Uses

Dactinomycin is used in curative, combined treatment of Wilms' tumor, Ewing's sarcoma, rhabdomyosarcoma, and gestational choriocarcinoma. It is an active drug in testicular tumors, lymphomas, melanomas, and sarcomas, although its use in most of these malignancies has been supplanted by other agents.

Adverse Reactions

The major side effects of dactinomycin are severe nausea, vomiting, and myelosuppression. Maximal depression of WBCs and platelet formation occurs 7 to 14 days after drug administration. Mucositis, diarrhea, and alopecia may occur. Radiation recall reactions may be manifested by severe erythema and desquamation of the skin in areas previously irradiated. The drug is immunosuppressive and carcinogenic.

Preparation and Dosage

Dactinomycin (*Cosmegen*) is supplied in vials containing 0.5 mg for IV injection. The drug is light-sensitive. The usual dosage is 15 μg/kg, or 0.5 mg/sq m IV daily for 5 days, which is repeated every 3 to 4 weeks. Extravasation should be avoided, since the drug is a potent vesicant.

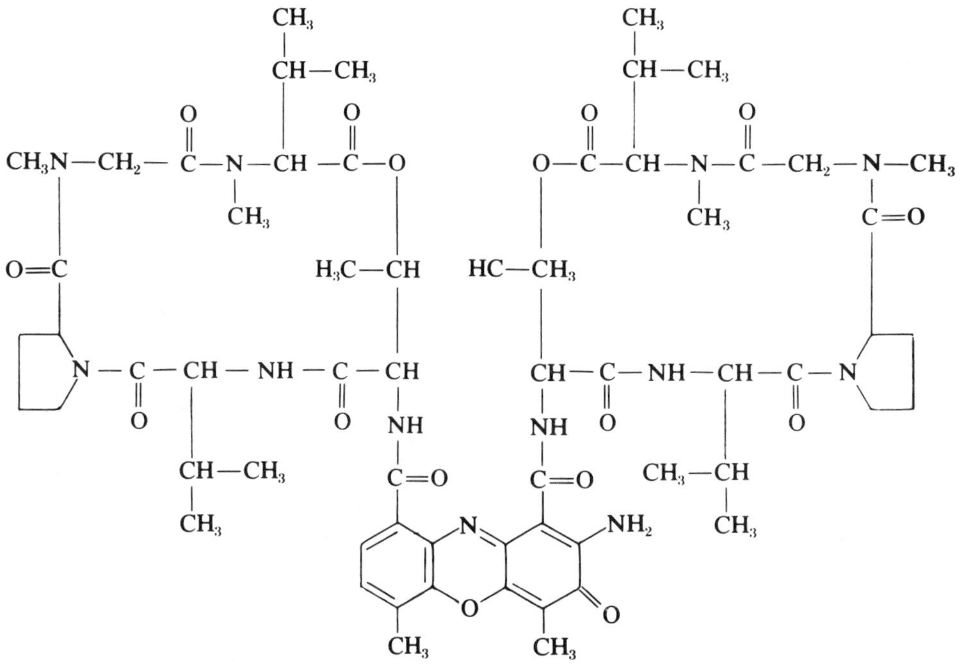

Figure 62-10. Dactinomycin.

Plicamycin

Plicamycin (mithramycin) is one of the chromomycin group of antibiotics produced by *Streptomyces tanashiensis.* Very little is known about the distribution, metabolism, and excretion of plicamycin. Because of its severe toxicity, the drug has limited clinical utility.

Mechanism of Action
Plicamycin binds to DNA and inhibits transcription. It also inhibits resorption of bone by osteoblasts, thus lowering serum calcium levels.

Clinical Uses
The major indication for plicamycin therapy is in the treatment of life-threatening hypercalcemia associated with malignancy. A single injection of 25 μg/kg will lower the serum calcium level within 25 to 48 hr. The duration of this effect is variable, but it usually lasts 3 to 5 days, at which time the injection can be repeated. Plicamycin also can be used in the palliative therapy of metastatic testicular carcinoma when all other known active drugs have failed.

Adverse Reactions
At the dosages used to treat hypercalcemia, plicamycin produces only mild nausea and occasional thrombocytopenia. The higher dosages used in testicular cancer are

very toxic, with up to 25 percent treatment-related mortality from hemorrhage, thrombocytopenia, and azotemia. Prothrombin times are prolonged and epistaxis, ecchymoses, and gastrointestinal bleeding may develop. Severe hepatic and renal damage can contribute to the drug-induced lethality. Decreased serum calcium and phosphorus may result in tetany or seizures. Other common side effects at higher dosages include severe nausea, fever, malaise, facial flushing, headache, and irritability.

Preparation and Dosage
Plicamycin (*Mithracin*) is available in vials containing 2.5 mg of the drug for IV injection. Injection must be IV, since extravasation will produce tissue necrosis. The dosage for treatment of hypercalcemia is 12.5 to 25 μg/kg. For advanced testicular cancer, 25 to 50 μg/kg can be given daily for 5 days or every other day for 1 week. If necessary, treatment can be repeated every 4 weeks.

Plant-Derived Products

Three classes of plant-derived drugs are used in cancer chemotherapy, the vinca alkaloids (vincristine and vinblastine), the epipodophyllotoxins (etoposide and teniposide), and the taxanes (paclitaxel and taxotere). These classes differ in their structures and mechanisms of action, but share the multidrug resistance mechanism, since they are all substrates for the multidrug transporter, P-glyco-protein.

Vinca Alkaloids

Vincristine and Vinblastine

The alkaloids vincristine and vinblastine are both produced by the leaves of the periwinkle plant, *Vinca rosea L.,* also known as *Catharanthus roseus* (Fig. 62-11). Despite their structural similarity, there are significant differences between them in regard to clinical usefulness and toxicity.

Mechanism of Action

The vinca alkaloids *bind avidly to tubulin,* a class of proteins that form the mitotic spindle during cell division. The drugs cause arrest in metaphase of cells entering mitosis, and cell division cannot be completed. The microtubular proteins function in many other processes within the cell, including motility, phagocytosis, secretion, and intracellular transport.

The vinca alkaloids usually have been regarded as M-phase-specific in the cell cycle. However, some mammalian cells are most vulnerable in the late S-phase. *Resistance* to vinca alkaloids has been correlated with a decreased rate of drug uptake or increased drug efflux from these tumor cells. Cross-resistance usually occurs with anthracyclines, dactinomycin, and podophyllotoxins (see Drug Resistance, Chap. 61).

Distribution, Metabolism, and Excretion

Both vincristine and vinblastine are extensively bound to tissues, and only very small amounts of the drug are distributed to the brain or CSF. In humans, the plasma disappearance of vinblastine is triphasic, with half-lives of 4 and 53 min, and 20 hr. Desacetyl vinblastine has been identified as a major metabolite. Similar clinical pharmacokinetics have been noted with vincristine.

Biliary excretion is the major route of drug excretion. In studies using vincristine, 69 percent of the dose was excreted in feces in 72 hr, 40 percent as metabolites.

Clinical Uses

Vincristine is an important component of curative combination chemotherapy for acute lymphoblastic leukemia as well as Hodgkin's disease (the MOPP regimen) and non-Hodgkin's lymphomas. It is also used in several regimens for pediatric solid tumors, including Wilms' tumor, Ewing's sarcoma, rhabdomyosarcoma, and neuroblastoma, and in adult tumors of the breast, lung, and cervix, and sarcomas. Its relative lack of myelosuppression makes it more attractive than vinblastine for use in combination with myelotoxic drugs.

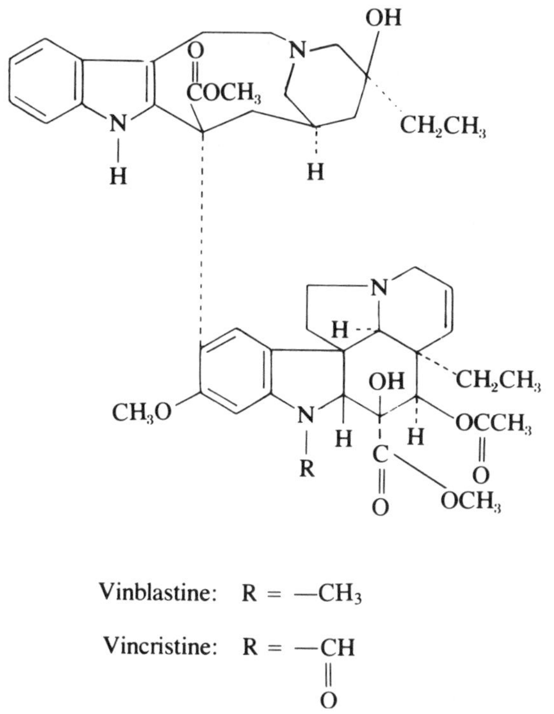

Vinblastine: R = —CH$_3$

Vincristine: R = —CH
                         ‖
                         O

Figure 62-11. The vinca alkaloids, vinblastine and vincristine.

Vinblastine is especially useful in testicular carcinomas, producing cures in the majority of patients when combined with bleomycin and cisplatin. It is also active in Hodgkin's disease and other types of lymphomas as well as breast cancer and renal cell carcinoma.

Adverse Reactions

Neurological toxicity is the major dose-limiting toxicity of vincristine, whereas bone marrow toxicity is limiting for vinblastine. The neurological toxicity of vincristine can take many forms, but it is most commonly seen as a mixed sensorimotor peripheral neuropathy. All patients treated with the drug will develop decreased or absent Achilles and other tendon reflexes, and most will have paresthesias of fingers and toes. Severe generalized weakness may develop, especially in older patients. Autonomic nervous system involvement commonly results in constipation, mild abdominal pain, and urinary retention; patients should be advised to take bulk-forming agents and laxatives prophylactically. Cranial nerve toxicity may be manifested as diplopia, hoarseness, ptosis, or facial weakness. Paroxysmal jaw pain may occur after the first dose of the drug, but it does not usually recur with subsequent doses. A few cases of severe orthostatic hypotension have been reported.

Central neurotoxicity occurs uncommonly and may

include mental depression, insomnia, and, rarely, seizures. Hyponatremia and inappropriate release of antidiuretic hormone also have been observed.

The neurological toxicity of vincristine is only partially reversible even months or years after cessation of therapy. Occurrence of peripheral neuropathy is to be expected and should not be an indication for discontinuing therapy unless the toxicity is exceptionally severe, especially if a treatment regimen is potentially curative for the patient's cancer.

Neurological toxicity is usually much less severe with vinblastine, although generalized myalgias and the other symptoms mentioned previously may occur with high doses. Severe leukopenia is the major side effect of vinblastine, occurring 4 to 7 days after treatment, with recovery by 14 to 18 days. Platelets are affected to a lesser extent. Nausea, vomiting, diarrhea, and alopecia also may be produced. These drugs are potent local vesicants and will produce tissue necrosis if extravasated.

Preparations and Dosage

Vincristine sulfate (*Oncovin*) is available in ampules containing 1 and 5 mg for IV injection. The usual dosage is 1.4 mg/sq m weekly, with a maximum single dose of 2 mg.

Vinblastine sulfate (*Velban*) is supplied in ampules containing 10 mg for IV injection. The usual dosages are 0.1 to 0.2 mg/kg/week, depending on blood counts.

Because of the importance of biliary excretion and hepatic metabolism in the disposition of these agents, dosages should be reduced for patients with extensive liver disease or biliary obstruction.

Epipodophyllotoxins

Etoposide

Etoposide is a semisynthetic derivative of podophyllotoxin that is produced in the roots of the American mandrake, or May apple.

Mechanism of Action

The mechanism of action is poorly understood. Unlike podophyllotoxin and vinca alkaloids, etoposide does not bind to microtubles. Etoposide forms a complex with the enzyme topoisomerase II, which results in a single-strand breakage of DNA. It is most lethal to cells in the S- and G_2-phases of the cell cycle. Drug *resistance* to etoposide is thought to be caused by decreased cellular drug accumulation by means of the pleiotropic or multidrug cross-resistance mechanism.

Pharmacokinetics

Pharmacokinetic studies of etoposide indicate a biphasic plasma decay, with an elimination half-life of 11.5

hr; 44 percent of the dose is excreted in the urine in 72 hr. The drug is more effective when given daily for 3 to 5 days, compared to a single injection every 3 weeks.

Clinical Uses and Adverse Reactions

Etoposide is most useful against testicular and ovarian germ cell cancers, lymphomas, small-cell lung cancers, and acute myelogenous and lymphoblastic leukemia. The clinical toxicities include mild nausea, alopecia, allergic reaction, phlebitis at the injection site, and bone marrow toxicity. Dose-limiting leukopenia occurs 8 to 10 days after administration, with recovery within 3 weeks.

Preparation and Dosage

Etoposide (*VePesid*) is available in vials containing 100 mg of drug for infusion. The route of administration is IV, with dosages ranging from 50 mg/sq m daily for 5 days to 250 mg/sq m as a single dose every 3 weeks. The drug should be infused over 30 to 45 min to avoid hypotension.

Teniposide

Teniposide (VM-26, *Vumon*) is closely related to etoposide in structure, mechanisms of action and resistance, and adverse effects. It is more lipophilic and approximately three-fold more potent than etoposide. Its major uses have been in pediatric cancers, particularly in acute lymphoblastic leukemias. Teniposide (*Vumon*) is available in vials containing 50 mg of the drug for IV infusion. Various doses and schedules of teniposide have been used in combination with other agents (cytarabine, vincristine, and prednisone) for patients with childhood acute lymphoblastic lymphomas who have had relapses after other therapies.

Taxanes

Paclitaxel

Chemistry

Paclitaxel (*Taxol*) is a highly complex, organic compound isolated from the bark of the Pacific yew tree, *Taxus brevifolia*.

Mechanism of Action

Paclitaxel binds to tubulin dimers and microtubulin filaments, promoting the assembly of filaments and preventing their depolymerization. This increase in the stability of microfilaments results in disruption of mitosis and cytotoxicity, and disrupts other normal microtubular functions such as axonal transport in nerve fibers. The antitubulin mechanism of paclitaxel is in contrast to vinca alkaloids, which bind to tubulin but inhibit assembly of microtubules.

Drug Resistance

The major mechanism of resistance that has been identified for paclitaxel is transport out of tumor cells, which leads to decreased intracellular drug accumulation. This is mediated by the multidrug transporter, P-glycoprotein, so that taxol shares cross-resistance with the other drugs in the multidrug resistance phenotype (anthracyclines, vinca alkaloids, epipodophyllotoxins, dactinomycin, mitoxantrone). Mutations in tubulin structure have also been identified that contribute to resistance to paclitaxel in cellular models, but the clinical significance of such tubulin mutations is not known.

Absorption, Metabolism, and Excretion

The elimination half-life of paclitaxel after 1-hr or 6-hr infusion IV varies from 5 to 17 hr. The large volume of distribution, 40 to 160 L/sq m, indicates extensive binding to various tissues. The drug is extensively metabolized by the liver, and doses must be reduced in patients with abnormal liver function or with extensive liver metastases. Very little of the drug (less than 10%) is excreted in the urine.

Clinical Uses

Paclitaxel is among the most active of all anticancer drugs, with significant efficacy against carcinomas of the breast, ovary, lung, and head and neck. It is combined with cisplatin in the therapy of ovarian and lung carcinomas, and with doxorubicin in breast cancer.

Adverse Reactions

The major side effect of Taxol is myelosuppression. Neutrophils are affected more than lymphocytes, platelets or red blood cells. The effect on blood counts is maximal at 10 to 12 days after therapy, with recovery by day 17 to 21. The myelosuppression is more common in patients who have had prior chemotherapies or radiation therapy, and may be ameliorated by reduction in the dose of paclitaxel or by treatment with bone marrow growth factors. Alopecia results in all patients who have had paclitaxel therapy. Peripheral neuropathy occurs frequently, is dose related, is reversible, and is primarily sensory. Most patients experience mild numbness and tingling of the fingers and toes beginning a few days after treatment and abating before the next cycle. Mild muscle and joint aching (myalgias and arthralgias) may also occur beginning 2 or 3 days after therapy and lasting a few days. Nausea is usually mild or absent when Taxol is used as a single agent, in contrast to most anticancer drugs.

Severe hypersensitivity reactions, consisting of dyspnea, hypotension, and chest pains, occur in 1 or 2 percent of patients. These abate with discontinuation of the drug and may require therapy with bronchodilators, epinephrine, antihistamines, and corticosteroids. These reactions were more common (15–20% of courses) before the use of pretreatment regimens with corticosteroids and antihistamines.

Cardiovascular side effects, consisting of mild hypotension and bradycardia, have been noted in up to 25 percent of patients. These are usually not symptomatic and do not require continuous monitoring or treatment. However, a history of symptomatic heart disease, including congestive heart failure and cardiac conduction abnormalities, is a relative contraindication for therapy with paclitaxel.

Preparations and Dosage

Paclitaxel (*Taxol*) is supplied in vials containing 30 mg of drug for intravenous infusion. Because the drug is lipophilic, it is dissolved in a nonaqueous solution containing 50% polyoxy-ethylated castor oil (*Cremophor*) and 50% ethanol. Taxol is administered intravenously by infusions that range in duration from 3 to 96 hr. The usual dose ranges from 135 to 250 mg/sq m every 3 weeks. The higher dose level of 250 mg/sq m should be followed by a course of therapy with filgrastim (G-CSF, *Neupogen*) to ameliorate the severe myelosuppression. Pretreatment with corticosteroid and antihistamines to prevent hypersensitivity reactions is recommended in all patients. A typical prophylactic treatment would consist of dexamethasone, 20 mg orally 12 and 6 hr before paclitaxel, and diphenhydramine, 50 mg IV, and cimetidine, 300 mg IV (or ranitidine, 75 mg IV) 30 minutes before paclitaxel. The formulation and poor solubility of paclitaxel require special precautions for reconstitution and administration; these are detailed in the product information sheet.

Enzymes

L-Asparaginase

The enzyme L-asparaginase has a very specific antitumor effect against acute lymphocytic leukemias and certain lymphomas. The enzyme currently used clinically is derived from the bacteria *Escherichia coli* and *Erwinia carotovora*.

Mechanism of Action

L-Asparaginase catalyzes the hydrolysis of L-asparagine to aspartic acid and ammonia. L-Glutamine also can undergo hydrolysis by this enzyme, and during therapy, the plasma levels of both amino acid substrates fall to zero. Tumor cells sensitive to L-asparaginase are deficient in the enzyme asparagine synthetase and therefore cannot synthesize asparagine. *Depletion of exogenous asparagine and glutamine inhibits protein synthesis in cells lacking asparagine syn-*

thetase, with subsequent inhibition of nucleic acid synthesis and cell death.

Distribution, Metabolism, and Excretion

The half-life of L-asparaginase in human plasma is 6 to 30 hr. The drug remains primarily in the intravascular space, so its volume of distribution is only slightly greater than the plasma volume. Metabolism and disposition are thought to occur through serum proteases, the reticulo-endothelial system, and (especially in patients with prior exposure to the drug) binding by antibodies. It is not excreted in urine, and very little appears in the CSF.

Clinical Uses

The major indication for L-asparaginase is in acute lymphoblastic leukemia; complete remission rates of 50 to 60 percent are possible. Lack of cross-resistance and bone marrow toxicity make the enzyme particularly useful in combination chemotherapy. L-Asparaginase also can be used in the treatment of certain types of lymphoma. It has no role in the treatment of nonlymphocytic leukemias or other types of cancer.

Adverse Reactions

Since it is a foreign protein, L-asparaginase may produce various hypersensitivity reactions, including urticarial skin rashes, in 10 to 20 percent of cases, and severe anaphylactic reactions in 5 to 10 percent. For this reason, patients should be hospitalized during treatment and pretreated with antihistamines; epinephrine and hydrocortisone should be readily available.

One third of patients will experience symptoms of nausea, anorexia, weight loss, and mild fever. Almost all patients will develop elevated serum transaminases and other biochemical indices of hepatic dysfunction, including decreased levels of plasma albumin and clotting factors during, and for a few days after, treatment. Severe hepatic toxicity occurs in fewer than 5 percent of cases. Marked elevation in blood ammonia levels is produced by the enzyme, but in most patients this is not associated with symptoms of cerebral dysfunction. However, about 30 percent of patients receiving L-asparaginase develop symptoms of CNS toxicity, including drowsiness, confusion, impaired mentation, and even coma. The mechanism involved in this toxicity is not known. Neurotoxicity is much more common in adults than in children.

Pancreatitis occurs in 5 to 10 percent of cases. Hyperglycemia, possibly due to inhibition of insulin synthesis, also may occur. Elevations in blood urea nitrogen (BUN) may occur, usually without severe impairment of renal function. *Asparaginase differs from most cytotoxic drugs in its lack of toxicity to bone marrow, gastrointestinal tract, and hair follicles.*

Preparations and Dosage

Asparaginase (*Elspar*) is supplied in vials containing 10,000 units for IV or IM injection. Several dosage regimens are employed in various protocols.

Because of the probability of immune sensitization with this foreign protein, the commercially available *E. coli* L-asparaginase should be used for only one induction course. If a second course is necessary, an antigenically distinct L-asparaginase produced by *E. carotovora* can be used.

Hormonal Agents

The rationale for the use of hormones in cancer treatment stems from the observation, in 1941, that cancer of the prostate gland regresses after estrogen treatment, or after removal of androgen stimulation by castration. Since then, the growth of many cancers has been shown to be inhibited by some hormones and stimulated by others. Glucocorticosteroids, such as prednisone, are toxic to lymphocytes and have antitumor activity in acute and chronic lymphocytic leukemia, the lymphomas, and multiple myeloma. Since prednisone is not toxic to normal bone marrow, it is particularly useful in combination chemotherapy of these diseases.

The use of hormones in some neoplasms may provide relatively nontoxic palliative therapy. Thus, up to 80 percent of patients with metastatic prostatic carcinoma will obtain symptomatic improvement with estrogens. Progestins are useful in endometrial cancer in 35 to 40 percent of cases and in about 15 percent of renal carcinomas. In breast cancer, several hormonal agents may cause temporary regressions, including antiestrogens, progestins, glucocorticoids, androgens, and, in postmenopausal women, high-dose estrogens.

The advantage of hormonal therapy is the lack of severe toxicity to normal tissues and occasional prolonged remissions. The pharmacology of the various hormones is presented elsewhere in this book (see Chaps. 66 to 68).

Tamoxifen

Tamoxifen (see Chap. 67, Fig. 67-3) is a synthetic antiestrogen used in the treatment of breast cancer.

Mechanism of Action

Normally, estrogens act by binding to a cytoplasmic protein receptor. The hormone-receptor complex is translocated into the nucleus and induces the synthesis of ribosomal RNA (rRNA) and messenger RNA (mRNA) at specific sites on the DNA of the target cell. Different protein receptors have been identified for the different classes of steroid hormones and are present in various target tissues and tumors.

Tamoxifen avidly binds to estrogen receptors within cells and competes with endogenous estrogens for these critical sites. The drug-receptor complex has little or no estrogen-agonist activity. Tamoxifen directly inhibits in vitro growth of human breast cancer cells that contain estrogen receptors, but has no effect on cells without such receptors.

Absorption, Metabolism, and Excretion

Tamoxifen is slowly absorbed, and maximum serum levels of 0.1 μg/ml are achieved 4 to 7 hr after oral administration. *The drug is concentrated in estrogen target tissues,* such as the ovaries, uterus, vaginal epithelium, and breasts. Serum levels or radioactivity after a single dose of the radiolabeled drug are still detectable after 2 weeks; excretion occurs primarily in the feces. Hydroxylation and glucuronidation of the aromatic rings are the major pathways of metabolism.

Clinical Uses

The presence of estrogen receptors (ER) in biopsies of breast cancers is a good predictor of response to tamoxifen therapy: 60 percent of women with ER-positive tumors will have a remission, as opposed to fewer than 10 percent with ER-negative tumors. Overall, 35 to 40 percent of women with breast cancer will respond to some degree, with antitumor effects lasting an average of 9 to 12 months. Complete remissions may occur in 10 to 15 percent of patients and may last several months to a few years. Therapy should be continued for at least 6 weeks to establish efficacy.

Adverse Reactions

Tamoxifen administration is associated with few toxic side effects, most frequently hot flashes (in 10–20% of patients) and, occasionally, vaginal dryness or discharge. Mild nausea occurs in 10 percent of patients. Some patients with bone metastases will experience exacerbation of bone pain and hypercalcemia during treatment; serum calcium levels should be monitored in these patients.

Preparation and Dosage

Tamoxifen citrate (*Nolvadex*) is available as 10-mg tablets. The usual dosage is 10 to 20 mg twice a day.

Estramustine

Estramustine phosphate sodium (*Emcyt*) is a hybrid structure combining estradiol and nornitrogen mustard in a single molecule. The drug has been approved for use in prostatic carcinomas and will produce clinical remissions in one third of patients who have failed to respond to previous estrogen therapy. The mechanism of action of estramustine is not well defined, but it does not appear to require either alkylation of DNA or the presence of estrogen receptors in tumor cells. Nonetheless, the toxicities of the drug are similar to those of estrogen therapy: breast tenderness and enlargement (gynecomastia), fluid retention, mild nausea, and an increased risk of thrombophlebitis and pulmonary embolism. The drug is not myelosuppressive. It is supplied as capsules containing 140 mg of estramustine phosphate. The usual dosage is 14 mg/kg/day in three or four divided doses.

Flutamide

Flutamide is a nonsteroidal antiandrogen compound that competes with testosterone for binding to androgen receptors. The drug is well absorbed on oral administration. It is an active agent in the hormonal therapy of cancer of the prostate, and has been shown to complement the pharmacological castration produced by the gonadotropin releasing hormone (LH-RH) agonist leuprolide. Flutamide prevents the stimulation of tumor growth that may occur as a result of the transient increase in testosterone secretion after the initiation of leuprolide therapy. The most common side effects of flutamide are those expected with androgen blockade: hot flashes, loss of libido, and impotence. Mild nausea and diarrhea occur in about 10 percent of patients.

Flutamide (*Eulexin*) is available as capsules containing 125 mg of the drug. The usual dose is two capsules three times a day.

Buserelin and Leuprolide

Buserelin and leuprolide are peptide analogues of the hypothalamic hormone LH-RH (luteinizing hormone-releasing hormone). Chronic exposure of the pituitary to these agents abolishes gonadotropin release and results in markedly decreased estrogen and testosterone production by the gonads.

These agents are active in prostatic carcinomas and breast cancers. Their major clinical use is in the palliative hormonal therapy of cancer of the prostate. Leuprolide has a plasma half-life of 3 hr after subcutaneous injection. It is a potent LH-RH agonist in the first several days to a few weeks after initiation of therapy and therefore initially stimulates testicular and ovarian steroidogenesis. After 2 to 4 weeks of therapy, LH and follicle-stimulating hormone (FSH) secretion by the pituitary gland are inhibited. Because of the initial stimulation of testosterone production, it is recommended that patients with prostatic cancer be treated concurrently with leuprolide and the antiandrogen flutamide (see above). Leuprolide is generally well tolerated, with hot flashes being the most common side effect, occurring in approximately half of the patients.

Leuprolide acetate (*Lupron*) is available in a 2.8-ml multiple-dose vial containing 5 mg/ml of leuprolide acetate. The usual dose is 1 mg/day administered as a single SC injection. It is also available as a depot suspension (*Lupron Depot*) in a vial containing 7.5 mg of leuprolide for monthly IM administration.

Somatostatin Analogue

Octreotide acetate is a synthetic peptide analogue of the hormone somatostatin. Octreotide shares the 4–amino acid sequence essential for the actions of somatostatin. These actions include inhibition of pituitary secretion of growth hormone and inhibition of pancreatic islet cell secretion of insulin and glucagon. Unlike somatostatin, which has a plasma half-life of a few minutes, octreotide has a plasma elimination half-life of 1 to 2 hr. Excretion of the drug is primarily renal.

Octreotide is useful in inhibiting the secretion of various autacoids and peptide hormones by metastatic carcinoid tumors (serotonin) and islet cell carcinomas of the pancreas (gastrin, glucagon, insulin, vasoactive intestinal peptide). The diarrhea and flushing of carcinoid syndrome are improved in 70 to 80 percent of the patients treated with octreotide. The side effects of octreotide are usually mild and include nausea and pain at the injection site in fewer than 10 percent of patients. Mild transient hypo- or hyperglycemia may result from alterations in insulin, glucagon, or growth hormone secretion by octreotide.

Octreotide acetate (*Sandostatin*) is available as ampules containing 50, 100, or 500 μg of the drug. The suggested daily dose is 100 to 600 μg/day injected SC in two to four divided doses.

Miscellaneous Agents

Hydroxyurea

This simple derivative of urea (Fig. 62-12) can reduce high circulating granulocyte counts in chronic myelocytic leukemia. Its use in the treatment of other malignancies, however, remains very limited.

Mechanism of Action

Hydroxyurea inhibits the enzyme *ribonucleotide reductase* and thus depletes intracellular pools of deoxyribonucleotides, resulting in a specific impairment of DNA synthesis. The drug, therefore, is an S-phase–specific agent

Figure 62-12. Miscellaneous antineoplastic agents.

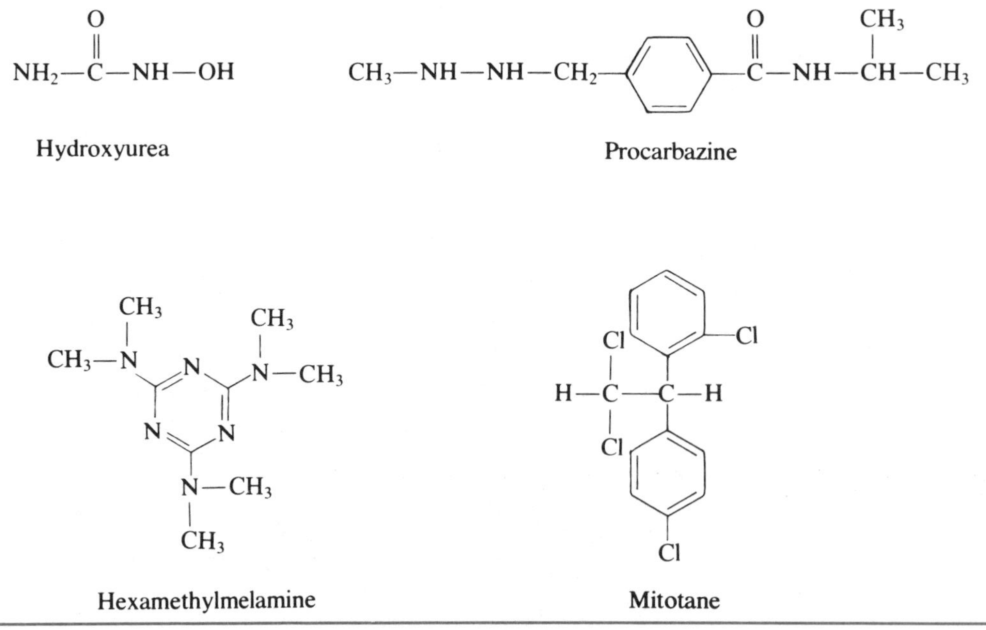

whose action results in an accumulation of cells in the late G_1- and early S-phases of the cell cycle.

Absorption, Metabolism, and Excretion

Hydroxyurea is rapidly absorbed after oral administration, with peak plasma levels achieved approximately 1 to 2 hr after drug administration. Its elimination half-life is 2 to 3 hr. The primary route of excretion is renal, with 30 to 40 percent of a dose excreted unchanged.

Clinical Uses

Hydroxyurea is used for the rapid lowering of blood granulocyte counts in patients with chronic granulocytic leukemia. The drug also can be used as maintenance therapy for patients with the disease who have become resistant to busulfan. Only a small percentage of patients with other malignancies have had even brief remissions induced by hydroxyurea administration.

Adverse Reactions

Hematological toxicity, with WBCs affected more than platelets, may occur typically 4 to 7 days after a 2-week course of treatment with 50 mg/kg/day. Megaloblastosis of the bone marrow also may be observed. Recovery is rapid, generally occurring within 10 to 14 days after discontinuation of the drug. Some skin reactions, including hyperpigmentation and hyperkeratosis, have been reported with chronic treatment.

Preparation and Dosage

Hydroxyurea (*Hydrea*) is available as 500-mg capsules. Two common therapy schedules have been used: 80 mg/kg as a single oral dose every third day and 25 to 50 mg/kg/day in two divided doses. The drug should be used with caution in patients with impaired renal function.

Procarbazine

Procarbazine (see Fig. 62-12) has proved useful against lymphomas and small-cell anaplastic (oat cell) lung cancers.

Mechanism of Action

Procarbazine may autooxidize spontaneously to form azoprocarbazine, and during this reaction hydrogen peroxide and hydroxyl free radicals are generated. These highly reactive products may degrade DNA and may be one mechanism of procarbazine-induced cytotoxicity. Cell toxicity also may be the result of a transmethylation reaction that can occur between the *N*-methyl group of procarbazine and the N7 position of guanine. Procarbazine administration produces a high degree of chromosomal breakage, and the compound is mutagenic, teratogenic, and carcinogenic in experimental systems.

Absorption, Metabolism, and Excretion

Procarbazine is rapidly absorbed after oral administration and has a plasma half-life in humans of only 10 min. The drug crosses the blood-brain barrier, reaching levels in CSF equal to those obtained in plasma. Metabolism is extensive and complex. An initial conversion to azoprocarbazine occurs both spontaneously and by enzymatic means. The hydrazine portion of the molecule may then undergo *N*-hydroxylation and *N*-demethylation. Urinary excretion accounts for 70 percent of the procarbazine and its metabolites lost during the first 24 hr after drug administration.

Clinical Uses

When originally tested as a single agent in advanced Hodgkin's disease, procarbazine produced tumor regression in 53 percent of patients. Unfortunately, these responses were brief, usually lasting only 1 to 3 months. The combination of procarbazine with mechlorethamine, vincristine, and prednisone in the MOPP regimen, however, resulted in an 81 percent complete remission rate in Hodgkin's disease. The majority of these patients are considered cured. Procarbazine is also incorporated into various combination chemotherapy protocols for non-Hodgkin's lymphomas and small-cell anaplastic (oat cell) carcinoma of the lung. Limited antitumor effects have been observed against multiple myeloma, melanoma, and non–oat cell lung cancers.

Adverse Reactions

The major side effects associated with procarbazine therapy are nausea and vomiting, leukopenia, and thrombocytopenia. Skin rashes have been reported as well as rare cases of allergic interstitial pneumonia. Procarbazine is a potent carcinogen in animals, although the magnitude of risk in humans has not been determined.

Drug Interactions

Procarbazine may potentiate the effects of tranquilizers and hypnotics. Hypertensive episodes may result if procarbazine is administered simultaneously with adrenomimetic drugs or tyramine-containing foods. Rarely, a reaction to alcohol similar to that provoked by disulfiram may occur, characterized by headaches, flushing, and diaphoresis.

Preparation and Dosage

Procarbazine hydrochloride (*Matulane*) is marketed as 50-mg capsules.

Mitotane

The observation that mitotane (see Fig. 62-12), a derivative of the insecticide DDT, could produce adrenocortical necrosis in animals led to its use in the palliation of inoperable adrenocortical adenocarcinomas. A reduction in both tumor size and adrenocortical hormone secretion can be achieved in about half of the patients taking the drug. Because normal adrenocortical cells also are affected, endogenous glucocorticoid production should be monitored and replacement therapy administered when appropriate.

Mitotane is incompletely absorbed from the gastrointestinal tract after oral administration. Once absorbed, it tends to accumulate in adipose tissue. Mitotane is slowly excreted and will appear in the urine for several years. The major toxicities associated with its use are anorexia, nausea, diarrhea, lethargy, somnolence, dizziness, and dermatitis.

Mitotane (*Lysodren*) is available as 500-mg tablets. Treatment should be initiated with 2 gm daily in divided doses, followed by a gradual increase to 8 to 10 gm, depending on gastrointestinal and neurological tolerance.

Hexamethylmelamine

Chemistry

The structural similarity of triethylenemelamine to the ethylenimonium ions of the nitrogen mustards led to the antitumor testing of several melamine analogues. Of these, hexamethylmelamine (see Fig. 62-12) proved to be the most active.

Mechanism of Action

Both DNA and RNA synthesis are inhibited in cells exposed to hexamethylmelamine, but the molecular mechanisms of these effects are not known.

Absorption, Metabolism, and Excretion

Hexamethylmelamine is readily absorbed after oral administration, with peak plasma levels achieved after 1 hr. The drug is readily metabolized to form a number of demethylated metabolites, of which only pentamethylmelamine retains some antitumor activity. Urinary elimination is the primary route of drug excretion.

Clinical Uses

Hexamethylmelamine is useful for the treatment of ovarian adenocarcinoma and is frequently combined with cyclophosphamide, cisplatin, and doxorubicin for this tumor. It also has some activity against small-cell lung cancer.

Adverse Reactions

Nausea and vomiting are the major toxicities associated with hexamethylmelamine administration. Myelosuppression is mild, with prompt recovery 2 to 3 weeks after cessation of treatment. Peripheral neuropathy, both sensory and motor, has occurred in 5 to 10 percent of patients undergoing prolonged daily drug administration.

Preparation and Dosage

Hexamethylmelamine is only available as 100-mg capsules. Dosages of 4 to 12 mg/kg/day over a several-month period are tolerated when the drug is given as a single agent. Cyclic combination regimens for ovarian and small-cell lung carcinomas employ dosages of 100 to 200 mg/sq m daily for 7 to 14 days every 3 to 4 weeks.

Cisplatin

Cisplatin is an inorganic coordination complex, with a planar configuration (Fig. 62-13). Cisplatin has a broad range of antitumor activity and is especially useful in the treatment of testicular and ovarian cancer.

Mechanism of Action

Cisplatin binds to DNA at nucleophilic sites, such as the N7 and O6 of guanine, producing alterations in DNA structure and inhibition of DNA synthesis. Adjacent guanine residues on the same DNA strand are preferentially cross-linked. This "platinating" activity is analogous to the mode of action of alkylating agents. Cisplatin also binds extensively to proteins. It does not appear to be phase-specific in the cell cycle.

Pharmacokinetic Properties

Cisplatin shows a biphasic plasma decay after its rapid intravenous infusion; there is a distribution phase half-life of 25 to 49 min and a prolonged elimination half-life of 2 to 4 days. More than 90 percent of the drug is bound to plasma proteins, and binding may approach 100 percent during prolonged infusion. Cisplatin does not cross the blood-brain barrier. Excretion is predominantly renal and is incomplete, with only 27 to 45 percent of the admin-

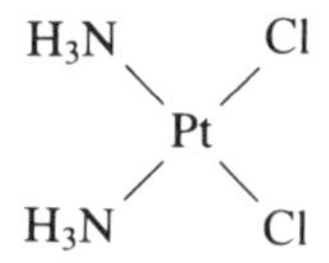

Figure 62-13. Cisplatin.

istered drug appearing in urine during the first 5 days after treatment; traces of platinum are detectable in fluids and tissues for up to 4 months. Information concerning cisplatin metabolites and breakdown products is sparse. The chloride atoms of the molecule are capable of exchanging with water molecules to form positively charged hydrated products. The antitumor activity of these materials is not known.

Clinical Uses

Cisplatin combined with bleomycin and vinblastine or etoposide produces cures in the majority of patients with metastic testicular cancer, as well as germ cell cancers of the ovary. It is a major agent in combination chemotherapy of ovarian adenocarcinomas. Cisplatin also shows some activity against carcinomas of the head and neck, bladder, cervix, prostate, lung, and osteogenic sarcoma.

Adverse Reactions

Renal toxicity is the major potential toxicity of cisplatin. The histopathological changes include degeneration of the proximal convoluted tubules. The toxicity is dose-related and cumulative; increases in BUN and creatinine occur within a few days of treatment. Proteinuria and excretion of renal tubular cells and enzymes also may be evident during the first few days after treatment. The renal toxicity can be avoided by vigorous hydration and diuresis of patients before, during, and after treatment.

The severe nausea and vomiting that accompany cisplatin administration may necessitate hospitalization. The nausea can persist for several days despite antiemetic therapy and may be severe enough to cause a patient to refuse to undergo further cisplatin treatment.

Cisplatin has mild bone marrow toxicity, with both leukopenia and thrombocytopenia occurring after 2 to 3 weeks; recovery is usually complete 3 to 5 weeks after drug administration. Anemia commonly occurs and may require transfusions of red blood cells. Anaphylactic allergic reactions shortly after cisplatin treatment have been described. Hearing loss in the high frequencies (4,000 Hz) may occur in 10 to 30 percent of patients. Less commonly, this ototoxicity may impair the ability to hear normal conversational tones.

Other toxicities that have been reported include peripheral neuropathies with paresthesias, leg weakness, and tremors. Excessive urinary excretion of magnesium may occur in up to half the patients, manifested by a hypomagnesemia with associated tetany and weakness.

Contraindications

Cisplatin therapy should not be initiated in patients with compromised renal function. A creatinine clearance should be performed before each dose; a value greater than 50 mg/min generally is required to allow treatment. Vigorous hydration and use of mannitol diuresis have reduced the incidence of renal toxicity to 5 percent or less.

Preparations and Dosage

Cisplatin (*Platinol*) is available in vials containing 10 or 50 mg of drug. The dosage is 50 to 100 mg/sq m every 3 to 4 weeks, delivered by IV infusions of 1- to 24-hr duration. Daily injections of 20 mg/sq m for 5 days every 3 to 4 weeks also have been used.

Carboplatin

Carboplatin is an analogue of cisplatin in which the chlorides have been replaced with a cyclobutane dicarboxylato leaving group. Aquation of this compound (replacement of the leaving group by water molecules) proceeds at a much slower rate than for cisplatin, but the resulting active species and DNA cross-linking mechanism are similar. The plasma half-life of carboplatin after initial distribution is 3 to 5 hr, without significant protein binding of the parent drug. The major route of excretion is renal.

Despite its lower chemical reactivity, carboplatin has antitumor activity that is similar to that of cisplatin against ovarian carcinomas, small-cell lung cancers, and germ cell cancers of the testis. Most tumors that are resistant to cisplatin are cross-resistant to carboplatin.

The major advantage of carboplatin over cisplatin is a markedly reduced risk for toxicity to the kidneys, peripheral nerves, and hearing, and less nausea and vomiting associated with its administration. However, carboplatin is more myelosuppressive than cisplatin, with a greater effect on platelets than WBCs; recovery usually occurs by 28 to 35 days after treatment. Other adverse effects include anemia, abnormal liver function tests, and occasional (2% of patients) allergic reactions.

Carboplatin (*Paraplatin*) is available in vials for IV injection containing 50, 150, or 450 mg. The usual dosage in patients with normal renal function is 300 to 400 mg/sq m repeated every 4 to 5 weeks. Dose reductions are required for patients with impaired renal function, with a 25 percent reduction if the creatinine clearance is 41 to 59 ml/min and a 50 percent reduction if the clearance is 16 to 40 ml/min.

Mitoxantrone

Mitoxantrone is a synthetic anthraquinone that is structurally and mechanistically related to the anthracyclines. It intercalates with DNA and produces single-strand DNA breakage. It is cross-resistant with doxorubicin in multidrug-resistant cells and in patients who have failed doxorubicin therapy.

Mitoxantrone is active against breast carcinomas, leukemias, and lymphomas. Its antitumor efficacy in patients with breast cancer is slightly lower than that of doxorubicin. Its major toxicity is myelosuppression, primarily affecting the WBCs, with recovery of blood counts by days 21 to 28. Mucositis and diarrhea may occur. Mitoxantrone produces less nausea and alopecia than doxorubicin, as well as a decreased risk for cardiac toxicity.

Mitoxantrone (*Novantrone*) is available in vials containing 20, 25, or 30 mg of drug for IV injection. The usual dosage is 10 to 14 mg/sq m IV every 3 to 4 weeks. Mitoxantrone is a mild vesicant, so that extravasation out of a vein may be painful but is not associated with severe tissue damage.

Monoclonal Antibodies

Monoclonal antibodies may be regarded as an important new class of anticancer drugs whose clinical role is being studied. Most monoclonal antibodies are murine proteins produced by immunizing mice with an antigen of interest (e.g., human cancer cells). The sensitized splenic B lymphocytes of the mouse are then fused with a murine myeloma cell line, and the resulting hybrid cells are screened for the production of the desired antibodies, which can be purified and produced in unlimited quantities. They can then be used in various diagnostic applications, such as radioimmunoassays, histochemical analysis, and tumor imaging, and can also provide therapeutic reagents for modern "serotherapy."

Clinical trials of monoclonal antibody intravenous infusion have been initiated in several tumors, including lymphomas, leukemias, melanoma, and colorectal carcinomas. Tumor remissions have been observed in a few patients.

While therapeutic trials have elucidated several problems with such an approach, monoclonal antibodies offer the possibility of a major increase in the specificity of cancer treatments. These applications include use of monoclonal antibodies as delivery systems for potent biological toxins, or conjugated to radioisotopes for targeted systemic radiotherapy.

Immunomodulating Agents

Levamisole

Levamisole (*Ergamisol*) is an antiparasitic drug that has been found to enhance T-cell function and cellular immunity. The drug has been shown to improve survival of patients with resected colorectal cancers (Duke's stage C), when combined with 5-fluorouracil. The mechanism for this interaction with 5-fluorouracil is not known, although the immunostimulation produced by levamisole is likely to be involved. Levamisole does not have antitumor activity against established or metastatic cancer, and has not been found useful in the adjuvant therapy of cancers other than colorectal cancer.

The major adverse effects of levamisole are nausea and anorexia, which occur in 5 to 10 percent of patients. Skin rashes, itching, flulike symptoms, or fevers have been observed in 1 to 2 percent of cases. Levamisole (*Ergamisol*) is supplied as 50-mg tablets. The usual dosage is 50 mg orally every 8 hr for 3 days, repeated every 2 weeks.

Interferons

Interferon alfa-2b is a recombinant DNA product derived from the interferon alfa-2b gene of human WBCs. It is a protein of approximately 19 kilodaltons molecular mass. The mechanism of antitumor action of interferons involves binding to a plasma membrane receptor but is otherwise poorly understood. The serum half-life of the drug is 2 to 3 hr after intramuscular or subcutaneous injection.

Interferon alfa-2b is useful in the treatment of a rare form of chronic leukemia, hairy cell leukemia, in which it produces remissions in 60 to 80 percent of patients. Despite extensive testing, the drug has minimal antitumor activity in most human cancers. Remissions lasting a few months have been observed in 10 to 20 percent of patients with lymphomas, multiple myeloma, melanoma, renal cell carcinoma, and ovarian carcinoma. The adverse effects of interferon alfa-2b include fever and a flulike syndrome of muscle ache, fatigue, headache, anorexia, and nausea, which occur in the majority of patients to some degree. Other less common side effects include leukopenia, diarrhea, dizziness, and skin rash.

Interferon alfa-2b (*Intron A*) is available in vials containing 3, 5, 10, or 25 million IU for injection. Interferon alfa-2a (*Roferon-A*) is available in vials containing 3 or 18 million IU for injection. The recommended dose for hairy cell leukemia is 2 to 3 million IU/sq m IM or SC, daily for several weeks and then three times per week. Injection SC rather than IM is recommended for patients with low platelet counts.

Interleukins

Aldesleukin

Aldesleukin (IL-2, *Proleukin*) is a human recombinant interleukin-2 protein. This lymphokine is produced using a genetically engineered strain of the bacterium *E. coli*. It differs from native human IL-2 by the absence of glycosylation and an N-terminal amine, and by the substitution of a serine for cysteine at amino acid position 125. The mechanism of action of IL-2 is thought to include multiple effects on the immune system, such as enhancement of T-lymphocyte cytotoxicity, induction of natural killer cell activity, and induction of interferon-γ production. Aldesleukin has been utilized alone as well as in combination with lymphokine activated killer (LAK) cells or tumor-infiltrating lymphocytes (TIL) cells, which are harvested from patients and reinfused after incubation with aldesleukin.

The drug produces remissions in 15 percent of patients with renal cell carcinoma, with median durations of remission of 18 to 24 months. Several serious toxicities have been observed, with a fatality rate of 5 percent in the initial studies. The major adverse effect is severe hypotension in as many as 85 percent of patients, which may lead to myocardial infarctions, pulmonary edema, and strokes, and requires continuous monitoring during therapy in an intensive care unit. This hypotension is thought to be due to a capillary leak syndrome resulting from extravasation of plasma proteins and fluid into extravascular space, as well as loss of vascular tone. Patients with significant cardiac, pulmonary, renal, hepatic, or central nervous system conditions should not receive therapy with aldesleukin. Other adverse reactions include nausea and vomiting, diarrhea, stomatitis, anorexia, altered mental status, fevers, and fatigue.

Aldesleukin (*Proleukin*) is supplied in vials containing 1.1 mg (18 million units) of the drug. A typical course of therapy consists of two 5-day treatment cycles, with 600,000 units infused IV over 15 min, every 8 hr for 14 doses, followed by a 9-day interval. A rest period of 7 weeks is recommended between courses.

Cellular Growth Factors

Filgrastim

Filgrastim (*Neupogen*) is a human recombinant granulocyte colony stimulating factor (G-CSF) produced by recombinant DNA technology from *E. coli*. It acts on pre-cursor hematopoietic cells in the bone marrow by binding to specific receptors that stimulate cellular proliferation and differentiation into neutrophils. It is also able to enhance some neutrophil functions, including phagocytosis and antibody-dependent killing. Filgrastim is used to accelerate recovery of neutrophils after chemotherapy, both to prevent infections and to shorten the duration of neutropenia in patients in whom infections have developed. The drug is generally well tolerated, with the major adverse reaction being mild to moderate bone pain secondary to stimulation of bone marrow proliferation (mostly low back and pelvic discomfort).

Filgrastim (*Neupogen*) is supplied in single-dose vials containing 300 μg or 480 μg of the drug. The usual dose is 5 μg/kg/day as a single daily injection, either subcutaneously or by short intravenous infusion. Treatment is usually begun at least one day after completion of a course of chemotherapy, to avoid stimulating bone marrow proliferation while coadministering cytotoxic agents.

Sargramostim

Sargramostim (GM-CSF, *Leukine, Prokine*) is a human recombinant granulocyte and macrophage colony stimulating factor. It is produced by expression of the transfected human gene in yeast cells, *Saccharomyces cerevisiae*, and therefore is glycosylated, unlike recombinant proteins produced in *E. coli*. Sargramostim stimulates the production and potentiates the function of both granulocytes and macrophages from hematopoietic progenitor cells. It is used to accelerate bone marrow repopulation after high-dose chemotherapy and radiation therapy, and bone marrow transplantation. Adverse effects with sargramostim therapy include bone pain in bone marrow sites (similar to filgrastim), as well as a higher incidence of other systemic symptoms than with filgrastim, including fatigue, fevers, skin rash, malaise, and fluid retention.

Sargramostim (*Leukine, Prokine*) is available in vials containing 250 μg or 500 μg of the drug. The usual dose is 250 μg/sq m daily as a 2-hr IV infusion for up to 21 days.

Supplemental Reading

Chabrier, B.A., and Collins, J.M. (eds.). *Cancer Chemotherapy: Principles and Practice*. Philadelphia: Lippincott, 1990.

DeVita, V.T., Hellman, S., and Rosenberg, S.A. (eds.). *Cancer—Principles and Practice of Oncology* (4th ed.). Philadelphia: Lippincott, 1993.

63

Immunomodulating Drugs

Daniel Wierda and *Leonard J. Sauers*

Immunopharmacology is the study of the use of pharmacological agents as modulators of immune responses. The principal applications involve the use of *immunosuppressive agents,* that is, compounds that suppress undesirable immune responses, and *biological response modifiers,* that is, drugs, microorganisms, or biological products that enhance or augment immune responses.

Three major therapeutic indications for immunointervention are autoimmune diseases, organ transplantation, and primary immunodeficiency diseases.

Autoimmunity

The body's immune system cells can, on occasion, react against normal endogenous proteins and thereby effect a reaction against certain body tissues. This abnormal immune response is termed *autoimmunity.* Ordinarily, a complex network of feedback loops keeps autoimmune reactions in check. Under certain circumstances, however, normal control is lost and the aberrant immune reaction will result in disease.

Myasthenia gravis is an example of an autoimmune disease in which antibodies are produced against the acetylcholine receptors in the neuromuscular junction. The abnormal immune response results in the breakdown of junctional receptors, ultimately rendering patients weak and unable to move voluntary muscles. Rheumatoid arthritis is another autoimmune disease in which antibodies are secreted against a component of an individual's own immunoglobulins. These antibody-immunoglobulin conjugates (immune complexes) form precipitates in the joints of affected individuals. Phagocytic cells are, in turn, attracted to these sites, where they release enzymes that destroy surrounding tissue (inflammation). Immunomodulating agents are often employed in debilitating cases of autoimmune disease to curb the production of autoantibodies.

Organ Transplantation

Suppression of the immune system is a virtual requirement during organ transplantation due to the propensity of the recipient to reject the foreign tissue by immunological mechanisms. Since transplantation is usually performed in patients with a poor prognosis for survival, the use of immunosuppressive agents has potentially great therapeutic benefit, because it provides the only real hope of continued life for many individuals. Immunosuppression can be a valuable form of therapy in persons suffering from diseases with autoimmune components (Table 63-1).

In the past, immunosuppression could only be achieved through the use of *nonspecific* cytotoxic drugs (e.g., cyclophosphamide or azathioprine) which are particularly toxic to rapidly proliferating cells such as those of the bone marrow, gonadal tissue, and gastrointestinal tract. Consequently, serious side effects, including bone marrow depression, overwhelming infections, and sterility, limited their usefulness as immunosuppressants. The concurrent use of corticosteroids with the immunosuppressants increased the risk of additional toxicity. With the development of the immunosuppressant cyclosporine, and more recently FK506, it is now possible to avoid much of this toxicity. Because of its relatively low degree of toxicity, cyclosporine has revolutionized the field of transplantation. It is now possible to successfully transplant tissues not previously considered as candidates for transplantation.

Primary Immunodeficiency Diseases

Primary immunodeficiency diseases (PIDs) are defects of the immune system that are due to genetic abnormali-

Table 63-1. Some Autoimmune Disorders in Which Immunosuppressive Therapy Has Been Utilized

Autoimmune hemolytic anemia
Myasthenia gravis
Cranial arteritis
Idiopathic thrombocytopenic purpura
Membranous glomerulonephritis
Childhood nephrosis
Polymyalgia rheumatica
Polymyositis
Psoriatic arthropathies
Rheumatoid arthritis
Systemic lupus erythematosus
Ulcerative colitis
Uveitis
Wegener's granulomatosis

ties or some failure in normal embryological development. They are usually apparent at birth or develop shortly thereafter. Approximately 36 PIDs have been described, including those specific for humoral immunity (e.g., X-linked agammaglobulinemia, immunoglobulin A [IgA] deficiency), cellular immunity (e.g., DiGeorge syndrome), or a combination of the two (e.g., severe combined immunodeficiency syndrome).

The clinical manifestations of PIDs vary and depend on the aspect of the immune system affected. In general, due to the role of antibodies in protection against bacterial infections, individuals with deficiencies in humoral immunity are more prone to infections from *Streptococcus pneumoniae* and *Haemophilus influenzae*. These individuals are also more prone to infections of the respiratory, gastrointestinal, and urinary tracts due to the protective role of IgA in secretions.

Individuals with defects in cellular immunity are more prone to fungal, protozoal, and viral infections such as *Candida albicans,* cytomegalovirus, and *Pneumocystis carinii* since cell-mediated immune responses are the primary defenses against these types of infection. Due to the role of cell-mediated immunity in tumor surveillance, these individuals will also demonstrate an increased incidence of malignancy if they survive long enough.

The treatment of a PID is based on the aspect of the immune system that is lacking. For those with deficiencies in humoral immunity, the only effective treatment currently available is antibody replacement (e.g., gamma globulin) and medical management of infections. For those with deficiencies in cell-mediated immunity, there is no effective pharmacological treatment. Medical management of infections is usually the only recourse aside from a fetal thymus transplant for those afflicted with DiGeorge syndrome.

General Principles of Immunosuppressive Therapy

Before describing individual drugs, it is important to consider three general principles of immunosuppressive therapy. (1) *Primary immune responses are more readily inhibited than are secondary responses.* Therefore, components of the primary phase of the immune response such as processing, proliferation, and differentiation will be the most sensitive to drug action. Consequently, drugs that are effective in suppressing an immune response in an unsensitized person generally will show much less of an effect, if any, in a sensitized individual. Once a population of memory cells has been established, immunosuppressive drugs show little effectiveness. (2) *Not all immune responses are equally affected by suppressive drugs.* Cellular and humoral immunity may be affected differentially. Additionally, the different classes of immunoglobulins in a humoral response may be variably affected. (3) *Beneficial effects, other than immunosuppression, may result from therapy with these drugs.* In particular, the antiinflammatory properties possessed by certain of these drugs may be valuable, because inflammation often accompanies the immune response. If only an inflammatory reaction is present, a true antiinflammatory drug that is devoid of the many side effects of immunosuppressive agents should be used.

The focus in the next section is on those immunosuppressants that have been shown to be clinically useful. Others that may hold promise in the future are mentioned briefly.

Individual Drugs Used in Organ Transplantation

Corticosteroids

Corticosteroids have been used alone or in combination with other agents in the treatment of autoimmune disorders and for the prevention of allograft rejection. However, the toxicity associated with their use requires prudent administration. The most commonly used of these drugs are prednisone and prednisolone.

Chemistry

The chemistry of the corticosteroids is presented in Chap. 66.

Mechanism of Action

Corticosteroids have immunosuppressive properties, but it is not clear to what extent this activity contributes to their therapeutic effectiveness. A rapid, but transient, reduction in blood lymphocytes occurs following a large single dose of corticosteroids. This lymphopenia is due to the redistribution of lymphocytes, possibly into the bone marrow, rather than to a lympholysis and occurs within 4 to 6 hr of administration. By 24 hr, blood lymphocytes have returned to normal levels. Corticosteroids may affect humoral immune responses by inhibiting antibody synthesis and by interfering with the binding of antibodies to target cells. Since cellular immunity is also impaired by corticosteroids, care must be taken to avoid the occurrence of an infection in the patient.

Although corticosteroids possess immunosuppressive properties, their real value is in controlling the inflammation that can accompany transplantation and autoimmune disorders. Virtually all phases of the inflammatory process are affected by these drugs. Details on the mechanisms of their antiinflammatory properties can be found in Chap. 43.

Clinical Use

Corticosteroid therapy alone is successful in only a limited number of autoimmune diseases, such as idiopathic thrombocytopenia and polymyalgia rheumatica. Numerous side effects result from high-dose, chronic corticosteroid therapy. These drugs have been used in combination with immunosuppressants for the treatment of allograft rejection. A major advantage of the concomitant use of cyclosporine is that the corticosteroids now can be used at lower dosages than was previously possible when they were coadministered with the cytotoxic immunosuppressants.

Adverse Reactions

Although corticosteroids have significant value in immunosuppressive therapy, the problems associated with long-term administration limit their usefulness. These problems include an increased tendency for infections, formation of ulcers, induction of hyperglycemia, and osteoporosis. Additional adverse effects are discussed in Chap. 66.

Preparations and Dosage

The corticosteroids that are used most widely in combination immunosuppressive therapy are prednisone (*Deltasone, Meticorten*) and *prednisolone*. Numerous dosage regimens have been utilized but, in general, initial dosages of 2 to 10 mg/kg/day are employed, tapering to less than 1 mg/kg/day within a few weeks or months. During rejection episodes, daily dosages of up to 1,000 mg/kg can be given for short periods.

Cyclosporine

Cyclosporine is a potent inhibitor of antibody- and cell-mediated immune responses and is the immunosuppressant of choice in the therapy for the prevention of transplant rejection. It also has application in the treatment of autoimmune diseases.

Chemistry

Cyclosporine is a highly stable 11-amino acid cyclic polypeptide (Fig. 63-1). The molecule is very lipophilic and, essentially, is not soluble in water. It is administered intravenously in an ethanol vehicle or orally dissolved in olive oil and ethanol.

Absorption, Metabolism, and Excretion

After oral administration, cyclosporine is absorbed slowly and incompletely with great variation occurring among individuals. Peak plasma concentrations are reached in 3 to 4 hr and the plasma half-life is between 10 and 27 hr. The drug is extensively metabolized by hepatic mixed-function oxidase enzymes and is excreted principally by means of the bile into the feces. At least 18 metabolites have been identified, about 6 percent of which are excreted in the urine. Metabolism results in inactivation of the immunosuppressive activity. Agents that enhance or inhibit the mixed-function oxidase enzymes will alter the therapeutic response to cyclosporine.

Mechanism of Action

Cyclosporine exhibits a high degree of specificity in its actions on T cells without significantly impairing B-cell activity. It can inhibit the T-cell–dependent limb of antibody production by lymphocytes by preventing differentiation of B cells into antibody-secreting plasma cells. It is not lymphotoxic; rather, the drug inhibits the production and acquisition of responsiveness to interleukins (particularly interleukin-2) in T cells. Because T cells appear to require interleukin-2 stimulation for continuous growth, cyclosporine impairs the proliferative response of T cells to antigens. Once T cells have been stimulated by antigens to synthesize interleukin-2, cyclosporine can no longer suppress the proliferation of T cells induced by this cytokine.

Clinical Effects

Cyclosporine has been approved for use in kidney, liver, heart, and heart-lung transplant patients. For example, its use in cadaveric kidney transplantation produces a patient survival rate of 95 percent and a graft sur-

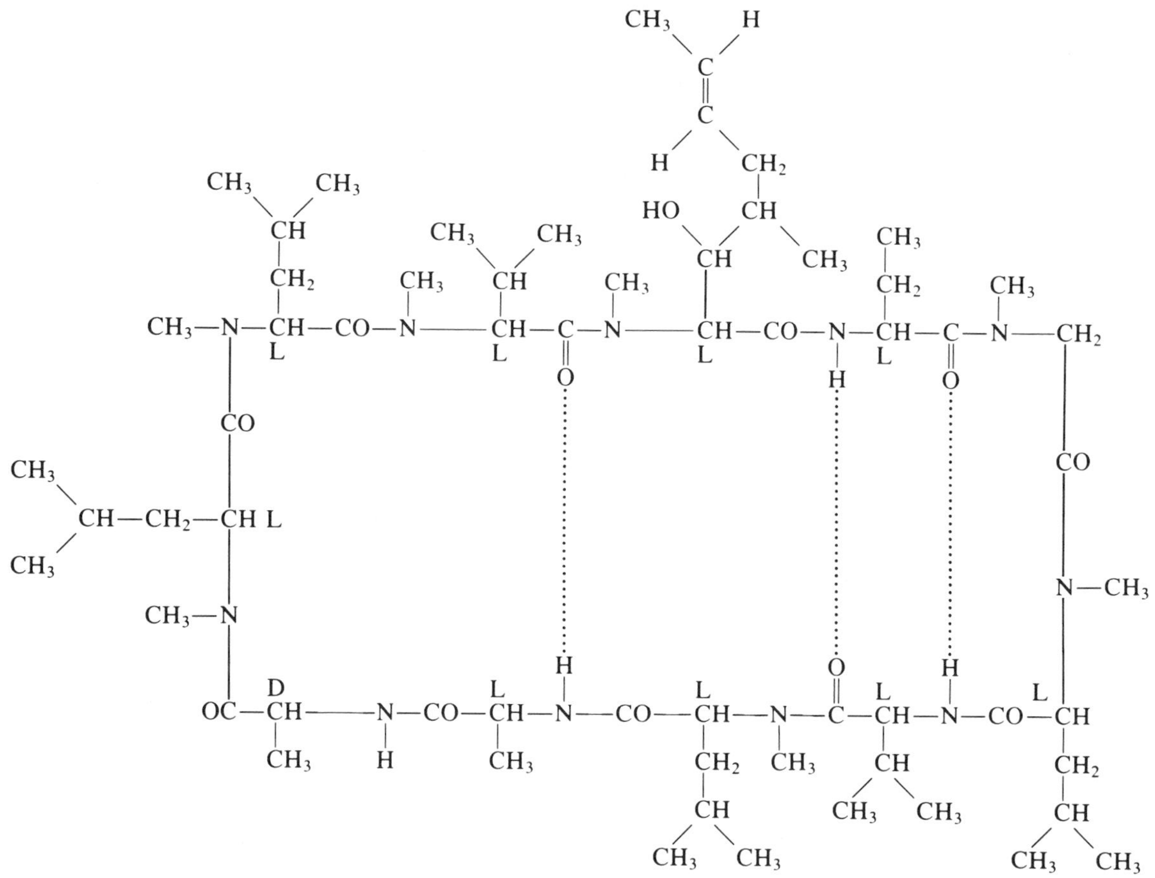

Figure 63-1. Cyclosporine.

vival rate of almost 80 percent. It is currently under study for use in pancreas, bone marrow, single lung, and heart-lung transplant procedures; the results to date are promising. Its use is particularly encouraging in transplantation procedures in children. It is recommended that corticosteroids be used concomitantly, although at half or less of their usual dose. Cyclosporine is not recommended for use with other immunosuppressants. However, patients being treated with azathioprine and steroids can be successfully switched to cyclosporine and steroids if side effects develop. Cyclosporine inhibits both the primary and secondary phases of the *cell-mediated* immune response. While effective in the primary *antibody-mediated* response, cyclosporine is relatively ineffective in the secondary phase.

Numerous studies have shown that cyclosporine is a more effective immunosuppressant than previously available drugs. There are fewer rejections, fewer side effects, and a better incidence of patient survival. Success almost equal to that of first-time recipients has been achieved with retransplantation procedures in patients who have

previously rejected grafts following conventional immunosuppressive therapy.

Cyclosporine is an inhibitor of chronic or immune-mediated inflammation. Consequently, it appears to have promise in the treatment of autoimmune disease. It has a beneficial effect on the course of rheumatoid arthritis, uveitis, insulin-dependent diabetes, systemic lupus erythematosus, and psoriatic arthropathies in some patients. Toxicity is more of a problem in these conditions than during use in transplantation since higher doses of cyclosporine are often required to suppress autoimmune disorders. It is too early to tell whether cyclosporine will become as useful in autoimmune conditions as it is in transplantation procedures.

Adverse Effects

Compared with previously available therapy, the adverse effects associated with cyclosporine are much less severe, but still are worthy of concern. Myelosuppression does not occur, and patients do not become neutropenic or thrombocytopenic. Bacterial infections are not a problem and, with the possible exception of reactivation of Epstein-Barr virus, viral infections have not been an area of concern. Nephrotoxicity is the major side effect, with reactions, after high doses, occurring in 25 to 40 percent of transplant patients. Effects range from severe tubular necrosis to chronic interstitial nephropathy. This effect is generally reversible with dosage reduction. Vasoconstriction appears to be an important aspect of cyclosporine-induced nephrotoxicity. Hypertension occurs in 25 percent of the patients and more frequently in those patients with some degree of renal dysfunction. Reversible hepatotoxicity has been observed in a small percentage of patients.

Preparations and Dosage

Cyclosporine (*Sandimmune*) is available as an oral solution in 50-ml bottles (100 mg/ml) and in 5-ml sterile ampules (50 mg/ml).

FK506

FK506 is a second-generation immunosuppressive agent with properties similar to those of cyclosporine A. It is a macrolide antibiotic extracted from the fermentation broth of the soil fungus *Streptomyces tsukubaensis*. Both cyclosporine A and FK506 selectively inhibit transcription of a specific set of lymphokine genes in T lymphocytes (e.g., interleukin-2, interleukin-4, and interferon-γ). How these drugs specifically suppress gene expression is not clear. Both drugs bind to cytoplasmic proteins in lymphocytes. Although these binding proteins (cytophilins) are different, they share similar functions in that they are important for the intracellular folding of proteins. It is speculated that these proteins are important in regulating gene expression in T lymphocytes and that both drugs somehow interfere in this process. Experimentally, FK506 is about 100 times more potent than cyclosporine A in prolonging graft survival. FK506 has also been shown to be effective when given intermittently, in contrast to cyclosporine A, which requires daily dosing to be effective. FK506 does not display the nephrotoxic side effect of cyclosporine A, and therefore it is being used as a replacement for cyclosporine when kidney immunosuppression is required.

Cytotoxic Drugs

Drugs that are capable of killing immunologically competent cells have been used widely in immunosuppressive therapy. These cytotoxic agents preferentially destroy rapidly dividing cells, thus explaining their effectiveness as immunosuppressive agents. Unfortunately,

any cell that is replicating is a target for their action. This lack of specificity leads to serious side effects and a less than optimal success rate for immunosuppressive therapy. Until recently, the cytotoxic drugs, in combination with corticosteroids, provided virtually the only mode of treatment with any chance of success. Although a number of cytotoxic drugs have immunosuppressive properties, only **azathioprine** and **cyclophosphamide** have been used extensively.

Cytotoxic drugs have been classified as being either *phase-specific* or *cycle-specific*. Phase-specific drugs are toxic during a specific phase of the mitotic cycle, usually the S-phase, when DNA synthesis is occurring. Therefore, these drugs are most effective against rapidly proliferating cells. Azathioprine, 6-mercaptopurine, and methotrexate belong to this class. Cycle-specific drugs can kill both cycling and intermitotic cells, resulting in a general depletion of immune cells. These drugs, however, show preference for proliferating cells. Cyclophosphamide is the major cycle-specific drug used for immunosuppression.

Azathioprine

Azathioprine, in combination with corticosteroids, has historically been used more widely than any other drug in immunosuppressive therapy.

Chemistry

Azathioprine is classified as a purine antimetabolite. It is a derivative of 6-mercaptopurine, containing an imidazole radical attached to the sulfur atom in the 6 position (Fig. 63-2).

Mechanism of Action

Azathioprine is a phase-specific drug that is toxic to cells involved in nucleic acid synthesis. It is converted in vivo to thioinosinic acid, which competitively inhibits the synthesis of inosinic acid, the precursor to adenylic acid and guanylic acid. The major consequence of this action is the inhibition of DNA, rather than RNA and protein, synthesis. Both cell-mediated and humoral immune responses are suppressed by azathioprine.

Azathioprine is a relatively powerful antiinflammatory agent. Although its beneficial effect in various conditions is principally attributable to its direct immunosuppressive action, the antiinflammatory properties of the drug play an important role in its overall therapeutic effectiveness.

Absorption, Metabolism, and Excretion

Azathioprine is well absorbed following oral administration, with peak blood levels occurring within 1 to 2 hr. It is rapidly and extensively metabolized to 6-mercaptopurine, which is further converted in liver and erythrocytes to a variety of metabolites, including 6-thiouric acid.

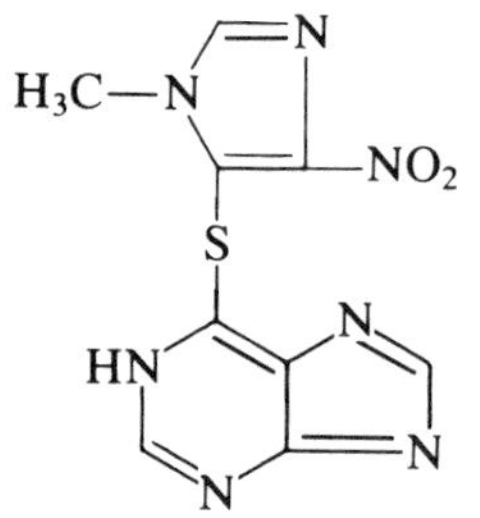

Figure 63-2. Azathioprine.

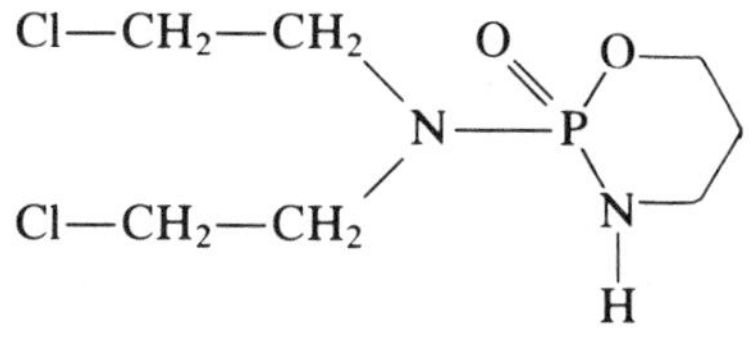

The route of excretion of metabolites is in the urine. The half-life of azathioprine and its metabolites in the blood is about 5 hr. Although both azathioprine and 6-mercaptopurine have immunosuppressive activity, the better oral absorption of azathioprine is the reason for its more widespread clinical use.

Clinical Uses

Azathioprine has been used widely in combination with corticosteroids to inhibit rejection of organ transplants, particularly kidney and liver allografts, and in certain disorders with autoimmune components, most commonly rheumatoid arthritis. It is as effective as cyclophosphamide in the treatment of Wegener's granulomatosis. It has largely been replaced by cyclosporine in immunosuppressive therapy.

Adverse Effects

The therapeutic use of azathioprine has been limited by the number and severity of adverse effects associated with its administration. Bone marrow depression resulting in leukopenia or thrombocytopenia, or both, may occur. Gastrointestinal toxicity may be a problem as well. It is also mildly hepatotoxic. Because of its immunosuppressive activity, azathioprine therapy can lead to serious infections. It has been shown to be mutagenic in animals and humans and carcinogenic in animals.

Preparations and Dosage

Azathioprine (*Imuran*) is available as 50-mg tablets and as a 20-ml vial containing the equivalent of 100 mg azathioprine as the lyophilized sodium salt to be used for IV administration following reconstitution.

Cyclophosphamide

Cyclophosphamide is most commonly used as an antineoplastic agent. However, in combination with corticosteroids, it has been used with some success in immunosuppressive therapy. Chapter 62 contains more detailed information on this drug.

Figure 63-3. Cyclophosphamide.

Chemistry

Cyclophosphamide is chemically related to the nitrogen mustards. It contains a cyclic phosphamide group (Fig. 63-3).

Mechanism of Action

Cyclophosphamide is a cycle-specific drug that can kill both replicating and nonreplicating cells. Its administration results in the cross-linking of DNA by metabolites of the parent drug. Cyclophosphamide is toxic to both T cells and B cells, but because their rate of recovery is slower, the effect on B cells is more pronounced. Consequently, the drug is most effective at suppressing humoral immune responses. Cell-mediated responses are more variable; some are inhibited while others are enhanced. The drug's toxicity toward T suppressor lymphocytes may explain the augmented cellular responses.

Absorption, Metabolism, and Excretion

Cyclophosphamide is well absorbed from the gastrointestinal tract and from parenteral sites of administration. It requires metabolic activation to become immunosuppressive (see Chap. 62).

Clinical Use

Cyclophosphamide is generally not effective in preventing allograft rejection reactions and is therefore not a treatment of choice in these situations. It has, however, been used successfully in combination with corticosteroids in several autoimmune disorders, including Wegener's granulomatosis, idiopathic thrombocytopenic purpura, childhood nephrosis, and severe rheumatoid arthritis. This result is probably due to its effectiveness in suppressing ongoing immune responses. Unlike azathioprine, it has little or no antiinflammatory activity. As for azathioprine, its use as an immunosuppressant has essentially been replaced by cyclosporine.

Adverse Effects

Great care should be exercised in using cyclophosphamide because of its toxicity to replicating cells. Bone marrow depression that results in severe leukopenia and thrombocytopenia may result, predisposing the patient to serious infections. Anorexia, nausea, or vomiting may occur as a result of its gastrointestinal toxicity. Alopecia is a possible side effect. Hemorrhagic or nonhemorrhagic cystitis may result from the toxic metabolites of cyclophosphamide that are present in the urine. Interstitial pulmonary fibrosis and gonadal suppression, resulting in infertility or sterility, also have been reported. In addition, secondary malignancies have developed in some patients treated with cyclophosphamide during antineoplastic therapy.

Preparations and Dosage

Cyclophosphamide (*Cytoxan*) is available as 25- and 50-mg tablets and vials for injection containing 100, 200, and 500 mg.

Other Cytotoxic Drugs

Although azathioprine and cyclophosphamide are the most popular cytotoxic drugs used for immunosuppression, others have been employed. Among these is methotrexate, a phase-specific agent that acts by inhibiting folate metabolism. It is highly toxic and appears to offer no advantages over azathioprine. Chlorambucil, an alkylating agent, has actions similar to those of cyclophosphamide. In contrast, its adverse effects are fewer in that alopecia and gastrointestinal intolerance are almost never encountered. Although its potency as an immunosuppressive agent is considerably less than that of cyclophosphamide, it may prove to be a suitable alternative in certain disorders. See Chap. 62 for further details on these agents.

Antibodies

Antiserum can be raised against lymphocytes or thymocytes by the repeated injection of human cells into an appropriate recipient, usually a horse. The use of such antiserum or the immunoglobulin fraction derived from it has been used to produce immunosuppression. Although antilymphocytic serum has been shown to suppress cellular and often humoral immunity against a variety of tissue graft systems, the responses are variable, particularly from one batch of serum to another.

Antithymocyte Globulin

Antithymocyte Globulin (ATG) is purified immunoglobulin from hyperimmune serum of horses immunized with human thymus lymphocytes. It has been used successfully alone and in combination with azathioprine and corticosteroids in the prevention of renal allograft rejection. Although it has benefit prophylactically, its use during rejection episodes may be its greatest value.

Antithymocyte globulin binds to circulating T lym-phocytes in the blood, which are subsequently removed from the circulation by the reticuloendothelial system. It also reduces the number of T lymphocytes in the thymus-dependent areas of the spleen and lymph nodes.

Since the preparations are raised in heterologous species, reactions may occur against the foreign proteins, leading to serum sickness and nephritis. The concomitant use of corticosteroids may alleviate this response.

The antibody is usually administered in dosages of 10 to 30 mg/kg body weight daily for approximately 14 days.

Orthoclone OKT3

Orthoclone OKT3 (muromonab-CD3) is a mouse monoclonal antibody used for the prevention of kidney or hepatic transplant rejection and as prophylaxis in cardiac transplantation. It is also used to deplete T cells in marrow from donors before bone marrow transplantation.

OKT3 alters the cell-mediated immune response by binding to the CD3 (cluster of differentiation antigen, T3) glycoprotein on T lymphocytes. CD3 is located next to the antigen recognition complex on T lymphocytes. Because of the close proximity of both cell surface glycoproteins, OKT3 blocks the antigen recognition site after binding to CD3. These T cells are unable to recognize foreign antigen and cannot participate in rejecting an organ graft. Within minutes of the first OKT3 injection, total circulating T cells are rapidly depleted from the blood. They later reappear, devoid of CD3 and antigen recognition complexes.

Experimentally, OKT3 is being used in combination with cyclosporine A. It is hoped that the two agents will act synergistically, allowing for lower doses of cyclosporine A. This in turn should lower the incidence and severity of adverse side effects from cyclosporine A therapy.

Adverse side effects include fever, pulmonary edema, vomiting, headache, and anaphylaxis. These symptoms usually appear within 45 to 60 min after the initial administration. Neutralizing antibodies may develop over time, which necessitate adjusting the dosage upward to compensate for loss of therapeutic activity. Infection can become a problem during chronic therapy.

OKT3 is usually given intravenously at a dose of 5 mg/kg/day for 10 to 14 days.

Biological Response Modifiers

A number of disorders can be treated with immunomodulating agents called *biological response modifiers* (BRMs), that is, drugs that have the ability to enhance the body's immune response. These disorders include immu-

Table 63-2. Biological Response Modifiers

MICROORGANISMS

Bacillus Calmette-Guérin
Muramyl dipeptides
Streptococcal components
Klebsiella pneumoniae (Biostim)
Propionibacterium components
Nocardia components
Pseudomonas components
Salmonella components

FUNGAL OR YEAST DERIVATIVES

Bestatin
Cyclosporine
FK506
MTP-PE

PEPTIDES

Dialyzable leukocyte extract
Neuropeptides
Thymic factors
Tuftsin

CYTOKINES

Colony stimulating factors
Interferons
Interleukins
Tumor necrosis factor

SYNTHETIC COMPOUNDS

ABPP (U-54461) AS-101
ADA-202-718
Azimexon
Cimetidine
CL-246, 738
CL-259, 763
Hydroetranol (NPT-15392)
Imuthiol (DTC)
Isoprinosine (inosiplex)
Levamisole
Pimelantide (RP-40639)
Therafectin

OTHERS

Forphenicol
Retinoids
Vitamin A (calcitriol)

nodeficiency diseases, cancer, some types of viral and fungal infections, and certain autoimmune disorders. These drugs may work on cellular or humoral immune systems, or both. Due to the limited response capacity of the immune system, BRMs generally are more effective when the disease entity (viruses, bacteria, fungi, tumor cell, tumor mass) is quantitatively small. Therefore, these agents work best when antibiotics already have been used or when chemotherapy has been undertaken, or when tumors have been removed by surgery.

BRMs are nonspecific in action, causing a general stimulation of the immune system. A wide variety of agents are capable of general potentiation of the immune system (Table 63-2). Although a number of these agents have been studied in humans, only those discussed below have gained widespread use. In most cases, the pharmacology of these compounds has not been well described.

Bacillus Calmette-Guérin

Bacillus Calmette-Guérin (BCG) and its active component, muramyl dipeptide, are bacterial products that require an intact immune system to produce their effects. BCG immunotherapy has been most successful in the treatment of bladder cancers. In one large multicenter study, BCG immunotherapy significantly reduced the incidence of bladder tumor recurrence when compared with no treatment or chemotherapy with thiotepa or doxorubicin. BCG is effective by intravesicular treatment of carcinoma in situ that is confined to the bladder.

Chemistry

BCG is a viable attenuated strain of *Mycobacterium bovis*. Nonviable strains of the bacterium also have been shown to augment the immune response. The smallest active compound derived from BCG thus far has been identified as muramyl dipeptide.

Mechanism of Action

The T cell is a principal target for BCG. It also appears to stimulate natural killer cells, which, in turn, can kill malignant cells. It has been suggested that BCG cross-reacts immunologically with tumor cell antigens.

Adverse Effects

The most dangerous complication of BCG therapy is severe hypersensitivity and shock. Chills, fever, malaise, and immune complex and renal disease are among the other side effects noted. The route of administration influences the nature of the side effects.

Preparations and Dosage

BCG is available in three types of preparations: live unlyophilized, live lyophilized, and killed lyophilized. Administration may be by oral, intradermal, intravenous, intralesional, or intrapleural injection, or by scarification.

The dosage is not standardized, but varies according to the route of administration. For example, 10^8 viable organisms have been administered by scarification, while 10^7 bacilli have been applied intralesionally.

Thymic Factors

The thymic factors are a group of polypeptides that have been isolated from the thymus and are used in T-lymphocyte immunodeficiency states.

Chemistry

A number of thymic preparations are available. These include thymic humoral factor, a dialyzable fraction of calf thymus extract, thymosin fraction 5, and thymodulin. Each is a mixture of several polypeptides from calf thymus extract: serum thymic factor, a nonapeptide secreted by thymic epithelium, and thymopoietin, a protein with a molecular weight of 5,260 daltons.

Mechanism of Action

Thymic factors are used to enhance T-lymphocytic functions. Therefore, to be effective, patients must have some precursor T lymphocytes. Thymic factors to date do not activate selective T-lymphocyte subsets, and their activity depends on the nature of the thymic extract preparation, the dosage used, and the patient's T-lymphocyte subsets available as targets.

Clinical Uses

Thymic factors have been used with some success in clinical trials in patients with severe combined immunodeficiency, DiGeorge or Nezelof syndrome, and viral disorders. Studies with thymodulin show promise in treating symptoms in asthmatics and patients with allergic rhinitis. The primary consideration for potential use of thymic factors in these immunodeficiency states is the presence of T-lymphocyte precursors.

Adverse Effects

Few major side effects have been reported, especially with purer forms produced by genetic engineering. Crude thymic preparations have produced allergic side effects in some patients.

Preparation

For most thymic factors no standard dosage or preparation is available yet.

Cytokines

An exciting application of immunomodulating therapy is in the use of cytokines (*lymphokines, monokines*). As mentioned earlier in this chapter, immune cell function is regulated by cytokines produced by leukocytes or other supporting cells. With the advent of genetic engineering, cytokines can be produced in pure form and in large quantities.

Interleukin-2

Interleukin-2 (IL-2) is a cytokine that promotes the proliferation, differentiation, and recruitment of T and B lymphocytes, natural killer cells, and thymocytes.

Chemistry
Human recombinant interleukin-2 (rIL-2) is a 15,500 kilodalton glycoprotein. It was originally designated as T-cell growth factor because of its capability of stimulating T helper and T cytotoxic cells.

Mechanism of Action
rIL-2 binds to IL-2 receptors on responsive cells and induces proliferation and differentiation of T helper cells and T cytotoxic cells. rIL-2 also can induce B-lymphocyte proliferation, activate macrophage activity, and augment the cytotoxicity of natural killer cells.

Clinical Uses
rIL-2 is administered systemically as an immunopotentiating agent in patients with acquired immunodeficiency disease (AIDS) and to augment specific antitumor immunity. Patients with renal cell carcinoma or melanoma have been effectively treated with rIL-2 in combination with adoptive transfer immunotherapy. The latter refers to the injection of the patient's own cytokine-activated killer cells or tumor-infiltrating lymphocytes that were previously placed in tissue culture for several weeks in the presence of rIL-2.

Adverse Effects
Systemic administration of rIL-2 causes symptoms of fever, nausea, vomiting, fatigue, and malaise. Other symptoms include flushing, diarrhea, rigors, rash, edema, and symptomatic hypertension. These tend to occur at increased dosage levels and are attenuated by reducing the dosage.

Preparation and Dosage
Optimum dosages are still being evaluated. The maximum tolerated dose is reported to be 1 million units/sq m.

Interferon-α and Interleukin-1

Two other cytokines, human recombinant interferon-α (rIFN-α) and recombinant interleukin-1 (rIL-1), also show promise as immunopotentiators, principally as adjuvants in the treatment of viral and malignant disorders. rIFN-α is produced by leukocytes and has the ability to inhibit viral DNA and RNA replication. At lower doses, rIFN-α can stimulate macrophages, T lymphocytes, and natural killer cell activity. rIL-1 is produced by macrophages in the host and is necessary for activation and development of immune cells. Intravenous administration of rIL-1 is associated with the general augmentation of immune responses.

Additional cytokines being evaluated as immunomodulators include recombinant tumor necrosis factor and colony stimulating factors. Clinical trials are characterizing the antitumor effect of tumor necrosis factor and the ability of colony stimulating factors to augment hematopoiesis in patients after chemotherapy.

Immune Globulin

Immune globulin is isolated from pooled human plasma either from donors in the general population or from hyperimmunized donors. It is used principally in the treatment of certain immune deficiencies.

Chemistry

Standard immune globulin solutions contain a distribution of all immunoglobulin subclasses with antibody titers for most major bacterial, viral, and fungal pathogens.

Absorption, Metabolism, and Excretion

Immune globulin is given intramuscularly or intravenously. It has an in vivo half-life of about 3 weeks.

Clinical Uses

Immune globulin is recommended in the treatment of primary humoral immunodeficiency, congenital agammaglobulinemias, common variable immunodeficiency, severe combined immunodeficiency, idiopathic thrombocytopenic purpura, autoimmune hemolytic anemia, hepatitis, and measles. It is also used in the prevention of infection in chronic lymphocytic leukemia and Kawasaki disease.

Autoimmune hemolytic anemia can arise as a result of the destruction of red blood cells coated with autoantibodies. Intravenous infusion of immune globulin can rapidly reverse the immune-mediated blood cell depletion. It is believed that immune globulin protects by binding to macrophage receptors (Fc), which then mediate the red cell destruction.

Adverse Effects

The principal side effects noted are possible anaphylactoid reactions and severe hypotension.

Preparations and Dosage

Immune globulin is supplied in 10- to 200-ml single-dose vials. Monthly dosages of 100 to 200 mg/kg are recommended.

Myeloid Colony Stimulating Factors

Recombinant granulocyte-macrophage colony stimulating factor (GM-CSF) and *granulocyte stimulating factor (G-CSF)* are cytokines, or growth factors, that support the survival, clonal expansion, and differentiation of hematopoietic cells. These factors are normally produced in the body by monocytes, fibroblasts, and endothelial cells. GM-CSF induces bone marrow progenitor cells, belonging to the granulocyte or macrophage lineage, to divide and differentiate into mature cells. G-CSF induces the maturation of granulocyte progenitor cells.

In general these recombinant cytokines are indicated for the acceleration of the recovery of circulating white blood cells in patients who have depressed hematopoiesis, either as a result of chemotherapy or of congenital disor-

Table 63-3. Indications for the Use of Myeloid Colony Stimulating Factors

Clinical indications	
GM-CSF, G-CSF	Chemotherapy-induced neutropenia
GM-CSF	Human immunodeficiency virus (HIV) infection
GM-CSF	Autologous bone marrow transplantation
G-CSF	Congenital neutropenia
GM-CSF, G-CSF	Cyclic neutropenia
GM-CSF	Myelodysplastic syndromes
GM-CSF	Aplastic anemia
Experimental indications	
GM-CSF, G-CSF	Myelosuppressive therapy in HIV infection
GM-CSF	Stimulation of peripheral blood stem cells obtained for bone marrow transplant
G-CSF	Escalating dose chemotherapy
G-CSF	Compromised host, e.g., burn patients
GM-CSF, G-CSF	Chemosensitization of myeloid leukemias

ders of hematopoiesis. A list of indications for the use of GM-CSF and G-CSF is provided in Table 63-3.

Adverse effects for both cytokines are those commonly observed following the administration of molecules produced by biotechnological means and include diarrhea, asthenia, rash, malaise, fever, headache, bone pain, chills, and myalgia. Many of these effects can be ameliorated by the administration of analgesics and antipyretics.

The recommended dosage for GM-CSF is 250 μg/m^2/ day for 21 days as a 2-h IV infusion. Doses for G-CSF range from 3 to 69 gm/kg; it can be given subcutaneously for 14 to 28 days.

Supplemental Reading

Borel, J.F., et al. Pharmacology of cyclosporine (Sandimmune®). *Pharmacol. Rev.* 41:240, 1989.

Clark, J.W. Biological Response Modifiers. In H.M. Pinedo, D.L. Longo, and B.A. Chabner (eds.), *Cancer Chemotherapy and Biological Response Modifiers.* New York: Elsevier, 1988.

Fauci, A.S., et al. Immunomodulators in clinical medicine. *Ann. Intern. Med.* 106:421, 1987.

Ruszala-Mallon, V., et al. Low molecular weight immunopotentiators. *Int. J. Immunopharmacol.* 10:497, 1988.

VII

Drugs Affecting the Endocrine System

64

Introduction to Endocrine Pharmacology

John A. Thomas

Endocrine pharmacology concerns itself with the therapeutic use of hormones, hormone-like substances, or drugs that can act either by suppressing or enhancing the metabolism of certain glands of internal secretion. *Endocrine replacement therapies* involve the physiological use of hormones to supplement low or deficient levels of endogenous hormones, such as occurs in Addison's disease and diabetes mellitus. Supraphysiological (i.e., pharmacological) amounts of hormones also can be used for their antiinflammatory properties, such as when certain adrenocortical steroids are used to treat rheumatoid arthritis and other collagen-related diseases (see Chap. 43). In addition, hormones themselves can be used in the diagnosis of some endocrine disorders. Various milestones in endocrine therapy are highlighted in Table 64-1.

Endocrine pharmacology not only involves the therapeutic and diagnostic use of hormones but also is concerned with drugs that can suppress or influence secondarily the organs of internal secretion. Antithyroidal drugs possess no inherent hormonal properties, but they can be effective inhibitors of thyroxine synthesis. Still other drugs that are used entirely for nonendocrine therapies can affect hormonal levels and the endocrine system. Drugs that are used in certain cancer therapies adversely affect rapidly dividing cells and can be deleterious to gonadal function. Some drugs that act on the nervous system but have no inherent hormonal activity can still affect the endocrine system, leading to disturbances in the menstrual cycle and infertility.

In addition to drugs that can exert unwanted effects on endocrine end organs (e.g., gonads) or on central nervous system (CNS) areas involved in hormonal regulation, there are agents that can either influence the hepatic biotransformation of hormones or interfere with their plasma binding.

Hormones of Low Molecular Weight

Steroids (e.g., androgens, estrogens, and corticoids), either natural or synthetic, are hormones of relatively low molecular weight that are used to treat a variety of endocrine and nonendocrine diseases. *Thyroxine* is a small molecule used extensively in the treatment of myxedema as well as in certain other nonthyroid disorders (see Chap. 69). Usually, hormones with low molecular weights (i.e., about 300) are chemically complexed in the blood to large carrier proteins. For example, thyroxine binds reversibly to a plasma globulin (thyroxine-binding globulin, TBG), while cortisol can bind to corticosteroid-binding globulin (CBG). These *carrier proteins not only provide a mechanism for extending the biological half-life of the smaller hormones but also provide a circulating reservoir of hormone* that the body can draw on as the physiological need arises.

Use of Supraphysiological Dosages of Hormones

When hormone treatments are used to supplement low levels of endogenous hormones, bringing them up to normal physiological levels, the likelihood of producing toxic side effects or creating further endocrine imbalances is minimal. On the other hand, many hormone therapies involve the use of *supraphysiological* dosages. With elevated amounts of hormone circulating in the blood, the potential for the appearance of unwanted effects is much greater.

Table 64-1. Some Milestones in Endocrine Therapy

Approximate year(s)	Event	Investigators
1906	Discovery of uterine-stimulating properties of posterior pituitary extracts	Dale
1909-1911	Use of posterior pituitary extracts	Bell; Hofbauer
1914	Isolation of thyroxine	Kendall et al.
1921	Discovery of insulin	Banting & Best
1925	Use of parathyroid extracts	Collip et al.
1928	Discovery of gonadotropin substitutes	Aschheim & Zondek, Cole & Hart
1930s	Elucidation of androgen-estrogen antagonism	Huggins et al.
1940s	Therapeutic use of adrenocortical steroids	Hench et al.
1942	Advent of oral hypoglycemic agents	Jambon et al.
1945	Discovery of antithyroidal drugs	Astwood et al.
1947	Discovery of hypothalamic releasing hormones	Green & Harris
1950s	Synthesis of orally active steroids	Pincus; Rock et al.
1953	Synthesis of oxytocin	du Vigneaud et al.
1950-1960	Isolation and synthesis of ACTH molecule	Evans & Li; Hoffmann; others
1970s	Purification of hypothalamic releasing hormones and development of radioimmunoassay	Guillemin, Schally, Yalow
1978-1979	rDNA human insulin developed	Villa-Komaroff et al., Goeddell et al.
1979	rDNA human growth hormone developed	Goeddell et al.
1980	Clinical use of rDNA human insulin	Keen et al.
1980	First dose of human rDNA insulin administered	
1981	Clinical trials of human rDNA growth hormone	
1982	FDA approves use of human rDNA insulin	
1984	Somatomedin C expressed from *Escherichia coli*	
1984	Human FSH and LH cloned	
1985	FDA approves use of human rDNA growth hormone	
1988	Clinical trials of erythropoietin	
1989	FDA approves use of erythropoietin	
1991	FDA approves use of GnRH agonists	

Key: ACTH = adrenocorticotropic hormone; rDNA = recombinant DNA; FSH = follicle-stimulating hormone; LH = luteinizing hormone; GnRH = gonadotropin-releasing hormone.

Chemical Suppression of Endocrine Secretions

Hormones can be administered in order to suppress endocrine secretions. Pharmacological doses of either natural or synthetic steroids can inhibit endocrine secretions of the adenohypophysis. Synthetic progestins effectively block the release of pituitary gonadotropins, inhibiting ovulation. In addition, substances without inherent hormonal properties can also affect endocrine function. For example, the thioamide-type agents (see Chap. 69) interfere with thyroxine biosynthesis and hence are effective antithyroidal drugs, useful in the management of thyrotoxicosis. In general, drugs that inhibit gonadal steroidogenesis are toxic and therefore of limited clinical utility. Although certain adrenal adenocarcinomas have been treated with drugs that inhibit steroidogenesis, such agents are not without undesirable effects.

Drug-Hormone Interactions

Although all of the mechanisms by which drugs and hormones affect one another's actions are not clearly understood, a number of such interactions have been identified as having clinical importance. For instance, the chronic administration of certain drugs (e.g., long-acting barbiturates and anticoagulants) stimulates the formation of increased amounts of hepatic drug-metabolizing enzymes. These enzymes are, in part, responsible for metabolizing steroids as well as nonsteroid drugs. Increasing the activity of hepatic enzymes can lead to an acceleration of steroid metabolism and thereby shorten the biological half-lives and physiological effects of these hormones.

The potential for drug-hormone interaction also exists when both drug and hormone can bind to the same plasma protein. In this case, one substance might displace the other from its binding site, thereby increasing the proportion of unbound material in the blood. Such an interaction has been demonstrated between salicylates (e.g., aspirin) and thyroxine. If salicylates are administered after thyroxine, they can dislodge the hormone from its plasma albumin binding sites and increase the concentration of free thyroxine in the blood.

Several other drug-hormone interactions have been described. Administration of a number of different drugs can affect standard laboratory tests of endocrine function. For example, drugs may, by interfering with the ability of thyroxine to bind to plasma proteins, give erroneous results when thyroxine levels are used for the evaluation of thyroid gland function. Also, morphine and certain antipsychotic drugs (also marijuana) can transiently suppress pituitary gonadotropins and lead to infertility and impotence.

Regulation of Hormone Receptors

There are a number of clinical conditions in which blood levels of certain hormones are markedly elevated but in which the expected physiological response is not seen. This apparent decrease in responsiveness is most likely due to some change in the target tissues rather than to any inherent change in the hormone itself.

Hormones must first bind to specific receptors, often located on the surface of the target tissue cells, before the cells can respond appropriately to them. It is possible that high circulating concentrations of hormones can induce changes in the surface receptors that render them less able to bind hormone molecules. Thus, cells may have a control mechanism to prevent any overreaction to elevated hormone concentrations. Although the exact mechanism by which the receptors on the cell surface bind less hormone in the presence of prolonged, excessive hormone levels is not known, the decreased binding has been thought to involve an actual loss in the total number of receptors available.

Several possible mechanisms to account for receptor loss have been proposed: The receptors could be degraded metabolically, they could change their three-dimensional conformation in such a way that binding is less efficient or impossible, or they could translocate to deeper sites in the lipid membrane, where they would no longer be available for hormone binding.

That tissue hormone receptors may have the ability to alter their responsiveness in the presence of prolonged and increased concentrations of their specific hormone (and perhaps other hormones as well) may have profound implications for clinical medicine as well as for the field of endocrine physiology. These changes in tissue responsiveness are likely to be important control mechanisms. For example, one cause of so-called insulin resistance purportedly is a target cell receptor defect(s).

Insulin resistance is a metabolic state in which normal or high concentrations of insulin produce a less than normal biological response. Insulin resistance can be due to three causes: (1) abnormal β-cell secretory product, (2) circulating insulin antagonists, or (3) target tissue defects (i.e., postreceptor or postbinding defects). Target tissue defects are believed to cause insulin resistance in non–insulin-dependent diabetes mellitus (NIDDM).

At present, much of the information regarding the regulation of hormone receptors must still be considered speculative and awaits further elucidation.

Supplemental Reading

Barsano, C.P., and Thomas, J.A. Endocrine disorders of occupational and environmental origin. *Occup. Med. State Art Rev.* 7:479, 1992.
Del Valle, J., and Yamada, T. The gut as an endocrine organ. *Ann. Rev. Med.* 41:447, 1990.
DeVries, C.P., et al. The insulin receptor. *Diabetes Res.* 11:155, 1989.
Galloway, J.A., et al. Biosynthetic human proinsulin. *Diabetes Care* 15:666, 1992.
Getzenberg, R.H., Pienta, K.J., and Coffey, D.S. The tissue matrix: Cell dynamics and hormone action. *Endocr. Rev.* 11:399, 1990.
Moghissi, K.S. Clinical applications of gonadotropin-releasing hormones in reproductive disorders. *Endocrinol. Metabol. Clin. North Am.* 21:125, 1992.
Orth, D.N. Corticotropin-releasing hormone in humans. *Endocr. Rev.* 13:164, 1992.
Thomas, J.A. Toxic Responses of the Reproductive System. In M.O. Amdur, J. Doull, and C.D. Klaassen (eds.), *Toxicology—The Basic Science of Poisons* (4th ed.). New York: Pergamon, 1991. Pp. 484–520.
Thomas, J.A., and Keenan, E.T. *Principles of Endocrine Pharmacology.* New York: Plenum, 1986.

65

Hypothalamic and Pituitary Gland Hormones

Priscilla S. Dannies

The hormones of the pituitary gland participate in the control of reproductive function, body growth, and cellular metabolism; deficiency or overproduction of these hormones disrupts this control. Therefore, the regulation of their secretion and the use of these hormones in replacement therapy are therapeutically significant. Clinical use in the past was limited by several factors. Since pituitary hormones from other species are usually not effective in humans, preparations used clinically have had to come from human material, such as pituitary glands or urine, which has limited available supplies. In addition, these hormones are not effective when taken orally because they are proteins, which are digested. The ability to prepare at least some of these hormones in large quantities by recombinant DNA techniques and the development of stable analogues that can be injected in depot form or taken nasally have permitted increased and more effective clinical use of these hormones.

Anterior Pituitary Hormones

Six major hormones are secreted by the adenohypophysis, or anterior pituitary gland (Fig. 65-1). Cells in the anterior pituitary gland also synthesize and secrete small amounts of a variety of other proteins, including renin, angiotensinogen, sulfated proteins, fibroblast growth factor, and other mitogenic factors. The physiological significance of these other secretory products is not known, but they may participate in autocrine regulation of the gland.

The secretion of anterior pituitary hormones is controlled in part by hypothalamic regulatory factors, which are stored in the hypothalamus and are released into the adenohypophyseal portal vasculature. Hypothalamic regulatory factors so far identified are peptides, with the exception of dopamine. Secretion of anterior pituitary hormones is also controlled by factors produced more distally that circulate in the blood. Predominant control of hormone production may be relatively simple, as with thyroid-stimulating hormone (TSH), the production of which is primarily stimulated by thyrotropin releasing hormone (TRH) and inhibited by thyroid hormones, or it may be complex, as with prolactin, the production of which is affected by many different neurotransmitters and hormones.

All anterior pituitary hormones are released in a pulsatile manner into the bloodstream; the secretion of many also varies with time of day or physiological conditions, such as exercise or sleep. At least part of the pulsatility of anterior pituitary hormone secretion is caused by pulsatile secretion of hypothalamic regulatory hormones. Understanding the rhythms that control hormone secretion has led to better uses of hormones in therapy.

Growth Hormone

Growth hormone, or somatotropin, is a protein with a molecular weight of 22,000 and a structure that is similar to that of prolactin and placental lactogens. Growth hormone stimulates linear body growth in children and regulates cellular metabolism in a variety of tissues in adults as well as children. Growth hormone causes stimulation of lipolysis, enhanced production of free fatty acids, elevated blood glucose, and a positive nitrogen balance. Many of its anabolic actions are mediated by enhanced production of an insulin-like growth factor (IGF-1), a protein produced in the liver and peripheral target tissue in response to growth hormone.

The episodic release of growth hormone is the most pronounced of the pituitary hormones. Serum levels between bursts of release are usually low (<5 ng/ml) and

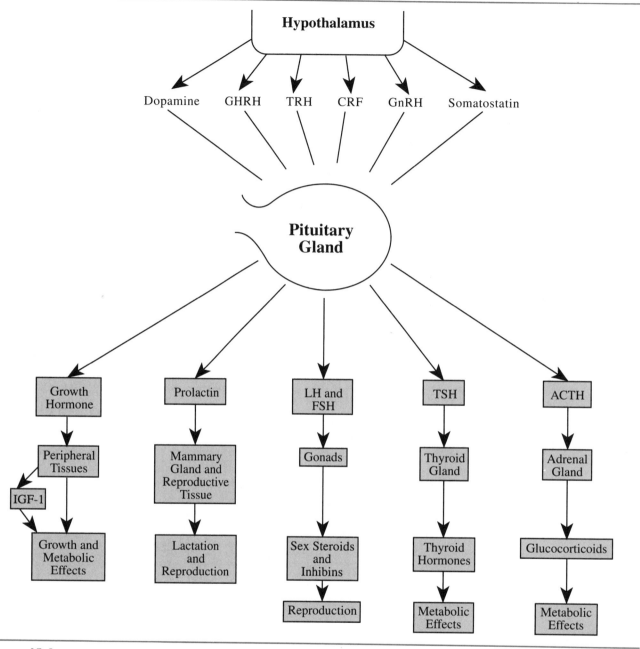

Figure 65-1. Hormones of the hypothalamus and the anterior pituitary gland. Hormones released from the hypothalamus represent one of the major means of controlling secretion from the anterior pituitary gland. GHRH = growth hormone releasing hormone; TRH = thyrotropin releasing hormone; CRF = corticotropin releasing hormone; GnRH = gonadotropin releasing hormone; LH = luteinizing hormone; FSH = follicle-stimulating hormone; TSH = thyroid-stimulating hormone; ACTH = adrenocorticotropic hormone; IGF-1 = insulin-like growth factor 1.

increase over 10-fold when release is elevated. The marked variation in serum levels may be the result of strong controls in opposite directions by two hypothalamic hormones, growth hormone releasing hormone (GHRH) and somatostatin. Growth hormone is released during sleep, with maximum release occurring one hour after the onset of sleep. Growth hormone is also released after exercise, by hypoglycemia and in response to arginine and levodopa (L-dopa).

Growth hormone deficiency in children results in short

stature; there are no obvious problems in growth hormone–deficient adults. Excessive secretion of growth hormone results in gigantism in children and in acromegaly in adults. Long bones will not grow in adults because the epiphyses are closed, but the bones in the extremities (hands, feet, jaw, and nose) will enlarge. Measurements of serum growth hormone levels are used for diagnosis of deficiency or excess secretion, but random measurements are not useful because large variations in growth hormone levels occur normally. Growth hormone deficiency is best demonstrated by lack of response to provocative stimuli, such as after administration of L-dopa or arginine. Excessive secretion is demonstrated by elevated serum levels of IGF-1 and an inability of oral glucose to suppress serum growth hormone levels to less than 2 ng/ml.

Growth hormone deficiency is treated by injections of growth hormone. The original source for the hormone was human pituitary glands, but use of hormone from this source was suspended when several cases of Creutzfeldt-Jakob disease were associated with its use. Fortunately, human growth hormone from recombinant sources became available at the time that use of the pituitary source was discontinued. Supplies were limited when the only source was pituitary glands from cadavers, but the supply of recombinant growth hormone is unlimited, allowing research into other possible uses, such as wound and fracture healing.

Two forms of recombinant growth hormone are available: recombinant somatotropin (*Humatrope*), which has the same amino acid sequence as pituitary-derived growth hormone, and recombinant somatrem (*Protropin*), which has an N-terminal methionine that pituitary-derived growth hormone does not have. Early reports that antibodies developed frequently to this form were later shown to be due to the presence of contaminants; current preparations are cleaner and antibodies develop less frequently. Subcutaneous injections each evening are more effective than the original regimen of intramuscular injections three times a week and are also preferred by patients. Part of the reason for the increased effectiveness may be that injections in the evening mimic the natural surge that occurs after sleep. Stimulation of growth is most effective when treatment begins early, and injections can be continued until the epiphyses close. Since no known problems are associated with growth hormone deficiency in adults, there is no reason to continue injections after induction of growth can no longer occur.

The primary treatment of acromegaly is surgery. Pharmacotherapy is used in conjunction with radiation therapy when surgery is too risky or not successful and is given to patients with excessive GHRH secretion. There are two drugs that are useful. One is bromocriptine, a dopamine agonist (see Chap. 38). Although dopamine stimulates growth hormone release in normal individuals, it inhibits growth hormone release in up to 50 percent of acromegalics. This drug has the advantage of being taken orally. The second drug is an analogue of somatostatin, octreotide, described in the section on hypothalamic regulatory hormones. Octreotide is effective in 80 to 90 percent of acromegalics, but must be injected. The two drugs in combination may be more effective than either alone.

Prolactin

Human prolactin is similar in structure to human growth hormone and both are good lactogens. Human prolactin was not identified as a separate hormone until the 1970s. Prolactin has diverse actions in different species. It exerts osmoregulatory influences in some species by enhancing sodium reabsorption, and in other species it stimulates ovarian and testicular steroidogenesis. In women, prolactin acts with other hormones on the mammary gland during pregnancy to develop and, afterward, to maintain lactation. Prolactin also must have a role in functions involving reproduction, because hyperprolactinemia causes impotency in men and amenorrhea and infertility in women. Chronically elevated levels of circulating prolactin are associated with suppression of 17β-estradiol and testosterone production in the ovaries and testes.

In women, prolactin serum levels increase during pregnancy and, at least initially after birth, during suckling. In both men and women, prolactin increases after sleep starts and continues to increase during the night, and it increases markedly during stress. Prolactin release is episodic during the day. Over 30 hormone and neurotransmitters affect prolactin production, but the dominant physiological control appears to be negative, mediated by dopamine released from the hypothalamus. Dopaminergic agonists inhibit prolactin release and antagonists, such as the antipsychotic drugs, increase release.

There is currently no known therapeutic use for prolactin, but serum levels are measured for diagnostic purposes. Elevated prolactin levels (>100 ng/ml) in the absence of stimulatory factors, such as antipsychotic drugs, are an indication of pituitary adenoma. Approximately one third of women who need treatment for infertility have high serum prolactin levels. Galactorrhea, or inappropriate lactation, is sometimes, but not always, associated with high prolactin levels. Hyperprolactinemia caused by microadenomas is treated successfully in most cases by the long-acting dopaminergic agonist, bromocriptine. Macroadenomas can be treated with bromocriptine before surgery to reduce their size. The doses given, usually 5 mg/day, are lower than those used to treat acromegaly and Parkinson's disease, and therefore the side effects, usually nausea and postural hypotension, are less likely to cause problems. Bromocriptine is also used to end lactation when it is not desired after parturition.

Thyroid-Stimulating Hormone

Thyroid-stimulating hormone, or thyrotropin, is a glycosylated protein of two subunits, α and β. The structure of this hormone is very similar to that of luteinizing hormone (LH) and follicle-stimulating hormone (FSH). The α chain is homologous in all three hormones; the β chain of each confers specificity. TSH stimulates the thyroid gland to produce thyroid hormones. Deficiencies are treated by giving thyroxine itself, which can be taken orally. TSH (*Thyropin*) is available for diagnostic purposes to differentiate between pituitary and thyroid gland failure as causes of hypothyroidism.

Gonadotropins

Follicle-stimulating hormone, LH, and human chorionic gonadotropin (hCG) are glycoproteins that are similar in structure to TSH; they contain α and β subunits. The glycosylation is not identical among the different hormones and the type of glycosylation influences the half-life of the hormone. A sulfated N-acetylgalactosamine attached to LH, but not FSH, causes LH to be much more rapidly metabolized; the half-life of LH is 30 min and that of FSH is 8 hr.

Luteinizing hormone and FSH are pituitary hormones that are secreted approximately every hour. In women before menopause, this pattern is superimposed on much larger changes that occur during the normal menstrual cycle. FSH is released in substantial amounts during the follicular phase of the menstrual cycle, and is required for proper development of ovarian follicles and for estrogen synthesis from the granulosa cells of the ovary. The major secretion of LH occurs in an abrupt burst just before ovulation. Luteinizing hormone is required for progesterone synthesis in the luteal cells and androgen synthesis in the thecal cells of the ovary. In men, FSH stimulates spermatogenesis and synthesis of androgen-binding protein in the Sertoli cells of the testes. Luteinizing hormone stimulates testosterone production from the Leydig cells. Production of these hormones is controlled by gonadotropin releasing hormone (GnRH) from the hypothalamus and by feedback control from target organs through steroids and forms of a protein, inhibin.

Injections of these hormones are used to treat infertility in women and men. These hormones are not yet available by recombinant techniques, because their structure, with subunits and glycosylation, is so much more complex than that of growth hormone. Sources of gonadotropins are therefore still from human urine. Human menopausal gonadotropin (hMG, *Pergonal*) is isolated from the urine of postmenopausal women and contains both FSH and LH. Because FSH is more stable, the primary activity in this preparation is FSH. A purified preparation of FSH from the same source (*Urofollitropin*) is also available. Luteinizing hormone and hCG bind to the same gonadal receptors and have the same actions, but hCG is more stable. hCG is produced in large amounts during early pregnancy by the trophoblast of the placenta. Preparations of hCG (*A.P.L., Follutein, Pregnyl, Profasi HP*) from the urine of pregnant women are therefore used for LH activity.

Therapy with gonadotropins is used to treat infertility in women who have potentially functional ovaries and who have not responded to other treatments. The therapy is designed to simulate changes that occur in the normal menstrual cycle, as far as is practical. A common protocol is injections of hMG (75 units of FSH and LH) per day for 9 to 12 days, until estradiol levels are equal to that in a normal woman, followed by a single large dose of hCG (5,000–10,000 units) to induce ovulation. Two problems with this treatment are risks of ovarian hyperstimulation and of multiple births. Ovarian hyperstimulation is characterized by sudden ovarian enlargement associated with an increase in vascular permeability and rapid accumulation of fluid in peritoneal, pleural, and pericardial cavities. The incidence of ovarian hyperstimulation induced by gonadotropin therapy is 0.5 to 2.0 percent. To prevent such occurrences, ovarian development is monitored during treatment by ultrasound techniques and by measurements of serum levels of estradiol.

Purified FSH is used to prepare follicles for in vitro fertilization, because LH activity might cause premature ovulation. Purified FSH is also used to treat infertility in women with polycystic ovarian disease; in this disease LH and androgen production may be elevated already.

Gonadotropins are used to induce spermatogenesis in hypogonadotropic hypogonadal men; a lengthy treatment is required to obtain mature sperm. hCG is injected for several weeks to increase testosterone levels; this is followed by injections of hMG for several months. Prepubertal cryptorchidism can be treated by injections of hCG for up to several weeks.

Adrenocorticotropic Hormone

Adrenocorticotropic hormone (ACTH), or corticotropin, is a peptide of 39 amino acids, synthesized as a larger precursor and cleaved. ACTH stimulates production of glucocorticords from the adrenal cortex. Release of ACTH is dependent on diurnal rhythms; serum levels are highest in the early morning. Secretion of this peptide also increases under stress. It is easier and less expensive to treat patients with adrenocortical insufficiency with glucocorticoid replacement therapy than to use ACTH. Therefore, although ACTH (*Acthar*) is available, its use is restricted to diagnosis; a shorter 24 amino acid analogue (*Cosyntropin*) is also used. Intravenous administration of ACTH should result in peak plasma levels of glucocorticords within 30 to 60 min if the adrenal gland is functional. Prolonged administration of ACTH in a repository form, however, may be necessary to stimulate steroid production, because ACTH has long-term trophic effects on adrenal cells in addition to the rapid stimulation of steroid production. If the cause of steroid deficiency is at the level of the pituitary gland, ACTH should eventually stimulate steroid production.

Hypothalamic Regulatory Hormones

Five peptides isolated from the hypothalamus regulate release of one or more pituitary hormones. In addition, dopamine released from the hypothalamus is one of the major factors that controls prolactin release by inhibiting it. All the peptides are synthesized as parts of larger precursors and then processed into the mature forms.

Somatostatin

Somatostatin (or somatotropin release inhibiting factor, SRIF) occurs primarily as a 14 amino acid peptide, although a 28 amino acid form also exists. Somatostatin was originally isolated from the hypothalamus based on its ability to inhibit the release of growth hormone. It was later found in many locations, including cortex, brainstem, spinal cord, gut, urinary system, and skin, and was found to inhibit the secretion of many substances in addition to growth hormone (Table 65-1).

Somatostatin has a half-life of 23 min and is therefore not useful clinically. An 8 amino acid analogue of somatostatin with 2 D-amino acids substituted for the naturally occurring L-amino acids is more stable, and has a half-life of 90 min. This analogue, called *octreotide,* is used successfully to counteract unpleasant effects caused by overproduction of secreted bioactive substances by certain tumors.

Table 65-1. Effects of Somatostatin

Inhibition of secretion of:
  Growth hormone
  Thyroid-stimulating hormone
  Prolactin
  ACTH
  Insulin
  Glucagon
  Pancreatic polypeptide
  Gastrin
  Cholecystokinin
  Secretion
  Vasoactive intestinal peptide
  Glucagon
  Exocrine pancreas secretion
Inhibition of bile flow
Inhibition of mesenteric blood flow
Decreased gastrointestinal motility

Subcutaneous injections reduce growth hormone secretion from pituitary tumors, hyperinsulinemia from insulinomas, and secretions from gastrointestinal endocrine tumors and carcinoid tumors that cause severe diarrhea. Octreotide may also control severe diarrhea associated with acquired immunodeficiency syndrome (AIDS) that has not responded to other treatments.

There are some transient side effects of gastrointestinal discomfort and decreased glucose tolerance that usually last only a few weeks after initiation of therapy. The most significant side effect of octreotide is formation of gallstones, resulting from reduced bile flow, which occurs with prolonged use.

Growth Hormone Releasing Hormone

GHRH is a peptide of 40 amino acids that stimulates release of growth hormone. It is presently used for investigational diagnostic purposes. The development of stable analogues may allow these compounds to be used in place of growth hormone therapy.

Thyrotropin Releasing Hormone

Thyrotropin releasing hormone, or protirelin, was the first releasing hormone to be characterized and consists of three amino acids. It was isolated based on its ability to stimulate TSH release, but, once isolated, it was found to be equally potent in stimulating prolactin release. So many hormones and neurotransmitters affect prolactin release that it is difficult to sort out which are involved in any particular physiological situation, and the times when TRH is important in prolactin release, if it is at all physiologically, are not known. Prolactin levels are elevated in mild hypothyroidism, suggesting that the increased secretion of TRH that would be expected under these conditions is also stimulating prolactin release.

Thyrotropin releasing hormone (*Relefact TRH, Thypinone*) is used to test pituitary responsiveness during the diagnosis of thyroid disease. An injection of TRH causes a rise in TSH that peaks in about 30 min in a normal person. In primary hypothyroidism, the defect is in the thyroid gland and, thus, TSH levels are elevated; TSH levels will increase further in response to TRH. In secondary hypothyroidism, the defect is in the pituitary gland; TSH levels are low and there is little response to TRH. In mild hyperthyroidism or hypothyroidism, thyroid hormone levels may still fall within the normal range, but the TSH response to TRH is suppressed in hyperthyroidism and enhanced in hypothyroidism.

Gonadotropin Releasing Hormone

Gonadotropin releasing hormone (gonadorelin, luteinizing hormone releasing hormone [*LHRH*]) is a deca-

Table 65-2. Biological Actions of GnRH Agonists and Antagonists

Drug	Dose and regimen	Effect
Agonist	Low, pulsatile	Pituitary and gonadal stimulation
Agonist	High, constant	Initial pituitary and gonadal stimulation followed by suppression within 2 weeks
Antagonist	Constant	Pituitary and gonadal suppression

Table 65-3. Clinical Application of GnRH or Analogues

Pituitary stimulation
Induction of ovulation
Hypogonadotropic hypogonadism
Cryptorchidism
Delayed puberty
Pituitary inhibition
Prostate cancer
Endometriosis
Uterine leiomyomas
Polycystic ovarian disease
In vitro fertilization

peptide that stimulates the production of LH and FSH. It is released in bursts from the hypothalamus at approximately hourly intervals, although in women the interval may lengthen in the luteal end of the menstrual cycle. The pituitary gland responds to these regular pulses by producing LH and FSH. The pattern of LH and FSH in cycling women, including the large burst of LH release before ovulation, can be stimulated by regular administration of GnRH pulses. The large burst of LH from the pituitary gland appears to be induced by complicated feedback by steroids and other products of the gonads that change the response of pituitary gland to the GnRH pulses, rather than to large changes in the amounts of GnRH secreted. The stimulatory response to GnRH is critically dependent on the timing of the pulses (Table 65-2). Continual administration of GnRH does not have the same effects as pulsatile administration; although production of LH and FSH is first stimulated, within a few days it is suppressed. Part of this desensitization to GnRH is caused by a decrease in the number of pituitary receptors for GnRH; additional postreceptor mechanisms are also important in this complete suppression.

Gonadotropin releasing hormone itself has a short half-life, 7 min, if given intravenously. Structural variations of the decapeptide have resulted in the development of more stable agonists with higher affinity for the GnRH receptor; a common modification is to substitute a D-amino acid for the sixth amino acid, glycine, in GnRH. Antagonists are also being developed, but are not clinically available as yet.

In situations in which stimulation of gonadotropin production is needed (Table 65-3), the pituitary gland usually is capable of responding to GnRH when administered appropriately, even in cases of hypogonadotropic hypogonadism, when LH and FSH levels are always low. Therefore, GnRH therapy can be substituted for gonadotropin therapy by administering GnRH (*Factrel*) pulses intravenously using an indwelling pump. GnRH itself is used since the short half-life is important to prevent accumulation between pulses. The advantage of this procedure compared to intramuscular injections of gonadotropins for treating infertility is that normal levels of LH and

FSH should be maintained because of feedback from the gonads. In women, there should be a decreased risk of ovarian hyperstimulation and multiple births because the procedure should not stimulate inappropriately high levels of gonadotropins.

For uses that involve pituitary inhibition and long-term suppression of gonadotropin production, several stable potent derivatives of GnRH are available, including leuprolide (*Lupron*), goserelin (*Zoladex*), and buserelin (*Suprafact*). These differ at the sixth and tenth amino acids, but all behave in an essentially identical fashion to suppress gonadotropin secretion. To avoid multiple injections, they are formulated so that they can be inhaled nasally several times a day or injected only once a month in a long-lasting depot form.

Androgens stimulate growth of prostatic cancer, and reducing androgens is used for palliative treatment. Methods of reducing androgens are treatment with estrogenic compounds, which suppress gonadotropin release, or castration, which removes the source of androgens. Estrogens increase mortality in men as a result of cardiovascular complications, unlike the cardioprotective effect estrogens have in women, and castration is not popular. Treatment with GnRH analogues to suppress gonadotropin release is therefore favored. Signs and symptoms of prostatic cancer may increase shortly after initiation of therapy, because initially stimulation of the pituitary gland occurs.

Uterine leiomyomas, polycystic ovarian disease, and endometriosis all regress when gonadotropin secretion is decreased. GnRH agonists all relieve these conditions, but the relief usually lasts only as long as the GnRH agonist is administered, and the conditions generally return within a few months after the therapy ceases. GnRH agonists are sometimes given along with FSH when stimulating follicles for in vitro fertilization to prevent premature ovulation caused by release of pituitary LH.

The main side effect, once the pituitary gland is suppressed, is occasional hot flashes (sudden sweating). Long-term use may result in decreased bone density, as occurs in menopause. If clinically useful GnRH antagonists are developed, they will have the advantage of not causing initial stimulation of gonadotropin production.

Corticotropin-Releasing Factor

This hormone consists of 41 amino acids and stimulates ACTH release. It is used for investigational purposes.

Hormones of the Posterior Pituitary Gland

Antidiuretic hormone (ADH) and oxytocin are synthesized in the supraoptic and paraventricular nuclei in the brain and are transported in secretory granules through axons to the posterior lobe. These hormones are cyclic peptides of eight amino acids. Each is synthesized as a larger precursor, which is processed into the hormone, plus a protein that binds the hormone, called neurophysin. Antidiuretic hormone and oxytocin have different amino acids at positions 3 and 8.

Antidiuretic Hormone

Antidiuretic hormone (or vasopressin) is released in response to increases in plasma osmolarity or decreases in blood volume. It produces its antidiuretic activity in the kidney, causing the cortical and medullary parts of the collecting duct to become permeable to water, thereby increasing water reabsorption, reducing osmolarity, and increasing volume. It causes this effect by binding to a subset of vasopressin receptors (Table 65-4), called V_2, that have relatively high affinity for the hormone. ADH also has actions at sites other than the kidney; V_2 receptors mediate an increase in circulating levels of two proteins involved in blood coagulation: factor VIII and von Willebrand's factor. At higher concentrations, ADH interacts with V_1 receptors to cause general vasoconstriction by smooth muscle contraction of most blood vessels.

Several preparations are available. One is vasopressin, or ADH, itself (*Pitressin*), which is available for injection. Lypressin (*Diapid*) is a natural analogue that comes from pigs, and differs from human vasopressin in that it has a lysine instead of an arginine. It has less pressor activity than vasopressin and can be administered nasally. Both have half-lives of about 15 min. Desmopressin (*DDAVP*) is a more stable analogue without an amine group at the first amino acid, and with D-arginine instead of L-arginine.

Table 65-4. Actions of ADH

Receptor type	Response
V_1	Pressor
V_2	Antidiuretic
	Hemostatic

Table 65-5. Uses of ADH and Analogues

diabetes insipidus
nocturnal enuresis
hemostatic disorders
experimental uses in controlling bleeding

It has very little pressor activity. It can be given subcutaneously or nasally, and the effects last for 12 hr.

Desmopressin is preferred for treatments when the pressor effect is not desired because it is stable. The primary indication for therapy (Table 65-5) is diabetes insipidus, a disorder that results when ADH secretion is reduced, that is characterized by polydipsia, polyuria, and dehydration. Desmopressin is used to reduce primary nocturnal enuresis, or bedwetting, in children. It is also given to people with mild hemophilia A or with some types of von Willebrand's disease in which von Willebrand's factor is quantitatively low, but not abnormal. In these cases, desmopressin is given when excessive bleeding occurs, or before surgery to help reduce bleeding indirectly by increasing the amounts of the coagulation factors. A possible adverse effect of desmopressin is water intoxication if too much is taken.

Vasopressin is used in experimental conditions to control bleeding after surgery. It is sometimes applied locally; if it is given systemically, the pressor effects may cause angina due to coronary vasoconstriction.

Oxytocin

Oxytocin causes milk release (milk letdown) by stimulating contraction of the myoepithelial cells of the milk ducts in lactating mammary glands, which forces milk from the alveoli of the breast. Oxytocin release is stimulated by suckling and also by auditory and visual stimuli, such as the baby's cry. Oxytocin also stimulates contraction of uterine smooth muscle in late phases of pregnancy. The physiological role of oxytocin in induction of parturition is uncertain because serum levels normally increase only in the later stages of labor. It is used clinically, however, to induce labor when appropriate and to augment labor, if necessary.

Indications for induction of labor are medical, such as placental insufficiency or premature rupture of membranes; the decision is made by balancing the risk to the fetus and mother against the risks that will occur if pregnancy is continued. Oxytocin should not be used if marked cephalopelvic disproportion or fetal distress is present. Excessive administration may cause tetanic uterine contractions that can cause fetal distress and uterine rupture. To induce labor, synthetic oxytocin (*Pitocin*) is given by intravenous infusion. The effective dose varies widely. A common regimen is to begin with a very low dose, such as 1 mU/min, and increase the dose by 1-mU increments every 15 to 30 min to avoid overstimulation of the uterus. Oxytocin is also used in incomplete or therapeutic abortions and to control postpartum uterine bleeding. Oxytocin is also available as a nasal spray (*Syntocinon*), which is used as an aid to lactation when milk ejection is impaired.

Supplemental Reading

Casper, R.F. Clinical uses of gonadotropin-releasing hormone analogues. *Can. Med. Assoc. J.* 144:153, 1991.

deVos, A., Ultsch, M., and Kossiakoff, A.A. Human growth hormone and extracellular domain of its receptor: Crystal structure of the complex. *Science* 255:306, 1992.

Fiete, D., et al. A hepatic reticuloendothelial cell receptor specific for SO_4-4 GalNAcβ1,4GlcNAcβ1,2 Manα that mediates rapid clearance of lutropin. *Cell* 67:1103, 1991.

Hurst, R.D., and Modlin, I.M. The therapeutic role of octreotide in the management of surgical disorders. *Am. J. Surg.* 162:499, 1991.

Jorgensen, J.O.L. Human growth hormone replacement therapy: Pharmacological and clinical aspects. *Endocr. Rev.* 12:189, 1991.

Klibanski, A., and Zervas, N.T. Diagnosis and management of hormone-secreting pituitary adenomas. *N. Engl. J. Med.* 324:822, 1991.

Martin, K., et al. Management of ovulatory disorders with pulsatile gonadotropin-releasing hormone. *J. Clin. Endocrinol. Metab.* 71:1081A, 1990.

Adrenocortical Hormones and Drugs Affecting the Adrenal Cortex

Ronald P. Rubin

The therapeutic use of steroids began in the early 1930s, even before the identity of adrenocortical hormones was known. P. S. Hench, working at the Mayo Clinic, made the astute clinical observation that the symptoms of female arthritics were alleviated when they became pregnant. He reasoned that remission of these symptoms was the result of adrenocortical hypersecretion during pregnancy. However, at the time only crude adrenal extracts were available, and his theory could not be tested. After World War II, when synthetically produced corticosteroids became available, they were tested in acute arthritis by Hench and his coworkers. Fortunately, adequate dosages were employed and the clinical response was dramatic. These observations immediately evoked a wide interest. The year after the first published report of the efficacy of cortisone in the treatment of rheumatoid arthritis, the Nobel Prize for medicine was jointly awarded to Hench and to Kendall and Reichstein for their efforts in isolating and synthesizing adrenal corticosteroids.

However, enthusiasm evoked by these first reports was soon tempered by a more sober evaluation of the toxic effects of administering high doses of steroids over a long period of time. The predominant side effect noted at the time was salt retention with edema. Chemists have spent decades attempting to alter the steroid structure to decrease sodium-retaining activity and to increase antiinflammatory glucocorticoid activity.

The steroidal nature of cortical hormones was established in 1937 when desoxycorticosterone was synthesized by Reichstein. Eventually, it was clearly established that the adrenal cortex elaborated a number of hormones, and that these compounds differed in the amount of inherent metabolic (*glucocorticoid*) and electrolyte-regulating (*mineralocorticoid*) activity each possessed. The actions of these hormones extend to almost every cell in the body. In humans, *hydrocortisone (cortisol)* is the main carbohydrate-regulating steroid, and *aldosterone* is the main electrolyte-regulating steroid.

Steroid Physiology

Anatomy of the Adrenal Cortex

The mammalian adrenal cortex is divided into three concentric zones: the *zona glomerulosa, zona fasciculata,* and *zona reticularis.* The zona glomerulosa produces hormones, such as aldosterone, that are responsible for regulating salt and water metabolism; the zona fasciculata produces glucocorticoids; and the zona reticularis produces adrenal androgens. While secretion by the two inner zones is controlled by pituitary adrenocorticotropic hormone (ACTH), aldosterone produced by the zona glomerulosa is principally controlled by the renin-angiotensin system. Desoxycorticosterone, a mineralocorticoid produced in the zona fasciculata, is under ACTH control.

Steroid Biosynthesis

Although the adrenal cortex is primarily involved in the synthesis and secretion of corticosteroids, it is also capable of producing and secreting such steroid intermediates as progesterone, androgens, and estrogens. The adrenal gland synthesizes steroids from cholesterol, which is derived from plasma lipoproteins via the low-density lipoprotein (LDL) and high-density lipoprotein (HDL) pathways. Additionally, cholesterol is released extramitochondrially from cholesterol esters catalyzed by a cholesterol ester hydrolase; this enzyme is activated by phosphorylation brought about by a cyclic adenosine monophosphate (cAMP)-dependent protein kinase. The ACTH-dependent stimulation of cholesterol ester hydro-

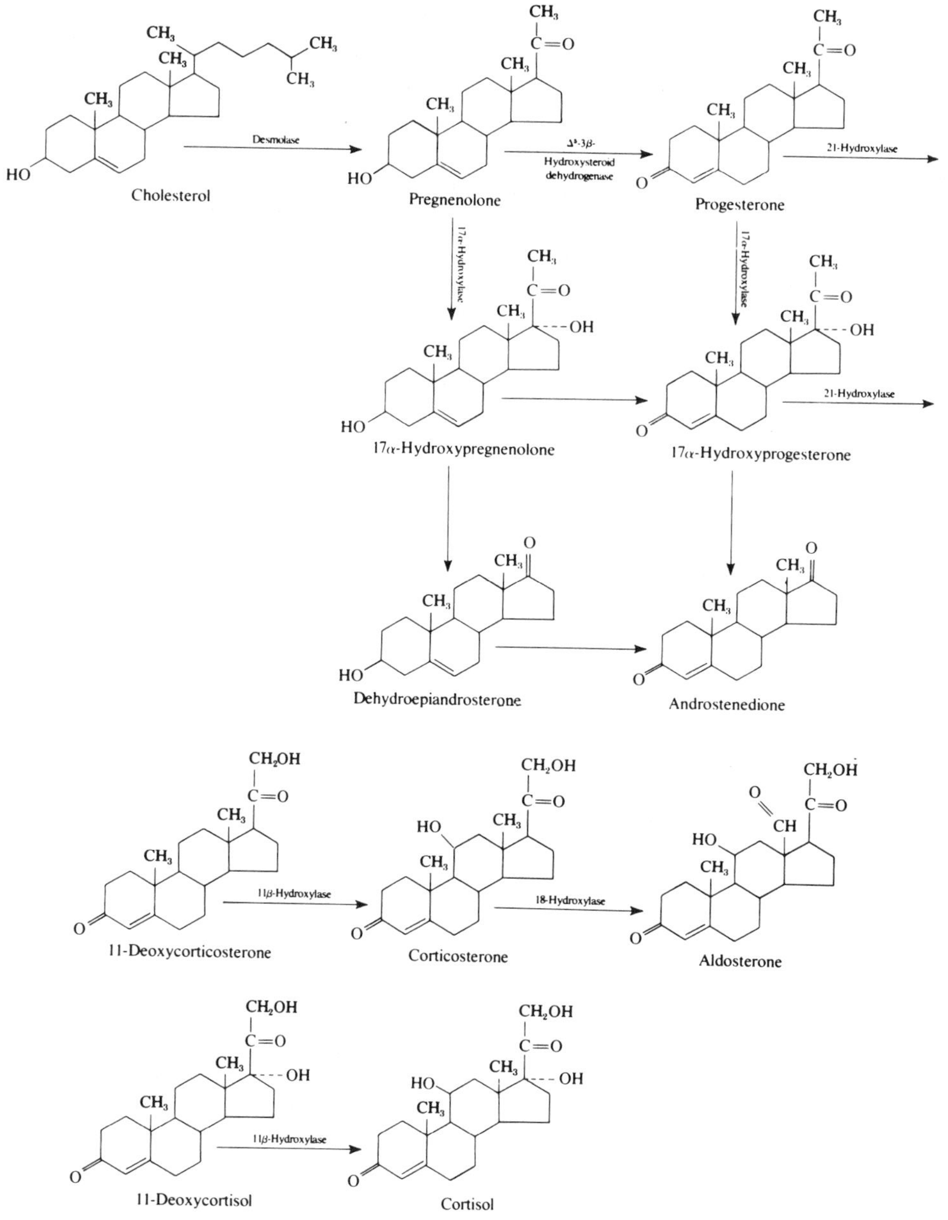

Figure 66-1. Metabolic pathways of corticosteroid biosynthesis.

lase activity provides an additional source of cholesterol for steroidogenesis.

Cholesterol is transported into the mitochondria of steroidogenic tissue, where side chain cleavage (SCC) is carried out. In common with other mixed-function oxidase systems, the cholesterol side chain cleavage requires NADPH and O_2 and a specific cytochrome P450$_{SCC}$. *The rate-limiting step in steroid biosynthesis is the conversion of cholesterol to pregnenolone* (Fig. 66-1). ACTH also stimulates this step, perhaps by enhancing the binding of cholesterol to the cytochrome P450$_{SCC}$ system present in the inner mitochondrial membrane.

Pregnenolone then leaves the mitochondria to become the obligatory precursor of corticosteroids and adrenal androgens. The biosynthetic pathway next branches into two separate routes: One route passes through progesterone and corticosterone to aldosterone, while the other proceeds from 17-α-hydroxyprogesterone and 1-deoxycortisol to yield cortisol. Thus, steroid intermediates are converted to steroid end products by sequential 17-, 21-, and 11-hydroxylation reactions. The steroid hydroxylase system has the characteristics of a mixed-function oxidase since two substrates—steroid and NADPH—are oxidized. All hydroxylases seem to be associated with a specific cytochrome P450. Glucocorticoids are synthesized mainly by $P450_{11\beta}$, whereas aldosterone production is catalyzed by $P450_{c18}$ from deoxycorticosterone.

The 17- and 21-hydroxylase enzymes are associated with microsomes, whereas the 11-β-hydroxylase has a mitochondrial origin. Since the last-named enzyme is not detectable in other steroid-producing tissues, the term *11-oxygenated steroids* is considered synonymous with adrenal steroids. Aldosterone synthesis involves an essential 18-hydroxylation step, with corticosterone as the precursor; this reaction also takes place within the mitochondria.

Steroid Transport in Blood

Glucocorticoids secreted into the systemic circulation are reversibly bound to a specific alpha globulin known as *transcortin* or *corticosteroid-binding globulin* (CBG). This binding system has a high affinity and low capacity for corticosteroids, which contrasts with the low-affinity binding of these compounds to plasma albumin. Approximately 80 percent of the normal cortisol content in human plasma (12 $\mu g/dl$) is bound to CBG, while 10 percent is bound to serum albumin; the remaining 10 percent is the biologically active unbound hormone.

Transcortin acts as a reservoir from which a constant supply of unbound cortisol may be provided to target cells. In addition, when serum albumin levels are low, less circulating cortisol becomes bound, thus yielding a greater physiological effect. Not only does protein binding control the amount of biologically active cortisol available, but it also reduces the rate at which steroids are cleared from the blood and thus limits steroid suppression of ACTH release from the pituitary gland. In addition to regulating the concentration of free hormone, transcortin may subserve additional functions since receptors for transcortin exist on plasma membranes of cells.

The binding affinity of human transcortin is not limited to corticoids. Progesterone and the synthetic glucocorticoid prednisone also can bind to this macromolecule. High estrogen states (pregnancy, estrogen administration, and use of oral contraceptives) greatly increase circulating transcortin levels. Thyroxine also stimulates transcortin formation, while androgen administration will decrease transcortin levels and the amount of bound glucocorticoids.

Steroid Metabolism

Most of the cortisol circulating in the blood will be metabolized before its excretion. The metabolism of adrenal steroids occurs primarily in the liver, and when metabolic processes are altered, as occurs in liver disease, the half-life of cortisol may increase from 100 min to 7 hr.

Two major steps are involved in the metabolism of cortisol. The first involves a reduction of double bonds and the introduction of a hydroxyl group in the A ring to form tetrahydro derivatives; this pathway accounts for 20 to 30 percent of the cortisol excreted. The second step is a glucuronic acid or sulfate conjugation to form more soluble derivatives that are poorly bound to plasma proteins and readily pass into the urine.

Adrenal androgens also are excreted, primarily as sulfates; they constitute about two-thirds of the total urinary 17-ketosteroids excreted. In the male, the other third is contributed by gonadal secretions.

Knowledge of corticosteroid metabolism is important clinically, since *alterations in adrenocortical function can be determined by measuring the amounts of 17-hydroxycorticosteroids.* However, radioimmunoassay of urinary free cortisol (and plasma cortisol) is supplanting measurements of urinary metabolites, despite the fact that less than 1 percent of total cortisol secreted by the adrenal is excreted unchanged.

Knowledge of the metabolic pathways of steroid metabolism also is mandatory for effective and safe use of these compounds when other agents are administered concomitantly. For example, since the metabolism of steroid hormones occurs, in part, through the action of the hepatic oxidative drug-metabolizing enzymes, concomitant administration of anticonvulsant drugs (e.g., phenytoin and carbamazepine), which are potent inducers of glucocorticoid metabolism, will augment the elimination of methylprednisolone severalfold. Also, since a steroid such as prednisone lacks glucocorticoid activity until it is converted to prednisolone by hepatic enzymes, patients with liver disease should receive prednisolone rather than prednisone.

Actions of the Corticosteroids

The pharmacological actions of steroids are generally an extension of their physiological effects. Adrenal corticosteroids exert effects on almost every organ in the body. In normal physiological concentrations, they are essential for homeostasis, for coping with stress, and for the very maintenance of life.

The designation "glucocorticoid activity" is arbitrary, since naturally occurring glucocorticoids, such as cortisol, also possess mineralocorticoid activity, and the principal mineralocorticoid, aldosterone, when administered in very high doses, has glucocorticoid activity. Moreover, hydrocortisone, as well as certain synthetic glucocorticoids such as prednisone and dexamethasone, binds to mineralocorticoid receptors. However, the distinction between these two groups serves a useful purpose when dissociation of the basic actions becomes crucial for optimizing steroids' therapeutic efficiency.

Carbohydrate, Protein, and Fat Metabolism

The glucocorticoids increase blood glucose and liver glycogen levels by stimulating gluconeogenesis. The source of this augmented carbohydrate production is protein, and the protein catabolic actions of the glucocorticoids result in a negative nitrogen balance. *The inhibition of protein synthesis by glucocorticoids brings about a transfer of amino acids from muscle and bone to liver, where amino acids are converted to glucose.* The nitrogen released during these transamination reactions is converted to urea by the liver. In contrast to the catabolic actions of glucocorticoids on protein synthesis in muscle and anabolic effects in liver, there is little effect on protein metabolism in brain and cardiac tissue.

Supraphysiological concentrations of glucocorticoids will induce the synthesis of specific proteins in various tissues. For instance, glucocorticoids stimulate the synthesis of enzymes involved in glucose and amino acid metabolism, including glucose 6-phosphatase and tyrosine transaminase. The production of these hepatic enzymes requires the biosynthesis of new enzyme protein. The relation of this action of glucocorticoids to their overall effects on general metabolic processes remains obscure, although the latency of their therapeutic actions implies that synthesis of new protein is a pivotal component of the mechanism of action of corticosteroids.

Glucocorticoids not only break down protein but also stimulate the catabolism of lipids in adipose tissue and enhance the actions of other lipolytic agents. This occurrence results in an increase in plasma free fatty acids and an enhanced tendency to ketosis. The mechanism of this lipolytic action is unknown; it is particularly puzzling why lipid is lost from some tissues and not from others.

The net effect of all the biochemical changes induced by the glucocorticoids is an antagonism of the actions of insulin. These biochemical events promote hyperglycemia and glycosuria, conditions not dissimilar to the diabetic state.

Electrolyte and Water Metabolism

Another major function of the adrenal cortex is in the regulation of water and electrolyte metabolism. The principal mineralocorticoid, *aldosterone,* can increase the rate of sodium reabsorption and potassium excretion severalfold. This will occur physiologically in response to sodium or volume depletion, or both. The primary site of this effect is the distal tubule (see Chap. 21). The steroid-binding specificity of mineralocorticoid and glucocorticoid receptors overlaps in the distal cortical cells and collecting tubules, so that glucocorticoids may mediate mineralocorticoid-like effects. Glucocorticoids also decrease the intestinal transport of calcium by antagonizing the action of 1,25-dihydroxyvitamin D_3 and promote calcium excretion by the kidney (see Chap. 70).

Cardiovascular Function

The importance of glucocorticoids in the maintenance of normal cardiovascular function is underscored by the fact that hypotension in adrenal insufficiency may require glucocorticoid therapy even after fluid and electrolytes are replaced. Glucocorticoids are also capable of directly stimulating cardiac output and potentiating the responses of vascular smooth muscle to the pressor effects of catecholamines and other vasoconstrictor agents. Such actions on vascular smooth muscle may be secondary to effects mediated through the central nervous system or on circulating volume. However, the presence of steroid receptors on vascular smooth muscle suggests a direct effect on vasomotor activity. Thus, corticosteroids appear to play an important role in the regulation of blood pressure by modulating vascular smooth muscle tone, by having a direct action on the heart, and through stimulating renal mineralocorticoid and glucocorticoid receptors.

Immune and Defense Mechanisms

The inflammatory response is a highly complex process that involves a number of cell types of the reticuloendothelial system and a number of chemical mediators, including prostaglandins, leukotrienes, kinins, and biogenic amines. *The inhibitory effects of glucocorticoids on inflammatory and immunological responses constitute the basis for their therapeutic efficacy.* All steps of the inflammatory process are blocked: There is a diminution in heat, erythema, swelling, and tenderness. Both the early components (edema, fibrin deposition, neutrophil migration, and phagocytosis) and late components (collagen synthesis and deposition) may be retarded.

A prominent histological feature of glucocorticoid action on the late-phase response to bronchial inhalation challenge with antigen is an inhibition of the influx of polymorphonuclear leukocytes, eosinophils, basophils, mononuclear cells, and lymphocytes into tissues (Fig. 66-2). The ability of glucocorticoids to alter reticuloendothelial cell traffic is one of the most prominent antiinflammatory actions of glucocorticoids. This action probably occurs by impairing the adherence of migrating cells to the vascular endothelium before their egress from the circulation into the tissues. Leukocyte accumulation at the inflammatory site may be suppressed for up to 12 hr after a single dose of corticosteroid. Glucocorticoids not only inhibit the entry of monocytes into tissue but their subsequent differentiation to become macrophages. In addition to their ability to inhibit the adherence of inflammatory cells to the vascular endothelium, steroids are effective vasoconstrictors. This action would further impede cell migration into tissues. However, glucocorticoids do not suppress antibody production.

While there is an increase in the number of polymorphonuclear leukocytes in the circulation, corticosteroids cause the involution and atrophy of all lymphoid tissue and decrease the number of circulating lymphocytes. The striking lymphocytopenia is caused in large part by an in-

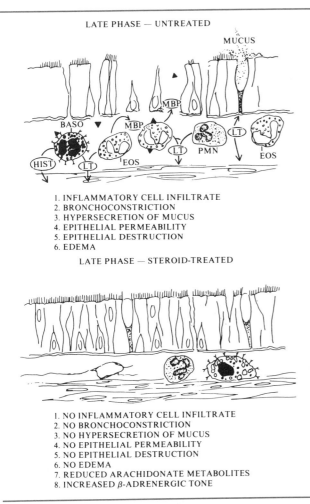

LATE PHASE — UNTREATED

1. INFLAMMATORY CELL INFILTRATE
2. BRONCHOCONSTRICTION
3. HYPERSECRETION OF MUCUS
4. EPITHELIAL PERMEABILITY
5. EPITHELIAL DESTRUCTION
6. EDEMA

LATE PHASE — STEROID-TREATED

1. NO INFLAMMATORY CELL INFILTRATE
2. NO BRONCHOCONSTRICTION
3. NO HYPERSECRETION OF MUCUS
4. NO EPITHELIAL PERMEABILITY
5. NO EPITHELIAL DESTRUCTION
6. NO EDEMA
7. REDUCED ARACHIDONATE METABOLITES
8. INCREASED β-ADRENERGIC TONE

Figure 66-2. Model of steroid action on the late-phase response to bronchial inhalation challenge with antigen. Steroid therapy *(bottom)* prevents the inflammatory cell infiltrate and concomitant sequelae usually observed in response to the antigen challenge *(top)*. BASO = basophils; EOS = eosinophils; PMN = polymorphonuclear leukocytes; HIST = histamine; LT = leukotrienes; MBP = major basic protein. (Reproduced with permission from R.P. Schleimer, The mechanisms of antiinflammatory steroid action in allergic disease. *Annu. Rev. Pharmacol. Toxicol.* 25:400; 1985. © 1985 by Annual Reviews Inc.)

hibition of lymphocyte proliferation, although diminished growth with preferential accumulation of cells in the G_1-phase of the cell cycle is followed by cell death. Steroids selectively affect a subclass of lymphocytes, the helper cells, rather than the suppressor cells. The biochemical basis of the receptor-mediated responses in lymphoid cells that ultimately results in the lymphocytolytic effect is not yet understood, but probably involves alterations in the production of interleukin-2, as well as its receptor binding and expression.

Glucocorticoids also inhibit cell proliferation in a variety of cell culture systems and inhibit cell growth by al-

tering the production of growth factor–like molecules. Under certain conditions, glucocorticoids will inhibit the growth of stromal fibroblasts and reduce the amount of tissue collagen, not only by reducing synthesis but also by enhancing its degradation.

Other Endocrine Organs

Since the synthesis and release of cortisol is regulated by pituitary ACTH, removal of the pituitary gland both in humans and experimental animals results in decreased function and subsequent atrophy of the zona fasciculata and zona reticularis. Infusion of supraphysiological concentrations of cortisol will suppress ACTH secretion from the pituitary and will markedly decrease circulating ACTH levels. This occurrence implies a negative feedback control for ACTH and corticosteroid release.

In addition to the humoral control of ACTH release, there also is direct nervous control, mediated through the median eminence of the hypothalamus. Nerve terminals in the median eminence store and release various hormones and neurotransmitters, including *corticotropin releasing factor (CRF)*; CRF is under the control of higher neural centers. During stress, CRF is released into the pituitary portal system to stimulate ACTH release. Activation of the hypothalamic-pituitary system also accounts for the diurnal, or circadian, nature of cortisol secretion; plasma cortisol concentrations reach a maximum between 6 and 8 A.M. and then slowly decrease through the afternoon and evening. Human and animal studies suggest the existence of an early (fast feedback) and more prolonged (delayed feedback; >2 hr) feedback of ACTH suppression. Both inhibitory systems are operative at the hypothalamic and pituitary levels. The fast-feedback effect of cortisol, which is absent in depressed patients, involves higher brain centers such as the hippocampus.

Corticosteroids also affect adrenomedullary function. In higher animals, the adrenal cortex surrounds the medulla, which harbors the catecholamine-producing chromaffin cells. Blood passing through the cortical sinuses comes into intimate contact with the chromaffin cells, so that they are exposed to high concentrations of steroid. Glucocorticoids can increase epinephrine production by exerting a stimulatory action on two of the enzymes that regulate catecholamine synthesis: tyrosine hydroxylase (the rate-limiting enzyme) and phenylethanolamine *N*-methyltransferase (which catalyzes the conversion of norepinephrine to epinephrine). Glucocorticoid receptors present in adrenomedullary chromaffin cells regulate phenylethanolamine *N*-methyltransferase activity by inducing enzyme messenger RNA (mRNA).

Steroids also are able to influence the metabolism of circulating catecholamines by inhibiting their uptake from the circulation by nonneuronal tissues (i.e., extraneuronal uptake; see Chap. 11); this effect of corticoids may explain their permissive action in potentiating the hemodynamic effects of circulating catecholamines.

Finally, steroids can exert suppressive actions on certain endocrine systems. Glucocorticoids inhibit thyroid-stimulating hormone (TSH) pulsatility and the nocturnal surge of this hormone by depressing thyrotropin releasing hormone (TRH) secretion at the hypothalamic level. In addition to hypercortisolism being associated with insulin resistance, glucocorticoids are inhibitors of linear growth and skeletal maturation in humans. Although the pathogenesis of this inhibition may involve impaired action of somatomedin and/or release of growth factors, a pivotal component is the depression of growth hormone secretion. The anticalcemic effect of the glucocorticoids, which is associated with an amplification of the actions of parathyroid hormone, also may retard bone growth. The inhibitory action of high levels of glucocorticoids on reproductive function is likely due both to an attenuation of luteinizing hormone (LH) secretion and to a direct action on the reproductive organs. The actions of glucocorticoids on growth hormone and LH secretion occur at the level of the hypothalamus.

General Pharmacology of Corticosteroids

Structure-Activity Relationships

Natural Corticosteroids

Within the basic structure of the steroid molecule (Fig. 66-3), a 4,5, double bond and a 3-ketone group are needed for typical steroid activity. A hydroxyl group on C11 is needed for glucocorticoid activity (corticosterone) but is not required for sodium-retaining activity (desoxycorticosterone). The addition of a hydroxyl group on C17, which converts corticosterone to cortisol, also increases glucocorticoid activity.

Synthetic Corticosteroids

Ring A

The addition of a double bond at the 1,2 position of cortisol or cortisone yields prednisone or prednisolone, respectively, and increases the ratio of carbohydrate to sodium-retaining potency. Prednisone is inactive and must be converted to prednisolone in the liver by reduction at the 11-keto position.

Ring B

The inclusion of an α-methyl group in position 6 of prednisolone will yield 6-α-methylprednisolone, a com-

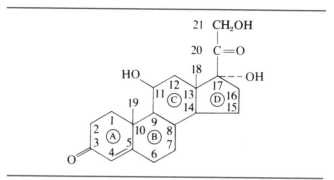

Figure 66-3. Basic corticosteroid nucleus.

pound with slightly greater glucocorticoid potency. This small structural modification greatly diminishes the binding of methylprednisolone to transcortin.

Ring C

The addition of a fluoride group on the 9 position of cortisol to give 9-α-fluorocortisol will greatly increase all biological activity.

Ring D

Hydroxylation or methylation at the 16 position of α-fluoroprednisolone to give triamcinolone, dexamethasone, or betamethasone increases antiinflammatory potency and drastically diminishes sodium-retaining activity.

The relative antiinflammatory potency of each of the synthetic analogues is compared with cortisol in Table 66-1 and is roughly correlated with its biological half-life. The major determinants of potency are the affinity for glucocorticoid receptors over a short time interval and clearance rates over a protracted time course. Hydrocortisone is considered a short-acting steroid; triamcinolone and prednisolone, intermediate-acting; and betamethasone and dexamethasone, long-acting. Thus, 5 mg prednisone, 0.75 mg dexamethasone, and 20 mg hydrocortisone should possess equal glucocorticoid potency.

The synthetic analogues (except 9-α-fluorocortisol) share an advantage over hydrocortisone in that sodium retention is not as marked at equipotent antiinflammatory doses. However, all of the other undesirable side effects of supraphysiological concentrations of hydrocortisone have been observed with the synthetic analogues.

Steroid Preparations

Glucocorticoids are available in a wide range of preparations, so they can be administered parenterally, orally, topically, or by inhalation. Orally administered steroids

Table 66-1. General Classification of Glucocorticoids

Steroid	Carbohydrate potency* (mg)	Antiinflammatory potency	Sodium-retaining potency	Biological half-life (hr)
Cortisol	20	1	1	8–12
Prednisolone (Δ^1-cortisone)	5	4	0.5	12–36
6-α-Methylprednisolone	4	5	0.5	12–36
9-α-Fluorocortisol	0.1	10	125	12–36
Triamcinolone (9-α-fluoro-16-hydroxyprednisolone)	4	5	0.1	12–36
Betamethasone (9-α-16-β-methylprednisolone)	0.6	25	0.05	36–54
Dexamethasone (9-α-fluoro- 16-α-methylprednisolone)	1	30	0.05	36–54

*Carbohydrate action of glucocorticoids is defined as the stimulation of glucose formation, diminution of its utilization, and promotion of its storage as glycogen.

are, obviously, the preferred mode of administration for prolonged therapy. However, parenteral administration is required in certain circumstances. Intramuscular injection of a water-soluble ester (phosphate or succinate)—formed by esterification of C21 steroid alcohol—produces peak plasma steroid levels within 1 hr. Such preparations are useful in emergency situations. By contrast, acetate and tertiary butylacetate esters are insoluble; they must be injected locally as suspensions that are slowly absorbed from the injection site, thereby prolonging the duration of effectiveness to approximately 8 hr. Local injections of such long-acting preparations may ameliorate symptoms associated with inflamed joints.

Steroids also are available in ointment form for topical administration. Topical preparations usually contain relatively insoluble steroids, such as clobetasol proprionate, triamcinolone acetonide, or triamcinolone diacetate. Side effects of this mode of drug application are usually milder and more transient than those seen after systemically administered steroids. However, potent topical corticosteroids such as clobetasol propionate (*Temovate*) can suppress adrenal function when used in large amounts for a long time, especially when the skin surface is denuded or when occlusive dressings are employed. Since the high-potency topical preparations carry a higher risk of local side effects, their use should be held in reserve. The introduction of inhaled glucocorticoid preparations such as betamethasone diproprionate and betamethasone valerate has provided an effective alternative to systemic steroids in the treatment of chronic asthma (see Chap. 45). Inhaled drug is delivered directly to the target site in relatively low doses, but with the potential for more frequent administration. Moreover, inhaled glucocorticoids are metabolized in the lung before they are absorbed, thereby reducing their systemic effects. In asthma, spray is inhaled through the mouth while in rhinitis, glucocorticoids are sprayed into the nasal passage.

Adverse Effects

General Considerations

Short-term glucocorticoid therapy of life-threatening diseases, such as status asthmaticus, provides dramatic improvement with few complications. However, when administered in pharmacological doses for prolonged periods, steroids generally produce serious toxic effects that

Table 66-2. Complications of Glucocorticoid Therapy

Hematologic and immunologic	Central nervous system
Leukocytosis	Insomnia
Lymphopenia	Depression
Eosinopenia	Nervousness
Altered inflammatory response	Psychosis
Gastrointestinal	Fluid and electrolyte
Peptic ulceration	Na^+ retention
Fatty liver	K^+ loss
Pancreatitis	Negative Ca^{2+} balance
Nausea, vomiting	Hypertension
Metabolic	Endocrinologic
Hyperglycemia	Suppression of HPA axis*
Protein wasting	Antagonisms with insulin, parathyroid, thyroid
Hyperlipidemia	Skin
Obesity	Thinning of skin
Musculoskeletal	Striae purpura
Myopathy	Ecchymoses
Growth failure	Acne
Osteopenia	Hirsutism
Ocular	General
Posterior subcapsular cataracts	Cushingoid features
Increased intraocular pressure	Truncal obesity
	Withdrawal syndrome

*Hypothalamic-pituitary-adrenocortical axis.

are extensions of their pharmacological actions. No route or preparation is free from the diverse side effects (Table 66-2), although individuals receiving comparable doses of glucocorticoids exhibit variations in side effects.

Glucocorticoid use has been cautiously reinstituted in various disease states such as rheumatoid arthritis, although it still should be regarded as adjunctive rather than the primary treatment in the overall management scheme. The toxic effects of steroids are of sufficient severity that a number of factors must be considered when their prolonged use is contemplated.

The first point is that *treatment with steroids is generally palliative rather than curative,* and only in a very few diseases, such as leukemia and nephrotic syndrome, do corticosteroids alter prognosis. One must also consider which is worse, the disease to be treated or a possible iatrogenically induced Cushing's disease (hypercortisolism). The patient's age can be an important factor, since such toxic effects as hypertension are more apt to occur in old and infirm individuals, especially those with underlying cardiovascular disease.

Once steroid therapy is decided upon, the lowest possible dose that can still provide the desired therapeutic effect should be employed. Relationships of dosage, duration, and host responses are essential elements in determining adverse effects.

The Infectious Process

The influence of glucocorticoids on host resistance is complex and controversial. Steroids can alter host-parasite interactions, suppress fever, decrease inflammation, and change the usual character of the symptoms produced by most infectious organisms. *There is a heightened susceptibility to serious bacterial, viral, and fungal infections.* Localized infections may become reactivated and spread, and infections acquired during the course of therapy may become more severe and even more difficult to recognize. This untoward effect of steroids may make it mandatory to administer antibiotics with the steroids, especially when there is a history of a chronic infectious process (e.g., tuberculosis). On the other hand, individuals with normal defenses who are treated with low to moderate doses of glucocorticoids are not at great risk of infection.

Effects on Gastric Mucosa

Steroid administration can lead to the formation of peptic ulcers, with hemorrhage or perforation, or it can reactivate a previously healed ulcer. Risk of this side effect increases if the duration of therapy is prolonged. Steroids may not be the primary offender, but owing to their ability to induce tissue atrophy, glucocorticoids probably en-

hance the ulcerogenic potential of environmental factors and other drugs such as the nonsteroidal antiinflammatory drugs (NSAIDs). Steroid-treated patients who are at particularly high risk for gastric mucosal injury include (1) those who require high doses of steroids and long-term therapy, (2) those with a history of peptic ulcer disease, and (3) arthritic patients receiving steroids and concomitant aspirin therapy. The use of H_2-receptor antagonists may prove beneficial in the treatment of steroid-induced gastric mucosal damage.

Hyperglycemic Action

In about one-fourth to one-third of the patients receiving prolonged steroid therapy, the hyperglycemic effects of glucocorticoids lead to decreased glucose tolerance, decreased responsiveness to insulin, and even glycosuria. Ketoacidosis occurs very rarely. Pharmacological concentrations of steroids only rarely precipitate frank diabetes in normal individuals but may unmask diabetes in those with low insulin reserve.

Osteoporosis

The most damaging and therapeutically limiting adverse effect of long-term glucocorticoid therapy is osteoporosis. Osteoporosis is a common side effect seen in older patients with advanced rheumatoid arthritis who have been treated with glucocorticoids for long periods. A majority of patients receiving chronic steroid therapy will develop osteoporosis and over 50 percent will experience a bone fracture. The overall effects appear to be due to direct actions of glucocorticoids on osteoblasts and to indirect effects such as impaired Ca^{2+} absorption and a compensatory increase in parathyroid hormone secretion. There is a particular loss of trabecular bone. Inhibition of bone growth is a well-known side effect of long-term systemic glucocorticoid therapy in children with bronchial asthma, even in those receiving alternate-day therapy. Medroxyprogesterone acetate, which is a glucocorticoid antagonist at the level of osteoblast function, may prove promising for relieving this untoward effect of glucocorticoids. Deflazacort, a methyl oxazoline derivative of prednisolone, may become the drug of choice in growing individuals. It diffuses less readily into bone tissue and is more rapidly cleared than prednisone, and therefore may produce comparable therapeutic responses with less bone loss.

Ophthalmic Effects

Glucocorticoids induce cataract formation, particularly in patients with rheumatoid arthritis. An increase in intraocular pressure, related to a decreased outflow of aqueous humor, is also a frequent side effect. Glaucoma may occur in as many as 40 percent of patients after ocular or systemic steroid administration.

Central Nervous System Effects

Despite the demonstration of hypercortisolemia in depressed patients, treatment with steroids may initially evoke euphoria. This reaction can be a consequence of the salutary effects of the steroids on the inflammatory process or it may be due to a direct effect on the psyche. The expression of the unpredictable and often profound effects exerted by steroids on mental processes generally reflects the personality of the individual; the effects produced may also at least partly relate to the direct actions of elevated steroid levels. Restlessness and early-morning insomnia may be forerunners of severe psychotic reactions. In such situations, cessation of treatment might be considered, especially in patients with a history of personality disorders. In addition, patients may become psychically dependent on steroids due to their euphoric effect, and withdrawal of the treatment may precipitate an emotional crisis, with suicide or psychosis as a consequence.

The hippocampus is a principal neural target for glucocorticoids. It contains high concentrations of glucocorticoid receptors and has a marked sensitivity to these hormones. Prolonged exposure to glucocorticoids or persistent stress may promote damage to hippocampal neurons during aging.

Fluid and Electrolyte Disturbances

In the normal subject, sodium and water retention may occur with steroid therapy, although the synthetic steroid analogues represent a lesser risk in this regard. Prednisolone produces some edema in doses greater than 30 mg; triamcinolone and dexamethasone are much less liable to elicit this side effect. Glucocorticoids may also produce an increase in potassium excretion. Muscle weakness and wasting of skeletal muscle mass frequently accompany this potassium-depleting action. The expansion of the extracellular fluid volume produced by steroids is secondary to sodium and water retention; this action of steroids results in hypertension. However, the presence of specific steroid receptors in vascular smooth muscle suggests that glucocorticoids are also more directly involved in the regulation of blood pressure. A separate entity, "steroid myopathy," is also improved by decreasing steroid dosage. The steroid-induced hypercalciuria can be corrected by thiazide diuretics, which decrease the renal excretion of calcium relative to that of sodium.

Pseudorheumatism

In certain patients, whose large dosages of corticosteroids for rheumatoid arthritis are gradually diminished, new symptoms develop that may be mistaken for a flareup of the joint disease. These can include emotional lability, fever, muscle aches, and general fatigue. It is tempting to increase the dosage of steroid in this situation, but continued maintenance at the lower dosage with a subsequent gradual decrease in the dose usually improves symptoms.

Additional Effects

Other side effects include acne, striae, truncal obesity, deposition of fat in the cheeks ("moon face") and upper part of the back ("buffalo hump"), and dysmenorrhea. Topical administration may produce local skin atrophy. In patients with acquired immunodeficiency syndrome (AIDS) who are treated with glucocorticoids, Kaposi's sarcoma becomes activated or progresses more rapidly.

Iatrogenic Adrenal Insufficiency

In addition to the potential dangers associated with long-term use of corticosteroids in supraphysiological concentrations, there are problems associated with the *withdrawal* of steroid therapy. After only 1 to 2 weeks of steroid therapy, high levels of steroids in the blood will depress hypothalamic and pituitary activity and will result in a decrease in endogenous adrenal steroid secretion and eventual *adrenal atrophy*. Adrenal suppression may persist for up to 1 year after steroid therapy is withdrawn. Long-acting steroids, such as dexamethasone and betamethasone, suppress the hypothalamic-pituitary axis more than do other steroids.

Alternate-day therapy will relieve the clinical manifestations of the inflammatory diseases while allowing for a day for the reactivation of endogenous corticosteroid output, thereby causing less severe and less sustained hypothalamic-pituitary suppression. This is feasible with doses of shorter-acting corticosteroids such as prednisolone. The usual daily dose is doubled and is given in the early morning to simulate the natural circadian variation that occurs in endogenous corticosteroid secretion. This method, which is usually employed only after the disease is controlled by maintenance therapy, will lessen the suppression of the hypothalamic-pituitary axis and may expedite the ultimate withdrawal from steroid therapy. The benefits of alternate-day therapy are seen only when steroids are used for a prolonged period.

Although not always predictable, the degree to which a given corticosteroid will suppress pituitary activity is related to the route of administration, the size of the dose, and the length of treatment. The parenteral route causes the greatest suppression, followed by the oral route, and finally topical application. Hypothalamic-pituitary suppression also may result if large doses of a steroid aerosol spray are used to treat bronchial asthma. Patients given high concentrations of steroids for long periods and subsequently exposed to undue stress (e.g., severe infection, surgery) face the danger of adrenal crisis. These patients must be given supplemental steroids to compensate for their lack of adrenal reserve and to sustain them during the crisis.

Acute adrenal insufficiency will, of course, occur from an abrupt cessation of steroid therapy. Symptoms of fever, myalgia, arthralgia, and malaise may be difficult to distinguish from reactivation of rheumatic disease. *Steroid treatment should be reduced gradually over several months to avoid this potentially serious problem.* Also, continued suppression may be avoided by administering daily physiological replacement doses (5 mg prednisone) until adrenal function is restored. The order of recovery is firstly the hypothalamus, then the pituitary, and lastly the adrenal cortex.

An additional problem associated with glucocorticoid therapy is that certain side effects can also be caused by the diseases for which glucocorticoids are administered. Thus, osteoporosis can be a sequela of rheumatoid arthritis, and the physician is left to determine whether the untoward effect is iatrogenically induced or is merely a symptom of the disease process being treated.

In addition to these problems, the physician must also be aware of the patient's natural reluctance to reduce the dose of steroid because of its salutary effects, both on the inflammatory process and on the psyche. Thus, the problems associated with withdrawal from long-term steroid therapy in rheumatoid arthritis are additional reasons why steroid treatment should be initiated only after rest, physiotherapy, and nonsteroidal antiinflammatory drugs, or gold, D-penicillamine, and methotrexate have been utilized.

Therapeutic Uses of Steroid Hormones

Replacement Therapy

In certain disease states, adrenocortical hormones are secreted in insufficient quantities to maintain homeostatic mechanisms. Adrenal insufficiency may result from hypofunction of the adrenal cortex (*primary adrenal insufficiency, Addison's disease*) or from a malfunctioning of the hypothalamic-pituitary system (*secondary adrenal insufficiency*). In treatment of primary adrenal insufficiency, one should administer enough cortisol to diminish hyperpig-

mentation and abolish postural hypotension; these are the cardinal signs of Addison's disease.

Although patients may require varying amounts of replacement steroid, 20 to 30 mg/day of cortisol supplemented with the mineralocorticoid 9-α-fluorocortisol (0.1 mg/day) is generally adequate. Aldosterone, the naturally occurring mineralocorticoid, is not employed since it is not effective orally. A doubling of the cortisol dose may be required during minor stresses or infections. In patients who require high-dose supplementation, prednisone can be substituted for cortisol to avoid fluid retention.

In the treatment of secondary adrenocortical insufficiency, lower doses of cortisol are generally effective, and fluid and electrolyte disturbances do not have to be considered since patients with deficient ACTH secretion generally do not have abnormal function of the zona glomerulosa.

Inflammatory States

Since glucocorticoids possess a wide range of effects on virtually every phase and component of the inflammatory and immune responses, they have assumed a major role in the treatment of a wide spectrum of diseases with an inflammatory or immune-mediated component. Rheumatoid arthritis is the original condition for which antiinflammatory steroids were employed. Although steroids offer symptomatic relief from this disorder by abolishing the swelling, redness, pain, and effusions, they do not effect a cure. Progressive deterioration of joint structures continues, and the disease process may be exacerbated after steroid therapy is terminated (for further information on this topic, see Chap. 43).

Because inflammation plays an important role in the pathogenesis of asthma, glucocorticoids are the treatment of choice in chronic asthma. Based on the concept that asthma is an inflammatory disease that leads to airway obstruction, a combined regimen can be employed in acute asthma, involving systemic glucocorticoids with an inhaled brochodilator such as a beta-adrenergic agonist. However, in recent years, the need for systemic glucocorticoid therapy has been replaced by the concomitant use of potent inhalation corticosteroids, which are associated with fewer side effects. The available inhaled glucocorticoids in the United States, beclomethasone dipropionate, triamcinolone acetonide, and flunisolide, have similar potency and are administered by a metered-dose inhaler.

Steroids are used in other collagen diseases such as lupus erythematosus; in hypersensitivity or allergic states, such as asthma, nephrotic syndrome, ulcerative colitis, and Crohn's disease; in granulomatous disease such as sarcoid; and in a wide range of dermatological and ophthalmological conditions. Steroids also serve a valuable function in the prevention and treatment of organ transplant rejection and in the improvement of muscle function in polymyositis.

Glucocorticoids also exert a facilitatory action on neuromuscular transmission that may contribute to their efficacy in several neuromuscular disorders, including polyradiculoneuropathies and Bell's palsy. Although only limited success can generally be expected in prescribing glucocorticoids in renal disease, the clinical benefits in idiopathic nephrosis in children have been established. In fact, response to steroids can be used as a diagnostic, as well as a prognostic, indicator in nephrotic syndrome.

Although infections are generally thought to be more frequent and possibly more severe in patients treated with steroids, they have been used on a short-term basis to reduce the severe symptoms associated with such bacterial infections as miliary tuberculosis and brucellosis, and in viral infections such as viral hepatitis and infectious mononucleosis. Under no condition should steroids be administered in such situations for more than 7 days.

Glucocorticoids are also used in the treatment of human immunodeficiency virus (HIV)-related disorders, including mucocutaneous exanthema, lymphoid interstitial pneumonitis, and demyelinating peripheral neuropathies. *Pneumocysts carinii* pneumonia is the commonest life-threatening infection associated with AIDS. Glucocorticoids are used as adjuvant therapy in this disorder to decrease the inflammatory response and allow time for antimicrobial agents to exert their effects.

Leukemia

Steroids are important components in the treatment of hematopoietic malignancies. Their efficacy in chronic lymphocytic leukemia and multiple myeloma stems from their lympholytic effects. A complication of chronic lymphocytic leukemia, autoimmune hemolytic anemia, also responds favorably to steroids. However, the development of resistance may limit the effectiveness of steroid therapy.

Shock

Prompt intensive treatment with corticosteroids may be lifesaving in conditions in which an excessive inflammatory reaction has resulted in septic shock. A massive infusion of corticosteroids can restore cardiac output and reverse hypotension by sensitizing the response of adrenergic receptors in the heart and blood vessels to the stimulating action of catecholamines. This protective role of steroids may be due to a direct effect on vascular smooth muscle. The ability of glucocorticoids to augment the in-

crease in cyclic adenosine monophosphate (AMP) elicited by dopamine in vascular smooth muscle cells may provide the mechanistic basis for the combination of glucocorticoids and dopamine therapy to preserve renal blood flow during shock. Alternatively, the antishock effects of steroids may stem from an inhibition of the synthesis and release of chemical mediators, free radicals, and lysosomal enzymes.

Congenital Adrenal Hyperplasia

Congenital enzymatic defects in the adrenal biosynthetic pathways lead to diminished cortisol and aldosterone production and release. In these conditions, ACTH secretion is increased, and adrenal hyperplasia occurs, accompanied by an enhanced secretion of steroid intermediates, especially adrenal androgens. By far the most common type of congenital adrenal hyperplasia is 21-hydroxylase deficiency, which accounts for over 90 percent of cases. Treatment of this condition requires administration of adequate amounts of glucocorticoid to normalize the patient's corticosteroid levels and (if needed) a mineralocorticoid preparation. It also may be necessary to suppress enhanced ACTH secretion with larger amounts of corticoids.

Proposed Mechanism of Steroid Action

One approach to understanding the mechanism of glucocorticoid action is to determine whether the primary locus of action is on the surface or the interior of the cell. Glucocorticoid receptors have been studied in a wide variety of tissues and, like aldosterone receptors, they are found *intracellularly*. Steroids transported by transcortin enter the target cell by diffusion and then form a complex with its cytosolic receptor protein (Fig. 66-4). The steroid-receptor complex undergoes an irreversible activation (transformation) process that results in its migration to the nucleus. The complex binds to specific DNA regions near or at some distance from the promoter. The interaction of the steroid-receptor complex with specific target DNAs, called the hormone response elements, stimulates or represses gene transcription and the production of mRNA to modify protein synthesis. The pivotal role that the glucocorticoid receptor plays in hormone action is illustrated by the fact that the magnitude of induction of a regulatable gene and cellular responsiveness is directly proportional to the number of occupied receptors. Furthermore, steroid resistance is accompanied by a decrease in receptor number.

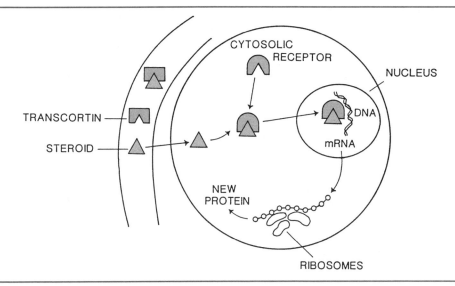

Figure 66-4. Schematic model of the mechanism of action of glucocorticoids.

The mechanisms that alter the production of proteins translated have significant implications for steroid therapy. Because there is a requirement for macromolecular synthesis, there is generally a lag of several hours before the effects of steroids are manifest. Moreover, the duration of various responses can endure after steroid levels fall. This may account for the fact that side effects elicited by steroids can be minimized by alternate-day therapy.

A key development in our understanding of the basic mechanism of the antiinflammatory actions of glucocorticoids emerged with the discovery of phospholipase inhibitory proteins, which are synthesized and secreted in response to glucocorticoid interactions with their cytoplasmic receptors. Metabolites of arachidonic acid (including prostaglandins, thromboxanes, and leukotrienes) are considered strong candidates as mediators of the inflammatory process. Tissue levels of free arachidonic acid are increased by the action of the enzyme phospholipase A_2. Thus, steroids may exert a primary effect at the inflammatory site by inducing the synthesis of a group of proteins called *lipocortins,* which suppress the activation of phospholipase A_2, thereby decreasing the release of arachidonic acid and the production of pro-inflammatory eicosanoids. This action of steroids contrasts with that of NSAIDs (see Chap. 43), which are thought to inhibit the enzymes that catalyze the synthesis of arachidonic acid metabolites. However, the question still remains open as to whether lipocortins represent an important clue to the development of antiinflammatory drugs with fewer side effects. Nevertheless, the concept that attributes the multiplicity of glucocorticoid effects to their ability to induce the synthesis of a family of regulatory proteins is not only consistent with their widespread actions but also reconciles the physiological and pharmacological actions of ste-

roids. (For further information on this topic, see Chap. 43.)

Inhibition of the production and effects of the cytokine interleukin-1 may also contribute to the antiinflammatory and immunosuppressive effects of glucocorticoids. In fact, a balance between the antiinflammatory effects of glucocorticoids and the pro-inflammatory effects of interleukin-1 appears to be a basic mechanism regulating host responses to infection and injury.

Drugs Used in the Diagnosis or Treatment of Adrenocortical Abnormalities

Corticotropin

Chemistry

Corticotropin (ACTH) is an open-chain polypeptide that consists of 39 amino acid residues, the first 24 of which are essential for its biological activity. The remainder of the amino acids are also clinically important, however, since they may be involved in stimulating antibody formation and causing allergic reactions. This is especially true when corticotropin of animal origin is injected into humans. Commercially available corticotropin is prepared from animal pituitary glands.

Absorption, Metabolism, and Excretion

Corticotropin is rapidly inactivated by gastrointestinal proteolytic enzymes and therefore must be administered parenterally. It is rapidly removed from the circulation (half-life of 15 min) and is probably inactivated in body tissues, since no intact compound is found in the urine.

Clinical Uses

The rationale for using corticotropin instead of pharmacological concentrations of glucocorticoids stems from the fact that corticotropin provides enhanced amounts of all endogenously secreted adrenocortical hormones, including androgens. However, obvious disadvantages are associated with the use of this polypeptide: (1) It must be given daily parenterally; (2) it is quite expensive; and (3) it is antigenic and thus can produce resistance and hypersensitivity reactions. Corticotropin is used as a diagnostic tool for the identification of primary adrenal insufficiency or as a method for evaluating the hypothalamic-pituitary-adrenal axis before surgery in patients previously treated with glucocorticoids.

Adverse Reactions

Aside from the already mentioned hypersensitivity and allergic reactions, corticotropin administration has been associated with electrolyte disturbances and masculinization in women.

Preparations

Corticotropin for injection (ACTH, *Acthar, Cortrophin Gel ACTH*) is available as a solution, a lyophilized powder, and a suspension. To achieve a satisfactory therapeutic result, the dosage must be individualized.

Cosyntropin

Cosyntropin is a polypeptide that consists solely of the first 24 amino acids of corticotropin. It appears to offer an advantage over the naturally occurring hormone in that it has a longer duration of action and lacks the antigenic portion of corticotropin. Although hypersensitivity reactions are rare following its administration, caution still should be exercised in giving cosyntropin to patients who are hypersensitive to corticotropin. Cosyntropin (*Cortrosyn*) is available as a lyophilized powder for parenteral use.

Metyrapone

Mechanism of Action

Metyrapone produces its primary pharmacological effect by inhibiting 11-β-hydroxylase, thus causing a diminished production and release of cortisol. The resulting reduction in the negative feedback of cortisol on the hypothalamus and pituitary causes an increase in ACTH release and an increase in the secretion of precursor 11-deoxysteroids.

Clinical Uses

Metyrapone is used in the differential diagnosis of both adrenocortical insufficiency and Cushing's disease (hypercortisolism). The drug tests the functional competence of the hypothalamic-pituitary axis under conditions in which the adrenals are able to respond to ACTH, that is, when primary adrenal insufficiency has been ruled out. A single measurement of plasma cortisol does not permit a reliable assessment of hypothalamic-pituitary-adrenal function because cortisol release is pulsatile and thus may appear within the normal range because of episodic secretion. For diagnosis of secondary adrenal insufficiency, the metyrapone test (or insulin hypoglycemia or cosyntropin stimulation tests) will provide more meaningful information.

After metyrapone administration, a patient with a disease of pituitary origin cannot achieve a compensatory increase in the urinary excretion of 17-hydroxycorticosteroids or 11-deoxysteroids. Moreover, if pituitary ACTH is suppressed by an autonomously secreting adrenal carcinoma, there will be no increase in response to metyrapone. On the other hand, if pituitary ACTH secretion is maintained, as occurs in adrenal hyperplasia, the inhibition of corticoid synthesis produced by metyrapone will stimulate ACTH secretion and the subsequent release of metabolites of precursor urinary steroids, which can be measured as 17-hydroxycorticosteroids. Metyrapone is now used less frequently in the differential diagnosis of Cushing's disease because of the ability to measure plasma ACTH directly.

The steroid-inhibiting properties of metyrapone have also been taken advantage of in the treatment of Cushing's disease, and it remains one of the more effective drugs used to treat this syndrome. However, the compensatory rise in ACTH levels in response to falling cortisol levels tends to maintain adrenal activity. This requires that glucocorticoids be administered concomitantly to suppress hypothalamic-pituitary activity. Although metyrapone inhibits the synthesis of aldosterone, it may not cause mineralocorticoid deficiency because of the compensatory increased production of 11-desoxycorticosterone.

Adverse Reactions

Side effects associated with the use of metyrapone include gastrointestinal distress, dizziness, headache, sedation, and the appearance of an allergic rash. The drug should not be used in cases of adrenocortical insufficiency or those in which hypersensitivity reactions can be expected. When administered to pregnant women during the second or third trimesters, the drug may impair steroid biosynthesis in the fetus.

Preparations and Dosage

Metyrapone (*Metopirone*) and metyrapone tartrate injection (*Metopirone Ditartrate*) are marketed commercially as 250-mg tablets or 10-ml ampules.

Aminoglutethimide

Aminoglutethimide, an amino derivative of the hypnotic agent glutethimide, was originally introduced as an anticonvulsant. It is no longer used for this purpose because it was found to produce adrenal insufficiency. Aminoglutethimide is a competitive inhibitor of desmolase, the enzyme that catalyzes the conversion of cholesterol to pregnenolone; it inhibits 11-hydroxylase activity as well. This drug also reduces estrogen production; it blocks the conversion of androstenedione into estrone by inhibiting the aromatase enzyme complex in peripheral (skin, muscle, fat) and in steroid target tissues. The net effect of this drug is to produce a medical adrenalectomy; that is, there is a diminished production of all steroid hormones, including aldosterone, cortisol, and adrenal sex hormones.

Such a medical adrenalectomy is an efficacious treatment for metastatic breast and prostate cancer, since it diminishes the levels of circulating sex hormones. However, because inhibition of steroid synthesis by aminoglutethimide can be overcome by enhanced ACTH release, glucocorticoids are administered concomitantly to suppress pituitary activity. Cortisol is preferable to dexamethasone in this situation because aminoglutethimide, as with phenytoin and phenobarbital, markedly enhances the hepatic microsomal metabolism of dexamethasone.

Aminoglutethimide (*Cytadren*) is suitable for use in Cushing's disease that results from adrenal carcinoma, and in congenital adrenal hyperplasia, in which it protects the patient from excessive secretion of endogenous androgens. The drug is not curative and relapse occurs when treatment is terminated. In more than half of the patients treated with this drug, adverse reactions, such as drowsiness, skin rashes, and nausea, can be expected, as well as leukopenia and even agranulocytosis (an idiosyncratic reaction). These symptoms occasionally diminish in severity, probably as a result of aminoglutethimide-induced acceleration of its own metabolism via hepatic enzyme induction. Aminoglutethimide and metyrapone are frequently used in combination as an adjunct to radiation or surgical therapy.

Mitotane

Mitotane (*Lysodren*) produces a selective atrophy of the zona fasciculata and zona reticularis, which results in a decrease in the secretion of 17-hydroxycorticosteroids; it also enhances the extraadrenal metabolism of cortisol. Mitotane is capable of inducing remission of Cushing's disease, but only at the price of severe gastrointestinal distress. Moreover, more than half of the patients relapse following cessation of therapy. Other side effects include lethargy, mental confusion, skin rashes, and altered hepatic function.

Mitotane is the drug of choice for treatment of primary adrenal carcinoma when surgery or radiation therapy is not feasible (see Chap. 62 for additional details, as well as information on preparations and dosage). However, it is problematic as to whether mitotane treatment influences patient survival. Its effectiveness in curtailing adrenal activity is due to an action on adrenocortical mitochondria to impair cytochrome P450 steps in steroid biosynthesis. Measurement of serum mitotane levels to ensure adequate therapeutic levels (>14 mg/liter) is advised.

In patients whose conditions do not respond to mitotane, metyrapone or aminoglutethimide, or both, can be employed to control steroid hypersecretion. Mitotane, being closely related to the organochlorine insecticides, shares their inductive effects on the liver microsomal drug-metabolizing enzyme system; its use may thus alter the requirement for concomitantly administered drugs that are also metabolized by this pathway.

Ketoconazole

Ketoconazole, an orally effective broad-spectrum antifungal agent (see Chap. 59), has proved beneficial in the treatment of Cushing's disease. This drug blocks hydroxylating enzyme systems by interacting with cytochrome P450 at the heme iron site to inhibit steroid and androgen synthesis in adrenals and gonads. Ketoconazole can be used as palliative treatment for Cushing's disease in patients undergoing surgery or receiving pituitary radiation, or in those in whom more definitive treatment is still contemplated. Ketoconazole can normalize glucocorticoid function in Cushing's disease both in short-term and chronic therapy. At doses of 200 to 1,000 mg/day, ketoconazole may prove useful as an alternative to steroid inhibitors that elicit side effects. Although an increase in plasma ACTH is usually not observed during the ketoconazole-induced decrease in plasma and urinary cortisol, a compensatory increase in ACTH may occur during prolonged therapy. Thus, constant vigilance for both hypocortisolism and hepatotoxicity is essential.

Trilostane

Trilostane (*Modrastane*) is a synthetic steroid that is a competitive inhibitor of the 3-beta hydroxysteroid dehydrogenase enzyme system. Its administration results in a decrease in the synthesis of cortisol, aldosterone, and androstenedione. The net effect is a lowering of steroid synthesis without an irreversible impairment of adrenal function. This drug is also available for treatment of Cushing's disease, but it can cause gastrointestinal symptoms, headache, suppression of gonadal function, and hypocortisolism.

Dexamethasone

The overnight dexamethasone suppression test offers a valuable diagnostic tool for Cushing's disease, and once the diagnosis is established, the prolonged (high-dose) dexamethasone suppression test is useful in distinguishing between excessive ACTH secretion and primary hypercortisolism.

When Cushing's disease is suspected, in addition to measuring the 24-hr urinary excretion of free cortisol, 0.75 to 1.0 mg dexamethasone is given to the patient in the late evening; plasma cortisol levels are determined the following day. Failure of dexamethasone to depress endogenous cortisol levels is indicative of Cushing's disease.

The simultaneous measurement of plasma ACTH and cortisol by radioimmunoassay is also useful as an adjunct to the prolonged dexamethasone suppression test. If the ACTH concentration is high in the presence of an above-normal cortisol concentration, Cushing's disease is likely to be due to excessive ACTH secretion. If a high cortisol concentration is observed in the presence of suppressed plasma ACTH, an adrenal tumor is likely.

Supplemental Reading

Baxter, J.D. Minimizing the side effects of glucocorticoid therapy. *Ann. Intern. Med.* 35:173, 1990.

Cook, D.M. Safe use of glucocorticoids. *Postgrad. Med.* 91:145, 1992.

Holland, E.G., and Taylor, A.T. Glucocorticoids in clinical practice. *J. Fam. Pract.* 32:512, 1991.

Nelson, D.H. New aspects of adrenal cortical disease. *Endocinol. Metab. Clin. North Am.* 20:247, 1991.

Szefler, S.J. Glucocorticoid therapy for asthma; clinical pharmacology. *J. Allergy Clin. Immunol.* 88:147, 1991.

67

Estrogens, Progestins, and Antiestrogens

Jeannine S. Strobl

The Natural Steroid Hormones

Structure and Biosynthesis

The structure common to all steroid hormones is the steroid nucleus (Fig. 67-1), a lipophilic tetracyclic hydrocarbon. All estrogens that occur naturally in animals have an aromatic A ring and one additional carbon atom at the 18 position of the steroid nucleus; this is called the *estrane nucleus.* The *pregnane nucleus* is common to all naturally occurring progestins. Progestins possess four additional carbon atoms at positions 18, 19, 20, and 21 of the common steroid nucleus. The varying biological activities and pharmacological properties of different estrogens and progestins are determined by the presence of various substituents on the estrane and pregnane nucleus, respectively.

Some biologically important natural estrogens and progestins include estradiol, estrone, estriol, and progesterone. Estradiol-17β is the most potent estrogen that is found naturally in women. Estrone is 10 times less biologically active than estradiol. Estriol is the weakest of the three; estriol is present at high levels in the urine of pregnant women and serves as an index of fetal viability. Progesterone is the most important naturally occurring progestin.

The major site of estrogen and progestin biosynthesis in nonpregnant, premenopausal women is the ovary. In pregnant women, the fetoplacental unit is the major source of estrogens and progestins. Peripheral sites of estrogen synthesis include the liver, kidney, brain, adipose tissue, skeletal muscle, and testes; small amounts of progesterone are secreted by the testes and adrenal gland. The combined estrogen and progestin production by all of these peripheral sites amounts to 10 percent or less of ovarian synthesis in normal premenopausal women. However, peripheral estrogen biosynthesis accounts for all estrogen that is present in males and postmenopausal women.

Ovarian biosynthesis of estrogens and progestins originates from cholesterol and from acetate. Cholesterol undergoes side chain cleavage and oxidation to form pregnenolone, the precursor for all steroid hormones. Progesterone is directly synthesized from pregnenolone while estrogen biosynthesis proceeds by means of the conversion of pregnenolone to androstenedione and testosterone. These last two androgens are precursors of estrogens. Androstenedione and testosterone undergo hydroxylation (C19 position) and then go through a series of reactions that are catalyzed by an aromatase enzyme complex leading to aromatization of the A ring of the steroid nucleus. The major steroid pathway in the ovary proceeds through testosterone on to the formation 17β-estradiol. Peripheral estrogen biosynthesis proceeds primarily through androstenedione and results in the production of estrone.

Metabolism and Excretion

Estrogens and progestins are extensively metabolized, leading to the production of compounds that are less physiologically active and also more water soluble than the parent hormones. These water-soluble estrogen and progestin metabolites are primarily excreted in the urine, although a small fraction of estrogen metabolites enter the bile, where they may undergo enterohepatic circulation before elimination. Normally 10 percent or less of estrogen and progestin metabolites are excreted in the feces.

The major site of estrogen and progestin metabolism is the liver, with metabolites also formed in the gastrointestinal tract, brain, skin, and other steroid target tissues. The principal pathways of estrogen and progestin metabolism are hydroxylation, O-methylation, and conjugation with either glucuronic acid or sulfate. Estrone, estriol, 2-methoxyestrone, and their respective glucuronide or sulfate conjugates are the most abundant estrogen urinary metab-

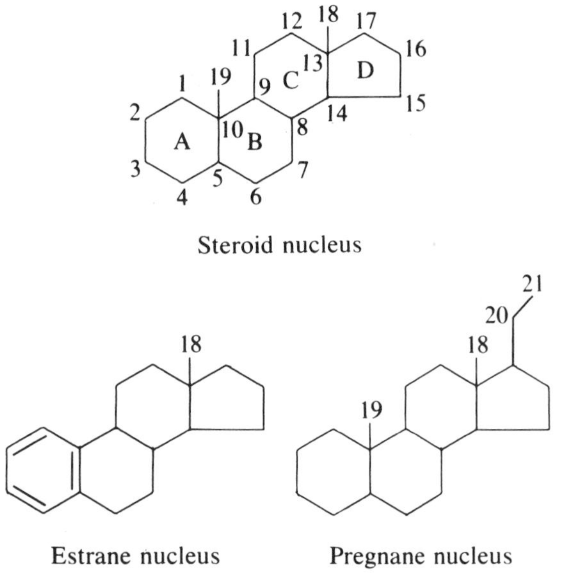

Steroid nucleus

Estrane nucleus   Pregnane nucleus

Figure 67-1. The steroid nucleus, indicating rings and positions, the estrane nucleus, and the pregnane nucleus.

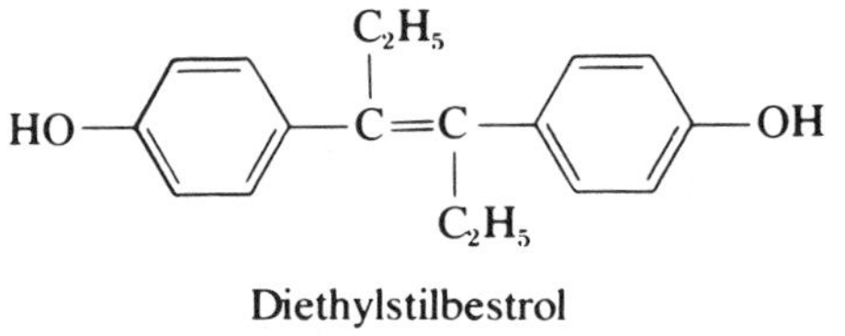

olites. Progesterone is excreted as pregnanediol or the pregnanediol conjugate.

Synthetic Estrogens and Progestins

Synthetic steroid hormones retain the common steroid nucleus, but they may contain novel substituents that affect their pharmacological activity. The two most widely used synthetic steroid estrogens are ethinyl estradiol and mestranol.

Approximately 50 percent of a dose of mestranol is demethylated to ethinyl estradiol. Ethinyl estradiol also can be deethinylated. Subsequently, the metabolism of these two synthetic estrogens proceeds by means of the same pathways as the natural steroid hormones. The principal metabolites of mestranol and ethinyl estradiol are hydroxylated derivatives that are conjugated with either glucuronic acid or sulfate. The synthetic steroid estrogens, in contrast to the natural estrogens, are excreted primarily in the feces.

One chemical class of synthetic progestins is derived from testosterone and is referred to as the 19-nortestosterones. These compounds have reduced androgenic activity and increased progestational activity. Norethindrone and norethindrone acetate are two synthetic progestins derived by the addition of an ethinyl group to the C17 position of 19-nortestosterone. There is little difference in the pharmacological activity of norethindrone and norethindrone acetate because the acetate group is

Figure 67-2. Diethylstilbestrol.

very readily cleaved to yield norethindrone in humans. Norethindrone is metabolized by means of hydroxylation and conjugation just as the natural progestins. The majority of the 19-nortestosterone metabolites are conjugates that are excreted in the urine.

A second chemical class of synthetic progestins contains the pregnane nucleus structure of progesterone along with some additional substitutions. Alkyl chain additions to the C17 position increase the biological half-life of these compounds. Modifications at positions C6 and C7 increase their progestational activity. Examples of these synthetic progestins include medroxyprogesterone and megestrol acetate. These compounds are metabolized in the same manner as progesterone and are excreted in the urine.

Nonsteroidal Estrogens

A large number of chemicals that lack the steroid ring structure exhibit estrogenic activity. The critical structural determinants for estrogenic activity are two nucleophilic sites, in which one is a phenolic hydroxyl group, lying in a single plane separated by 10 to 12 Å.

Diethylstilbestrol (DES) is a nonsteroidal molecule (Fig. 67-2) with potent estrogenic activity. Metabolism of DES proceeds through a variety of pathways that are also utilized by the natural estrogens, including aromatic ring hydroxylation, O-methylation, and conjugation reactions. Conjugates of DES frequently undergo enterohepatic recirculation. DES is excreted primarily in the feces.

Antiestrogens

Antiestrogens are compounds that, when given before or simultaneously with estrogens, antagonize some of the effects of the estrogens. Interestingly, when so-called antiestrogens are administered in the absence of estrogens, these compounds can elicit some estrogenic responses. Two antiestrogens are in extensive clinical use: clomiphene citrate and tamoxifen citrate (Fig. 67-3). Neither

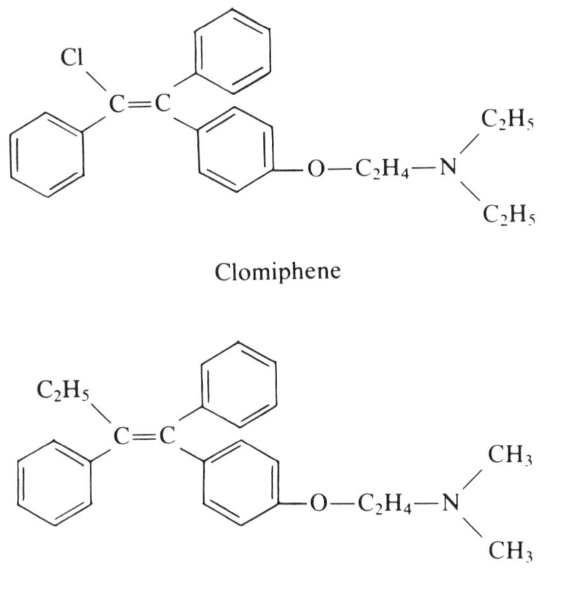

Clomiphene

Tamoxifen

Figure 67-3. Antiestrogens.

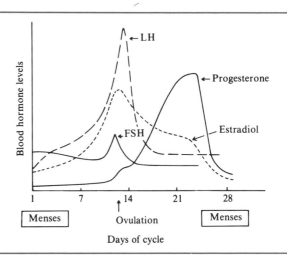

Figure 67-4. Blood hormone levels of ovarian hormones and gonadotropins in women during a normal menstrual cycle. LH = luteinizing hormone; FSH = follicle-stimulating hormone.

contains the steroid nucleus. Clomiphene and tamoxifen structurally resemble the nonsteroidal estrogen DES more than the natural estrogens.

Tamoxifen and clomiphene are orally active. Biliary excretion is the major route of drug elimination, with 80 to 90 percent of a dose being excreted in the feces.

See Chap. 62 for a detailed discussion of the use of tamoxifen in breast cancer.

Effects and Uses of Agents

Physiological Actions of Estrogens and Progestins

Adenohypophyseal-Gonadal Interactions

A basic knowledge of the normal relationships that exist between the hypothalamus, the anterior pituitary, and the female reproductive tract is needed to understand the therapeutic actions and side effects of hormone administration.

Secretion of gonadotropin releasing hormone (GnRH) from the hypothalamus stimulates the release of follicle-stimulating hormone (FSH) and luteinizing hormone (LH) from the anterior pituitary. FSH and LH regulate the production of estrogen and progesterone by the ovary. Ovarian estrogen and progesterone secretion proceeds in a cyclical manner. It is this cyclical release of estrogen and progesterone that determines the regular hormonal

changes in the uterus, vagina, and cervix associated with the menstrual cycle. Cyclical changes in blood levels of estrogen and progesterone, together with FSH and LH, modulate the development of ova, ovulation, and the corpus luteum in the ovary.

Control of Ovarian Steroidogenesis

During the first, or *follicular*, phase of the menstrual cycle, FSH stimulates the development of granulosa cells within the ovarian follicles. In the ovarian theca cells, LH stimulates the production of androgens, the precursors for estrogen biosynthesis. These androgens diffuse into the nearby granulosa cells. FSH and androgens can stimulate aromatase enzyme activity in the granulosa cells causing the testosterone to be converted to 17β-estradiol. Through this metabolic process, estradiol blood levels rise slowly during the early phase of the menstrual cycle and then fall quite rapidly (Fig. 67-4). Estradiol blood levels peak around midcycle (i.e., days 12–14) and are thought to be important in triggering a midcycle surge of LH and FSH secretion. Estrogens have a biphasic effect on LH and FSH release, with high levels of estrogen at midcycle triggering LH and FSH release; subsequently they suppress LH and FSH secretion. This suppression is mediated by inhibition of GnRH release from the hypothalamus.

The *luteal* phase of the menstrual cycle follows the LH and FSH surge (see Fig. 67-4). The brief elevation of LH levels stimulates production of the ovarian corpus luteum. The high levels of estradiol and FSH at midcycle inhibit aromatase activity in the granulosa cells. As a consequence, during the luteal phase, estrogen production is reduced and androgens produced by the ovarian theca cells accumulate. Androgens, together with low levels of FSH, stimulate the production of progesterone by the granulosa cells in the corpus luteum. The menstrual cycle ends about 14 days later, with the regression of the corpus luteum and a concomitant fall in estrogen and progesterone production. The triggering mechanism for this regression may involve both estrogens and prostaglandins. In the event that pregnancy occurs, human chorionic gonadotropin secretion by the embryo maintains the corpus luteum through stimulation of progesterone and estrogen synthesis.

Reproductive Tract Changes During the Menstrual Cycle

Ovary

During the follicular phase of the menstrual cycle, one or more follicles are prepared for ovulation. FSH and estrogens are the most important hormones for this developmental process. Complete follicular maturation cannot occur in the absence of LH. Rupture of a mature follicle follows the midcycle peak of LH and FSH by about 24 hr. In humans, usually one mature ovum is released per cycle. During the luteal phase of the menstrual cycle and under the influence of LH, the ovarian granulosa cells of the corpus luteum become vacuolated and accumulate a yellow pigment called lutein.

Uterus

The lining of the uterus, that is, the endometrium, consists of a layer of epithelial cells overlying a layer of vascularized stromal cells. Under the influence of estrogen and progesterone, the endometrium undergoes cyclical changes that prepare it for the implantation of a fertilized ovum. The follicular phase of the menstrual cycle also may be called the *proliferative phase* when referring to changes that occur in the uterus. Estrogens induce endometrial cell division and growth.

During the luteal phase, when the uterus is exposed to high concentrations of progesterone and moderate estradiol levels, the mitotic activity in the endometrial cells is suppressed. The action of progesterone on the endometrium converts it from a proliferative state to a secretory state. The epithelial cell structure assumes a more glandular appearance. Vascularization of the stroma increases and some stromal cells begin to look like the decidual cells of early pregnancy. Estrogens and progesterone are key hormones in the maintenance of pregnancy.

When implantation of the ovum does not occur, estrogen and progesterone levels fall late in the luteal phase and menstrual bleeding ensues. The endometrial lining, but for a single layer of epithelial cells, is shed.

Vaginal Epithelium

Estrogens stimulate proliferation of the vaginal epithelium. However, proliferation of the vaginal epithelium is checked by the cyclical exposure to progesterone during the luteal phase.

Endocervical Glands

The composition of the cervical mucus that is secreted by these glands is regulated by estrogens and progestins. Under the influence of high levels of estrogen or progesterone, the physiochemical composition of cervical mucus may reduce sperm motility and provide a barrier to fertilization.

Breasts

Estrogens stimulate proliferation of the ductal epithelial cells in breast tissue. Progesterone mediates lobuloalveolar development at the ends of these mammary ducts. Minor cyclical changes in the breast occur during the cyclical variation of estrogen and progesterone levels during the menstrual cycle. The effects of estrogens and progesterone on breast development are most noticeable during puberty and pregnancy.

Growth and Development

Estrogens cause the growth of the uterus, fallopian tubes, and vagina. Estrogens also are responsible for the expression of female secondary sex characteristics during puberty. These include breast enlargement, the female distribution of body hair, female body contours as determined by subcutaneous fat deposition, and skin texture.

Estrogens can stimulate the release of growth hormone and exert a positive effect on nitrogen balance. These effects contribute to the growth spurt during puberty. Closure of the bone epiphyses signaling the end of long bone growth is also estrogen-mediated. Estrogens maintain bone mass by inhibiting bone resorption. This action of estrogen may be mediated by stimulating calcitonin production. Additionally, progestins antagonize loss of bone.

In males, estrogens stimulate the growth of the stromal cells in the accessory sex organs.

Cardiovascular Effects

Estrogens may protect against atherosclerosis and myocardial infarction, since the incidence of heart attacks in premenopausal women is several times lower than in men of similar ages. Further, the incidence of heart attacks in postmenopausal women reaches that of men. The reason for this so-called protective effect of estrogen is not clearly established, but estrogens do lower serum cholesterol by stimulating the formation of high-density lipoproteins and reducing low-density lipoproteins.

During the normal menstrual cycle, estrogens and progestins may cause sodium retention, breast engorgement, and, rarely, mild edema. During pregnancy, in the presence of high circulating levels of estrogens and progesterone, there is an increased risk of thromboembolic diseases. This risk may be due to associated increases in the synthesis of blood clotting factors by the liver.

The Brain

Estrogen and progesterone have marked effects on female sexual behavior in certain mammals. Such behavioral changes can be elicited by the direct application of estrogen or progesterone to areas in the hypothalamus. The biosynthesis of estradiol from testosterone in the hypothalamus is also thought to contribute to male sexual behavior in rodents.

Other Actions

The high levels of estrogens and progesterone associated with pregnancy may alter liver function and glucose metabolism. High circulating levels of estrogen can cause mild glucose intolerance. Estrogens increase the synthesis of many liver proteins including transferrin, sex hormone–binding globulin (SHBG), corticosteroid-binding globulin, and thyroid-binding globulin. Reductions in serum albumin and antithrombin III synthesis can occur in the presence of elevated female sex steroids.

Pharmacology

The naturally occurring estrogens and progestins are ineffective orally due to their rapid metabolic inactivation within the gastrointestinal tract and in the liver. The synthetic steroids containing an ethinyl substitution are metabolized more slowly. Thus, synthetic steroid hormones have improved oral absorption properties and extended biological half-lives compared to the natural estrogens and progesterone.

Another factor that influences the pharmacological activity of the estrogens is their binding to plasma proteins. More than 90 percent of blood estradiol is protein bound, with SHBG being the major serum estrogen-binding moiety. Estrogens that are bound to SHBG are biologically inactive because of their high binding affinity while estrogens that are bound loosely to serum albumin are available for entry into tissues and are, therefore, biologically active.

Progesterone in plasma is 89 percent protein bound. Progesterone binds with a relatively high affinity to the serum protein, corticosteroid-binding globulin, and also to albumin.

DES is a very effective pharmacological agent, particularly since it is neither bound to SHBG nor rapidly metabolized.

Long-acting semisynthetic estrogens and progestins contain esterified lipophilic substituents. Esterification of these steroids prolongs their release from depot injection sites. Long-acting estrogens include estradiol benzoate and estradiol valerate. Hydroxyprogesterone caproate and medroxyprogesterone acetate are long-acting synthetic progestins.

Mechanism of Action

The specificity of action of the steroid hormones is due to the presence of intracellular receptors within target tissues.

Estrogens, such as estradiol, rapidly penetrate the cell membrane through simple diffusion, and then interact with a protein receptor. After some chemical modification, the estrogen-protein complex demonstrates increased affinity for nuclei and DNA. The metabolic responses to estradiol require an interaction between DNA and the estrogen-receptor complex. This interaction results in increased ribosomal and specific messenger RNA (mRNA) synthesis as well as increased protein synthesis. Thus, biochemical effects produced by steroid hormones ultimately involve the regulation of intracellular protein synthesis in target tissues.

Estradiol can augment target tissue responses to progesterone by inducing an increase in the concentration of progesterone receptors. Progesterone, on the other hand, appears to limit tissue responses to estrogen by decreasing the concentration of estrogen receptors.

Clinical Uses

The chief therapeutic uses of estrogens and progestins are as oral contraceptive preparations and in the treatment of menopausal symptoms. Estrogens, progestins, and antiestrogens are also important agents in the treatment of breast and endometrial cancer. A variety of other gynecological disorders are treated with estrogens, progestins, or both, including the management of infertility.

It is clear that hormone therapy is associated with a large number of side effects. The steroid hormones should, therefore, be given at their lowest effective dosages and for the shortest possible time to minimize adverse reactions.

Oral Contraception

Oral contraceptives are among the most effective forms of birth control (Table 67-1). The most widely used type of oral contraceptive in the United States today is the *combination* pill, that is, a combination of estrogen and progestin (Table 67-2). Users take a daily pill containing both estrogen and a progestin for 20 to 21 days of the menstrual cycle and then no pill or a placebo for the remainder of the cycle or the next 7 to 8 days. Withdrawal bleeding occurs 2 to 3 days after discontinuation of the pill regimen.

Table 67-1. Pregnancy Rates vs. Contraceptive Method

Method	Pregnancies (%)*
Male sterilization	0.15
Norplant System	0.2
Female sterilization	0.4
Oral contraceptives	3
Intrauterine device (IUD)	3
Condom	12
Diaphragm or sponge	18–28
Spermicide	21
None	85

*Accidental pregnancy rate during a 1-year period.
Source: Data from J. Trussell and K. Kost, *Stud. Fam. Plann.* 18:237, 1987.

Table 67-2. Some Oral Contraceptive Preparations Available in the United States, with Estrogen-Progestin Content

Estrogen	Progestin	Trade name
Ethinyl estradiol (20 μg)	Norethindrone acetate (1mg)	Loestrin
Ethinyl estradiol (30 μg)	Norgestrel (300 μg)	Lo-Ovral
Ethinyl estradiol (30 μg)	Levonorgestrel (150 μg)	Nordette, Levlen
Ethinyl estradiol (35 μg)	Norethindrone (0.5 mg)	Brevicon, Modicon
Ethinyl estradiol (50 μg)	Norgestrel (0.5 mg)	Ovral
Ethinyl estradiol (50 μg)	Ethynodiol diacetate (1 mg)	Demulen
Mestranol (50 μg)	Norethindrone (1 mg)	Ortho-Novum, Norinyl, Norethin
None	Norethindrone (0.35 mg)	Micronor, Nor-QD
None	Norgestrel (0.075 mg)	Ovrette

A variety of combination pills are available, which vary in the dose of synthetic estrogen and progestin that they contain. Ethinyl estradiol and mestranol are the only two estrogen constituents used for oral contraception in the United States. The use of ethinyl estradiol is favored. Mestranol is inactive until it is metabolized to ethinyl estradiol.

There are several different progestins used in combination-type pills. Norgestrel is a mixture of active and inactive enantiomers. Levonorgestrel is the active enantiomer. Levonorgestrel and norethindrone are the most

Table 67-3. Estrogen/Progestin Composition of Tri-Levlen 28, a Triphasic Oral Contraceptive

	Estrogen	Progestin	Days
Phase I	Ethinyl estradiol (30 μg)	Levonorgestrel (50 μg)	1–6
Phase II	Ethinyl estradiol (40 μg)	Levonorgestrel (75 μg)	7–11
Phase III	Ethinyl estradiol (30 μg)	Levonorgestrel (125 μg)	12–21
Blank tablets	0	0	22–28

potent synthetic progestins in oral contraceptive preparations.

Combination pills with the lowest effective concentrations of both the estrogen and progestin component should be prescribed. These preparations are referred to as low-dose oral contraceptive agents. Side effects due to both the estrogen and progestin components are minimized with the use of these agents.

Clinical experience with the low-dose combination pills indicates that the estrogen-to-progestin ratio is critical in achieving maximum contraceptive activity. In certain combination pills (e.g., *Tri-Norinyl, Tri-Levlen, Triphasil*), the estrogen-to-progestin ratio is varied in three phases over the initial 21 days by changing the progestin content of the tablets. An example of the estrogen and progestin doses found in this type of oral contraceptive is shown in Table 67-3.

Another type of oral contraceptive formulation that is available is the progestin-only, or *mini-pill*. The mini-pill consists of a low dose of either norethindrone or norgestrel (see Table 67-2). Due to an increased incidence of certain side effects and a slightly decreased contraceptive activity, progestin-only oral contraceptives are not extensively used.

The *Norplant System* for contraception consists of a series of levonorgestrel-filled silastic tubes. These tubes are implanted subcutaneously on the inside of the upper arm by a physician. One set of six tubes remains effective for up to 5 years, but the contraceptive effects are readily reversible by the removal of the implant. Side effects of the Norplant System are similar to those seen with other progestin-only contraceptives; however, accidental pregnancies are less frequent.

Mechanism of Action

Inhibition of ovulation is the primary mechanism involved in the contraceptive action of sequential and combination birth control pills. Ovulation is prevented by the suppression of the midcycle surge of FSH and LH. Estrogens are most active in inhibiting FSH release, but at high enough doses they also inhibit LH release. In low-dose combination pills, the progestin causes LH suppression.

The progestin component is also important in causing withdrawal bleeding at the end of the cycle.

The mechanism by which progestin-only pills inhibit fertility has not been clearly established, but ovulation is not consistently suppressed. The contraceptive action of progestins alone may result from changes in the cervical mucus, making it less permeable to sperm, or to effects on the endometrium that interfere with implantation.

Treatment of Menopausal Symptoms

The beginning of the female menopause is marked by the last menstrual cycle. This is the result of declining ovarian function and reduced synthesis of estrogens and progesterone. Estrogen production in postmenopausal women is usually about 10 percent of that in premenopausal women. Almost no progesterone is synthesized in postmenopausal women.

The four most common menopausal symptoms are vasomotor disorders, or "hot flashes," urogenital atrophy, osteoporosis, and psychological disturbances. A varying proportion of women may experience one or more of these symptoms. Vasomotor disorders are the most common complaint, affecting 70 to 80 percent of postmenopausal women. Twenty-five percent of postmenopausal women experience the more serious symptom, osteoporosis.

Conjugated equine estrogens are the most commonly used estrogens in the treatment of menopausal symptoms. *Premarin* is a mixture of estrogen sulfates, including estrone, equilin, and 17-α-dihydroequilin. The sulfate derivatives are orally active and are cleaved within the body to yield the active, unconjugated estrogen. Typical dosages of conjugated estrogens are 0.625 or 1.25 mg/day for the control of vasomotor symptoms or osteoporosis.

Norethindrone and *dl*-norgestrel are the progestins commonly given to postmenopausal women receiving estrogens. Both are orally active. Dosages of norethindrone (1.0–2.5 mg/day) and of *dl*-norgestrel (0.15 mg/day) are equally effective in the control of endometrial proliferation.

Vasomotor Symptoms

The cause of the vasomotor changes is unclear, but they appear to be associated with the release of LH after normal female estrogen levels have fallen. These symptoms occur with variable frequency but generally they disappear without treatment within 2 to 3 yr of their onset. Estrogen or progestin therapies are often effective in suppressing these vasomotor symptoms. With either hormone, individual titrations should be performed to determine the lowest effective dosage. Since these symptoms eventually disappear spontaneously, the need for continued therapy should be periodically assessed by withdrawing the hormone. Due to the risk of endometrial cancer

with estrogen administration, a preliminary endometrial biopsy should be performed before instituting therapy, and a biopsy should be repeated at 6- to 12-month intervals. Estrogens should be given in an intermittent fashion, 21 days on estrogen followed by at least 7 to 10 days of treatment with a progestin alone.

Urogenital Atrophy

The tissues of the distal vagina and urethra are of similar embryonic origin and both are sensitive to the trophic action of estrogens. Postmenopausal atrophy of these tissues may result in painful sexual intercourse, dysuria, and frequent genitourinary infections. Unlike the vasomotor complaints, these symptoms seldom improve if untreated. Treatment with a combination of minimally effective dosages of an estrogen and a progestin is recommended. Estrogen can be administered orally or in a topical preparation with equivalent efficacy. Progestins are given orally.

Osteoporosis

Osteoporosis is a decrease in bone mass and constitutes the most serious menopausal symptom. It has been estimated that following cessation of ovarian function, the loss of bone mass proceeds at a rate of 1 to 3 percent per year. As a result of osteoporosis, as many as 50 percent of women will develop spinal compression fractures by age 75, and 20 percent will suffer hip fractures by age 90. The physiology underlying the gradual reduction in bone mass beginning at age 40 to 50 is complex and involves falling levels of estrogen production as well as changes in absorption of dietary calcium, parathyroid hormone, calcitonin, and 1,25-dihydroxycholecalciferol secretion (see Chap. 70).

Hormone replacement therapies can slow bone loss but cannot reverse existing deficits. Estrogen treatment is the most effective therapy for osteoporosis and significantly reduces the incidence of bone fractures in postmenopausal women. Progestin administration also inhibits bone loss and the combination of both estrogen and progestin may constitute an even better therapy. Combination therapy with estrogens and progestins in osteoporosis will lessen the risk of endometrial cancer that might occur during treatment of this condition with estrogens alone.

Alternatives to steroid hormone replacement therapy for osteoporosis include calcitonin, biphosphonates, and calcium supplementation. In addition, long-term tamoxifen administration has recently been shown to delay bone loss in postmenopausal women.

Psychological Disturbances

It has not been proved that the depression and anxiety reported to occur in postmenopausal women are the result of estrogen deprivation. There is no clear indication for the use of estrogens in the treatment of psychiatric problems. The insomnia and fatigue experienced by many postmenopausal women may be related to reduced estrogen levels. There is a correlation between the incidence of nighttime hot flashes and waking episodes and low levels of estrogen. Effective control of these vasomotor symptoms by the administration of either estrogens or progestins may reduce insomnia.

Replacement Therapy

Oophorectomy causes many of the symptoms seen in menopause. The onset and intensity of vasomotor symptoms and osteoporosis, however, may be more severe than in women proceeding into the more gradual age-associated process of menopause. The regimens for estrogen-progestin replacement therapy in oophorectomized patients are comparable to those recommended for postmenopausal women.

There are several genetic conditions that lead to failure of ovarian development. These conditions include phenotypic females with an XO (Turner's syndrome) or an XY sex chromosome karyotype. Genetic defects also may appear in individuals with a normal XX sex chromosome karyotype; presumably genes on the autosomal as well as on the sex chromosomes are required for normal ovarian development. Pituitary hypogonadism is a consequence of inherited deficiencies in normal pituitary function. The adenohypophysis fails to produce LH, FSH, or both, and abnormal ovarian function results.

These genetic alterations lead to a failure in the synthesis of normal amounts of estrogen or progesterone. As a consequence, female secondary sex characteristics do not appear at puberty. Only with estrogen treatment is there a stimulation of the growth of the genitalia, breast enlargement, and development of female body contours and distribution of body hair. Some increases in body height also occur with estrogen therapy, but this is more marked after androgen treatment.

Treatment of Infertility

Anovulation is often related to altered estrogen-progestin ratios and can be treated with a variety of agents, including estrogen and progestin replacement, clomiphene citrate, bromocriptine, FSH, LH, human chorionic gonadotropin (hCG) and GnRH. Clomiphene citrate (see Fig. 67-3) and bromocriptine are currently the two most widely used agents.

Induction of Ovulation

Anovulation is often due to insufficient release of LH and FSH during the midphase of the menstrual cycle. Induction of ovulation by clomiphene citrate is thought to be mediated by means of a stimulation of FSH and LH release. The mechanism of this action is probably related to the *antiestrogenic* properties of clomiphene citrate. Although estrogens generally exert a negative feedback inhibition on FSH and LH secretion by means of a suppression of GnRH from the hypothalamus, clomiphene exerts its action by stimulating the secretion of these hormones. Antagonism of this feedback system results in a surge of FSH and LH secretion and, hence, ovulation.

Patients with normal or elevated estrogen levels and normal pituitary and hypothalamic function respond most frequently to treatment with clomiphene citrate. In this patient group, the ovulation rate following clomiphene citrate may be 80 percent. Clomiphene citrate is administered on a cyclical schedule. First, menstrual bleeding is induced; drug is then given orally for 5 days at a dose of 50 mg/day. Ovulation is expected 5 to 11 days after the last dose of clomiphene citrate. Pregnancy rates after six such treatment cycles approach 50 to 80 percent, with most pregnancies occurring during the first three clomiphene-treated cycles. Clomiphene is also used in conjunction with gonadotropins to induce ovulation for in vitro fertilization.

Treatment of Cancer

Certain tissues of the female and male reproductive tracts, which are subject to the trophic action of hormones, exhibit a high frequency of neoplasia. Cancer of the breast is the second most common form of cancer in American women. Prostatic cancer is a frequent cancer among American men. Both of these cancers, and, in addition, the rarer endometrial cancer in women, are often responsive to treatments with estrogens, antiestrogens, or progestins. The toxicity of these hormonal treatments compared with standard cancer chemotherapy is low.

Renal carcinoma has also been treated with the progestin, medroxyprogesterone acetate.

Breast Cancer

Early breast cancer is usually treated by surgery and local irradiation. Hormonal therapy is reserved for patients with advanced metastatic breast cancer. Breast cancer occurs in both premenopausal and postmenopausal women. Approximately one third of all patients will experience a complete or partial remission, with a mean duration of 9 to 12 months on treatment with hormones. Endocrine therapy of advanced breast cancer is not curative.

Normal breast growth is stimulated by estrogens. Therefore, it is not surprising that some breast tumors regress following treatment with antiestrogens. Breast cancer in premenopausal and postmenopausal women responds equally well to antiestrogen therapy. The antiestrogen tamoxifen is the drug of choice for this purpose. It is administered orally, twice daily, in daily dosages of 20 or 40 mg. The half-life of tamoxifen in the blood is approximately 1 week. Cancer remissions usually are not apparent until at least 1 month after treatment is initiated.

There is currently much interest in the use of tamoxifen as a chemopreventative in women with high risk for development of breast cancer. Women who have survived cancer in a single breast are at high risk for developing cancer in the contralateral breast. Daily tamoxifen has been shown to reduce the incidence of second breast cancers in these patients by 40 percent.

Paradoxically, breast cancer remissions follow high-dose estrogen therapy. The mechanism of this effect is completely unknown. In general, postmenopausal patients respond better than premenopausal women. DES is the estrogen most commonly used for this purpose.

Progestins have been used with some success in the treatment of breast cancer, although the response rate is lower than with either antiestrogen or high-dose estrogen therapy. Most clinical experience has been obtained using oral megestrol acetate.

The successful response rate of breast cancers to estrogen, antiestrogen, or progestin treatment is dependent on the presence of high-affinity receptors for estrogen or progesterone, or both. Fewer than 10 percent of mammary tumors that lack detectable estrogen receptor levels will respond to hormonal therapies. The response rate of tumors that exhibit estrogen receptors or both estrogen and progesterone receptors ranges from 60 to 80 percent; the higher response rate correlates with higher receptor levels. The best prognosis is for those patients whose tumors have high levels of both estrogen and progesterone receptors. Thus, determination of hormone receptor levels in tumor samples is highly recommended before selecting a therapy.

Endometrial Cancer

Progesterone administration induces remissions in approximately one third of patients with metastatic endometrial cancer. The mean duration of response is 27 months. Almost 60 percent of all endometrial adenocarcinomas contain progesterone receptors. Preliminary data show a correlation between progesterone receptor status and response rates in this disease. The mechanism of the effect of progesterone on endometrial cancer is not known.

Prostatic Cancer

Androgens cause growth of the prostate gland and stimulate proliferation of prostatic cancers. Estrogen treatment can induce remission in 50 to 80 percent of metastatic prostatic tumors. The average duration of remission is 15 months.

The mechanism of this effect is thought to be twofold. First, estrogens lower serum testosterone levels. Estrogens suppress hypothalamic release of GnRH, thereby inhibiting the release of LH, which stimulates androgen production by the testes. Second, estrogens are believed to antagonize androgen action in the prostate gland itself.

Daily doses of DES of 1 to 5 mg have been administered in the treatment of prostatic cancer, with the lower doses resulting in a decreased incidence of cardiovascular side effects.

Other Uses

Dysfunctional Uterine Bleeding

This is an abnormally heavy uterine bleeding that usually results from anovulation and insufficient progesterone production. Progesterone treatment alone may be sufficient to stop bleeding if therapy is initiated soon after the problem arises. If extensive bleeding has occurred, regulation of the succeeding menstrual cycles by treatment with combination-type oral contraceptive formulations is indicated.

Dysmenorrhea

Unusual pain during the bleeding period of the menstrual cycle may be related to ovulation. The administration of combination oral contraceptives to supplement endogenous female sex steroids may lead to a normalization of ovulating cycles and lessened dysmenorrhea.

Endometriosis

Endometriosis is a condition in which there is often extrauterine growth of the endometrial tissues of the uterus. This causes pain, extrauterine bleeding, and infertility. Treatment with progesterone can often inhibit proliferation of these tissues.

Lactation

Pharmacological dosages of estrogens and progesterone have been used to suppress postpartum milk production. These steroids are most effective when given soon after delivery. This use has been tempered by the risk of cardiovascular side effects.

Adverse Reactions

Common side effects associated with estrogen use include nausea, weight gain, and edema. Progestin use is associated with weight gain and mild depression. Tolerance to these effects usually develops over a period of several months.

Low-dose estrogen combination-type oral contraceptives in some patients result in irregular, midcycle bleeding episodes. High-progestin preparations, especially the progestin-only mini-pill, can result in irregular bleeding and prolonged amenorrhea.

Cancer

Endometrial Cancer

In premenopausal and postmenopausal women receiving estrogens alone, endometrial hyperplasia frequently develops. This reaction is generally regarded to be a premalignant state, because individuals reported to have endometrial hyperplasia later have a higher-than-normal incidence of endometrial carcinoma. Administration of estrogens only is associated with a 1.7- to 15-fold increased risk of endometrial carcinoma. The relative risk rises with increased dosage and duration of estrogen use. Women receiving progestins 10 days per month during estrogen therapy generally do not develop endometrial carcinoma. Women taking combination oral contraceptives have a slightly decreased risk of developing endometrial carcinoma than do nonusers. This occurrence possibly is related to constant exposure of the endometrium to both progestin and estrogen.

Breast Cancer

Despite the fact that estrogens stimulate breast epithelial cell proliferation, there is little evidence that either estrogen alone or estrogen and progestin administration results in an increased incidence of breast cancer. Most studies report no increase in breast cancer among individuals taking estrogen alone; a few report a very modest increase. The risk of developing breast cancer may increase when estrogen replacement therapy is continued for 10 years or more. The incidence of breast cancer among women who take combination oral contraceptives is lower than that in women using other methods (i.e., nonchemical) of birth control. The most recent studies indicate that benign breast disease does not predispose oral contraceptive users to breast cancer development, although this was previously a concern.

Ovarian Cancer

Oral contraceptive use appears to slightly lessen the incidence of ovarian cancer.

Hepatic Cancer

Hepatocellular carcinoma and benign hepatomas are rare complications of oral contraceptive use.

Cardiovascular Complications

Most, but not all, cardiovascular side effects are due to the estrogen constituent and not the progestin constituent. The problems generally are most severe or frequent when either of the synthetic estrogens, ethinyl estradiol or mestranol, is used. These preparations alter liver function more significantly than do the natural estrogens, such as the sulfate conjugates or esterified estrogens. Alterations in the synthesis of specific liver proteins are implicated in the etiology of several estrogen-dependent cardiovascular side effects.

Hypertension

Mild hypertension frequently occurs in oral contraceptive users. Systolic blood pressure is elevated 5 to 6 mm Hg; diastolic blood pressure increases are on the order of 1 to 2 mm Hg. Serum renin substrate and renin activity are increased in women who take oral contraceptives, but whether this is directly related to the elevations in blood pressure has not been proved. Hypertension is not commonly a problem in postmenopausal women receiving conjugated estrogens.

Thromboembolic Diseases

Earlier reports cited greater incidences of thrombophlebitis and pulmonary embolism formation among oral contraceptive users than are generally now regarded as true. Current estimates are that oral contraceptive use increases the overall risk of thromboembolic disease two- to threefold. The increased use in recent years of oral contraceptives with lower estrogen content probably contributes to the decreased risk. However, the risk is greater in women who smoke, who are over age 35, or who are diabetic.

Synthetic estrogens present in oral contraceptives are implicated in thromboembolic and blood clotting disorders. A number of the coagulation factors and fibrinogen are liver proteins whose synthesis is increased by synthetic estrogens and may contribute to thromboembolism formation. The effect of conjugated estrogens in thromboembolic disease is less certain. Most reports show no or little increased risk associated with their use.

Serum Lipid Profiles

Multiple changes in serum lipid profiles have been reported in association with estrogen and progestin therapy. There is a relationship between elevated levels of cholesterol, triglycerides, very low density lipoproteins (VLDL), low-density lipoproteins (LDL), and coronary artery disease. The elevation of high-density lipoproteins (HDL), in contrast, appears to be related to a reduced incidence of cardiovascular effects. The hormonal effects vary depending on the dosage, duration, route of administration, and particular preparation.

The synthetic progestins derived from 19-nortestosterone, such as levonorgestrel, norgestrel, norethindrone, and norethindrone acetate, elicit the greatest increases in serum HDL. Medroxyprogesterone acetate (10 mg/day) and megestrol acetate (0.5 mg/day), which are 17 α-hydroxyprogesterone derivatives, do not alter HDL levels. Progestins do not antagonize estrogen-induced rises in triglycerides.

When estrogen and progestin are administered concurrently, serum levels of HDL and triglycerides vary according to the relative strength of the estrogen and progestin in the preparation. Thus, the magnitude of serum lipid changes varies among oral contraceptive preparations.

Migraine Headaches

A 0.5 percent incidence of migraines has been reported among users of oral contraceptives. Migraine headaches may be a warning signal for an oncoming stroke, and immediate discontinuation of oral contraceptive use is recommended.

Teratogenesis

DES was once given for the prevention of spontaneous abortions, but it no longer has such a medical indication. There is a 0.01 to 0.1 percent incidence of rare vaginal and cervical clear cell adenocarcinoma among the female offspring of mothers who received DES during their first trimester of pregnancy. Progestins may be teratogenic during the first trimester of pregnancy. Therefore, if pregnancy is suspected, oral contraceptive use should not be initiated or use should be stopped promptly.

Fertility

There is some delay in the return of fertility after discontinuation of oral contraceptive use. Gonadotropin profiles should be normal 3 months after combination oral contraceptive use is stopped. The incidence of prolonged amenorrhea extending beyond 6 months is 2 to 3 percent. This reaction is especially a problem with the use of the progestin-only mini-pill.

Breast Feeding

The use of oral contraceptives may interfere with lactation. In addition, the hormones may be present in the mother's milk and thus be taken in by the nursing child. If breast feeding is planned, the use of oral contraceptives should be discontinued until after weaning.

Gallbladder Disease

In postmenopausal women receiving estrogens, there is a 2.5-fold increased incidence of gallbladder disease. This occurrence may be related to changes in plasma lipid metabolism.

Glucose Tolerance

Estrogen usage is associated with a mild decrease in glucose tolerance. Estrogens do not cause diabetes, but their concurrent use in the diabetic patient may require adjustment in insulin dosage.

Ocular Toxicities

There have been reports of optic neuritis and retinal thrombosis associated with oral contraceptive use, but the incidence of these effects is low.

Antiestrogen-Associated Toxicity

Clomiphene Citrate

Ovarian enlargement is the most common side effect of clomiphene use. The occurrence of multiple births following ovulation induction with clomiphene is 4 to 9 percent; 90 percent of these multiple births are twins. Since clomiphene is teratogenic, therapy should be discontinued if there is a chance that conception has occurred. Rarely, nonreversible ocular toxicities have been reported with clomiphene use.

Tamoxifen Citrate

Nausea, vomiting, and hot flashes may accompany tamoxifen administration. Tamoxifen may cause a transient flare of tumor growth and increased pain due to bone metastases. These reactions are thought to be due to an initial estrogenic action of this drug. Mild or transient depression of platelet counts often occurs in patients receiving tamoxifen. At very high doses, not generally used in cancer treatment now, ocular toxicity has been reported. Chronic administration of tamoxifen causes liver tumors in rats. The risk of hepatocellular carcinoma in humans receiving long term (5–10 yr) therapy has not yet been ascertained. Long-term tamoxifen administration is associated with a slightly (0.4%) elevated incidence of endometrial cancer.

Contraindications

The contraindications to the use of estrogens, progestins, or estrogen-progestin combinations are presented in Table 67-4. Additionally, these natural and synthetic hor-

Table 67-4. Contraindications for Drug Use

Formulation	Contraindicated if present
Estrogens	Breast* or endometrial cancer
	Pregnancy
	Hepatic dysfunction or liver cancer
	Preexisting cardiovascular disease
Progestins	Pregnancy
	Depression
Oral contraceptives	Pregnancy
	Smokers over age 35
Antiestrogens	Pregnancy
	Endometrial cancer

*Except the therapeutic use of high-dose estrogens for breast cancer management.

Table 67-5. Preparations and Dosages of Estrogens

	Trade name	Dosage preparations
Estradiol	Estrace	1-, 2-mg tablets; vaginal cream 0.01%
	Estraderm	Skin patch delivery system
Polyestradiol phosphate	Estradurin	40-mg for IM injection
Piperazine estrone sulfate	Ogen	0.75-, 1.5-, 3-, 6-mg tablets; vaginal cream
Ethinyl estradiol	Estinyl	0.02-, 0.05-, 0.5-mg tablets
Quinestrol (3-cyclopentylethinyl estradiol)	Estrovis	100-μg tablets
Chlorotrianisene	TACE	12-, 25-mg capsules
Diethylstilbestrol	Diethylstil-bestrol, USP; Stilphostrol	1-, 5-mg tablets 50-mg tablets, IV solution
Dienestrol	Ortho Dienestrol Cream	Vaginal cream 0.01%
Conjugated estrogens	Premarin	0.3-, 0.625-, 0.9-, 1.25-, 2.5 mg tablets; vaginal cream 0.06%; 25-mg vials for IV or IM injection
Esterified estrogens USP/ methyltestosterone	Estratest	1.25/2.5-mg and 0.625/1.25-mg tablets

Table 67-6. Preparations and Dosages of Progestins

	Trade name	Dosage preparations
Medroxyprogesterone acetate	Provera, Amen, Cycrin	2.5-, 5-, 10-mg tablets
	Depo-Provera	100-, 400-mg/ml for injection
Megestrol acetate	Megace	20-, 40-mg tablets
Norethindrone	Norlutin	5-mg tablet
Norethindrone acetate	Aygestin, Norlutate	5-mg tablet

Table 67-7. Preparations and Dosages of Antiestrogens

	Trade name	Dosage preparations
Tamoxifen citrate	Nolvadex	10-mg tablets
Clomiphene citrate	Clomid, Serophene	50-mg tablets

tion for binding sites on plasma proteins, and enhanced excretion.

Preparations and Dosages

Tables 67-5 and 67-6 present summaries of estrogen and progestin preparations used in the treatment of gynecologic disorders and malignancies. Common antiestrogens are listed in Table 67-7.

mones should not be used in patients with congenital hyperlipidemia and are best avoided in patients with diabetes mellitus. Steroids also should be used with discretion in patients with migraine, hypertension, depression, epilepsy, and leiomyoma of the uterus.

Drug Interactions

Certain concomitantly administered drugs may interfere with the effectiveness of the oral contraceptives or lead to an increased incidence of breakthrough bleeding. These include rifampicin, isoniazid, ampicillin, neomycin, penicillin V, chloramphenicol, sulfonamides, nitrofurantoin, phenytoin, barbiturates, primidone, analgesics, and phenothiazines.

The oral contraceptives also may decrease the effectiveness of anticoagulants, anticonvulsants, tricyclic antidepressants, guanethidine, and hypoglycemic agents. The causes of such drug interactions include alterations in hepatic microsomal drug-metabolizing enzymes, competi-

Supplemental Reading

Chappel, S.C., and Howles, C. Reevaluation of the roles of LH and FSH in the ovulatory process. *Hum. Reproduction* 6:1206, 1991.

Derman, R.J. An overview of the noncontraceptive benefits and risks of oral contraception. *Int. J. Fertil.* 37 (Suppl. 1):19, 1992.

Duursma, S.A., and Raymakers, J.A. Estrogen and bone metabolism. *Obstet. Gynecol. Surv.* 47:38, 1992.

Harlop, S. The benefits and risks of hormone replacement therapy: An epidemiologic overview. *Am. J. Obstet. Gynecol.* 166:1986, 1992.

Jordan, V.C., and Murphy, C.S. Endocrine pharmacology of antiestrogens as antitumor agents. *Endocr. Rev.* 11:578, 1990.

Khoo, S.K., and Chick, P. Sex steroid hormones and breast cancer: Is there a link with oral contraceptive and hormone replacement therapy? *Med. J. Aust.* 156:124, 1992.

Orme, M., and Bach, D.J. Oral contraceptive steroids—pharmacologic issues of interest to the prescribing physician. *Adv. Contraception* 7:325, 1991.

Seed, M. Sex hormones, lipoproteins and cardiovascular risks. *Atherosclerosis* 90:1, 1991.

Sonderheim, S.J. Update on the metabolic effects of steroidal contraceptives. *Endocrinol. Metab. Clin. North Am.* 20:911, 1991.

Staffa, J.A., et al. Progestins and breast cancer: An epidemiologic review. *Fertil. Steril.* 57:473, 1992.

Whitcroft, S.I., and Stevenson, J.C. Hormone replacement therapy: Risks and benefits. *Clin. Endocrinol.* 36:15, 1992.

68

Androgens and Anabolic Steroids

Frank L. Schwartz and *Roman J. Miller*

Androgens are steroid hormones that are secreted primarily by the testis but also by the adrenal gland and ovary. Testosterone, the principal androgen secreted by the testis, and other androgenic compounds possess virilizing activities that serve to regulate both differentiation and secretory function of the male sex accessory organs. Androgens also exhibit protein anabolic activity in skeletal muscle, bone, and kidneys. As a class, the androgens are reasonably safe drugs, having limited and relatively predictable side effects.

History

Several key developments that led to the great expansion of our knowledge of androgen physiology and biochemistry came in the 1930s. In that decade, various pure androgenic substances were extracted from urine, testosterone was isolated from the testes, and the successful synthesis of testosterone was accomplished. When androgens were noted to possess both virilizing and protein anabolic activities, efforts were devoted to separating these two properties. The steroids with the highest ratio of protein anabolic activity to virilizing activity are 19-nortestosterone and its derivatives.

In the 1940s, Huggins and associates initiated the first clinical approach to androgen antagonism by using estrogens in the treatment of prostatic cancer. Estrogens inhibited prostatic growth by several mechanisms, including suppression of luteinizing hormone (LH) and follicle-stimulating hormone (FSH) regulation of testosterone biosynthesis and direct antagonism of the actions of testosterone at the receptor level in the prostatic neoplasia. Various compounds have now been developed that inhibit androgen-sensitive tissues by interference with gonadotropin regulation of testicular synthesis (e.g., gonadotropin releasing hormone [GnRH] antagonists), direct blockade of testosterone synthesis (e.g., ketoconazole), or direct inhibition of the action of testosterone in target tissues (e.g., flutamide, spironolactone, and finasteride).

Chemistry and Biosynthesis

Nomenclature

The basic steroid nucleus (Fig. 68-1) is common to all steroid hormones. The addition of a hydrogen atom at position 5 and an angular methyl group at positions 18 and 19 establishes the basic chemical framework for the androgens (i.e., the androstane series).

Characterization of Plasma Androgens

In men, *testosterone* is the principal circulating androgen (Fig. 68-2), and the testes are the principal source of testosterone. Although the adrenal gland is capable of androgen synthesis, fewer than 10 percent of the circulating androgens are normally derived from this source in men. Testosterone is synthesized by the testes at the rate of about 8 mg/24 hr, providing a plasma concentration of 0.5 to 0.6 μg/dl.

Androstenedione (Fig. 68-2) is an androgen of secondary importance in men. Both the testes and adrenal cortex contribute significantly to plasma androstenedione levels; total daily production is 2 to 3 mg. The androstenedione production rate in women is about 3 mg/24 hr, and plasma levels are approximately 0.15 μg/dl. Androstenedione concentrations in women vary greatly in the normal population and throughout the menstrual cycle, with levels peaking in the luteal phase of the cycle. Both the ovaries and the adrenal glands are capable of androgen synthesis and, in premenopausal women, ovarian production contributes approximately one third of the total androgens synthesized.

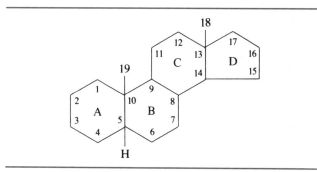

Figure 68-1. Basic cyclopentanoperhydrophenanthrene nucleus, showing four rings (A–D) with conventional numbering system for carbon atoms. Note the angular methyl groups at positions 18 and 19.

Dehydroepiandrosterone (DHEA) is an androgen (see Fig. 68-2) that is produced by the adrenal glands of both sexes. The total DHEA production rate is about 7 mg/24 hr, but owing to rapid hepatic clearance, the plasma concentration of DHEA is relatively low. The low plasma concentration, coupled with its low androgenic activity, relegates DHEA to only minor importance as an androgen.

Plasma androgen levels vary throughout the day, but whether such variation is simply random or fits a repeatable diurnal pattern is a matter of current debate. Certainly, when compared with the diurnal variation seen with cortisol, plasma testosterone concentrations are reasonably constant.

In humans, circulating testosterone is bound reversibly to two major plasma proteins: *albumin* and *gamma globulin.* Binding to albumin is a relatively nonspecific, low-affinity and high-capacity association, whereas binding to a specific gamma globulin fraction, called *sex hormone-binding globulin (SHBG)*, is a high-affinity, steroid-specific interaction. Under physiological conditions, 98 percent of testosterone is protein bound, 40 percent to albumin and 58 percent to SHBG. The 2 percent or less of circulating *free testosterone* reflects the amount that is biologically active and available for interaction with target cells.

SHBG levels are known to be influenced by a variety of conditions. Pregnancy and the use of oral contraceptives, both of which are associated with elevated estrogen levels, result in increased SHBG concentrations. Estrogens also may be responsible for the elevated levels of SHBG seen in cirrhotic patients and normal aging men. SHBG also is increased in hyperthyroidism, hypogonadism, and chronic bronchitis. Levels are suppressed in women treated with testosterone or chronic glucocorticoid therapy. It is important to note that elevations of SHBG do not necessarily result in a fall in free testosterone levels.

Plasma testosterone levels exhibit age-associated changes. The levels of the hormone are very low throughout childhood until early adolescence when, in boys, increasing testicular steroidogenesis precedes the onset of puberty. Beginning at about age 30, urinary 17-ketosteroid excretion declines steadily. This occurrence is due, in part, to decreased testicular production of testosterone. However, since there is a concomitant decline in the metabolic clearance rate of testosterone, the total plasma testosterone concentration remains relatively constant to well beyond the fifth decade and may only decline significantly after age 70. After the fifth decade, unbound testosterone levels decrease as a result of increased SHBG levels.

Urinary 17-ketosteroid excretion in women declines progressively after the age of 30. The decreased 17-ketosteroid level is due to a progressive decline in the adrenal synthesis of various steroids, including androstenedione, as well as to the reduction in ovarian steroidogenesis at menopause.

Steroidogenesis

The main steroidogenic components of the testis are the interstitial cells of Leydig found between the seminiferous tubules. The principal secretory product of Leydig cells, testosterone, is not stored to any significant degree within these cells.

Biochemical studies of Leydig cell steroidogenic function have shown that *testosterone synthesis begins with acetate derived either from glucose or products of lipid metabolism.* Acetate is converted into cholesterol through numerous reactions in or on the smooth endoplasmic reticulum. Cholesterol, once formed, is stored in lipid droplets in an esterified form. The cholesterol required for steroidogenesis is transferred into the mitochondria, where the side chain is cleaved by enzymes on the inner membranes to form pregnenolone. *This reaction is the rate-limiting step in testosterone biosynthesis and is the step stimulated by LH.* Pregnenolone is returned to the cytoplasm, where it serves as the principal precursor of testosterone.

Testosterone synthesis from pregnenolone can occur along two distinct metabolic pathways (delta-4 and delta-5; see Fig. 68-2). The names given to these two routes of metabolism refer to the position in the steroid molecule where an unsaturated bond is maintained. Thus, in the delta-4 pathway an unsaturated position is between C4 and C5 (see Fig. 68-1 for nomenclature) of ring A, whereas in the delta-5 pathway, the unsaturated position is between C5 and C6 of ring B. *In the human testis, the delta-5 pathway is the predominant (but not exclusive) one used for the biosynthesis of testosterone.*

The Sertoli cells are known to be important in spermatogenesis, in part through their synthesis of an *androgen-binding protein (ABP)*. ABP, when secreted into the lumen of the seminiferous tubules, selectively binds tes-

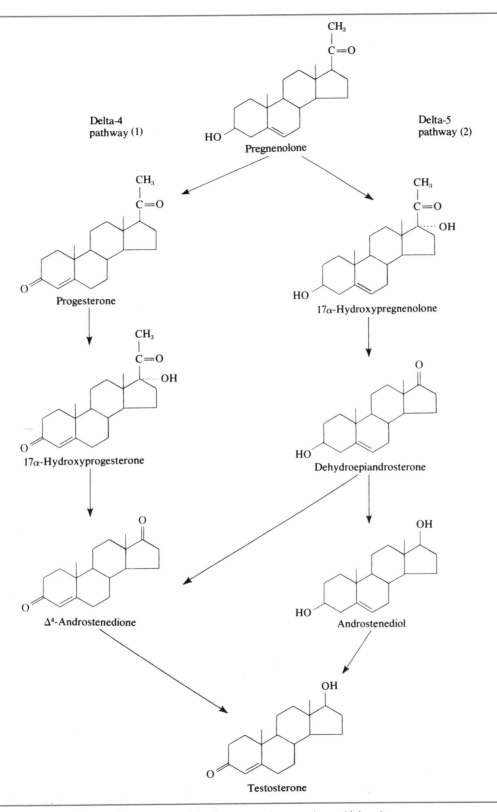

Figure 68-2. Synthetic pathways of testosterone. (1) Adrenostenedione pathway (delta-4); (2) dehydroepiandrosterone pathway (delta-5).

tosterone of Leydig cell origin and serves as a hormone reservoir and transport protein for the androgen.

Luteinizing hormone is the primary regulator of Leydig cell androgen synthesis. LH has been shown in animals to bind to specific receptors on the Leydig cell surface, where it activates adenylyl cyclase, with resultant increases in intracellular cyclic adenosine monophosphate (cAMP) levels and enhanced steroidogenesis. FSH is the prime regulator of Sertoli cell function.

Regulation of Plasma Testosterone

The regulation of plasma testosterone is accomplished through a dynamic feedback interaction among the hypothalamus, pituitary, and testis. The hypothalamus synthesizes and releases GnRH into the hypothalamohypophyseal portal system. GnRH stimulates release of pituitary gonadotropins, LH, and FSH, which traverse to the testes to regulate testosterone synthesis and spermatogenesis, respectively. The resultant increases in testosterone levels exert a negative feedback at both the hypothalamus and the pituitary level.

Recently, modulation of this complex interaction between GnRH, LH, FSH, and the gonadal steroids has been clarified. GnRH is released in a pulsatile manner by the hypothalamus. The pulse frequency is sex-specific with males exhibiting a 120-min frequency and females exhibiting a 60- to 90-min frequency. The pulse frequency of GnRH release modulates pituitary LH and FSH release. Androgens and estrogens can modulate gonadotropin release at both the hypothalamus and pituitary levels. In this regard, the gonadal steroids modulate GnRH pulse frequency and amplitude at the hypothalamus level while simultaneously modifying pituitary responses to GnRH by influencing GnRH receptor levels. Increasing GnRH receptor levels results in "upregulation" while decreases in GnRH receptors result in "downregulation." In the hypothalamus, the negative feedback of testosterone involves both the conversion to dihydrotestosterone (DHT) and aromatization into estradiol.

A protein hormone called *inhibin* also affects the secretion of one of the gonadotropins, FSH. Inhibin has been isolated both from testicular extracts and from antral fluid of ovarian follicles in females. Inhibin functions to inhibit the release of FSH from the pituitary. It does not affect hypothalamic production of GnRH. A proposed scheme for the regulation of GnRH, LH, FSH, inhibin, and testosterone is illustrated in Fig. 68-3.

The catabolism of plasma testosterone is performed primarily by the liver; this is outlined in Fig. 68-4. Androgens are metabolized into water-soluble compounds that are eliminated primarily as 17-ketosteroids in the urine.

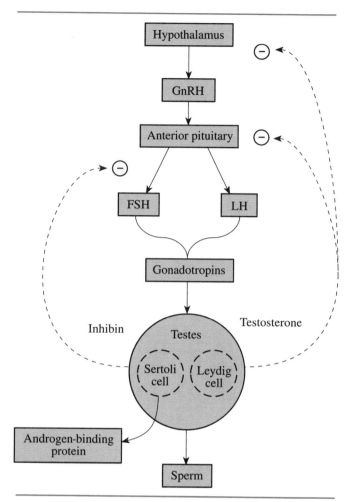

Figure 68-3. Hormonal interrelationships between the hypothalamus, anterior pituitary, and testes. Solid arrows indicate excitatory effects; dashed arrows indicate inhibitory effects. GnRH = gonadotropin releasing hormone; FSH = follicle-stimulating hormone; LH = luteinizing hormone. (Modified from Stuart Ira Fox, *Human Physiology* (3rd ed.). Copyright © 1990 Wm. C. Brown Publishers, Dubuque, Iowa. All Rights Reserved. Reprinted by permission.)

Mechanism of Action

Given the wide spectrum of androgen actions, it is reasonable to expect that the intracellular processes mediating these diverse effects may vary among different target tissues. Although these processes have been thoroughly characterized in the male sex accessory organs and central nervous system (CNS), those mediating protein anabolic effects in non-sex accessory tissues remain unclear.

The currently accepted hypothesis of androgen action in male sex accessory organs is depicted in Fig. 68-5. Testosterone diffuses from the blood across the plasma mem-

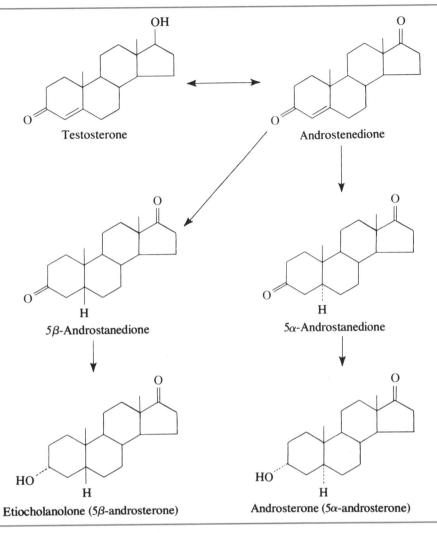

Figure 68-4. Primary pathways for testosterone catabolism.

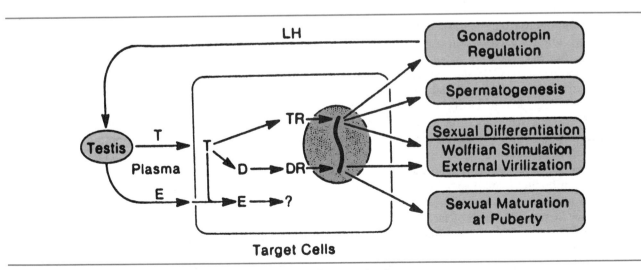

Figure 68-5. Schematic representation of the mechanism of action of androgen. T = testosterone; D = dihydrotestosterone; E = estradiol; R = receptor protein; LH = luteinizing hormone. (From J.D. Wilson, Androgen abuse by athletes. *Endocr. Rev.* 9:189, 1988. Copyright 1988 by The Endocrine Society.)

brane of the sex accessory organ cell, where it is rapidly metabolized to dihydrotestosterone (DHT) and androstanediol. In many sex accessory organs, DHT rather than testosterone is the primary intracellular androgen and, in most bioassay systems, is more potent than testosterone. Once formed, DHT preferentially binds to an androphilic receptor protein in the cytoplasm. This DHT-receptor complex is subsequently activated and transferred to the nucleus of the cell, where it associates with proteins on the nuclear matrix.

After the interaction with chromatin occurs, RNA synthesis is initiated, resulting in enhanced protein synthesis and cellular metabolism. If a sufficient androgen stimulation occurs, DNA synthesis and cellular division begin. When sex accessory organ cell growth reaches a certain magnitude, neither increases in the dosage nor prolongation of androgen therapy will produce further growth.

Non-sex accessory tissues that are targets for the protein anabolic actions of androgens possess low levels of endogenous hormone and minimal 5α-reductase activity. However, they do contain specific androgen receptors that probably mediate much of the androgenic protein anabolic actions. Androgens also compete for glucocorticoid receptors in these tissues; thus, much of the androgen's protein anabolic effect is actually an "antiglucocorticoid" effect.

Pharmacological Actions

Androgens produce a wide variety of effects within male sex accessory tissues as well as non–sex accessory tissues. These effects can be divided into virilizing and protein anabolic actions (Table 68-1). Some attempts have also been made to separate the organizational, or morphogenic, action of androgens from their excitatory, or maintenance, activity. The *morphogenic actions* are those irreversible effects that occur during embryogenesis and involve differentiation of the CNS and male reproductive tracts. In contrast, *excitatory actions* of androgens usually occur at puberty. A large percentage of the postpuberal or *maintenance actions* of androgens are reversible. Thus, male sexual behavior, libido, and reproductive functions will regress with androgen deficiency.

In addition to the effects on male reproductive functions, androgens influence a number of other systems, many of which are associated with "maleness." At puberty, there is an increased growth of facial, pubic, and body hair. Androgens also lower vocal pitch through laryngeal enlargement and through a thickening and lengthening of the vocal cords. At puberty, there is a significant (30%) increase in the rate of long-bone growth, which eventually is terminated by androgen-induced closure of epiphyseal plates in the mid- to late teens.

Table 68-1. Pharmacological Actions of Androgens

Virilizing effects
    Gonadotropin regulation
    Spermatogenesis
    Sexual dysfunction
    Sexual restoration and development
Protein anabolic effects
    Increased bone density
    Increased muscle mass
    Increased red blood cell mass

Androgens also have several other actions, not necessarily associated with maleness. Lymphoid tissue, such as tonsils, adenoids, thymus, and lymph nodes, which are maximal in size in the prepubertal boy, regress during puberty. Apart from the protein anabolic actions of androgens on bone and skeletal muscle, androgens induce some degree of anabolism in other tissues, including bone marrow, liver, kidney, and heart. Androgens are also potent, nonspecific stimulators of erythropoiesis. This action, which explains the higher hematocrit in males, is due at least in part to increased erythropoietin production by the kidney, as well as to a direct effect on bone marrow stem cell division.

Clinical Uses

The primary therapeutic use of androgens is for testicular deficiency (Table 68-2), in which induction and maintenance of male secondary sex characteristics are desired. Although replacement therapy is the primary use of androgen administration, these hormones also are useful in certain conditions not necessarily associated with hormone deficiency.

Hypogonadism

Testicular failure may develop prepuberally as eunuchoidism, or postpuberally, with symptoms of infertility, impotence, or decreased libido. Prepuberal hypogonadism is commonly unsuspected clinically until adolescence, when sexual maturation and increased growth fail to occur.

Prepuberal Hypogonadism

The eunuchoid phenotype is caused by absent or deficient androgenic induction of undifferentiated embryonic bipotential tissue into fully developed male sex accessory organs. Etiologies of this condition include deficient tes-

Table 68-2. Preparations and Dosage Schedules of Androgenic Steroids Used Primarily for Androgen Replacement

Agent (trade name)	Preparation	Adult dosage schedule
Testosterone (*Oreton, Neo-Hombreol F,* others)	Aqueous suspension, 25–50 mg/ml; 75-mg pellet	50 mg, 3 times/week IM; 4 pellets, every 4–6 months, SC
Testosterone propionate (*Neo-Hombreol, Oreton Propionate,* others)	Aqueous suspension, 25, 50, 100 mg/ml; 10-mg tablets	10–20 mg/day, buccally; 25 mg, 2–4 times/week, IM
Testosterone enanthate (*Delatestryl,* others)	Solution in oil, 100 and 200 mg/ml	100–400 mg, every 2–4 weeks, IM
Testosterone cypionate (*DEPO-Testosterone,* others)	Solution in oil, 50 and 200 mg/ml	100–400 mg, every 2–4 weeks, IM
Methyltestosterone (*Metandren, Neo-Hombreol*[M], others)	5-, 10-, 25-mg tablets	5–25 mg/day, buccally; 10–50 mg/day, PO
Fluoxymesterone *(Halotestin)*	2-, 5-, 10-mg tablets	2–20 mg/day, PO

ticular steroidogenesis (both congenital and acquired), target organ androgen insensitivity syndromes (receptor defects, 5α-reductase deficiency), deficient pituitary gonadotropic secretion, deficient hypothalamic GnRH, hyperprolactinemia, and unknown factors. Androgen replacement therapy is effective only in conditions in which end-organ androgen sensitivity is present; thus, certain forms of pseudohermaphroditism are unresponsive to androgen replacement.

The compounds most effective in bringing about masculinization are the long-acting enanthate, cypionate, or propionate esters of testosterone. Treatment is continued for 2 or 3 years or until adequate sexual maturation has occurred. Once sexual maturation is complete, lower maintenance levels of these compounds can be utilized. Owing to inconsistent drug absorption, oral androgen preparations, though more convenient, do not result in full sexual development in hypogonadotropic males. In addition, methyltestosterone has been implicated in cholestatic hepatitis after long-term administration. Mesterolone is a newer oral compound that does not cause hepatitis, but its clinical efficacy in inducing sexual maturation has not been demonstrated. A promising new compound is testosterone buciclate. This is a long-acting ester of testosterone; in one study a 600-mg injection was able to maintain androgen serum concentrations in the low-normal range for about 3 months in hypogonadal men.

Postpuberal Hypogonadism

Postpuberal hypogonadism can be classified as either hypergonadotropic primary or hypogonadotropic secondary hypogonadism. Hypergonadotropic hypogonadism occurs postpuberally as the result of surgical castration or testicular destruction (through orchitis, radiation, etc.). Hypogonadotropic testicular failure secondary to hypopituitarism in the adult is usually associated with complete destruction of the pituitary and also commonly results in serious deficiencies of thyroid and adrenal function. An-

drogen replacement in these individuals usually restores secondary male sexual characteristics, libido, and potency. In patients with hypopituitarism, androgens restore positive nitrogen balance, increase strength and erythropoiesis, and initiate a sense of well-being.

Oral preparations of methyltestosterone (*Metandren, Oreton Methyl*) or fluoxymesterone (*Halotestin*) are effective in postpuberal males; however, long-term use of methyltestosterone should be discouraged because of associated hepatotoxicity (see Adverse Reactions). Enanthate and cyclopentylpropionate esters also are effective as maintenance androgens.

Cryptorchidism

Failure of testicular descent into the scrotum is the most common anatomical developmental disorder observed in males (3% of all 1-year-old boys). The proper management of this disorder has been debated for years by both surgeons and endocrinologists. Nondescent of the testes may be secondary to mechanical obstruction in the inguinal canal or to an endocrine imbalance in which the hormonal stimulus necessary to induce testicular descent appears to be inadequate.

Treatment of cryptorchidism with human chorionic gonadotropin (hCG; *Antuitrin S, Follutein*) for at least 6 weeks has been effective in inducing testicular descent. Testosterone administration also has been used to stimulate testicular descent; however, the side effects of possible premature sexual development or closure of epiphyseal plates make the routine clinical application of testosterone unwise.

Aging and Impotence

The aging process in men is associated with decreased testicular function, which results in reduced testicular steroidogenesis, decreased free plasma testosterone levels, decreased 17-ketosteroid excretion, and increased gonadotropin levels. Decreased testicular function has been implicated as a cause of reduced libido, muscle mass, and strength in elderly men. However, these observations are so variable that a causal relationship between lowered androgen levels and these effects has not been established firmly. Furthermore, in elderly men, or during the *climacteric* (characterized by nervousness, depressed libido, decreased vasomotor stability, and depression), androgen replacement has not been demonstrated to be beneficial. In addition, it is wise to avoid the indiscriminate use of androgens in this age group because of the high incidence of related prostate neoplasms (benign and malignant).

Androgen administration in high dosages has proved to be moderately successful in increasing libido, sexual performance, and stimulation of spermatogenesis in younger men who have true testicular failure. An endocrine basis for impotence in men accounts for only a small segment of the total population evaluated for this problem. Psychological and neurological disorders (diabetes mellitus, peripheral vascular disease, spinal cord injury, etc.) are the principal underlying causes in most cases.

Short Stature

The rationale for androgen therapy in short stature is based on the fact that *androgens are the most potent compounds available for the stimulation of linear bone growth.* With the development of recombinant human growth hormone (rHGH) as the principal treatment of short stature, the indications for androgen therapy of short stature are very limited.

Anemia

Androgens are effective in the therapy of anemias that are secondary to endocrine hypofunction. In high dosages, these compounds have also been used in the treatment of other types of anemias, such as myeloid metaplasia, multiple myeloma, leukemia, lymphoma, anemia of chronic disease (e.g., chronic renal failure), and aplastic anemia. Androgen therapy in these disorders is effective only when adequate erythroid precursor cells exist in the bone marrow, and the beneficial effects of androgens usually require 3 to 6 months to become clinically apparent. Subsequent androgen stimulation of myeloid and megakaryocyte cells in the bone marrow also may occur during therapy, but these developments are observed much later than erythroid stimulation. Recombinant erythropoietin (rEPO) is now available and has replaced androgen therapy for the treatment of most forms of chronic anemia.

Therapeutic Use of Androgens in Women

Because of the antagonistic action of androgens in many estrogen-sensitive tissues, it would seem logical that androgens might be effective therapeutic agents in clinical situations of estrogen excess or in estrogen-dependent neoplasms. However, the virilizing side effects of these compounds has limited their use.

Breast Cancer

Although androgens have been used to treat advanced premenopausal and postmenopausal mammary cancers, beneficial effects occur in only about 20 percent of patients and, in all cases, the effects are merely palliative. In addition, androgens are no longer considered to be primary drugs in the therapy of premenopausal mammary tumors. If androgens are used at all, the rationale for use is based on their ability to suppress ovarian steroidogenesis that is secondary to an inhibition of pituitary LH secretion. *The use of androgens in postmenopausal women has largely been replaced by drugs that are antiestrogens (e.g., tamoxifen).* In comparison with androgens, the antiestrogens are much more effective in blocking the actions of adrenal estrogens.

Endometriosis

Endometriosis is the abnormal growth of endometrial tissue in the peritoneal cavity. Women with this disorder present with dysmenorrhea, dyspareunia, chronic pelvic pain, and infertility. Danazol (*Danocrine*) is a 2,3-isoxazol derivative of 17α-ethynyl testosterone (ethisterone) that has weak protein anabolic properties but is effective in endometriosis through its antigonadotropic action; it suppresses LH and FSH release, which, in turn, results in decreased ovarian steroidogenesis and a subsequent regression of endometriomas.

Danazol is also approved for use in fibrocystic breast disease and is being investigated for the treatment of hereditary angioneurotic edema, alpha-1 antitrypsin deficiency, gynecomastia, and systemic lupus erythematosus. The recommended dosage of danazol is 800 mg/day.

Female Hypopituitarism

Female hypogonadism, especially that caused by hypopituitarism, is an indication for androgen therapy. In females with hypopituitarism in whom all hormonal defi-

Table 68-3. Preparations and Dosage Schedules of Androgenic Steroids Used Primarily as Anabolic Agents

Agent (trade name)	Preparation	Adult dosage schedule
Ethylestrenol *(Maxibolin)*	Elixir, 2 mg/5 ml; 2-mg tablets	4–8 mg/day, PO
Methandrostenolone *(Dianabol)*	2.5-, 5-mg tablets	5 mg/day, PO
Nandrolone decanoate, USP *(Deca-Durabolin)*	Solution in oil, 50 and 100 mg/ml	50–100 mg, every 3–4 weeks, IM
Nandrolone phenpropionate, USP *(Durabolin)*	Solution in oil, 25 and 50 mg/ml	25–50 mg/week, IM
Oxandrolone, USP *(Anavar)*	2.5-mg tablets	5–10 mg/day, PO
Oxymetholone, USP *(Androyd, Anadrol)*	2.5-, 5-, 10-, 50-mg tablets	5–15 mg/day, PO
Stanozolol, USP *(Winstrol)*	2-mg tablets	2 mg, 3 times per day, PO

ciencies (thyroid, adrenal, growth hormone) have been corrected, normal sexual development and long-bone growth do not occur without sex hormone replacement. Estrogen administration during adolescence is necessary for the development of the breast, the gynecoid pelvis, and other female characteristics. However, maximal long-bone growth and development of axillary and pubic hair will not occur without androgen replacement. The use of *methyltestosterone* and *diethylstilbestrol* in combination has been demonstrated to be effective in inducing this development.

Protein Anabolic Actions of Androgens

Anabolic activities of testosterone, such as increases both in amino acid incorporation into protein and in RNA polymerase activity, have been demonstrated in skeletal muscle.

Apart from the direct anabolic effects in specific tissue, androgens antagonize the protein catabolic action of glucocorticoids. In fact, there is evidence to suggest that the anabolic action of androgens is due in part to a direct androgen antagonism of glucocorticoid binding to its cytoplasmic receptor in skeletal muscle. Thus, androgens may cause anabolism by antagonizing the catabolic action of glucocorticoids.

The androgen compounds with the greatest ratio of protein anabolic effects to virilizing effects are the *19-nortestosterone derivatives* (Table 68-3). Compounds that are used clinically include nandrolone phenpropionate (*Durabolin*), nandrolone decanoate (*Deca-Durabolin*), methandrostenolone (*Dianabol*), oxymetholone (*Anadrol, Androyd*), stanozolol (*Winstrol*), and oxandrolone (*Anavar*).

Clinically, these compounds may be useful in treating short stature in which long-bone growth stimulation is required, but where the side effects of masculinization are undesired. They are also used to treat the hypoprotein-

Table 68-4. Clinical Uses of Protein Anabolic Steroids

Protein catabolic states (burns, malnutrition, maintenance)
Short stature
Anemia
Endometriosis
Breast cancer
Osteoporosis

emia of nephrosis. Protein anabolic androgens also have been used in debilitated postoperative patients, burn patients, and premature infants, all of whom are in severe negative nitrogen balance (Table 68-4).

Anabolic Steroids in Athletes

The use and abuse of anabolic steroids by athletes and body builders of either sex to increase strength and muscle mass are widespread. Surveys indicate that in the United States 6 percent of high school athletes, 20 percent of college athletes, and more than 50 percent of professional athletes in certain sports use or abuse anabolic steroids at some time. Use of these compounds does result in increased muscle mass, strength, and endurance. However, much of this benefit is now thought to be due as much to enhanced training effort as it is to the protein anabolic effects of the androgens. Individuals who take these compounds typically use 100 to 200 times the normal dose and will "cycle or stack" multiple anabolic compounds together in an effort to enhance the biological effect.

Common endocrine side effects of these compounds include virilization in women, suppression of endogenous gonadotropins and hypogonadism (amenorrhea in women, impotence in men), and severe psychological disturbances (depression, mania, "roid-rage"). Other physiological side effects are hepatotoxicity, suppression of high-density lipoprotein (HDL) cholesterol, increased cardiovascular risk, insulin resistance, and decreased thyroid hormone production.

Adverse Reactions

Toxicity in Women

Although masculinization is a desired action of androgens in the treatment of men with testicular deficiencies, these effects can be quite distressing to women. The degree of virilization in women will vary and depends on the dosage, duration of therapy, and particular androgen preparation used. In women receiving high doses of androgen for any reason, facial hair growth may progress to generalized total body hair growth, baldness may develop, shrinkage of breast size may occur, and the voice may deepen to a lower pitch. In addition, clitoral hypertrophy, uterine atrophy, and menstrual irregularities may develop. Although some of the symptoms are reversible and disappear on cessation of therapy, several symptoms—baldness, growth of facial hair, clitoris enlargement, and deepening of the voice—are commonly irreversible. Steroids taken by pregnant women may cause pseudohermaphroditism in the genetically female fetus and may even cause its death.

Toxicity in Men

The administration of androgens to sexually mature males is associated with fewer untoward effects than those described for women or children. However, hypogonadal males, especially prepuberal ones, show enhanced sensitivity to administered androgens. Androgen administration to normal males inhibits the release of pituitary gonadotropins (FSH, LH) and, as a consequence, a decrease in the testicular production of testosterone occurs. Spermatogenesis is also reduced and if treatment is continued, azoospermia may result. Cessation of treatment normally allows the restoration of normal sperm levels, which may require 6 months or longer. Androgen therapy in elderly men, especially those with known prostatic neoplasms, is contraindicated because of the likelihood of stimulating the growth of prostatic tumors.

Toxicity in Both Sexes

Androgen administration to male or female adults, especially at high dosages, results in fluid retention and may produce edema or exacerbate the edema associated with congestive heart failure, cirrhosis, renal failure, nephrotic syndrome, and hypoalbuminemia of any etiology. Androgen-induced fluid retention is due to sodium and chloride retention, similar to that caused by estrogen administra-

tion, but it may also be caused by the protein anabolic actions of androgens that promote tissue protein synthesis over albumin synthesis. Since androgens stimulate the activity of sebaceous glands, oily skin and acne are found in some individuals who are receiving anabolic therapy. A change in cholesterol levels also has resulted from androgen therapy in that decreased levels of high-density lipoprotein cholesterol and increased levels of low-density lipoprotein cholesterol have been found. This change in the distribution of cholesterol may contribute to coronary artery disease, especially in persons who are exposed for long periods of time to high levels of anabolic steroids.

As many as 80 percent of the individuals treated with those androgens that have a 17-methyl substitution on the steroid molecule have developed liver disorders, including hyperbilirubinemia, elevation of plasma levels of glutamicoxaloacetic transaminase, glutamic-pyruvic transaminase, and alkaline phosphatase. Although these changes are ordinarily reversed if steroid treatment is discontinued, further treatment may induce obstruction of the bile canals, resulting in jaundice. Hepatic cholestasis, which may occur, typically disappears within 3 months after discontinuing steroid treatment. The responsible steroid compounds include oxymethalone, stanozolol, and 17-methyl-19-nortestosterone. Neither testosterone nor any of its ester derivatives is associated with these liver disorders. Intermittent administration of 17-methyl compounds has been demonstrated to lower the incidence of these symptoms and appears to be a useful method of androgen administration.

Long-term androgenic treatment of anemia, hypopituitarism, and impotence has been associated with liver tumors. Although some tumor-associated deaths have been reported, most hepatocellular carcinomas are slow to develop and quick to atrophy when steroid therapy is discontinued. Also associated with steroid treatment is a rare liver disorder involving the development of blood-filled sacs in the tissue (peliosis hepatis). Subsequent rupturing of the sacs results in severe hemorrhaging and liver failure.

Additional effects resulting from anabolic steroid treatment have been described. Obstructive sleep apnea syndrome has been associated with testosterone administration; however, the symptoms disappeared with the discontinuation of androgen therapy. Signs related to superior sagittal sinus thrombosis—seizures, facial palsy, hemiplegia, stupor, and coma—have been associated with androgen therapy for hypoplastic anemia. Again, the discontinuation of hormone therapy leads to a general subsidence of these symptoms. Finally, several psychological changes have been associated with anabolic steroid treatment, including increased aggressive behavior, elevation or depression in mood, alterations in sex drive, and occasional psychotic episodes.

Preparations and Dosage

Preparations and dosages of most commonly used androgens and anabolic steroids are summarized in Tables 68-2 and 68-3. Although various products are currently available that combine androgens with numerous other substances, ranging from estrogens to sedatives, their use is not advised pharmacologically. If several drugs are indicated for the therapy of a particular problem, each drug should be administered at its optimal dosage rather than at the fixed doses found in combination preparations.

Male Antifertility Agents

In spite of a continuing need, no reversible chemical agent that can adequately control male fertility without inducing toxic side effects is yet available. Two drugs currently under examination as antifertility compounds are discussed in this section.

Gossypol

Gossypol is a phenolic compound that occurs naturally in the seeds and roots of cotton plants (Fig. 68-6). Its potential as an antifertility agent was first considered when investigators linked the observations of a Chinese village that lacked a single childbirth for an entire decade with the fact that during the same time period members of the village used cottonseed oil for cooking purposes. Subsequent animal experiments revealed that Sertoli cells, pachytene spermatocytes, and late spermatids were the primary cellular targets for gossypol, the active compound in cottonseed oil.

Although its mechanism is not completely understood, gossypol causes vacuolization and breakage of tight junctions in Sertoli cells as well as a decreased formation of androgen-binding protein. In spermatic cells, plasma and inner mitochondrial membranes are the postulated subcellular sites of action, since gossypol is known to inhibit adenylate cyclase activity and to uncouple oxidative phosphorylation.

Clinical trials involving over 8,000 male subjects have been conducted in China and Latin America. In the Chinese study, gossypol treatment resulted in an antifertility rate of 99.07 percent. A range of symptoms from increased nonmotile sperm to azoospermia was found in the ejaculates of treated men. Following cessation of gossypol treatment, length of recovery of normal ejaculates varied from 3 months to 4 years, although in some subjects re-

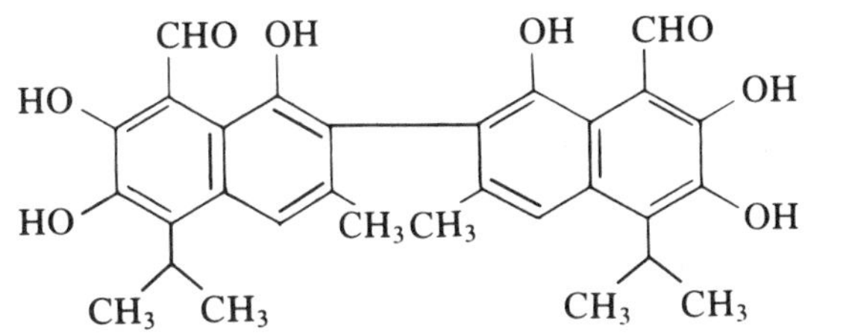

Figure 68-6. Gossypol.

covery was incomplete, indicating the potential irreversibility of the antifertility effect.

Side effects were generally mild and included change in appetite, fatigue, dryness of mouth, diarrhea, and a subjective decrease in libido and potency. An important side effect, which involved symptoms of hypokalemic paralysis, was found in fewer than 1 percent of the treated subjects. However, treatment with potassium salts in the early stages of therapy prevented paralysis.

Although gossypol is extremely effective in its antifertility actions, further studies on its possible toxicity are needed.

19-Nortestosterone

A European clinical study examined the effectiveness of an anabolic steroid, *19-nortestosterone,* as a male antifertility agent. Intramuscular injections of 19-nortestosterone, in dosages of 100 mg/week for 3 weeks, followed by 10 more weeks of 200 mg/week, resulted in an azoospermia that persisted 4 to 14 weeks after the last injection. Libido and potency were unaffected, although serum testosterone, FSH, and LH declined with the treatment. No serious side effects were seen and all seminal parameters returned to normal by 30 weeks posttreatment. Due to the effectiveness and apparent lack of toxicity associated with 19-nortestosterone administration, further investigation appears to be warranted.

Gonadotropin Releasing Hormone (and Analogues)

Gonadotropin releasing hormone and many of its synthetic analogues (also called LHRH [luteinizing hormone releasing hormone] analogues) are rapidly gaining therapeutic application in a variety of endocrine disorders (see Chap. 65). GnRH analogues can induce "chemical castration" by suppressing LH and FSH release. Administration of these compounds results in a reduction in sperm counts,

Table 68-5. Dosage Schedules and Clinical Uses of Antiandrogens

Agent (trade name)	Dose	Major use
Gonadotropin antagonists		
Leuprolide acetate *(Lupron Depot)*	3.75–7.5 mg IM per month	Prostate cancer
Androgen receptor antagonists		
Spironolactone *(Aldactone)*	25–200 mg 2 times per day	Hirsutism
Flutamide *(Eulexin)*	250 mg 3 times per day	Benign prostate hypertrophy
		Prostate cancer
Testosterone biosynthesis inhibitors		
Ketoconazole *(Nizoral)*	800–1,600 mg/day	Precocious puberty
5α-Reductase inhibitors		
Finasteride *(Proscar)*	5 mg/day	Benign prostatic hypertrophy
		Prostate cancer

sperm density, and circulating testosterone levels, which results in decreased libido and impotence. These compounds are administered subcutaneously and require testosterone supplementation.

Antiandrogens

By definition, antiandrogens are substances that prevent or depress the action of male hormones in their target organs. Potential actions include gonadotropin suppression, inhibition of androgen synthesis, and androgen receptor blockade. Clinical uses of antiandrogens include situations of androgen excess, for example, precocious puberty, androgen-secreting tumors, and adrenogenital syndromes (Table 68-5). In women, antiandrogens are effective in the treatment of hirsutism, premenstrual syndrome, and severe cystic acne. In men, they are also used in the treatment of benign and malignant neoplasms of the prostate.

Gonadotropin Antagonists

Estradiol and other estrogens such as diethylstilbestrol have been used extensively in the past for the treatment of advanced carcinoma of the prostate (see Chap. 67). Estrogens inhibit androgen-sensitive tissues through several mechanisms, including LH suppression, inhibition of testicular steroidogenesis, and androgen receptor antagonism. These compounds, however, increase the risk of cardiovascular complications and cause gynecomastia.

Gonadotropin releasing hormone analogues are compounds that effectively suppress LH and FSH secretion in the pituitary, which results in suppression of testosterone synthesis and spermatogenesis by the testis (see Chap. 65).

Several of these compounds are used in the treatment of LHRH-dependent central precocious puberty of either sex and metastatic carcinoma of the prostate.

Androgen Biosynthesis Inhibitors

Ketoconazole (*Nizoral*) is a broad-spectrum antifungal agent (see Chap. 59) that, in very high doses, inhibits several steps in the biosynthesis of both adrenal and gonadal steroids. While the normal antifungal dose is 200 mg/day, testosterone biosynthesis in both the adrenal and testis is completely abolished by doses of 800 to 1,600 mg/day.

Androgen Receptor Antagonists

Spironolactone (*Aldactone*) is a compound originally developed as a mineralocorticoid antagonist and is used as a diuretic/antihypertensive agent (see Chap. 21). However, at high doses spironolactone competes for both androgen and progesterone receptors. It is a weak androgen antagonist, but is now used to treat hirsutism and premenstrual syndrome in women and precocious puberty in either sex.

Flutamide (*Eulexin*) is a nonsteroidal androgen receptor antagonist that inhibits nuclear androgen receptor binding. It is effective in reducing normal male sex accessory tissue function and is now approved for the treatment of prostatic carcinoma at a dose of 250 mg three times a day. It has to be used in combination with a GnRH antagonist (e.g., leuprolide acetate) for maximum effectiveness. It will eventually be used for treatment of hirsutism and male pattern baldness, perhaps in a topical preparation.

Cyproterone acetate is a progestational antiandrogen that blocks androgen receptor binding and suppresses androgen-sensitive tissues. It is available in Europe.

5α-Reductase Inhibitors

Finasteride (*Proscar*) is a 5α-reductase inhibitor that blocks the conversion of testosterone to dihydrotestosterone. Since dihydrotestosterone is the major intracellular androgen in most target tissues, finasteride is effective in suppressing male sex accessory function without interfering with libido. It is now approved for the treatment of benign prostatic hyperplasia but may also have application in the treatment of hirsutism and male pattern baldness.

Supplemental Reading

Behre, H.M., and Nieschlag, E. Testosterone buciclate (20 Aet-1) in hypogonadal men: Pharmacokinetics and pharmacodynamics of the new long-acting androgen ester. *J. Clin. Endocrinol. Metab.* 75:1204, 1992.

Forest, M.G. (ed.). *Androgens in Childhood: Biological, Physiological, Clinical, and Therapeutic Aspects.* New York: Karger, 1989.

Griffin, J.E. Male Reproductive Function. In J.E. Griffin and S.R. Ojeda (eds.), *Textbook of Endocrine Physiology.* New York: Oxford University Press, 1992. Pp. 169–188.

Kochakian, C.D. History of anabolic-androgenic steroids. *NIDA Research Monograph* 102:29, 1990.

Kuipers, H., et al. Influence of anabolic steroids on body composition, blood pressure, lipid profile, and liver functions in body builders. *Int. J. Sports Med.* 12:413, 1991.

Parker, M.G. (ed.). *Nuclear Hormone Receptors.* New York: Academic, 1991.

Pryor, J.P., and Lipschultz, (eds.). *Andrology.* Boston: Butterworth, 1987.

Sherman, M.R., and Stevens, J. Structure of mammalian steroid receptors: Evolving concepts and methodological developments. *Ann. Rev. Physiol.* 46:83, 1984.

Smith, D.A., and Perry, P.J. The efficacy of ergogenic agents in athletic competition. Part I: Androgenic-anabolic steroids. *Ann. Pharmacother.* 26:520, 1992.

Strauss, R.H., and Yesalis, C.E. Anabolic steroids in the athlete. *Annu. Rev. Med.* 42:449, 1991.

Uzych, L. Anabolic-androgenic steroids and psychiatric-related effects: A review. *Can. J. Psychiatry* 37:23, 1992.

69

Thyroid and Antithyroid Drugs

John M. Connors

The hormones synthesized and released by the thyroid gland (other than calcitonin; see Chap. 70) affect such fundamental processes as oxygen consumption, heat production, and metabolism of carbohydrates, fats, and proteins. Thyroid hormones are recognized as the regulators of the metabolic level in most tissues (notable exceptions include adult brain, spleen, and testis) and are required for normal growth and differentiation.

Thyroxine (T$_4$, tetraiodothyronine) and *triiodothyronine* (T$_3$, liothyronine) are the principal thyroid hormones. They are amino acids with a unique diphenyl ether structure that contains the element iodine. Although they are stored within the thyroid gland as integral units within the large protein *thyroglobulin,* the thyroid hormones exist in the blood, noncovalently bound to plasma proteins. T$_4$, the major secretory product, has a relatively long half-life and its actions lead to slow steady hormone action. T$_3$ is secreted by the thyroid gland and also arises from the extrathyroidal metabolism of T$_4$.

The thyroid hormones have important, but not necessarily identical, effects on most tissues in the body. They appear to be required for the optimal functioning of other hormones, such as the catecholamines, corticosteroids, and antidiuretic hormone. Inadequate or excessive secretion of these hormones results in the clinical conditions called *hypothyroidism* and *hyperthyroidism,* respectively. Thyroid dysfunction can produce dramatic changes in the pattern of growth and development and in the functioning of the cardiovascular, gastrointestinal, skeletal, neuromuscular, and reproductive systems.

Thyroid disorders are among the most frequently occurring endocrine diseases confronting the general physician. Severe cases of thyroid dysfunction are readily recognized. The diagnosis of more subtle forms of thyroid disease requires an understanding of the pathophysiology of clinical features and the use of modern laboratory tests. Once the diagnosis is established, therapy is usually straightforward and generally successful.

Biosynthesis, Storage, and Metabolism

The thyroid hormones are biosynthesized from tyrosine and iodine. An adequate dietary intake of iodine is necessary for optimal production of thyroid hormones. Dietary iodine (I$_2$) is reduced to the oxidative level of iodide (I$^-$) before absorption, which is virtually complete in the small intestine. The conversion of inorganic iodide to thyroid hormone involves a series of biochemical steps in the thyroid gland that include the following (Fig. 69-1):

1. Active transport of iodide
2. Thyroglobulin synthesis
3. Iodination of tyrosyl residues in thyroglobulin
4. Coupling of iodotyrosines within thyroglobulin to form T$_4$ and T$_3$
5. Proteolysis of thyroglobulin, with release of free iodotyrosines and iodothyronines
6. Deiodination of iodotyrosines within the thyroid and neutralization of the liberated iodide

These steps may be compromised in disease and can be blocked selectively by a variety of chemicals and drugs.

Iodide Trapping

The first step in thyroid hormone synthesis is the active transport and concentration of inorganic iodide in the thyroid epithelial cells. The iodide concentration mechanism, or "iodide trap," requires energy to actively transport iodide across the epithelial cell membrane; this action results in an intrathyroidal iodide concentration some 30 times greater than that found in plasma. As are all subsequent steps, the trapping of iodide is stimulated by *thyroid-stimulating hormone* (TSH, thyrotropin) from the anterior

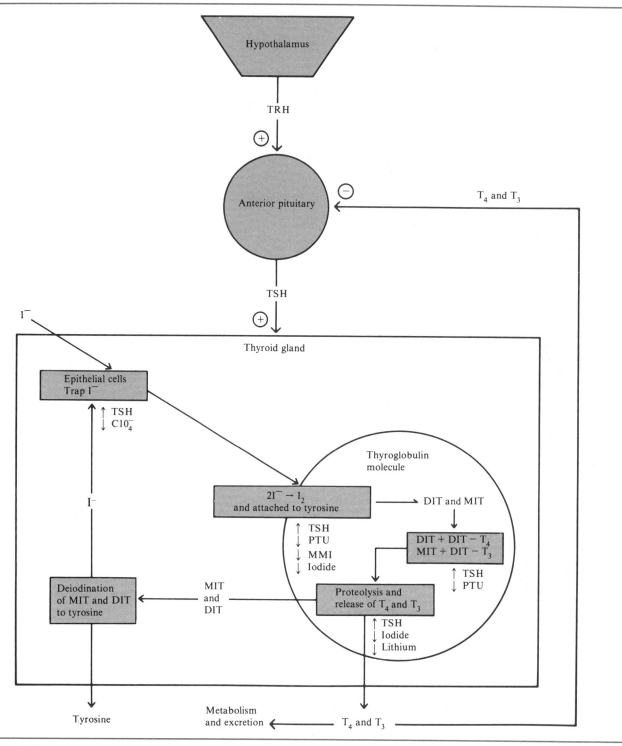

Figure 69-1. Adenohypophyseal-thyroid-iodine relationships: (+) indicates a stimulatory effect; (−) indicates inhibition. TRH = thyrotropin releasing hormone; TSH = thyroid-stimulating hormone; MIT = monoiodotyrosine; DIT = diiodotyrosine; PTU = propylthiouracil; MMI = methimazole. (See text for a description of the various processes.)

pituitary. This step is competitively inhibited by inorganic ions, such as thiocyanate and perchlorate; this inhibition accounts for the antithyroid action of these compounds.

In addition, exposure of the thyroid gland to excess iodide suppresses hormone formation and secretion and reduces the capacity of the gland to accumulate further iodide. These effects are exerted at several levels of thyroid follicular cell metabolism, including iodide transport and organification (the Wolff-Chaikoff effect), intermediary metabolism, adenylyl cyclase activity, and proteolysis and hormone release.

Thyroglobulin Synthesis

Thyroglobulin is a glycoprotein with a molecular weight of approximately 600,000 that plays a central role in the ability of the thyroid to synthesize T_4 and T_3. It contains 120 tyrosyl groups, and those are the sites at which iodination takes place. Iodination probably occurs either during or after the secretion of thyroglobulin into the follicular lumen. It is in the lumen that thyroglobulin becomes a part of the intrafollicular colloid.

Oxidation, Iodination, and Coupling

Once iodide (I^-) has been trapped by the thyroid gland, it is rapidly oxidized, in a peroxidase-dependent reaction, to iodine (I_2). Thyroid peroxidases also catalyze the iodination of tyrosyl residues in the large thyroglobulin molecule to form monoiodotyrosine (MIT) and diiodotyrosine (DIT). This process occurs at the surface of the microvilli, which are located at the apical border of the thyroid follicular cells and, possibly, more deeply into the follicular lumen.

T_3 (3,5,3'-triiodo-L-thyronine) is formed as a result of the coupling of MIT and DIT through an ether linkage; T_4 (3,5,3',5'-tetraiodo-L-thyronine) is formed through the coupling of two DIT molecules. Despite the large number of potential iodination sites within the thyroglobulin molecule (i.e., 120 tyrosyl groups), coupling only takes place at a few specific locations. On average, each thyroglobulin molecule contains three molecules of T_4 and a lesser amount of T_3. Coupling occurs in the thyroglobulin molecule. Oxidation, iodination, and coupling are inhibited by thiourea derivatives.

Hormone Storage

The thyroid gland is unique among endocrine glands in its large hormone storage capacity and relatively slow release of hormone. T_4 and T_3 are stored in the colloid of the thyroid follicles as part of the gland's thyroglobulin.

Proteolysis and Release of Hormone

Since both T_4 and T_3 are stored in the thyroid gland in peptide linkage within thyroglobulin and are released into the bloodstream as free hormones, it is apparent that their secretion must be preceded by proteolysis of the thyroglobulin. Release of hormone from the thyroid involves uptake of thyroglobulin from the colloid by endocytosis. The engulfed droplets fuse with lysosomes and are hydrolyzed.

T_4 and T_3 are released into the circulation, while iodotyrosines (MIT and DIT) are deiodinated. Iodide from deiodination of iodotyrosines contributes to the intracellular iodide pool from which reincorporation into hormone can occur. *The proteolysis of thyroglobulin and subsequent release of T_4 and T_3 are stimulated by TSH.* The most important agent acting on secretion is *iodide* itself, which causes a pronounced inhibition of hormone release. Lithium ion has a similar, but less pronounced, inhibitory effect on thyroid hormone release.

The active circulating thyroid hormones are T_4 and T_3. Circulating T_4 is derived solely from thyroid secretion, whereas T_3 arises from thyroid secretion and peripheral monodeiodination of T_4. Under normal conditions, only 15 to 20 percent of the circulating T_3 arises from thyroid secretion; the remainder arises peripherally. The T_3/T_4 ratio may increase significantly in both hyperthyroidism and hypothyroidism. A small amount of reverse T_3 (rT_3, or 3,3',5'-triiodo-L-thyronine) is also secreted by the thyroid gland, with a portion arising from monodeiodination of T_4. At physiological levels, rT_3 is essentially without thyromimetic activity.

Thyroid Hormone Transport and Metabolism

Both T_4 and T_3 are rapidly and extensively bound to plasma proteins following their release from the thyroid gland. The major fraction of both T_4 and T_3 is bound to *thyroxine-binding globulin (TBG)*. A secondary blood protein carrier of T_4 is *transthyretin* (formerly called thyroxine-binding prealbumin, or TBPA). Albumin binds both T_4 and T_3 weakly. Approximately 0.03 percent of T_4 and 0.30 percent of T_3 circulates in the unbound, or free, state. *It is currently thought that only the free hormone is physiologically active.*

The half-life of circulating thyroxine is approximately 5 to 7 days in humans. T_3 turns over much more rapidly, with a half-life of approximately 1 day. Under normal conditions, 70 to 90 μg of T_4 are secreted and disposed of each day. The turnover of T_3 is about 25 to 30 μg/day. Since T_3 is three to five times more active than T_4, the conversion of T_4 to T_3 represents a process of hormone activation.

Most of the T_4 and T_3 is deiodinated; the rest is deaminated, decarboxylated, or excreted unchanged in the feces. Loss of one or more iodine atoms from each aromatic ring results in metabolites with little or none of the biological activity of thyroid hormone; such deiodination can limit the duration and effectiveness of thyroid hormones. The iodide released by deiodination of T_3 or T_4 either recycles through the body, including the thyroid, or is excreted in the urine.

The major metabolic pathways of T_4 and T_3 leave the diphenyl ether structure intact. Oxidative deamination of T_4 and T_3 results in the formation of tetraiodothyroacetic acid (*tetrac*) and 3,5,3'-triiodothyroacetic acid (*triac*), respectively. Both metabolites are conjugated with β-glucuronide and, to a lesser extent, with sulfate, and excreted in bile. Tetrac and triac possess less than 10 percent of the biological effectiveness of T_4 in humans.

Control of Thyroid Activity

Feedback Control

The thyroid and pituitary exist in a negative-feedback control loop, the activity of which is driven by the peripheral consumption of thyroid hormones and modulated by hypothalamic control of pituitary responsiveness (see Fig. 69-1).

The primary control of thyroid hormone synthesis and secretion results from the action of TSH. Once secreted, TSH travels through the blood and is subsequently bound to specific receptors on the plasma membrane of thyroid follicular cells. TSH acts as a "first messenger" to the thyroid cells, but it does not enter the cell. The TSH bound to its receptor activates a membrane-bound enzyme, adenyl cyclase, which stimulates the formation of intracellular adenosine 3',5'-cyclic adenosine monophosphate (cAMP). All the steps in thyroidal iodide metabolism and hormonogenesis are stimulated by the intracellular "second messenger," cAMP.

The secretion of TSH is regulated by two factors, the net positive input from the hypothalamus (due to the interaction of at least three hypothalamic hormones: *thyrotropin releasing hormone, somatostatin,* and *dopamine*), and a negative input by thyroid hormones. Thyrotropin releasing hormone (TRH) binds to the pituicyte membrane on specific receptor sites and causes increased synthesis and secretion of TSH. TRH-induced TSH secretion is not initially dependent on protein synthesis. In contrast, T_4 and T_3 exert feedback on the pituicyte through a mechanism that involves synthesis of RNA and protein. The stimulatory effect of TRH and the inhibitory effect of thyroid hormones are delicately balanced at the pituitary level; an excess of one can overcome the effects of the other.

The second major influence on the activity of the thyroid is the level of intrathyroidal iodine stores. There is much evidence that the thyroid has an intrinsic ability to acclimate to iodide excess or deficiency independent of the pituitary. Ingestion of very large quantities of iodide results in the thyroidal binding of greater-than-normal amounts in the form of organic iodine. However, there is a progressive increase in the amount of iodide released from the thyroid that is not bound as hormone or hormone precursors. This "iodide leak" buffers the gland against production of excess quantities of hormone and possible hypermetabolism.

The gland also responds to iodide deficiency. Under conditions of decreased dietary iodine intake, a greater amount of MIT is produced in proportion to DIT within thyroglobulin. An increased frequency of coupling of MIT-DIT results, producing an increased ratio of T_3/T_4. Since T_3 is metabolically more active than T_4, this coupling helps to maintain homeostatic thyroid function in the face of moderate iodine deficiency.

Physiological Effects of Thyroid Hormones

There is no generally accepted unifying theory that explains the multifaceted actions of thyroid hormones. The actions of thyroid hormones are understood largely in terms of the metabolic alterations that occur in the hypothyroid or hyperthyroid state. Thyroid hormones exert specific actions on protein, carbohydrate, and lipid metabolism, and on growth and development, and they interact with various other hormones. In addition, they help to maintain reproductive, cardiac, gastrointestinal, and hematopoietic functions.

One of the long-known effects of thyroid hormone is its *thermogenic* or *calorigenic* action. Thyroid hormone appears to stimulate oxygen consumption as a consequence of the additive effects of small changes in the levels of numerous rate-limiting enzymes. Thus, thyroid hormones act to maintain or stimulate the basal metabolic rate (BMR).

Virtually all of the physiological effects of thyroid hormone are thought to be initiated by the binding of T_3 to DNA-binding proteins termed *T_3 receptors* (T_3R). Positive or negative effects on gene transcription may be generated by the thyroid hormone-receptor-DNA complex, depending on the specific gene and target tissue. T_4 is also specifically bound to the receptors, but with an affinity that is an order of magnitude lower. Since the intranuclear T_4 concentrations are lower than those of T_3, virtually all thyroid hormone specifically bound to the T_3R proteins is T_3. Thus, the intranuclear T_3 concentration determines the thyroid status of the cells.

Management of Hypothyroid States

Causes of Hypothyroidism

Hypothyroidism refers to the exposure of body tissues to a subnormal amount of thyroid hormone. Thyroid hormone deficiency may result in a wide variety of physiological and clinical disturbances involving virtually every organ system (see Clinical Manifestations of Hypothyroidism). Inadequate production of thyroid hormone can result from a wide variety of causes.

Primary hypothyroidism results from the inability of the thyroid gland itself to produce sufficient hormone. This occurrence may be due to spontaneous degeneration of glandular tissue (idiopathic hypothyroidism), chronic autoimmune thyroiditis (Hashimoto's disease), radiation damage caused by iodine 131, total or subtotal thyroidectomy, or thyroid dysgenesis (sporadic nongoitrous cretinism) in the first months or years of life.

Biosynthetic defects in thyroid hormonogenesis also may result in a deficit in thyroid hormone. Biosynthetic defects may be due to inherited enzymatic deficiencies, dietary iodide deficiency, or naturally occurring or therapeutically administered antithyroid agents. In most instances, primary hypothyroidism is accompanied by an elevated serum concentration of TSH. Goiter (enlargement of the thyroid) may or may not be present.

Secondary hypothyroidism, or pituitary hypothyroidism, is less common than primary hypothyroidism and is a consequence of TSH deficiency. TSH deficiency may result from any type of pituitary disease. The most common causes in adults are pituitary tumors or postpartum infarctions (Sheehan's syndrome). Most hypothyroid patients with pituitary disease exhibit undetectable or inappropriately low serum TSH concentrations. Usually there is an impaired secretion of TSH in response to exogenous TRH administration.

A deficiency in the release of TRH by the hypothalamus also may result in hypothyroidism (*tertiary hypothyroidism*). TRH deficiency is characterized by inappropriately low levels of serum TSH, which increase upon administration of TRH.

Clinical Manifestations of Hypothyroidism

The symptoms and signs of hypothyroidism (*myxedema*) in the adult are many and include the following: dry skin; puffiness of the hands, feet, and face; pallor; thinning, dryness, or loss of hair; lethargy; fatigue; slow speech, poor memory, anxiety, nervousness; decreased reflexes; hypothermia; reduced systolic and increased diastolic blood pressure; bradycardia; hoarseness; weight gain; constipation; and menstrual abnormalities. The clinical manifestations of hypothyroidism involve virtually every organ system. In general, there is a slowing of physical and mental activity and of cardiovascular, gastrointestinal, and neuromuscular function.

Hypothyroidism in infants during the first months or year of life leads to many signs and symptoms, including some of those noted. The most serious consequences of thyroid hormone deficiency at this stage are on mental and physical development. If uncorrected, there is progressive impairment of mental development, with delay in reaching major developmental milestones, and neurological disturbances. Brain growth and myelination are impaired, as are linear body growth and skeletal development. The result is *cretinism* (an infant with myxedema and neurological, mental, and physical retardation).

Indications for Treatment

Early diagnosis and treatment are essential for achieving therapeutic success in the management of cretinism. *Regardless of the etiology or severity of hypothyroidism, replacement therapy with thyroid hormone is necessary.*

Thyroid hormone preparations may be beneficial in the treatment of large multinodular goiter and chronic lymphocytic (Hashimoto's) thyroiditis, since hormone replacement suppresses TSH secretion and therefore may result in a reduction in the size of the goiter. Similarly, in some cases of thyroid carcinoma, thyroid hormone therapy may be used to minimize TSH stimulation. Vague symptoms suggesting hypometabolism should not be treated indiscriminately with thyroid hormone.

Appropriate therapy for hypothyroidism leads to restoration of the euthyroid state. For the majority of patients, therapy means lifelong replacement of thyroid hormones from an exogenous source. Thyroid hormone replacement is reliable, nonallergenic, inexpensive, and indistinguishable from endogenous secretion in its effects.

Adverse Reactions

Adverse effects (i.e., symptoms of hyperthyroidism) are almost invariably the result of drug overdosage and include cardiac palpitation and arrhythmias, tachycardia, weight loss, tremor, headache, insomnia, and heat intolerance. Symptoms will subside if medication is withheld for several days; therapy can then be reinstituted at a lower maintenance level.

Hypothyroid patients respond rapidly to replacement dosages of thyroid hormones. In patients with atherosclerosis or myocardial disease, the dosage must be increased gradually so that the capacity of the heart to handle the increased metabolic demands is not exceeded. When hypothyroidism and adrenal insufficiency coexist, as occurs in pituitary insufficiency (i.e., secondary hypothyroidism), an appropriate corticosteroid must be given before the initiation of thyroid hormone replacement therapy. This is done to prevent the development of acute adrenocortical insufficiency that could occur as a result of a thyroid hormone-induced increase in metabolic clearance of adrenocortical hormones.

Thyroid hormones increase the catabolism of vitamin K-dependent clotting factors and thereby enhance the effects of coumarin anticoagulants. During concomitant therapy, the dosage of the latter may have to be reduced.

Initiation of thyroid hormone therapy in patients with diabetes mellitus may increase the requirement for insulin or oral hypoglycemic agents. Similarly, thyroid hormone therapy may increase the need for digoxin in digitalized patients.

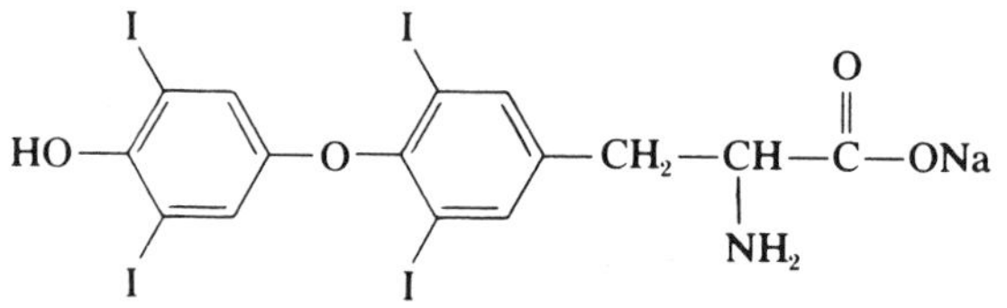

Figure 69-2. Levothyroxine sodium.

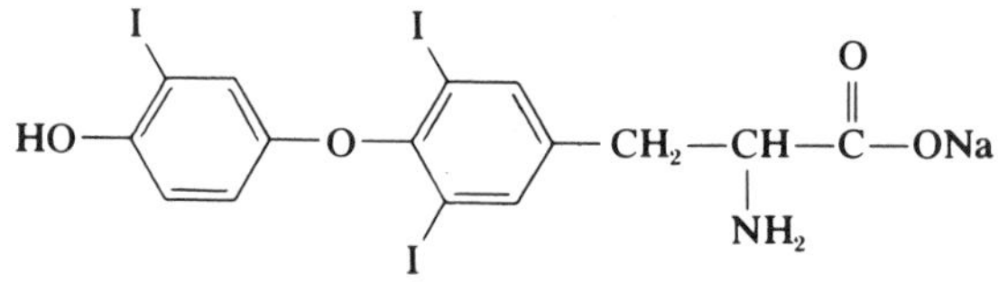

Figure 69-3. Liothyronine sodium.

Drugs

Levothyroxine Sodium

Levothyroxine sodium (Fig. 69-2) is the sodium salt of the naturally occurring levorotatory isomer of T_4. Administration of levothyroxine alone may produce normal levels of both T_4 and T_3.

Levothyroxine is most commonly used as replacement therapy in hypothyroidism. Other uses include the treatment of simple nonendemic goiter, chronic lymphocytic (Hashimoto's) thyroiditis, and thyrotropin-dependent thyroid carcinoma. It also can be used to prevent the goitrogenic effects of other therapeutic agents (e.g., lithium, aminosalicylic acid, and some sulfonamide compounds).

Levothyroxine is the drug of choice. It can be administered either orally or intravenously. In general, the intravenous dosage for levothyroxine is one-half the oral dosage. It is less completely absorbed from the gastrointestinal tract than is liothyronine and has a slower onset of action when given orally.

Levothyroxine sodium (generic, *Levothroid, Levoxine, Synthroid*) is available as either oral tablets (25–300 μg) or as a lyophilized powder (200–500 μg with 10 to 15 mg mannitol) for reconstitution in saline.

Liothyronine Sodium

Liothyronine sodium (Fig. 69-3) is the sodium salt of the naturally occurring levorotatory isomer of T_3.

Synthetic T_3 (liothyronine sodium) is generally not preferred for maintenance therapy because of its relatively short half-life and duration of action. However, some physicians prefer liothyronine for initial therapy in myxedema and myxedema coma because of its short half-life and its better absorption from the gastrointestinal tract (80–100% absorbed compared to 50–70% for levothyroxine).

It is active orally, and approximately 90 percent of an administered dose is absorbed from the gastrointestinal tract. It has a relatively rapid onset of action, and its peak effect and duration of action are shorter than those of T_4 (i.e., levothyroxine sodium). Monitoring is difficult because blood levels fluctuate after each dose. It is not generally used in replacement therapy because of its short duration of action.

Liothyronine does find some use in T_3 suppression tests to differentiate hyperthyroidism from euthyroidism and for short-term suppression of a solitary thyroid nodule before radioactive iodine scanning or when thyroid therapy must be interrupted periodically, as in patients with thyroid cancer who require ablative radioiodine therapy. Liothyronine also is used occasionally as an initial form of therapy in patients with cardiac disease.

The adverse reactions and contraindications are generally the same as those for levothyroxine.

Liothyronine sodium (*Cytomel*, generic) is commercially available in tablet (5, 25, and 50 μg) form. Liothyronine is not recommended for intravenous use.

Liotrix

Liotrix is a 4:1 mixture of levothyroxine sodium and liothyronine sodium. The mixture is equivalent to, but offers no other therapeutic advantages over, levothyroxine alone, since conversion of T_4 to T_3 in peripheral tissues results in a near-normal ratio of the two hormones in the circulation. Its indications, adverse reactions, and contraindications are the same as those described for levothyroxine.

Liotrix (*Euthroid* -½, -1, -2, and -3; *Thyrolar* -¼, -½, -1, -2, -3) is available as oral tablets containing, respectively, levothyroxine sodium and liothyronine sodium: 30:7.5, 60:15, 120:30, and 180:45 μg (*Euthroid*) and 12.5:3.1, 25:6.25, 50:12.5, 100:25, and 150:37.5 μg (*Thyrolar*). It should be noted also that the same potency designations (corresponding to equivalent grains of desiccated thyroid) used by the two manufacturers indicate different quantities of hormones. These variations should be taken into consideration when substituting one brand for the other.

Thyroid, USP

Thyroid, USP, is derived from dried and defatted thyroid glands of domestic animals (bovine, ovine, or porcine). The thyroid hormone content varies somewhat from one species to another. For example, the T_4/T_3 ratio of bovine preparations may range from about 3 to nearly 5. Porcine T_4/T_3 ratios are somewhat lower and range from 2.5 to 3.6. Thyroid preparations are therefore standardized on the basis of their iodine content because of variations in the actual T_4/T_3 ratio. Approximately 0.20 percent of the preparation's weight should be represented by the iodine content. Since much of the iodine present in the thyroid is present in a metabolically inactive form (i.e., iodothyronines, MIT, and DIT), a given preparation may satisfy the *USP* iodine assay requirements and yet not contain sufficient amounts of T_4 and T_3 to produce the desired metabolic effect. *Thyrar* (a beef extract) and *Armour Thyroid* tablets (a pork extract) are evaluated by additional biological assays to help ensure constant potency from one batch to another. Although these products are less variable than those assayed on the basis of iodine content alone, they are not as uniform as synthetic products.

Thyroid, USP, has the same indications, adverse reactions, and precautions as levothyroxine. However, desiccated thyroid is now usually prescribed only for individuals who have been maintained for years on this product, and many of these patients may benefit from a substitution in therapy. Desiccated thyroid is not recommended for initial therapy in newly diagnosed patients.

Thyroid hormone should be taken on an empty stomach to enhance absorption. For replacement therapy, the dosage must be determined on an individual basis by the clinical response and results of laboratory tests.

Thyroid, USP, is available generically and under trademark (*Thyrar, Armour Thyroid Tablets, S-P-T, Thyroid Strong*). It is marketed as oral tablets (15–325 mg), enteric-coated tablets (32–130 mg), and capsules (65–325 mg).

Thyroglobulin

Thyroglobulin is an orally active, partially purified extract of frozen porcine thyroid. It contains T_3 and T_4 and conforms to the *USP*-required iodine content specifications; it also has been assayed and standardized biologically for metabolic potency. Thyroglobulin is slightly more expensive and offers no particular therapeutic advantage over thyroid, USP; on a milligram-for-milligram basis it is equipotent with the desiccated product. Its clinical use, adverse reactions, and cautions also are similar. Initiating therapy with thyroglobulin is no longer recommended.

Thyroglobulin is available generically (tablets, 60 mg) and under trademark (*Proloid*, 32-, 65-, 100-, 130-, and 200-mg tablets, corresponding to ½, 1, 1½, 2, and 3 grains of thyroid, *USP*, respectively).

Drug Interactions

Several drugs can interfere with thyroid gland activity. The nature of the various drug-hormone interactions differs among the various compounds. Some agents produce alterations in the circulating levels of thyroid-binding globulin (e.g., estrogen) while others may compete with thyroxine for binding sites on serum proteins (e.g., salicylates). When large dosages of thyroid hormones are given in association with adrenomimetic amines (as has occurred in the now unacceptable method of treating obesity), serious and even life-threatening signs of cardiovascular toxicity have been produced.

Drugs containing significant quantities of iodine may also affect thyroid function. For example, the antiarrhythmic drug amiodarone contains 37% iodine by weight and is structurally similar to the thyroid hormones. The drug inhibits hepatic 5'-iodothyronine monodeiodinase, resulting in increases in serum T_4 and rT_3, whereas serum T_3 is decreased. There is a significant incidence of either hypo- or hyperthyroidism in patients being treated with this drug. This is largely due to the effects of iodine released from metabolism of the drug during chronic therapy; in susceptible individuals amiodarone may unmask autoimmune thyroid disease.

Management of Hyperthyroidism (Thyrotoxicosis)

Causes and Manifestations

The term *hyperthyroidism* refers to any condition in which the body tissues are exposed to supraphysiological amounts of thyroid hormones. There are various types of hyperthyroidism, although only two are common: *toxic adenoma* and *Graves' disease*. Less common causes include toxic multinodular goiter, thyroiditis, and single hyperfunctioning thyroid nodules, among others.

Thyrotoxicosis is manifested by effects on temperature regulation (e.g., increased heat production; warm, moist, flushed skin; and heat intolerance), changes in the cardiovascular system (e.g., tachycardia, widened pulse pressure, arrhythmias, and possibly angina), skeletal muscle weakness, and possibly wasting, tremor, emotional instability, nervousness, insomnia, frequent bowel movements (occasionally diarrhea), and often weight loss despite increased appetite.

Several eye signs are also often noted in thyrotoxicosis, irrespective of the underlying cause. These include retraction of the upper eyelid, evident as the presence of a rim of sclera between the lid and the limbus, and lid lag, in which the globe lags behind the upper lid when the patient gazes slowly upward. These ocular manifestations appear to be due largely to increased adrenergic stimulation and are ameliorated by adrenergic antagonists; they are reversed promptly upon successful treatment of the thyrotoxicosis. It is important to differentiate these ocular symptoms, which occur in all forms of thyrotoxicosis, from those of infiltrative ophthalmopathy, which are more serious and specific for Graves' disease. Not every patient presents the total spectrum of symptoms listed.

Graves' disease, the most common form of hyperthyroidism, is an autoimmune disease that is characterized by the presence of autoantibodies for the thyrotropin (TSH) receptor on thyroid follicular cells. These thyroid receptor antibodies (TRAb) mimic TSH in stimulating the thyroid gland, and their presence leads to the hypersecretion of thyroid hormones in Graves' disease. In such patients, the serum concentrations of T_4, T_3, and TRAb may be elevated while TSH is suppressed.

In addition to hyperthyroidism, additional symptoms include diffuse toxic goiter, infiltrative ophthalmopathy (*exophthalmos*), and occasional infiltrative dermopathy. The infiltrative ophthalmopathy specific to Graves' disease occurs in about 50 percent of cases and is characterized by increased retroorbital tissue, producing exophthalmos, and by lymphocytic infiltration of the extraocular muscles, producing a spectrum of ocular muscle weakness. The infiltrative ophthalmopathy associated with Graves' disease follows a course that is commonly independent of the thyrotoxic aspect and is, to a large extent, uninfluenced by drug treatment.

Thyroid Storm

A potentially fatal thyrotoxic crisis may occur in hyperthyroid patients spontaneously or following trauma, infection, or inadequate preparation for surgery. Symptoms include hyperthermia, extreme tachycardia with arrhythmias, profound asthenia, marked behavioral changes, vomiting, dehydration, high-output heart failure, syncope, or coma. Treatment involves sedation, oxygen administration, measures to reduce body temperature, and administration of antithyroid medication, iodine, corticosteroids, and fluids and electrolytes. β-Blockers are administered as necessary. Treatment should be initiated before laboratory confirmation of diagnosis is obtained.

Therapy

Treatment of hyperthyroidism is directed at reducing the excessive secretion of thyroid hormones. This action can be accomplished by *reducing the amount of functional thyroid tissue* (through subtotal thyroidectomy or ablation of thyroidal tissue with ^{131}I), or by *inhibiting thyroidal secretion* through the use of antithyroid drugs, or both. Since many of the signs and symptoms of hyperthyroidism reflect increased cellular sensitivity to adrenergic stimulation, a beta-adrenergic antagonist, such as propranolol, can be used adjunctively.

Treatment with either radioiodine or subtotal thyroidectomy often leads to the development of hypothyroidism. This fact constitutes the major argument for the use of such antithyroid drugs as *propylthiouracil* and *methimazole*. Unfortunately, only a small proportion of those patients treated with antithyroid drugs obtain long-term remission of hyperthyroidism. It is generally accepted that 1 or 2 years of control of hyperthyroidism is probably required for a reasonable expectation of the patient's remaining in remission when medication is stopped. Relapse after one course of antithyroid drug therapy usually indicates the need for alternative forms of treatment (i.e., radioiodine or subtotal thyroidectomy).

Inhibitors of Thyroid Hormone Synthesis

Thiourea Derivatives

Derivatives of thiourea are among the primary drugs used to decrease thyroid hormone production. The clinical effects of these drugs are not apparent until the body's stored supply of thyroid hormone has been utilized, and several weeks may pass before signs of decreased thyroid activity are observed. The propyl- and methylthiouracil preparations also are effective antithyroid drugs.

Mechanism of Action

The antithyroid action of the thioamides involves their ability to interfere with the incorporation of iodide into

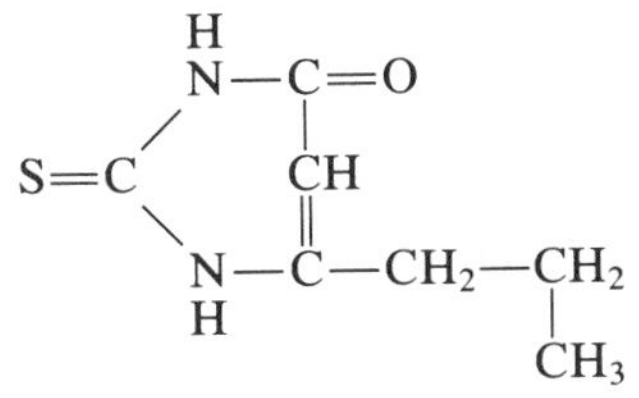

Figure 69-4. Propylthiouracil.

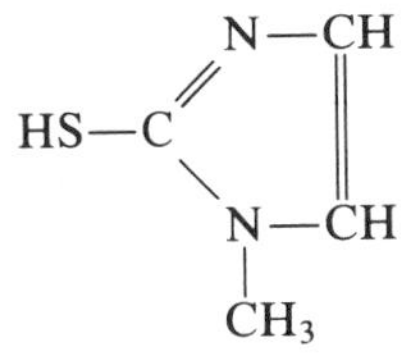

Figure 69-5. Methimazole.

thyroglobulin. Propylthiouracil also appears to inhibit the coupling of iodotyrosine to form T_3 and T_4. The thioamides have little or no effect on the breakdown or release of thyroid hormone that has already been synthesized and stored in the gland. Propylthiouracil also inhibits the peripheral monodeiodination of T_4.

Absorption, Metabolism, and Excretion

The thioamides are usually well absorbed from the gastrointestinal tract and have short plasma half-lives (1–9 hr). However, their duration of action is relatively long and therefore the interval between doses should be no more than 8 hr, particularly during initial therapy. Thioamide derivatives are excreted in the urine conjugated to glucuronide, although a small amount appears in the urine unchanged. Glucuronide conjugates also are found in bile, but little is found in feces. This occurrence implies the existence of an enterohepatic circulation for these agents.

Clinical Uses

The thioamide derivatives, of which propylthiouracil (Fig. 69-4) is the prototype, are used in the management of existing hyperthyroidism (with or without radioactive iodine), for thyrotoxic crisis, and for preparing individuals for subtotal thyroidectomy.

Adverse Reactions

The most frequently observed side effect is the development of a skin rash, which occurs in about 5 percent of the patients. Arthralgia, myalgia, cholestatic jaundice, lymphadenopathy, drug fever, psychosis, and a lupus-like syndrome also have been reported. The most serious problems, however, are granulocytopenia and agranulocytosis. Serious agranulocytosis occurs in about 0.5 percent of the patients and usually occurs within 3 months of starting therapy. It is rapid in onset and usually will not be diagnosed by differential white cell counts at clinic visits.

Prolonged drug administration may result in goiter formation, since an increased secretion of TSH may occur as a result of the inhibition of T_3 and T_4 synthesis. This goitrogenic action is usually the result of overtreatment and necessitates an adjustment in the dosage regimen. Therapeutic failures or remissions are not uncommon and may necessitate the institution of other measures, including thyroidectomy.

Although the drugs can be used for hyperthyroidism complicated by pregnancy, they should be given in minimally effective doses to avoid inducing goiter, cretinism, or both, in the developing fetus.

Preparation and Dosage

Propylthiouracil is given in higher doses initially and is administered until the patient is euthyroid; then approximately one-half that dose is given for maintenance. Routine evaluation of the therapy is advised, with adjustment of dosage as required.

For *preoperative* preparation of the thyroidectomy patient, the drug is given to adults and children in the same dosages used for hyperthyroidism until euthyroidism is attained; iodine is then added to the regimen before surgery (see the following discussion). For *thyrotoxic crisis* in adults, 600 mg to 1.2 gm is given daily in divided doses. The initial dose is followed by iodine administration within a few hours.

Propylthiouracil is available generically as 50-mg tablets.

Methimazole

Methimazole (Fig. 69-5) has similar actions and indications as propylthiouracil, but it does not inhibit peripheral conversion of T_4 to T_3 and is approximately 10 times more potent. The plasma half-life is longer than that of propylthiouracil and effectiveness can sometimes be achieved with less frequent administration.

Methimazole (*Tapazole*) is available for oral use as 5- and 10-mg tablets.

Potassium Perchlorate

Potassium perchlorate ($KClO_4$) interferes with iodide transport into the thyroid gland; it is an inhibitor of the anionic pump. Because this drug can cause fatal aplastic anemia, it is no longer considered to be therapeutically useful. At one time, it was considered to be an alternative form of therapy for patients in whom a hypersensitivity to the thioamides had developed.

Iodides

The effects of iodide on the thyroid gland are complex. Pharmacological amounts of iodide appear to transiently inhibit organic iodine formation and to block hormone release. Iodide has long been used, usually in combination with a thioamide, in the immediate preoperative care of patients about to undergo subtotal thyroidectomy for Graves' disease.

Another use of iodide has been in the management of the hyperthyroidism that occurs after a therapeutic dose of ^{131}I has been given. The response to radioiodine may be delayed for several weeks and during this time the thyroid gland is particularly sensitive to the quieting effect of iodide and does not escape readily from that influence. Management of thyrotoxicosis with iodine alone frequently results in the phenomenon of *iodine escape,* which leads to an exacerbation of the hyperthyroidism.

Administration of potassium iodide can block the accumulation of radioiodine by the thyroid gland. In the event of an accident at a nuclear power plant, large quantities of radionuclides, including isotopes of radioiodine, could be released into the atmosphere. Thyroid blockade by iodides would be the most effective means of limiting the thyroidal uptake of radioiodine. The use of iodine during pregnancy is not recommended because it is transported across the placenta, and fetal goiter and hypothyroidism may result.

Adverse Reactions and Precautions

Iodine reactions can be divided into two categories: (1) Intrathyroidal—Iodine-induced thyrotoxicosis (Jod-Basedow's phenomenon) may occur in patients with nontoxic nodular goiter at low doses (<25 mg/day). At higher doses (50–500 mg/day) iodide goiter or hypothyroidism, or both, may develop, but this usually requires prolonged exposure to high doses of iodine. (2) Extrathyroidal—Sore mouth and throat, hypersalivation, painful sialadenitis, acne and other rashes, diarrhea, and productive cough may occur.

Routes, Usual Dosage, and Preparations

Oral

In preparation for thyroidectomy in adults and children, it is common practice to administer strong iodine solution (two to six drops 3 times daily) or potassium iodide solution (five drops 3 times daily) for 10 days before surgery. For thyrotoxic crisis, 1 hr after antithyroid drugs and as part of the medical emergency treatment, two drops of strong iodide solution or 50 to 100 mg potassium iodide solution, USP, should be administered every 12 hr.

Intravenous

For thyrotoxic crisis, 250 to 500 mg sodium iodide is administered daily after an antithyroid drug and propranolol have been given.

Potassium iodide is available generically as 300-mg tablets. In addition, 130-mg tablets (*Thyro-Block*) are available, but only to state and federal agencies.

Potassium iodide solution (21 mg per drop in 30-ml containers) is available only to state and federal agencies.

Sodium iodide is available generically in bulk (crystals, granules, powder) and in solution (100 mg/ml in 10-ml containers and 200 mg/ml in 20-ml containers).

Strong iodine solution (Lugol's solution) is available generically. The solution contains 5% iodine and 10% sodium iodide.

Lithium Carbonate

Lithium carbonate had been in use for some years in the treatment of manic-depressive states (see Chap. 33) before it was realized that it suppressed thyroid gland activity. Lithium appears to act in a manner similar to that of iodide in preventing the release of both hormonal and nonhormonal iodine from the thyroid gland. Lithium offers no particular advantage over drugs of the thioamide class.

Since lithium causes an accumulation of thyroidal iodide, and since such an accumulation leads to an eventual iodine escape, there is probably no therapeutic place for this agent in the long-term management of thyrotoxicosis.

Radioiodine

Iodine 131 is a safe and effective compound for the management of thyrotoxicosis due to toxic adenoma or toxic multinodular goiter. There is no evidence that ^{131}I increases the incidence of leukemia or thyroid carcinoma. A major disadvantage associated with the therapy is the possibility of increased incidence of hypothyroidism. Microcurie amounts of ^{131}I are used for diagnostic evaluation of thyroid function, whereas millicurie quantities are used for the selective destruction of thyroid cells. ^{131}I exerts its therapeutic effect primarily through beta-particle emissions, which destroy thyroid tissue.

Treatment of Graves' disease patients with ^{131}I results in the inevitable development of hypothyroidism due to a combination of irradiation-induced latent nuclear damage of thyroid follicular cells, with loss of reproductive integrity, and the natural history of eventual autoimmune-mediated hypothyroidism.

Route, Usual Dosage, and Preparations

Oral

Sodium iodide I 131 (generic, *Iodotope I-131*) is available for oral administration in the form of capsules (0.8–10 mCi) and solutions (3.5–15 mCi/ml) in the form of carrier-free sodium iodide. Information on the label includes activity (at a specified hour and date), the name and quantity of any added substance (preservative, dye, or stabilizing agent), the intended use (diagnostic or therapeutic; oral or IV), and the recommended dosage.

Propranolol Hydrochloride

The pharmacology of propranolol (*Inderal*) is discussed in some detail in Chap. 13. This β-blocker is effective in alleviating many of the signs and symptoms of thyrotoxicosis. Propranolol may reduce hyperthyroid-induced tachycardia, tremor, sweating, heat intolerance, and anxiety. Therefore, it is a useful adjunct to other appropriate therapy for thyrotoxicosis. Propranolol has proved to be useful for short-term management of certain thyrotoxic neonates and in thyrotoxic crises, but for long-term management of hyperthyroid states, it is inferior to the thioamides. Generally, propranolol is not used alone.

Propranolol is contraindicated in the thyrotoxic patient with obstructive airway disease, since it impairs bronchodilation. The hyperglycemia resulting from propranolol administration would also limit its usefulness in diabetic patients with thyrotoxicosis. For further discussion of adverse reactions, precautions, and preparations, see Chap. 13.

Supplemental Reading

Brent, G.A., Moore, D.D., and Larsen, P.R. Thyroid hormone regulation of gene expression. *Ann. Rev. Physiol.* 53:17, 1991.

Farrar, J.J., and Toft, A.D. Iodine-131 treatment of hyperthyroidism: Current issues. *Clin. Endocrinol.* 35:207, 1991.

Helfand, M., and Crapo, L.M. Monitoring therapy in patients taking levothyroxine. *Ann. Intern. Med.* 113:450, 1990.

McDougall, R. Graves' disease: Current concepts. *Med. Clin. North Am.* 75:97, 1991.

Schimke, R.N. Hyperthyroidism: The clinical spectrum. *Postgrad. Med.* 91:229, 1992.

Surks, M.I., et al. American Thyroid Association guidelines for use of laboratory tests in thyroid disorders. *J.A.M.A.* 263:1529, 1990.

Wolf, P.G., and Meek, J.C. Practical approach to the treatment of hypothyroidism. *Am. Fam. Physician* 45:722, 1992.

70

Parathyroid Hormone, Calcitonin, and Vitamin D

Frank L. Schwartz

The primary hormones involved in calcium metabolism and bone remodeling are *parathyroid hormone* (PTH), *calcitonin* (CT), and various *metabolites of vitamin D*. However, other hormones, such as thyroid hormones, growth hormone, androgens, estrogens, and the glucocorticoids, can influence mineral homeostasis in both normal and pathological conditions.

PTH is secreted from the parathyroid gland in response to a decrease in the plasma concentration of ionized calcium. PTH action in bone leads to the transfer of labile calcium stores into the bloodstream. In the intestine PTH increases rates of dietary calcium absorption, and in the kidney it increases calcium reabsorption and inhibits calcium excretion. The release of CT is normally inhibited by low calcium levels. The opposite effect occurs when serum calcium concentrations are high, that is, PTH release is inhibited, and CT secretion is enhanced during hypercalcemia.

Vitamin D, through its active metabolite, 1,25-dihydroxycholecalciferol [1,25-$(OH)_2D_3$], also plays an important role in maintaining calcium homeostasis by enhancing intestinal calcium absorption, by increasing PTH-induced mobilization of calcium from bone, and by promoting calcium reabsorption in the kidney.

Mineral Metabolism

Calcium and phosphate are the principal extracellular electrolytes that are regulated by PTH, CT, and vitamin D. These ions have distinct intracellular and extracellular functions, which appear to be regulated by separate, though related, mechanisms. *Extracellular* calcium is involved in muscle contraction, hormone action, neurotransmitter secretion, and exocrine and endocrine secretion. Extracellular calcium also serves as a cofactor in various enzymatic reactions. *Intracellular* phosphorus is a component of ribonucleic acid phosphate polymers, phospholipids, glycolytic pathway intermediates, and phosphorylated nucleotides as well as being a major component of intracellular phosphate buffer systems.

Despite the significant plasma concentrations of both calcium and phosphorus, 99 percent of all body calcium and 85 percent of all body phosphorus reside in the *hydroxyapatite* crystals of bone. Although dietary intake is the usual source of most plasma calcium and phosphorus, if either intestinal absorption is inadequate or renal excretory loss is great, bone becomes the principal source of these two minerals.

Plasma calcium exists in three forms: *ionized* (50%), *protein bound* (46%), and *complexed* to organic ions (4%). The plasma calcium concentration is normally in the range of 4.5 to 5.7 mEq per liter (L). In contrast, phosphorus levels can vary widely depending on the individual's age, diet, and hormonal status.

Calcium Homeostasis

The regulation of serum calcium concentration is a complex process that requires coordinated responses among a variety of hormones and their target tissues. The model shown in Fig. 70-1 consists of three "wings," depicting overlapping feedback loops that represent the interactions between bone (wing 1), intestinal (wing 2), and renal (wing 3) contributions to calcium homeostasis. The left side of the model (A loops) describes events that increase blood calcium and are physiological responses to *hypocalcemia*, whereas the right side (B loops) describes events that decrease blood calcium and are physiological responses to *hypercalcemia*.

Hypocalcemia results in a direct increase in PTH synthe-

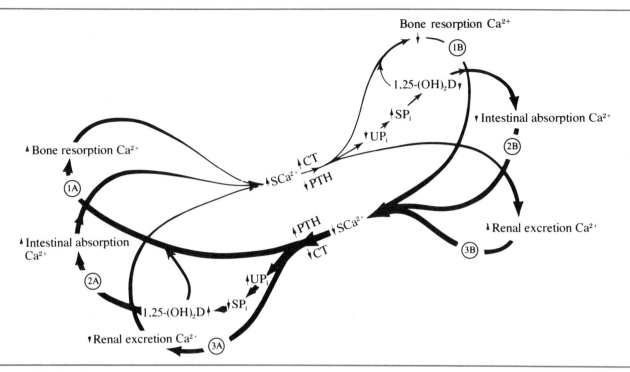

Figure 70-1. The "butterfly model" of calcium homeostasis. The model consists of three overlapping control loops (negative feedback) that interlock and relate to one another through the level of blood concentrations of ionic calcium, parathyroid hormone (PTH), and calcitonin (CT). The loops are numbered 1, 2, and 3; the limbs of the three loops that describe physiological events that increase blood concentrations of calcium are designated A (left), and the limbs that describe events that decrease blood concentrations of calcium are designated B (right). UP_i = urinary phosphate, SP_i = serum phosphate, SCa^2 = serum calcium. (From C. D. Arnaud, *Calcium homeostasis: Regulatory elements and their integration.* Fed. Proc. 37:2557, 1978.)

sis and release, which, in turn, causes an indirect increase in $1,25-(OH)_2D_3$ production through the renal actions of PTH. CT release is inhibited during hypocalcemia.

In states of *hypercalcemia*, CT release is augmented, while PTH release is inhibited. In hypercalcemia, bone resorption is reduced due to a direct action of CT on osteocyte activity. In the intestine, reduced levels of $1,25-(OH)_2D_3$ result in less calcium absorption. Within the kidney, CT directly induces an initial phosphate diuresis, which is followed by increased calcium, sodium, and phosphate excretion. The mechanism by which PTH and CT exert opposite biological effects on calcium reabsorption and bone mineralization is incompletely understood. It appears that PTH and CT activate enzyme systems within different cell populations in these common target organs. For instance, it is currently believed that in renal tissue, specificity of hormone action for both PTH and CT is due to the stimulation of anatomically separate tubule cells. These cells are presumed to have opposing functions with regard to calcium and phosphorus reabsorption. In this way, the occurrence of reabsorption or diuresis would depend on which specific cell population was activated.

Parathyroid Hormone

PTH is comprised of a single-chain polypeptide, composed of 84 amino acid residues, devoid of disulfide bonds, and having a molecular weight of 9,500 (Fig. 70-2). Biological activity of the human hormone resides primarily in the amino terminal end of the protein (i.e., amino acids 1–34). This portion of PTH has full biological activity, both in vivo and in vitro. Various synthetic fragments, as well as precursors, of PTH are undergoing pharmacological evaluation for use as therapeutic agents.

Synthesis and Secretion

Plasma calcium concentration is the principal factor regulating PTH synthesis and release. The increases in PTH synthesis and secretion induced by hypocalcemia are believed to be mediated through an activation of parathyroid gland adenylate cyclase and a subsequent increase in intracellular cyclic adenosine monophosphate (cAMP). Augmented PTH synthesis is the end result of increased gene tran-

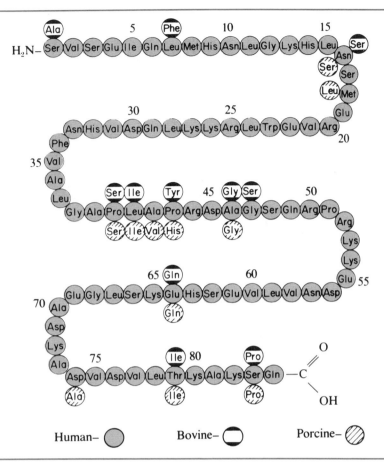

Figure 70-2. Comparison of the amino acid sequence of human, bovine, and porcine PTH. The human hormone is shown by the backbone sequence; substitutions found in the bovine and porcine hormones are indicated by circles alongside. (From H. T. Keutmann et al., Complete amino acid sequence of human parathyroid hormone. *Biochemistry* 17:5723, 1978.)

scription (synthesis of messenger RNA [mRNA] from DNA).

Formation of PTH begins with the synthesis of several precursor molecules. *PreproPTH* is the initial peptide that is synthesized within the parathyroid gland, and it serves as a precursor to both proPTH and PTH. PreproPTH appears to be formed within the rough endoplasmic reticulum and is then transported into the cisternal space where proteolytic cleavage of a segment results in the formation of proPTH. The proPTH polypeptide is thought to aid in the transport of the hormone into the cisternal space where another proteolytic cleavage occurs, forming PTH. Although PTH is the predominant peptide released by the parathyroid gland in response to hypocalcemia, precursors of PTH and smaller fragments also are released. These components also may have biological activity.

Although serum calcium appears to be the principal regulator of PTH synthesis and release, these processes can be influenced by other factors as well. For instance, parathyroid cells contain specific adrenoceptors that re-

spond in vitro to norepinephrine and epinephrine administration by releasing PTH. Vitamin D_3 also may influence PTH synthesis and release. This action is brought about through an interaction with $1,25\text{-}(OH)_2D_3$ receptors located within parathyroid gland tissue.

Mechanism of Action

As is common with many other peptide hormones, one of the earliest effects of PTH in bone and kidney is the activation of the enzyme adenylyl cyclase and the generation of cAMP. Specific plasma membrane receptors for PTH have been demonstrated within target organs, and interactions of PTH with these receptors have been directly linked to adenylyl cyclase activity and concomitant expression of hormone activity.

PTH has three principal actions in bone. First, PTH induces transformation of osteoprogenitor cells into osteoclasts; the latter cells increase bone turnover. Second,

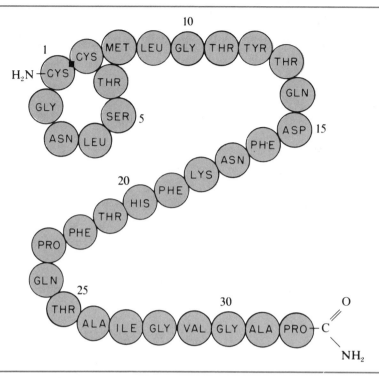

Figure 70-3. Amino acid sequence of human calcitonin. (From R. Neher et al., Human calcitonin. *Nature* 220:984, 1968.)

PTH stimulates deep osteocytes to mobilize calcium from perilacunar bone. And, third, PTH causes stimulation of surface osteocytes to increase the outward flux of calcium ion from bone. During brief periods of hypocalcemia, PTH release results in mobilization of calcium from labile areas of bone that lie adjacent to osteoclasts. This stimulation normally is not associated with any significant bone resorption. However, during prolonged hypocalcemia, such as occurs in renal osteodystrophy or malabsorption syndromes, PTH mobilizes deep osteocytes in perilacunar bone and results in significant bone resorption.

PTH stimulates the conversion of 25-(OH)D$_3$ into 1,25-(OH)$_2$D$_3$ within the kidney. Intrarenal 1,25-(OH)$_2$D$_3$ causes an amplification of the PTH-induced calcium reabsorption, whereas plasma 1,25-(OH)$_2$D$_3$ enhances PTH action in bone. PTH has no direct effect on intestinal calcium absorption; its actions are indirect through induction of 1,25-(OH)$_2$D$_3$ synthesis and release from the kidney.

Calcitonin

Chemistry

The *calcitonins* are single-chain polypeptides composed of 32 amino acid residues with a molecular weight of approximately 3,600 (Fig. 70-3). A cysteine disulfide bridge at the 1-7 position of the amino terminal end of the peptide is essential for biological activity; it appears that the entire amino acid sequence is required for optimal activity.

Synthesis and Secretion

The regulation of CT synthesis and release from the parafollicular C cells of the thyroid gland is calcium dependent. *Hypercalcemia is the principal stimulus responsible for CT synthesis and release.* Compounds such as glucagon, prolactin, thyroid-stimulating hormone (TSH), thyroxine, adrenergic agents, gastrin, pancreozymin, and serotonin also can stimulate adenylyl cyclase activity and CT release. Although CT has been isolated in tissues other than the parafollicular C cells (parathyroid, pancreas, thymus, adrenal), it is not known whether this material is biologically active.

Secretagogues, such as gastrin and pancreozymin, may contribute significantly to the regulation of endogenous CT. In fact, it has been postulated that gastrin-induced CT release following meals may inhibit postprandial hypercalcemia. Such an action may be one of the primary physiological functions of CT. CT does not directly affect calcium absorption.

A calcitonin precursor has been identified within the thyroid parafollicular C cells. It is thought to function in a manner analogous to the proPTH, that is, to facilitate intracellular transport and secretion of the hormone. The metabolic degradation of CT appears to occur in both the liver and kidney.

Although blood CT levels are normally very low, excessive levels have been found in association with medullary carcinoma of the thyroid and, more rarely, with carcinoid tumors of the bronchus and stomach.

Mechanism of Action

CT is thought to require an interaction with specific plasma membrane receptors within target organs in order to initiate biological effects. This interaction has been directly linked to the generation of cAMP via adenylate cyclase activation.

Vitamin D_3 (Cholecalciferol)

Chemistry

Vitamin D is a sterol in which the B ring of the steroid nucleus is replaced by a diene bridge. Cholecalciferol is derived from cholesterol; however, for biological activity it must undergo further metabolic transformation and should be considered a *prohormone*. There are three principal metabolites of vitamin D that possess biological activity: 25-hydroxycholecalciferol [25-(OH)D_3], 1,25-dihydroxycholecalciferol [1,25-(OH)$_2$D$_3$], and 24,25-dihydroxycholecalciferol [24R,25-(OH)$_2$D$_3$].

Synthesis and Secretion

The primary supply of vitamin D_3 in humans is not obtained from the diet, but rather is derived from the ultraviolet photoconversion of 7-dehydrocholesterol to vitamin D_3 in skin. Thus, there are seasonal variations in vitamin D_3 synthesis. Vitamin D_3 is a prohormone and requires further metabolic conversion to exert biological activity in its target organs (Fig. 70-4). The liver and the kidney are the major sites of metabolic activation of this endogenous sterol hormone. The initial transformation of the native vitamin D_3 molecule occurs in the liver and is catalyzed by the enzyme 25-OH-D_3-hydroxylase to form 25-(OH)D_3, which is the primary circulating form (10–80 μg/ml) of vitamin D_3. It, as well as the other vitamin D_3 metabolites, circulates in the blood bound to a specific transport globulin.

Circulating 25-(OH)D_3 is converted in the kidney to the most active form of vitamin D_3, 1,25-(OH)$_2$D$_3$, by a PTH-dependent 1-(OH)-D_3-hydroxylase enzyme system. Blood concentrations of 1,25-(OH)$_2$D$_3$ are approximately 1/500 those of 25-(OH)D_3. Further metabolic conversion of 1,25-(OH)$_2$D$_3$ occurs, and one metabolite, 24R,25-(OH)$_2$D$_3$, is capable of suppressing parathyroid secretion. Its role in calcium homeostasis remains undefined at present.

The biogenesis of 1,25-(OH)$_2$D$_3$ is under feedback control. Hypocalcemia results in the enzymatic activation of 1,25-(OH)$_2$D$_3$ through the renal 25-(OH)$_2$D$_3$-1-hydroxylase system (see Fig. 70-4). Parathyroidectomy abolishes 1,25-(OH)$_2$D$_3$ release in response to hypocalcemia, whereas PTH administration restores enzyme activity, indicating that this is a PTH-dependent process.

In addition to the endogenous metabolites, there are exogenous sterols that possess activity similar to that of vitamin D. Ergocalciferol (vitamin D_2) is derived from the plant sterol, ergosterol, and may act as a substrate for both the 25-hydroxylase and the 1-hydroxylase enzyme systems of the liver and kidney to form 25-(OH)D_2 and 1,25-(OH)$_2$D$_2$, respectively. Dihydrotachysterol is another sterol that is used as a therapeutic agent; it also functions as a substrate for the hydroxylase enzyme in the liver and kidney.

Mechanism of Action

Great progress has been made in elucidating the precise cellular mode of action of 1,25-(OH)$_2$D$_3$ in target tissues (Fig. 70-5). Similar to steroid hormones, this compound exerts its influence within target tissues, such as the intestine, bone, kidney, and parathyroid gland, through sterol-specific, high-affinity cytoplasmic receptor proteins. The receptor serves to translocate the hormone from the cell cytoplasm to the nucleus, where biological response is initiated.

Thus, 1,25-(OH)$_2$D$_3$ is believed to exert its biological activity within target tissues through an interaction with specific intracellular receptor proteins. This results in the generation of specific gene products, which then facilitate calcium transport (absorption, reabsorption, and influx) within the appropriate target organs.

Summary

PTH, CT, and vitamin D_3 work in concert to regulate plasma calcium levels. PTH and CT act directly on bone and kidney to increase or decrease, respectively, plasma calcium levels. PTH and CT effects on intestinal calcium absorption are indirectly mediated by changes in plasma 1,25-(OH)$_2$D$_3$ levels (see Fig. 70-1). In addition, both substances can influence the rate of 1,25-(OH)$_2$D$_3$ release from the kidney.

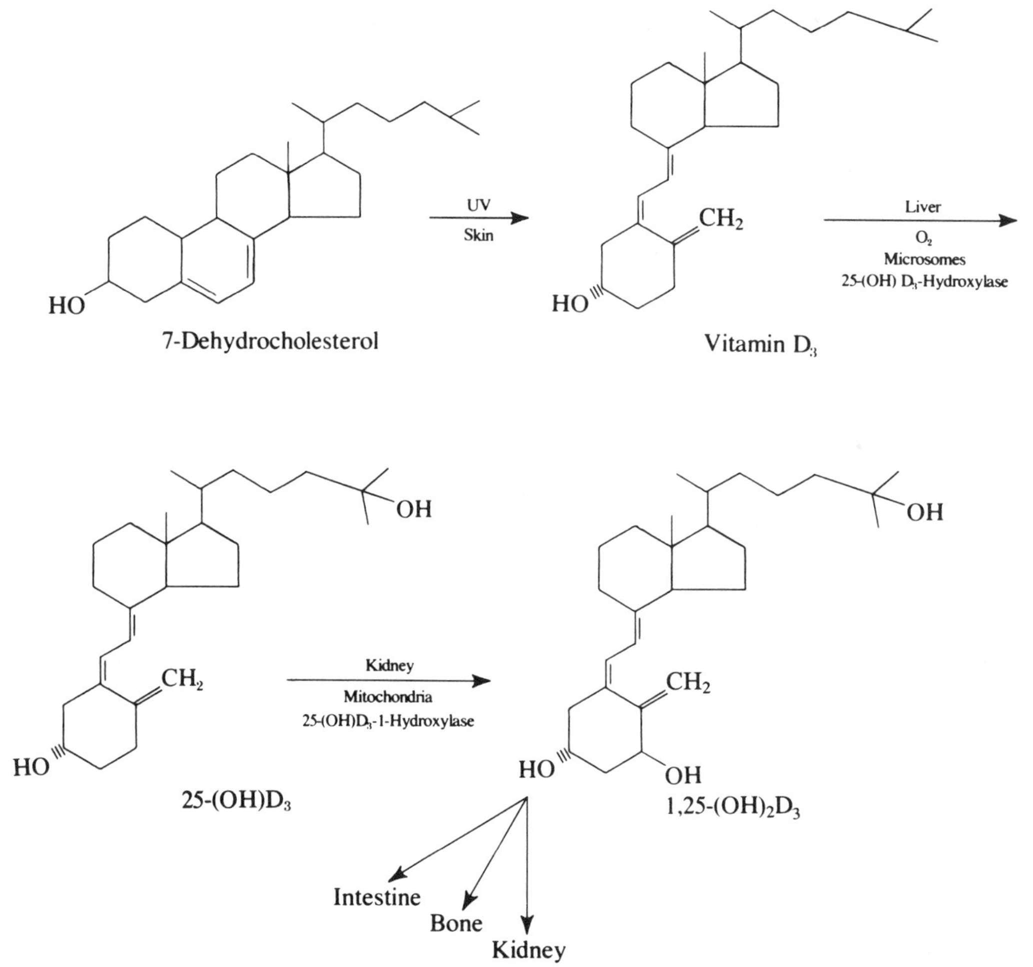

Figure 70-4. Functional metabolism of vitamin D, including its biosynthesis by photolysis reaction in skin. (From H.F. DeLuca, Vitamin D metabolism and function. *Arch. Intern. Med.* 138:836, 1978.)

Apart from the feedback relationship that exists between plasma calcium and the release of PTH, CT, and vitamin D_3, the local ionic concentrations of phosphate and magnesium within the bone, kidney, and intestine also influence the rate and direction of calcium flux.

Clinical Uses of Parathyroid Hormone, Calcitonin, and Vitamin D

Therapy for disorders in calcium and phosphorus metabolism usually involves ablation of glandular tissues in situations of hormone excess and replacement of specific hormones in conditions of deficiency. However, during conditions of acute calcium excess or deficiency, adjunc-

tive measures for the control of plasma calcium and phosphorus levels are important and supersede hormonal manipulation as the primary form of therapy.

Clinical Disorders

Hypoparathyroidism

Hypoparathyroidism, either postsurgical or idiopathic, is characterized by hypocalcemia and, frequently, hyperphosphatemia. The result is the development of tetany and cardiac arrhythmias. Serum calcium levels must be restored immediately. In addition to the absence of PTH in hypoparathyroidism, there is a partial deficiency of circulating $1,25\text{-}(OH)_2D_3$ caused by the diminished PTH-induced formation of $1,25\text{-}(OH)_2D_3$.

Following emergency restoration of plasma calcium

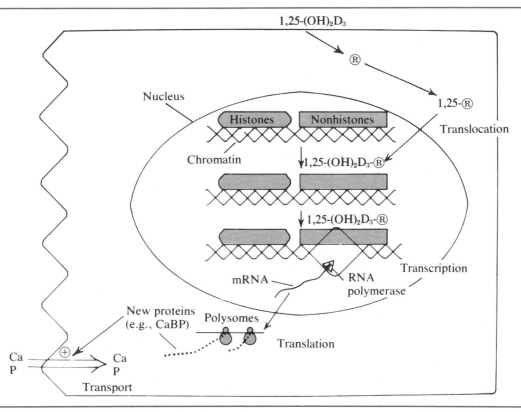

Figure 70-5. Proposed molecular mechanism of action of 1,25-(OH)$_2$D$_3$ in an intestinal mucosa cell. ® = receptor protein; CaBP = calcium-binding protein. (From M.R. Haussler and T.A. McCain, Basic and clinical concepts related to vitamin D metabolism and action. I. *N. Engl. J. Med.* 297:974, 1977.)

levels with intravenous calcium gluconate, successful maintenance of normal blood calcium levels is usually achieved by treating patients with oral calcium supplements and a vitamin D preparation such as ergocalciferol.

The incidence of iatrogenic hypercalcemia, secondary to hypervitaminosis D, is much less common with specific metabolite therapy than with vitamin D$_3$ or vitamin D$_2$ (ergocalciferol) administration because of the shorter half-lives of the metabolites. Dihydrotachysterol, which also is capable of restoring normocalcemia, was the drug of choice before the advent of specific metabolite therapy, because it had a shorter duration of action than vitamin D$_3$. Recombinantly produced human PTH is now being tested in clinical trials.

Pseudohypoparathyroidism

Pseudohypoparathyroidism is a rare condition in which there is end-organ insensitivity to PTH action at the PTH receptor level. In this condition, affected individuals appear to have hypoparathyroidism; however, PTH levels are either high or inappropriately normal. Serum calcium levels are low secondary to the end-organ resistance to PTH. Although difficult to treat, a correction of the hypocalcemia, along with improvement of bone responsiveness to endogenous PTH, can sometimes be accomplished with 1,25-(OH)$_2$D$_3$ or 1α-(OH)D$_3$.

Severe Hypercalcemia

Hypercalcemia is a medical emergency that is a relatively frequent clinical problem. Various modalities are now used to treat this condition; IV hydration and loop diuretics (furosemide) are important supportive measures. Several compounds with pharmacological action on mineral metabolism also are helpful.

Calcitonin is effective in reducing serum calcium levels rapidly in life-threatening hypercalcemia. Subcutaneous administration of salmon (*Calcimar*) or human (*Cibacalcin*) calcitonin results in a lowering of serum calcium levels within 3 to 5 days in 75 to 90 percent of all malignant hypercalcemia.

Biphosphonates are compounds structurally related to pyrophosphate that bind to the hydroxyapatite of bone and inhibit resorption. Etidronate and Pamidronate are infused intravenously. The major side effect of these compounds is a transient increase in creatinine and phosphate levels.

Plicamycin (*Mithracin*), an inhibitor of RNA synthesis in osteoclasts, is effective when infused over a 4- to 6-hr period every 3 to 4 days. The major side effect of this compound is bone marrow suppression.

Osteoporosis

Osteoporosis is a very common disorder, particularly in postmenopausal women. It is characterized by a decrease in bone density that often results in an increased frequency of skeletal fractures of the wrist, hip, and axial skeleton. Factors that are especially predisposing to this condition are premature menopause, hypogonadism, malabsorption syndrome, thin habitus, positive family history, cigarette smoking, and heavy alcohol ingestion.

The most effective treatment of osteoporosis is prevention. In menopausal women, the greatest amount of bone density is lost during the first 5 years after onset of menopause. Premenopausal women who are at increased risk, therefore, should be placed on a regimen of estrogen replacement therapy, calcium supplementation, and vitamin D at the onset of menopausal symptoms. However, the benefits (increased bone density, decreased cardiovascular risk, decreased vaginal atrophy) must be weighed against risks (increased incidences of breast and endometrial cancer) before initiation of therapy.

Once bone loss is severe enough to result in compression fractures and pain, therapy is much less effective. CT injections (100–200 units SC or IM daily) are effective in promoting fracture healing and reducing pain. Also, small increases in bone density have been reported following CT administration. Sodium fluoride given cyclically along with calcium supplements can induce a modest increase in bone density once osteoporosis has occurred. However, fluoride-stimulated increases in bone density are not normal bone, and the claimed reduction in fracture rates is not proved.

Rickets and Osteomalacia

Rickets and osteomalacia are metabolic bone diseases that develop in children and adults, respectively, as a result of inadequate bone mineralization. Prevention of these two diseases requires the presence of normal physiological levels of serum calcium and phosphate to allow adequate bone mineralization. Rickets in children was quite widespread during the Industrial Revolution, when inadequate exposure to ultraviolet light impaired the synthesis in skin of vitamin D_3 from 7-dehydrocholesterol. Although supplementing food with vitamin D has reduced the incidence of rickets in the United States, it is still a worldwide health problem.

The treatment and prevention of rickets and osteomalacia involve relatively simple procedures today. Administration of *ergocalciferol* (vitamin D_2) or *cholecalciferol* (vitamin D_3) is usually adequate for treatment.

Vitamin D-Resistant Rickets

Although 33 forms of vitamin D–resistant rickets have been described, the most common form is an X-linked dominant hypophosphatemic condition, which is characterized by low plasma phosphorus, normal calcium levels, low or normal PTH levels, and increased renal phosphate excretion. It is currently believed that this condition is not due to a specific defect in vitamin D metabolism but rather to a defect in phosphate transport. Current therapy involves administration of 1.0 to 1.5 gm of oral phosphate in divided doses in addition to 1α-(OH)D_3 or 1,25-(OH)$_2$D$_3$ (1 μg/day, orally).

Vitamin D-Dependent Rickets

This disease is an autosomal recessive condition that results in rickets despite normal intake of vitamin D. Children with this disease present clinically with rickets, hypocalcemia, hypophosphatemia, elevated serum alkaline phosphatase, and aminoaciduria. The defect may be in the renal 25-(OH)D_3-1-hydroxylase enzyme system. Therefore, either 1,25-(OH)$_2$D$_3$ or pharmacological amounts of 25-(OH)D_3 are effective. Using this approach, there is evidence of bone healing within 7 days of beginning therapy.

Drug-Induced Osteopenia

Chronic administration of the anticonvulsant drugs phenytoin and phenobarbital is known to produce rickets or osteomalacia, whereas chronic glucocorticoid therapy can result in rather severe bone loss. These drugs appear to induce changes in bone density through suppression of intestinal calcium absorption, with a subsequent induction of secondary hyperparathyroidism. In addition, corticosteroid administration increases bone turnover by altering osteoblast differentiation. The corticosteroids are also capable of inhibiting collagen synthesis, which results in decreased bone matrix and reduced bone mass.

Vitamin D can increase calcium absorption in patients receiving anticonvulsant or glucocorticoid drugs. Recent studies using 25-(OH)D_3 in patients receiving moderate dosages of corticosteroids also have demonstrated increased rates of calcium absorption. This increased absorption occurred much earlier than that seen after vitamin D_2 (ergocalciferol) administration. In addition, the chances of inadvertent hypervitaminosis and hypercalcemia are reduced when 25-(OH)D_3 is given. The symptoms of anticonvulsant-induced osteomalacia are thought to respond to treatment with 25-(OH)D_3.

Renal Osteodystrophy

Patients with chronic renal failure develop hyperphosphatemia, hypocalcemia, and secondary hyperparathyroidism. In addition, chronic dialysis results in an abnormal deposition of aluminum in bone. The combination of secondary hyperparathyroidism and aluminum deposition results in severe metabolic bone disease. The hyperparathyroidism is thought to be due to a decreased renal 1,25-$(OH)_2$ hydroxylase activity and resultant decreased 1,25-$(OH)_2$ formation. Therefore, 1,25-$(OH)_2D_3$ therapy along with oral phosphate-binding agents and calcium supplementation has become important in the treatment of renal osteodystrophy.

Paget's Disease

Paget's disease of bone is a common disorder in individuals over the age of 50. It can affect any bone of the body; however the skull, humerus, and tibia are most commonly affected. It is characterized by mixed lytic and sclerotic bone changes and results in pain, deformity, and fractures of affected bones. The biphosphonates (etidronate) and calcitonins are most commonly used in the treatment of this disease; however, plicamycin and gallium nitrate are also effective. Long-term use of etidronate can cause osteomalacia by directly impairing new bone formation; thus, patients treated for Paget's disease are usually given this drug for 3- to 6-month cycles.

Other Clinical Disorders

Disorders such as celiac sprue, Crohn's disease, pancreatic insufficiency, cirrhosis, cholestatic liver disease, and diabetes mellitus can lead to osteomalacia secondary to impaired calcium absorption. The malabsorption not only affects the calcium ion itself, but in situations in which bile acids are also deficient, vitamin D will be poorly absorbed. Most patients respond to daily doses of 4,000 to 12,000 IU of oral vitamin D_3 or vitamin D_2.

Adverse Reactions

With the exception of the possible development of hypervitaminosis, which is associated with high-dose administration of vitamin D_2 and D_3, the three hormones discussed in this chapter are relatively safe compounds. However, edema, urticaria, nausea, and tenderness at the site of injection have been described for calcitonin and PTH. Anaphylactoid reactions to injections of these foreign proteins have also occurred.

Vitamin D toxicity is characterized by hypercalcemia, which, if prolonged, can lead to a deposition of calcium salts in soft tissue, primarily the kidney. Nephrolithiasis or diffuse nephrocalcinosis (or both) may result. Treatment of vitamin D intoxication involves immediate cessation of vitamin administration along with efforts directed at reducing calcium absorption from the intestine. Because vitamin D is a fat-soluble sterol that is readily stored in tissues, therapy may require several weeks or months to be effective. Administration of glucocorticoids can be useful in blocking the intestinal absorption of calcium in this situation.

Preparations and Dosage

Parathyroid Hormone

Parathyroid injection (*Paroidin*) is an extract prepared from bovine parathyroid tissue that contains both PTH and fragments of PTH. Administration can be SC, IM, or IV, although IM injections are preferred. Human recombinant PTH is currently being clinically tested.

Calcitonin

Calcitonin (*Calcimar*) is a synthetic 32-amino acid polypeptide that is identical to salmon calcitonin. Activity is stated in terms of international units. It is supplied as a lyophilized powder (200 IU/ml in 2-ml containers), which is to be diluted with a sterol gelatin solution (*Calcimar Diluent*). Administration is SC or IM. Bovine, porcine, and human calcitonin (*Cibacalcin*) also are available.

Vitamin D

Vitamin D comes in many different formulations, including multivitamin preparations, fish liver oils with or without vitamin A, combinations with calcium salts, and vitamin D preparations alone. In therapy, vitamin D is obtained by the ingestion of cholecalciferol (D_3) or ergocalciferol (D_2).

Cholecalciferol is pure vitamin D_3 derived from the ultraviolet conversion of 7-dehydrocholesterol to cholecalciferol. It can be chemically synthesized or derived from the irradiation of food. It is supplied in 25,000- and 50,000-IU capsules.

Ergocalciferol (vitamin D_2) is a sterol derived from yeast and fungal ergosterol and is supplied in 25,000- and 50,000-IU capsules (*Deltalin, Drisdol*, calciferol, vitamin D) or as a solution of 8,000 IU/ml.

Calcitriol [*Rocaltrol*, 1,25-$(OH)_2D_3$] is the metabolically active vitamin D_3 compound and is supplied in 0.25- and 0.5-μg tablets.

Dihydrotachysterol is a synthetic compound that may act somewhat more quickly than either vitamin D_2 or D_3.

It is supplied as 0.125-, 0.2-, and 4-mg tablets; 0.125-mg capsules (*Hytakerol*); or as a solution in oil (0.25 mg/ml).

Supplemental Reading

Bilczikian, J.P. Management of acute hypercalcemia. *N. Engl. J. Med.* 326:1196, 1992.

Broadus, A.E., et al. Humoral hypercalcemia of cancer: Identification of a novel parathyroid hormone–like peptide. *N. Engl. J. Med.* 319:556, 1988.

DeLuca, H.F. The vitamin D story: A collaborative effort of basic science and clinical medicine. *FASEB J.* 2:224, 1988.

Minghetti, P.P., and Norman, A.W. 1,25(OH)$_2$-vitamin D$_3$ receptors: Gene regulation and genetic circuitry. *FASEB J.* 2:3045, 1988.

Pak, C., et al. Safe and effective treatment of osteoporosis with intermittent slow release sodium fluoride. *J. Clin. Endocrinol. Metab.* 68:150, 1989.

Pecila, A. (ed.). *Calcitonin, Chemistry, Physiology, Pharmacology and Clinical Aspects.* Amsterdam: Excerpta Medica, 1985.

Recker, R.R. Current therapy for osteoporosis. *J. Clin. Endocrinol. Metab.* 76:14, 1993.

Reichel, H., Koeffler, H.P., and Norman, A.W. The role of the vitamin D endocrine system in health and disease. *N. Engl. J. Med.* 320:980, 1989.

Insulin, Glucagon, Somatostatin, and Orally Effective Hypoglycemic Drugs

John A. Thomas and *Michael J. Thomas*

Glucose Homeostasis

Glucose serves as a major energy source for all cells. It is particularly important for the cells of the central nervous system (CNS), since they depend almost exclusively on bloodborne glucose for their minute-to-minute energy needs. The glucose present in the blood penetrates most tissues slowly unless insulin is present to facilitate its transport. CNS cells, capillary endothelial cells, gastrointestinal epithelial cells, pancreatic β cells, and renal medullary cells, however, are freely permeable to glucose.

The *islets of Langerhans,* which are the endocrine portion of the pancreas, consist of cordlike groupings of cells that are found along pancreatic capillary channels. Microscopic techniques have revealed two principal types of secretory cells within the islets: α cells, which are involved in the synthesis and storage of glucagon, and β cells, which synthesize and store insulin. Other types of cells, including C cells, D cells, E cells, and F(X) cells, are also present in the mammalian pancreas, but their functions have not been entirely defined. Somatostatin and pancreatic polypeptide are found in the D and F cells, respectively.

The β cells generally monitor changes in the availability of small calorigenic molecules, such as glucose, amino acids, ketone bodies, and fatty acids, and they will appropriately alter their rates of insulin secretion in response to those fluctuations. *Glucose plays the dominant role in regulating β cell insulin secretion.* Pancreatic α cells also secrete glucagon in response to increases in amino acid and fatty acid levels; their secretion, however, is inhibited by glucose. The function of the β cells is to prevent hypoglycemia, and their rate of secretion is largely dependent on blood glucose concentrations. When glucose levels fall, glucagon secretion is augmented. This hormone has powerful glycogenolytic effects on the liver and thus plays a central

role in ensuring that adequate amounts of glucose reach tissues both during minor fluctuations in blood glucose levels and during severe glucose deprivation.

Blood glucose concentrations are maintained within homeostatic limits by a variety of biochemical and physiological control mechanisms. Circulating glucose levels are determined by the balance established between cellular glucose production and utilization, rate of gastrointestinal glucose absorption, and rate of loss of glucose from the kidney. *Glucagon* and *insulin* are the two most important hormonal factors that aid in bringing blood glucose levels back to normal should its concentration be altered.

Insulin

Approximately 100 years have passed since von Mering and Minkowski first demonstrated that pancreatectomized dogs exhibited signs and symptoms characteristic of diabetes mellitus. Shortly thereafter, Banting and Best used pancreatic extracts to reverse these symptoms in patients suffering from severe diabetes. This work provided the basis for establishing a cause-and-effect relationship between insulin deficiency and diabetes. Insulin was subsequently isolated, crystallized, and eventually synthesized in the laboratory. Insulin replacement therapy has been used in the clinical management of diabetes mellitus for over 50 years. In 1982, recombinant DNA (rDNA)-derived *human insulin* was used clinically to treat diabetics.

Chemistry

The insulin molecule is a simple protein that consists of 51 amino acids arranged as two polypeptide chains (an A chain and B chain) connected by disulfide bonds (Fig.

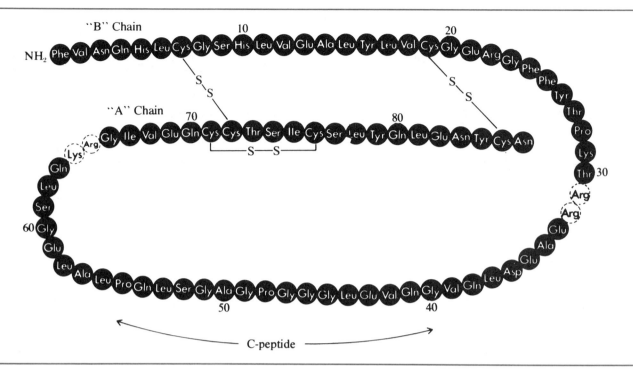

Figure 71-1. Chemical structure of human insulin, showing amino acid sequence and bond types between "A" and "B" chains.

71-1). Destruction of the disulfide linkages reduces biological activity. The hormone can exist, at least in vitro, in different states of polymerization (monomer, dimer, or hexamer), depending on temperature, pH, and concentration of zinc. In its monomeric, or active, form, insulin has a molecular weight of about 6,000. Although the amino acid sequence and composition of animal insulins, such as bovine, ovine, and porcine insulin, may differ from human insulin, their biological actions are similar. Fortunately, the immunological differences between animal and human insulin are minimal.

Biosynthesis

The insulin molecule is not formed separately from A and B chains but rather as a larger, single-chain polypeptide, called *proinsulin*. Proinsulin is derived from a larger precursor, *preproinsulin;* the latter substance is rapidly converted to proinsulin in the rough endoplasmic reticulum of the β cell. Once proinsulin has been formed, it is proteolytically cleaved, either in the Golgi apparatus of β cells or in newly formed secretory granules, to form insulin. The hormone is then packaged and stored within secretory granules. Proinsulin has little inherent biological activity and must be converted to insulin by the action of several proteases. The end result of these cleavage reactions is the formation of insulin and a C-terminal basic

residue called the *C peptide.* Both materials are stored in the β cell granules and both are liberated during β cell secretion. The C-peptide facilitates the correct folding of the A and B chains and maintains the alignment of the disulfide bridges before cleavage.

Secretion

The specific stimulus for insulin secretion involves elevations in circulating levels of glucose and, to a much lesser extent, other substrates. It has been proposed that the β cell membrane contains specific glycoreceptors that recognize D-glucose (Fig. 71-2). Stimulation of these receptors activates an adenylyl cyclase system and causes an influx of calcium ions. The now-altered ionic balance within the β cells facilitates a contraction of the subcellular microtubule-microfilament system, which is involved in the migration of insulin-containing secretory granules into contact with the cell membrane. Fusion of the granule and cell membranes permits the granule contents to be released (*exocytosis*).

Insulin secretion is a continuous process but following a meal rich in carbohydrates, the blood levels of the hormone can increase severalfold. The rate of secretion of insulin in normal human subjects is about 1 to 2 mg/24 hr. Hepatic insulinases destroy about one half of this secreted insulin.

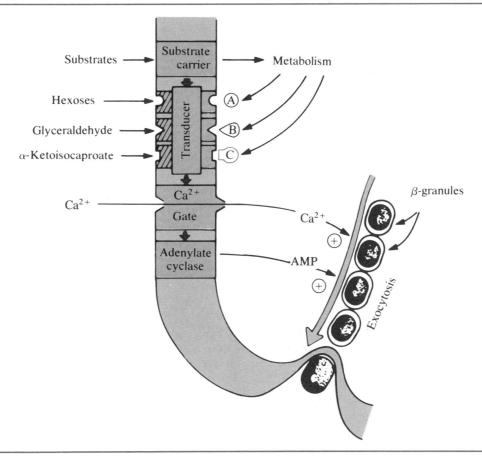

Figure 71-2. Hypothetical mechanisms in pancreatic islet cells. The cell membrane of the islet cell contains five coupled systems: (1) the substrate carriers; (2) a receptor-transducer complex with receptors for hexoses (primarily glucose), glyceraldehyde, and α-keto-isocaproate on the outside and sites for various metabolites and cofactors (e.g., A, B, C) and the inside of the membrane; (3) a Ca^{2+} gate that controls Ca^{2+} entry; (4) an adenylyl cyclase system; and (5) the secretory complex comprised of microtubules and secretory granules involved in the process of exocytosis driven by Ca^{2+} and cyclic adenosine monophosphate (cAMP). (From F.M. Matschinsky et al., Metabolism of Pancreatic Islets and Regulation of Insulin and Glucagon Secretion. In L.J. DeGroot et al. (eds.), *Endocrinology*. vol. 2. New York: Grune & Stratton, 1979.)

Although insulin that is stored in the granules of the β cell is constantly being secreted into the blood (Fig. 71-3), under appropriate conditions these granules can be rapidly mobilized and their contents released into the blood. Although glucose itself seems to be the most important physiological stimulus, several substances can stimulate the release of this pancreatic hormone. Mannose and ribose as well as arginine and leucine are effective stimuli for the secretion of insulin. The actions of hormones, such as glucagon, adrenocorticotropic hormone (ACTH), growth hormone, secretin, gastrin, cholecystokinin, and pancreozymin, can also enhance insulin release either directly or indirectly. It is quite likely that the gastrointestinal hormones, acting in concert, are particularly important in promoting insulin release following the ingestion of glucose. In contrast, somatostatin acts directly on the β cell to prevent insulin release. The secretion of insulin is also dependent on several electrolytes, with calcium playing the most critical role.

Information on the control of glucagon secretion is much less complete, although exocytosis also is thought to be involved. In contrast to its effects on β cells, *glucose suppresses glucagon secretion from pancreatic cells.*

The autonomic nervous system also participates in the regulation of the rate of insulin secretion. The islets of Langerhans receive both cholinergic and noradrenergic innervation input. Insulin secretion will be enhanced by vagal stimulation (or cholinergic agonists) and will be diminished by sympathetic nerve stimulation (or by directly acting α-adrenoceptor agonists).

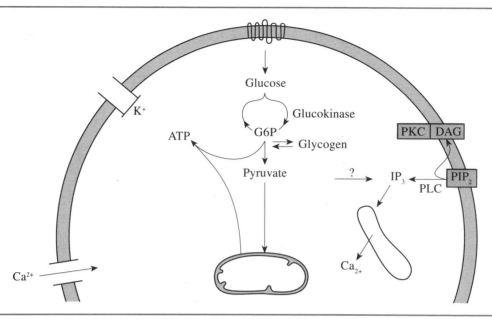

Figure 71-3. Diagram of the major steps leading to glucose-induced insulin secretion. Glucose enters the β cell through a glucose transporter (GLUT2). It is phosphorylated by glucokinase, then undergoes metabolism and oxidation to carbon dioxide and water. An offshoot of this process, probably a rising adenosine triphosphate/adenosine diphosphate (ATP-ADP) ratio, closes the ATP-sensitive K^+ channel, leading to cellular depolarization, opening of voltage-dependent Ca^{2+} channels, and an influx of Ca^{2+}. The rise in intracellular Ca^{2+}, along with a variety of other second messengers, leads to granule recruitment and extrusion. (From J.L. Leahy et al., Beta-cell dysfunction induced by chronic hyperglycemia. Reprinted with permission from *Diabetes Care,* vol. 15, p. 446. Copyright © 1992 by American Diabetes Association, Inc.)

Mechanism of Action

The effects of insulin are mediated through its interaction with specific high-affinity receptors (Fig. 71-4) located on the outer surface of cell plasma membranes. The initial step in the action of insulin involves binding to its receptor. The insulin receptor is comprised of an α subunit (135,000 daltons) and a β subunit (90,000 daltons). The insulin receptor is very specific for insulin. The hormone-receptor interaction is reversible, and the insulin molecule apparently is not chemically altered during its contact with the receptor. The hormone-receptor complex, once formed, is internalized by an endocytotic mechanism, with the insulin molecule eventually being metabolized and the insulin receptor being recycled to the membrane for use again.

Conditions associated with elevated insulin levels in the blood (e.g., obesity) appear to result in a decrease in the number of insulin receptors on cell membranes ("*downregulation*"). Decreases in circulating insulin concentration (e.g., diabetes) may lead to "*upregulation.*" The implications of such an upregulation in the numbers of insulin receptors in the diabetic state would be a shift to the left of the insulin dose-response curve such that less insulin would be needed to produce a given biological effect.

The extent to which receptor regulation participates in adjustments to changing physiological conditions has not been definitively established.

Once the insulin-receptor complex is formed, the hormone can initiate a large number of biochemical actions. An early event probably involves the triggering of the oxidation of specific sulfhydryl groups located in the plasma membrane that may be involved in glucose and amino acid transport. Several of the rapid actions of insulin, including the stimulation of hexose transport and changes in certain enzyme activities, do not depend on the synthesis of new proteins or nucleic acids.

A sudden activation of the insulin receptors results in a biphasic release of the hormone. An initial rapid secretion is followed by a secondary, more slowly decaying release. Whether this pattern results from the secretion of insulin from two separate subcellular sites is not clear, although the latter, more prolonged secretion appears to depend on the synthesis of new hormone protein.

Pharmacological Actions

The biochemical actions of insulin are complex, and involve an integration of carbohydrate, protein, and lipid

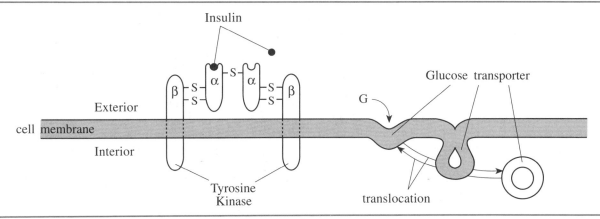

Figure 71-4. Schematic model of the insulin receptor. The receptor is a heterotetramer and consists of two α subunits that are extracellular and two β subunits that are membrane-spanning; the β subunits contain tyrosine kinase. The subunits are linked to each other by disulfide bonds. Intracellular activities are mediated through cAMP-independent phosphorylation. The glucose transporter is translocated to the plasma membrane in reponse to a signal produced by insulin binding to its receptor. It is later translocated back to the intracellular fluid.

metabolism. The actions of insulin (and glucagon) must be orchestrated, so that homeostasis of all these metabolic pathways is coordinated and maintained.

Effects on Hepatic Glycogen Metabolism

Insulin decreases the efflux of glucose from the liver in several ways. First, the hepatic outflow of glucose is diminished through insulin's ability to *inhibit glycogenolysis.* Second, insulin appears to promote hepatic glucose storage by *stimulating glycogen synthesis* through a stimulation of glycogen synthetase activity and an inhibition of glycogen phosphorylation. Although plasma glucose levels appear to influence the total amount of glucose eventually accumulated in the liver, plasma insulin concentrations seem to be the final determinant as to whether storage will occur at all.

Effect on Hepatic Gluconeogenesis

Insulin markedly impairs the hepatic conversion of a variety of noncarbohydrate substances into glucose (*gluconeogenesis*). This reaction is accomplished, in part, by decreasing the amount of circulating gluconeogenic substrates (e.g., plasma amino acids, glycerol) available for conversion. Insulin also appears to inhibit directly the intrahepatic conversion of these substrates into glucose.

Effect on Lipolysis

Insulin is a potent *antilipolytic agent* and is capable of profoundly inhibiting peripheral lipolysis. This is accomplished, in part, through an inhibition of cyclic adenosine monophosphate (cAMP)-sensitive lipase activity, thereby decreasing the flow of free fatty acids (FFA) and glycerol to the liver. FFA are precursors of the ketone bodies, acetoacetate and beta-hydroxybutyrate. Any reduction in circulating FFA levels will reduce the ketogenesis and acidosis that are often associated with the diabetic state. Insulin also may be antiketogenic through a direct action on the liver.

In contrast, under conditions of hypoinsulinemia (e.g., diabetes mellitus), glucagon, through its *lipolytic action,* may play a significant role in stimulating ketogenesis.

Effect on Protein Metabolism

Insulin can reduce the concentration of plasma amino acids by promoting their active transport into cells, especially muscle. These amino acids are now available for incorporation into cellular protein leading to a *net positive nitrogen balance.*

In diabetes mellitus, the lack of insulin results in elevated blood levels of amino acids, reduced protein synthesis, and augmented hepatic gluconeogenesis. The end result is an elevation in plasma glucose levels.

Absorption, Metabolism, and Excretion

Since the liver removes substantial amounts (40–50%) of the hormone, only relatively small amounts of the total endogenous insulin that are secreted each day ever reach peripheral tissues. Although a number of tissues accumulate small amounts of insulin, *the liver and kidney are the principal sites of hormone uptake and degradation.*

Insulin metabolism is accomplished both through the actions of an insulin-specific protease, which is found in

Table 71-1. Some Commonly Used Insulin Preparations

Type	Source	Relative effect* on blood glucose (hr)		
		Onset	Peak	Duration
Regular insulin	B,P,H	½–1	1–2	5–7
Insulin zinc, prompt	B,P	½–1	1–2	12–16
Isophane (NPH)	B,P,H	1½–2	8–12	20–28
Insulin zinc	B,P,H	1½–2	8–12	18–24
Protamine zinc	B,P	3 –4	8–12	36
Insulin zinc, extended	B,P,H	3 –4	8–14	36

Key: B = beef; P = pork; H = human.
*The effects are only representative and will vary depending on the dosage and the severity of the disease.

the cytosol of many tissues, and by the reductive cleavage of the insulin disulfide bonds by glutathione-insulin transhydrogenase. Following its glomerular filtration, insulin is almost completely reabsorbed and metabolized within the proximal convoluted tubules of the nephron.

When used as a drug, insulin is commonly administered either subcutaneously or intramuscularly. Being a polypeptide hormone, it is readily inactivated if administered orally. In emergency situations, such as diabetic coma or severe diabetic acidosis, insulin can be given intravenously. The plasma half-life of intravenously administered insulin is less than 10 min.

Some of the pharmacokinetic properties of different commercially available insulin preparations are depicted in Table 71-1. These preparations can be divided according to their duration of action. So-called *fast-acting* preparations (e.g., regular crystalline or prompt insulin zinc suspension [*Semilente Insulin*]) begin to exert their hypoglycemic effects as early as 30 min after administration. *Intermediate-acting* preparations have a more delayed onset of action, but they act longer (e.g., isophane insulin suspension [NPH insulin] or insulin zinc suspension [*Lente Insulin*]). Protamine zinc and extended insulin zinc suspension (*Ultralente*) are often referred to as *long-acting* insulin preparations.

Insulin pumps are a rather recent drug delivery technology that can be used to treat the diabetic patient. These pumps may contain a microcomputer to regulate the flow of insulin.

Adverse Reactions to Insulin Therapy

The most common side effects associated with insulin therapy are hypoglycemia, hypokalemia, and varying degrees of allergic reactions. Mild allergic reactions are not uncommon and are due to the injection of foreign proteins (i.e., insulin of animal origin). In essentially all patients treated with exogenous insulin, including human

insulin, insulin-binding immunoglobulin G (IgG) antibodies develop.

Hypoglycemia may result in such CNS symptoms as tremors, nervousness, stimulation of the autonomic nervous system, and convulsions or unconsciousness. Alterations in electrocardiogram tracings due to excessive insulin treatment are related to the resultant hypokalemia.

Other complications arising from insulin therapy include lipodystrophy, insulin lipoma, and localized infections at the site of injection. The occurrence of lipodystrophy can be diminished both by frequent changes in the site of injection and by use of an intramuscular rather than a subcutaneous route of administration.

The long-term use of insulin preparations sometimes results in *insulin resistance,* and insulin-neutralizing antibodies have been detected in the blood of treated diabetics. Autoantibodies against the insulin receptor have been detected in the serum of patients with acanthosis nigricans type B, who exhibit severe insulin resistance. In addition to immunological causes, a number of metabolic or pathological states have been associated with insulin resistance. Such resistance may result from alterations in excessive nonpancreatic hormonal secretory activity, as found in Cushing's disease (corticosteroids), acromegaly (growth hormone), thyrotoxicosis (thyroxine), and pregnancy (estrogens).

Diabetes Mellitus

Diabetes currently affects approximately 5 percent of the population, and it is estimated that the number of diabetics will double every 15 years. Although insulin treatment has greatly increased the life expectancy of the diabetic patient and diet control and hypoglycemic drugs are useful, diabetes remains the third leading cause of death by disease and the second leading cause of blindness in the United States.

Forms of Diabetes Mellitus

Diabetes mellitus is a disorder of carbohydrate, protein, and lipid metabolism. Its central disturbance appears to involve an abnormality either in the secretion of, or the effects produced by, insulin, although other factors also may be involved.

Diabetes mellitus has been classified into *insulin-dependent* diabetes mellitus (IDDM), also known as type I (IDDM was formerly called juvenile-type diabetes mellitus), and *non-insulin-dependent* diabetes mellitus (NIDDM), also known as type II. NIDDM was formerly known as maturity-onset diabetes mellitus. Table 71-2 identifies some of the more salient differences between IDDM and NIDDM.

Table 71-2. Some Characteristics of IDDM (Insulin-Dependent, Type I) and NIDDM (Non–Insulin-Dependent, Type II) Diabetes Mellitus

Characteristic	IDDM (juvenile form)	NIDDM (maturity-onset)
Onset (age)	<30 yr	Approximately 40 yr
Type of onset	Abrupt	Gradual
Nutritional status at onset	Usually undernourished	Usually obese
Clinical symptoms	Polydipsia, polyphagia, polyuria	Often none
Ketosis	Frequent, unless diet, insulin, and exercise are properly coordinated	Infrequent (except in the presence of infection or stress)
Endogenous insulin	Negligible	Present, but relatively ineffective because of obesity
Related lipid abnormalities	Hypercholesterolemia frequent, particularly when control is suboptimal; all lipid fractions elevated in ketoacidosis	Cholesterol and triglycerides often elevated; carbohydrate-induced hypertriglyceridemia common
Insulin therapy	Required	Required in only 20–30% of patients
Hypoglycemic drugs	Should not be used	Clinically indicated
Diet	Mandatory along with insulin for blood glucose control	Diet alone frequently sufficient to control blood glucose

Source: From J.A. Thomas and E.J. Keenan, *Principles in Endocrine Pharmacology,* New York: Plenum, 1986.

Etiology

Three major metabolic abnormalities contribute to hyperglycemia in NIDDM, including defective glucose-induced insulin secretion, increased hepatic glucose output, and inability of insulin to stimulate glucose uptake in peripheral target tissues. These abnormalities involve the cellular glucose transport in β cells, liver, adipose tissue, and skeletal muscle, and may be the result of alterations in glucose transporter isoforms (GLUT) (Fig. 71-4). There are at least five isoforms of the glucose transporter: GLUT1 (e.g., red blood cells, kidney), GLUT2 (e.g., liver, β cell), GLUT3 (e.g., brain, placenta), and GLUT5 (e.g., small intestine). In the liver, hepatocyte glucose transport via GLUT2 probably plays only a permissive role in sustaining increased glucose efflux. GLUT4 appears to play an important role in the mechanism of insulin resistance. Many new insights into the pathogenesis of NIDDM may be related to the role of these transporter isoforms. A *genetic (hereditary) component* has been recognized in a portion of the diabetic population. Because the incidence of diabetes is higher in the families of persons with diabetes than in other families, it is generally agreed that the predisposition to diabetes is genetically determined.

The risk of developing diabetes increases with *age*. Although diabetes is relatively infrequent in children, its occurrence is 10 times greater in persons over 45 years of age than in those younger.

Viruses may be instrumental in causing at least one type of diabetes. Epidemiological studies have associated the appearance of certain viral infections with the subsequent development of IDDM. The most likely candidates appear to include the mumps virus, the rubella virus, and members of the Coxsackie virus family.

Glucagon is a potent hepatic glycogenolytic agent and produces a marked hyperglycemia and hypoaminoacidemia. It promotes lipolysis and stimulates the adenyl cyclase-AMP system in a number of tissues. Glucagon may play a deleterious role in some of the metabolic aberrations seen in the patient with diabetes mellitus. It has been proposed that in IDDM some β cells lose their glucose-sensing capacity and therefore insulin therapy cannot completely stabilize the metabolic balance between the two hormones. Theoretically, a glucagon-suppressing agent that does not enhance glucose utilization might have therapeutic benefit.

Although insulin levels are low in diabetes, glucagon is normally present in excess. Several investigators now believe that glucagon may be even more important than insulin in the maintenance of normal blood glucose concentrations. Furthermore, glucagon appears to regulate the oxidation of fatty acids in the liver and therefore may be importantly involved in the production of ketoacidosis. Thus, a reduction in circulating glucagon levels may alleviate the symptoms of diabetes.

Since *somatostatin* (see the following discussion), a hypothalamic releasing factor, can inhibit the pancreatic release of both glucagon and insulin, alterations in its circulating levels also must be considered as being contributory to the development of diabetes.

Changes in the plasma levels of adrenal hormones (cortex and medulla), thyroid hormones, and the hormones of the anterior pituitary can alter the body's requirements for insulin. Epinephrine causes hepatic glycogenolysis and a transient hyperglycemia. A so-called steroid diabetes (see

Chap. 66), often caused by the overzealous use of antiin-flammatory steroids, also can result in hyperglycemia. Thyrotoxicosis is accompanied by an increased blood glucose level and hence an increase in the requirement for insulin. Physiological or psychological stress also can increase insulin requirements.

Finally, it has been suggested that, especially in NIDDM, where the pancreas produces normal quantities of insulin, the essential problem may be a reduced sensitivity of fat and muscle cells to the effects of insulin (i.e., *insulin resistance.*) It is now well known that there are specific receptor sites on cellular membranes where insulin and glucagon interact to regulate glucose metabolism. A major cause of NIDDM is believed to involve a defect in insulin binding to its normal cellular receptors.

Diabetes mellitus is a highly complex disorder, and the simple concept that its pathogenesis is due solely to insulin deficiency is no longer tenable.

Metabolic Disturbances of the Diabetic State

There are only two major sources of blood glucose: *exogenous,* or the ingestion of dietary carbohydrate, and *endogenous,* which is that contributed by hepatic and renal gluconeogenesis and by the breakdown of hepatic glycogen stores. Diabetes mellitus is a metabolic disorder in which carbohydrate metabolism is reduced while that of proteins and lipids is increased.

Dietary glucose, as well as glucose that has been mobilized from body stores, is not utilized effectively and accumulates in the blood (*hyperglycemia*). As blood sugar levels increase, the amount of glucose filtered by the glomeruli eventually will exceed the reabsorption capacity (T_m, transport maximum) of the proximal tubule cells and glucose will appear in the urine (*glucosuria*). The hyperglycemia and glucosuria that are associated with the diabetic state generally will persist even in the fasting individual.

Since some cells are quite permeable to glucose and do not require insulin to facilitate glucose entry, prolonged hyperglycemia will result in these cells having glucose concentrations that approach those found in the blood. These tissues generally metabolize glucose to *fructose* and *sorbitol,* both of which may be retained in the cells even after blood glucose is returned to normal concentrations. Such an accumulation of carbohydrates will lead to tissue edema and electrolyte imbalance. The appearance of a sorbitol-induced cataract in the lens of the eye and eventual blindness (i.e., retinopathy) also may occur. Sorbitol accumulation can occur in peripheral nerves and result in alterations in sensation.

Protein catabolism and the rate of nitrogen excretion are increased when blood insulin falls to low levels. In ad-

dition, new hepatic glucose is formed from amino acids (*gluconeogenesis*). The breakdown of lipids and fatty acids is also accelerated by decreased levels of insulin, and excessive amounts of so-called *ketone bodies,* such as acetoacetic acid, beta-hydroxybutyric acid, and acetone, are formed. The glomerular filtration of large quantities of glucose and associated water, nitrogenous substances, and ketone bodies causes the sequelae of electrolyte depletion, dehydration, hunger, and thirst. Severe, uncontrolled diabetic ketoacidosis can result in coma and death.

Clinical Management of Diabetes

Dietary control is the cornerstone of the management of diabetes, independent of the severity of the symptoms. Treatment regimens that have proved effective include diet in combination with exogenous insulin or orally effective hypoglycemic drugs. Exercise is also a useful adjunct to the overall therapy. Starch blockers (e.g., acarbose) and aldose reductase inhibitory agents have recently been added to the therapeutic approach to managing diabetes. However, since diet, exercise, and oral hypoglycemic drugs will not always achieve the clinical objectives of controlling the symptoms of diabetes, insulin remains universally important in the therapeutic management of the disorder. *There is little or no justification for the combined use of oral hypoglycemic drugs and insulin.*

The administration of insulin is recommended for the treatment of IDDM as well as for the treatment of diabetic coma and ketoacidosis. Insulin also is recommended for the pregnant diabetic and in the diabetic patient before surgery. Since early diagnosis and treatment are essential in cases of life-threatening ketoacidosis, it is generally recommended that all patients with diabetes, and especially those who are prone to ketoacidosis, should carry an identification card or bracelet indicating their diabetic condition.

Because the spectrum of patients with diabetes extends from the totally asymptomatic individual to one with a life-threatening ketoacidosis, *therapeutic management must be highly individualized.* The important objective is to maintain a glucose level that is as close to normal as possible without producing hypoglycemia or overly restricting the patient's lifestyle. Untreated diabetics who are prone to ketoacidosis commonly require an intermediate-acting insulin preparation. Unstable or ketoacidosis-prone diabetics are usually difficult to maintain with only a single daily dose of either an intermediate- or long-acting insulin preparation. Dividing the daily dosage so that three fourths is given in the morning and the remainder either before dinner or at bedtime may be effective. The use of varying combinations of fast-acting and long-acting insulin (see the following discussion) is also helpful.

Insulin Preparations and Dosage

Insulin preparations that are commercially available differ in their relative onset of action, maximal activity, and duration of action (see Table 71-1). Conjugation of the insulin molecule with either *zinc* or *protamine*, or both, will convert the normally rapidly absorbed parenterally administered insulin to a preparation with a more prolonged duration of action. The various formulations of insulin are usually classified as *short-acting* (0.5–14 hr), *intermediate-acting* (1–28 hr), and *long-acting* (4–36 hr). The duration of action can vary, however, depending on such factors as injection volume, injection site, and blood flow at the site of administration.

Insulin injection (regular insulin, crystalline zinc insulin, *Regular Iletin I*) is a rapidly acting preparation with a short duration of action. It can be administered IV as well as SC. Although its primary use is to supplement intermediate- and long-acting insulin preparations, it is also the preparation of choice for IDDM or when trauma, shock, or concomitant infection occurs in the labile diabetic. It is marketed as solutions containing either 40, 80, or 100 units/ml. Bovine, porcine, or mixed bovine-porcine sources are available. Of the available insulin preparations, highly purified porcine insulin is the least antigenic. *Regular (Concentrated) Iletin II* is a high-dose form for use in patients in whom some degree of insulin resistance has developed.

Insulin, zinc suspension, prompt (*Semilente Iletin I, Semilente Insulin*), is also a rapidly acting form of insulin, which is used to supplement intermediate- and long-acting preparations. It is administered SC as a suspension containing either 40, 80, or 100 units/ml. Bovine, porcine, or mixed bovine-porcine sources are used.

Isophane insulin suspension (NPH insulin, NPH *Iletin I*) is an intermediate-acting insulin preparation whose rate of absorption from subcutaneous sites has been slowed by conjugating the hormone with protamine. It is used in treating all diabetic states except for the initial management of diabetic ketoacidosis or diabetic emergencies. It is provided as a suspension containing 40, 80, or 100 units/ml.

Insulin zinc suspension (*Lente Iletin I, Lente Insulin*) is an intermediate-acting mixture of prompt insulin zinc suspension (30%) and extended insulin zinc suspension (70%). It is used similarly to isophane insulin suspension and is supplied as a suspension containing 40, 80, or 100 units/ml insulin of bovine, porcine, or mixed bovine-porcine origin.

Insulin suspension, protamine zinc (*Protamine, Zinc & Iletin I*), is a long-acting preparation whose effects have been extended by incorporating more protamine and zinc in the mixture than is found in isophane insulin suspension. Its approximate duration of action is 36 hr. It is supplied as a suspension containing 40, 80, or 100 units/ml.

Insulin zinc suspension, extended (*Ultralente Iletin I, Ultralente Insulin*), is quite similar to protamine zinc insulin suspension, except that it does not contain protamine. It is available as a suspension containing either 40, 80, or 100 units/ml.

Human insulin (rDNA and semisynthetic) can be synthesized using porcine insulin as starting material, followed by chemical modification of the threonine and alanine residues. This results in the amino acid composition of human insulin. rDNA human insulin is synthesized in *Escherichia coli* and is available in several formulations: neutral regular human insulin (*Humulin R, Novolin R*), NPH human insulin, and isophane-type (*Humulin N*). *Insulatard NPH Human* is a suspension of isophane and purified human (semisynthetic) insulin (100 units/ml). *Velosulin Human* is a semisynthetic purified human insulin (100 units/ml).

Human insulins, while possessing an onset, peak, and duration of action that are comparable to those of animal insulins, are more costly and, unfortunately, not entirely devoid of immunological reactions.

Oral Hypoglycemic Agents

Although insulin has the disadvantage of having to be injected, it is without question the most uniformly effective treatment of diabetes mellitus available. Although insulin remains the drug of choice in severe cases of diabetes and in IDDM, some milder forms of diabetes mellitus that do not respond to diet management alone can be treated with oral hypoglycemic agents. The success of oral hypoglycemic drug therapy is usually based on a restoration of normal blood glucose levels and the absence of glycosuria.

There are two major chemical classes of oral hypoglycemic drugs: the *sulfonylurea drugs* and the *biguanide derivatives*. The only biguanide that had been used extensively, phenformin, has been withdrawn from the United States market because of the increased incidence of severe lactic acidosis associated with its use.

Linogliride, an oral hypoglycemic that is structurally unrelated to the sulfonylureas. While limited in clinical usage, its mechanism of action involves amplifying a cellular signal generated during β cell activation. It appears to have a secretagogue-like action.

Sulfonylureas

Chemistry

During the last two decades, literally thousands of sulfonamide-related agents have been synthesized and tested

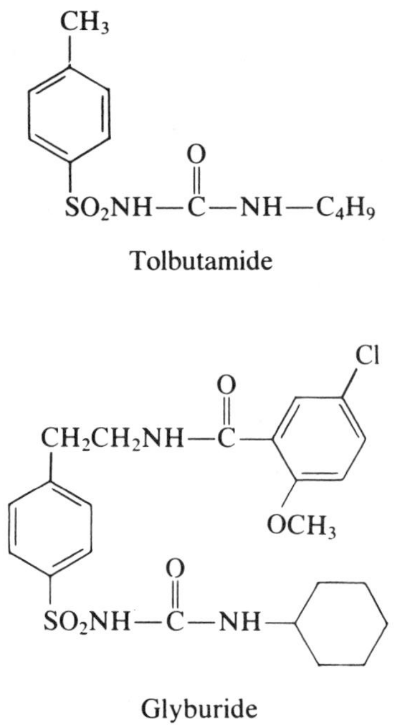

Figure 71-5. Two sulfonylurea oral hypoglycemic agents.

with the hope of discovering the ideal oral hypoglycemic drug, but only a few are used to any extent in the United States.

The chemistry of two representative sulfonylurea drugs is depicted in Fig. 71-5, and their structural similarities to the sulfonamide antibacterial agents are readily apparent (see Chap. 48). The sulfonylureas possess no antibacterial activity.

Mechanism of Action

The primary mechanism of action of the sulfonylureas involves *a direct stimulation of insulin release from the β cells* of the islets of Langerhans in the pancreas. In the presence of viable β cells, that is, insulin-secreting cells, the sulfonylurea drugs enhance the release of endogenous insulin, thereby producing a hypoglycemia. The sulfonylureas, particularly at high dosages, also can cause a reduced outflow of glucose from the liver. In normal subjects, but not diabetics, these agents may enhance the peripheral utilization of glucose, possibly through extrapancreatic effects. These mechanisms are summarized in Table 71-3.

The sulfonylureas are *ineffective* in the management of severe diabetes or in IDDM, since the number of viable β cells in these forms of diabetes is sparse. Severely obese diabetics respond poorly to the sulfonylureas, possibly because of the insulin resistance that often accompanies obesity.

Table 71-3. Potential Mechanisms of Hypoglycemic Action of Sulfonylureas

Site	Mechanism
Pancreatic	Improved insulin secretion
	Reduced glucagon secretion
Extrapancreatic	Improved tissue sensitivity to insulin
	Direct
	Increased receptor binding
	Improved postbinding action
	Indirect
	Reduced hyperglycemia
	Decreased plasma free fatty acid
	concentrations
	Reduced hepatic insulin extraction

Source: From J.E. Gerich, Oral hypoglycemic agents. *N. Engl. J. Med.* 321:1231, 1989.

Absorption, Metabolism, and Excretion

There are seven sulfonylurea compounds now available for use in the treatment of diabetes mellitus. These compounds are acetohexamide, chlorpropamide, gliclazide, glipizide, glyburide, tolazamide, and tolbutamide. They all are readily absorbed from the gastrointestinal tract and can be given orally. Their biological half-lives vary from about 3 hr (glipizide) to 36 hr (chlorpropamide).

The degree and the rate of metabolism vary with the particular sulfonylurea. The pharmacological profile of the sulfonylurea drugs is depicted in Table 71-4. Approximately 75 percent of an administered dose of tolbutamide is oxidized in the liver to an inactive metabolite, carboxytolbutamide. Acetohexamide is rapidly reduced to several derivatives, the principal metabolite being the biologically active hydroxyhexamide. Tolazamide has a slower rate of absorption than do the other sulfonylureas, and it is metabolized to at least three compounds, each of which has less hypoglycemic potency than the parent drug. Chlorpropamide has a relatively long biological half-life because of its minimal biotransformation and slow rate of excretion.

Glipizide, gliclazide, and glibenclamide (glyburide), the so-called second generation of orally effective sulfonylurea hypoglycemic agents, are well absorbed in the gastrointestinal tract. These drugs are metabolized in the liver and their duration of action is approximately 24 hr.

Adverse Reactions

The frequency and severity of side effects associated with the acute administration of the sulfonylurea drugs are not great. Hypoglycemic reactions have been reported

Table 71-4. Pharmacokinetic Properties of Sulfonylurea Agents

Drug	Half-life (hr)	Effect duration (hr)	Daily dose (mg)	No. of dosages/day	Activity of metabolites
Acetohexamide	0.8–2.4*	12–18	250–1500	2	+
Chlorpropamide	24–48	24–72	100–500	1	+
Gliclazide	6–15	10–15	40–320	1–2	−
Glipizide	1–5	14–16	2.5–20	1 (–2)	−
Glyburide	2–4	20–24	2.5–20	1–2	−/+
Tolbutamide	3–28	6–10	500–3000	2–3	−
Tolazamide	4–7	16–24	100–1000	1–2	+

Key: + = active; − = inactive.
*Elimination half-life of the active metabolite is ≈4–6 hr.
Source: From L.C. Groop, Sulfonyl ureas in NIDDM. Reprinted with permission from *Diabetes Care*, vol. 15, p. 7400. Copyright © 1992 by American Diabetes Association, Inc.

after the use of each of the seven compounds. Because of its relatively long biological half-life, chlorpropamide-induced hypoglycemia may last several days and require frequent administration of dextrose. Other adverse reactions include muscular weakness, ataxia, dizziness, mental confusion, skin rash, photosensitivity, blood dyscrasias, and cholestatic jaundice. Fortunately, cross-reactions are not too common among the sulfonylureas, and therefore one hypoglycemic drug can be substituted for another in an attempt to achieve better therapeutic results while minimizing a particular side effect. They are not recommended for use during pregnancy.

Aside from the more commonly seen side effects of the sulfonylureas, some studies have indicated a higher mortality in diabetic patients receiving oral hypoglycemic drugs compared to those receiving insulin. The predominant cause of death seems to be of cardiovascular origin.

Cautions and Drug Interactions

Since diabetic patients with renal or hepatic disease are more vulnerable to hypoglycemia, the sulfonylurea compounds should not be used in these individuals. Caution also is necessary when coadministering these drugs with thiazide diuretics, since the latter agents can exacerbate the diabetic condition. A decrease in alcohol tolerance also has been observed in patients taking sulfonylurea compounds. The following drugs may potentiate the hypoglycemic action of the sulfonylurea drugs: sulfonamides, propranolol, salicylates, phenylbutazone, chloramphenicol, probenecid, and alcohol. Since the sulfonylureas are highly bound to plasma proteins and extensively metabolized by microsomal enzymes, coadministered drugs capable of either displacing them from their protein-binding sites or inhibiting their metabolism may induce a severe hypoglycemia.

Preparations and Dosage

Acetohexamide (*Dymelor*) is the only sulfonylurea possessing uricosuric activity and therefore it has particular value in diabetics with gout. It is available as 250- and 500-mg tablets.

Chlorpropamide (*Diabinese*) has a relatively slow onset of action, with its maximal hypoglycemic potential often not reached for 1 or 2 weeks. Similarly, several weeks may be required to eliminate the drug completely after discontinuation of therapy. It is marketed as 100- and 250-mg tablets.

Tolazamide (*Tolinase*) is an orally effective hypoglycemic drug that causes less water retention than do the other compounds in this class. It is available as 100-, 250-, and 500-mg tablets.

Tolbutamide (*Orinase*) is a relatively short-acting compound whose indications are similar to those of the other orally effective hypoglycemic drugs. Although it is used primarily in tablet form (500 mg), an IV preparation of tolbutamide sodium (1-gm powder) is available for diagnostic purposes.

Glyburide (*DiaBeta, Micronase*) is comparable to chlorpropamide and tolazamide. Its average duration of action is about 24 hr. It is available as 1.25-, 2.5-, and 5.0-mg tablets.

Glipizide (*Glucotrol*) has a duration of action that is similar to that of chlorpropamide and tolazamide. It is available as 5- and 10-mg tablets.

Biguanides

A second group of oral hypoglycemic agents that are chemically distinct from the sulfonylureas are the biguanides. The Food and Drug Administration (FDA) has banned the sale of the only biguanide (phenformin hydrochloride, *DBI*), and it can now be used only on approval by the FDA.

Aldose Reductase Inhibitors

A number of aldose reductase inhibitors have been introduced for the treatment of diabetic neuropathy and retinopathy. Aldose reductase, an enzyme that converts sugars to polyols, has been implicated in basement membrane changes in diabetes mellitus. Aldose reductase inhibitory agents presumably prevent the thickening in retinal capillaries. *Alconil, Sorbinil,* and *Tolrestal* have undergone limited clinical trials. Side effects include hypersensitivity, skin rash, fever, chills, myalgia and lymphadenopathy.

Somatostatin

In the search for a hypothalamic releasing factor for growth hormone, a contaminating substance was discovered that actually caused an inhibition of somatotropin release. This tetradecapeptide was named *growth hormone release inhibiting hormone* (GH-RIH), *somatotropin release inhibiting factor* (SRIF), or *somatostatin* (see Chap. 65).

Somatostatin inhibits the secretion of *both* insulin and glucagon and can reduce fasting hyperglycemia in insulin-deficient juvenile diabetics. Elevated levels of growth hormone that are seen in patients with acromegaly also can be reduced by somatostatin.

Natural and synthetic somatostatin have similar biological actions. The biological half-life of both natural and synthetic somatostatin is very brief (about 5 min) since it is quickly inactivated in the plasma. A host of somatostatin analogues [e.g., Des-(Ala^1)-somatostatin, Des-(Ala^1-Gly^2-Asn^5)-somatostatin, D-Trp^8-somatostatin, etc.] have been synthesized in an effort to extend its biological half-life and hence make it an even more potent inhibitor of growth hormone release. None of the currently available compounds possesses significantly longer durations of action than the parent polypeptide.

The therapeutic indications for somatostatin appear to be in the management of acromegaly, pancreatic islet cell tumors, and diabetes mellitus. In diabetes, *somatostatin can acutely improve fasting and postprandial hyperglycemia in insulin-requiring diabetics through its ability to suppress glucagon secretion.* Because growth hormone has been implicated in the genesis of diabetic retinopathy, the suppression of growth hormone secretion may reduce ocular changes. It is also possible that somatostatin may ameliorate the severity of diabetic ketoacidosis.

Clearly, the clinical implications for somatostatin have not been fully realized, but an understanding of the role that this polypeptide plays in the management of diabetes mellitus represents an important challenge to the physician.

Supplemental Reading

Bailey, C.J. Biguanides and NIDDM. *Diabetes Care* 15:755, 1992.

DeVries, C.P., et al. The insulin receptor. *Diabetes Res.* 11:155, 1989.

Efendic, S., Kindmark, H., and Berggren, P.O. Mechanisms involved in the regulation of the insulin secretory process. *J. Int. Med.* 229 (Suppl. 2):9, 1991.

Elsas, L.J., and Longo, N. Glucose transporters. *Ann. Rev. Med.* 43:377, 1992.

Francisco, G.E. Antidiabetic agents. *Primary Care* 17:499, 1990.

Galloway, J.A., et al. Biosynthetic human proinsulin. *Diabetes Care* 15:666, 1992.

Gerich, J.E. Oral hypoglycemic agents. *N. Engl. J. Med.* 321:1231, 1989.

Groop, L.C. Sulfonylureas in NIDDM. *Diabetes Care* 15:737, 1992.

Karam, J.A. Diabetes mellitus: Perspectives on therapy. *Endocrinol. Metab. Clin. North Am.* 2:1, 1992.

Klip, A., and Leiter, L.A. Cellular mechanism of action of metformin. *Diabetes Care* 13:696, 1990.

Philippe, J. Structure and pancreatic expression of the insulin and glucagon genes. *Endocr. Rev.* 12:252, 1991.

Sara, V.R., and Hall, K. Insulin-like growth factors and their binding proteins. *Physiol. Rev.* 70:591, 1990.

Skyler, J.S. Strategies in diabetes mellitus. *Postgrad. Med.* 89:45, 1991.

VIII

Additional Important Drugs

Histamine and Histamine Antagonists

Richard J. Head and *Knox Van Dyke*

Histamine

One of every 10 Americans suffers from some allergic problem. These allergic conditions, which frequently result from disturbances of the immunoinflammatory system, include sinus problems, hay fever, bronchial asthma, hives, eczema, contact dermatitis, food allergies, and reactions to drugs. These conditions are associated with the release of histamine as well as other autacoids, such as serotonin and the prostaglandins.

Histamine is an endogenous substance that is widely distributed in body tissues and can, on release from its storage sites, exert a variety of pharmacological effects of varying intensity. These effects range from mild irritation and itching to anaphylactic shock and eventual death. Although the physiological role of this biogenic amine is not clearly understood, its release is frequently associated with the existence of various inflammatory states, and therefore its release has been proposed as playing a role in response to noxious stimuli, especially in conditions in which its release is uncontrolled. Histamine release may be increased in urticarial reactions, mastocytosis, and basophilia. Also, histamine appears to have a neurotransmitter role in the central nervous system (CNS).

Distribution

The presence of histamine in human and animal tissues has been known for decades, and the precise concentrations of histamine within tissues or biological fluids is well documented. The largest concentrations of histamine are present in the skin, lungs, and gastrointestinal mucosa. Smaller concentrations can be found in many other organs and tissues (Table 72-1), including an association within or near blood vessels. Histamine is present in human plasma at relatively low concentrations (usually < 0.5 ng/ml), in contrast to whole blood, in which the histamine concentrations can be as much as 30-fold greater. Substantial quantities of histamine are present in urine, with excretion rates approximating 10 to 40 μg/24 hr.

Virtually all the histamine found in individual organs and tissues is synthesized locally and then stored in subcellular organelles. The two principal sites of storage of histamine are *mast cells* within tissues and *basophils* in blood. In both of these cell types, histamine is synthesized and then bound in the presence of *heparin* into a storage complex in subcellular granules. The ubiquitous distribution of histamine in tissues and organs can be explained largely on the basis of the frequent presence of mast cells in many tissues. Likewise, the high concentrations of histamine in blood as compared to plasma reflect the localization of histamine in basophils.

From the standpoint of a site of histamine storage and release, the mast cell and basophil can, with reservation, be considered to be equivalent. It should be emphasized, however, that mast cell populations vary from one tissue to another, whereas all organs are constantly perfused with bloodborne histamine stored within basophils.

In all probability, histamine can be found in structures other than mast cells or basophils. In particular, it is believed that histamine may be present in neurons as well as in mast cells in the CNS. In selected tissues in the periphery, histamine also may be present in non-mast cell sites as a consequence of local synthesis.

Synthesis

Histamine shares, along with many other biogenic amines (e.g., serotonin and catecholamines), the property that its synthesis and pharmacological activity are consequences of decarboxylation of an amino acid precursor (Fig. 72-1). Histamine is synthesized from the amino acid histidine by an action of the enzyme *histidine decarboxylase.*

Table 72-1. Histamine Content of Human Tissues

Tissue	Histamine content
Lung	33 ± 10 µg/g*
Mucous membrane (nasal)	15.6 µg/gm
Stomach	14 ± 4.0 µg/gm*
Duodenum	14 ± 0.9 µg/gm*
Skin	6.6 µg/gm (abdomen)
	30.4 µg/gm (face)
Pancreas	4.8 ± 1.5 µg/gm*
Spleen	3.4 ± 0.97 µg/gm*
Kidney	2.5 ± 1.2 µg/gm*
Liver	2.2 ± 0.76 µg/gm*
Heart	1.6 ± 0.07 µg/gm*
Thyroid	1.0 ± 0.13 µg/gm*
Skeletal muscle	0.97 ± 0.13 µg/gm*
Central nervous tissue	0–0.2 µg/gm
Whole blood	16–89 µg/L
Plasma	2.6 µg/L
Basophils	1,080 µg/10^9 cells
Eosinophils	160 µg/10^9 cells
Neutrophils	3.0 µg/10^9 cells
Lymphocytes	0.6 µg/10^9 cells
Platelets	0.009 µg/10^9 platelets

*Mean ± standard error.
Source: From P.P. Van Arsdel, Jr. and G.N. Beall, The metabolism and functions of histamine. *Arch. Intern. Med.* 106:192, 1960. Copyright © 1960 by the American Medical Association.

Enzymes that catalyze the decarboxylation of histidine are widespread in nature, a finding that may account for the presence of histamine in some foodstuffs.

Release of Histamine from Storage Sites

Histamine can be released from mast cell granules in two ways, both of which have pharmacological importance. Endogenous or exogenous compounds can promote an *exocytotic* release of histamine without cell destruction or lysis. Alternatively, histamine can be released from mast cells by a variety of *nonexocytotic* processes including mast cell lysis, modification of mast cell membranes, and physical displacement of histamine. Establishing the precise nature by which histamine release from mast cells occurs is extremely complex.

When considering adverse drug reactions that involve histamine release, both exocytotic and nonexocytotic mechanisms of release should be considered. It should be stressed again that histamine is only one of several potent pharmacological agents that can be released from mast cells. In addition to histamine, mast cell granules contain such pharmacologically active substances as kinins and other vasoactive peptides. These substances, in turn, also contribute to the overall response seen during mast cell degranulation.

Antigen-Mediated Release of Histamine

If an individual has been immunologically sensitized by a foreign substance (*antigen*), further contact with that antigen can lead not only to a secondary augmentation of the immune response, but also to the appearance of tissue-damaging reactions. These reactions can occur immediately or their appearance may be delayed up to several days.

Tissue mast cells and blood basophils are the principal cells involved in immediate hypersensitivity reactions. It is from these organelles that histamine release is initiated through an antigen-antibody reaction. This interaction triggers a series of events, culminating in the fusion of the histamine-containing storage granule membrane with the cell membrane and the eventual expulsion of the granular contents. From the standpoint of the immunoinflammatory response, attention should be directed toward exocytotic release of histamine and, in particular, antigen-mediated release of histamine.

Antigenic substances that are capable of producing an allergic response bring about the synthesis of various antibodies, some of which are of the immunoglobulin G (IgE) class (*reaginic antibodies*). These antibodies attach themselves to the outer surface of the mast cell membrane (Fig. 72-2). This process initiates a series of biochemical events (which may involve activation of proteolytic enzymes, methylation of phospholipids, cellular influx of calcium, and phosphorylation reactions) that ultimately culminate in the release of the mast cell granule contents.

The process of histamine release is started by a sensitization of the mast cells, that is, by the binding of the antibody molecules to the mast cell membrane. There are two antigen-combining sites on each IgE antibody. Once the antibodies are attached to the outside of the mast cells, they are ready to capture specific antigens. The attachment of the antigen or allergen serves as a signal to initiate a release of the granule contents (see Fig. 72-2).

The exocytotic release of the contents of mast cell granules mediated by specific antigens is the basis of the *immediate hypersensitivity reaction*. Although antigens are generally large molecules, drugs, particularly after their association with endogenously occurring larger-molecular-weight molecules, also may promote the sensitization process and the release of mast cell granule contents on subsequent drug exposure.

Intrinsic Regulation of Histamine Release

It has been known for decades that certain endogenous compounds can modulate the antigen-mediated release of histamine from sensitized tissues. Recent findings point to

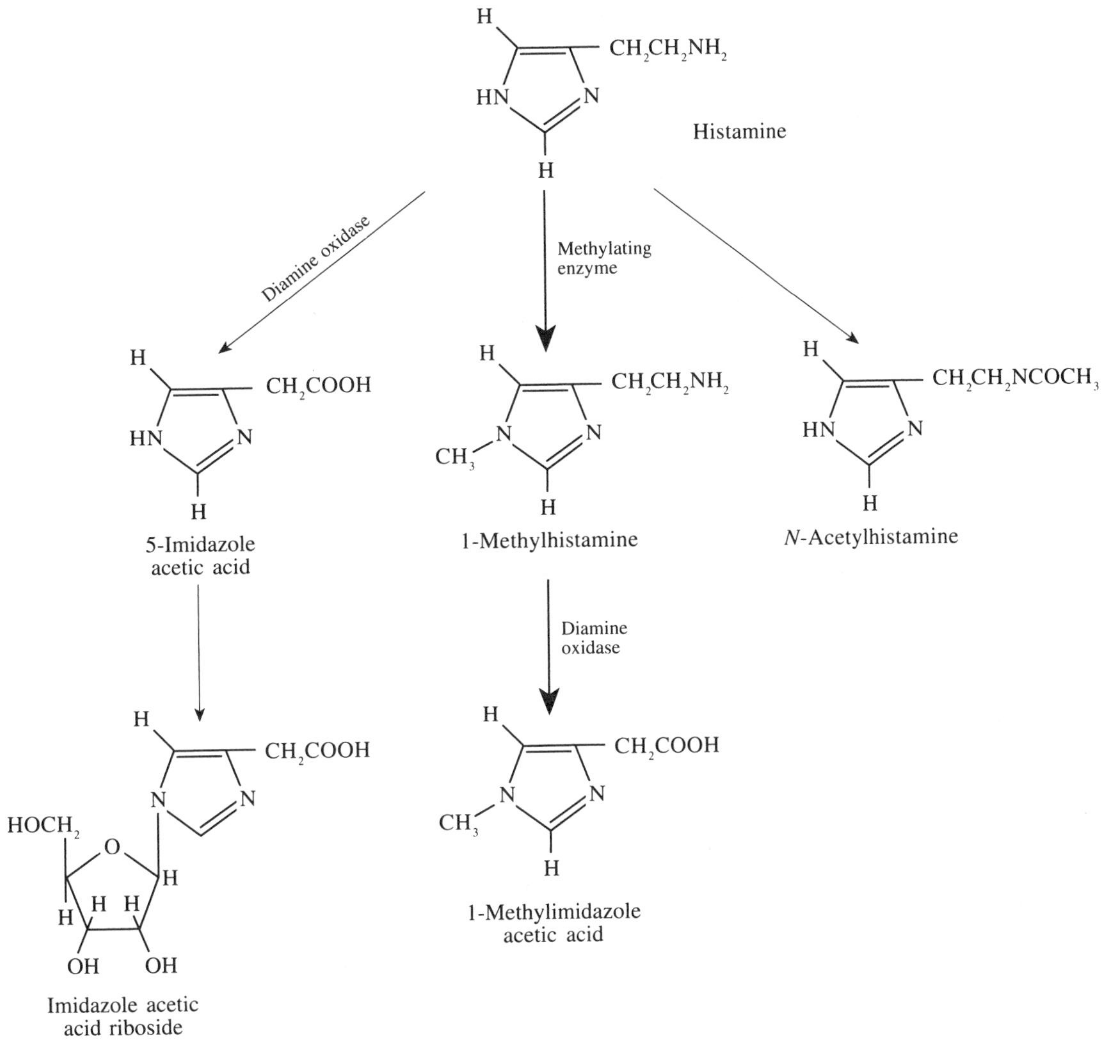

Figure 72-1. Metabolism of histamine. Broad arrows indicate major routes. The formation of N-acetylhistamine is observed only after oral ingestion of histamine.

the existence of receptors on mast cells and that occupation of receptors can regulate the release of mast cell mediators. For example, it is believed that there are histamine receptors (of the H_2 subclass) on mast cells, which, when activated, inhibit the release of mast cell granule contents.

Isoproterenol and epinephrine can inhibit antigen-induced histamine release from sensitized tissue. This catecholamine-induced inhibition is a consequence of activation of β_2-receptors. In contrast, acetylcholine enhances the release of the contents of mast cell granules; this action also is thought to be mediated by activation of mast cell receptors.

These observations suggest that the antigen-mediated release of mast cell granular contents may be autoregulated by histamine as well as modulated by compounds prominent in the autonomic nervous system.

Non-Antigen-mediated Release of Histamine

Histamine may be released from mast cells by mechanisms that do not involve the immune system. Release of histamine can be induced by various drugs, high-molecular-weight proteins, venoms, or other processes that damage or disrupt cell membranes. Any physical stress of sufficient intensity (e.g., thermal or mechanical stress) also will result in histamine release.

Drugs or chemicals may cause secretion of histamine from mast cells by physically displacing histamine from granules. Alternatively, compounds may be cytotoxic and release histamine during disruption of cell membranes. As a generalization, basic chemicals and basic peptides can cause the release of histamine from mast cells. The hista-

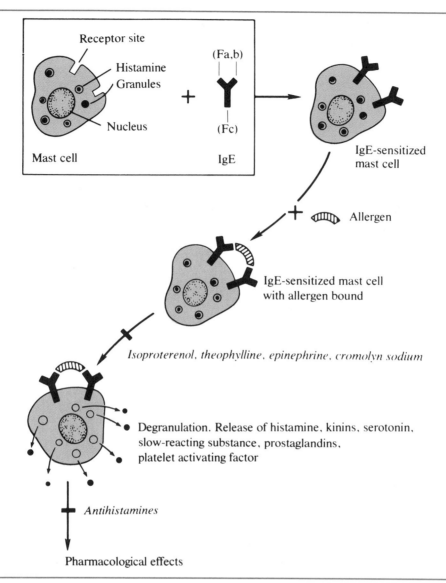

Figure 72-2. The process of histamine release. Inset shows an intact mast cell with histamine stored in granules. An IgE antibody molecule is depicted adjacent to the mast cell. Two IgE molecules combine with a mast cell (sensitization). The attachment of an antigen (allergen) to the previously sensitized mast cell initiates release of histamine (and other substances) from the mast cell. This degranulation can be prevented by such agents as isoproterenol, theophylline, epinephrine, and cromolyn sodium. H_1 antihistamines do not interfere with degranulation but, instead, prevent actions of histamine at various pharmacological receptors.

mine-liberating compound 48/80, morphine, codeine, *d*-tubocurarine, guanethidine, bradykinin, neurotensin, substance P, and somatostatin all have the ability to release histamine from mast cells. In addition, chlorpromazine may cause the release of histamine from mast cells by a cytotoxic mechanism.

An indirect immunological release of histamine from mast cells may be mediated through the actions of *ana-phylatoxins*. Activation of complement leads to the production of polypeptides (anaphylatoxins) that can promote the release of histamine from mast cells.

Other diverse agents also may promote the release of histamine. Venoms contain basic polypeptides as well as the histamine releasing enzyme phospholipase A. Radiation and x-ray contrast media also can liberate histamine from mast cells.

Inactivation of Released Histamine

The inactivation of histamine is achieved both by enzymatic metabolism of the amine and by transport processes that reduce the concentration of the compound in the region of its receptors. There is evidence suggesting that histamine can utilize the catecholamine uptake processes in selected tissues.

Histamine metabolism occurs primarily through two pathways (see Fig. 72-1). *Histamine methyltransferase* catalyzes the transfer of a methyl group from *S*-adenosyl-1-methionine to one of the imidazole nitrogen substitutions, forming 1-methylhistamine. The enzyme is present in tissues but not in blood. Histamine is also oxidatively deaminated by the enzyme *diamine oxidase (histaminase)* to form imidazole acetic acid. Diamine oxidase is present in tissues and in blood and is inhibited by antimalarial drugs. Diamine oxidase plays a role in metabolizing the histamine that may be present in quite large concentrations in food.

A minor metabolic pathway utilizes diamine oxidase to form 5-imidazole acetic acid from histamine, with a subsequent conjugation with ribose at the N1 position of the ring to produce 1-imidazole acetic acid riboside. An additional product, *N*-acetylhistamine (a conjugate of acetic acid and histamine), can occur if histamine is ingested orally. This metabolite may be the result of metabolism by gastrointestinal tract bacteria. Because of its rapid breakdown after oral administration, histamine produces few systemic effects when given by this route.

The kidney can metabolize and sequester histamine derived from the circulation. It should be remembered that the kidney also can synthesize histamine and that histamine has an influence on the renal circulation. Determining the precise contribution of the kidney to the removal of histamine from the body has proved to be difficult.

Histamine Receptors

Histamine brings about its effects through the activation of at least *two* separate receptor populations: H_1 and H_2. These receptors can be distinguished on the basis of their differing sensitivities to agonists (e.g., 2-methylhistamine for H_1 and 4-methylhistamine for H_2 receptors) and antagonists (e.g., pyrilamine for H_1 and cimetidine for H_2 receptors). H_3 receptors have been found in the brain and are thought to play an autoregulatory role.

Histamine, as with many neurotransmitters, stimulates the formation of cyclic adenosine monophosphate (cAMP) in a variety of tissues. This effect is mediated by both H_1 and H_2 receptors. Some tissues have predominantly one receptor type, while others contain a mixture of the two. Intestinal and bronchiolar smooth muscle primarily contains H_1 receptors, whereas gastric secretion is mediated almost exclusively through H_2-receptor activation. Blood vessels possess both H_1 and H_2 receptors in varying proportions, although receptor activation results in vasodilation in both instances. In general, when both receptor types are present in a single tissue, the effects of H_1 stimulation usually predominate. One exception to this generalization is that vasodilation of human temporal arteries results from H_2 activation.

Physiological Role

Many of histamine's biological actions are mediated by activation of histamine receptors. The two types of histamine receptors (H_1 and H_2) mediate physiological functions that are either additive or opposing in nature. A summary of the distribution of histamine receptors as well as tissue and organ responses is shown in Table 72-2.

Most of our knowledge concerning the distribution of receptors, as well as organ responses to histamine, has

Table 72-2. Distribution of H_1 and H_2 Receptors in Different Organ Systems

Organ	Type of receptor	Histamine-mediated response
Uterus	H_2	Relaxation
Stomach	H_2	Stimulation of gastric acid production
Ileum	H_1 (predominant)	Contraction
	H_2 (small fraction)	Relaxation
Bronchi	H_1 (predominant)	Bronchoconstriction
	H_2 (small fraction)	Bronchoconstriction
Arteries		
Great	H_1	Contraction
Small	H_1 and H_2	Relaxation
Heart	H_2	Positive chronotropic effect
	H_2	Positive inotropic effect (ventricle)
	H_1	Positive inotropic effect (atrium)
	H_1	Prolongation of atrioventricular conduction time
	H_1 and H_2	Increase of coronary flow
Mast cells	H_2	Feedback control of histamine release
Sympathetic nervous system	H_2	Inhibition of sympathetic transmission
CNS	H_1	Sedation
	H_1 and H_2	Antiemetic effect

Source: From D. Reinhardt and U. Borchard, H_1-receptor antagonists: Comparative pharmacology and clinical use. *Klin. Wochenschr.* 60:983, 1982. Used with permission.

come from studies that are based on the addition of exogenous histamine to isolated tissues, a situation that is analogous to a pathological state in which tissues are exposed to high concentrations of histamine. It follows that care must be exercised in extrapolating the results of in vitro experiments to the normal physiological situation, where the magnitude of localized histamine release as well as its availability to interact with receptors is unknown.

Despite this qualification, it is likely that histamine plays a role in the regulation of the microcirculation. Histamine's actions in increasing gastric acid secretion suggest its importance in the physiological control of gastric acid secretion. As mentioned earlier, histamine is also thought to be a neurotransmitter in the CNS, where its function may relate to endocrine regulation. Recent findings implicate a role for histamine in the modulation of cellular immunity.

Pharmacological Effects

Histamine's principal pharmacological actions can be divided conveniently into its influence on receptor-mediated cellular events and whole-organ responses. Intracellular concentrations of cAMP and, in some instances, cyclic guanosine monophosphate (cGMP), often increase with occupation of cell surface histamine receptors. The cyclic nucleotides are regulated as second messengers, and the increase in their concentration initiates expression of cell function. In peripheral tissues, activation of H_1 receptors can produce an intracellular increase in cGMP concentrations. In contrast, occupation of H_2 receptors leads to elevation of cAMP concentrations. It should be noted that the foregoing conclusions are generalizations and have not been demonstrated exhaustively for all tissues and organs that respond to histamine.

Histamine's principal actions are on (1) the cardiovascular system, (2) the respiratory system, (3) glandular tissue, and (4) intradermal tissue.

Cardiovascular System

Histamine administration is characterized by a fall in blood pressure, a positive inotropic and chronotropic response, and a reddening of the skin of the face (due to vasodilation of cutaneous vessels), and the individual generally experiences a throbbing headache resulting from dilation of brain arterioles. Histamine dilates arterioles, capillaries, and venules by activation of both H_1 and H_2 receptors. The permeability of the walls of capillaries and small vessels is increased by histamine, resulting in an outward passage of fluid and protein into the extracellular space and an eventual edematous swelling of tissues.

Histamine's effects on blood pressure are quite complex. In general, histamine administration will cause a fall in blood pressure, the magnitude of which will depend on the concentration of histamine injected, the involvement of baroreceptor mechanisms, and the degree of histamine-induced release of adrenal catecholamines that occurs.

Respiratory System

Histamine stimulates bronchiolar smooth muscle contraction through activation of H_1 receptors. In addition, histamine is thought to stimulate secretory activity and prostaglandin formation in the respiratory tract. Circulating concentrations of histamine are elevated in acute and exercise-induced asthma. Asthmatics are generally more sensitive to the actions of histamine and therefore experience a more profound bronchiolar constriction than do nonasthmatics.

Glandular Tissue

Histamine administration promotes the release of catecholamines from the adrenal gland, the secretion of gastric acid and pepsin from the gastric mucosa, and secretions from the salivary glands. Its actions in releasing catecholamines are thought to be mediated by histamine receptors, although the receptor subtype has not been identified. Of course, histamine's pronounced vasodilator actions may, through augmentation of baroreceptor reflex mechanisms, induce adrenal catecholamine release. Secretion of acid from the gastric mucosa is a complex process that involves a stimulatory role of histamine and acetylcholine (of vagal nerve origin) on parietal cells. The ability of histamine receptor antagonists (i.e., H_2 blocking agents) to inhibit gastric secretion has led to the belief that histamine release is of major importance in the process of acid secretion.

Intradermal Tissue

The intradermal effects of histamine are well illustrated by the *Lewis triple response.* The intradermal injection of as little as 10 µg histamine produces three distinct effects:

1. Dilation of capillaries in the immediate vicinity of the injection, resulting in a localized red or blue region (*flush*).
2. Dilation of arterioles, resulting in a redness (*flare*) over an area that is generally wider than that due to the capillary dilation; the area affected will depend on the amount of histamine injected and on the degree of previous sensitization to the allergen. The cause of this diffuse flare or redness probably involves a neural mechanism, possibly an axon reflex, since cutting the nerves in the region abolishes the flare.

3. Appearance of swelling (*wheal*) in the area of capillary dilation. The increased permeability of the blood vessels in this region is responsible for the edema.

The intradermal injection of specific antigens in sensitized individuals will result in the appearance of a wheal and, as such, is a skin test that can, in part, be used to quantify the extent of allergic response of the individual. The exposure of intradermal tissue to histamine is invariably accompanied by transient pain and itching.

Anaphylaxis

In contrast to the release of mediators of inflammation that may produce discomfort (e.g., in hay fever), the rapid and extensive release of mediators in anaphylaxis may threaten the life of the individual. The introduction of a specific antigen, usually in food or in injected material, into a sensitized individual can cause the rapid release of mast cell contents, with a resultant decrease in blood pressure, impaired respiratory function, abdominal cramps, and urticaria. The most extreme and severe forms of anaphylaxis are life threatening and require prompt and continued treatment to abolish and reverse the actions of the mediators of anaphylaxis on various target tissues. While many of the cardiovascular abnormalities of septic shock are similar to those seen after histamine administration, blood concentrations of histamine are not elevated during septic shock.

Tachyphylaxis

Histamine has played a prominent role in experimental pharmacology in understanding the phenomenon of tachyphylaxis. *Tachyphylaxis can be viewed as a rapid diminution in response of a tissue to repeated drug administration.* Although the molecular basis for tachyphylaxis may have several origins, at least one mechanism has been well established. Tachyphylaxis may be expected after administration of a drug that produces its action by releasing histamine from mast cells (i.e., an indirectly acting compound). Clearly, once a drug-induced depletion of the granule histamine stores has occurred, the responses to subsequent drug administration will be reduced. Such a loss of pharmacological action after repeated drug dosing may help to explain a frequently observed rapid loss of clinical effectiveness of some indirectly acting compounds.

Clinical Uses

Histamine has only minor uses in clinical medicine. It may be helpful in distinguishing between pernicious and other forms of anemia. If pernicious anemia is present, histamine administration will fail to evoke the usually observed secretion of gastric hydrochloric acid. Histamine has been used to diagnose pheochromocytoma, since this tumor is especially responsive to histamine and will secrete excessive amounts of catecholamines after its injection. This procedure is hazardous and its use can no longer be sanctioned. Carcinoid tumors contain many biologically active molecules including histamine, which is elevated in patients with carcinoid syndrome.

The histamine analogue *betazole,* given either intravenously or subcutaneously, can be used for the same diagnostic purposes as histamine. Betazole is a pyrazole, rather than an imidazole, derivative. The advantage of betazole is that its administration is generally accompanied by fewer side effects than are seen after histamine injection. As with histamine, betazole may be dangerous in asthmatic patients.

Preparations and Dosage

Histamine phosphate is available in solutions for injection containing 0.275, 0.55, and 2.75 mg/ml. The usual dosage is 0.01 mg/kg of histamine base or 0.0275 mg/kg of the salt.

Betazole hydrochloride (*Histalog*) solution is given as a single subcutaneous or intramuscular dose of 0.5 mg/kg.

Histamine Antagonism and Histamine Antagonists

The effects of histamine on body tissues and organs can be diminished in four ways:

1. Histamine synthesis may be inhibited.
2. Histamine release from storage sites may be prevented.
3. Histamine receptors may be blocked by appropriate antagonists.
4. Pharmacological antagonists may be used to reverse the effects of histamine (e.g., epinephrine's ability to relax histamine-induced bronchial constriction).

Of the approaches listed, only the inhibition of histamine synthesis has not been employed clinically. Since histamine is thought to be involved both as a potential neurotransmitter and as a partial mediator of tissue growth and repair, inhibition of total body histamine synthesis appears to be undesirable. It is for this reason that impairment of histamine synthesis is not predicted to be of therapeutic utility.

H_1-Receptor Antagonists

Chemistry

Chemically, H_1-receptor antagonists can be depicted as substituted ethylamine compounds that possess the general structure shown in Fig. 72-3. In comparison with histamine, the H_1 antagonists contain no imidazole ring and have substituents on the side chain amino group. The main characteristic that differentiates one H_1 antagonist from another is the particular X group that is attached to the side chain. Varying the X groups results in an altered biological response, and one that is related to the drug's antihistaminic properties. Two common H_1 antagonists are shown in Fig. 72-4.

Mechanism of Action

The vast majority of histamine antagonists are H_1-receptor blocking agents. These drugs are equilibrium-competitive inhibitors of H_1 receptor–mediated responses. They have no ability to block histamine release.

Absorption, Metabolism, and Excretion

Antihistamines are well absorbed (less than 30 min) after oral administration, with peak drug blood levels occurring within 1 hr. The therapeutic effect will last 4 hr, unless the drug is in a time-release dosage form; the latter permits an activity of up to 10 to 12 hr. The H_1 antagonists are generally metabolized in the liver through hydroxylation. The lessened therapeutic effectiveness that is

often seen when individual drugs are given for prolonged periods is probably related to an induction of hepatic drug-metabolizing enzymes. The parent compound and its metabolites are excreted in the urine.

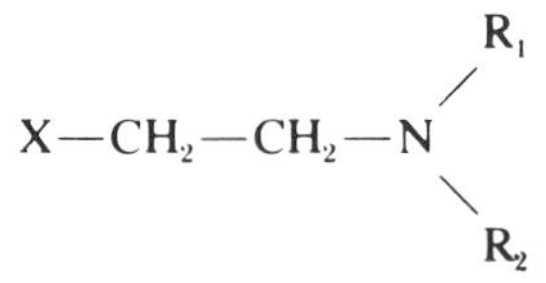

Clinical Uses

The H_1-receptor blocking drugs find their greatest use in the symptomatic treatment of allergic rhinitis. In mild allergy, the majority of patients report some degree of relief after their administration. As the allergy season progresses, or in cases of chronic allergic rhinitis in which nasal stuffiness is the major symptom, antihistamines become less effective. In these two instances, because of the development of tolerance, the dosage of the drug frequently must be increased to maintain effectiveness. H_1 antagonists are also more useful in the acute, rather than the chronic, form of urticaria (e.g., hives).

Another important use of H_1 antagonists is in the treatment of motion sickness (from any mode of transportation). *Diphenhydramine, dimenhydrinate, cyclizine, and meclizine are the preferred antihistaminic agents for reducing the symptoms of motion sickness.* Diphenhydramine also is known to be at least partially effective in Parkinson's disease. It is possible that both the anti-motion sickness and the antiparkinsonian effects of the H_1 blocking agents are actually due to the anticholinergic properties they possess rather than to their antihistaminic actions.

The itch and pain associated with locally applied or released histamine (i.e., the Lewis triple response) can be markedly reduced by H_1-blocking drugs. This may be due, in part, to their local anesthetic activity. Pyrilamine and promethazine are especially active in this regard. Other allergic responses, such as those due to injection or ingestion of allergens, also can be partially relieved through antihistamine therapy. The usual allergic responses seen in susceptible individuals after intradermal injections of allergens (e.g., skin testing) can be prevented for several hours by prior administration of H_1 antagonists.

Some cases of asthma in children can be relieved by these H_1 antagonist drugs, but generally they are contra-

Figure 72-3. Generic structure of H_1-receptor antagonists.

Figure 72-4. Representative H_1 antagonists.

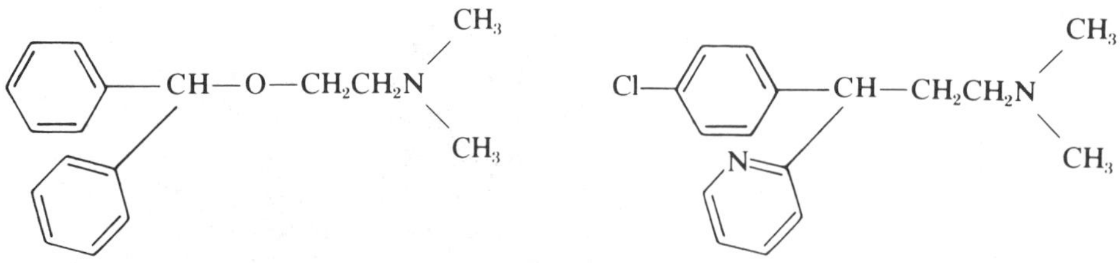

indicated in asthma because of their drying effect on bronchiolar secretions. The H₁ antagonists *are not drugs of choice* in acute anaphylactic emergencies; diseases of the skin, eyes, and nose; or the virally caused common cold.

Finally, *many H₁-receptor blocking drugs have sedative properties,* and some have been used in over-the-counter preparations for sleep induction. *The most widely used H₁ blocking drugs for sleep production are diphenhydramine, promethazine, and pyrilamine* (see also Chap. 33). For the rest of the H₁ compounds, the drowsiness they cause when they are administered for various allergic conditions constitutes an unwanted side effect (see the following discussion).

Nonsedating Antihistamines

Terfenadine is an H₁ histamine receptor antagonist (Fig. 72-5). Because of its low lipid solubility, terfenadine does not cross the blood-brain barrier. It therefore blocks H₁ receptors, which are almost exclusively found outside the CNS. The drug is well absorbed after oral administration with plasma levels peaking after about 2 hr. Terfenadine is extensively metabolized and has an elimination half-life of about 20 hr. Sixty percent is eliminated by the fecal route while the remainder appears in the urine. Terfenadine is primarily indicated for the relief of symptoms associated with seasonal allergic rhinitis including sneezing, rhinorrhea, pruritus, and tearing. It has relatively few side effects and is especially devoid of CNS actions. Terfenadine (*Seldane*) is usually given in a dosage of 60 mg twice a day.

Astemizole is a long-acting, nonsedating antihistamine that antagonizes histamine at H₁ receptors (see Fig. 72-5).

Like terfenadine it has limited lipid solubility and does not readily enter the CNS or cause drowsiness. It has minimal affinity for cholinergic, dopaminergic, and β-adrenergic receptors. After high doses there is evidence of antiserotonin and α-adrenoceptor blocking action. Astemizole is rapidly and completely absorbed from the gastrointestinal tract after oral administration, but the presence of food will interfere with its absorption. The drug undergoes extensive first-pass metabolism and at least nine metabolites have been identified. It is largely excreted in the feces. Enterohepatic recirculation of metabolites may contribute to its prolonged duration of effect. Its mean half-life ranges from 9 to 13 days after a single dose. Astemizole has a delayed onset of action and therefore is not as effective for acute allergic symptoms as is terfenadine. It should be useful, however, in maintenance and prophylactic therapy in patients with chronic allergic conditions who have difficulty in remembering to take their medication. Astemizole is relatively free of side effects, but increased appetite and weight gain do occur. Astemizole (*Hismanal*) is available as 10-mg tablets and the usual dose is one tablet daily.

Recently, a drug interaction has been identified following the concurrent use of erythromycin and terfenadine. This combination can cause arrhythmias and possibly death. The interaction with astemizole and erythromycin is unclear presently. However, both terfenadine and astemizole have caused lethal arrhythmias in children when given in high doses. Clearly, this is a caution in the use of these drugs. In addition, caution should be exercised when using terfenadine with any compound that inhibits hepatic drug metabolism, such as ciprofloxacin, cimetidine, or disulfiram.

Figure 72-5. Two nonsedating H₁ antagonists.

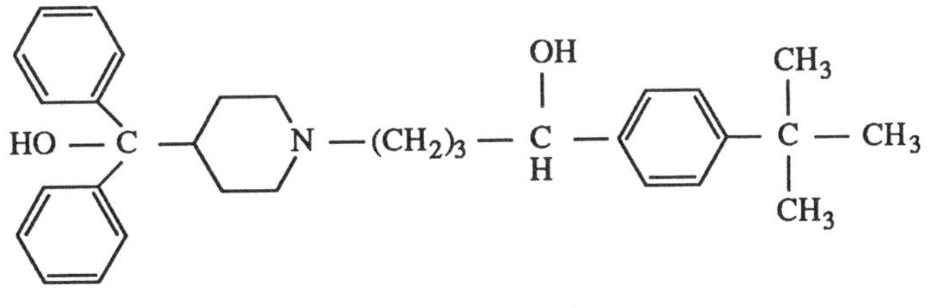

Terfenadine

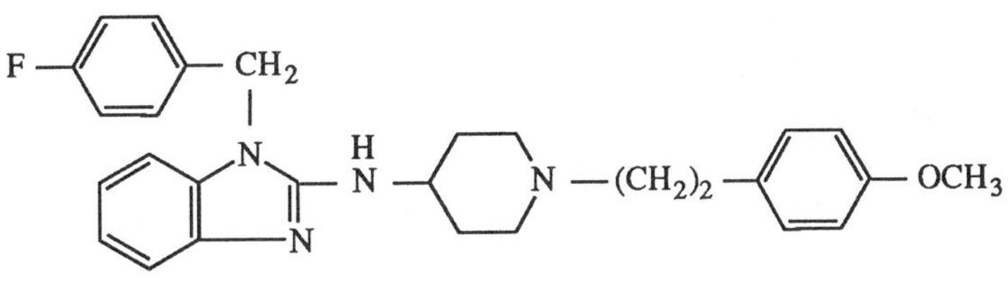

Astemizole

Table 72-3. Some Representative H$_1$ Antagonists

Class and generic name	Trade name	Adult dose	Degree of sedation produced*	Relative anti-motion sickness and antiemetic properties*	Dosage form
Ethanolamines					
Diphenhydramine hydrochloride	Benadryl	50 mg, q4–6h	3	2	Capsule, elixir, injectable
Dimenhydrinate	Dramamine	50 mg, q4–6h	3	2	Tablet, syrup, suppository, injectable
Ethylenediamines					
Tripelennamine citrate	Pyribenzamine Citrate	50 mg, q4–6h	2+	1	Tablet, delayed-action tablet, cream, ointment
Pyrilamine maleate	Dorantamin	25–50 mg, q4–6h	2+	1	Tablet, timed-release capsule
Alkylamines					
Chlorpheniramine maleate	Chlor-Trimeton	2–4 mg, q4–6h	2	1	Tablet, repeat-action tablet, syrup, injectable
Brompheniramine maleate	Dimetane	4–8 mg, q4–6h	2	1	Tablet, sustained-action tablet, elixir, injectable
Dexchlorpheniramine maleate	Polaramine	2 mg, q4–6h	2	1	Tablet, sustained-action tablet, syrup
Dexbrompheniramine maleate	Disomer	2 mg, q4–6h	2	1	Sustained-action tablet
Piperazines					
Cyclizine hydrochloride	Marezine Hydrochloride	50 mg, q4–6h	1	2	Tablet, suppository, injectable
Meclizine hydrochloride	Bonine, Antivert	25–50 mg, q24h	1	2	Tablet (chewable)
Phenothiazines					
Promethazine hydrochloride	Phenergan	25–50 mg, q4–6h	3	3	Tablet, syrup, suppository, injectable
Miscellaneous					
Cyproheptadine hydrochloride	Periactin	25–50 mg, qd	2+	1	Tablet, syrup

*1 = none or mild; 2 = moderate; 3 = potent.

Adverse Reactions

When used in the recommended amounts, antihistamines are surprisingly nontoxic. However, acute poisoning in children has been reported, with the most common symptoms being excitation and convulsions. Although children frequently suffer overdosage with antihistamines, acute poisoning is relatively rare. Symptomatic treatment for drug overdosage should not include the use of long-acting barbiturates for the control of convulsions, since additive CNS depression can occur.

In usual dosages (Table 72-3), the most prominent side effect is *drowsiness*. The degree of sleepiness induced by a given H$_1$ antagonist is related both to the dose administered and to the individual's sensitivity to the agent. Some people are affected by the sedative effect to such an extent that they would rather suffer the allergic symptoms than take the antihistamine. The sedative effect is additive with the effects of other depressants, such as alcohol. The combination of an antihistamine and alcohol has prob-ably been a causative factor in a number of highway accidents.

The anticholinergic actions that these compounds possess may result in a drying of both salivary and bronchial secretions to the point of local irritation. Their local anesthetic side effects may be put to use by incorporating the drugs into topical applications for the treatment of itching (antipruritic effect). Unfortunately, topical application can cause skin sensitization and is best avoided.

Cyclizine and chlorcyclizine cause teratogenic effects in rats and therefore, although they have been used to treat the nausea of pregnancy, they should be avoided in that condition. This side effect appears to be more related to the particular R group attached to the H$_1$ antagonist side chain than to the drug's antihistamine activity.

Preparations and Dosage

Table 72-3 contains a listing of many of the commercially available H$_1$ antagonists.

H₂-Receptor Antagonists

H₁ antagonists do not block the gastric secretory effects of histamine. Because inhibition of gastric secretion is of paramount importance in the treatment of peptic ulcer, attempts were made to synthesize histamine antagonists that would specifically block the H₂ receptors in the stomach. Cimetidine is discussed in greater detail than the others since it is a prototype. *These drugs compete with histamine specifically for H₂ receptors.* The H₂-receptor antagonists generally retain the imidazole ring (possibly methylated at position 5) and have a longer side chain than do the H₁ antagonists.

Cimetidine

Mechanism of Action

Cimetidine competitively and reversibly inhibits the actions of histamine on H₂ receptors, including those found in the stomach, heart, and smaller arteries. This action is relatively specific for the histamine H₂ receptor and finds its greatest use as a particularly effective inhibitor of gastric acid secretion. Recent research indicates that parietal cells of the stomach do not contain H₂ receptors. The cells that contain the receptors are just below the parietal cells in the lamina propria. These may be phagocytic/macrophage-like cells. Antibody-producing plasmacytes may also be involved. Cimetidine does not appear to have significant anticholinergic activity.

Absorption, Metabolism, and Excretion

Cimetidine is rapidly absorbed following oral administration and produces peak blood levels in 45 to 90 min. The drug remains effective in inhibiting basal gastric acid secretory activity for 4 to 5 hr and has a half-life of about 2 hr. Renal excretion of cimetidine and its metabolites (principally a sulfoxide derivative) serves as the primary route of drug elimination.

Clinical Uses

The major approved uses for cimetidine and other H₂ blockers include both the short-term and prophylactic treatment of active duodenal ulcers (see Chap. 73), short-term treatment of active benign gastric ulcer, and treatment of such hypersecretory conditions as Zollinger-Ellison syndrome, that is, ulcerogenic tumors of the pancreas. Additionally, there is a rationale for the use of cimetidine in hemorrhage from esophageal, gastric, or duodenal erosions; in esophageal reflux; and possibly in stress-induced gastric mucosal ulcers.

Adverse Reactions

Headache, tiredness, muscle pain, skin rash, dizziness, mental confusion, sexual dysfunction, diarrhea, and gynecomastia have all been reported. Although no cases of fatal agranulocytosis have been reported after cimetidine administration, agranulocytosis and thrombocytopenia have been seen. Most adverse effects are infrequent and rarely require discontinuance of the drug.

Preparations and Dosage

Cimetidine hydrochloride (*Tagamet*) is available as tablets (200 or 300 mg), liquid (5 ml contains 300 mg), and parenteral solutions (300 mg/2ml). Basal and nocturnal acid secretion is 90 percent inhibited by 300 mg for about 4 hr. Food or chemically induced (e.g., betazole, pentagastrin, caffeine) stimulation of gastric secretion will be inhibited by cimetidine by at least 50 percent for several hours.

Other H₂ Blocking Drugs

In addition to cimetidine, three other H₂ antagonists have been approved by the Food and Drug Administration (FDA) for treatment of active duodenal ulcer and for maintenance therapy after the ulcer has healed: ranitidine (*Zantac*), nizatidine (*Axid*), and famotidine (*Pepcid*).

All three compounds lack the imidazole group that previously was considered to be essential (see Fig. 73-3 for structure). Although their dosages are different, their clinical usefulness and uses appear to be very similar to those of cimetidine. Their clinical uses in the treatment of ulcers are covered extensively in Chap. 73.

Cimetidine and ranitidine may interfere with the hepatic metabolism of other drugs; this does not appear to be a problem with famotidine or nizatidine. Further, cimetidine antagonizes testosterone, causing gynecomastia in men, while the other H₂ blockers are without this effect.

Inhibition of Histamine Release

Cromolyn sodium inhibits degranulation and therefore prevents histamine release from the IgE-sensitized mast cells. Such an effect prevents the release of histamine and other autacoids from their mast cell granule storage sites (see Fig. 72-2). It is an important drug in the prophylaxis of severe bronchial asthma, especially from inhaled allergens (see Chap. 45).

The drug is administered by inhalation of the dry powder using a device known as a *Spinhaler*. Consequently, it is directed specifically toward the areas that contain large populations of sensitized mast cells, that is, bronchi and lungs. Cromolyn sodium is not effective in all types of asthma but can be quite helpful in selected cases of inflammation due to inhaled allergens and in cases of exercise-induced asthma. The protective effect of cromolyn sodium can last for up to 6 hr. In addition, cromolyn sodium can be inhaled intranasally for allergic rhinitis.

An ophthalmic preparation of cromolyn sodium (*Opticrom 4%*) has been marketed for the symptomatic treatment of a variety of ocular disorders that are probably the result of airborne allergens. Decreased ocular itching, tearing, redness, and discharge are said to be evident within a few days of institution of therapy. Studies involving instillation of cromolyn sodium 4% solution into the eyes of normal human volunteers indicates that only about 0.03 percent of the dose is absorbed systemically.

Additional information on cromolyn sodium can be found in Chap. 45.

Supplemental Reading

Safety of terfenadine and astemizole. *Med. Lett. Drugs Ther.* 34:9, 1992.

Watanabe, T., and Wada, H. *Histaminergic Neurons: Morphology and Function.* Boca Raton, Fla.: CRC, 1991.

73

Drugs Used in Gastrointestinal Disorders

Donald G. Seibert

The gastrointestinal tract consists of the esophagus, stomach, small intestine, and colon. It processes ingested boluses of food and drink, with eventual expulsion of waste material. The liver is a major site of metabolism for a number of compounds including bilirubin, lipoproteins, and many medications. It also secretes cholesterol, bile salts, and partially metabolized compounds into the biliary tree. Intervention by disease or pharmacological therapy may alter function of the gastrointestinal tract or liver.

From the midesophagus to the anus, smooth muscle surrounds the alimentary canal and is responsible for active movement and segmentation of intestinal contents. A thick circular smooth muscle layer is found beneath bands of longitudinal muscle. Longitudinal muscle shortens the bowel and helps mix intestinal contents; circular muscle contraction also provides mixing, but is primarily responsible for propulsive movement and segmentation.

From the gastric body to the colon, repetitive spontaneous depolarizations occur originating in the interstitial cells of Cajal from which they spread to the circular muscle layer and then to the longitudinal muscle layer. The rate of slow-wave contraction varies in different regions of the gastrointestinal tract, occurring approximately 6 per minute in the stomach, 12 per minute in the proximal intestine, and 8 per minute in the distal intestine. The increased frequency of contraction in the proximal intestine forms a gradient of contraction, and intestinal contents are therefore propelled distally. Though the stomach has fewer spontaneous contractions than does the small intestine, there is normally no retrograde spread of a depolarization wave from duodenum to stomach.

The underlying intrinsic smooth muscle motility is modulated by neurohormonal influences. The gut is innervated by afferent sensory neurons, extrinsic motor neurons, and intramural neurons. It also has mucosal sensory receptors for the monitoring of chemical, osmotic, or painful stimuli, and muscle receptors to monitor degrees of stretch.

Extrinsic gastrointestinal innervation is provided by both the parasympathetic and sympathetic nervous systems. Parasympathetic stimulation increases muscle contraction of the gut while sympathetic stimulation inhibits contractions. Stimulation of either α- or β-adrenoceptors will result in inhibition of contractions. The *intramural* nervous system consists of a myenteric (Auerbach's) plexus located between the circular and longitudinal muscle areas, and Meissner's plexus, which is a submucosal plexus found between the muscularis mucosa and the circular muscle layers. These two plexuses contain stimulatory cholinergic neurons.

Ingested liquids are rapidly emptied from the stomach into the intestine while digestible solids are first mechanically broken down in the stomach by peristaltic contractions. Stimulation of osmotic, carbohydrate, and fat receptors in the small bowel inhibits gastric peristaltic contractions and retards gastric emptying.

The small intestinal motility in the fed state consists of random slow-wave contractions that result in slower transit and longer contact of food with enzymes and absorptive surfaces. With fasting, an organized peristaltic wave, termed the *interdigestive migrating motor complex*, begins to cycle every 84 to 112 min. During the migrating motor complex, a peristaltic contraction ring travels from the stomach to the cecum at 6 to 8 cm/min. In the stomach the contractions sweep against a widely patent pylorus permitting the passage of nondigestible solids. In the small intestine this too clears the intestine of nondigested material and functions as an intestinal "housekeeper." The migrating motor complex appears to correlate with *motilin* hormonal levels and is modulated by vagal innervation.

Colonic motor function also has cyclic slow waves in the proximal colon. These contractions are primarily retrograde in the proximal colon allowing segmentation and liquid reabsorption. In the distal colon a propulsive mass movement occurs intermittently. This may be stimulated following food ingestion and is termed the *gastrocolonic reflex.*

Approximately 1.0 to 1.5 liters (L) fluid is ingested per day and, coupled with secretions from the stomach, pancreas, and proximal duodenum, approximately 8 L chyme enters the jejunum per day. Reabsorption of 6 to 7 L occurs within the small bowel, leaving a residual 1.5 L fluid, 90 percent of which is reabsorbed in the colon. This pattern of liquid reabsorption permits the elimination of fecal waste, containing an average of between 0.1 and 0.2 L fluid per day. *Diarrhea* occurs if there is an altered rate of intestinal motility, if mucosal function or permeability is altered, or if the fluid load entering the colon overwhelms colonic reabsorption. *Constipation* may occur if intestinal movement is inhibited or if there is a fixed obstruction.

Drugs that Improve Gastric Emptying

Symptoms of delayed gastric emptying may range from postprandial bloating and fullness to nausea and delayed vomiting of previously ingested foods. Gastric emptying time can be quantified by measurement of the passage of radiolabeled liquids, radiolabeled digestible solids, or radiopaque nondigestible solids from the stomach into the small bowel. Fifty percent of ingested liquid should be emptied within 30 min, and 50 percent of a digestible solid should be emptied within 2 hr. Radiopaque markers normally pass into the small intestine by 6 hr. Since indigestible material does not readily pass the pylorus without a migrating motor complex, the latter test may be the best assay for an intact interdigestive motor complex.

Emptying time can be prolonged as a result of an autonomic neuropathy seen with long-standing diabetes mellitus. Pseudo-obstruction due to an idiopathic intestinal muscle disease or an intestinal neuropathy may also cause delays in gastric emptying as well as intestinal transit. In addition, delays occur secondary to Chagas' disease, muscular dystrophy, scleroderma, and infiltrative diseases such as amyloidosis. A reduced gastric emptying can occur acutely following electrolyte disorders and gastroenteritis. In addition, anticholinergics, tricyclic antidepressants, levodopa, and β-adrenergic agonists inhibit gastric emptying and gastric contractions. Emptying may be enhanced by metoclopramide, domperidone, cisapride, and cholinergic stimulation.

Metoclopramide Hydrochloride

Metoclopramide stimulates upper gastrointestinal tract motility without augmenting biliary, gastric, or pancreatic secretions. It has both a central and a peripheral effect. Centrally, it is a dopamine antagonist, an action that is im-

portant both for its antiemetic and its side effects. Peripherally, it stimulates the release of intrinsic postganglionic stores of acetylcholine and sensitizes the gastric smooth muscle to muscarinic stimulation. The ability of metoclopramide to antagonize the inhibitory neurotransmitter effect of dopamine on the gastrointestinal tract results in increased gastric contraction and enhanced gastric emptying and small bowel transit.

Pharmacokinetics

Metoclopramide is rapidly absorbed following an oral dose in a patient with intact gastric emptying. Peak plasma concentration is achieved within 40 to 120 min. With normal renal function plasma half-life is about 4 hr. Twenty percent of an oral dose is eliminated unchanged in the urine, while 60 percent is eliminated as sulfate or glucuronide conjugates. After intravenous administration, a response occurs within 1 to 30 min.

Clinical Uses

Improved gastric emptying will frequently alleviate symptoms in patients with diabetic, postoperative, or idiopathic gastroparesis. Since metoclopramide also can decrease the acid reflux into the esophagus that results from slowed gastric emptying or lower esophageal sphincter pressure, the drug can be used in the treatment of peptic esophagitis.

Adverse Effects

Side effects include fatigue, insomnia, and altered motor coordination. Parkinsonian side effects and acute dystonic reactions also have been reported. Metoclopramide stimulates prolactin secretion causing galactorrhea and menstrual disorders. Extrapyramidal side effects seen following administration of the phenothiazines, thioxanthines, and butyrophenones may be accentuated by metoclopramide.

Preparations and Dosage

Metoclopramide hydrochloride (*Reglan*) is available in tablet, syrup, and injectable forms. The oral dose is 10 mg 30 min before meals and at bedtime. The intravenous dose for gastroparesis is identical. It can also be given by subcutaneous, intramuscular, and intraperitoneal routes.

Agents in Development

Domperidone (*Motilium*), another drug used to decrease gastric emptying time, has the identical clinical uses as metoclopramide. It has not been released for general use in the United States. Domperidone functions primarily as a peripheral dopamine antagonist. Since it does not readily cross the blood-brain barrier, it has few central side effects. Peak plasma blood levels are achieved from 10 to 30 min after intramuscular or oral administration, and 1 to 3 hr after rectal dosing. Following oral administration 31 percent of the drug is excreted in the urine. The elimination half-life is 7.5 hr if normal renal function is present.

Extrapyramidal reactions and parkinsonian side effects have not been noted with the use of domperidone. Galactorrhea and menstrual disorders have been noted secondary to induced rises in serum prolactin levels. Because cardiac arrhythmias were noted following parenteral administration, further studies using this route of administration have been stopped in the United States.

Cisapride is a potent stimulant of gastric emptying. When used for gastroparesis, patients will frequently respond to this agent even though they have failed to respond to metoclopramide therapy. Small intestinal and colonic effects allow improved transit in patients with small intestinal pseudo-obstruction and chronic constipation.

Cisapride appears to act by facilitating the release of acetylcholine from the myenteric plexus. It has no antiadrenergic, antidopaminergic, or cholinergic side effects. Following oral administration, peak plasma levels occur in 1.5 to 2.0 hr; the drug's half-life is 10 hr. The most frequent side effect has been diarrhea. In a few patients seizure activity has occurred that was reversible after medication was discontinued.

Because *cholinergic agonists* may enhance the effect of metoclopramide, combined therapy with these two agents may help patients who have failed to respond adequately to metoclopramide alone. Cholinergic stimulation by acetylcholine analogues (e.g., bethanechol) or a cholinesterase inhibitor (e.g., neostigmine) results in combined gastric and duodenal contractions, which do not, by themselves, improve gastric emptying.

Pharmacological Modulation of Diarrhea

Diarrhea is the frequent passage of watery unformed stools. Its causes are many and include irritable bowel syndrome, infectious disorders, thyrotoxicosis, malabsorption or maldigestion, and laxative abuse. Medications used to treat other disorders also may induce diarrhea. For example, xanthines (e.g., theophylline preparations) cause diarrhea secondary to alteration of mucosal cyclic adenosine monophosphate (cAMP). Antihypertensive drugs, such as reserpine and guanethidine, may induce diarrhea by changing gut neuronal input and reducing noradrenergic-mediated relaxation. The dose of quinidine is frequently limited by diarrhea.

Attempts to treat diarrhea should first focus on the patient's list of medications followed by a quick search for an underlying systemic disorder. If specific therapy (i.e., treatment of thyrotoxicosis, inflammatory bowel, a malabsorptive disease) is not possible, both adsorbent powders and opiates may reduce diarrhea irrespective of the cause. Opiates should not, however, be utilized indiscriminately in bloody diarrhea since their use in inflammatory bowel disease involving the colon may increase the risk for megacolon and their use in infectious enterocolitis may promote intestinal perforation.

Adsorbent Powders

In the treatment of diarrhea, kaolin powder and other hydrated aluminum silicate clays, often combined with pectin (a complex carbohydrate), are the most widely used adsorbent powders (e.g., *Kaopectate*).

Kaolin is a naturally occurring hydrated aluminum silicate that is prepared for medicinal use as a very finely divided powder. The rationale behind its use in acute nonspecific diarrhea stems from its ability to adsorb some of the bacterial toxins that often cause the condition. It is almost harmless and is effective in many cases of diarrhea if taken in large enough doses (2–10 gm initially, followed by the same amount after every bowel movement). The adsorbents are generally safe. Because they may interfere with the absorption of some drugs from the gastrointestinal tract, it is generally recommended that other therapeutic agents be given 2 to 3 hr before or after the adsorbent powder.

Bismuth subsalicylate (*Pepto-Bismol*) also binds intestinal toxins and may coat irritated mucosal surfaces. This compound is a salicylate and may, therefore, produce signs of salicylism (e.g., ringing of the ears) if taken chronically, especially if given with aspirin. Bismuth is radiopaque and may interfere with radiological examinations. Its use may cause temporary gray-black discoloration of the stool and brown pigmentation of the tongue.

Activated charcoal is the most effective substance known for adsorbing poisons and for this reason is the treatment of choice after an ingested poison or drug overdosage has been partially retrieved with gastric lavage or induced emesis. It is no longer used widely in the treatment of diarrhea.

Hydrophilic substances (polycarbophil, methylcellulose, and various psyllium seed derivatives) that bind water and bile salts may be useful in controlling diarrhea that is associated with the passing of excessively watery stools.

Opiates

Most of the opiates have a constipating action; morphine was used in the treatment of diarrhea before it was used as an analgesic. Unfortunately, many of the opium preparations, while effectively relieving diarrhea and dysentery, also produce such objectionable side effects as respiratory depression and addiction. The opiates are capable of altering the motility pattern in all parts of the gastrointestinal tract. These compounds usually produce an increase in segmentation and a decrease in the rate of propulsive movement of the gut contents. The feces become dehydrated as a result of their longer stay in the gastrointestinal tract. The tone of the internal anal sphincter is increased, and the subjective response to the stimulus of a full rectum is reduced by the central action of the opiates. All of these actions produce constipation.

The dangers of dependency and addiction clearly preclude the use of such compounds as morphine, meperidine, and methadone as treatment for diarrhea. Antidiarrheal specificity, therefore, is of paramount importance in choosing among the synthetic opiates and their analogues (e.g., diphenoxylate and loperamide).

Diphenoxylate (marketed in combination with atropine as *Lomotil* in the United States and as *Reasec* in most European countries) is chemically related to both analgesic and anticholinergic groups of compounds. It is as effective in the treatment of diarrhea as the opium derivatives, and at the doses usually employed there is a low incidence of central opiate actions. Diphenoxylate is rapidly metabolized by ester hydrolysis to the biologically active metabolite diphenoxylic acid. *Lomotil* is recommended as adjunctive therapy in the management of diarrhea. It is contraindicated in children under 2 years old and in patients with obstructive jaundice. Adverse reactions are often caused by the atropine in the preparation and can include anorexia, nausea, pruritus, dizziness, and numbness of the extremities. *Lomotil* is supplied as tablets and liquid (2.5 mg diphenoxylate hydrochloride; 0.025 mg atropine sulfate).

Loperamide hydrochloride (*Imodium*) structurally resembles both haloperidol and meperidine. In equal doses, loperamide protects against diarrhea longer than does diphenoxylate. It reduces the daily fecal volume, and decreases intestinal fluid and electrolyte loss. Loperamide produces a rapid and sustained inhibition of the peristaltic reflux through depression of longitudinal and circular muscle activity. The drug also possesses antisecretory activity, presumably through an effect on intestinal opiate receptors. Loperamide is effective against a wide range of secretory stimuli and can be utilized in the control and symptomatic relief of acute diarrhea that is not secondary to bacterial infection. Adverse effects associated with its use include abdominal pain and distention, constipation, dry mouth, hypersensitivity, and nausea and vomiting. Loperamide is supplied as 2-mg capsules.

Opium tincture (10% opium) is a rapidly acting preparation for the symptomatic treatment of diarrhea. The more widely used paregoric (camphorated opium tincture) is equally effective and is frequently used in combination with other antidiarrheal agents. Codeine also has been used for short-term symptomatic treatment.

Pharmacological Modulation of Constipation

Constipation is defined as the infrequent passage of stool. It may be secondary to a sluggish colon in which soft stool is seen throughout the colon or to difficulties with evacuation in which firm stool is seen primarily in the sigmoid and rectum. There is a great deal of variability in bowel habits from person to person; a normal stool frequency may vary from three stools per week up to three stools per day.

The dangers of excessive purging are salt and fluid loss as well as a gradually increasing desensitization of the bowel to normal stimuli; the latter effect forces the laxative user to employ larger and larger doses.

Cathartics are used to increase stool frequency and reduce stool viscosity. They are also used before radiological, endoscopic, or abdominal surgical procedures. Here preparations are desired that will quickly empty the colon of fecal material. Cathartics, saline laxatives, and nonabsorbable hyperosmolar solutions are utilized. Even with long-term use, bulk laxatives and pure osmolar laxatives (lactulose) do not predispose patients to formation of a cathartic-type colon and should be the initial agents utilized for chronic constipation after a structural obstructing lesion has been excluded.

Classification and comparison of representative laxatives are provided in Table 73-1.

Bulk-Forming Laxatives

The bulk-forming laxative group includes *methylcellulose* and *carboxymethylcellulose, agar* and *tragacanth, psyllium seed* (plantago, *Metamucil*), and *bran.* All act by increasing the bulk of the feces, part of this action being due to their capacity to attract water, thus forming a hydrogel. The increased volume of feces stretches the walls of the gastrointestinal tract and stimulates peristalsis. Their action may not be evident for 2 to 3 days after starting treatment. Because they all bring about an increased water content in the feces, the patient should be advised to drink adequate amounts of water; otherwise dehydration may result.

The use of *high-fiber diets* has recently received a great deal of publicity, and many claims have been made for the value of such diets. Fiber in the diet is derived entirely from plant material—either from fruit and vegetables or from cereals, the latter being known as *bran.* The fiber content in each case is a complex carbohydrate in the form

Table 73-1. Classification and Comparison of Representative Laxatives

Type of laxative-cathartic effect and latency		
Softening of formed stool (1–3 days)	Soft semifluid stool (6–12 hr)	Watery stool (2–6 hr)

Bulk-forming agents
  Dietary fiber
  Methylcellulose
  Psyllium preparations
  Calcium polycarbophil
Docusate salts
  Sodium, potassium, or calcium salts
    of dioctylsulfosuccinate
Lactulose
	Saline laxatives (low dose)
	  Milk of magnesia
	  Magnesium sulfate
	Diphenylmethane derivatives
	  Phenolphthalein
	  Bisacodyl
	Anthraquinone derivatives
	  Senna
	  Cascara sagrada
	  Danthron
		Saline laxatives (high dose)
		  Milk of magnesia
		  Magnesium citrate
		  Magnesium sulfate
		  Sodium phosphates
		  Sodium sulfate
		Castor oil

Source: From *AMA Drug Evaluations* (5th ed.). Chicago: American Medical Association, 1983.

of cellulose, pectin, and lignin. These fibers pass through the gastrointestinal tract relatively unaltered by enzymes (herbivorous animals have a cecum in which bacterial action breaks this material down).

A high-fiber diet is effective in the prevention of constipation and diverticulitis. Fiber, 10 gm/day, accompanied by a low-cholesterol diet, has been shown to lower total serum cholesterol by 15 percent. In addition, insulin control of diabetes can be improved since postprandial hyperglycemia is lessened. Claims also have been made that such diets prevent cancer of the colon; these claims are made on the basis that cancer of the colon is much less prevalent in Third World populations that eat a very high-fiber diet. The explanation advanced is that intestinal flora act on bile salts to produce carcinogens and that the presence of bran changes the intestinal flora and decreases the mucosal contact time of carcinogens that are ingested or synthesized. These claims require further study.

Since clear advantages accrue from a high-bran diet (a reduction in both constipation and diverticulitis), and since no undesirable side effects or toxic actions are generally seen, *a bulk-forming laxative is the laxative of choice in patients who suffer from constipation.*

Osmotic Laxatives

Lactulose syrup (*Cephulac, Chronulac*) functions as an osmotic cathartic. It is a synthetic disaccharide that is poorly absorbed from the gastrointestinal tract since there is no mammalian enzyme capable of hydrolyzing it to its monosaccharide components. It therefore reaches the colon unchanged and is metabolized by colonic bacteria to lactic acid and to small quantities of formic and acetic acids. Colonic lumen osmolality increases and fluid movement occurs secondary to osmotic pressure. Since lactulose does contain galactose, it is contraindicated in patients

Table 73-2. Commonly Used Salts and Their Official Doses

Salt	Preparation and dose
Magnesium	Magnesium sulfate (Epsom salt), 15 gm; magnesium hydroxide (milk of magnesia), 15 ml; magnesium citrate solution, 200 ml
Sodium	Sodium phosphate (disodium hydrogen phosphate), 4–8 gm; sodium sulfate (Glauber's salt), 15 gm
Potassium	Potassium sodium tartrate (Rochelle salt), 10 gm; potassium sodium bicarbonate–tartaric acid (Seidlitz powder), 10 gm

who require a galactose-free diet. Metabolism of lactulose by intestinal bacteria may result in increased formation of intraluminal gas and abdominal distention.

Saline Laxatives

Saline laxatives are soluble inorganic salts that contain multivalent cations or anions (Table 73-2). These charged particles do not readily cross the intestinal mucosa and therefore tend to remain in the lumen of the gastrointestinal tract, where they help retain fluid through the osmotic effect exerted by the nonabsorbed ions. The volume in the gastrointestinal tract is increased, distending the colon and producing a physiological stimulus for peristalsis through activation of stretch receptors. This explanation of the mechanism by which the saline cathartics exert their effects, however, may be too simplistic since active secretion of fluid into the gut lumen has been documented following the administration of magnesium-containing agents.

Most saline purgatives have an unpleasant salty taste that makes them unpalatable. This drawback may be overcome by flavoring or formulating them into effervescent powders. These salts should always be given with substantial amounts of water; otherwise the patient may be purged at the expense of body water, resulting in dehydration. Saline cathartics should not be used in patients with congestive heart failure since there may be an excessive absorption of sodium. Similarly, in cases of renal failure, magnesium or phosphate-containing products should not be utilized since the loss of a renal clearance of these ions may result in cumulative toxic levels despite their minimal absorption.

Enemas may contain water, saline, soaps, mineral detergents (docusate potassium) or hypertonic (sorbitol, sodium phosphate–biphosphate) fluids. These are convenient and generally safe for short-term use. Many of these solutions irritate the mucosa and may produce excessive mucus in the stool. Excessive use of these enema products may result in water intoxication and hyponatremia. These preparations should be administered only when there is a clear indication for their use.

Iso-osmotic Electrolyte Colonic Lavage Solutions

GoLYTELY and *Colyte* contain polyethylene glycol, sodium sulfate, sodium bicarbonate, sodium chloride, and potassium chloride as an iso-osmotic solution. Four liters is ingested over 2 to 3 hr either orally or through a nasogastric tube. There is minimal net absorption or excretion of fluid or electrolytes and the patient has repeated liquid stools until the administered solution has been expelled. If gastric emptying is slow, patients may have abdominal distention with vomiting. This preparation should not be utilized if a bowel obstruction or an impaired gag reflex is present. It is used primarily to clear the bowel before radiological or endoscopic procedures, and is also occasionally employed to assist with evacuation in a patient who has a sluggish colon. After such purging, the patient should be placed on a regular regimen of bulk laxatives, lactulose, or both.

Fecal Softeners

Fecal softeners are substances that are not absorbed from the alimentary canal and act by increasing the bulk of the feces and softening the stool so that it is easier to pass. Two fecal softeners are in common use.

The first is *liquid paraffin (mineral oil)*, which has been in use for many years, either as the oil or as a white emulsion. Available in many proprietary forms, it is a mixture of liquid hydrocarbons. Its use has been criticized for many reasons: It dissolves the fat-soluble vitamins and prevents their absorption, it is itself absorbed slightly and appears in the mesenteric lymph nodes, and if it is inhaled

into the lungs (which it may be in elderly or debilitated patients), it may produce inflammatory responses such as lipoid pneumonia. Its continual use, therefore, is contraindicated, although its occasional administration in otherwise well patients is not harmful. It is employed primarily in patients who must avoid straining at stool, including persons with hemorrhoids and other painful anal lesions. Leakage of mineral oil past the anal sphincter may occur, leading to soiling of clothing.

Docusate sodium, formerly called dioctyl sodium sulfosuccinate (*Colace, Doxinate*), is a surface-active agent that produces fecal softening in 1 or 2 days. By means of its detergent properties, docusate sodium allows water to penetrate and soften colonic contents when it is administered as a retention enema. Orally ingested docusate sodium may, in addition, act as a stool softener by stimulating the secretion of water and electrolytes into the intestinal lumen. Docusate sodium has been used both alone and in combination with other laxatives. Although, by itself, it appears to be relatively nontoxic, it may, when taken in combination with other laxatives (e.g., oxyphenisatin, anthraquinones), increase their absorption and lead to liver toxicity. Caution also should be taken when docusate sodium is prescribed together with liquid paraffin, since the absorption of the mineral oil is increased by the detergent.

Agents Acting on the Mucosa

This group of compounds contains a variety of drugs whose exact mode of action is not known, although it is thought that they act on the mucosa of the intestine to stimulate peristalsis either by irritation or by exciting reflexes in the myenteric plexuses.

The group includes the anthraquinones (cascara, aloe, senna, rhubarb), castor oil, and a group of chemicals, which include phenolphthalein and bisacodyl. All act in the lumen of the gastrointestinal tract and are inactive if given parenterally. They produce irritation of the mucosa if given in large doses, and this irritation affects water and ion transport. However, a direct local irritation may not be essential to the action of these agents, since the purgative effects are prevented if the mucosa has been anesthetized with a local anesthetic before drug administration. For this reason it is suggested that these drugs may act by stimulating afferent nerves to initiate a reflex increase in gut motility.

Anthraquinone derivatives are among the oldest laxatives known. They act on the colon rather than on the ileum and produce evacuation 8 to 10 hr after administration. This makes them particularly suitable for dosage overnight. Phenolphthalein is partially absorbed (about 15% of a given dose) and then reexcreted in the bile; hence, if it is taken constantly, it will accumulate and exert too drastic an action. It inhibits active sodium and glucose absorption in the bowel.

Castor oil is a bland oil but is hydrolyzed in the gut, with the resultant production of ricinoleic acid, which is the active purging agent. This hydrolysis requires the presence of bile, a fact that is sometimes overlooked when castor oil is given as a laxative before x-ray in biliary obstruction. The ricinoleic acid acts on the ileum and colon to induce an increased fluid secretion and colonic contraction. Castor oil and castor oil, emulsified, are sold in capsule and liquid formulations.

Bisacodyl (*Dulcolax*) is available as 10-mg enteric-coated tablets and as 10-mg suppositories. It causes colonic contraction and inhibits water absorption in the small and large intestine.

Cascara sagrada is one of the mildest of the anthraquinone-containing laxatives and is supplied as a 300-mg tablet and as a plain or aromatic fluid extract.

Pharmacological Modulation of Vomiting

Vomiting is a complex series of integrated events, culminating with the forceful expulsion of gastric contents through the mouth. The sequence of events frequently begins with nausea, which may be accompanied by increased salivation, pupillary dilation, sweating, and pallor. Duodenal and jejunal tone is increased while gastric tone and peristalsis are diminished, tending to cause a reflux of duodenal contents into the stomach. Nausea is followed by retching, during which contractions of the abdominal musculature occur with simultaneous attempts at inspiration against a closed glottis. The gastric antrum contents and gastric contents begin to move into the esophagus. During vomiting, which is the third and final stage, there is sustained contraction of the diaphragm and abdominal musculature. The resultant high intragastric pressure moves more gastric contents into the esophagus and, with continued force, contents are expelled out the mouth.

These events are coordinated by the *emetic center,* which is located within the lateral reticular formation of the medulla oblongata close to the respiratory and salivatory centers. Electrical stimulation by microelectrodes of this area produces emesis. In the intact organism stimulation may occur from peripheral sites, the cortex, and the chemoreceptor trigger zone (Fig. 73-1). Peripheral stimulation, which is mediated by vagal and sympathetic nerves, may originate from the vestibular system (as is seen in motion sickness), from the coronary arteries (seen in cardiac ischemia), or from distention and inflammation of sites in the gastrointestinal tract.

The *chemoreceptor trigger zone* (CTZ) is responsive to chemical (particularly dopamine) stimulation and, through the fasciculus solitarius, is connected to the emetic center. Direct stimulation of the CTZ by microelectrodes does not result in vomiting. Most drug-induced emesis, including emesis induced by apomorphine, levodopa, cardiac glycosides, the majority of cancer chemotherapeutic agents, and nicotine, appears to be mediated by this route. Cytotoxic chemotherapy also stimulates the release of serotonin from enterochromaffin cells of the upper gastrointestinal tract. Vomiting may then be induced through serotonergic stimulation of enteric vagal afferents or possibly through direct central nervous system stimulation. Unpleasant memories and anticipatory vomiting before repeat chemotherapy as well as corticoelectrical stimulation producing emesis suggest that the cerebral cortex, acting through the emetic center, may also initiate vomiting.

Emetics

The most commonly used emetics are ipecac and apomorphine. Induced emesis is the preferred means of emptying the stomach in awake patients who have ingested a toxic substance or have recently taken a drug overdose. Emesis should not be induced if the patient has central nervous system depression or has ingested certain volatile hydrocarbons and caustic substances.

Ipecac syrup is prepared from the dried rhizome and roots of *Cephaelis ipecacuanha* or of *C. accuminata,* plants from Brazil and Central America that have the alkaloid *emetine* as their active principal ingredient. It acts directly on the CTZ and also indirectly by irritating the gastric mucosa. In adults ipecac syrup is administered as a 15- to 30-ml dose with 300 to 400 ml water. If vomiting has not occurred within 20 min, a second dose can be administered. Ipecac is cardiotoxic if absorbed and can cause cardiac conduction disturbances, atrial fibrillation, or a fatal myocarditis. If emesis does not occur, gastric lavage using a nasogastric tube must be performed.

Apomorphine, a derivative of morphine, acts directly on the CTZ. It also is more effective if water is first administered before oral or subcutaneous dosing. Excessive dosage may cause respiratory depression and circulatory collapse. Narcotic antagonists such as naloxone usually will reverse the depressant actions of apomorphine. Because of the possibility of respiratory depression, apomorphine is infrequently used as an emetic.

Antiemetics

Antiemetics may prevent emesis by blocking the CTZ or by preventing peripheral or cortical stimulation of the emetic center.

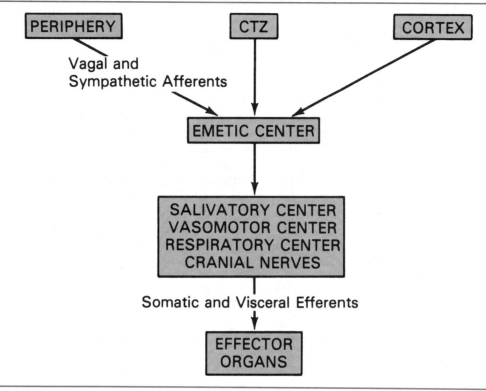

Figure 73-1. Schematic representation of reflex pathways for vomiting initiated by pharmacologic agents. Pharmacologically induced vomiting can be triggered at one (or more) of three sites: the chemoreceptor trigger zone (CTZ), the pharynx and gastrointestinal tract (periphery), and the supramedullary loci (cortex). Afferent impulses from the three trigger sites are integrated at the medullary emetic center. When the vomiting threshold is exceeded, the emetic center programs the vomiting act through neighboring medullary control centers and somatic and visceral efferent nerves. (Reprinted with permission from L.J. Seigel and D.L. Longo, The control of chemotherapy-induced emesis. *Ann. Intern. Med.* 95:352,1981.)

Antihistamines

The antihistamines appear to block peripheral stimulation of the emetic center. They are therefore most effective in motion sickness and inner ear dysfunction as is seen in Ménière's syndrome, labyrinthitis, and streptomycin ototoxicity. Dimenhydrinate, diphenhydramine, and meclizine hydrochloride are the three antihistamines primarily used in the prevention of nausea from inner ear stimulation. Each drug produces some degree of drowsiness. Because of its slower onset of effect, meclizine should be administered at least 1 hr before expected travel. Its use also may result in blurred vision, dry mouth, and fatigue. A more complete discussion of the H$_1$ antihistamines can be found in Chap. 72.

Anticholinergics

Because of the induction of vertigo, dry mouth, drowsiness, blurred vision, and tachycardia, oral preparations of scopolamine hydrobromide are no longer utilized. The transdermal adhesive form of scopolamine (*Transderm Scōp*) provides up to 72 hr of antimetic production when applied to the postauricular area. Similar side effects are found as with oral scopolamine but are milder. There is no pediatric formulation of this agent.

Benzodiazepines

Benzodiazepines and their congeners may help prevent central cortical-induced vomiting. A prominent side effect is drowsiness. Discussions of these agents are found in Chap. 33.

Cannabinoids

The antiemetic site of action of tetrahydrocannabinol (dronabinol, THC, *Marinol*) is unknown although it appears to affect the central cerebral cortex axis. Relief may occur in patients refractory to other antiemetics. It is less effective in the elderly, primarily because of its side effects. The antiemetic effect is associated with a "high" and this appears to be better tolerated in the young. Sedation is seen in approximately 30 percent of patients. Ataxia, drowsiness, dry mouth, or orthostatic hypotension may be seen in up to 35 percent of the older patient population. Gastrointestinal absorption is variable though blood levels correlate with efficacy. The bioavailability is not as variable if the agent is smoked. The coadministration of prochlorperazine may prevent some of the central nervous side effects seen with the use of tetrahydrocannabinol.

Dopamine Antagonists

As dopamine antagonists, domperidone and metoclopramide centrally inhibit stimulation of the CTZ. By improving gastric emptying, they also decompress the stomach, thereby decreasing a peripherally associated stimulation of the emetic center. Domperidone does not have central nervous system side effects while metoclopramide may precipitate extrapyramidal reactions and sedation. Domperidone is not available commercially in the United States and because of cardiac dysrhythmias is no longer provided in this country in an intravenous dosage form. Both of these agents were discussed in some detail earlier under Drugs that Improve Gastric Emptying.

Phenothiazines

Phenothiazines, which include prochlorperazine, promethazine, thiethylperazine, and trimethobenzamide, act at the CTZ by inhibiting dopaminergic transmission. They also decrease vomiting caused by gastric irritants, suggesting that they inhibit stimulation of peripheral vagal and sympathetic afferents. Sedation will frequently occur following their administration. Patients also may have problems with acute dystonic reactions, orthostatic hypotension, cholestatic hepatitis, and blood dyscrasias.

Other Drugs with Antiemetic Action

Corticosteroids, including dexamethasone and methylprednisolone, may inhibit emesis that is associated with cancer chemotherapeutic drugs. The mechanism of this effect is not known. Patients taking the corticosteroids may have problems with lethargy, weakness, fluid retention, or facial rash.

Both haloperidol (*Haldol*) and droperidol (*Inapsine*) block stimulation of the CTZ. They may be more effective in the treatment of chemotherapy-associated nausea than are the phenothiazines. The major side effect associated with their use is an extrapyramidal reaction; sedation and hypotension occur infrequently.

Ondansetron (*Zofran*) is a potent antagonist of serotonin (5-HT) receptors of the 5-HT$_3$ type. It can interrupt serotonergic initiation of the vomiting reflex. It has a half-

life of 3.0 to 3.5 hr. Ondansetron produces diarrhea in 22 percent of patients and headache in 16 percent.

Drugs Used in the Treatment of Peptic Ulcer Disease

Gastric Secretion

Functionally, the gastric mucosa is divided into three areas of secretion. The *cardiac gland area* secretes mucus and pepsinogen. The *oxyntic (parietal) gland area,* which corresponds to the fundus and body of the stomach, secretes hydrogen ion, pepsinogen, and bicarbonate. The *pyloric gland area,* located in the antrum, secretes gastrin and mucus.

The parietal cells secrete H$^+$ in response to gastrin, cholinergic, and histamine stimulation (Fig. 73-2). Both cholinergic- and gastrin-induced stimulation bring about a receptor-mediated rise in intracellular calcium, an activation of intracellular protein kinases, and eventually an increased activity of the H$^+$-K$^+$ pump leading to acid secretion into the gastric lumen. Following histamine stimulation, a guanine nucleotide–binding protein (G$_s$) activates adenyl cyclase leading to an increase in intracellular levels of the second messenger, cAMP. Activation of cAMP-dependent protein kinases then initiates the stimulation of the H$^+$-K$^+$ pump.

Acid secretion by the stomach can be modulated by the cephalic-vagal axis, gastric distention, and local mucosal chemical receptors. The smell, taste, sight, or discussion of food may result in cephalic-vagal postganglionic cholinergic stimulation of target parietal cells and enhanced antral gastrin release. After food is ingested, gastric distention initiates vagal stimulation as well as short intragastric neural reflexes, both of which increase acid secretion. Proteins present in ingested meals also stimulate acid secretion. Evidence from animal studies suggests that after protein amino acids are converted to amines, gastrin is released.

Gastric acid secretion is inhibited in the presence of acid itself. A negative feedback occurs when the pH approaches 2.5 such that further secretion of gastrin is inhibited until the pH rises. Ingested carbohydrates and fat also inhibit acid secretion after they reach the intestines; several hormonal mediators for this effect have been proposed. The secretion of pepsinogen appears to parallel the secretion of H$^+$ while the patterns of secretion of mucus and bicarbonate have not been well characterized.

The integrity of the mucosal lining of the stomach and proximal small bowel is, in large part, determined by the mucosal cytoprotection provided by mucus and bicarbonate secretion from the gastric and small bowel mucosa. Mucus retards diffusion of the H$^+$ from the gastric lumen

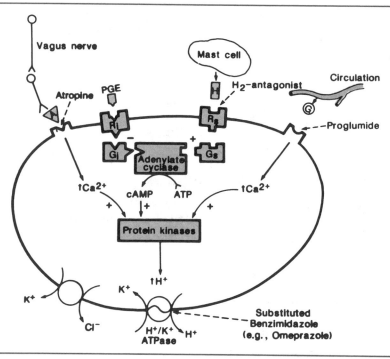

Figure 73-2. Schematic representation of a parietal cell, showing the pathways by which secretagogues are believed to stimulate hydrogen ion generation and secretion. Also shown (*dashed arrows*) are the sites of action of various antisecretory agents. A = atropine; PGE and E = series of prostaglandins; H = histamine; G = gastrin; R_i and R_s = inhibitory and stimulatory receptor-binding sites; G_i and G_s = inhibitory and stimulatory catalytic subunits; ATP = adenosine triphospate; ATPase = adenosine triphosphatase. It is unknown whether increases in cytosolic calcium (Ca^{2+}) represent a mobilization from intracellular stores or an influx of calcium from extracellular sites. (From M.M. Wolfe and A.H. Soll, The physiology of gastric acid secretion. Reprinted with permission from *N. Engl. J. Med.* 319:1707,1988.)

back to the gastric mucosal surface. In addition, the bicarbonate that is secreted into the layer between the mucus and epithelium permits a relatively higher pH to be maintained in the region next to the mucosal surface. If any H^+ does diffuse back to the level of the mucosal surface, both the local blood supply and the ability of the local cells to buffer this ion will ultimately determine whether peptic ulceration will occur.

Medications that raise intragastric pH or enhance mucosal cytoprotection are used to treat peptic ulcer disease. Many of these agents are discussed in the following sections.

Antacids

The rationale for the use of antacids in peptic ulcer disease lies in the assumption that buffering of H^+ in the stomach permits healing. The use of both low and high doses of antacids is effective in peptic ulcer as compared to placebo. Healing rates are comparable to those observed after the use of histamine (H_2) blocking agents. The buffering agents present in the various antacid preparations consist of combinations of ingredients that include *sodium bicarbonate, calcium carbonate, magnesium hydroxide,* and *aluminum hydroxide* (Table 73-3).

A variety of adverse effects have been reported following the use of antacids. For example, if sodium bicarbonate is absorbed it may cause systemic alkalinization and sodium overload. Calcium carbonate may induce a hypercalcemia and a rebound increase in gastric secretion secondary to the elevation in circulating calcium levels. Magnesium hydroxide may produce an osmotic diarrhea, and the excessive absorption of Mg^{2+} in patients with renal failure may result in central nervous system (CNS) toxicity. Aluminum hydroxide is associated with constipation; serum phosphate levels also may become depressed because of phosphate binding within the gut. The use of antacids, in general, may interfere with the absorption of a number of antibiotics and other medications.

The dosage recommended for most of the antacid preparations is either 1 to 2 tsp or one to four tablets, 1 and 3 hr after meals and before bedtime. There is wide variation in acid-neutralizing capacity of the products on the mar-

Table 73-3. Antacids

Trade name	Contents	Dose	mEq H$^+$ buffer/dose
ALternaGEL	Aluminum hydroxide	5–10 ml	16–32
Amphojel	Aluminum hydroxide	10 ml	20
Basaljel	Aluminum carbonate	10 ml	23
Di-Gel liquid	Aluminum hydroxide, magnesium hydroxide, simethicone	10 ml	18
Gelusil M	Aluminum hydroxide, magnesium hydroxide, simethicone	10 ml	24
Gelusil-II	Aluminum hydroxide, magnesium hydroxide, simethicone	10 ml	48
Maalox	Aluminum hydroxide, magnesium hydroxide	10–20 ml	27–54
Maalox TC Suspension	Aluminum hydroxide, magnesium hydroxide	5–10 ml	28.3–56.6
Maalox TC Tablets	Aluminum hydroxide, magnesium hydroxide	1 tablet	28.3
Mylanta-II	Aluminum hydroxide, magnesium hydroxide, simethicone	5–10 ml	25.4–50.8
Riopan	Magaldrate	5–10 ml	15–30
Riopan Tablets	Magaldrate	1 tablet	13.5
Titralac	Calcium carbonate	5 ml	19
Tums	Calcium carbonate	1 tablet	10

ket (see Table 73-3), and it is recommended that a high-potency antacid be utilized. If diarrhea occurs or if there is renal failure, a magnesium-based preparation should be discontinued. The agents are generally safe, but there is occasional patient resistance because some of the formulations are unpalatable and expensive.

H$_2$-Receptor Antagonists

The histamine receptor (H$_2$) antagonists marketed in the United States are cimetidine, ranitidine, famotidine, and nizatidine. Although there are substantial differences in their relative potency, 70 to 85 percent of duodenal ulcers are healed during 4 to 6 weeks of therapy with any of these agents. Since nocturnal suppression of acid secretion is particularly important in healing, nighttime-only dosing has been made available by each manufacturer. Only cimetidine and ranitidine have been approved by the Food and Drug Administration (FDA) for use in the treatment of gastric ulceration.

The incidence of healing of gastric ulceration after 6 to 8 weeks of therapy approaches 60 to 80 percent with the use of cimetidine or ranitidine. After the initial healing of an acute duodenal ulcer or a gastric ulcer there is a high likelihood of recurrence if the medication is discontinued. Continued maintenance therapy, therefore, is often recommended in some patients after acute therapy is completed. This is characteristically at one-half the dose employed for acute ulcer disease therapy. Cimetidine and ranitidine also are approved for the treatment of peptic esophageal disorders.

Cimetidine

Cimetidine, like histamine, contains an imidazole ring structure (Fig. 73-3). It is well absorbed following oral ad-

ministration with peak blood levels occurring 45 to 90 min after drug ingestion. Blood levels remain within therapeutic concentrations for approximately 4 hr after a 300-mg dose. Following oral administration, 50 to 75 percent of the parent compound is excreted unchanged in the urine; the rest appears primarily as the sulfoxide metabolite.

Cimetidine may, infrequently, cause diarrhea, nausea, vomiting, or mental confusion. A rare association with granulocytopenia, thrombocytopenia, and pancytopenia has been reported. Gynecomastia has been demonstrated in patients receiving either high-dose or long-term therapy. This occurs because cimetidine has a weak antiestrogen effect. Since cimetidine is, in part, metabolized by the cytochrome P450 system, coadministered drugs such as the benzodiazepines, theophylline, and warfarin, which are also metabolized by this system, may accumulate if their dosage is not adjusted.

Cimetidine hydrochloride (*Tagamet*) is available as 200-, 300-, 400-, and 800-mg tablets.

Ranitidine

Ranitidine has a thiazole ring (see Fig. 73-3). Oral doses are well absorbed, with a peak plasma level achieved 1 to 3 hr after ingestion. Twenty-five percent of the oral dose is excreted into the urine unchanged and approximately 50 percent of the dose is eliminated by hepatic metabolism. The half-life of elimination is 2.5 to 3.0 hr.

Ranitidine, like cimetidine, has a low incidence of toxicity associated with its use. Relatively infrequently reported side effects include cardiac arrhythmias related to intravenous dosing, confusion, and an anicteric drug-induced hepatitis. Ranitidine does not alter cytochrome P450 activity or the pharmacokinetics of other drugs metabolized by this pathway.

Ranitidine hydrochloride (*Zantac*) is available as tablets

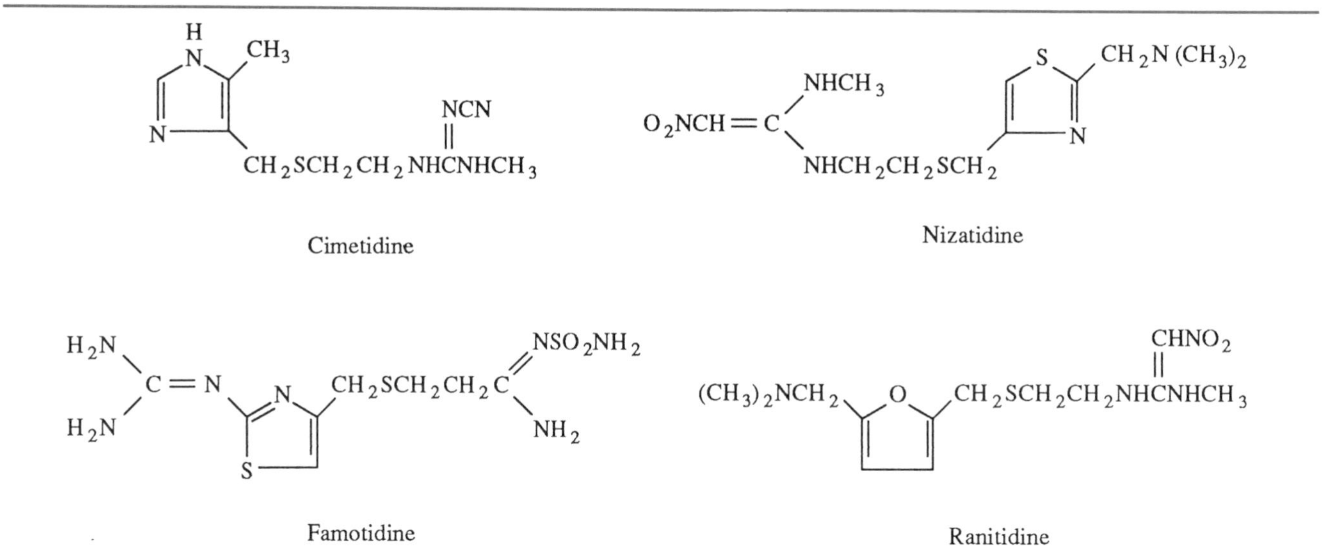

Figure 73-3. Structures of H_2-receptor antagonists.

(150 and 300 mg) and as an injectable solution. With renal dysfunction or hepatic dysfunction, the dosage should be reduced by half.

Famotidine

Famotidine (*Pepcid*) contains a furan ring structure (see Fig. 73-3). After oral administration the onset of effect occurs within 1 hr, and inhibition of gastric secretion is present for the next 10 to 12 hr. Elimination is by renal (65–70%) and metabolic (30–35%) routes. There appears to be no problem with drug interactions. Gynecomastia has not been reported. In general, side effects are similar to those found with other H_2-receptor blockers. The recommended adult oral dose is 20 mg twice a day or 40 mg at bedtime.

Nizatidine

Nizatidine (*Axid*) is the newest H_2-receptor antagonist (see Fig. 73-3). It contains a thiazole ring and a side chain identical to that found in ranitidine, and a relative potency twice that of cimetidine. Ninety percent of an oral dose is absorbed. Following a 300-mg oral dose, the peak plasma concentration occurs in 0.5 to 3.0 hr, and inhibition of gastric secretion is present for up to 10 hr. The elimination half-life is 1 to 2 hr and more than 90 percent of an oral dose is excreted in the urine. Most side effects are similar to those seen with the other H_2-receptor antagonists; gynecomastia has occurred rarely. Nizatidine does not alter the microsomal cytochrome P450 metabolism of other drugs. It has been reported to increase serum salicylate concentrations when high doses are utilized. In the presence of renal insufficiency, a reduction in dosage is recommended.

Anticholinergic Drugs

Pirenzepine (*Gastrozepine*) is a newly developed agent of relative gastrointestinal specificity and possesses fewer CNS, ocular, and salivary anticholinergic side effects than other agents of its type. It is not currently available in the United States. For a general discussion of the pharmacology of the antimuscarinic drugs, see Chap. 15.

Prostaglandins

Prostaglandins of the A, E, and I type inhibit gastric acid secretion. The mechanism for this inhibition has been discussed previously (see Chap. 42). Prostaglandins also stimulate increased mucous and bicarbonate secretion by gastric mucosa.

Misoprostol (*Cytotec*), which is a 15-deoxy-15-hydroxy-16-methyl analogue of prostaglandin E_1, has been approved for use in the prevention of nonsteroidal anti-inflammatory drug–induced ulceration. It also is approved in other countries for the treatment of peptic ulcer disease. Misoprostol is absorbed rapidly after oral administration and is hydrolyzed to the active compound. It is metabolized by the liver and excreted mainly in the urine. Adverse effects include crampy abdominal pain, a dose-related diarrhea, and uterine contractions. The last-named side effect may result in its being used as an abortifacient. Enprostil, an analogue of prostaglandin E_2, is expected to be commercially available shortly.

Omeprazol

Omeprazol (*Prilosec*) is a substituted benzimidazole that causes marked inhibition of gastric acid secretion.

Peptic ulcers and erosive esophagitis that are resistant to conventional therapy will frequently heal when this agent is utilized. It is absorbed from the small intestine at an alkaline pH, but is converted to an inactive form when exposed to acid. It must therefore be administered as an enteric-coated preparation or as a buffered suspension.

In the parietal cell it is converted to its active form only in those cells that are actively secreting acid. This active form binds to H^+-K^+-adenosine triphosphatase (ATPase), irreversibly inactivating the hydrogen pump. Peak absorption occurs 3 to 4 hr after drug administration, and though the drug is absent from plasma, inhibition of gastric acid secretion persists for up to 3 days. Bioavailability improves with repeated dosing, probably as a function of rising gastric pH.

Few side effects have been noted so far, although patient numbers are not large since this is still an investigational agent. Hypergastrinemia has been noted as a reaction secondary to the marked reduction in acid secretions. Gastric carcinoid tumors have developed in rats, but not in mice or in human volunteers. The usual dose is 20 mg taken orally each day.

Sucralfate

Sucralfate is an aluminum hydroxide sulfated sucrose complex that is only minimally absorbed from the gastrointestinal tract. It is also used in the treatment of duodenal peptic ulcer disease. After exposure to gastric acid the compound becomes negatively charged creating a viscous ulcer adherent complex. This complex is believed to inhibit back-diffusion of H^+. Other drug effects noted are a direct reduction in pepsin activity and a slight rise in tissue prostaglandin levels. A stimulation of a cytoprotection mechanism may, therefore, assist mucosal healing. The drug has no acid-buffering capacity.

Constipation is the main side effect associated with its use. As with other aluminum compounds, the drug may bind phosphorus, resulting in a secondary hypophosphatemia. Binding to a number of other coadministered medications may result in a significant reduction in their bioavailability.

Sucralfate (*Carafate*) is usually given in a 1-gm oral dose before meals. It readily dissolves into a suspension and can be ingested as a slurry.

Carbenoxolone

Carbenoxolone sodium (*Biogastrone, Biorex*) is synthesized from naturally occurring substances found in licorice root. It has been used effectively in Europe for the treatment of both gastric and duodenal ulceration. It appears to act through cytoprotective mechanisms, since it does not alter gastric acid secretion or have any acid-buf-

fering capacity. Its actions include an alteration in gastrointestinal mucous composition and an increased survival time of gastric mucosal cells. Because it causes significant fluid retention, hypokalemia, and hypertension, it is unlikely to be available commercially in the US in the near future.

Additional Useful Agents

Colloidal bismuth effectively promotes healing of gastric and duodenal ulcers. Colloidal bismuth suspensions available are tripotassium dicitrate bismuthate (*deNol*) and bismuth subsalicylate (*Pepto-Bismol*). As with sucralfate, the agents form an adherent coat over an active ulcer base. A second mechanism involved in the healing process may be the complete eradication of the organism *Campylobacter pylori* from the gastroduodenum.

These compounds are not readily absorbed, especially after short-term administration, but following chronic therapy serum bismuth concentrations rise as does bismuth urinary output. Chronic therapy may be associated rarely with an encephalopathy. There is also the potential for renal tubular injury.

Treatment of Inflammatory Bowel Disease

Idiopathic inflammatory bowel disease includes ulcerative colitis and Crohn's disease. *Ulcerative colitis* is characterized by a relapsing inflammatory condition involving variable lengths of the colon with symptoms of bleeding, urgency, diarrhea, and tenesmus. The endoscopic and radiographic appearance may demonstrate multiple diffuse erosions or ulcerations. On biopsy, distorted crypt abscesses and diminished goblet cells are seen. When involvement is limited to the distal colon, it is termed idiopathic proctitis. *Crohn's disease* may involve the gut from esophagus to anus; however, the small bowel and/or colon are the major areas of involvement. If the colon is predominantly involved, the symptoms and presentation are quite similar to those of ulcerative colitis. Small bowel involvement may give more symptoms of obstruction and abscess formation. Normal areas of gut may be found between areas of inflamed mucosa.

The present primary mode of therapy for these diseases involves the use of corticosteroids and sulfasalazine. In Crohn's disease azathioprine, 6-mercaptopurine, or metronidazole also has been utilized. These agents may enhance healing of fistulas or anal disease and are primarily employed for their ability to permit either a reduction in the dose of, or a withdrawal from, corticosteroids. The pharmacology of the corticosteroids (Chap. 66) and met-

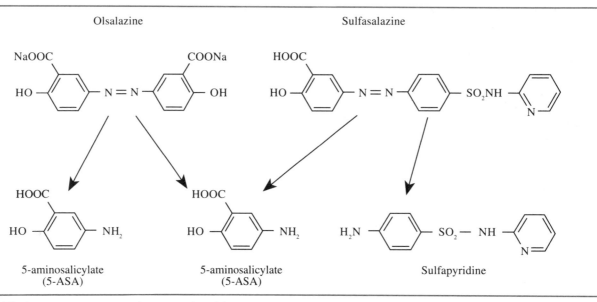

Figure 73-4. Two preparations that are used to deliver 5-aminosalicylate (5-ASA) to small intestine and colon.

ronidazole (Chap. 56) and the immunosuppressive drugs (Chap. 63) is discussed elsewhere.

Sulfasalazine

Sulfasalazine was first introduced in 1940 as a treatment for rheumatoid arthritis. It was found that a number of patients with coexistent inflammatory bowel disease showed improvement of their gastrointestinal symptoms, and the drug has subsequently been used extensively for the treatment and maintenance therapy of patients with inflammatory bowel disease.

Clinical Uses

With mild to moderate ulcerative colitis sulfasalazine treatment alone results in an 85 percent remission rate. The drug can then be continued at a reduced maintenance dose level since 90 percent of those in remission will remain so if sulfasalazine is continued. Termination of therapy leads to an 80 percent relapse within the next year. In Crohn's disease sulfasalazine acts primarily on involved colonic mucosa, although remission of ileal disease also has been reported. The National Cooperative Crohn's Disease Study found sulfasalazine to be better in the treatment of colonic involvement while corticosteroids were judged better in the treatment of involved small bowel. Since sulfasalazine does not prevent relapse of Crohn's disease once remission is achieved, maintenance therapy is not characteristically utilized.

Pharmacokinetics

Sulfasalazine is composed of sulfapyridine and 5-aminosalicylate (5-ASA) linked by an azo bond (Fig. 73-4). Following oral administration, 30 percent of the sulfasalazine is absorbed from the small intestine. Because the majority of the compound that is absorbed is later excreted into the bowel, between 75 and 85 percent of the administered oral dose eventually reaches the colon intact. Bacteria in the colon then split the azo linkage, liberating sulfapyridine and 5-ASA. The sulfapyridine is absorbed, then acetylated, hydroxylated, and conjugated to glucuronic acid in the liver. The major portion of the sulfapyridine molecule and its metabolites is excreted in the urine. The 5-ASA stays in the colon, eventually reaching extremely high fecal levels.

Mechanism of Action

Sulfapyridine has no effect on the inflammatory bowel disease and instillation of this agent into the colon does not result in healing of colonic mucosa. This metabolite is, however, responsible for most of sulfasalazine's side effects. 5-ASA is the active metabolite and may inhibit the synthesis of mediators of inflammation. 5-ASA enemas are effective in treating distal and local disease.

Adverse Effects

Nausea, vomiting, and headaches are the most common side effects and are related to the blood level of sulfapyridine. If the dose is reduced, symptoms frequently improve. Fever, rash, aplastic anemia, and autoimmune hemolysis are hypersensitivity reactions to the medication. These occur less commonly and are not dose related. Despite the appearance of hypersensitivity reactions (e.g., fever and rash) in some patients, the need for the medication may require reinstitution of drug therapy at very low doses along with attempts at desensitization. Sulfasalazine should not be used in patients with hypersensitivity agranulocytosis or aplastic anemia.

Drug Interactions

Sulfasalazine inhibits the absorption of folic acid and therefore patients may become folate deficient during long-term therapy. Sulfasalazine decreases the bioavailability of digoxin. Cholestyramine reduces the metabolism of sulfasalazine.

Preparations and Dosage

Sulfasalazine (*Azulfidine*) is available as 500-mg tablets, 500-mg enteric-coated tablets, and a 250-mg/5 ml suspension.

5-ASA Preparations

A preparation (*Rowasa*) that contains 5-ASA (also called mesalamine) can be administered as an enema for distal colonic disease (see Fig. 73-4). The usual dose is one 4-gm enema per day. 5-ASA also has been formulated in a slow-release oral form (*Pentasa, Asacol*). One third of the 5-ASA contained in this preparation is released in the small intestine and two thirds is made available in the colon. The response of ulcerative colitis to this formulation appears to be identical to that seen after sulfasalazine. No side effects have been noted with use of *Pentasa*.

Olsalazine sodium (*Dipentum*) is a compound that links two 5-ASA molecules with an azo linkage. Following cleavage of the azo linkage in the colon, two 5-ASA molecules are then released. Subjects given 1 gm olsalazine had the same cecal level of 5-ASA as patients given 2.3 gm sulfasalazine. With higher doses, diarrhea may result. Olsalazine may have some clinical efficacy in ulcerative colitis.

Agents Used for Gallstone Dissolution

In the United States, approximately 1 million people are found each year to have gallstones. In symptomatic

cases, a cholecystectomy has been the predominant form of therapy. With asymptomatic or mildly symptomatic patients, controversy exists over the need for cholecystectomy or gallstone dissolution therapy. Ninety percent of these gallstones are cholesterol stones, while the remaining 10 percent are black or brown pigmented stones. *Pharmacological dissolution therapy has only been effective when treating cholesterol stones.*

When cholesterol stones are found, bile is frequently supersaturated with cholesterol and a high cholesterol-to-bile salt-lecithin ratio is present. Supersaturation is increased by prolonged fasting or poor gallbladder emptying. Since some intermittent supersaturation occurs normally, stone formers are also likely to be lacking inhibitors of nucleation.

Cholesterol stones can be identified by their lack of calcium seen on abdominal film or computed tomography of the abdomen. These stones also tend to float during oral cholecystography and ultrasound examination of the gallbladder.

Oral dissolution therapy has included the use of chenodeoxycholic acid (chenodiol, *Chenix*) and ursodeoxycholic acid (*Actigall*). Both of these compounds are naturally occurring bile acids, although only trace amounts of ursodeoxycholic acid are usually found in bile. While the mechanism by which they induce stone dissolution is unknown, both agents can markedly decrease the secretion rate of cholesterol, thereby desaturating the bile. The bile salt secretion rate is not increased. Dissolution is more likely to occur in patients who are nonobese, have a gallbladder that concentrates iodine dye during oral cholecystography, and have stones that contain noncalcified stones of less than 1.7 cm in diameter.

Chenodeoxycholic acid at 12 to 15 mg/kg/day or ursodeoxycholic acid at 8 to 12 mg/kg/day completely dissolves 20 to 60 percent of gallstones within 2 years of initiating therapy. After complete dissolution is documented, therapy should be continued for 1 to 3 months to dissolve particles that may be too small to be seen on ultrasound. Fifty percent of completely dissolved gallstones will later recur. Chenodeoxycholic acid, but not ursodeoxycholic acid, is associated with diarrhea, increases in hepatic enzyme levels, and rare hepatic injury. In addition, plasma low-density lipoprotein (LDL) cholesterol may increase slightly. Studies involving primary biliary cirrhosis and primary sclerosing cholangitis suggest that ursodeoxycholic acid is somewhat protective against hepatic injury from chronic hepatic cholestasis.

Methyltert-butyl ether (MTBE) will dissolve cholesterol gallstones within hours of its instillation into the gallbladder. It requires the insertion of a percutaneous transhepatic catheter that is itself resistant to dissolution; caution is required since placement may precipitate hemorrhage or infection. During instillation there is a disagreeable odor, a risk of explosion, and a dose-dependent nausea and vomiting. MTBE is a duodenal irritant and the solvent should not be permitted to drain out of the bile duct. Because of these drawbacks, the use of MTBE outside the gallbladder on common bile duct stones has been limited.

Monooctanoin (*Moctanin*) is a monoglyceride detergent that will completely dissolve common duct stones in 25 to 30 percent of patients and decrease stone size in another 20 percent. This occurs within 1 to 3 weeks of drug perfusion through a postsurgical T tube or through an endoscopically placed nasobiliary drain. During treatment, patients frequently complain of nausea, vomiting, diarrhea, and abdominal pain. Though this agent is not as fast-acting as MTBE and does not dissolve stones as completely, it is technically easier to use. Partial dissolution of stones also may allow easier endoscopic or radiological extraction of smaller stones that have been made softer, obviating a common bile duct surgical exploration.

Supplemental Reading

Carmichael, J.M., and Reddy, A.N. Rational approach to long-term use of H_2-antagonists. *Am. J. Med.* 82:796,1987.

Furness, J.B., and Costa, M. *The Enteric Nervous System.* New York: Churchill Livingstone, 1987.

Kromer, W. Endogenous and exogenous opioids in the control of gastrointestinal motility and secretion. *Pharmacol. Rev.* 40:87,1988.

Metoclopramide (*Reglan*) for gastroesophageal reflux. *Med. Lett. Drugs Ther.* 27:21,1985.

Misoprostol. *Med. Lett. Drugs Ther.* 31:21,1989.

Nizatidine (*Axid*). *Med. Lett. Drugs Ther.* 30:77,1988.

Porreca, F., Galligan, J.J., and Burks, T.F. Central opioid receptor involvement in gastrointestinal motility. *Trans. Pharmacol. Sci.* 7:104,1986.

Sachs, G., et al. Gastric H, K-ATPase as therapeutic target. *Annu. Rev. Pharmacol. Toxicol.* 28:269,1988.

Stenson, W.F. (ed.). Gastrointestinal pharmacology. *Gastroenterol. Clin. North Am.* 21:511,1992.

Urosodiol for dissolving cholesterol gallstones. *Med. Lett. Drugs Ther.* 30:81,1988.

74

Vitamins

Suzanne Barone

Vitamins are a group of unrelated chemical substances that are essential in small amounts for the regulation of normal metabolism, growth, and function of the human body. Not all the vitamins can be synthesized in the body and therefore some vitamins must be obtained from outside sources. A proper well-balanced diet provides a healthy person with an adequate supply of vitamins.

Vitamins become a pharmacological concern when there is an imbalance in the body's vitamin supply. Deficiency diseases can result from insufficient vitamin ingestion, irregular absorption, or impaired metabolic utilization of these nutrients. Hypervitaminosis, that is, the ingestion or administration of excessive quantities of vitamins, also may be pharmacologically significant since toxicity associated with vitamin overdosage may occur.

This chapter focuses on the pharmacological and toxicological properties of vitamins. A brief summary of the function and dietary sources of the various vitamins is given. The concept of a recommended dietary allowance and vitamin supplementation is outlined, followed by a discussion of deficiency diseases; the therapeutic use of vitamins; the adverse reactions associated with vitamin administration, including the toxicity of hypervitaminosis; and the potential systemic interaction of vitamins with therapeutic agents. The final portions of the chapter discuss anemia, a nutritional disease that can be induced by many drugs.

Physiological Function and Dietary Sources

Vitamins are usually classified as either fat-soluble (vitamins A, D, E, and K) or water-soluble (vitamins B and C) compounds. The fat-soluble vitamins are generally metabolized slowly and are stored in the liver. In contrast, the water-soluble vitamins are rapidly metabolized and are readily excreted in the urine.

Fat-Soluble Vitamins

Vitamin A

Vitamin A, or retinol, plays a role in a variety of physiological processes. This vitamin is essential for the proper maintenance of the functional and structural integrity of epithelial cells, and it plays a major role in epithelial differentiation. Bone development and growth in children have also been linked to adequate vitamin A intake. Vitamin A, when reduced to the aldehyde 11-*cis*-retinal, combines with opsin to produce the visual pigment *rhodopsin*. This pigment is present in the rods of the retina, and is partly responsible for the process of dark adaptation.

Principal dietary sources of vitamin A are milk fat (cheese and butter) and eggs. Since it is stored in the liver, inclusion of liver in the diet also provides vitamin A. A plant pigment, *carotene,* is a precursor for vitamin A and is present in highly pigmented vegetables, such as carrots, rutabaga, and red cabbage.

Vitamin D

Vitamin D is the collective term for a group of compounds formed by the action of ultraviolet irradiation on sterols. Cholecalciferol (vitamin D_3) and calciferol (vitamin D_2) are formed by the irradiation of the provitamins 7-dehydrocholesterol and ergosterol, respectively. The conversion to vitamin D_3 occurs in the skin. The liver is the principal storage site for vitamin D, and it is here that the vitamin is hydroxylated to form 25-hydroxyvitamin D. Additional hydroxylation to form 1,25-dihydroxyvitamin D occurs in the kidney in response to the need for calcium and phosphate. A discussion of the role of vitamin D in calcium homeostasis is provided in Chap. 70.

The major source of vitamin D in humans is sunlight irradiation of the skin. Milk, a major dietary source of calcium, has been fortified with vitamin D to facilitate the intestinal absorption of calcium.

Table 74-1. The B Vitamins

Vitamin	Active form	Role
Thiamine (B_1)	Thiamine pyrophosphate	Carbohydrate metabolism
Riboflavin (B_2)	Flavin adenine dinucleotide; flavin mononucleotide	Carbohydrate metabolism
Nicotinic acid (niacin)	Nicotinamide adenine dinucleotide	Dehydrogenation of proteins in cellular respiration
Pyridoxine (B_6)	Pyridoxal phosphate Pyridoxamine phosphate	Amino acid transformations
Pantothenic acid	Coenzyme A	Transfer of acetyl groups
Cyanocobalamin (B_{12})	—	Nucleic acid synthesis
Biotin	—	Fatty acid synthesis
Folic acid (folacin)	Pteroylglutamic acid–containing coenzymes	Nucleic acid synthesis, protein metabolism

Vitamin E

Vitamin E is a potent antioxidant that is capable of protecting polyunsaturated fatty acids from oxidative breakdown. This vitamin also functions to enhance vitamin A utilization. Although several other physiological actions have been suggested, to date no unifying concept exists to explain these actions.

Vitamin E (alpha tocopherol) is found in a variety of foodstuffs, the richest sources being plant oils, including wheat germ and rice, and the lipids of green leaves.

Vitamin K

Vitamin K activity is associated with several quinones, including phylloquinone (vitamin K_1), menadione (vitamin K_3), and a variety of menaquinones (vitamin K_2). These quinones promote the synthesis of proteins that are involved in the coagulation of blood. These proteins include prothrombin, factor VII (proconvertin), factor IX (plasma thromboplastin), and factor X (Stuart factor). A detailed discussion of blood coagulation is found in Chap. 27.

The vitamin K quinones are obtained from three major sources. Vitamin K_1 is present in various plants, especially green vegetables. The menaquinones that possess vitamin K_2 activity are synthesized by bacteria, particularly gram-positive organisms; the bacteria in the gut of animals produce useful quantities of this vitamin. Vitamin K_3 is a chemically synthesized quinone that possesses the same activity as vitamin K_1.

Water-Soluble Vitamins

Vitamin B

This vitamin group is made up of different substances that tend to occur together in foods and are given the collective name *vitamin B complex.* The vitamins of the B group usually have to be converted to an active form, and most of them play a vital role in intracellular metabolism. These vitamins are listed in Table 74-1.

The distribution of the vitamin B complex is widespread. The B vitamins are obtained from both meat and vegetable products, except for vitamin B_{12}, which occurs only in animal products. The richest source of the B vitamin group is seeds, including the germ of wheat or of rice.

Vitamin C

Vitamin C (ascorbic acid) is essential for the maintenance of the ground substance that binds cells together and for the formation and maintenance of collagen. The exact biochemical role it plays in subserving these functions is not known, but it may be related to its ability to act as an oxidation-reduction system.

Vitamin C is found in fresh fruit and vegetables. It is very water soluble, is readily destroyed by heat, especially in an alkaline medium; and is rapidly oxidized in air. Enzymes present in organelles of fruit and vegetables can catalyze the oxidation of vitamin C, especially if the plants have been damaged. For this reason, fruit and vegetables that have been stored in air, cut or bruised, washed or cooked, may have lost much of their vitamin C content.

Recommended Dietary Allowances and Vitamin Supplementation

Recommended dietary allowances (RDAs) are the levels of intake of essential nutrients that are considered to be adequate to meet the known nutritional needs of practically all healthy persons. The allowances were revised in 1989 by the Food and Nutrition Board of the National

Academy of Sciences–National Research Council. These allowances exceed the minimum requirement that is necessary to prevent deficiencies in healthy populations. In addition to allowances for vitamins, RDAs were developed for essential minerals, including calcium, phosphorus, magnesium, iron, zinc, iodine, and selenium. A varied diet containing a wide range of foodstuffs provides more than the RDA of each vitamin, and *supplementing these amounts will have no beneficial effect and may result in the toxicity associated with hypervitaminosis.* Since these recommendations are given for healthy populations in general and not for individuals, special problems, such as premature birth, inherited metabolic disorders, infections, chronic disease, and use of medications, are not covered by the RDAs. Separate RDAs have been developed for pregnant and lactating women. Vitamin supplementation may be required in patients with these special conditions as well as in groups who do not consume an appropriate diet.

Deficiency Diseases

Medical personnel who work in affluent areas are unlikely to see large numbers of people suffering from vitamin deficiency diseases. However, certain groups of the population are particularly at risk, such as low-income families. An awareness of both the symptoms and the vulnerable groups will facilitate the recognition of these diseases.

The classic symptoms of any vitamin deficiency disease, as observed in laboratory animals, are often blurred in humans. In most cases, the nutritional deficiency is not confined to one specific substance. The clinical picture is often complicated by deficiencies of other vitamins, minerals, calories, and protein, and the presence of infections and parasite infestations, which usually accompany longstanding malnutrition.

It is the nonspecific nature of the early symptoms that makes a diagnosis of vitamin deficiency difficult. Biochemical, physiological, and behavioral changes can occur in the marginal deficiency state, without or before the appearance of more specific symptoms. Since the nonspecificity of these changes makes them difficult to detail, this section focuses on the symptoms associated with individual vitamin deficiency diseases.

Vitamin A

An early sign of hypovitaminosis A is night blindness. This condition is related to the role of vitamin A as the prosthetic group of the visual pigment rhodopsin. The night blindness may progress to *xerophthalmia* (dryness and ulceration of the cornea) and blindness. Other symptoms of vitamin A deficiency include cessation of growth and skin changes due to hyperkeratosis.

Since vitamin A is a fat-soluble vitamin, any disease that results in fat malabsorption and impaired liver storage brings with it the risk of vitamin A deficiency; these conditions include biliary tract disease, pancreatic disease, sprue, and hepatic cirrhosis. One group at great risk are children from low-income families, who tend to lack fresh vegetables (carotene) and dairy products (vitamin A) in the diet.

Vitamin B

Thiamine

Severe thiamine (vitamin B_1) deficiency results in a disease known as *beriberi.* The symptoms vary widely and can include growth retardation, muscular weakness, apathy, edema, and heart failure. Neurological symptoms, such as personality changes and mental deterioration, also may be present in severe cases. Because of the role played by thiamine in metabolic processes in all cells, a mild deficiency may occur when energy needs are increased.

Since thiamine is widely distributed in food, beriberi is rare except in communities existing on a single staple cereal food. The disease does occur with some frequency in alcoholics, whose poor diet may lead to an inadequate daily intake of thiamine.

Riboflavin

Riboflavin (vitamin B_2) deficiency results in a localized seborrheic dermatitis that may be limited to the face and scrotum. Other symptoms of *ariboflavinosis* include angular stomatitis, cheilitis, and glossitis. Specific ocular signs include vascularization of the cornea and keratitis.

This deficiency usually occurs in association with deficiency of other B complex vitamins.

Nicotinic Acid

Niacin deficiency results in the appearance of the symptoms of *pellagra.* The clinical picture progresses from an initial phase of general malaise to symptoms including photosensitivity, sore and swollen tongue, gastritis, and diarrhea. Neurological disturbances, depression, and apathy also may occur.

Both niacin and the amino acid tryptophan can be converted to diphosphopyridine nucleotide (NAD) and triphosphopyridine nucleotide (NADP). These reactions require the presence of thiamine, riboflavin, and pyridoxine. Therefore, treatment of the symptoms of pellagra should include, in addition to B complex vitamin supplementation, an intake of dietary proteins to provide adequate amounts of tryptophan.

Pyridoxine

Pyridoxine (vitamin B_6) deficiency symptoms vary, but generally they are expressed as alterations in the skin, blood, and central nervous system (CNS). Symptoms include sensory neuritis, mental depression, and convulsions. A hypochromic, sideroblastic anemia also may result. Since pyridoxine is required for the conversion of tryptophan to NAD and NADP, pellagra-like symptoms can occur with vitamin B_6 deficiency. This deficiency is found most often in conjunction with other B complex deficiencies.

Pantothenic Acid

The symptoms of pantothenic acid deficiency have not been clinically described. Since pantothenic acid is a ubiquitous vitamin, isolated deficiency is unlikely. However, marginal deficiency may exist in persons with generalized malnutrition.

Cyanocobalamin

Cyanocobalamin (vitamin B_{12}) deficiency results in pernicious anemia that is characterized by megaloblastic anemia and neuropathies. Since this vitamin is found in almost all animal products, dietary deficiencies are rare, except in some strict vegetarians. Vitamin B_{12} is recycled by an effective enterohepatic circulation and thus has a very long half-life.

Absorption of vitamin B_{12} from the gastrointestinal tract requires the presence of gastric *intrinsic factor*. This factor binds to the vitamin, forming a complex that can now be absorbed in the terminal ileum. Lack of this factor results in pernicious anemia. Following a gastrectomy, patients must be given vitamin B_{12} parenterally.

Biotin

Biotin deficiency is characterized by anorexia, nausea, vomiting, glossitis, depression, and dry, scaly dermatitis. Biotin deficiency occurs when *avidin,* a biotin-binding glycoprotein, is present. Avidin, which is found in raw egg whites, binds the biotin, making it nutritionally unavailable.

Folic Acid

Folic acid deficiency symptoms include megaloblastic anemia, glossitis, diarrhea, and weight loss. The requirement for this vitamin increases during pregnancy and lactation.

Vitamin C

The deficiency disease associated with a lack of ascorbic acid is called *scurvy*. Early symptoms include malaise and follicular hyperkeratosis. Capillary fragility results in hemorrhages, particularly of the gums. Abnormal bone and teeth development can occur in growing children. The body's requirement for vitamin C increases during periods of stress such as pregnancy and lactation.

Vitamin D

The principal disorder that is associated with inadequate vitamin D intake is *rickets*. The low blood calcium and phosphate levels that occur during vitamin D deficiency stimulate parathyroid hormone secretion to restore calcium levels (see Chap. 70). In children, this deficiency leads to the formation of soft bones that become deformed easily; in adults, osteomalacia results from the removal of calcium from the bone.

Vitamin D deficiency may occur in patients with metabolic disorders, such as hypoparathyroidism and renal osteodystrophy. The requirement for vitamin D is slightly higher in members of darker-pigmented races, since melanin interferes with the irradiation that produces vitamin D_3 in the skin.

Vitamin E

Deficiency of vitamin E is characterized by low serum *tocopherol* levels and a positive hydrogen peroxide hemolysis test. This deficiency is believed to occur in patients with biliary, pancreatic, or intestinal disease that is characterized by excessive steatorrhea. Premature infants with a high intake of fatty acids exhibit a deficiency syndrome characterized by edema, anemia, and low tocopherol levels. This condition is reversed by giving vitamin E.

Vitamin K

Vitamin K deficiency results in an increased bleeding time. This hypoprothrombinemia may lead to hemorrhage from the gastrointestinal tract, urinary tract, and nasal mucosa. In normal, healthy adults, deficiency is rare. The two groups at greatest risk include newborn infants and patients receiving anticoagulant therapy. Hypoprothrombinemia preexists in these two groups. Any disease that causes the malabsorption of fats may lead to deficiency. Inhibition of the growth of intestinal bacteria from extended antibiotic therapy will result in a decreased vitamin K synthesis and possible deficiency. Proper dietary vitamin K intake is required under these conditions.

Vitamin Deficiency Disease— Therapeutic Uses

All of the vitamins are used as specific treatments for their respective deficiency diseases. The dosages required will vary according to the severity of the disease and the vitamin involved. It must be stressed that administration of high dosages of vitamins, especially fat-soluble vitamins, for prolonged periods may lead to toxicity.

Cancer

Vitamin A can suppress many chemically induced tumors in the laboratory. Epidemiological evidence suggests that foods rich in carotenes or vitamin A are associated with a lower risk of cancer. However, the National Research Council Committee on Diet, Nutrition and Cancer argues against the use of vitamin A supplementation because of the toxicities produced by large amounts of this vitamin.

The antioxidant properties of vitamins C and E can inhibit the formation of some carcinogens. However, the data are not sufficient to draw conclusions about the vitamins' effects on human cancers.

Miscellaneous Uses

Vitamin A and its retinoid analogues have gained popularity in the treatment of acne and other dermatological diseases. Chapter 46 presents an in-depth discussion of the various analogue preparations, their uses, and side effects.

Vitamin K supplements are given to neonates until normal intestinal bacteria that are capable of producing the vitamin develop.

Niacin has been used clinically to lower serum cholesterol levels. Nicotinic acid is used as adjunctive therapy in patients with hyperlipidemia. It is one of the drugs of first choice for patients who do not respond adequately to diet and weight loss.

Vitamin Toxicity

Toxic effects have been observed when large dosages of some vitamins are ingested. Generally the water-soluble vitamins are less toxic, since excess quantities are usually excreted in the urine. Excessive amounts of fat-soluble vitamins, however, are stored in the body, thus making toxic levels of these vitamins easier to obtain.

Vitamin A

Acute hypervitaminosis A results in drowsiness, headache, vomiting, papilledema, and a bulging fontanel in infants. The symptoms of chronic toxicity include scaly skin, hair loss, brittle nails, and hepatosplenomegaly. In children, anorexia, irritability, and swelling of the bones have been seen. Retardation of growth also may occur. Vitamin A is teratogenic in large amounts; therefore, dosages that exceed the RDA should not be given during a normal pregnancy.

Vitamin D

The hypercalcemia that develops with the condition of hypervitaminosis D is responsible for the toxic symptoms. Muscle weakness, bone pain, anorexia, ectopic calcification, hypertension, and cardiac arrhythmias may occur. Toxicity in infants can result in mental and physical retardation, renal failure, and death.

Vitamin E

Large dosages of vitamin E over a long period of time may result in the symptoms of muscle weakness, fatigue, headache, and nausea. This toxicity can be reversed by discontinuing the large-dose supplementation.

Vitamin K

Toxicity of vitamin K has not been well defined. Jaundice may occur in a newborn if large dosages of vitamin K are given to the mother before birth. Although kernicterus may result, this can be prevented by using vitamin K_1.

Vitamin B Complex

Pyridoxine

Large dosages of pyridoxine have been reported to cause peripheral neuropathies. Ataxia and numbness of the hands and feet as well as impairment of the senses of pain, touch, and temperature may result.

Nicotinic Acid

Excessive niacin intake may result in flushing, pruritus, and gastrointestinal disturbances. These symptoms are due to niacin's ability to cause the release of histamine. Large dosages of nicotinic acid can result in hepatic toxicity.

Table 74-2. Primary Intestinal Absorptive Defects Induced by Drugs

Drug	Use	Malabsorption or fecal nutrient loss	Mechanism
Mineral oil	Laxative	Carotene, vitamins A, D, K	Physical barrier Nutrients dissolve in mineral oil and are lost ↓ Micelle formation
Phenolphthalein	Laxative	Vitamin D, Ca	Intestinal hurry K depletion Loss of structural integrity
Neomycin	Antibiotic to "sterilize" gut	Fat, nitrogen, Na, K, Ca, Fe, lactose, sucrose, vitamin B_{12}	Structural defect ↓ Pancreatic lipase Binding of bile acids (salts)
Cholestyramine	Hypocholesterolemic agent Bile acid sequestrant	Fat, vitamins A, K, B_{12}, D, Fe	Binding of bile acids (salts) and nutrients, e.g., Fe
Potassium chloride	Potassium repletion	Vitamin B_{12}	↓ Ileal pH
Colchicine	Antiinflammatory agent in gout	Fat, carotene, Na, K, vitamin B_{12}, lactose	Mitotic arrest Structural defect Enzyme damage
Biguanides (metformin, phenformin)	Hypoglycemic agents (in diabetes)	Vitamin B_{12}	Competitive inhibition of vitamin B_{12} absorption
p-Aminosalicylic acid	Antituberculosis agent	Fat, folate, vitamin B_{12}	Mucosal block in vitamin B_{12} uptake
Salicylazosulfapyridine (sulfasalazine, *Azulfidine*)	Antiinflammatory agent in ulcerative colitis and regional enteritis	Folate	Mucosal block in folate uptake

Source: From D.A. Roe, *Drug-Induced Nutritional Deficiencies.* Westport, Conn.: AVI Publishing Co., 1978. Table 5.1, p. 130.

Vitamin C

Megavitamin intake of vitamin C may result in diarrhea due to intestinal irritation. Since ascorbic acid is partially metabolized and excreted as oxalate, renal oxalate stones may form in some patients.

Vitamin–Drug Interactions

Drug interactions and the adverse effects that can result are of special concern to members of the medical profession. Although vitamins are not always thought of as being drugs, these nutrients can interact with drugs and result in a variety of effects. Vitamin–drug interactions can produce either a decrease or an increase in the effectiveness of the drug or, conversely, the intake of drugs can affect the disposition of vitamins in the body. A common site of interaction is the gastrointestinal tract. Many drugs can produce vitamin malabsorption, resulting in a drug-induced nutrient depletion and hypovitaminosis. Table 74-2 lists some common vitamin absorptive defects produced by drugs. Both fat-soluble and water-soluble vitamins can be affected by drug intake. Some of the more common drug–vitamin interactions are examined in this section.

Vitamin A

Vitamin A absorption from the small intestine requires the presence of dietary fat and pancreatic lipase to break down retinyl esters and bile salts to promote the uptake of retinol and carotene. Drugs, such as mineral oil, neomycin, and cholestyramine, that can modify lipid absorption from the gastrointestinal tract can impair vitamin A absorption. Several mechanisms involved in such interactions are listed in Table 74-2. The use of oral contraceptives can significantly increase plasma vitamin A levels.

Since alcohol dehydrogenase is required for the conversion of retinol to retinal, excessive and prolonged ethanol ingestion can impair the physiological function of vitamin A. The decreased conversion of retinol to retinal results from a competitive utilization of the enzyme by alcohol. Night blindness may result, since the visual cycle is a retinol-dependent physiological process.

Vitamin D

Many drugs can affect the absorption or metabolism of vitamin D. Laxatives and agents that bind bile salts inhibit the gastrointestinal absorption of vitamin D. The glucocorticoids in high dosages may interfere with the hepatic metabolism of vitamin D. Prolonged administration of hepatic microsomal enzyme inducers such as phenobarbital, phenytoin, primidone, and glutethimide can lead to an accelerated degradation of vitamin D_3 to form inactive metabolites. The synthesis of vitamin D_3 can be impaired by physical and chemical barriers to ultraviolet light (e.g., sunscreens).

Vitamin K

In addition to the drugs listed in Table 74-2 that inhibit vitamin K absorption, the most common group of drugs that produce vitamin K deficiency are the coumarin anticoagulants. The hypoprothrombinemic effects of dicumarol can be overcome by administration of vitamin K.

Vitamin C

Oral contraceptives decrease the plasma levels of ascorbic acid. Aspirin has also been shown to decrease tissue levels of vitamin C. The renal excretion of acidic and basic drugs may be altered when administered with large doses of vitamin C.

Vitamin B Complex

Folic Acid

Many drugs interact with folate to affect its absorption, antagonize its biochemical activity, or increase its loss from the body. These drugs include ethanol, phenytoin, and oral contraceptives. Salicylates can compete with folic acid for plasma protein binding. Methotrexate, a cytotoxic agent, is a folate antagonist that inhibits the biosynthesis of this coenzyme.

Pyridoxine

Many drug classes have been shown to act either as vitamin B_6 antagonists or to increase vitamin B_6 turnover. Alcohol decreases the production of pyridoxal phosphate, the coenzyme formed from vitamin B_6. Hydrazines, such as isoniazid (INH), act as coenzyme inhibitors. Cycloserine, an antitubercular drug, and penicillamine, a chelating agent, inactivate the coenzyme. Steroid hormones, such as those present in oral contraceptive preparations, compete with the coenzyme. Pyridoxine can decrease the efficacy of levodopa, an antiparkinsonian drug, by stimulating the decarboxylation of dopa to dopamine in peripheral tissues. Phenobarbital and phenytoin serum levels may be decreased following pyridoxine supplementation.

Vitamin B$_{12}$

Four groups of drugs have been shown to affect the absorption of vitamin B_{12}. These drugs include the oral hypoglycemic biguanides, colchicine, ethanol, and aminosalicylic acid.

Niacin

Drug-induced niacin deficiency has resulted from the use of isonicotinic acid hydrazide, which interferes with the conversion of niacin from tryptophan. Administration of alcohol as well as the antimetabolites 6-mercaptopurine and 5-fluorouracil also may lead to niacin deficiency. Niacin can decrease the effectiveness of several drugs. The uricosuric effects of sulfinpyrazone and probenecid may be inhibited by nicotinic acid.

Riboflavin

Riboflavin absorption is decreased by hypermotility of intestinal contents. Drugs that increase motility or those that induce diarrhea may decrease riboflavin absorption. Hyperthyroidism and the administration of thyroxine also reduce riboflavin absorption.

Thiamine

The main drug to interact with thiamine, resulting in deficiency, is alcohol. Alcoholics may have both a decreased intake and absorption of thiamine. The presence of liver disease can prevent the formation of the active coenzyme.

Anemia

Anemia occurs when the hemoglobin concentration of blood is reduced below normal levels. This condition may result from chronic blood loss, abnormal hemolysis, or nutritional deficiency. Many therapeutic agents can induce this change in hemoglobin as an unwanted side effect.

There are many different classifications of anemia. The physiological classification categorizes the different types of anemia according to the pathophysiological factor involved in inducing the decreased hemoglobin concentration. Anemias due to cell hypoproliferation include aplastic anemia and iron deficiency anemia. Hemolytic anemia results from excessive destruction of red blood cells. Megaloblastic anemia, sideroblastic anemia, and iron deficiency anemia result from an abnormality in the maturation of red blood cells.

This section focuses on the nutritional anemias, including iron deficiency anemia, megaloblastic anemia, and sideroblastic anemia. Treatment of these conditions involves replacement of the deficient compound.

Iron Deficiency Anemia

Iron is a constituent of hemoglobin, and iron deficiency will lead to a decrease in hemoglobin synthesis. Since iron is conserved by the body, deficiency usually results from acute or chronic loss of blood or insufficient iron intake during physiological stress. Infants, children, and premenopausal women require more iron than do men because of the increased demand that occurs during growth, pregnancy, and loss of blood during menstruation. In tropical climates, bleeding due to an infestation by the hookworm parasite is a common cause of iron deficiency.

The symptoms of iron deficiency anemia include fatigue, weakness, shortness of breath, and soreness of the tongue. Therapeutic iron supplementation is used to treat this type of anemia. Oral administration of ferrous salts (generic ferrous sulfate, *Feosol, Fero-Gradumet*) is preferred, but parenteral iron (iron dextran, *Imferon*) can be given if oral therapy fails. Toxic reactions occur more frequently after parenteral iron administration. Gastrointestinal disturbances are common following oral dosages. Health care providers should counsel patients that iron supplements are toxic and should be kept out of the reach of children. In 1991, Poison Control Centers reported 11 deaths of children following accidental ingestion of iron-containing preparations.

Megaloblastic Anemia

Megaloblastic anemia is characterized by large cells in the bone marrow and blood due to a defective maturation of hematopoietic cells. Folic acid or vitamin B_{12} deficiency will result in this type of anemia. Malabsorption, impaired utilization, chronic infections, and drugs can lead to folic acid or vitamin B_{12} deficiency.

Folic acid or folate salts (*Folvite*) are administered to correct folate-deficient megaloblastic anemia. Vitamin B_{12}–deficient patients receive cyanocobalamin supplements. Vitamin B_{12} deficiency due to a lack of gastric intrinsic factor results in pernicious anemia. This type of megaloblastic anemia results in neurological damage if it is not treated. Parenteral injections of vitamin B_{12} or oral preparations containing both vitamin B_{12} and intrinsic factor (*Biopar Forte*) must be given.

Sideroblastic Anemia

Sideroblastic anemia is characterized by excessive iron in the cells that cannot be incorporated into porphyrin to form heme. Although it is rare, the most common cause of sideroblastic anemia is alcoholism and pyridoxine deficiency. Pyridoxine is required for the formation of pyridoxal phosphate, a coenzyme in porphyrin synthesis.

Supplemental Reading

Bender, D.A. *Nutritional Biochemistry of the Vitamins.* Cambridge: Cambridge University Press, 1992.

Combs, G.F. *The Vitamins: Fundamental Aspects in Nutrition and Health.* San Diego, Calif. Academic Press, 1992.

Food and Nutrition Board, National Research Council. *Recommended Dietary Allowances* (10th ed.). Washington, D.C.: National Academy Press, 1989.

Gaby, S., et al. *Vitamin Intake and Health: A Scientific Review.* New York: Marcel Dekker, 1991.

Udall, J.N., and Greene, H.L. Vitamin update. *Pediatr. Rev.* 13:185, 1992.

75

Drugs for the Control of Supragingival Plaque

Angelo Mariotti and *Arthur F. Hefti*

The periodontium, which is responsible for the retention of teeth in the maxilla and mandible, consists of four different tissue types. *Cementum* and *alveolar bone* are the hard tissues to which the fibrous *periodontal ligament* anchors the tooth into the skeleton, and the *gingiva* is the covering tissue of the periodontium (Fig. 75-1). The gingiva is a unique body tissue in that it allows the penetration of calcified tissue (i.e., teeth) into an intact mucosa, while protecting the underlying periodontal tissues. The accumulation of microorganisms on the tooth surface can alter the structure and function of the gingiva, inducing an oral inflammatory disease called gingivitis.

During adolescence the occurrence of gingivitis is almost universal and in adulthood affects approximately 50 percent of the population. Because of the frequent appearance of gingivitis, this disease remains a principal concern for the dentist since it can be converted to other, more destructive, forms of periodontal disease. Hence, the prevention or cure of gingivitis is of particular interest.

The most common method of eliminating gingivitis is by the mechanical removal of the microorganisms found in plaque via toothbrush and floss. However, effective mechanical removal of plaque is a tedious, time-consuming process that is affected by an individual's gingival architecture, tooth position, dexterity, and motivation. Consequently, incomplete removal of dental plaque by mechanical means allows for the induction or continued progression, or both, of gingivitis. Therefore, pharmacological agents that prevent or reduce plaque can aid the dentist by effectively preventing or eliminating gingival inflammation. Accordingly, the development of safe and effective, topically applied liquid antimicrobial agents will help in the maintenance of healthy gingival tissues. This chapter examines the relationship of supragingival plaque to gingivitis and the unique pharmacokinetic characteristics of common antiplaque rinsing agents.

The Role of Supragingival Plaque in the Initiation of Gingivitis

Many different types of materials will accumulate on teeth. By far the most ubiquitous and important deposit is plaque. Plaque consists primarily of microorganisms in an organized matrix of organic and inorganic components. Bacteria account for at least 70 percent of the mass of plaque. In fact, one cubic millimeter of dental plaque contains more than 100 million bacteria consisting of as many as 400 different species. The organic matrix of plaque consists of polysaccharide, protein, and lipid components while the inorganic matrix is comprised principally of calcium and phosphorous ions.

Dental plaque can be separated into two distinct, but dependent, categories depending on location of plaque in relation to the gingiva. The dental plaque found above the gingival margin of the tooth is designated as supragingival and the dental plaque found below the gingival margin (i.e., in the gingival sulcus) is called subgingival. There is indisputable evidence that supragingival plaque is responsible for gingivitis. Numerous studies have demonstrated that gingivitis can be experimentally induced in a noninflamed periodontium by allowing the unimpeded accumulation of supragingival plaque, and is reversed by the thorough and complete removal of supragingival plaque.

Gingivitis is due principally to the accumulation and retention of plaque coronal to the gingival margin. The accumulation of supragingival plaque is also a prime influence in the development of subgingival plaque. As undisturbed plaque matures, it changes in composition and becomes more complex. A bacterial succession occurs whereby microorganisms associated with gingival health, that is, gram-positive rods and cocci, are replaced by microorganisms associated with gingivitis, that is, gram-

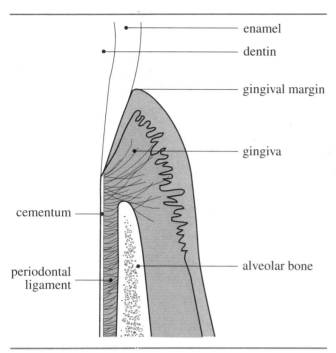

enamel

dentin

gingival margin

gingiva

cementum

alveolar bone

periodontal
ligament

Figure 75-1. Diagram of anatomic landmarks in the periodontium.

negative cocci and rods, as well as spiral-shaped organisms and spirochetes. As a consequence of the change in microflora, the inflammation-induced changes in the gingiva cause an increase in epithelial cell turnover and connective tissue degradation, resulting in anatomical changes that tend to expose the gingival sulcus to the oral environment. This change in the subgingival environment provides a new niche for bacteria to grow because it is continually bathed by exudate from the gingival crevice and end products from the supragingival plaque. Hence, control of supragingival plaque will also have a profound influence on the developing composition of periodontitis-associated subgingival plaque.

Pharmacokinetics of the Oral Cavity

The therapeutic outcome of topically applied liquid agents (i.e., rinses) used to control oral infections will depend on the characteristics of drugs that take advantage of the unique physiologic and anatomic circumstances found in the oral cavity. Listed in this section is a broad overview of important oral pharmacokinetic principles.

Absorption

The vascularity of the oral cavity, combined with a thin epithelial lining, allows for the absorption of drugs at a rapid rate. Nonionized drugs, such as nitroglycerin, take advantage of these tissue characteristics and diffuse rapidly across the oral mucosa into the bloodstream. Unlike most drugs, for which the principal objective is to introduce the agent into the bloodstream rapidly, the goal of rinsing agents is to be retained in the oral cavity for as long as possible. Thus, the rapid passage of an agent from its site of action in the oral cavity into the bloodstream is a distinct disadvantage in controlling plaque levels, since absorption can lead to toxic effects elsewhere in the body and a significant reduction of the free drug in the oral cavity. Therefore, agents with a very low degree of membrane permeability are best suited for oral retention and control of supragingival plaque levels. In most instances, the drugs used to restrain plaque levels are highly ionized and, therefore, are generally unable to penetrate the oral mucosa.

Distribution

Once an agent is topically applied in the oral cavity, the free drug can act at the primary site (i.e., bacteria in the plaque) or it can be partitioned to compartments where the drug binds nonspecifically. These drug reservoirs include the enamel, dentin and/or cementum of the tooth, the gingiva and alveolar mucosa, the organic and inorganic components of plaque, and salivary proteins.

The fraction of the administered dose that is nonspecifically bound to oral reservoirs is highly dependent on the concentration, amount of time, and chemical nature of the agent used. For example, a 1-minute rinse with 0.2% chlorhexidine will result in approximately 30 percent of the total amount dispensed being retained, whereas a 3-minute rinse with 0.1% sodium fluoride will result in less than 1 percent of the administered dose being found in the oral cavity after one hour. The ability of oral agents to nonspecifically and reversibly bind to oral reservoirs is an important quality in order for a sustained release of drugs to occur.

Metabolism

In the oral cavity, drug metabolism occurs in mucosal epithelial cells, microorganisms, and enzymes found in the saliva, as well as in renal and hepatic tissue once the drug is swallowed. Although biotransformation of agents in the oral cavity is potentially an important aspect of reducing effective drug concentrations, quantitatively it accounts only for a small percentage of drug inactivation.

Excretion

In most cases, drugs are cleared from the oral cavity by expectoration and salivary flow. In fact, salivary flow is

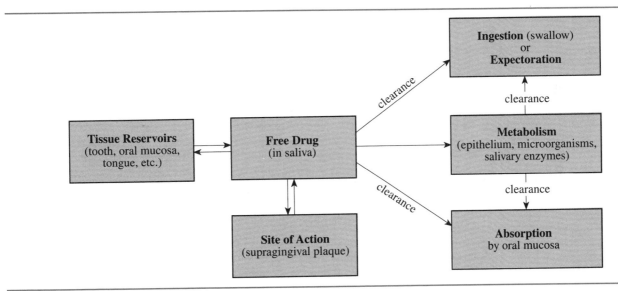

Figure 75-2. Schematic representation of pharmacokinetic factors that affect substantivity of rinsing agents.

extremely important in the removal of many agents from the oral cavity. Human saliva has a diurnal flow that varies between 500 and 1,500 ml in the daytime to less than 10 ml of secretion at night. For instance, 1 gm sucrose placed in the mouth at night would remain three times longer in the oral cavity than the same amount placed in the mouth in the morning. The rate of clearance of a drug from the oral cavity is, therefore, of profound importance in determining the duration of time a drug is in contact with the tooth surface.

Substantivity

The period of time that a drug is in contact with a particular substrate in the oral cavity is defined as *substantivity*. Drugs that have a prolonged duration of contact are considered to have high substantivity. Substantivity in the oral cavity depends on two important pharmacokinetic features: the degree of reversible, nonspecific binding to oral reservoirs and the rate of clearance by salivary flow (Fig. 75-2).

Oral reservoirs are an important source for the continued release of drugs. The oral compartments that accumulate a drug must be able to reversibly bind large portions of the administered dose and release therapeutic concentrations of free drug to the site of action over long periods of time. Therefore, effective antiplaque rinsing agents with high substantivity ideally would not bind irreversibly or with high affinity to oral reservoirs.

Salivary flow also will significantly affect the substantivity of topically applied liquid agents. The clearance of an agent from the oral cavity is directly proportional to the rate of salivary flow. Hence, during periods of high salivary flow there would need to be a greater release of drug from oral reservoirs in order to maintain therapeutic concentrations. Strategies that utilize natural or drug-induced periods of low salivary flow can increase the substantivity of an oral agent.

Antimicrobial Rinsing Agents

Chlorhexidine

In 1954, it was discovered that certain bisbiguanides had broad-spectrum antibacterial activity. One particular bisbiguanide, chlorhexidine, was found to have significant bacteriostatic and bactericidal properties. Subsequently, it was used as a skin disinfectant as well as in the treatment of dermatological infections. In 1962, it was introduced into experimental dentistry as a potential inhibitor of calculus formation. It was soon found, however, that chlorhexidine had an even more striking effect as an inhibitor of plaque formation.

General Properties

Chlorhexidine is a symmetrical cationic molecule consisting of two 4-chlorophenyl rings and two biguanide groups connected by a central hexamethylene chain. It is a strong base and is most stable as a salt; the highly water-soluble digluconate is the most commonly used preparation. Because of its cationic properties, it binds strongly to hydroxyapatite (the mineral component of tooth enamel), the organic pellicle on the tooth surface, salivary proteins, and bacteria. Much of the chlorhexidine binding in the

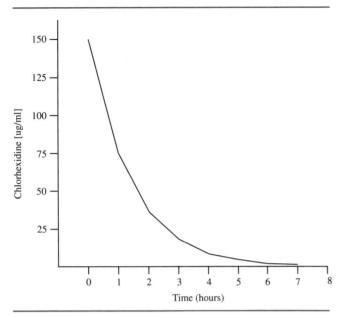

Figure 75-3. The clearance of chlorhexidine from oral cavity.

mouth occurs on the mucous membranes, such as the alveolar and gingival mucosa, from which sites it is slowly released in active form.

Pharmacokinetics

The rate of clearance of chlorhexidine from the mouth after one mouth rinse with 10 ml of a 0.2% aqueous solution follows approximately first-order kinetics, with a half-life of 60 min and initial concentration of 150 mg/ml (Fig. 75-3). This means that following application of a single rinse with a 0.2% chlorhexidine solution, the concentration of the compound exceeds the minimum inhibitory concentration (MIC) for oral streptococci (5 mg/ml) for almost 5 hr. The pronounced substantivity, as well as the relative susceptibility of oral streptococci, may account for the great effectiveness of chlorhexidine in inhibiting supragingival plaque formation.

Mechanisms of Action

Comparable to other disinfectants, chlorhexidine's spectrum of antibacterial activity is broad and not specific. Although chlorhexidine affects virtually all bacteria, gram-positive bacteria are more susceptible than gram-negative bacteria. Furthermore, *Streptococcus mutans* and *Actinomyces viscosus* seem to be particularly sensitive. *Streptococcus mutans* has been associated with the formation of carious lesions in fissures and on interproximal tooth surfaces, and has been identified in large numbers in plaque and saliva samples of subjects with high caries activity.

Applications of chlorhexidine as a 0.2% mouthwash have therefore been suggested to be a valuable measure in caries prevention.

Low concentrations of chlorhexidine are bacteriostatic, and high concentrations are bactericidal. Bacteriostasis is the result of chlorhexidine binding to the negatively charged bacterial cell wall (e.g., lipopolysaccharides), where it interferes with membrane transport systems. Oral streptococci take up sugars via the phosphoenolpyruvate-mediated phosphotransferase (PEP-PTS) system. The PEP-PTS is a carrier-mediated, group translocating process in which a number of soluble and membrane-bound enzymes catalyze the transfer of the phosphoryl moiety of PEP to the sugar substrate with the formation of sugar phosphate and pyruvate. Chlorhexidine is known to abolish the activity of the PTS at bactericidal concentrations. High chlorhexidine concentrations cause intracellular protein precipitation and subsequent cell death. Despite its pronounced effect on plaque formation, no detectable changes in resistance of plaque bacteria were found in a 6-month longitudinal study of mouth rinses.

Clinical Use

Initially, chlorhexidine was used in studies examining the inhibition of calculus formation. The investigators observed that a 0.1% solution of chlorhexidine diacetate almost completely inhibited new formation of calcified supragingival plaque, with few, if any, side effects at drug concentrations as low as 0.05%. The advantage of chlorhexidine rinses in preventing supragingival plaque formation was subsequently established in numerous short- and long-term clinical studies.

The previous routine treatment for cases of severe chronic gingivitis consisted of calculus and plaque removal, and oral hygiene instructions. Subsequent resolution of the gingival inflammation was largely dependent on the successful daily plaque control by the patient. However, the use of a 0.1 to 0.2% chlorhexidine mouthwash supplementing daily plaque control will facilitate the patient's effort to fight new plaque formation and to resolve gingivitis. Consequently, use of chlorhexidine is indicated in the following situations: in disinfection of the oral cavity before dental treatment; as an adjunct during initial therapy, especially in cases of rapidly progressive periodontitis and localized juvenile periodontitis; following periodontal surgery; and in handicapped patients.

Adverse Effects and Toxicity

The most conspicuous side effect of chlorhexidine is the development of a yellow to brownish extrinsic stain on the teeth and soft tissues in some patients. The discoloration on tooth surfaces is extremely tenacious, and a professional tooth cleaning using strong abrasives is necessary to remove it completely. The staining is dose dependent and variation in severity is pronounced between individuals. The side effect is attributed to the cationic nature of the antiseptic. Desquamative soft tissue lesions have also been reported with use of drug concentrations exceeding 0.2%, or after prolonged application. A frequently observed side effect is impaired taste sensation. It was reported that rinsing with a 0.2% aqueous solution of chlorhexidine digluconate resulted in a significant and selective change in taste perception for salt, but not for sweet, bitter, and sour.

In vitro, chlorhexidine can adversely affect gingival fibroblast attachment to root surfaces. Furthermore, protein production in human gingival fibroblasts is reduced at chlorhexidine concentrations that would not affect cell proliferation. Such findings corroborate earlier studies showing delayed wound healing in standardized mucosal wounds after rinsing with 0.5% chlorhexidine solution.

As an oral rinsing agent, no toxic systemic effects of chlorhexidine have been reported to date. Since chlorhexidine is poorly absorbed in the oral cavity and gastrointestinal tract, little if any enters the bloodstream. Furthermore, the formation of metabolic carcinogens has not been reported and long-term studies have not demonstrated teratogenicity.

Preparations

In the United States, chlorhexidine (*Peridex*) is sold by prescription as a 0.12% mouthwash. Other countries allow higher concentrations and the drug is available over the counter.

Benzophenanthridine Alkaloids

Sanguinarine is a benzophenanthridine alkaloid extract from the blood root plant *Sanguinaria canadensis*. Similar cationic compounds are found, for example, in Nigerian chew sticks, which have a reputation for being plaque inhibiting. Sanguinarine has a broad spectrum of activity against gram-positive and gram-negative oral bacteria, especially species associated with gingivitis and advanced forms of periodontal disease. A commercially available product containing sanguinarine is *Viadent* mouthwash, with an active compound concentration of 150 mg/ml. Similar to chlorhexidine, sanguinarine shows pronounced affinity for bacterial plaque, but unlike chlorhexidine it is not very effective in inhibiting plaque formation in vivo. This is probably the result of the high binding affinity of the compound to oral reservoirs, which, therefore, prevents drug concentrations in saliva from reaching therapeutic levels. In addition, the initial concentration found in *Viadent* rinses may not be sufficient to result in effective plaque inhibition.

Clinical studies, using an experimental gingivitis model, described plaque reductions induced by sanguinarine that were significantly superior to placebo rinses, but were clearly inferior to chlorhexidine. In clinical terms, the available information suggests some plaque-inhibiting properties for sanguinarine, but the effect is minimal if compared to chlorhexidine.

Side effects from *Viadent* oral rinses are few. A burning sensation has occasionally been reported and has likely been due to metal ions that are incorporated in the commercially available product.

Viadent mouthwash does not have acceptance by the American Dental Association (ADA) Council on Dental Therapeutics as a plaque-reducing agent.

Phenolic Compounds

A mixture of essential oils, consisting of thymol (0.06%), eucalyptol (0.09%), methyl salicylate (0.06%), and menthol (0.04%) in an alcohol-based vehicle (26.9%), represents the components that provide the plaque-inhibiting properties of rinsing agents such as *Listerine*.

Essential oils may reduce plaque levels by inhibiting bacterial enzymes and reducing pathogenicity of plaque by decreasing the amount of endotoxin; the alcohol present is probably responsible for denaturing bacterial cell walls. The substantivity of *Listerine* appears to be quite low and, therefore, it must be used at least twice a day to be effective. A variety of clinical studies have demonstrated that *Listerine* is capable of reducing plaque and gingivitis over extended periods; however, the degree of reduction is variable. Depending on which 6-month study is examined, *Listerine* will reduce plaque and gingivitis anywhere from 14.9 to 20.8 percent or 6.5 to 27.7 percent, respectively.

Adverse reactions to *Listerine* include a bitter taste and burning sensation in the oral cavity. Regular use of high-alcohol rinses can aggravate existing oral lesions and desiccate mucous membranes. Recent information from the National Institutes of Health has suggested that an association exists between the chronic use of high-alcohol mouthwashes (>20% ethanol) and certain oral cancers. At this time the link between alcohol-containing rinses and cancer is not conclusive and does not necessitate changing rinsing agents.

Fluorides

Fluorides are widely used in caries prevention, for which they have been highly effective. Systemic application via drinking water (1 mg/L), tablets (0.25–1 mg), or drops (0.125–0.5 mg), or topical application by mouth-

Table 75-1. Comparison of Antiplaque Agents in Oral Rinses

Rinse	Active agent	Concentration (%)	Pharmacologic actions	Effect on plaque	Effect on gingivitis	Dispensed	Side effects
Peridex	Chlorhexidine	0.12	Interferes with sugar transport Disrupts cell membranes Precipitates intracellular proteins	↓↓↓	↓↓↓	P	Extrinsic tooth staining Altered taste sensation Enhanced calculus formation Oral ulcers
Viadent	Sanguinarine	0.01	Suppresses bacterial enzymes	↓	↓	OTC	Burning sensation Bitter taste
Listerine[a]	Essential oils[b] Alcohol	0.25 26.9	Inhibits bacterial enzymes Reduces amount of endotoxin Denatures bacterial cell walls	↓	↓/o	OTC	Bitter taste Burning sensation Desiccation of mucous membranes
Act[c]	Fluoride	0.23	Inhibits bacterial glycolysis	o	o	OTC	Mild tooth staining
Proxacol[a]	Hydrogen peroxide	3.00	Releases oxygen as an active intermediate	o	o	OTC	Oral ulcers Carcinogen?
Plax[a]	Sodium benzoate? Sodium lauryl sulfate?	Unknown Unknown	Dissolves plaque?	o	o	OTC	None reported

Key: ↓ = decrease; o = no change; P = prescription; OTC = over the counter.
[a]*Listerine*, *Proxacol*, and *Plax* are trade name examples; other similar generic rinsing agents are commercially available.
[b]Essential oils contain eucalyptol, methyl salicylate, thymol, and menthol.
[c]Suggested use of fluoride rinses at these concentrations is for control of carious lesions.

washes (200–1,000 mg/L), gels for home use (900 mg/kg), and professional use (9,000–19,000 mg/kg), and dentifrices (1,000 mg/kg) is available for caries prevention. In contrast to the efficacy of fluorides in preventing carious lesions, these agents have relatively poor antibacterial properties. The weak therapeutic benefit of fluorides on gingivitis is due to a modest inhibition of glycolysis in plaque bacteria. Sodium fluoride, monofluorophosphate, and stannous fluoride are the compounds used in oral rinses.

A few well-controlled clinical studies suggested a potential plaque-inhibiting effect for oral rinses containing stannous fluoride. However, these results were not consistently reproducible. A possible reason for the inconsistency between these studies may be the presence of the stannous ion. It is conceivable that the plaque-inhibiting capability is due to the stannous ion rather than to fluoride and that the stannous ion is not stable over prolonged periods.

Mild tooth staining has been observed after use of stannous fluoride products. The ADA Council on Dental Therapeutics endorses fluorides for their caries-inhibiting effect but not for plaque inhibition.

Oxygenating Agents

As an adjunct to oral hygiene procedures, oxygenating agents have a long history of use. The promise of these compounds is their ability to kill bacteria by releasing oxygen as an active intermediate or by the direct oxidation of microorganisms. Nonetheless, the application of oxygenating agents, such as hydrogen peroxide, as a treatment modality against oral microorganisms has provided little success. Although hydrogen peroxide is poorly absorbed by oral tissues, it also has poor substantivity. The effects of hydrogen peroxide on supragingival plaque and gingivitis demonstrate no clinical benefits. In fact, the chronic use of hydrogen peroxide raises serious questions of safety because of its ability to induce oral ulcers and its role as a possible carcinogen.

Prebrushing Rinses

The topical application of a liquid rinse before brushing to aid in the mechanical removal of supragingival plaque is a novel therapeutic idea. Since the introduction of the first prebrushing rinse, there has been a rapid increase in the number of generic products that claim to physically loosen or remove plaque. Prebrushing rinses usually contain a plethora of ingredients, and it is not known which constituent is the active chemical. It has been suggested that sodium benzoate may behave as an antiplaque agent and that sodium lauryl sulfate acts as a detergent to dislodge or loosen the plaque on teeth. Presently, when prebrushing rinses were tested against placebo rinses, prebrushing rinses appeared to have no effect on plaque reduction. A summary of antiplaque agents in oral rinses is given in Table 75-1.

Future Directions

Today, prevention of gingivitis and periodontitis is achieved principally through mechanical plaque control; however, a dentition free of supragingival and subgingival plaque is extremely difficult to accomplish and to maintain. On an annual basis, Americans spend over three quarters of a billion dollars on oral rinsing agents, although few *effective,* plaque-inhibiting oral rinses are available at this time and many are associated with side effects that prohibit long-term use.

The goal of future product development is not so much an improvement in the antiplaque performance of the existing, effective compounds, but rather a lessening of their side effects and a development of better delivery systems. Products that combine various known compounds with well-established plaque-inhibiting properties are currently under investigation. Among the most promising products are the combination of amine fluoride and stannous fluoride, or the combination of copper sulfate and hexetidine. In the future, chemoprevention of supragingival plaque will depend on products that are effective, substantive, and safe.

Index

Index

Aarane. *See* Cromolyn sodium
ABP. *See* Androgen-binding protein
Absence seizures, 414
  ethosuximide in, 420
  valproic acid in, 419
Absorption, 19–32
  from alimentary tract, 24–25
  cell membrane in, 19–21
  in elderly, 39
  food and, 26
  gastrointestinal, 25–26
  lungs in, 26–27
  oral or first-order, 57–58
  parenteral administration and, 27–28, 70
  percutaneous, 69, 523
  physiological barriers to, 31–32
  plasma protein binding and, 29–30
  rate of, 65, 66
  rectal administration and, 68
  selective accumulation in, 30–31
  skin and, 27
  from solutions, 67
  transport mechanisms in, 22–24
    active transport and, 22–24
    bulk flow and, 22, 23
    endocytosis and, 23, 24
    facilitated diffusion and, 23, 24
    filtration and, 22, 23
    ion-pair transport and, 23, 24
    passive diffusion and, 22, 23
Abstinence syndrome, 439–440
  in drug abuse, 459
  in hypnotics and antianxiety withdrawal, 465
  narcotic antagonist and, 462
  psychomotor stimulants and, 382
Abuse of drugs. *See* Drug abuse
Accupril. *See* Quinapril
Accutane. *See* Isotretinoin
ACE inhibitors. *See* Angiotensin-converting enzyme inhibitors
Acebutolol, 140
  actions of, 301
  characteristics and preparations of, 138
  structure of, 137
Acetaldehyde
  disulfiram and, 456
  ethanol metabolism and, 452
Acetaminophen
  as analgesic, 433, 436
  antidote for, 77
  covalent binding of, 45
  glutathione conjugation and, 39
  hepatic necrosis and, 74
  pH and, 21

toxicity of, 73, 74
  volume of distribution of, 28
Acetanilid, 436
Acetazolamide
  as anticonvulsant, 421
  in carbonic anhydrase inhibition, 222–223
Acetic acid, 659
Acetic acid derivatives, 433
Acetohexamide, 806–807
Acetophenetidin, 436
Acetyl-β-methylcholine, 145
Acetylated streptokinase-plasminogen activator complex, 322
N-Acetylation, 38–39
Acetylcholine, 328
  acetylcholinesterase and, 161, 162
  actions of, 146–147
  blockade of, 181–182
  blood-brain barrier and, 336
  chemical structure of, 146
  cholinomimetics and, 145
  cholinoreceptors and, 112
  clinical uses of, 147
  diastolic depolarization and, 279
  end-plate receptors for, 179–180
  epinephrine and, 17
  ganglionic action potential and, 171
  ganglionic blocking agents and, 244
  histamine release and, 813
  muscarinic blocking drugs and, 151
  in muscle contraction, 9–10
  in neurotransmission, 104, 108–109
  phenoxybenzamine and, 132
  preganglionic neurons and, 169
  release of
    depression of, 178–179
    enhancement of, 177–178
  sympathetic nervous system impairment and, 236
  synthesis and storage of, 107
  vagal stimulation and, 260
Acetylcholine analogues, 825
Acetylcholine chloride, 147
Acetylcholinesterase, 161
  acetylcholine and, 109
  insecticides and, 82
Acetyl-CoA. *See* Acetylcoenzyme A
Acetylcoenzyme A, 38, 108–109
N-Acetylcysteine, 77, 270
Acetylhydrazine, 589
N-Acetylprocainamide, 288
Acetylsalicylic acid. *See* Aspirin
N-Acetyltransferase, 233
ACh. *See* Acetylcholine
AChE. *See* Acetylcholinesterase

Achromycin. *See* Tetracyclines
Acid as disinfectant, 659
Acidosis
  in methanol ingestion, 456
  with myocardial insufficiency, 257
  in salicylate intoxication, 435
Acne, 843
  corticosteroids and, 739
  isotretinoin in, 527
  mupirocin in, 530
  tetracyclines in, 577
  tretinoin in, 528
Acquired immunodeficiency syndrome, 607–616
  clinical drug testing for, 89
  diseases related to, 614–616
    clofamazine in, 615
    foscarnet in, 615
    ganciclovir in, 615–616
    pentamidine in, 615
  infectious process in, 607, 609, 610
  sequential blockade and synergism in, 613–614
  treatment of, 608–613
    azidothymidine in, 608–611
    dideoxycytidine in, 612–613
    dideoxyinosine in, 611–612
    human recombinant interleukin-2 in, 713
    steroid therapy in, 739, 741
Acrolein, 668
Acromegaly, 725
Acrylamide, 75
Actamer. *See* Bithionol
ACTH. *See* Adrenocorticotropic hormone
Acthar. *See* Corticotropin
Actigall. *See* Ursodeoxycholic acid
Actinic keratoses, 528
Actinomycosis, 560
Actinoplanes tecihomyceticus, 584
Action potential
  anticholinesterase agents and, 165
  calcium and, 10
  generation of, 282
  lidocaine and, 292
Activase, 322
Activated charcoal, 825
Active transport, 22–24
Active tubular reabsorption, 49–50
Active tubular secretion, 48–49
Acute dystonic reaction, 391
Acyclovir
  antiviral properties of, 604–605
  in herpes infection, 614
Acylmonoglucuronide, 505

Adalat. *See* Nifedipine
Adaptive cytoprotection, 481
Addiction
  defined, 459
  naltrexone for, 447
  psychomotor stimulants in, 382
Addison's disease, 740
Adenine, 501
Adenine arabinoside. *See* Vidarabine
Adenocard. *See* Adenosine
Adenohypophyseal-thyroid-iodine
  relationships, 776
Adenoma
  in hyperthyroidism, 782
  prolactin and, 725
Adenosine
  in arrhythmias, 309–310
  in coronary autoregulation, 265
  methylxanthines and, 384
Adenosine deaminase, 685
Adenosine monophosphate, cyclic. *See* Cyclic
  adenosine monophosphate
Adenosine triphosphate
  blocking agents and
    adrenergic, 240
    ganglionic, 244
  conversion of, 10–11
  as neuromodulator, 104
  sympathetic nervous system impairment
    and, 236
Adenosylmethionine, 39
Adenylate cyclase
  calcitonin and, 791
  catecholamines and, 123–124
  G proteins and, 10
  parathyroid hormone and, 788, 789
  tricyclic antidepressants and, 399
ADH. *See* Antidiuretic hormone
Adipex-P. *See* Phentermine hydrochloride
Adipose tissue
  blood perfusion rate in, 29
  catecholamines and, 123–124
  drug accumulation in, 30
  glucocorticoids and, 733–734
Adjuvant chemotherapy, 671
Administration of drugs, 65–72
  bioavailability and bioequivalence in, 65,
    66
  biophase in, 12
  in cancer chemotherapy, 669–670
  chronic, 58–60
  intravenous. *See* Intravenous drugs,
    administration of
  nonoral, 68–70
    buccal and sublingual, 68
    inhalation in, 69
    intramuscular, 68
    intravenous and intraarterial, 68
    percutaneous absorption in, 69
    rectal, 68
    subcutaneous, 68–69
  oral, 65–68
    capsules in, 67
    drug concentration-curve in, 58
    solutions in, 67
    suspensions in, 67
    tablets in, 67–68
  prolonged-release, 70–72
    oral, 70
    parenteral, 27–28, 70–71
    prodrugs in, 71–72
  rectal, 25
  sublingual, 24

Adrenal gland
  atrophy of
    mitotane and, 744
    steroid therapy and, 739
  congenital hyperplasia of, 741
  cortex of
    anatomy of, 731
    angiotensins and, 191
    electrolyte and water metabolism and,
      734
    hormones of. *See* Adrenocortical
      hormones
  drug metabolism and, 34, 35
  insufficiency of
    corticotropin in, 743
    metyrapone in, 743
    steroids and, 739–740
  medulla of, 106–107
Adrenalectomy, 44
Adrenalin chloride. *See* Epinephrine
Adrenaline. *See* Epinephrine
Adrenergic agonists. *See* Adrenomimetic
  drugs
Adrenoceptor antagonists, 104, 129–143,
  238–240
  adrenoceptors and, 129–130
  α-receptor blocking agents and, 131–136
    haloalkylamines in, 131–133
    imidazoline derivatives in, 133–135
    quinazoline derivatives in, 135–136
  as antihypertensives, 238–240
  in autonomic hyperreflexia, 174
  β-adrenoceptor blocking agents and, 136–
    142
    acebutolol as, 140
    atenolol as, 140
    betaxolol as, 140
    carteolol as, 140
    characteristics and preparations of, 138
    esmolol as, 140
    metoprolol as, 139–140
    nadolol as, 140
    pindolol as, 140–141
    propranolol as, 139
    timolol as, 140
  classification of, 130–131
  combination β and α, 142–143
Adrenoceptors, 104, 112–113, 129–130
  adrenomimetic drugs and, 115–116
  amphetamines and, 382
  G proteins and, 11
  presynaptic, 113
  smooth muscle and
    bronchial, 106
    vascular, 122–123
Adrenocortical hormones, 731–745
  adverse effects of, 737–740
  aminoglutethimide in, 744
  corticotropin in, 742–743
  cosyntropin in, 743
  dexamethasone in, 745
  ketoconazole in, 744
  mechanism of, 741–742
  metyrapone in, 743–744
  mitotane in, 744
  physiology of, 731–736
    biosynthesis in, 731–733
    carbohydrate, protein, and fat
      metabolism in, 733–734
    cardiovascular function in, 734
    electrolytes and water metabolism in,
      734
    endocrine organs and, 735–736

    immune and defense mechanisms in,
      734–735
    metabolism in, 733
  preparations of, 736–737
  structure-activity relationships of, 736
  therapeutic uses of, 740–741
  transport of, 733
  trilostane in, 745
Adrenocorticotropic hormone, 726–727
  angiotensinogen and, 189
  in gout, 508
  insulin secretion and, 799
Adrenomimetic drugs, 115–128
  adrenoceptors and, 129
  α blockade by, 238
  in asthma, 514–517
  calcitonin and, 790
  chemistry of, 115, 116
  clinical uses of, 124–125
  cyclic adenosine monophosphate and, 263
  dobutamine in, 127
  dopamine in, 124
  effects of, 118–124
    central nervous system, 123
    metabolic, 123–124
    potassium homeostasis and, 124
    smooth muscle, 122–123
    vascular, 118–122
  ephedrine in, 127–128
  mechanism of action of, 115–118
  phenylephrine, metaraminol, and
    methoxamine in, 126–127
  terbutaline and albuterol in, 127
  thyroid hormone interactions with, 781
Adriamycin. *See* Doxorubicin
Adrucil. *See* 5-Fluorouracil
Adsorbent powders, 825
Advertisement of drugs, 86–87
Advil. *See* Ibuprofen
AeroBid. *See* Flunisolide
Aerosols
  absorption of, 27
  corticosteroid, 517, 519
  for drug inhalation, 69, 70
Aerosporin. *See* Polymyxins
Afferent arteriole, 213–214
Afferent fiber, 236
Affinity, term, 16
Aflatoxin, 79
African trypanosomiasis, 618, 622, 623
Afterdepolarization, 280
Agar, 541, 826
Age, drug metabolism and, 39–40
Aged. *See* Elderly
Agent Orange
  cytochrome P450 and, 41
  exposure to, 78
Agonists
  competitive antagonists and, 17
  defined, 10
  partial, 15, 138
  structure-activity relationship of, 12
Agranulocytosis
  clozapine and, 395
  procainamide and, 289
  tocainide and, 296
AIDS. *See* Acquired immunodeficiency
  syndrome
Air pollution, 78–79
Airway
  asthma and, 509–510
  general anesthesia and, 344
Akathisia, 391

Alanine, 332
Albumin
   drug binding to, 29–30
   liver disease and, 61
   quinidine and, 286
   serum, 39
   testosterone and, 762
Albuterol, 127, 514–516
Alcohol, 44. *See also* Ethanol
   aliphatic
      ethanol as, 451–456
      isopropanol as, 457
      methanol as, 456–457
      oxidation of, 36
   antihistamines and, 820
   as disinfectant, 659
   drug metabolism and, 41
   γ-aminobutyric acid and, 330
   metronidazole and, 619
   microbial spectrum of, 658
   as muscle relaxant, 184
   oral anticoagulants and, 318
   oral hypoglycemics and, 807
   placental barrier and, 32
   vitamins and, 845
Alcohol dehydrogenase, 36, 452
Alcoholic cardiomyopathy, 455
Alcoholism, 451, 455, 466
Alconil. *See* Aldose reductase inhibitors
Aldactazide, 225
Aldactone. *See* Spironolactone
Aldesleukin, 703
Aldomet. *See* Methyldopa
Aldose reductase inhibitors, 808
Aldosterone
   angiotensins and, 191
   antagonists of, 224–225
   in electrolyte and water metabolism, 734
   in potassium regulation, 217
   renal perfusion and, 219
   in sodium reabsorption, 216
Aldrin, 81
Aleran. *See* Melphalan
Alfenta. *See* Alfentanil
Alfentanil, 445
   as analgesic, 360
   with propofol, 359
Alferon N. *See* Interferons
Alimentary tract. *See also* Gastrointestinal
      system
   acetylcholine and, 146
   adrenoceptors and, 113
   aminoglycosides and, 570
   chemotherapeutic toxicity and, 667–668
   drug absorption and, 24–25
   ganglionic blockade and, 174
   innervation of, 106
   isoproterenol and, 516
   norepinephrine and, 147
   salicylates and, 435, 488
Aliphatic alcohols. *See* Alcohol, aliphatic
Aliphatic phenothiazines, 388
Aliphatic solvents, 79, 80
Alkaline glutaraldehyde, 658
Alkaline phosphatase, 684
Alkaloids, 145
   acetylcholine and, 112
   belladonna, 151, 155
   benzophenanthridine, 851
   emetine and dehydroemetine as, 619–620
   muscarine as, 149
   oxotremorine as, 149
   pilocarpine as, 149

in respiratory disorders, 157
   vinca, 693–694
Alkyl sulfonates, 680
Alkylamines, 820
Alkylating agents, 673–681
   alkyl sulfonates as, 680
   ethylenimines as, 680–681
   menstrual irregularities and, 669
   nitrogen mustards as, 673–678
      chlorambucil and, 678
      cyclophosphamide and, 675–677
      ifosfamide and, 677
      mechlorethamine and, 673–675
      melphalan and, 677–678
   nitrosoureas in, 678–680
      carmustine, lomustine, and semustine
         and, 678–679
      streptozocin and, 679–680
   pulmonary toxicity and, 668
   resistance to, 666
   spermatogenesis and, 77
   in sterilization, 660
   triazenes in, 681
Alkylation, receptor, 132
Allergens, 77
Allergic contact dermatitis, 76
Allergic reaction
   to antimicrobial agents, 541
   cutaneous, 76
   eicosanoids and, 479–480
   epinephrine and, 124
   immunotoxicity and, 75
   to local anesthetics, 366
Allergic rhinitis, 818
Allopurinol
   cyclophosphamide and, 677
   in gout, 506–508
   mercaptopurine and, 685
   oral anticoagulants and, 318
Allyl formate, 74
Allylamines, 648
Aloe, 828
Alopecia
   cyclophosphamide and, 676
   mechlorethamine and, 675
   methotrexate and, 683
   paclitaxel and, 695
   valproic acid and, 419
α_1-acid glycoprotein
   plasma protein drug binding and, 30
   quinidine and, 286
   renal disease and, 62
α_1-adrenoceptors, 112
α_2-adrenoceptors, 112
α-blockers. *See* α-receptor blocking agents
α-cell, 797
α-receptor, 130–131
α-receptor blocking agents, 131–136, 238
   haloalkylamines in, 131–133
   imidazoline derivatives in, 133–135
   phenothiazines and, 391
α-reductase inhibitors, 773
Alpha tocopherol. *See* Vitamin E
Alprazolam, 371, 372, 373
Alprostadil, 482
Altace. *See* Ramipril
Altepase, 322
Alternagel. *See* Aluminum hydroxide
Aluminum carbonate, 833
Aluminum hydroxide, 832, 833
Aluminum silicate clay, 825
Aluminum sucralfate, 481
Alveolar-arterial tension gradient, 340

Alveolus
   drug absorption and, 26
   hepatotoxin and, 74
   inhalational general anesthesia and, 340–
      344
Alvosulfon. *See* Dapsone
Amantadine, 429, 601
Ambenonium, 166, 167
Amcil. *See* Ampicillin
Amdinocillin, 555, 556, 557
Amebiasis, 617–618
   chloroquine in, 630
   paromomycin in, 625
Amen. *See* Medroxyprogesterone acetate
Amenorrhea
   mechlorethamine and, 675
   progestin and, 755
American mandrake, 694
Amicar. *See* Aminocaproic acid
Amidate. *See* Etomidate
Amides, 361
Amikacin, 571–572
Amikin. *See* Amikacin
Amiloride, 225
   as antihypertensive, 231
   with hydrochlorothiazide, 226
Amine fluoride mouth rinse, 853
Amines, 367–368
   histamine as, 811
   metal interactions with, 79
   thyroid hormone and, 781
Amino acids
   conjugation of, 39
   excitatory, 330–331
   glucocorticoids and, 734
   neurotransmission and, 330
   parathyroid hormone and, 789
p-Aminobenzoic acid, 364, 545, 546
γ-Aminobutyric acid, 330
   barbiturates and, 375
   benzodiazepines and, 370
   blood-brain barrier and, 336
   ethanol and, 453
   ivermectin and, 641
   valproic acid and, 419
γ-Aminobutyric acid receptor, 331, 380
Aminocaproic acid, 323
Aminoglutethimide, 318, 744
Aminoglycoside-aminocyclitol antibiotics,
      569–574
   neuromuscular blockade and, 182
   procainamide and, 289
   spectinomycin in, 573
   streptomycin in, 569–573
   in tuberculosis, 590
6-Aminopenicillanic acid, 555, 556
Aminophylline, 383, 384
   in asthma, 513
   dosage of, 385
Aminopyridines, 177–178, 179
Aminopyrine
   cardiac disease and, 62
   half-life of, 40
4-Aminoquinoline antimalarials, 497–
      498
5-Aminosalicylate, 836, 837
Aminosalicylic acid
   in tuberculosis, 590–591
   vitamin interactions with, 844, 845
Amiodarone, 304–306
   anticoagulants and, 318
   iodine and, 781
   pulmonary toxicity of, 74

Amitriptyline
  chemical structure of, 398
  dosage and serum concentration of, 403
  guanethidine and, 242
Amlodipine
  preparations and dosage of, 254
  selectivity of, 249
Ammonia, 552, 553
Amnesia, 372
Amobarbital, 377
Amodiaquine
  dosage of, 635
  in malaria, 631
Amoxapine, 398
  adverse effects of, 402
  dosage and serum concentration of, 403
Amoxicillin
  absorption of, 558
  clavulanate potassium and, 557
  in gonococcal infection, 560
  volume of distribution of, 28
Amoxil. *See* Amoxicillin
Amphetamine, 381–383
  actions of, 128
  enterohepatic recirculation and, 51
  lung and, 31
  norepinephrine and, 116
  partial pressure–minimum alveolar
    concentration and, 339
Amphetamine sulfate, 383
Amphojel. *See* Aluminum hydroxide
Amphophile, 451
Amphotericin B, 647–649
  in leishmaniasis, 626
  liposomal, 649
  in mycosis, 614
Ampicillin
  in gonococcal infection, 560
  in *Haemophilus influenzae* infections, 560
  in paratyphoid fever, 578
  placental barrier and, 32
  streptomycin and, 571
  volume of distribution of, 28
Amrinone
  in myocardial insufficiency, 263
  propranolol and, 303
Amyl nitrite, 82
Amytal. *See* Amobarbital
Anabolic steroids, 761–773
  adverse reactions to, 769, 770
  antiandrogens and, 772–773
  anticoagulant interaction with, 318
  athletes and, 769
  chemistry and biosynthesis of, 761–764,
    765
  clinical uses of, 766–769
  gonadotropin releasing hormone and
    analogues and, 771–772
  inhibitors of, 772
  male antifertility agents and, 771
  mechanism of action of, 764–766
  nomenclature of, 761, 762
  preparations and dosage of, 771
Anadrol. *See* Oxymetholone
Analeptic stimulants, 380–381
Analgesics, 431–450
  anesthesia and, 345
  antitussive, 449–450
  central skeletal muscle relaxants with, 184
  clinical drug testing and, 88
  nonopioid, 432–437
    aniline derivatives as, 436–437
    arylalkanoic acids as, 437

    diclofenac as, 437
    fenamates as, 437
    indomethacin as, 437
    piroxicam as, 437
    salicylates and derivatives as, 432–436
  opioid, 437–446
    alfentanil as, 445
    chemistry of, 438–439
    codeine as, 444, 445
    dextropropoxyphene as, 446
    fentanyl as, 445
    heroin as, 444
    hydromorphone as, 444
    levorphanol as, 444
    mechanism of action of, 439
    meperidine as, 444–445
    methadone as, 446
    morphine as, 440–444
    sufentanil as, 445
    tolerance and physical dependence of,
      439–440
  opioid agonist-antagonists in, 447–449
    buprenorphine as, 449
    butorphanol as, 448
    nalbuphine as, 448
    pentazocine as, 447–448
  opioid antagonists as, 446–447
    nalmefene as, 447
    naloxone as, 446–447
    naltrexone as, 447
Anaphylatoxin, 814
Anaphylaxis, 76
  amphotericin B and, 649
  bleomycin and, 690
  cisplatin and, 701
  histamine and, 817
  penicillins and, 562
Anaprox. *See* Naproxen
Anavar. *See* Oxandrolone
Ancef. *See* Cefazolin
Ancobon. *See* Flucytosine
Ancylostoma duodenale
  mebendazole and, 643
  pyrantel pamoate and, 641
  thiabendazole and, 642
Androgen-binding protein, 762
Androgen receptor antagonists, 772
Androgens, 761–773
  adverse reactions to, 770
  antiandrogens in, 772–773
  anticoagulant interaction with, 318
  athletes and, 769
  chemistry and biosynthesis of, 761–764,
    765
  clinical uses of, 766–769
  gonadotropin releasing hormone and, 728,
    771–772
  history of, 761
  inhibitors of, 772
  male antifertility agents in, 771
  mechanism of action of, 764–766
  nomenclature of, 761, 762
  plasma, 761–762
  preparations and dosage of, 771
  in prostatic cancer, 755
  toxicity of, 770
Androstenedione, 747, 761, 763
Androyd. *See* Oxymetholone
Anectine. *See* Succinylcholine
Anemia
  androgens and anabolic steroids in, 768
  busulfan and, 680
  chloramphenicol and, 90, 579

  cisplatin and, 701
  immune globulin in, 714
  mitomycin and, 691
  nematode-induced, 639
  sulfonamides and, 546
  tocainide and, 296
  types of, 846
  vitamin deficiencies in, 842, 845–846
Anesthesia
  γ-aminobutyric acid and, 330
  analgesia and, 345
  anticholinesterase agents and, 166
  apnea and, 346
  apparatus for, 343–344
  balanced, 351
  barbiturates in, 376
  benzodiazepines in, 372
  caudal, 365
  classic, 345–346
  concentration of agents in
    lung, 339–340
    tissue, 338
  excitement in, 345
  extremity block and, 365
  gases in, 350–351
  Henry's law and, 337–338
  ideal, 353
  infiltration, 364
  inhalational, 337–344. *See also* Inhalational
    anesthesia
  intravenous drugs in, 353–360
  local, 361–368
    adverse reactions to, 366
    in channel blockade, 180
    chemistry of, 361
    clinical uses of, 364–366
    differential blockade for, 362–363
    eutectic mixture of, 368
    mechanism of action of, 361–362
    model structure of, 362
    in pain control, 431–432
    pharmacokinetics of, 363–364
    vasoconstrictors with, 366
  lumbar epidural, 365
  muscarinic blocking drugs and, 156
  norepinephrine in, 125
  regional block, 364–365
  signs and stages of, 345–346
  spinal, 365
  surgical, 346
  sympathetic block, 365
  topical, 364
  volatile liquids in, 347–349
ANF. *See* Atrial natriuretic factor
Angel dust, 470
Angina pectoris, 265–267
  β-blockers in, 139, 263
  bretylium and, 304
  calcium channel blockers in, 250, 252
  nitrates in, 271
  verapamil in, 308
Angioplasty, 319
Angiotensin I
  chemistry of, 190
  converting enzyme and, 187
Angiotensin II, 187
  aldosterone synthesis and, 191
  chemistry of, 190
  converting enzyme and, 187
  myocardial insufficiency and, 257
  renin release and, 188
Angiotensin II receptor antagonists, 194
Angiotensin III, 190

Angiotensin-converting enzyme inhibitors, 264
Angiotensinogen, 189
Angiotensins
  antagonists of, 191–194
  chemistry of, 190
  clinical uses of, 191
  in ganglionic blockade, 171, 172
  hypertension and, 231
  synthesis and structures of, 188
Angle-closure glaucoma, 167
Aniline derivatives, 436–437
Animal
  dander of, 79
  research ethics and, 95
Anionic detergents, 661
Anions
  in body fluids, 212
  elimination of
    biliary, 50
    renal, 48–49
Anisindione, 316, 317, 318
Anistreplase, 322
Anopheles, 627, 628
Anorexia
  cestode infection and, 637
  cyclophosphamide and, 710
  levamisole and, 702
  renal disease and, 61
  trematode infection and, 643
Anovulation, 754
Ansaid. *See* Flurbiprofen
Anspor. *See* Cephradine
Antacids
  anticoagulants and, 318
  dideoxyinosine and, 611
  in peptic ulcers, 156
  phenytoin and, 415
  renal disease and, 61
Antagonism, 10, 16–18
  of antimicrobial agent, 538
  calcium, 249–251
Antagonists. *See specific antagonists*
Anterior pituitary hormones, 723–729
  adrenocorticotropic hormone in, 726–727
  gonadotropins in, 726
  growth hormone in, 723–725
  prolactin in, 725
  thyroid-stimulating hormone in, 726
Anterograde amnesia, 372
Anthelmintic drugs, 637–645
  benzimidazoles as, 642–643
  cestodes and, 637–639
  nematodes and, 639–642
  trematodes and, 643–645
Anthracyclines, 687–689
  doxorubicin and daunorubicin as, 687–689
  idarubicin as, 689
  multidrug resistance and, 666
Anthralin, 533
Anthraquinone derivatives, 827, 828
Anthraquinones, 828–829
Antiandrogens, 772–773
Antianginal drugs, 265–274
  β-blocking agents as, 271–274
  calcium entry blockers as, 274
  dipyridamole as, 271
  organic nitrates as, 267–271
  oxygen supply and demand and, 266
  therapeutic objectives for, 267
Antianxiety drugs. *See* Anxiolytic drugs
Antiarrhythmic drugs, 275–311
  adenosine as, 309–310

amiodarone as, 304–306
bretylium as, 303–304
cardiac electrophysiology and, 275–283
  automaticity in, 278–280
  conduction in, 278–280
  ionic basis in, 277–278
  transmembrane potential in, 275–276
classification of, 283–284
digitalis glycosides as, 309
diltiazem as, 309
disopyramide as, 289–291
flecainide as, 297–299
iodine and, 781
lidocaine as, 292–294
magnesium sulfate as, 310
mexiletine as, 296–297
moricizine as, 291–292
phenytoin as, 294–296
procainamide as, 287–289
propafenone as, 299–300
propranolol as, 300–303
quinidine as, 284–287
sotalol as, 306–307
tocainide as, 296
verapamil as, 307–309
Antibiotics
  aminoglycoside-aminocyclitol, 569–574
    neuromuscular blockade and, 182
    procainamide and, 289
    spectinomycin as, 573
    streptomycin as, 569–573
  antineoplastic, 687–692
    anthracyclines in, 687–689
    bleomycins in, 689–692
  antiprotozoal, 625–626
  bacitracin in, 583–584
  β-lactam, 555–568
    cephalosporins as, 563–566
    cephems and penems as, 566–567
    monobactams as, 567
    penicillins as, 555–563. *See also*
      Penicillins
  chloramphenicol in, 577–579
  defined, 537
  in dermatological disorders, 530
  glycopeptide, 584–585
  host resistance and, 543
  lincosamides in, 581–582
  macrolide, 417, 579–581
    in *Mycobacterium* infections, 589
    in neuromuscular blockade, 182
  neuromuscular blockade and, 182
  polymyxins in, 585–586
  tetracyclines in, 575–577
Antibody
  antinuclear, 143
  in histamine release, 812
  immunoglobulin E, 812
  in malaria, 627
  monoclonal, 702
  organ transplantation and, 711
  penicillin, 562
Anticholinergic drugs, 151. *See also*
    Muscarinic blocking drugs
  adverse reactions of, 158
  as antiemetics, 830
  in asthma, 517
  in gastrointestinal disorders, 834
  in irritable bowel syndrome, 156–157
  in ophthalmology, 156
  in Parkinson's disease, 157, 429
  in peptic ulcers, 156
  in urology, 157

Anticholinesterase agents, 165, 179
Anticoagulants, 315–319
  absorption, metabolism, and excretion of, 316, 317
  adverse reactions to, 316, 317
  barbiturates and, 376
  chemistry of, 315, 316, 317
  contraindications and cautions for, 316, 317–318
  gemfibrozil and, 207
  hemostatic mechanisms and, 313–315
  indications for, 318–319
  mechanism of action of, 315, 317
  phenobarbital and, 418
  preparations and dosage of, 316, 318
  salicylates and, 435–436
  thyroid hormone and, 780
  vitamins and, 845
  xanthines and, 385
Anticonvulsant drugs, 413–424
  benzodiazepines as, 420–421
  carbamazepine as, 416–417
  clonazepam as, 420
  in epilepsy, 413–414
  ethosuximide as, 420
  in febrile seizures, 423
  general principles of, 422–423
  indications for, 421–422
  mephobarbital and metharbital as, 418
  osteopenia and, 794–795
  phenobarbital as, 417–418
  phenytoin as, 414–416
  pregnancy and, 423
  primidone as, 418–419
  quantal dose-response curve and, 13
  in status epilepticus, 423–424
  valproic acid as, 419
Antidepressants
  anticholinergic poisoning and, 158
  levodopa and, 428
  sedative-hypnotic effects of, 374–375
  tricyclic, 397–404
    adrenergic transmission and, 114
    adrenomimetic drugs and, 116
    adverse reactions of, 400–402
    anticoagulants and, 318
    in anxiety, 375
    central nervous system and, 398–399
    chemistry of, 397–398
    contraindications and cautions for, 158
    guanethidine and, 242
    mechanism of action of, 399–400
    monitoring of, 402–403
    pharmacokinetics of, 403–404
    physostigmine and, 379
    platelet function and, 320
    selective serotonin reuptake inhibitors versus, 405
Antidiuretic hormone, 214–215, 216, 729
Antidotes for toxic drugs and chemicals, 77
Antidromic firing, 165
Antiemetics, 829–831
Antiestrogens, 748–749
  in breast cancer, 768
  contraindications for, 757
Antifertility agents, 771
Antifibrinolytic drugs, 321, 323
Antifreeze, 457
Antifungal drugs, 647–656
  amphotericin B as, 647–649
  azoles as, 651–654
  in dermatologic disorders, 530–531
  flucytosine as, 650–651

Antifungal drugs (*cont.*)
  griseofulvin as, 650
  liposomal amphotericin B as, 649
  naftifine hydrochloride as, 654–656
  nystatin as, 649–650
Antigen
  in asthma, 509
  histamine release and, 812
Antihistamines
  anticholinergic poisoning and, 158
  as antiemetics, 830
  antiinflammatory properties of, 485
  in motion sickness, 157, 818
  sedative-hypnotic effects of, 374
Antihypertensives, 229–248
  adrenergic neuron-blocking drugs as, 240–
    242
  adrenoreceptor antagonists as, 238–240
  centrally acting hypotensive drugs as, 244–
    248
  contraindications to, 240
  diarrhea from, 825
  diuretics as, 219, 230–231
  ganglionic blocking agents as, 244
  mechanism of action of, 232, 239
  in myocardial insufficiency, 264
  norepinephrine and, 242–244
  sympathetic nervous system function and,
    236–238
  triple combination of, 233
  vasodilators as, 231–236
Antiinflammatory drugs, 485–500
  4-aminoquinoline antimalarials as, 497–
    498
  in asthma, 511
  azathioprine as, 709
  cytostatic-cytotoxic and antimetabolite
    drugs as, 498
  gold preparations as, 494–495, 496
  in gout, 504
  methotrexate as, 498–499
  nonsteroidal, 486–494. *See also*
    Nonsteroidal antiinflammatory drugs
  penicillamine as, 499
  in rheumatoid arthritis, 485–486, 487
  steroidal, 495–497
Antilepromatous drugs, 595–596
Antilipolytic agent, 801
Antilirium. *See* Physostigmine
Antimalarial drugs, 627–636
  4-aminoquinoline as, 497–498
  amodiaquine as, 631
  chloroquine as, 629–630
  cloroguanide as, 633
  dapsone as, 634
  in dermatological disorders, 529–530
  in development, 634
  hydrochloroquine as, 630–631
  malarial parasite and, 627–628, 629
  mefloquine as, 634
  primaquine as, 631
  pyrimethamine as, 632–633
  quinacrine as, 633–634
  quinine as, 633
  selection of, 634–636
  therapeutic considerations in, 628–629
Antimetabolites, 681–687
  in connective tissue disease, 498
  folate antagonists as, 681–683
  purine analogues as, 683–685
    cladribine as, 685
    fludarabine as, 685
    mercaptopurine as, 684–685

  pentostatin as, 685
  thioguanine as, 683–684
  pyrimidine analogues as, 685–687
    cytarabine as, 685–686
    fluorouracil as, 686–687
    ftorafur and floxuridine as, 687
  vitamin interactions with, 845
Antimicrobial drugs
  combination therapy and, 542–543
  laboratory aspects of, 541–542
  prophylactic use of, 543
  rinsing agent, 847–853
  synthetic organic, 545–553
    methenamine as, 552–553
    nalidixic acid as, 550–552
    nitrofurans as, 549–550
    sulfonamides as, 545–548
    trimethoprim as, 548–549
  use and selection of, 542
Antiminth. *See* Pyrantel pamoate
Antimonials, 624–625
Antimuscarinic drugs, 151–152
Antineoplastic agents, 673–703
  alkylating agents as, 673–681
    alkyl sulfonates as, 680
    ethylenimines as, 680–681
    nitrogen mustards as, 673–678
    nitrosoureas as, 678–680
    triazenes as, 681
  antibiotics as, 687–692
    anthracyclines as, 687–689
    bleomycins as, 689–692
  antimetabolites as, 681–687
    folate antagonists as, 681–683
    purine analogues as, 683–685
    pyrimidine analogues as, 686–687
  carboplatin as, 701–702
  cellular growth factors as, 703
  cisplatin as, 700–701
  enzymes as, 695–696
  hexamethylmelamine as, 700
  hormonal agents as, 696–698. *See also*
    Hormonal agents, antineoplastic
  hydroxyurea as, 698–699
  immunomodulating agents as, 702–703
  mitotane as, 700
  mitoxantrone as, 702
  monoclonal antibodies as, 702
  plant-derived, 692–695
    epipodophyllotoxins as, 694
    taxanes as, 694–695
    vinca alkaloids as, 693–694
  procarbazine as, 699–700
  toxicity of, 667–669
Antinuclear antibody, 143
Antioxidants, 843
Antiparkinsonian drugs, 158
Antiplatelet drugs, 319–320
  coagulation systems and, 315
  hemostatic mechanisms and, 313–315
Antiprotozoal drugs, 617–626
  in amebiasis and balantidial dysentery, 617–
    618
  antibiotics as, 625–626
  antimonials as, 624–625
  arsenicals as, 623
  diloxanide furoate as, 625
  eflornithine as, 622–623
  emetine and dehydroemetine as, 619–620
  iodoquinol as, 620–621
  in leishmaniasis and trypanosomiasis, 618
  metronidazole in, 618–619
  nifurtimox in, 623–624

  pentamidine in, 621
  quinacrine in, 624
  suramin in, 621–622
  in trichomoniasis and giardiasis, 617–618
Antipsychotic drugs, 387–395
  anticholinergic poisoning and, 158
  clozapine as, 394–395
  haloperidol as, 393–394
  lithium carbonate as, 395
  loxapine as, 394
  molindone as, 394
  in parkinsonism, 425
  phenothiazine derivatives as, 388–392
  psychosis and, 387
  sedative-hypnotic effects of, 374–375
  in tardive dyskinesia, 430
  thioxanthenes as, 392–393
  use of, 335, 336
Antipyresis, 432
Antipyrine
  half-life of, 40
  renal disease and, 62
  smoking and, 42
Antirheumatic drugs, 485–500
  4-aminoquinoline antimalarials as, 497–
    498
  cytostatic-cytotoxic and antimetabolite
    drugs as, 498
  gold preparations as, 494–495, 496
  methotrexate as, 498–499
  new approaches in, 499–500
  nonsteroidal antiinflammatory drugs and,
    486–494. *See also* Nonsteroidal
    antiinflammatory drugs
  penicillamine as, 499
  in rheumatoid arthritis, 485–486, 487
  steroidal antiinflammatory drugs and, 495–
    497
Antiseptics, 657–662
  alkylating agents as, 660
  dehydrating agents as, 659
  evaluation of, 658–659
  oxidizing agents as, 659
  permeability and, 661–662
  sterilization principles and, 657–658
  sulfhydryl combining agents as, 660–661
Antiserum, 77
Antisialagogue, 156
Antispasmodics, 158
Antispasticity agents, 182–184
Antithymocyte globulin, 711
Antithyroid drugs, 780–781
  in breast milk, 52
  drug interactions of, 781
  in hyperthyroidism, 781–782
  hypothyroidism from, 779
  thyroid hormone inhibitors as, 782–784
Antitussives, 449–450
  benzonatate as, 450
  dextromethorphan as, 449
  levopropoxyphene as, 449
  morphine as, 440
  noscapine as, 449
Antiviral drugs, 599–606
  acyclovir as, 604–605
  amantadine hydrochloride as, 601
  cytarabine as, 603
  in dermatological disorders, 531–532
  idoxuridine as, 603–604
  immune globulin and, 600–601
  interferons as, 605–606
  ribavirin as, 602–603
  vidarabine as, 601–602

viral infection stages and, 600
zidovudine as, 602
Antuitrin S. *See* Human chorionic
gonadotropin
Anturane. *See* Sulfinpyrazone
Anxiety, 369
barbiturates in, 376
benzodiazepines in, 371, 372
β-adrenoceptor blocking agents in, 141
Anxiolytic drugs, 369–377
abuse of, 464–465
antihistamines as, 374
antipsychotics and antidepressants as, 374–375
azapirones as, 369–377
barbiturates as, 375–377
benzodiazepines as, 369–373
β-adrenoceptor blocking agents as, 374
chloral hydrate as, 377
nonprescription, 377
propanediol carbamates in, 377
Aplastic anemia, 90, 579
Apnea
anesthesia and, 346
theophylline in, 384
Apomorphine, 829
Apparent volume of distribution, 28–29
Apresoline. *See* Hydralazine
Aprotinin, 196
APSAC. *See* Acetylated streptokinase-plasminogen activator complex
AquaMEPHYTON. *See* Phytonadione
Aquaretics, 222
Aquatag. *See* Benzthiazide
Aquatensen. *See* Methyclothiazide
Ara-A. *See* Vidarabine
Ara-C. *See* Cytarabine
Arabinosylhypoxanthine, 602
Arachidonic acid
eicosanoids and, 477
glucocorticoids and, 742
Arachnoiditis
cytarabine and, 686
methotrexate and, 683
Aralen. *See* Chloroquine
Aramine. *See* Metaraminol
Area postrema, 336
Area under drug concentration-time curve,
58
Arfonad. *See* Trimethaphan
Arginine, 799
Ariboflavinosis, 841
Armour Thyroid. *See* Thyroid, USP
Aromatic solvents, 79, 80–81
Arrhythmias, 275
amiodarone in, 304, 306
β-adrenoceptor blocking agents in, 301
calcium channel blockers in, 252
cardiac glycosides in, 261
chlorpromazine and, 390
flecainide in, 298
levodopa and, 427
local anesthetics and, 365–366
mexiletine in, 297
propranolol in, 303
reentry in, 281
trichloroethylene and, 80
tricyclic antidepressants and, 401
Arsenic
antidote for, 77
cancer and, 79
immunotoxicity and, 76
toxicity of, 80

Arsenicals, 618, 623
Arsine gas, 80
Artane. *See* Trihexyphenidyl
Artemether, 634
Artemisinin, 634
Arteries. *See* Blood vessels
Artesunate, 634
Arthralgia, 527
Arthritis
arylalkanoic acids in, 437
gouty
colchicine in, 503
phagocytosis in, 502–503
uric acid levels in, 502
rheumatoid, 485–486, 487
autoimmunity in, 705
azathioprine in, 710
chloroquine in, 630
corticosteroids and, 739
glucocorticoid therapy in, 738, 740
gold preparations in, 494–495, 496
methotrexate in, 498–499, 683
new approaches to, 499–500
penicillamine in, 499
Arthropan. *See* Choline salicylate
Aryl and heteroarylalkanoic acid–type drugs,
490–494
diclofenac as, 493
etodolac as, 493
fenoprofen as, 492
flurbiprofen as, 493
ibuprofen as, 491–492
indomethacin as, 490–491
ketoprofen as, 492–493
nabumetone as, 493–494
naproxen as, 492
sulindac as, 491
tolmetin as, 492
Arylalkanoic acids, 433, 437
5-ASA. *See* 5-Aminosalicylate
Asacol. *See* 5-Aminosalicylate
Asbestos
pneumoconiosis and, 79
pulmonary toxicity and, 74
Ascariasis, 639
mebendazole in, 643
piperazine in, 640
pyrantel pamoate in, 641
thiabendazole in, 642
Ascites, 219
Ascorbic acid, 840, 843
Ascriptin. *See* Aspirin
Asendin. *See* Amoxapine
L-Asparaginase
antineoplastic properties of, 695–696
bone marrow and, 667
methotrexate and, 683
neurotoxicity of, 669
Aspartic acid, 330–332, 336
Aspartylaminopeptidase, 190
Aspergillus, 647, 654
Aspirin, 432
as analgesic, 433, 434
as antiinflammatory, 487, 488
as antiplatelet, 319, 321
in arthritis, 489
in breast milk, 52
interaction with
anticoagulant, 318
vitamin, 845
for pain, 434–435
platelet cyclooxygenase and, 480–481
pregnancy and, 480

sulfate conjugation and, 38
volume of distribution of, 28
Astemizole, 819
Asthma, 509–521
adrenomimetic drugs in, 115, 127, 514–517
anticholinergics in, 517
β-blockers and, 141
bethanechol and, 148
bronchodilators in, 512–513
corticosteroids in, 517–519
cromolyn sodium in, 519–520
eicosanoids and, 479–480
glucocorticoids in, 740
nedocromil sodium in, 520
occupational, 76
steroid-sparing drugs in, 520–521
sulfuric acid and sulfur dioxide toxicity and,
79
theophylline in, 71
treatment strategy in, 510–511
xanthines in, 384
Atabrine. *See* Quinacrine
Atarax. *See* Hydroxyzine
Ataxia
amiodarone and, 306
fluorouracil and, 687
Atenolol, 140
actions of, 301
in angina pectoris, 273
characteristics and preparations of, 138
structure of, 137
ATG. *See* Antithymocyte globulin
Atherosclerosis, 750
Athletes, anabolic steroids and, 769
Ativan. *See* Lorazepam
Atonic seizure, 414
Atony, 167
ATP. *See* Adenosine triphosphate
Atracurium besylate, 182
Atrial fibrillation
amiodarone in, 306
β-adrenoceptor blocking agents in, 301
diltiazem in, 309
oral anticoagulants and, 318–319
procainamide in, 288
quinidine in, 286
Atrial flutter
β-adrenoceptor blocking agents in, 301
diltiazem in, 309
quinidine in, 286
Atrial natriuretic factor, 257
Atrial tachyarrhythmia
adenosine in, 310
β-adrenoceptor blocking agents in, 301
calcium channel blockers in, 252
procainamide in, 288
verapamil in, 308
Atrioventricular block
adenosine and, 310
amiodarone and, 306
moricizine and, 291
procainamide and, 288
quinidine and, 287
Atrioventricular node
amiodarone and, 305
bretylium and, 303
calcium channel blockers and, 252
disopyramide and, 289
flecainide and, 298
lidocaine and, 292
moricizine and, 291
phenytoin and, 294

Atrioventricular node (*cont.*)
  propafenone and, 299
  propranolol and, 302
  quinidine and, 285
  sotalol and, 307
  verapamil and, 308
Atrium
  amiodarone and, 305
  bretylium and, 303
  disopyramide and, 289
  flecainide and, 297–298
  innervation of, 105
  lidocaine and, 292
  moricizine and, 291
  propafenone and, 299
  propranolol and, 302
  sotalol and, 307
  verapamil and, 308
Atromid-5. *See* Clofibrate
Atrophy
  adrenal
    mitotane and, 744
    steroid therapy and, 739
  urogenital, 753
Atropine
  absorption, metabolism, and excretion of,
    155
  adverse reactions of, 158
  anticholinesterase agents and, 166
  in asthma, 517
  blood vessels and, 154
  carbachol and, 148
  in carotid sinus syncope, 155–156
  central nervous system and, 154
  in channel blockade, 180
  cholinergic transmission and, 114
  as equilibrium-competitive antagonist, 17
  ether and, 347
  heart and, 154
  as muscarinic blocking drug, 151
  in myocardial infarction, 156
  nicotinic receptors and, 147
  in ophthalmology, 154, 156
  as poisoning antidote, 77, 149, 157
  as preanesthetic medication, 156
  side effects of, 154
  structure of, 153
  uses of, 155
Atropine sulfate
  action of, 153
  in anticholinesterase poisoning, 168
Atrovent. *See* Ipratropium
Attention deficit disorder, 382
AUC. *See* Area under drug concentration-
    time curve
Augmentin. *See* Clavulanate potassium
Auranofin, 494, 496
Aureomycin. *See* Chlortetracycline
Aurothioglucose, 494, 496
Autacoid, 171
Autoimmune disease, 708
Autoimmune reaction, 75
Autoimmunity, 705
Autoinduction, 417
Autologous bone marrow transplantation, 667
Automaticity, 278–280, 291
Autonomic ganglia
  blocking of, 173
  receptors in, 169
Autonomic hyperreflexia, 174
Autonomic nervous system, 101–114
  adrenal medulla and, 106–107
  adrenoceptor antagonists and, 129–143. *See
    also* Adrenoceptor antagonists

adrenomimetic drugs and, 115–128. *See also*
    Adrenomimetic drugs
cholinesterases and cholinesterase inhibitors
    and, 161–168
cholinomimetics and, 145–149
effector cell receptors and, 112–114
ganglia in, 102–103
ganglionic blocking agents and, 169–175
muscarinic blocking drugs and, 151–159.
    See also Muscarinic blocking drugs
neurotransmission in, 107–112, 177–184
  acetylcholine and, 108–109, 177–179
  acetylcholine end-plate receptors and,
    179–182
  alcohol and, 184
  antispasticity agents and, 182–184
  catecholamine metabolism and, 110–112
  channel blockade and, 180
  chlorpromazine and, 184
  depolarization and desensitization and,
    180–181
  fentanyl and, 184
  fonazine mesylate and, 184
  norepinephrine and, 109–110, 111
  pharmacological intervention of, 114
  transmitters in, 103–104
organ innervation and, 104–106
phenothiazines and, 390
preganglionic-postganglionic ratio in, 103
sinoatrial node and, 278
somatic nervous system versus, 101, 102
tricyclic antidepressants and, 401
Autonomic neurovegetative syndrome, 174
Autonomy in bioethical analysis, 93
Aversion therapy in alcoholism, 455
Avidin, 842
Axid. *See* Nizatidine
Axon
  degeneration of
    anticholinesterase agents and, 168
    insecticides and, 82
  varicosity of, 107, 108
Aygestin. *See* Norethindrone
Azactam. *See* Aztreonam
Azapirones, 373–374
Azathioprine, 709–710
  allopurinol and, 507–508
  anticoagulants and, 318
  as antiinflammatory, 498
  in dermatologic disorders, 532, 533
  immune response and, 666
  immunotoxicity and, 76
  in inflammatory bowel disease, 835
Azidothymidine, 602, 608–611
  in human immunodeficiency virus, 607
Azithromycin, 579
Azlin. *See* Azlocillin
Azlocillin, 561
Azmacort. *See* Triamcinolone
Azoles, 651–654
  antifungal action of, 648
  imidazoles as, 651–654
  triazoles as, 654
Azolid. *See* Phenylbutazone
Azoprocarbazine, 699
AZT. *See* Azidothymidine
Aztreonam, 567
Azulfidine. *See* Sulfasalazine

B663. *See* Clofazimine
B cell, 710
Bacampicillin, 558
Bacillus anthracis, 584
Bacillus Calmette-Guérin, 712–713

Bacillus polymyxa, 585
Bacillus subtilis, 583
Bacitracin, 583–584
  in dermatologic disorders, 531
  neomycin and, 571
Baclofen, 183
Bacteremia, 560, 561
Bacteria
  aminoglycosides and, 570
  antimicrobial sensitivity of, 538–539
  antiseptics and disinfectants and, 658
  glucocorticoids and, 738
  penicillins and, 555, 560
Bacterial endocarditis, 561
Bacterial meningitis, 559
Bacteriostatic effect, 537
Bacteroides fragilis
  chloramphenicol in, 578
  penicillin resistance and, 560
Bactocill. *See* Oxacillin
Bactrim. *See* Trimethoprim-sulfamethoxazole
Balanced anesthesia, 351
Balantidial dysentery, 617–618
Balantidium coli, 617
Barbital, 22
Barbiturates, 375–377
  absorption and metabolism of, 375–376
  abuse of, 464
  adverse reactions to, 376
  in analeptic stimulant overdose, 381
  as anesthetic, 356–357
  anticoagulants and, 318
  in breast milk, 52
  central nervous system and, 363
  in channel blockade, 180
  chemistry of, 375
  clinical use of, 376
  drug interactions of, 376
  γ-aminobutyric acid and, 330, 370
  mechanism of action of, 375
  partial pressure–minimum alveolar
    concentration and, 339
  phenobarbital as, 417
  preparation and dosage of, 376–377
Baroreceptors, 105
Basal ganglia disorders, 430
Basaljel. *See* Aluminum carbonate
Baseballing, in cocaine abuse, 466
Basolateral membrane, 502
Basophil, 811
BCG. *See* Bacillus Calmette-Guérin
BCNU. *See* Carmustine
Beclomethasone, 518, 519, 740
Beclovent. *See* Beclomethasone
Beef tapeworm, 639
Behavioral problems
  attention deficit disorder and, 382
  clonazepam in, 420
Belladonna alkaloids, 151
  absorption, metabolism, and excretion of,
    155
  as anticholinergics, 429
  poisoning by, 147–148, 158
Bell's palsy, 741
Benadryl. *See* Diphenhydramine
Bendroflumethiazide, 224
Beneficence in bioethical analysis, 93–94
Benemid. *See* Probenecid
Benign prostatic hypertrophy, 134–135, 290
Benzalkonium chloride, 661
Benzapril, 103, 192, 193–194
Benzedrine. *See* Amphetamine sulfate
Benzene
  exposure to, 80–81

immunotoxicity and, 76
metabolism of, 36–37
Benzethonium chloride, 661
Benzimidazoles, 642–643
Benzocaine, 367
Benzodiazepine receptor, 370
Benzodiazepine receptor antagonists, 370
Benzodiazepines, 44, 369–373
  absorption, distribution, and metabolism of,
    370–371, 372
  adverse effects of, 372–373
  in alcohol withdrawal, 372, 455
  as anesthetics, 357, 360
  antacids and, 833
  in anticholinergic poisoning, 158
  as anticonvulsants, 420–421
  as antiemetics, 830
  in anxiety, 371, 372
  central nervous system and, 363
  chemistry of, 369, 370
  chloride movement and, 380
  clonazepam as, 420
  drug interactions with, 373
  in epilepsy and seizures, 372
  γ-aminobutyric acid and, 330
  in insomnia, 371–372
  mechanism of action of, 369–370
  in muscle relaxation, 183, 372
  preparations and dosage of, 373
  in sedation, amnesia, and anesthesia,
    372
Benzoic acid, 659
Benzomorphans, 439
Benzonatate, 450
Benzophenanthridine alkaloids, 851
Benzopyrine, 41
Benzothiadiazides, 218, 223–224, 264
Benzothiadiazide derivatives, 235
Benzoyl peroxide, 533
Benzthiazide, 224
Benztropine mesylate, 429
Benzylpenicillin, 559, 562
Beriberi, 841
Beryllium
  allergic contact dermatitis and, 76
  as carcinogen, 79
  toxicity of, 74, 80
β-adrenoceptor blocking agents, 136–142
  absorption, metabolism and excretion of,
    272–273
  acebutolol in, 140
  adverse reactions of, 141–142, 273
  with α-adrenergic blockers, 238
  in angina, 265, 267, 271–274
  as antihypertensives, 238–240
  atenolol as, 140
  barbiturates and, 376
  betaxolol as, 140
  carteolol as, 140
  class II antiarrhythmic drugs and, 284
  clinical uses of, 141, 239–240, 273
  contraindications to, 240
  diazoxide and, 235
  esmolol as, 140
  with hydralazine, 233
  in hyperthyroidism, 785
  mechanism of action of, 239, 272
  metoprolol as, 139–140
  nadolol as, 140
  pindolol as, 140–141
  preparations and dosage of, 138, 273–274
  propranolol as, 139
  sedative-hypnotic effects of, 374
  in thyroid storm, 782

timolol as, 140
  with vasodilators, 231
  verapamil and, 308
β-adrenoceptors, 112
  sinoatrial node and, 278
  tricyclic antidepressants and, 399
β-blockers. *See* β-adrenoceptor blocking
  agents
β-carotene, 528
β-cells, 797, 798
β-glucuronidase, 38
β-lactam antibiotics, 555–568
  cephalosporins as, 563–566
  cephems and penems as, 566–567
  monobactams as, 567
  penicillins in, 555–563
    adverse reactions of, 561–563
    antibacterial spectrum of, 557
    β-lactamase inhibitors and, 556–557
    chemistry of, 555, 556, 557
    clinical uses of, 559–561
    mechanism of action of, 555–557, 558
    pharmacokinetics of, 557–559
    preparations of, 563
β-lactamase inhibitors, 556–557
β-lactamases
  cephalosporins and, 563–564
  penicillins and, 555
β-receptors, 130
Betadine. *See* Povidone-iodine
Betaloc. *See* Metoprolol
Betamethasone
  in asthma, 518
  structure-activity relationships of, 736
Betamethasone diproprionate, 737
Betamethasone valerate, 737
Betapace. *See* Sotalol
Betaxolol, 138, 139, 140
Betazole, 817
Bethanechol, 148
  chemical structure of, 146
  as choline ester, 145
  metoclopramide with, 825
  pharmacological actions of, 147
Biaxin. *See* Clarithromycin
Bicarbonate, 211, 212
  in antacids, 832, 833
  in methanol poisoning, 456
  peptic ulcer disease and, 831
Bicillin. *See* Penicillin G
Bicuculline, 330
Bidirectional block, 283
Biguanides, 807–808, 844, 845
Bile
  amiodarone and, 306
  drug excretion and, 50
  macrolides and, 580
  tetracyclines and, 576
Bile acid sequestrant, 208
  in hypolipidemia, 203
  lovastatin with, 206
  niacin with, 205
  vitamin interactions with, 844
Biliary colic, 384
Bilirubin
  microsomal enzyme activity and, 42
  sulfonamides and, 546–548
Biltricide. *See* Praziquantel
Binding
  drug-receptor, 11–12
  glomerular filtration rate and, 48
  to plasma proteins, 29–30
Binding insensitive drug, 61
Binding sensitive drug, 61

Bioavailability
  in administration of drugs, 65, 66
  of calcium channel blockers, 253
  of digoxin, 67
Biocef. *See* Cephalexin
Bioequivalence, 65, 66
Biogastrone. *See* Carbenoxolone
Biological agents in air pollution, 78
Biological response modifiers, 711–714
  bacillus Calmette-Guérin in, 712–
    713
  cytokines as, 713–714
  immune globulin in, 714
  thymic factors as, 713
Biomedical ethics, 93–97
  application of, 93–94
  research subjects and, 95
  science, industry, and conflicts of interest
    in, 95–97
  scientific misconduct and, 94–95
Biopar Forte. *See* Intrinsic factor
Biorex. *See* Carbenoxolone
Biotin, 840, 842
Biotransformation, 33–36
Biphosphonates
  in hypercalcemia, 793
  in Paget's disease, 795
  steroid replacement therapy and, 753
Bipolar disorder, 387
  haloperidol in, 393
  lithium carbonate in, 408–411
  mood-stabilizing agents in, 411
Bipyridyl herbicides, 81, 82
Birth defects, anticonvulsants and, 423
Bis-quaternary amines, 166
Bisacodyl, 828, 829
Bismuth, 835
Bismuth subsalicylate, 825, 835
Bispectral index, 355
Bisphenols, 662
Bithionol, 638, 644–645
Bitolterol, 514
Black beauties, 466
Black tar, 461
Bladder
  acetylcholine and, 146
  adrenoceptors and, 113
  anticholinesterase agents and, 167
  bacillus Calmette-Guérin and, 712
  catecholamines and, 123
  choline esters and, 147
  cyclophosphamide and, 676
  ganglionic blockade and, 174
  ifosfamide and, 677
  muscarinic blocking drugs and, 154
Blastomyces dermatitidis, 647
Blastomycosis, 648
Bleeding, uterine, 755
Blenoxane. *See* Bleomycin sulfate
Bleomycin sulfate, 689–690
Bleomycins, 689–692
  bleomycin sulfate as, 689–690
  bone marrow and, 667
  dactinomycin as, 691–692
  in dermatologic disorders, 533
  mitomycin as, 690–691
  plicamycin as, 692
  pulmonary toxicity and, 74, 668
Blindness
  chloroquine and, 630
  methanol ingestion and, 456
  nematode-induced, 639
Blink reflex in parkinsonism, 425
Blocadren. *See* Timolol

Block
extremity, 365
regional, 364–365
sympathetic, 365
Blocking agents. *See* Adrenoceptor
antagonists
Blood
body water and electrolytes and, 212–214
drug concentration in, 55–56
area under, 58
intravenous infusion and, 59, 60
volume of distribution and, 60–61
steroid transport and, 733
Blood-air partition coefficient, 26–27
Blood-brain barrier, 333–336, 669
Blood dyscrasia
gold therapy and, 495
phenothiazines and, 392
Blood flow
absorption and, 62
β-blockers and, 139
calcium channel blockers and, 251
drug distribution and, 28
lidocaine and, 293
myocardial insufficiency, 257
oxygen supply and, 265, 266
uterine, 32
Blood fluke, 643
Blood glucose
glucocorticoids and, 733
glucose homeostasis and, 797
Blood perfusion rate, 29
Blood-placental barrier, 452
Blood pressure
adrenomimetic drugs and, 115
antihypertensives and, 229
β-blockers and, 139
calcium channel blockers and, 251
catecholamines and, 120–121, 122
labetalol and, 142
oral contraceptives and, 756
phenothiazines and, 390
phenoxybenzamine and, 132–133
sympathetic nervous system and, 237
Blood smear in malaria, 627
Blood-testis barrier, 32
Blood urea nitrogen
nephrotoxicity and, 75
tetracyclines and, 577
Blood vessels
adrenoceptors and, 113
catecholamines and, 120–121
ganglionic blockade and, 174
innervation of, 104–105
muscarinic blocking drugs and, 154
Blood volume replacement, 135
Blue angels, 464
Blurred vision
amiodarone and, 305
benzodiazepines and, 372
flecainide and, 299
mexiletine and, 297
phenothiazines and, 390
Body water, 211–218
blood supply and, 212–214
diuretics and, 218–220
ethanol and, 451–452
glomerular filtration and, 212
nephron segments and, 213–215
potassium regulation and, 216–218
sodium conservation and, 215–216
total volume of, 28
tubular reabsorption and secretion of, 212

Bolus, intravenous
blood concentration of drug in, 59, 60
determination of, 63
Bone
drug accumulation in, 31
eicosanoids and, 481
lincosamides and, 581
pain in, 703
parathyroid hormone and, 789
progestins and, 750
tetracyclines and, 577
Bone marrow
azathioprine and, 710
chemotherapeutic toxicity and, 667
chlorambucil and, 678
chloramphenicol and, 578, 579
cyclophosphamide and, 676, 710
cytarabine and, 686
hydroxyurea and, 699
melphalan and, 677
sargramostim and, 703
transplantation of, 667
Boric acid, 659
Botulinum toxin, 77, 178–179
cholinergic transmission and, 114
as food contaminant, 79
Bowel disease, 835–837
Bowman's capsule, 213
Brachial plexus block, 364
Bradycardia
adenosine and, 310
autonomic nervous system and, 104
cholinesterase inhibitors and, 165
muscarinic blockers and, 154
norepinephrine and, 121
paclitaxel and, 695
propranolol and, 302
Bradykinesia, 425
Bradykinin, 194
cardiac actions of, 196
chemistry of, 195
in ganglionic blockade, 172
histamine release and, 814
inflammation and, 479
Brain
antipsychotic drugs and, 389
in blood-brain barrier, 333–336
blood perfusion rate in, 29
central nervous system stimulants and, 385
drug metabolism and, 34, 35
estrogens and progestins and, 751
tetracyclines and, 576
Brainstem reticular system, 388
Branhamella, 579
Breast cancer
aminoglutethimide in, 744
androgens and anabolic steroids in, 768
buserelin and leuprolide in, 697
chlorambucil in, 678
cyclophosphamide in, 676
estrogens and progestins in, 754–755, 756
fluorouracil in, 687
hormonal agents in, 696
melphalan in, 677
methotrexate in, 682–683
mitoxantrone in, 702
paclitaxel in, 695
tamoxifen in, 696, 697
thiotepa in, 680
Breast feeding
amiodarone and, 306
drug elimination and, 52–53
oral contraceptives and, 757

Brethaire. *See* Terbutaline
Brethine. *See* Terbutaline
Bretylium, 303–304
Bretylol. *See* Bretylium
Brevibloc. *See* Esmolol
Brevicon. *See* Norethindrone
Brevital Sodium. *See* Methohexital
Bricanyl. *See* Terbutaline
Brofaramine, 407
Bromide, 414
Bromine, 79
Bromocriptine
in acromegaly, 725
in anovulation, 754
in hyperprolactinemia, 725
in Parkinson's disease, 429
Bromophos, 81
5-Bromouracil, 23
Brompheniramine, 820
Bronchial inhalation challenge, 734, 735
Bronchial smooth muscle
acetylcholine and, 146
adrenoceptors and, 113
catecholamines and, 123
Bronchial tree, 106
Bronchitis
penicillins in, 559
trimethoprim in, 549
Bronchoconstriction
acetylcholine and, 146
β-blockers and, 139, 141, 240
platelet activating factor and, 482
Bronchodilation
acetylcholine and, 147
epinephrine and isoproterenol and, 123
Bronchodilators, 511, 512–513
Bronchospasm, 79
Brucellosis
streptomycin in, 571
trimethoprim in, 549
Brugia malayi, 640
BSP. *See* Sulfobromophthalein
Buccal mucosa, 24
Buccal tablet, 68
Bufferin. *See* Aspirin
Bulk flow, 22, 23
Bulk laxatives, 826–829
Bumetanide, 226–228
as antihypertensive, 230–231
preparations of, 228
Bumex. *See* Bumetanide
BUN. *See* Blood urea nitrogen
Bundle branch block
flecainide and, 299
procainamide and, 289
α-Bungarotoxin, 179
Bupivacaine, 364, 367
Buprenorphine, 449, 463
Bupropion
in depression, 408
dosage and serum concentration of, 403
Burkitt's lymphoma
cyclophosphamide in, 676
methotrexate in, 682
Burns
ethylene oxide and, 660
mafenide acetate in, 546
nitrofurazone in, 550
Buserelin, 697–698, 728
BuSpar. *See* Buspirone
Buspirone, 373–374

Busulfan, 680
  interstitial fibrosis and, 668
  toxicity of, 74
Butanols, 457
Butazolidin. *See* Phenylbutazone
Butorphanol, 448
Butyrophenones, 824
Butyrylcholinesterase, 161
Bypass graft, 319

C cell, 791
Cadmium, 74, 79, 80
Caffeine, 383–385
  in breast milk, 52
  central skeletal muscle relaxants with, 184
  cyclic adenosine monophosphate and, 263
Calan. *See* Verapamil
Calciferol, 839
Calcimar. *See* Calcitonin
Calcitonin
  calcium homeostasis and, 787–788
  chemistry of, 790
  human, 793
  in hypercalcemia, 793
  mechanism of action of, 791
  mineral metabolism and, 787
  in Paget's disease, 795
  steroid replacement therapy and, 753
  synthesis and secretion of, 790–791
Calcitriol, 795
Calcium
  antagonism to, 249–251
  antiarrhythmic drugs and, 284
  ethanol and, 453
  extracellular, 787
  glucocorticoids and, 734
  in homeostasis, 787–788
  in hyperkalemia, 218
  "L type" channel of, 277
  in muscle contraction, 10
  myocardial insufficiency and, 257
  parathyroid hormone and, 788
  regulation of, 250
  in renal osteodystrophy, 795
  second messenger system and, 117–118, 119
  steroid replacement therapy and, 753
  triggered activity and, 280
  verapamil and, 308
Calcium carbonate, 832, 833
Calcium channel blockers, 249–254
  in angina, 265, 267, 274
  in arrhythmia, 252, 262
  calcium antagonism and, 249–251
  cardiac oxygen supply and demand and, 273
  in coronary vasospasm, 267
  in hypertension, 229, 232, 252
  in ischemic heart disease, 252
  nadolol with, 273
  nifedipine as, 273
  pharmacokinetics of, 253
  preparations and dosage of, 253–254
  selectivity of, 250–251
  toxicity of, 253
  uses of, 250, 252–253
  vascular effects of, 251–252
Calcium disodium edetate, 77
Calcium polycarbophil, 827
Calcium salts of dioctylsulfonosuccinate, 827
Calculus, dental, 847–853
Calor, in inflammation, 478
Camoquin. *See* Amodiaquine
cAMP. *See* Cyclic adenosine monophosphate

Camphorated opium tincture, 826
Campylobacter, 580
Cancer. *See also specific cancers*
  acquired immunodeficiency syndrome-associated, 614–615
  clinical drug testing for, 89
  cure rates in, 664
  diethylstilbestrol and, 90
  drug metabolism and, 43
  estrogens and progestins in, 754–755, 756
  vitamin A in, 843
Cancer chemotherapy, 663–672
  combination, 670–671
  drug resistance in, 665–666
  future of, 671–672
  immune system and, 666
  log-cell kill hypothesis in, 665
  pharmacokinetics in, 669–670
  toxicology in, 667–669
  tumor cell biology in, 663, 664
  tumor growth and growth fraction in, 665
  vomiting and, 829
Candidal infection
  in acquired immunodeficiency syndrome, 614
  amphotericin B in, 648
  cellular immunity defects and, 706
  clotrimazole in, 652
  flucytosine in, 651
  miconazole in, 653
  nystatin in, 649
  tetracyclines in, 577
Cannabinoids, 830–831
Canrenone, 225
Cantharidin, 532
Capastat. *See* Capreomycin
Capillary
  bulk flow and, 22
  drug distribution and, 28
  glomerular, 47
Capoten. *See* Captopril
Capreomycin, 594
Capsaicin, 533
Capsule
  Bowman's, 213
  oral administration of, 67
Captopril, 192–193, 264
Carafate. *See* Sucralfate
Carbacephem, 566–567
Carbachol
  actions of, 147
  bethanechol and, 148
  chemical structure of, 146
  as choline ester, 145
  ophthalmic solution of, 148
Carbamate insecticides, 81, 82
Carbamates, 162–163, 165
Carbamazepine, 416–417
  anticoagulants and, 318
  in manic illness, 411
  properties of, 421, 422
Carbamoylation, 679
Carbamylcholine, 10, 145
Carbapenem, 566–567
Carbenicillin
  absorption of, 558
  aminoglycosides and, 572
Carbenoxolone, 835
Carbidopa, 426, 428
Carbocaine Hydrochloride. *See* Mepivacaine
Carbohydrates, glucocorticoids and, 733–734
β-Carbolines, 330
Carbon disulfide, 75

Carbon monoxide
  antidote for, 77
  toxicity of, 75, 78
Carbon tetrachloride, 74
Carbonic anhydrase inhibitor, 167, 222–223
Carboplatin, 701–702
Carboprost tromethamine, 482
Carboxyhemoglobin, 78
Carboxyl group, 79
Carboxymethylcellulose, 826
Carcinogenesis, 76
  biotransformation and, 45
  chemotherapeutic toxicity and, 669
  covalent bonding and, 11
  metals and, 79
Carcinoma. *See* Cancer
Cardene. *See* Nicardipine
Cardenolides, 255
Cardiac action potential, 249
Cardiac glycosides, 255–264
  biliary elimination of, 50
  chemistry of, 258
  cholinergic effects of, 260–261
  clinical uses of, 261–262
  heart and, 255–257
  mechanism of action of, 259–261
  in myocardial insufficiency, 257–264
  pharmacokinetics of, 258
  preparations and dosage of, 263
  side effects of, 262–263
  therapeutic index for, 14
  vomiting and, 829
Cardiac muscle, 255–257
Cardiac output
  angiotensins and, 190
  catecholamines and, 120–121
  digoxin and, 259
  disopyramide and, 290
  dopamine and, 124
  ganglionic blocking agent and, 174
  in hypertension, 229
  in myocardial insufficiency, 257
  phenoxybenzamine and, 132
  in pulmonary excretion, 51–52
  quinidine and, 286
  sotalol and, 307
Cardioactive steroids, 255
Cardiogenic shock
  disopyramide and, 290
  flecainide and, 299
  mexiletine and, 297
  moricizine and, 291
  propafenone and, 300
Cardiomyopathy
  alcoholic, 455
  verapamil in, 252
Cardioselective blockers, 138, 139
Cardiovascular system. *See also* Heart
  acetylcholine and, 146, 147
  adrenomimetic drugs and, 120–122
  angiotensins and, 190–191
  antianginal drugs and, 265–274. *See also* Antianginal drugs
  antiarrhythmic drugs and, 275–311. *See also* Antiarrhythmic drugs
  anticholinesterase agents and, 165
  anticoagulants and, 315–319
  antihypertensives and, 229–248. *See also* Antihypertensives
  antiplatelet drugs and, 319–320
  calcium channel blockers and, 251–252
  cardiac glycosides and, 255–264. *See also* Cardiac glycosides

Cardiovascular system (*cont.*)
  cholesterol and hypocholesterolemic drugs and, 197–209. *See also* Cholesterol
  choline esters and, 147
  epinephrine and, 514–515
  fibrinolytic system and, 320–321
  histamine and, 816
  innervation of, 105
  labetalol and, 142
  local anesthetics and, 363
  marijuana and, 471
  morphine and, 440
  muscarinic blocking drugs and, 153
  nicotine and, 172
  phenothiazines and, 390
  plasma kinins and, 194–196
  renin and, 187–190
  renin-angiotensin system antagonists and, 191–194
  thrombolytic drugs and, 32–323
  water and electrolyte metabolism and, 211–228. *See also* Electrolytes
Cardizem. *See* Diltiazem
Cardovar. *See* Trimazosin
Cardura. *See* Doxazosin
Carisoprodol, 184
Carmustine, 678–679
β-Carotene, 839
Carotid sinus syncope, 155–156
Carteolol, 138, 140
Cascara, 828–829
Castellani's paint, 531
Castor oil, 828, 829
Cataplexy, 382
Catapres. *See* Clonidine
Cataract
  cholinesterase inhibitors and, 167
  glucocorticoids and, 738
  PUVA therapy and, 529
Catechol, 110
Catechol-O-methyltransferase
  adrenomimetic drugs and, 117
  norepinephrine and, 110–111
Catecholamines, 115–125
  adrenoceptors and, 129
  adverse reactions of, 125
  β-adrenergic blocking agents and, 139, 238–239
  bretylium and, 304
  cardiovascular effects of, 118–122
  chemical structures of, 115, 116
  clinical uses of, 124–125
  dopamine and, 124
  halothane and, 348
  imidazolines and, 133
  metabolism of, 110–112, 123
  methoxyflurane and, 349
  methyldopa and, 246
  metyrosine and, 244
  potassium homeostasis and, 124
  propranolol and, 302
  small intensely fluorescent cells and, 170, 171
  smooth muscle and, 122–123
  steroids and, 735–736
Catharanthus roseus, 693
Cathartics, 826–829
Catheter infection, 586
Cation exchange resin, 218
Cationic detergents, 661
Cations
  in body fluids, 212

elimination of
  biliary, 50
  renal, 48–49
Caudal anesthesia, 365
Caudate nucleus, 389
CBG. *See* Corticosteroid-binding globulin
CD3, 711
Ceclor. *See* Cefaclor
Ceepryn. *See* Cetylpyridinium chloride
Cefaclor, 564
Cefadroxil, 564
Cefadyl. *See* Cephapirin
Cefanex. *See* Cephalexin
Cefazolin, 564
Cefixime, 564
Cefotan. *See* Cefotetan
Cefotaxime, 564
Cefotetan, 564, 565
Cefoxitin, 564
Cefpodoxime, 564
Ceftazidime, 564
Ceftin. *See* Cefuroxime
Ceftriaxone, 564
  in gonorrhea, 565
  in Lyme disease, 566
Cefuroxime, 564
Celiac sprue, 795
Cell cycle
  dacarbazine and, 681
  drugs and, 664
  tumor, 663
Cell proliferation
  glucocorticoids and, 735
  toxicity and, 76
Cellulose acetate phthalate–coated tablets, 68
Celontin. *See* Methsuximide
Central anticholinergic syndrome, 154
Central nervous system, 325–474
  adrenomimetic drugs and, 123
  angiotensins and, 190–191
  aniline derivatives and, 436
  anticholinesterase agents and, 165
  anticonvulsants and, 413–424. *See also* Anticonvulsant drugs
  antihypertensives and, 244–248
  antipsychotic drugs and, 387–395. *See also* Antipsychotic drugs
  barbiturates and, 375
  benzodiazepines and, 370
  depressants of
    clonazepam in, 420
    ethanol and, 456
    phenobarbital in, 417
  drug abuse and, 459–474. *See also* Drug abuse
  drug distribution and, 31
  ethanol and, 451–456
  general anesthetics and, 345–360. *See also* General anesthesia
  haloperidol and, 393
  indomethacin and, 491
  inhalational anesthetics and, 337–344. *See also* Inhalational anesthesia
  lithium carbonate and, 408–409
  local anesthetics and, 361–368. *See also* Local anesthetics
  methanol and, 456–457
  mood disorders and, 397–411. *See also* Mood disorders
  morphine and, 440
  muscarinic blocking drugs and, 153, 154
  muscle relaxants and, 183–184

nicotine and, 173
opioid and nonopioid analgesics and, 431–450. *See also* Analgesics
Parkinson's disease and, 425–429
pharmacology of, 327–336
  basic neuroscience in, 327–328
  blood-brain barrier in, 333–336
  methodology and, 333
  neurotransmitters and, 328–333
  practical consequences in, 335, 336
phenothiazines and, 389–390
salicylates and, 432–434
sedative-hypnotic and anxiolytic drugs and, 369–377. *See also* Sedative-hypnotic drugs
steroids and, 739
stimulants of, 379–385
  abuse of, 466–468
  analeptic, 380–381
  partial pressure–minimum alveolar concentration and, 339
  phenytoin in, 416
  psychomotor, 381–383
  xanthines in, 383–385
toxicity and, 75
tricyclic antidepressants and, 398–399, 401
xanthines and, 384
Centrax. *See* Prazepam
Cephalexin, 75, 564
Cephalosporins, 563–566
  adverse reactions of, 566
  antibacterial spectrum of, 564
  anticoagulants and, 318
  chemistry of, 563–564
  clinical uses of, 565–566
  pharmacokinetics of, 564–565
  preparations and dosage of, 566
Cephalosporium, 555
Cephalosporium acremonium, 563
Cephalothin, 564
  aminoglycosides and, 572
  nephrotoxicity of, 75
Cephapirin, 565
Cephems, 566–567
Cephradine, 564
Cephulac. *See* Lactulose
Ceptaz. *See* Ceftazidime
Cerebrospinal fluid
  cephalosporins and, 565
  drug distribution and, 31
Cerubidine. *See* Daunorubicin
Cestodes, 637–639
Cetylpyridinium chloride, 661
cGMP. *See* Cyclic guanosine 3′,5′-monophosphate
CGP38560A, 191
CGs. *See* Cardiac glycosides
Chagas' disease, 618, 624
Charcoal, activated, 825
Chelating agents, 495, 499
Chelation, 16
Chemical allergens, 77, 78
Chemical antagonism, 16
Chemical bonds, 11
Chemoprophylaxis
  for malaria, 634
  for tuberculosis, 589
Chemoreceptor trigger zone, 389, 829, 830
Chemotherapy, 537–715
  in acquired immunodeficiency syndrome, 607–616. *See also* Acquired immunodeficiency syndrome

adjuvant, 671
adverse effects of, 541
anthelminthic, 637–645. *See also*
    Anthelmintic drugs
aminoglycoside-aminocyclitol antibiotics
    in, 569–574
antifungal, 647–656. *See also* Antifungal
    drugs
antimalarial, 627–636. *See also* Antimalarial
    drugs
antimicrobial, 537, 540, 545–553. *See also*
    Antimicrobial drugs
antiprotozoal, 617–626. *See also*
    Antiprotozoal drugs
antiseptics, disinfectants, and sterilization
    in, 657–662
antiviral drugs in, 599–606
bacitracin in, 583–584
β-lactam antibiotics in, 555–568. *See also* β-
    lactam antibiotics
cancer, 663–672
    antineoplastic agents in, 673–703. *See
        also* Antineoplastic agents
    combination, 670–671
    drug resistance in, 665–666
    future of, 671–672
    immune system and, 666
    log-cell kill hypothesis in, 665
    pharmacokinetics in, 669–670
    toxicology of, 667–669
    tumor cell biology in, 663, 664
    tumor growth and growth fraction in,
        665
    vomiting and, 829
chloramphenicol in, 577–579
drug combinations in, 538
glycopeptides in, 584–585
host resistance and, 543
immunomodulating drugs in, 705–715. *See
    also* Immunomodulating drugs
in vivo measurements in, 542
in leprosy, 594–596
lincosamides in, 581–582
macrolide antibiotics in, 579–581
marijuana and, 472
microbial factors in, 540–541
patient compliance and, 543
pharmacological principles of, 539–540
polymyxins in, 585–586
prophylactic, 543
sensitivity tests and, 541–542
static and cidal effects in, 537, 540
tetracyclines in, 575–577
in tuberculosis, 587–594. *See also*
    Tuberculosis
Chenix. *See* Chenodeoxycholic acid
Chenodeoxycholic acid, 837
Chenodiol, 837
Chest pain
    adenosine and, 310
    sotalol and, 307
Chibroxin. *See* Norfloxacin
Child
    clinical drug trials and, 90
    tuberculin chemoprophylaxis for, 589
    tubular transport mechanism in, 49
"China White," 473
Chinese doctrine of signatures, 4
Chlamydial infection
    chloramphenicol in, 578
    sulfonamides in, 545, 546
    tetracyclines and, 575, 577

Chloral hydrate
    anticoagulants and, 318
    dosage of, 373
    sedative-hypnotic effects of, 377
Chlorambucil, 666, 678, 711
Chloramine-T, 659
Chloramphenicol, 577–579
    adverse effects of, 90
    anticoagulants and, 318
    microsomal enzyme activity and, 42
    newborn and, 37–38
    oral hypoglycemics and, 807
    phenytoin and, 295
Chlorcyclizine
    in lung, 31
    in monooxygenase enzyme induction,
        42
    teratogenic effects of, 820
Chlordane
    in monooxygenase enzyme induction, 42
    topical absorption of, 27
    toxicity of, 81
Chlordecone, 51, 81
Chlordiazepoxide, 369
    dosage of, 373
    half-life of, 40
    pharmacokinetics of, 372
    smoking and, 42
    solubility of, 68
Chlorhexidine, 849–851, 852
    in disinfection, 662
    microbial spectrum of, 658
    in oral cavity, 848
Chloride, 211, 212
    γ-aminobutyric acid receptor and, 380
    ethanol and, 453
    methylxanthines and, 384
Chlorinated solvents, 75
Chlorine
    as disinfectant, 659
    exposure to, 79
    microbial spectrum of, 658
Chlorine gas, 74
2-Chloro-deoxy-adenosine, 685
Chloroform, 349
    exposure to, 80
    hepatotoxicity of, 74
    nephrotoxicity of, 75
Chloroguanide hydrochloride, 633
Chloromycetin. *See* Chloramphenicol
Chlorophenoxy herbicides, 81, 82
Chloroprocaine, 364, 367
Chloroquine
    as antiinflammatory, 497
    in dermatologic disorders, 530
    eye and, 30
    in malaria, 629–630
    resistance to, 634–636
Chlorosalicylamide derivative, 637
Chlorothiazide, 223, 224
    as antihypertensive, 230
    cholestyramine and, 204
    in myocardial insufficiency, 264
Chlorotrianisene, 758
Chlorpheniramine, 818, 820
Chlorpromazine, 387, 388–392
    as α-receptor blocking agent, 131
    in anxiety, 374–375
    chemical structure of, 388
    eye and, 30
    hepatotoxicity of, 74, 75
    microsomal enzyme activity and, 42

as muscle relaxant, 184
smoking and, 42
Chlorpropamide, 806–807
Chlorprothixene, 392
Chlorpyrifos, 81
Chlortetracycline, 576
Chlorthalidone, 223, 224
Chlorzoxazone, 184
Cholecalciferol, 839
    adverse reactions to, 795
    cholesterol and, 791
    in rickets, 794
Cholecystokinin, 799
Cholera, 577
Cholestasis, 75, 795
Cholesterol, 197
    agents reducing, 197–209
        in combination therapy, 208–209
        diet versus, 201–202
        hypolipidemic, 202–203
        lipoproteins and, 197–199, 200, 201
        niacin in, 843
        in plasma cholesterol reduction, 203–206
        plasma lipid levels and, 200–201, 202
        in plasma triglyceride reduction, 206–
            208
    cholecalciferol and, 791
    dietary regulation of, 201–202, 827
    in gallstones, 837
    plasma, 203–206
    in plasma membrane, 21
    synthesis of, 731–732
Cholesterol ester hydrolase, 731–732
Cholestyramine, 203–204
    absorption, metabolism and excretion of,
        204
    adverse reactions to, 204
    anticoagulants and, 318
    clinical uses of, 204
    in combination therapy, 208
    mechanism of action of, 203–204
    preparations and dosage of, 204
    sulfasalazine and, 837
    vitamins and, 844
Cholestyramine resin, 204
Choline, 108–109
Choline esters, 145–148
    acetylcholine as, 146–147
    actions of, 147
    bethanechol as, 148
    carbachol as, 148
    chemical structures of, 146
    methacholine as, 147–148
Choline magnesium trisalicylate, 488
Choline salicylate, 488
Cholinergic agonists, 825
Cholinergic crisis, 166–167
Cholinergic receptors
    acetylcholinesterase and, 164
    poisoning symptoms and, 82
    postganglionic neurons and, 169
Cholinesterase inhibitors, 162–168
    absorption, metabolism, and excretion of,
        165
    adverse reactions of, 167–168
    chemistry of, 162–163
    clinical uses of, 166–167
    contraindications and cautions with, 168
    mechanisms of action of, 163
    metoclopramide with, 825
    pharmacological actions of, 164–165
    poisoning by, 157

Cholinesterases, 161–162
  acetylcholinesterase as, 162
  inhibitors of, 162–168. *See also*
    Cholinesterase inhibitors
Cholinoceptor antagonists, 104
Cholinoceptors, 104, 112
Cholinomimetic drugs
  directly acting, 145–149
    alkaloids as, 149
    choline esters as, 145–148
    ether and, 347
  indirectly acting, 161
Cholybar. *See* Cholestyramine resin
Chorea, 430
Chorionic gonadotropin, human, 726, 767
Chromium
  allergic contact dermatitis and, 76
  cancer and, 79
Chromomycosis, 651
Chromophore, 528
Chronic obstructive lung disease, 157
Chronulac. *See* Lactulose
Chrysotherapy in arthritis, 495
Chylomicrons, 197, 198, 199
Chymotrypsin, 26
Ciclopirox olamine, 648, 655
Cilastin, 567
Ciliary body, 105
Ciloxan. *See* Ciprofloxacin
Cimetidine, 821, 833
  anticoagulants and, 318
  flecainide and, 299
  lidocaine and, 294
  procainamide and, 289
  propafenone and, 300
  structure of, 834
  terfenadine and, 819
  theophylline and, 513
Cinchonism, 287, 633
Cinobac. *See* Cinoxacin
Cinoxacin, 550, 551
Cipro. *See* Ciprofloxacin
Ciprofloxacin, 551, 819
Circulation
  coronary collateral, 266
  electrolyte metabolism and, 212–214
  enterohepatic, 38, 50
  fetal, 31–32
  peripheral, 272
Cirrhosis
  drug metabolism and, 44
  ethanol and, 455
  hepatotoxin and, 74
  methotrexate and, 668, 683
  osteomalacia in, 795
Cisapride, 825
Cisplatin, 700–701
  bone and, 31
  nephrotoxicity of, 75
  neurotoxicity of, 669
  resistance to, 666
Citanest. *See* Prilocaine hydrochloride
Citrinin
  as food contaminant, 79
  nephrotoxicity of, 75
Cladribine, 685
Claforan. *See* Cefotaxime
Clarithromycin, 579–581
Clavulanate potassium, 557
Clavulanic acid, 556–557
Clear cell carcinoma, 90
Clearance
  creatinine, 57

defined, 56–57
  hepatic, 61
  in intravenous bolus, 63
  renal, 409
Cleft palate, 423
Cleocin. *See* Clindamycin
Clindamycin, 581–582
  in dermatologic disorders, 531
  in *Pneumocystis carinii* pneumonia, 614
Clinical testing in drug development, 88
Clinoril. *See* Sulindac
Clitocybe dealbata, 157
Clobetasol propionate, 737
Clofazimine, 596, 615
Clofibrate, 207–208
  anticoagulants and, 318
  gemfibrozil and, 207
  niacin with, 205
  in platelet function, 320
  volume of distribution of, 28
Clomid. *See* Clomiphene
Clomiphene, 748–749
  in anovulation, 754
  preparations and dosage of, 758
  toxicity of, 757
Clomipramine, 397
Clonazepam
  in epilepsy, 420
  in manic illness, 411
  properties of, 421, 422
  in seizures, 372
  in strychnine-induced convulsions, 381
  valproic acid and, 419
Clonic seizures, 414
Clonidine, 246–248
  chemical structure of, 241
  pressor response with, 131
  renin release and, 191
  transdermal patch, 247
  tricyclic antidepressants and, 403
  in withdrawal therapy, 463
Clonorchiasis, 644
Clonorchis sinensis, 630, 643
Cloquinol, 531
Clorazepate dipotassium, 373, 421
Clostridium botulinum, 179
Clostridium difficile infection
  lincosamides in, 582
  vancomycin in, 585
Clostridium perfringens, 584
Clostridium tetani, 584
Clotrimazole, 651–652
Cloxacillin, 557
Cloxapen. *See* Cloxacillin
Clozapine, 387, 394–395
Clozaril. *See* Clozapine
Coactin. *See* Amdinocillin
Coadministration of drugs
  biliary excretion and, 51
  drug metabolism and, 44
Coagulation, disseminated intravascular. *See*
    Disseminated intravascular coagulation
Coagulation disorders
  anticoagulants in, 315–319
  antiplatelets in, 319–320
  cephalosporins in, 566
Coal dust, 79
Coal tar, 529
Coal-tar analgesics, 436
Coated release beads, 70
Coated tablets, 68
Cocaine, 366–367, 368
  abuse of, 466–468

cardiovascular system and, 363
  discovery of, 361
  indirectly acting adrenomimetic drugs and,
    116
  metabolism and, 364
  neurotoxicity of, 75
  placental barrier and, 32
Coccidioides immitis, 647
Coccidioidomycosis, 614, 648
Cocoa, 383
Codeine, 438, 444, 445
  as analgesic, 434, 442
  for cough, 449
  histamine release and, 814
  microsomal enzyme activity and, 42
Coenzyme A, 452
Coffee
  caffeine content of, 383
  headache and, 385
Cogentin. *See* Benztropine mesylate
Cogwheel rigidity, in parkinsonism, 425
Coke, 466
Cola drinks, 383
Colace. *See* Docusate sodium
Colbenemid. *See* Probenecid
Colchicine
  allopurinol and, 507
  in dermatologic disorders, 532, 533
  in gout, 503–504
  vitamins and, 844, 845
Colestipol, 204
  in combination therapy, 208
  niacin with, 205
Colistimethate sodium, 586
Colistin, 585–586
Colitis
  lincosamides and, 581–582
  ulcerative, 835–837
Collecting ducts, 214–215
Colloidal bismuth, 835
Colonic lavage solutions, 828
Colorectal cancer, 702
Coly-Mycin. *See* Colistin
Colyte, 828
Coma
  ethanol consumption and, 454
  streptozocin and, 679
Combination chemotherapy, 538
  in acquired immunodeficiency syndrome,
    613
  aminoglycosides in, 572–573
  antimicrobial, 542–543
  in cancer, 670–671
  drug resistance and, 665–666
  in leprosy, 596
  in malaria, 632
  in tuberculosis, 587
Combination pill, 751–752
Comedogenic acne vulgaris, 528
Compazine. *See* Prochlorperazine
Competitive antagonism, 17
Complement in histamine release, 814
Compound 1080, 81
Compound 40/80, 814
COMT. *See* Catechol-O-methyltransferase
Conadil. *See* Sulthiame
Concentration, minimum inhibitory,
    541
Concentration effect, in general anesthesia,
    342–343
Concentration gradient
  across placenta, 32
  facilitated diffusion and, 23, 24

passive transfer and, 22
tubular lumen and, 48
Conduction, myocardial, 280–283
Condylomata acuminata, 531–532, 606
Conflict of interest, in research, 95–97
Confusion
    benzodiazepines and, 372
    tocainide and, 296
Congenital adrenal hyperplasia, 741
Congestive heart failure. *See* Heart failure
Conjugated equine estrogens, 753, 758
Conjugation reactions
    biliary excretion and, 51
    in drug metabolism, 37–39
Conjunctiva, 158
Constant fraction, 665
Constipation, 824
    calcium channel blockers and, 253
    morphine and, 440–441
    treatment of, 826–829
    verapamil and, 308
Contact dermatitis, 76, 158
Contaminant exposure, 79
Continuous infusion, in cancer
            chemotherapy, 669–670
Contraception, oral. *See* Oral contraceptives
Contractility
    calcium channel blockers and, 251, 252
    disopyramide and, 290
    oxygen supply and, 266
    phenoxybenzamine and, 132
    procainamide and, 288
Contrast media, 814
Control group, in human drug testing, 88
Controlled Substances Act, 460–461
Converting enzyme, 189–190, 191–194
Convulsants, 379
Convulsions
    central nervous system stimulants and, 381
    lidocaine and, 293
Coordinate covalent bond, 11
Coordination complex, 11–12
Copper sulfate and hexetidine mouth rinse,
            853
Coramine. *See* Nikethamide
Cordarone. *See* Amiodarone
Corgard. *See* Nadolol
Cornea
    amiodarone and, 305
    idoxuridine and, 603
Corns, 435
Coronary artery bypass graft, 319
Coronary artery disease, 266, 319
Coronary artery spasm, 267, 268
Coronary blood flow
    β-blockers and, 139
    bethanechol and, 148
    oxygen supply and, 265, 266
Corotrope. *See* Milrinone
Cortical focal seizure, 418
Corticosteroid-binding globulin, 733, 751
Corticosteroids, 731–745
    actions of, 733–734
    in adrenocortical abnormalities, 742–745
    adverse effects of, 737–740
    anticoagulants and, 318
    as antiemetics, 831
    antiinflammatory properties of, 495–497
    in asthma, 511, 517–519
    defense mechanisms and, 734–735
    drug metabolism and, 44
    endocrine organs and, 735–736
    in gout, 508

immunotoxicity and, 76
in inflammatory bowel disease, 835
insulin resistance and, 802
metabolism of, 733
natural, 736
in organ transplantation, 706–707
in osteopenia, 794–795
in rheumatoid arthritis, 496
synthetic, 736
in thyroid storm, 782
topical, 525–526
Corticotropin, 726–727, 742–743
    chlorpromazine and, 390
    in gout, 508
Corticotropin-releasing factor, 729, 735
Cortisol
    microsomal enzyme activity and, 42
    renal disease and, 62
Cortrophin. *See* Corticotropin
Cortrosyn. *See* Cosyntropin
Corynebacterium diphtheriae infection
    erythromycin in, 580
    glycopeptides in, 584
Cosmegen. *See* Dactinomycin
Cosolvent in drug solutions, 67
Cosyntropin, 743
Cotrimoxazole, 614
Cough, 449–450
    codeine for, 444
    morphine and, 440
Coumadin. *See* Warfarin
Coumarin
    phenytoin and, 416
    vitamins and, 845
Covalent bond, 11–12
    alkylating agents and, 673
    metabolites and, 45
Coxiella, 575, 577
Crack, 466
Cramping, 633
Craniosacral division, 102
Creatinine
    clearance of, 57
    nephrotoxicity and, 75
Cresols, 661
Cretinism, 779
Creutzfeldt-Jakob disease, 725
CRF. *See* Corticotropin-releasing factor
Crigler-Najjar syndrome, 38
Critical volume hypothesis, 337
Crohn's disease, 795, 835–837
Cromolyn sodium, 511, 519–520, 821–822
Cross-linkage, 673
Cross-sensitivity, 491–492
Cross-tolerance, 464
Crude petroleum distillates, 80
Cryptococcus neoformans infection
    in acquired immunodeficiency syndrome,
            614
    amphotericin B in, 647, 648
    flucytosine in, 651
    nystatin in, 649
Cryptorchidism, 767
Crystal, 466
Crystodigin. *See* Digitoxin
CTZ. *See* Chemoreceptor trigger zone
Cufor-hedake-Brane-Fude, 85
Cultural factors in pharmacology
            development, 4–5
Culture of *Plasmodium falciparum*, 627
Cuprimine. *See* Penicillamine
Curare, 181
    anticholinesterase agents and, 166

as blocking agent, 173
neuromuscular system and, 363
Curarelike drugs, 182
Cushing's disease
    aminoglutethimide in, 744
    dexamethasone in, 745
    ketoconazole in, 744
    metyrapone in, 743
Cutaneous allergic reaction, 76
Cyanide
    antidote for, 77
    exposure to, 82
Cyanocobalamin, 840
    deficiency of, 842
    in megaloblastic anemia, 846
Cyanosis
    in congestive heart failure, 256
    with myocardial insufficiency, 257
Cyclamate
    banning of, 79
    intestinal microflora and, 45
Cycle-specific drugs, 709
Cyclic adenosine monophosphate
    adrenomimetics and, 514
    calcitonin and, 791
    catecholamines and, 123–124
    diarrhea and, 825
    histamine and, 815, 816
    insulin and, 801
    kinases and, 10–11
    in myocardial insufficiency, 263–264
    parathyroid hormone and, 788, 789
    peptic ulcer disease and, 831
    in signal transduction, 117–118, 119
    theophylline and, 512
Cyclic guanosine 3′,5′-monophosphate
    histamine and, 816
    in hypertension, 229
Cyclinex. *See* Tetracyclines
Cyclizine
    in allergy, 820
    in motion sickness, 818
Cyclobenzaprine, 184
Cyclohexanone derivative, 357
Cyclohexylamine, 45
Cyclooxygenase
    arachidonic acid and, 477
    inflammation and, 479
Cyclopar. *See* Tetracyclines
Cyclopentolate
    adverse reactions of, 158
    in ophthalmology, 156
    uses for, 155
Cyclophosphamide, 710–711
    anticoagulants and, 318
    as antiinflammatory, 498
    antineoplastic properties of, 675–677
    in dermatologic disorders, 532, 533
    dose fractionation of, 669
    drug interactions with, 670
    hair loss and, 668
    immune response and, 666
    in immunosuppressive therapy, 710–711
    immunotoxicity and, 76
    lung and, 74
Cycloplegia, 154
Cycloplegics, 105, 158
Cyclopropane, 350–351
    adverse reactions of, 158
    anesthetic apparatus of, 343
    partition coefficients of, 340
    propranolol and, 302
    solubility of, 341

Cycloserine
  in tuberculosis, 593–594
  vitamin interactions with, 845
Cyclosporine
  in dermatologic disorders, 532, 533
  immunotoxicity and, 76
  nephrotoxicity of, 75
  in organ transplantation, 705, 707–709
Cycrin. *See* Medroxyprogesterone acetate
Cyklokapron. *See* Tranexamic acid
Cylert. *See* Pemoline
Cyproheptadine, 820
Cyproterone acetate, 772
Cyst, protozoal, 617
Cysteine, 332
Cysticercosis, 639
Cystitis
  cancer chemotherapy and, 668
  cyclophosphamide and, 676
  ifosfamide and, 677
Cytadren. *See* Aminoglutethimide
Cytarabine, 603, 669, 685–686
Cytochrome P450, 34–36
  ethanol metabolism and, 452
  ketoconazole and, 744
  liver and, 74
  in nephron, 75
Cytokines, 712, 713–714
Cytolysis, 76
Cytomegalovirus infection
  in acquired immunodeficiency syndrome,
    614
  cellular immunity defects and, 706
Cytomel. *See* Liothyronine sodium
Cytosar-U. *See* Cytarabine
Cytosine arabinoside, 603
Cytotec. *See* Misoprostol
Cytotoxic drugs
  in connective tissue disease, 498
  in dermatological disorders, 532–533
  first-order kinetics of, 665
  in organ transplantation, 709
Cytoxan. *See* Cyclophosphamide

D receptors, 124
Dacarbazine, 681
Dactinomycin, 691–692
  hair loss and, 668
  multidrug resistance and, 666
Dalmane. *See* Flurazepam
Danazol, 768
Dander, animal, 79
Danocrine. *See* Danazol
Dantrium. *See* Dantrolene
Dantrolene, 183
Dapsone
  in dermatological disorders, 529
  in leprosy, 595
  in malaria, 634
  in *Pneumocystis carinii* pneumonia, 614
Daraprim. *See* Pyrimethamine
Darvon. *See* Propoxyphene
Datura stramonium, 157
Daunorubicin, 687–689
DDAVP. *See* Desmopressin
DDC. *See* Dideoxycytidine
DDI. *See* Dideoxyinosine
DDT
  in monooxygenase enzyme induction, 42
  topical absorption of, 27
  toxicity of, 81
Dead space ventilation, 344

Deafness
  loop diuretics and, 228
  vancomycin and, 585
Dealkylation, 36
Deca-Durabolin. *See* Nandrolone decanoate
Decamethonium, 26
Decarboxylase inhibitors
  levodopa and, 426
  in parkinsonism, 428–429
Declaration of Helsinki, 95
Declomycin. *See* Demeclocycline
Deep vein thrombosis, 319
Deferoxamine, 77
Deflazacort, 738
Dehydrating agents, 659
7-Dehydrocholesterol, 839
Dehydroemetine, 619–620
Dehydroepiandrosterone, 762, 763
Delaney Clause, of 1958 Food Additives
    Amendment, 79
Delaxin. *See* Methocarbamol
Delayed afterdepolarization, 280
Delayed hypersensitivity, 76
Delirium
  in hypnotics and antianxiety withdrawal,
    465
  tricyclic antidepressants and, 401
Delirium tremens, 466
Delivery systems of drugs. *See* Administration
    of drugs
Deltalin. *See* Ergocalciferol
Deltasone. *See* Prednisone
Demecarium, 166, 167
Demeclocycline, 222, 576
Demerol. *See* Meperidine
Demethylation, 36
Demser. *See* Metyrosine
Demulen. *See* Norethindrone
deNol. *See* Tripotassium dicitrate bismuthate
Dental calculus, 847–853
Deoxy-6-thioguanosine-triphosphate, 684
Deoxycoformycin, 685
Deoxycytidine kinase, 685
Deoxyribonucleic acid
  alkylating agents and, 673
  fludarabine and, 685
  vidarabine and, 601–602
Deoxyribonucleic acid gyrase, 550
Depakene. *See* Valproic acid
Depen. *See* Penicillamine
Dephosphorylation, 163
Depo-Provera. *See* Medroxyprogesterone
    acetate
DEPO-Testosterone. *See* Testosterone
    cypionate
Depolarization
  blockade of, 180–181
  membrane action potential and, 277
  norepinephrine and acetylcholine and, 279
  phenytoin and, 294
Deprenyl. *See* Selegiline
Depressants, 417
Depression, 397–408
  bupropion in, 408
  buspirone in, 374
  monoamine oxidase inhibitors in, 406–407
  serotonin reuptake inhibitors in, 404–405
  trazodone in, 407–408
  tricyclic antidepressants in, 397–404
Depurination, 673
Dermatitis
  allergic contact, 76
  atropine and, 158

cancer chemotherapy and, 668
  gold therapy and, 495
  methotrexate and, 683
  penicillins and, 562
Dermatitis herpetiformis, 529
Dermatological disorders, 523–534
  antibiotics in, 530
  antifungal agents in, 530–531
  antimalarial drugs in, 529–530
  antiviral agents in, 531–532
  corticosteroids in, 525–526
  cytotoxic and immunosuppressive agents
    in, 532–533
  dapsone in, 529
  percutaneous absorption and, 523
  photochemotherapy and, 528–529
  photodynamic therapy in, 529
  retinoids in, 526–528
  scabies and lice and, 532
  skin structure and, 523, 524
  sunscreens in, 533–534
  topical drug therapy in, 523–525
Dermatophytes, 530
  clotrimazole and, 651–652
  griseofulvin and, 650
  miconazole and, 653
  nystatin and, 650
Dermis, 27, 523, 524
DES. *See* Diethylstilbestrol
Desacetyl vinblastine, 693
Desethylamiodarone, 306
Desethylchloroquine, 630
Desflurane, 340, 341, 349
Designer drugs, 473
Desipramine
  chemical structure of, 398
  dosage and serum concentration of, 403
  guanethidine interactions with, 242
Desmopressin, 729
Desoxyn. *See* Methamphetamine
Desyrel. *See* Trazodone
Detergents, 658, 661
Detrusor muscle
  adrenoceptors and, 113
  catecholamines and, 123
Dexamethasone
  in asthma, 518
  in Cushing's disease, 745
  structure-activity relationships of, 736
Dexbrompheniramine, 820
Dexchlorpheniramine, 820
Dexedrine. *See* Dextroamphetamine sulfate
Dextroamphetamine sulfate, 383
Dextromethorphan, 449
Dextropropoxyphene, 446
Dextrothyroxine, 318
DHEA. *See* Dehydroepiandrosterone
DHT. *See* Dihydrotestosterone
DiaBeta. *See* Tolbutamide
Diabetes insipidus, 729
Diabetes mellitus, 802–805
  β-blockers in, 139, 141
  calcium channel blockers in, 253
  diet in, 804
  estrogens and, 757
  glucocorticoids and, 738
  osteomalacia in, 795
  steroid diabetes and, 803–804
Diabinese. *See* Chlorpropamide
Diacetylmorphine. *See* Heroin
Diacylglycerol, 117–118, 119
Dialysis, in renal osteodystrophy, 795
Diamidines, 618

Diamine oxidase, 815
Diaminodiphenylsulfone. *See* Dapsone
Diamox. *See* Acetazolamide
Dianabol. *See* Methandrostenolone
Diapid. *See* Lypressin
Diarrhea, 824, 825–826
　bretylium and, 304
　cancer chemotherapy and, 667
　colchicine and, 504
　lincosamides and, 581
　mefenamic acid and, 490
　meperidine in, 445
　methotrexate and, 683
　morphine in, 441
　nalidixic acid in, 552
　penicillins and, 561
　polymyxins in, 585–586
　quinidine and, 287
　schistosomes and, 643
Diasone Sodium. *See* Sulfoxone sodium
Diazepam, 357
　aging and, 40
　as anticonvulsant, 420
　central nervous system and, 363
　dosage of, 373
　half-life of, 40
　ketamine with, 358
　metabolism and excretion of, 355
　pH and, 21
　pharmacokinetics of, 372
　in seizures, 372
　smoking and, 42
　solubility of, 68
　in status epilepticus, 423
　in strychnine-induced convulsions, 381
Diazinon, 81
Diazoxide, 235
　chemical structure of, 233
　in hypertension, 232
　as noncompetitive antagonist, 18
Dibenzodioxins, 76
Dibenzyline. *See* Phenoxybenzamine
Dibozane, 131
1,2-Dibromo-chloropropane, 77
2,4-Dichlorophenoxyacetic acid, 82
Diclofenac, 437
　as analgesic, 433
　antiinflammatory properties of, 493
　in arthritis, 489
Dicloxacillin, 557–558
Dicumarol, 44, 317–318
Dicyclomine, 155, 157
Dideoxycytidine, 607, 612–613
Dideoxyinosine, 607, 611–612
Dieldrin, 81
Dienestrol, 758
Dientamoeba fragilis, 620
Diet
　diabetic, 804
　drug metabolism and, 40
　high-fiber, 826–827
　iodine in, 775
　vitamins in, 839–840
Diethyl ether, 340
Diethylcarbamazine, 638, 640–641
Diethylstilbestrol, 772
　adverse effects of, 90
　preparations and dosage of, 758
　in prostatic cancer, 755
Diffusion
　in drug excretion
　　pulmonary, 51
　　renal, 48

facilitated, 23, 24
　passive, 22, 23
Diffusion constant, 523
Diffusion hypoxia, 343
Diflucan. *See* Fluconazole
Diflunisal
　as analgesic, 433, 434
　anticoagulants and, 318
　for pain, 434–435
Difluoromethyornithine, 622–623
DiGel liquid. *See* Aluminum hydroxide
Digestive system. *See* Gastrointestinal system
Digibind, 262
Digitalis, 255
　in arrhythmia, 309
　calcium channel blockers and, 252
　inspired tension of anesthetic gas and, 342
　intoxication of
　　hypokalemia and, 218
　　lidocaine in, 293
　　phenytoin and, 295
　　propranolol and, 303
　quinidine and, 286
　toxicity of, 262
Digitoxin
　barbiturates and, 376
　cholestyramine and, 204
　in myocardial insufficiency, 263
　pharmacokinetics of, 258
　serum concentration of, 262
Digoxin
　action of, 262
　amiodarone and, 306
　bioavailability of, 67
　cardiac output and, 259
　effects of, 309
　flecainide and, 299
　half-life of, 40
　in myocardial insufficiency, 261, 263
　pharmacokinetics of, 258
　propafenone and, 299
　quinidine and, 287
　serum concentration of, 58, 262
　solubility of, 68
　structural formula of, 258
　sulfasalazine and, 837
　toxicity of, 262
Dihydrofolate reductase, 548
　drug resistance and, 665–666
　methotrexate and, 681
Dihydrofolic acid, 548
Dihydrostreptomycin, 40
Dihydrotachysterol, 791, 793, 795–796
Dihydrotestosterone, 766
Dihydrouracil dehydrogenase, 687
Dihydroxyalcohols, 457
1,25-Dihydroxycholecalciferol, 51, 787, 791,
　　839
　in hypoparathyroidism, 792
　in osteopenia, 794
　pseudohypoparathyroidism and, 793
　in renal osteodystrophy, 795
　in rickets, 793, 794
　synthesis of, 790
Dihydroxyphenylalanine
　in norepinephrine synthesis, 109
　structural analogue of, 245
1,25-Dihydroxyvitamin D$_3$. *See* 1,25-
　　Dihydroxycholecalciferol
Diiodohydroxyquin, 620–621
Diiodotyrosine, 777
Dilacor. *See* Diltiazem
Dilantin. *See* Phenytoin

Diloxanide furoate, 625
Diltiazem
　in angina pectoris, 267
　in arrhythmia, 309
　chemical formula of, 250
　clinical uses of, 274
　pharmacokinetics of, 253
　preparations and dosage of, 253–254
　receptor-blocking properties of, 251
Diluents in capsules, 67
Dimenhydrinate, 820
　as antiemetic, 830
　in motion sickness, 818
Dimercaprol
　as arsenic antidote, 77
　chelation and, 16
Dimethyl tubocurarine, 182
Dimethylphenyl piperazinium, 171, 172
Dinitrate, 267
Dinoprost tromethamine, 482
Dinoprostone, 482
Dioctyl sodium sulfosuccinate. *See* Docusate
　　sodium
Diols, 457
Dioscorides, 5
Dioxin, 78, 82
Dipentum. *See* Olsalazine sodium
Dipetalonema perstans, 640
Diphenhydramine, 820
　as anticholinergic, 429
　as antiemetic, 830
　anxiolytic properties of, 374
　in motion sickness, 818
　sedative properties of, 819
　structure of, 818
Diphenoxylate, 445, 826
Diphenoxylate salts, 445
Diphenylhydantoin. *See* Phenytoin
Diphosphopyridine nucleotide, 841
Diphyllobothrium latum, 638, 639
Diprivan. *See* Propofol
Dipyridamole, 271
　adenosine and, 310
　as antiplatelet drug, 319
Diquat, 81, 82
Disalcid. *See* Salsalate
Disease
　Addison's, 740
　Chagas', 618, 624
　Creutzfeldt-Jakob, 725
　Crohn's, 795, 835–837
　Cushing's
　　aminoglutethimide in, 744
　　dexamethasone in, 745
　　ketoconazole in, 744
　　metyrapone in, 743
　drug metabolism and, 43–44
　Graves'
　　in hyperthyroidism, 782
　　radioiodine in, 784
　Hashimoto's, 779, 780
　Hodgkin's
　　carmustine in, 679
　　mechlorethamine in, 674
　　MOPP regimen in, 666
　　procarbazine in, 699
　　single agents in, 671
　Lyme, 566
　Paget's, 795
　Parkinson's, 425–429
　　amantadine in, 429
　　anticholinergic drugs in, 429
　　decarboxylase inhibitors in, 428–429

Disease, Parkinson's (*cont.*)
  dopamine agonists in, 429
  levodopa in, 426–428
  selegiline in, 429
 Raynaud's, 252
 von Willebrand's, 729
 Wilson's, 499
Disinfectants, 657–662
 agents affecting permeability in, 661–662
 alkylating agents as, 660
 dehydrating agents as, 660
 evaluation of, 658–659
 oxidizing agents as, 659
 sterilization principles and, 657–658
 sulfhydryl combining agents as, 660–661
Disintegrants in capsules, 67
Disodium hydrogen phosphate, 827
Disopyramide, 289–291
 cardiac disease and, 62
 electrophysiological actions of, 285
Disseminated intravascular coagulation, 319
Dissociative anesthesia, 357
Dissolution of drugs, 67
Distal tubule, 214–215
Distribution of drugs, 28–32
 in elderly, 39
 physiological barriers to, 31–32
 plasma protein binding and, 29–30
 selective accumulation in, 30–31
 volume of, 28–29
Disulfiram
 in alcoholism, 455, 456
 anticoagulants and, 318
 for periodic drinker, 466
 phenytoin and, 295
 terfenadine and, 819
DIT. *See* Diiodotyrosine
Diucardin. *See* Hydroflumethiazide
Diuresis
 chlorpromazine and, 390
 ethanol and, 453
 excessive, 221
 xanthines and, 384
Diuretics, 218–220
 absorption and elimination of, 223–224
 adverse reactions to, 224, 225, 226, 228
 anticoagulants and, 318
 as antihypertensives, 230–231
 benzothiazides as, 223–224
 carbonic anhydrase inhibitors as, 222–223
 clinical uses of, 224–228
 excessive diuresis from, 221
 guanethidine with, 242
 hydralazine with, 233
 loop, 226–228
  as antihypertensives, 230–231
  in myocardial insufficiency, 264
  in nephrotic syndrome, 220
  in pulmonary edema, 219
 mechanism of action of, 221
 in myocardial insufficiency, 264
 osmotic, 221
  in acute renal failure, 220
  intracranial pressure and, 219
 pharmacokinetics of, 225, 226, 227
 potassium-sparing, 224–226
  as antihypertensives, 231
  nonsteroidal, 226
 preparations of, 224
 as renin inhibitor, 191
 resistance to, 220–221
 response to, 223, 227
 thiazide
  with α-adrenergic blockers, 238

as antihypertensives, 230
 in ascites, 219
 with β-adrenergic blocking agents, 239
 in nephrotic syndrome, 220
 in premenstrual edema, 220
 sodium intake with, 219
 spironolactone and, 225
 urate, 504–506
 with vasodilators, 231
Diuril. *See* Chlorothiazide
Dizziness
 buspirone in, 374
 flecainide and, 298
 indomethacin and, 490
 mexiletine and, 297
 moricizine and, 291
 propafenone and, 300
DMPP. *See* Dimethylphenyl piperazinium
DNA. *See* Deoxyribonucleic acid
Dobutamine, 127, 263
Dobutrex. *See* Dobutamine
Docusate calcium, 827
Docusate potassium, 827, 828
Docusate sodium, 827, 828
Dolor, in inflammation, 478
Domperidone, 824–825, 831
Dopa, 109, 245
Dopa-decarboxylase, 109, 245
Dopamine, 328
 actions of, 124
 blood-brain barrier and, 336
 cellular locations of, 333
 chemical structure of, 116
 feedback control of, 778
 ganglionic action potential and, 171
 in myocardial insufficiency, 263
 in norepinephrine synthesis, 109
 in parkinsonism, 426
 preparations and dosage of, 125
 reserpine and, 243
 schizophrenia and, 387
 small intensely fluorescent cells and, 169
Dopamine agonists, 429
Dopamine antagonists, 831
Dopamine β-hydroxylase, 109
Dopamine receptors, 388, 389
Dopar. *See* Levodopa
"Dope," 461
Dopram. *See* Doxapram
Doryx. *See* Doxycycline
Dosage
 liquid, 67
 maximum, 70
 oral, 65–67
 in topical therapy, 523, 525
Dose-response curve, 13
Dose-response relationship, 12–16
 graded, 14–15
 potency and intrinsic activity and, 15–16
 quantal, 13–14
 receptors and, 10
Dosing interval, 64
Double-blind technique, 88–89
"Downs," 464
Doxapram, 380, 381
Doxazosin, 135, 136
Doxepin
 chemical structure of, 398
 dosage and serum concentration of, 403
Doxinate. *See* Docusate sodium
Doxorubicin, 687–689
 enterohepatic recirculation and, 51
 hair loss and, 668
 neurotoxicity of, 75

Doxychel. *See* Doxycycline
Doxycycline, 575
 in malaria, 635
 in renal disease, 576
Drisdol. *See* Ergocalciferol
Dronabinol, 472, 830–831
Droperidol, 355
Drowsiness
 benzodiazepines and, 372
 lidocaine and, 293
Drug abuse, 459–474
 alcoholism and, 466
 barbiturates in, 375
 central nervous system stimulants in, 466–468
 characteristics of, 459–460
 Controlled Substance Act and, 460–461
 ethanol in, 455
 hallucinogens in, 468–471
 history of, 459
 inhalants in, 472–473
 malaria and, 627
 marijuana in, 471–472
 opioids in, 461–464
 xanthines in, 384–385
Drug-blood level curve, in oral administration, 66
Drug delivery system, term, 65
Drug hangover, 372
Drug industry, 95–97
Drug-metabolizing enzymes
 allopurinol and, 507
 barbiturates and, 376
 benzodiazepines and, 371
 mitotane and, 744
 phenobarbital and, 418
 steroid metabolism and, 733
 vitamins and, 845
Drug testing, 85–91
 adverse reaction surveillance in, 90
 control groups in, 88
 informed consent in, 87–88
 institutional review boards in, 87
 legislation in, 85–87
 phases of, 89
 randomization in, 88
 special populations in, 89–90
 techniques in, 88–89
Drugs. *See also specific drugs*
 absorption and distribution of, 19–32
  after parenteral administration, 27–28
  alimentary tract and, 24–25
  formulation factors in, 26
  lungs and, 26–27
  metabolism and, 26
  physiological barriers in, 31–32
  plasma protein binding and, 29–30
  selective accumulation in, 30–31
  skin and, 27
  transport mechanisms in, 22–24
  volume of distribution and, 28–29
 advertisement of, 86–87
 blood concentration of, 55–56
  area under, 58
  intravenous infusion and, 59, 60
  volume of distribution and, 60–61
 cell cycle and, 664
 delivery systems of. *See* Administration of drugs
 development of, 88–89
 efficacy of, 86–87
 excretion of, 47–53
  biliary, 50–51
  breast milk and, 52–53

in elderly, 40
  hepatic, 61
  pulmonary, 51–52
  renal, 47–50
  sweat and saliva and, 52
half-life of, 70
labeling of, 86
marketing of, 96–97
mechanisms of action of, 9–18
  antagonism in, 16–18
  binding in, 11–12
  dose-response relationship and, 12–16
  equations in, 16
  receptors and, 9–11
metabolism of, 33–46. *See also* Metabolism,
  drug
nonoral. *See* Nonoral medication
oral. *See* Oral medication
origins of, 3
pharmacokinetics of, 55–64
  basic concepts in, 55–57
  chronic administration in, 58–60
  multicompartment models in, 60
  oral or first-order absorption in, 57–58
  physiological determinants in, 60–61
prolonged-release, 70–72
testing of. *See* Drug testing
therapeutic index of, 70
toxicity of. *See* Toxicity
volume of distribution and, 60–61
"Dry labbing," 94
Dry mouth, 390
DTIC. *See* Dacarbazine
Duct, renal collecting, 214–215
Dulcolax. *See* Bisacodyl
Durabolin. *See* Nandrolone phenpropionate
Duranest. *See* Etidocaine
Duricef. *See* Cefadroxil
Dust, coal, 79
Dwarf tapeworm, 639
Dyazide. *See* Triamterene
Dycil. *See* Dicloxacillin
Dymelor. *See* Acetohexamide
Dynacirc. *See* Isradipine
Dynapen. *See* Dicloxacillin
Dynorphins, 438
Dyphylline, 385
Dyrenium. *See* Triamterene
Dyscrasia, blood, 495
Dysentery
  balantidial, 617–618
  schistosome-induced, 643
Dyskinesia
  levodopa and, 427
  tardive, 430
Dysmenorrhea
  corticosteroids and, 739
  estrogens and progestins in, 755
  ibuprofen in, 437
  prostaglandins and, 480
Dysphagia, in cancer chemotherapy, 667
Dysphonia, 518
Dysphoria
  in lysergic acid diethylamide abuse, 469
  morphine and, 440
Dyspnea
  adenosine and, 310
  flecainide and, 299
  sotalol and, 307
Dystonia, 391
Dysuria, 676

E-Mycin. *See* Erythromycin
EAA. *See* Excitatory amino acids

Early afterdepolarization, term, 280
Echothiophate, 163, 166, 167
Econazole, 654
Ecotrin. *See* Aspirin
Eczematous eruption, 76
EDCF. *See* Endothelium-derived constricting
  factor
Edecrin. *See* Ethacrynic acid
Edema
  in congestive heart failure, 256, 257
  glucocorticoids and, 739
  of pregnancy, 220
  of premenstrual period, 220
  pulmonary, 219
EDRF. *See* Endothelium-derived relaxing
  factor
Edrophonium, 163
  acetylcholine receptor blockade and, 181–182
  metabolism of, 165
  uses of, 166
Effective dose, term, 14
Effective refractory period, 280
Effector cells
  in autonomic nervous system, 101
  receptors of, 112–114
Efficacy, 86–87
  clinical drug testing for, 89
  term, 16
Eflornithine, 622–623
Efudex. *See* Fluorouracil
Eicosanoids, 477–482
  asthma and allergic states and, 479–480
  biosynthesis of, 477–478
  fever and, 480
  hemostasis and, 480–482
  inflammation and, 478–479
  reproduction and, 480
  therapeutic, 482
Ejaculation, 390
Elavil. *See* Amitriptyline
Elderly
  clinical drug trials and, 90
  drug metabolism and, 39–40
  impotence and, 767–768
  parkinsonism and, 425
  phenylbutazone and, 489
  selective serotonin reuptake inhibitors and,
    405
  tubular transport mechanism in, 49
Electrical discharge of neuron, 413
Electrocardiography
  adenosine and, 310
  amiodarone and, 305
  disopyramide and, 289
  flecainide and, 298
  lidocaine and, 292
  moricizine and, 291
  phenytoin and, 294
  propafenone and, 299
  propranolol and, 302
  quinidine and, 286
  sotalol and, 307
Electrolytes
  adrenal cortex and, 734
  in iso-osmotic colonic lavage solutions, 828
  metabolism of, 211–218. *See also* Body
    water
    blood supply and, 212–214
    nephron segments and, 213–215
    potassium regulation and, 216–218
    sodium conservation and, 215–216
    tubular reabsorption and secretion of,
      212
  steroids and, 739

Electrophysiology of heart, 275–283
  adenosine and, 309–310
  amiodarone and, 305
  automaticity in, 278–280
  bretylium and, 303
  conduction in, 278–280
  disopyramide and, 289
  flecainide and, 297
  ionic basis of, 277–278
  lidocaine and, 292
  mexiletine and, 296–297
  moricizine and, 291
  phenytoin and, 294
  procainamide and, 287
  propafenone and, 299
  propranolol and, 300–302
  quinidine and, 284–285
  sotalol and, 307
  tocainide and, 296
  transmembrane potential in, 275–276
  verapamil and, 308
Elephantiasis, 639
Elimination rate constant, 55, 60
  in intravenous bolus, 63
  of lithium carbonate, 409–411
Elixophyllin. *See* Theophylline
Elspar. *See* L-Asparaginase
Embolism
  intravenous drug administration and, 28
  oral anticoagulants and, 318
Emcyt. *See* Estramustine
Emetics, 829
Emetine, 619–620
EMLA. *See* Eutectic mixture of local
  anesthetics
Enalapril, 192, 193–194
  in myocardial insufficiency, 264
  structure of, 193
Enalkiren, 191
Encephalitis lethargica, 425
Encephalopathy
  arsenicals and, 623
  methotrexate and, 683
  Wernicke's, 455
End-plate currents, in neuromuscular
  transmission, 177, 178
Endocarditis
  enterococcal, 571
  penicillins in, 561
  treatment of, 542
  vancomycin in, 584–585
Endocervical glands, 750
Endocrine system, 717–810
  angiotensins and, 191
  diabetes mellitus and, 802–805
  disorders of, 792–795
  hormones in
    adrenocortical, 731–745. *See also*
      Adrenocortical hormones
    androgens and anabolic steroids in, 761–
      774. *See also* Androgens
    calcitonin and, 790–791
    chemical suppression of, 720
    cholecalciferol and, 791–792
    drug interactions with, 720–721
    estrogens, progestins, and antiestrogens
      in, 747–759. *See also* Estrogens
    hypothalamic and pituitary gland, 723–
      730. *See also* Hypothalamic hormones
    low molecular weight, 719
    parathyroid, 788–790
    receptor regulation and, 721
    supraphysiological dosages of, 719
  hypoglycemic agents and, 805–808

Endocrine system (*cont.*)
  insulin and, 797–802. *See also* Insulin
  phenothiazines and, 389–390, 391
  steroids and, 735–736
  thyroid and antithyroid drugs and, 776–786. *See also* Thyroid hormones
Endocytosis, 23, 24
Endogenous opioid peptides, 332
Endometrial cancer, 696, 753, 755, 756
Endometriosis
  androgens and anabolic steroids and, 768
  estrogens and progestins and, 755
  gonadotropin releasing hormone and, 728
Endoplasmic reticulum
  drug metabolism and, 36
  enzymes in, 34
Endorphins, 9, 438
Endothelium
  enzymes in, 335
  vascular tone and, 122
Endothelium-derived constricting factor, 122
Endothelium-derived relaxing factor, 122, 151, 232
Enduron. *See* Methyclothiazide
Enema, 828
Enflurane, 349
  in neuromuscular blockade, 182
  partition coefficients of, 340
  solubility of, 341
Enkephalins, 9, 106, 438
Enoxacin, 551
Entamoeba histolytica, 617
Enteric coating, 68, 69
Enterobacter infection
  cephalosporins in, 564
  penicillins in, 557
Enterobius vermicularis infection
  mebendazole in, 643
  piperazine in, 640
  pyrantel pamoate in, 641
  thiabendazole in, 642
Enterococcal infection
  ampicillin in, 561
  penicillins in, 559
  trimethoprim in, 548
Enterocolitis, 584–585
Enterohepatic circulation, 38, 50
Enuresis, 729
Environmental Protection Agency, 78
Enzymes
  antineoplastic, 695–696
  in cerebral endothelium, 335
  cholinesterase in, 161
  drug-metabolizing, 33–36
    allopurinol and, 507
    barbiturates and, 376
    benzodiazepines and, 371
    induction of, 41–42
    mitotane and, 744
    phenobarbital and, 418
    steroids and, 720
    vitamins and, 845
  eicosanoids and, 477
  in hepatic clearance, 61
  hydralazine and, 233
  in inflammation, 479
  renin and, 189–190, 191–194
  toxicity of, 73
Eosinophil, 509
Eosinophilia, 690
EPA. *See* Environmental Protection Agency
Ephedrine, 127–128, 357

Epidermis, 27, 523, 524
Epidural anesthesia, 365
Epiglottitis, 560
Epilepsy
  anticonvulsant drugs in, 413–414
  barbiturates in, 376
  benzodiazepines in, 372
  febrile seizures and, 423
  in pregnancy, 423
Epinephrine, 328, 368
  acetylcholine and, 17
  adrenal medulla and, 106
  in asthma, 514–516
  blood-brain barrier and, 336
  cardiovascular effects of, 120
  chemical structure of, 116
  fungus ergot and, 130
  ganglionic action potential and, 171
  as hepatic glycogenolytic agent, 803
  histamine release and, 813, 817
  local anesthetics with, 366
  nicotinic receptors and, 172
  in open-angle glaucoma, 167
  pharmacodynamics of, 121, 122
  phenoxybenzamine and, 133
  preparations and dosage of, 125
  trichloroethylene and, 80
Epipodophyllotoxins, 694
Epogen. *See* Recombinant erythropoietin
Epoxide hydrolases, 73
Epoxides, 76
Epsom salt. *See* Magnesium sulfate
EPSP. *See* Excitatory postsynaptic potential
Equanil. *See* Meprobamate
Equilibration in drug absorption, 27
Equilibrium-competitive antagonism, 129
  of β-blockers, 138
  of imidazolines, 133
  of labetalol, 142
  of quinazoline derivatives, 135
Equilibrium-competitive bond, 17
Eramycin. *See* Erythromycin
Ergamisol. *See* Levamisole
Ergocalciferol, 495, 791, 793, 794
Ergosterol, 839
Ergot alkaloids, 130
ERP. *See* Effective refractory period
Ery-Tab. *See* Erythromycin
ERYC. *See* Erythromycin
Erypar. *See* Erythromycin
EryPed. *See* Erythromycin
Erythema, 528
Erythrityl tetranitrate, 267, 268, 271
Erythrocin. *See* Erythromycin
Erythrocyte cholinesterase, 161
Erythromycin, 579–581
  anticoagulants and, 318
  astemizole and, 819
  in dermatological disorders, 531
  in protozoal infection, 625
  serum concentrations of, 69
Erythropoietic protoporphyria, 528
Erythropoietin, 667, 768
Escherichia coli infection
  ampicillin in, 560
  penicillins in, 557
  sulfonamides in, 546
  trimethoprim in, 548
Eserine, 163
Esidrix. *See* Hydrochlorothiazide
Eskalith. *See* Lithium carbonate
Esmolol, 138, 140, 301

Esophagitis, 824
  doxorubicin and, 688
  muscarinic blocking agents and, 158
Esotropia, 167
Essential oils as mouth rinse, 851, 852
Esters, 361, 366–367
  of acetylcholinesterase, 162
  of ampicillin, 558
Estrace. *See* Estradiol
Estraderm. *See* Estradiol
Estradiol, 747, 772
  enterohepatic recirculation and, 51
  microsomal enzyme activity and, 42
  preparations and dosage of, 758
Estramustine, 697
Estrane nucleus, 747, 748
Estrogens, 747–759
  adenohypophyseal-gonadal interactions of, 749
  adverse reactions of, 755–757
  in cancer treatment, 754–755
  cardiovascular effects of, 750–751
  contraindications for, 757–758
  drug interactions of, 758
  drug metabolism and, 45
  in dysfunctional uterine bleeding, 755
  in dysmenorrhea, 755
  in endometriosis, 755
  as gonadotropin antagonists, 772
  in growth and development, 750
  hepatotoxicity of, 74, 75
  in infertility, 754
  insulin resistance and, 802
  lactation and, 755
  mechanism of action of, 751
  menopause and, 753
  menstrual cycle and, 750
  metabolism and excretion of, 747–748
  nonsteroidal, 748
  oral contraception and, 751–753
  ovarian steroidogenesis and, 749–750
  ovulation and, 754
  in premenstrual edema, 220
  preparations and dosages of, 758
  psychological disturbances and, 753–754
  in replacement therapy, 754
  structure and biosynthesis of, 747
  synthetic, 748
  tamoxifen as, 696–697
  thyroid-binding globulin and, 781
Ethacrynic acid, 226–228
Ethambutol, 587–588, 591–592
Ethanol, 451–456
  adverse reactions of, 454–455
  as antiseptic, 659
  benzodiazepines and, 372
  in breast milk, 52
  central nervous system and, 453
  chemistry of, 451
  cytochrome P450 and, 41
  in diazepam preparation, 357
  drug metabolism and, 41
  as ethylene glycol antidote, 77
  hepatotoxicity of, 74
  interactions with
    drug, 455–456
    vitamin, 845
  mechanism of action of, 453
  in methanol poisoning, 77, 456
  pharmacokinetics of, 451–453
  pulmonary excretion of, 51
  therapeutic uses of, 453–454
Ethanolamines, 820

Ethchlorvynol, 318
Ether, 347
    anesthetic apparatus and, 343
    in classic anesthesia, 345–346
    solubility of, 341
Ethics, 93–97
    application of, 93–94
    conflicts of interest in, 95–97
    research subjects and, 95
    scientific misconduct and, 94–95
Ethinyl estradiol, 748, 752
    preparations and dosage of, 758
    prolonged release of, 71
Ethionamide, 592–593
Ethosuximide, 420, 421, 422
Ethotoin, 416
Ethrane. See Enflurane
Ethril. See Erythromycin
Ethyl alcohol. See Ethanol
Ethylene glycol, 77, 457
Ethylene oxide
    microbial spectrum of, 658
    in sterilization, 660
Ethylenediamine, 76, 820
Ethylenimines, 680–681
Ethylestrenol, 769
Ethynodiol diacetate, 752
Etidocaine, 364, 367
Etidronate
    in hypercalcemia, 793
    in Paget's disease, 795
Etodolac, 489, 493
Etomidate
    as anesthetic, 358–359
    metabolism and excretion of, 355
Etoposide, 694
    in Kaposi's sarcoma, 614–615
    multidrug resistance and, 666
Etretinate, 527–528
Eulexin. See Flutamide
Eunuchoidism, 766
Euphoria
    glucocorticoids and, 739
    lysergic acid diethylamide and, 469
    morphine and, 440
Eutectic mixture of local anesthetics, 368
Euthroid. See Liotrix
Euthyroid state, 779
Excitatory amino acids, 330–331
Excitatory neurotransmitter, 327
Excitatory postsynaptic potential, 169–171,
        327
Excretion, 47–53
    biliary, 50–51
    breast milk and, 52–53
    in elderly, 40
    hepatic, 61
    pulmonary, 51–52
    renal, 47–50
    sweat and saliva and, 52
Exercise-induced asthma, 520
Exna. See Benzthiazide
Exocytosis, 109, 798
Exophthalmos, 782
Experimental method, 5–7
Exposure, nontherapeutic, 78–82
    air pollution in, 78–79
    cyanide in, 82
    food additives and contaminants in, 79
    metals in, 79, 80
    pesticides in, 81–82
    solvents in, 79–81
Extracellular fluid, 221

Extracorporeal photopheresis, 528
Extraneuronal uptake, 110, 112
Extrapyramidal syndrome, 393, 394
Extrapyramidal system, 391
Extrinsic asthma, 509
Eye
    acetylcholine and, 146
    adrenoceptors and, 113
    cholinesterase inhibitors and, 164, 167
    drug accumulation in, 30
    ganglionic blockade and, 174
    gentamicin and, 572
    glucocorticoids and, 738–739
    indomethacin and, 491
    innervation of, 105–105
    morphine and, 440
    muscarinic blocking drugs and, 153, 154
    oral contraceptives and, 757
Eyelid
    contact dermatitis of, 158
    idoxuridine and, 603

Facilitated diffusion, 23, 24
Factor VII, 840
Factor IX, 840
Factor X, 840
False transmitter, 245
Familial dysautonomia, 148
Famotidine, 834
    as histamine blocker, 821
    structure of, 834
Fansidar. See Pyrimethamine
Fasciola hepatica, 643, 644
Fasciolopsis buski, 638, 639
Fast excitatory postsynaptic potential, 169–
        171
Fast inward channels, 277
Fastin. See Phentermine hydrochloride
Fatigue
    estrogens and, 754
    methylxanthines in, 384
    sotalol and, 307
Fatty acids, 123–124
FDA. See Food and Drug Administration
Febrile convulsion, 418
Fecal softeners, 828
Federal Bureau of Chemistry, 86
Feedback control of thyroid hormones, 778
Felbamate, 421
Felbatol. See Felbamate
Feldene. See Piroxicam
Felodipine, 249
Female hypopituitarism, 768–769
Fenamates, 437
    as analgesic, 433
    antiinflammatory properties of, 490
Fenestrations, 28
Fenfluramine, 382, 383
Fenoprofen, 492
    as analgesic, 433, 437
    anticoagulants and, 318
    in arthritis, 489
Fentanyl, 438, 445
    as analgesic, 442
    anesthetic uses of, 360
Fenvalerate, 81
Feosol. See Ferrous sulfate
Fermentation, ethanol and, 451
Fero-Gradumet. See Ferrous sulfate
Ferrous sulfate, 846
Fertility
    oral contraceptives and, 757
    prostaglandins and, 480

Fetal alcohol syndrome, 455
Fetus
    cancer chemotherapy and, 669
    drug and chemical toxicity to, 76–77
    local anesthetics and, 364
    morphine and, 441
    phenytoin and, 416
    placental barrier and, 31–32
Fever
    allopurinol and, 507
    amphotericin B and, 649
    anticonvulsant drugs in, 423
    eicosanoids and, 480
FFA. See Free fatty acids
Fibrillation
    atrial
        amiodarone in, 306
        β-adrenoceptor blocking agents in, 301
        diltiazem in, 309
        oral anticoagulants and, 318–319
        procainamide in, 288
        quinidine in, 286
    ventricular
        β-adrenoceptor blocking agents in, 301
        bretylium and, 304
        lidocaine in, 293
Fibrin degradation products, 320
Fibrinogenolysis, 321
Fibrinolysis, 320
Fibrinolytic pathway, 313
Fibrinolytic system, 320–321
    antifibrinolytic drugs and, 323
    coagulation systems and, 315
    hemostatic mechanisms and, 313–315
Fibrosis
    cancer chemotherapy and, 668
    cyclophosphamide and, 676
    melphalan and, 677
Filarial worm, 639
Filgrastim, 703
Filtration, 22, 23, 47
Finasteride, 761, 772, 773
First-pass effect, 441
Fish oil, 201–202, 207
Fish tapeworm, 639
FK506, 705, 709
Flagyl. See Metronidazole
Flashbacks, 469
Flatworm, 637–639
Flavoprotein, 35
Flaxedil. See Gallamine triethiodide
Flecainide, 297–299, 306
Flexeril. See Cyclobenzaprine
Flora
    antibiotics and, 543
    biliary excretion and, 51
    drug metabolism and, 45
    neomycin and, 571
Floropryl. See Isoflurophate
Flosequinan, 263–264
Floxin. See Ofloxacin
Floxuridine, 687
Fluconazole, 654
    anticoagulants and, 318
    in cryptococcosis, 614
    in cutaneous fungal disease, 531
Flucytosine, 648, 650–651
Flufenamic acid, 204
Fluid intake
    allopurinol and, 507
    steroids and, 739
    sulfinpyrazone and, 506
Fluke, 643–645

Flunisolide, 519, 740
Fluoride, 794, 851–852
Fluorine, 79
Fluorocitrate, 687
Fluorocortisol, 736
5-Fluorocytosine, 650–651
Fluoroquinolones, 318
5-Fluorouracil, 686–687
    active transport of, 23
    cell cycle and, 664
    in dermatological disorders, 532, 533
    methotrexate and, 683
    vitamins and, 845
Fluothane. *See* Halothane
Fluoxetine, 403, 404–405
Fluoxymesterone, 767
Fluphenazine, 70, 388
Flurazepam, 372, 373
Flurbiprofen, 493
    as analgesic, 433, 437
    anticoagulants and, 318
    in arthritis, 489
Flushing
    adenosine and, 310
    calcium channel blockers and, 253
Flutamide, 697, 761, 772
Flutter, atrial. *See* Atrial flutter
Fluvoxamine, 404
Folate antagonists, 681–683
Folate deficiency
    anticonvulsants and, 423
    phenytoin in, 416
Folic acid, 840
    deficiency of, 842
    in drug interactions, 845
    in megaloblastic anemia, 846
    methotrexate and, 681
    sulfonamides and, 545
    trimethoprim and, 548
Follicle, hair, 668
Follicle-stimulating hormone, 726, 749, 764
Folliculitis, 530
Follutein. *See* Human chorionic gonadotropin
Fonazine mesylate, 184
Food
    drug absorption and, 26
    loracarbef and, 567
    macrolides and, 580
    penicillins and, 557
    tetracyclines and, 575
Food additives, 79
Food and Drug Administration, 86, 87
    on company-sponsored promotional
        activities, 97
    drug approval procedures of, 94, 95
    on multisource drugs, 58
Food coloring, 79
Food, Drug and Cosmetic Act, 86, 87
Forane. *See* Isoflurane
Formaldehyde
    methanamine and, 552
    in sterilization, 660
Formic acid, 456
Formoterol, 517
Formularies, 85
Formulation factors in drug absorption, 26
Fortaz. *See* Ceftazidime
Foscarnet
    in AIDS-related disease, 615
    in cytomegalovirus, 614
Fosinopril, 193
Fraction of unbound drug, 61
Fragrance chemicals, 77

Francisella tularensis, 571
Frank-Starling mechanism, 255–256
Free-basing, 466–467
Free fatty acids, 801
Free radicals, 689
Frequency distribution curve, 13–14
Fructose, 804
FSH. *See* Follicle-stimulating hormone
Ftorafur, 687
fu. *See* Fraction of unbound drug
5-FU. *See* 5-Fluorouracil
Fulvicin. *See* Griseofulvin
Functio laesa, 478
Functional antagonism, 16–17
Fungal contamination of food, 79
Fungal infection
    acquired immunodeficiency syndrome and,
        614
    antifungal drugs in, 647–656
        amphotericin B in, 647–649
        azoles in, 651–654
        cutaneous, 530–531
        flucytosine in, 650–651
        griseofulvin in, 650
        liposomal amphotericin B in, 649
        naftifine hydrochloride in, 654–656
        nystatin in, 649–650
    glucocorticoids and, 738
Fungizone. *See* Amphotericin B
Furacin. *See* Nitrofurazone
Furadantin. *See* Nitrofurantoin
Furamide. *See* Diloxanide furoate
Furazolidone, 619
Furosemide, 226–228
    as antihypertensive, 230
    in chronic renal failure, 220
    clearance of, 62
    in myocardial insufficiency, 264
    preparations of, 228
    proximal tubule and, 214
    volume of distribution of, 28

G-CSF. *See* Granulocyte colony stimulating
    factor
G_2-phase, 663
G proteins. *See* Guanine nucleotide-binding
    proteins
GABA. *See* γ-Aminobutyric acid
Gabapentin, 421
Galactorrhea, 725
Galen, 4–5
Gallamine triethiodide, 182
Gallbladder disease, 757
Gallstones, 727, 837–838
Gamastan. *See* Immune globulin
Gambian sleeping sickness, 618
Gambian trypanosomiasis, 621, 623
Gamete, mosquito, 628
Gametocyte, mosquito, 628
Gamma-aminobutyric acid. *See* γ-
    Aminobutyric acid
Gamma globulin, 600–601, 762
Gamminune. *See* Immune globulin
Ganciclovir
    in AIDS-related disease, 615–616
    in cytomegalovirus, 614
Ganglia, 101
    in autonomic nervous system, 102–103
    blockade of, 172
    receptors in, 147, 169
    stimulation of, 171–172
    transmission through, 169–171

Ganglionic action potential, 171
Ganglionic blocking agents, 169–175
    adverse reactions of, 174–174
    as antihypertensives, 244
    clinical uses of, 174
    excitatory and inhibitory potentials and,
        169–171
    mechanism of action of, 173
    nicotinic receptor stimulation and, 171–
        173
    pharmacological actions of, 173–174
    preparations and dosage of, 175
Ganglionic cell muscarinic receptor, 170
Garamycin. *See* Gentamicin
Gas gangrene, 560
Gases
    affinity of, 338
    alveolar uptake of, 340–342
    general anesthetic, 345–352
    nontherapeutic exposure to, 78–79
    partial pressure of, 337–338
    pulmonary excretion of, 51
    tissue concentration of, 338
Gastric emptying
    absorption and, 25–26
    drugs enhancing, 824–825
Gastric mucosa
    nonsteroidal antiinflammatory drugs and,
        481
    steroids and, 738
Gastric secretion
    drugs reducing, 831–832
    phentolamine or tolazoline and, 134
Gastrin
    calcitonin and, 790
    insulin secretion and, 799
Gastritis, 455
Gastroenteritis, 61
Gastrointestinal drugs, 823–838
    in constipation, 826–829
    in diarrhea, 825–826
    in gallstone dissolution, 837–838
    gastric emptying and, 824–825
    in inflammatory bowel disease, 835–837
    in peptic ulcer disease, 831–835
    in vomiting, 829–831
Gastrointestinal system
    acetylcholine and, 146
    adrenoceptors and, 113
    aminoglycosides and, 570
    anticholinesterase agents and, 165
    catecholamines and, 123
    choline esters and, 147
    disturbance of
        chemotherapy and, 667–668
        diquat and, 82
        levodopa and, 427
        mexiletine and, 297
        mitotane and, 744
        nonsteroidal antiinflammatory drugs and,
            486–487
        phentolamine and tolazoline and, 134
        quinidine and, 287
    eicosanoids and, 481
    ethanol and, 453, 455
    ganglionic blockade and, 174
    innervation of, 106
    isoproterenol and, 516
    lincosamides and, 581–582
    morphine and, 440–441
    muscarinic blocking drugs and, 153, 154
    nicotine and, 173
    norepinephrine and, 147

renal disease and, 61
salicylates and, 435, 488
Gastrozepine. *See* Pirenzepine
Gelusil. *See* Aluminum hydroxide
Gemfibrozil, 207
  anticoagulants and, 318
  in hypolipidemia, 203
  lovastatin with, 206
Gemonil. *See* Metharbital
Gender in drug metabolism, 44
Gene amplification, 666
General anesthesia
  γ-aminobutyric acid and, 330
  balanced, 351
  inhalational, 337–344
    alveolar uptake of gases in, 340–342
    anesthetic apparatus for, 343–344
    concentration effect in, 342–343
    diffusion hypoxia and, 343
    gases in, 350–351
    Henry's law and, 337–338
    partial pressure–minimum alveolar
      concentration in, 338–339
    pulmonary perfusion and, 341
    rate of concentration in, 339–340
    second gas effect of, 343
    solubility of agents for, 340–341
    upper airway and, 344
    volatile liquids in, 347–349
  intravenous drugs in, 353–360
    benzodiazepines as, 357
    distribution of, 354, 355
    etomidate as, 358–359
    ketamine as, 357–358
    metabolism and excretion of, 355
    narcotics as, 360
    pharmacokinetic properties of, 354–355
    propofol as, 359
    ultra–short-acting barbiturates as, 356–357
  signs and stages of, 345–346
Generation time, 663
Genetics in drug metabolism, 42–43
Genital herpes, 604
Genital warts, 532
Genitourinary system. *See* Urinary system
Genotoxicity, 76
Gentamicin, 571–572
  nephrotoxicity of, 75
  volume of distribution of, 28
Gentian violet, 531
Geocillin. *See* Carbenicillin
Geometric scale, 15
Geopen. *See* Carbenicillin
Geriatric patients. *See* Elderly
Germanin. *See* Suramin
Gestation, toxicity and, 77
GHRH. *See* Growth hormone releasing
  hormone
Giardia lamblia, 617–618
Giardiasis, 617–618, 634
Gingiva, 847–853
Gingival hyperplasia, 416
Gingivitis, 847–848
Gingkolide B, 482
Glandular tissue, histamine and, 816
Glauber's salt, 827
Glaucoma
  β-blockers in, 139, 141
  cholinesterase inhibitors in, 167
  disopyramide and, 290
  epinephrine in, 125
  glucocorticoids and, 739

muscarinic blocking agents and, 158
  pilocarpine in, 149
Glibenclamide, 806–807
Gliclazide, 806–807
Glipizide, 806–807
Globus pallidus, 389
Glomerular filtration, 47–48, 212
Glomerulus, 34, 213–214
Glossitis, 561
Glucagon
  anticoagulants and, 318
  calcitonin and, 790
  glucose and, 797, 799
  as hepatic glycogenolytic agent, 803
  insulin and, 799
  propranolol and, 303
  secretion of, 799
Glucocorticoids
  adverse effects of, 737–740
  angiotensinogen and, 189
  antiinflammatory properties of, 479, 496
  with etomidate, 359
  glucose-6-phosphatase and, 734
  in gout, 503
  mechanism of, 741–742
  in osteopenia, 794
  synthesis of, 733
  vitamins and, 795, 844
Gluconeogenesis
  in diabetes, 804
  hepatic, 801
Glucose
  in acetylcholine synthesis, 108–109
  blood
    glucocorticoids and, 733
    glucose homeostasis and, 797
  estrogens and, 751
  glucagon and, 799
  homeostasis and, 797
  insulin and, 799, 800
  oral contraceptives and, 757
  as oral hypoglycemic antidote, 77
Glucose-6-phosphatase,
  glucocorticoids and, 734
Glucose 6-phosphate,
  epinephrine and, 123
Glucose transporter isoforms, 800, 803
Glucosuria, 804
Glucotrol. *See* Glipizide
Glucuronic acid conjugates, 51
Glucuronide, 37–38, 782
GLUT. *See* Glucose transporter isoforms
Glutamic acid, 330–332, 336
Glutamine, 39
Glutaraldehyde, 660
Glutathione
  acetaminophen and, 45
  conjugation of, 39
Glutethimide
  aminoglutethimide and, 744
  anticoagulants and, 318
  in breast milk, 52
  codeine and, 465
  in monooxygenase enzyme induction, 42
  vitamins and, 845
Glyburide, 806–807
Glycerin, 222
Glycerol. *See* Glycerin
Glyceryl trinitrate, 24
Glycine, 330
  blood-brain barrier and, 336
  central nervous system and, 380

conjugation with, 39
  uric acid and, 501
Glycine xylidide, 293
Glycogen
  glucocorticoids and, 733
  hepatic metabolism of, 801
Glycogenolysis
  adrenoceptors and, 113
  epinephrine and, 123
  in hepatic glycogen metabolism, 801
  sympathetic nervous system and, 103
Glycols, 457
Glycopeptides, 584–585
Glycoproteins, 634–635. *See also* P-
  glycoprotein
Glycopyrrolate
  anticholinesterase agents and, 166
  as preanesthetic medication, 156
  uses for, 155
Glycosides. *See* Cardiac glycosides
GM-CSF. *See* Granulocyte-macrophage
  colony stimulating factor
GnRH. *See* Gonadotropin releasing hormone
GnRH antagonists. *See* Gonadotropin
  releasing hormone antagonists
Goeckerman regimen, 529
Goiter
  in hypothyroidism, 779
  levothyroxine sodium in, 780
  multinodular, 779
  thyroid hormone inhibitors in, 783
Gold preparations
  in asthma, 520–521
  in rheumatoid arthritis, 494–495, 496
Gold sodium thiomalate, 494, 496
GoLYTELY, 828
Gonadorelin, 727–728
Gonadotropin, human chorionic, 726, 767
Gonadotropin antagonists, 772
Gonadotropin releasing hormone, 726, 727–728, 749
  analogues of, 771–772
  in testosterone regulation, 764
Gonadotropin releasing hormone antagonists, 761
Gonococcal infection, 560
Gonorrhea
  ceftriaxone in, 565
  penicillins in, 560
  trimethoprim in, 549
"Goofballs," 464
Goserelin, 728
Gossypol, 771
Gout, 485, 501–508
  allopurinol in, 506–508
  colchicine in, 503–504
  indomethacin in, 508
  oxyphenbutazone in, 508
  phenylbutazone in, 508
  pyrazinamide in, 593
  renal urate homeostasis and, 502
  uric acid and, 501–502
  uricosuric drugs in, 504–506
Graded dose-response relationship, 14–15
Gram-negative infection
  aminoglycosides in, 570
  methanamine in, 552
  nitrofurans in, 550
  quinolones in, 551
  sulfonamides in, 546
  trimethoprim in, 548
Gram-positive infection
  nitrofurans in, 550

Gram-positive infection (*cont.*)
  sulfonamides in, 546
  trimethoprim in, 548
Grand mal epilepsy, 414
Granular uptake, 110
Granulocyte colony stimulating factor, 667
  azidothymidine and, 611
Granulocyte-macrophage colony stimulating
  factor, 667, 714
Granulomatosis, Wegener's, 710
Granulomatous disease, 606
"Grass," 472
Graves' disease
  in hyperthyroidism, 782
  radioiodine in, 784
Gray baby syndrome, 38, 579
Grifulvin. *See* Griseofulvin
Grisactin. *See* Griseofulvin
Griseofulvin
  anticoagulants and, 318
  antifungal action of, 531, 648
Growth factors, antineoplastic, 703
Growth fraction, 665
Growth hormone, 723–725
  herbicides and, 82
  insulin and, 799, 802
Growth hormone releasing hormone, 727
Guanabenz, 245–248
Guanadrel, 240
Guanethidine, 129–130, 240–242
  adrenergic transmission and, 114
  diarrhea and, 825
  histamine release and, 814
  indirectly acting adrenomimetic drugs and,
    117
  tricyclic antidepressants and, 403
Guanfacine, 245–248
Guanidine, 178
  in botulinum toxin poisoning, 179
  in myasthenic syndrome, 179
Guanine, 501
Guanine nucleotide-binding proteins, 10–11
  lithium carbonate and, 409
  in signal transduction, 117
Guanosine, 602
Guanosine 3′,5′-monophosphate, cyclic
  histamine and, 816
  in hypertension, 229
Guanosine triphosphate, 10
Guanylate cyclase, 232
Guedel stages of anesthesia, 345, 346
Guinea worm, 639
Gyne-Lotrimin. *See* Clotrimazole
Gynecomastia
  busulfan and, 680
  estramustine and, 697

Habituation in drug abuse, 459
Haemophilus influenzae infection
  cephalosporins in, 565
  chloramphenicol in, 578
  erythromycin in, 580
  humoral immunity deficiencies and, 706
  loracarbef in, 567
  macrolides in, 579
  penicillins in, 559, 560
  trimethoprim in, 549
Haemophilus vaginalis, 546
Hair follicle, 668
Hairy cell leukemia, 606
Halcion. *See* Triazolam
Haldol. *See* Haloperidol

Half-life, 33, 56, 70
  aging and, 40
  in intravenous bolus, 63
  in multicompartment pharmacokinetic
    model, 60
  steady state and, 59
Hallucinations
  in amphetamine abuse, 467
  benzodiazepines and, 372
Hallucinogens, 468–471
Haloalkylamines, 131–133, 136
  absorption, metabolism, and excretion of,
    133
  as antagonists, 17, 129, 238
  mechanism of action of, 132
Halogenated solvents, 78
Halogens
  as disinfectants, 659
  microbial spectrum of, 658
Haloperidol
  as α-receptor blocking agent, 131
  as antiemetic, 831
  antipsychotic effects of, 393–394
  in chorea, 430
Halotestin. *See* Fluoxymesterone
Halothane, 347–349
  anesthetic apparatus and, 343
  inspired tension of anesthetic gas and, 342
  in neuromuscular blockade, 182
  partial pressure–minimum alveolar
    concentration and, 339
  partition coefficients of, 340
  propranolol and, 302
  second gas effect and, 343
  solubility of, 341
  toxicity of, 74, 348
Hangover
  benzodiazepines and, 372
  ethanol, 454–455
Hashimoto's thyroiditis, 779, 780
Hashish, 471
Hazardous chemicals in workplace, 78
hCG. *See* Human chorionic gonadotropin
HCO₃. *See* Bicarbonate
HDL. *See* High-density lipoprotein
Headache
  amphotericin B and, 649
  buspirone in, 374
  calcium channel blockers and, 253
  catecholamines and, 125
  flecainide and, 299
  retinoids and, 527
  sotalol and, 307
  verapamil and, 308
  xanthines in, 384
Hearing loss
  aminoglycosides and, 572
  cisplatin and, 701
  loop diuretics and, 228
  vancomycin and, 585
Heart
  acetylcholine and, 146, 147
  adrenoceptors and, 113
  arrhythmias of. *See* Arrhythmias
  β-blockers and, 139
  blood perfusion rate in, 29
  bradykinin and, 196
  chemotherapeutic toxicity and, 668
  dopamine and, 124
  electrophysiology of, 275–283
    automaticity in, 278–280
    conduction in, 280–283

    ionic basis of, 277–278
    transmembrane potential in, 275–276
  estrogens and progestins and, 750–751,
    756–757
  innervation of, 104, 105
  isoproterenol and, 122
  labetalol and, 142–143
  monoamine oxidase inhibitors and, 407
  morphine and, 440
  muscarinic blocking drugs and, 154
  nitrates and, 273
  norepinephrine and, 121
  phentolamine and tolazoline and, 134
  physiology and pathophysiology of, 255–
    257
  prosthetic valves of, 318
  steroids and, 734
  tricyclic antidepressants and, 401
  xanthines and, 384
Heart block
  flecainide and, 299
  procainamide and, 288
Heart failure
  amiodarone and, 305
  β-blockers and, 141, 272
  carbachol and, 148
  cardiac glycosides in, 255–264. *See also*
    Cardiac glycosides
  disopyramide and, 290
  diuretics in, 218
  doxorubicin and, 688, 689
  ganglionic blocking agents in, 174
  methacholine and, 147
  muscarinic blocking agents and, 158
  myocardial insufficiency and, 255, 256
  pharmacokinetics in, 62
  procainamide and, 288
  propafenone and, 300
  propranolol and, 303
  quinidine and, 287
  theophylline in, 384
Heart rate
  angiotensins and, 190
  calcium channel blockers and, 251,
    252
  catecholamines and, 120–121, 122
  oxygen supply and, 266
  sotalol and, 307
Heavy drinker, term, 451
Heavy metals, 50
Helminthic infection, 637–645
  benzimidazoles in, 642–643
  cestodes in, 637–639
  nematodes in, 639–642
  trematodes in, 643–645
Hematoporphyrins, 529
Hemicholinium, 114
Hemodynamics
  adenosine and, 310
  amiodarone and, 305
  bretylium and, 304
  disopyramide and, 290
  flecainide and, 298
  lidocaine and, 292
  mexiletine and, 297
  moricizine and, 291
  phenytoin and, 294
  procainamide and, 288
  propafenone and, 299
  propranolol and, 302
  quinidine and, 286
  sotalol and, 307

tocainide and, 296
verapamil and, 308
Hemolytic anemia, 546–547
Hemophilia, 729
Hemorrhage
anticonvulsants and, 423
calcium channel blockers in, 252
cancer chemotherapy and, 668
epinephrine in, 125
glucocorticoids and, 738
phenobarbital and, 418
warfarin and, 82
Hemostatic mechanisms, 313–315
Henderson-Hasselbalch equations, 20
Henle's loop, 213–214
Henry's law, 337–338
HEPA filter. *See* High-efficiency particulate
air filter
Heparin, 315–316
absorption, metabolism, and excretion of,
316
adverse reactions to, 316, 321
aminoglycosides and, 572
anticoagulants and, 318
antidote for, 77
in arterial embolism, 318
contraindications and drug interactions
with, 316
histamine and, 811
low-molecular-weight fractions of, 319
mechanism of action of, 315
pharmacological actions of, 315, 321
preparations and dosage of, 316
volume of distribution of, 28
Heparin pump, 71
Hepatic gluconeogenesis, 801
Hepatic microsomal enzyme inducers, 845
Hepatitis
amiodarone and, 305
drug metabolism and, 44
erythromycin and, 580
glutaraldehyde and, 660
halothane and, 348
interferon in, 606
isoflurane and, 349
isoniazid and, 589
Hepatotoxicity, 74–75
of allopurinol, 507
of aniline derivatives, 437
of diquat, 82
of ketoconazole, 654
of mercaptopurine, 685
of monoamine oxidase inhibitors, 406, 407
of nonsteroidal antiinflammatory drugs,
481
of valproic acid, 419
Heptachlor, 81
Herbicides, 81, 82
Heroin, 438, 444
abuse of, 461–462
as analgesic, 442
placental barrier and, 32
Herpes infection
in acquired immunodeficiency syndrome,
614
acyclovir in, 604
mechlorethamine in, 675
vidarabine in, 602
Herplex Liquifilm. *See* Idoxuridine
Hetacillin, 558, 563
Hetrazan. *See* Diethylcarbamazine
Hexachlorobutadiene, 75

Hexachlorophene, 661, 662
Hexamethonium, 173
Hexamethylenetetramine, 552–553
Hexamethylmelamine, 669, 700
Hexane, 75, 80
Hexobarbital, 43
Hibiclens. *See* Chlorhexidine
Hiccup, 391
High-ceiling diuretics, 226–228. *See also*
Loop diuretics
High-density lipoprotein, 198, 201
High-efficiency particulate air filter, 657
High-fiber diets, 826–827
Hippocampus, 739
Hiprex. *See* Methenamine
Hirudin, 319
His-Purkinje system
activation and impulse transmission
through, 281
amiodarone and, 305
automaticity of, 279
bretylium and, 303–304
disopyramide and, 289
flecainide and, 298
lidocaine and, 292
moricizine and, 291
phenytoin and, 294
propafenone and, 299
propranolol and, 302
quinidine and, 285–286
sotalol and, 307
verapamil and, 308
Hismanal. *See* Astemizole
Histadine decarboxylase, 811–812
Histalog. *See* Betazole
Histaminase, 815
Histamine, 332, 811–817
antagonism of, 817–821
antigen and, 812
clinical uses of, 817
distribution of, 811
epinephrine and, 124
in ganglionic blockade, 172
inactivation of, 815
in inflammation, 479
inhibition of, 821–822
metabolism of, 813
non–antigen-mediated, 813–815
pharmacological effects of, 816–817
phenoxybenzamine and, 132
physiological role of, 815–816
preparations and dosage of, 817
regulation of, 812–813
synthesis of, 811–812
Histamine antagonists, 817–821, 833–834
absorption, metabolism and excretion of,
818, 821
adverse reactions to, 820, 821
anticholinergic poisoning and, 158
anxiolytic properties of, 374
chemistry of, 818
clinical uses of, 818–820, 821
mechanism of action of, 818, 821
motion sickness and, 157
in peptic ulcers, 156
preparations and dosage of, 820, 821
Histamine methyltransferase, 815
Histofluorescence, 333
Histoplasma capsulatum infection
amphotericin B in, 647
nystatin in, 649
Histoplasmosis, 614, 648

Histrionicotoxin, 179
HIV infection. *See* Human immunodeficiency
virus infection
hMG. *See* Human menopausal gonadotropin
Hodgkin's disease
acquired immunodeficiency syndrome and,
615
carmustine in, 679
mechlorethamine in, 674
MOPP regimen in, 666
procarbazine in, 699
single agents in, 671
Homeostasis
adrenomimetic drugs and, 124
autonomic nervous system in, 101
calcium metabolism and, 787–788
glucose, 797
lipid mediators of, 477–483
eicosanoids in, 477–482
platelet-activating factor in, 482
Hookworm, 641
Hormonal agents, antineoplastic, 696–698
buserelin and leuprolide as, 697–698
estramustine as, 697
flutamide as, 697
somatostatin analogue as, 698
tamoxifen as, 696–697
Hormone receptors, 721
Hormones
adrenocortical, 731–745
adverse effects of, 737–740
aminoglutethimide and, 744
corticotropin and, 742–743
cosyntropin and, 743
dexamethasone and, 745
ketoconazole and, 744
mechanism of, 741–742
metyrapone and, 743–744
mitotane and, 744
physiology of, 731–736
preparations of, 736–737
steroid biosynthesis and, 731–733
structure-activity relationships of, 736
therapeutic uses of, 740–741
transport of, 733
trilostane and, 745
anterior pituitary, 723–729
adrenocorticotropic hormone in, 726–
727
gonadotropins in, 726
growth hormone in, 723–725
prolactin in, 725
thyroid-stimulating hormone in, 726
drug interactions with, 720–721
growth, 723–725
herbicides and, 82
insulin and, 799, 802
hypothalamus, 727–729
anterior pituitary and, 723
corticotropin-releasing factor in, 729
gonadotropin releasing hormone in,
727–728
growth hormone-releasing hormone in,
727
somatostatin in, 727
thyrotropin releasing hormone in, 727
low molecular weight, 719
supraphysiological dosages of, 719
"Horse," 461
HPETE. *See* Hydroxyperoxyeicosatetranoic
acid
5-HT. *See* Serotonin

HTX. *See* Histrionicotoxin
Human calcitonin, 793
Human chorionic gonadotropin, 726, 767
Human growth hormone, recombinant, 768
Human immunodeficiency virus infection
  amphotericin B in, 648
  drug abuse and, 28, 460
  process of, 607, 609, 610
  steroid therapy in, 741
  tuberculosis and, 587
  zidovudine in, 602
Human insulin, 805
Human menopausal gonadotropin, 726
Humatin. *See* Paromomycin
Humatrope. *See* Somatotropin
Humorsol. *See* Demecarium
Humulin R. *See* Human insulin
Huntington's chorea, 430
Hydantoins, 416
Hydralazine, 232–234, 264
Hydration in topical therapy, 523, 525
Hydrazines, 845
Hydrea. *See* Hydroxyurea
Hydrocarbon toxicity, 79
Hydrochloroquine, 630–631
Hydrochlorothiazide, 224
  absorption of, 62
  amiloride with, 226
  as antihypertensive, 230
  triamterene with, 226
Hydrocodone, 442
Hydrocortisone
  as antiinflammatory, 496
  in asthma, 518, 519
  bacitracin and, 583
  structure-activity relationships, 736
Hydrodiuril. *See* Hydrochlorothiazide
Hydroflumethiazide, 224
Hydrogen bond, 12
Hydrogen exchange, 215
Hydrogen, in coronary autoregulation, 265
Hydrogen peroxide, 852–853
  as disinfectant, 659
  in inflammation, 479
Hydrogen-potassium pump, 831–832, 835
Hydrolases, peptidyldipeptide, 189–190
Hydrolysis
  acetylcholine, 162
  in drug metabolism, 36–37
  renal disease and, 62
Hydromorphone, 438, 442, 444
Hydromox. *See* Quinethazone
Hydrophilic substances, 825
Hydroxyapatite, 787
Hydroxychloroquine
  as antiinflammatory, 498
  in dermatological disorders, 530
  platelet function and, 320
4-Hydroxycoumarin derivatives, 316, 317
5-Hydroxyindoleacetic acid, 329
Hydroxyl free radical
  in inflammation, 479
  reperfusion injury and, 507
Hydroxylase deficiency, 741
Hydroxylation, 36
Hydroxynalidixic acid, 551
Hydroxyperoxyeicosatetranoic acid, 477
  asthma and, 480
  inflammation and, 479
4-Hydroxypropranolol, 139
Hydroxyquinolines, 531
5'-Hydroxytryptamine. *See* Serotonin
Hydroxyurea, 698–699

Hydroxyzine, 374
Hygroton. *See* Chlorthalidone
Hylorel. *See* Guanethidine
Hymenolepis nana, 638, 639
Hyperbilirubinemia, 37
Hypercalcemia, 787, 788
  calcitonin and, 790
  dideoxyinosine and, 612
  iatrogenic, 793
  parathyroid hormone and, 793–794
  plicamycin in, 692
Hypercholesterolemic drugs, 197–209
  in combination therapy, 208–209
  diet versus, 201–202
  hypolipidemic, 202–203
  lipoproteins and, 197–199, 200, 201
  niacin in, 843
  in plasma cholesterol reduction, 203–206
  plasma lipid levels and, 200–201, 202
  in plasma triglyceride reduction, 206–208
Hypercortisolemia, 739
Hyperexcitability, 379
Hyperglycemia
  in diabetes mellitus, 804
  morphine and, 440
  steroids and, 738
Hypergonadotropic primary hypogonadism, 767
Hyperkalemia, 218, 668
Hyperkinetic syndrome, 382
Hyperlipidemia, 197, 199, 843
Hyperlipoproteinemia, 197, 198, 199
Hyperosmolar solutions, 826
Hyperphagia, 382
Hyperphosphatemia, 668
Hyperpigmentation
  cortisol in, 740
  in PUVA therapy, 529
Hyperplasia
  congenital adrenal, 741
  gingival, 416
Hyperpolarization
  in γ-aminobutyric acid receptor-chloride interaction, 380
  in hypertension, 229
  of sinoatrial cells, 279
  vasodilator action and, 232
Hyperpyrexia, 407
Hyperreactivity of airway, 509–510
Hyperreflexia, 174
Hypersensitivity
  to aminosalicylic acid, 591
  anaphylactic, 76
  L-asparaginase and, 696
  immediate, 812
  paclitaxel and, 695
  to penicillins, 561–563
  to salicylates, 488
  to sulfonamides, 546
Hypersensitivity pneumonitis, 76
Hyperstat. *See* Diazoxide
Hypertension
  antihypertensives in, 229–248
    adrenergic neuron-blocking drugs as, 240–242
    adrenoreceptor antagonists as, 238–240
    calcium channel blockers as, 252
    centrally acting hypotensive drugs as, 244–248
    contraindications to, 240
    diarrhea and, 825
    diuretics as, 218–219, 230–231
    ganglionic blocking agents as, 174, 244

    mechanism of action of, 232, 239
    myocardial insufficiency and, 264
    norepinephrine and, 242–244
    pharmacological approaches to, 229–230
    quinazoline derivatives as, 135
    sympathetic nervous system function and, 236–238
    triple combination of, 233
    vasodilators as, 231–236
  cyclosporine and, 709
  defined, 229
  drug-induced, 105
  ocular, 139
  oral contraceptives and, 756
  pregnancy-induced, 480
  primary or essential, 229
  rebound, 247
Hypertensive crisis, 406
Hyperthermia, 389
Hyperthyroidism
  antithyroid drugs in, 781–782
  β-adrenoceptor blocking agents in, 141
  bethanechol and, 148
  from hypothyroidism therapy, 779–780
  thyroid hormones in, 775
Hypertonic fluid, 214
Hypertriglyceridemia, 206–208, 527
Hypertrophy, prostatic, 158
Hyperuricemia
  dideoxyinosine and, 612
  gout and, 501
  management of, 503
  probenecid in, 505
  pyrazinamide and, 593
Hypervitaminosis A, 843
Hypervitaminosis D, 793, 843
Hypnotic drugs, 369–377
  antihistamines as, 374
  antipsychotics and antidepressants as, 374–375
  azapirones as, 369–377
  barbiturates as, 375–377
  benzodiazepines as, 369–373
  β-adrenoceptor blocking agents as, 374
  chloral hydrate as, 377
  nonprescription, 699
  procarbazine and, 699
  propanediol carbamates as, 377
Hypocalcemia, 787–788
Hypochlorite, 659
Hypochlorous acid, 479
Hypoglycemia
  β-blockers in, 139, 141
  disopyramide and, 290–291
Hypoglycemic agents, 805–808
  absorption, metabolism and excretion of, 806
  adverse reactions to, 806–807
  anticoagulants and, 318
  antidote for, 77
  chemistry of, 805–806
  drug interactions with, 807
  mechanism of action of, 806
  preparations and dosage of, 807
  thyroid hormones and, 780
  vitamins and, 845
Hypoglycemic coma, 679
Hypogonadism, 754, 766–767
Hypogonadotropic secondary hypogonadism, 767
Hypokalemia, 217–218
  diuretics and, 224
  sotalol and, 307

Hypolipidemic drugs, 202–203
Hyponatremia
  cancer chemotherapy and, 668
  cyclophosphamide and, 676
Hypoparathyroidism, 792–793
Hypopituitarism, female, 768–769
Hypoplastic anemia, 296
Hypoprothrombinemia, 842
Hypotension
  aldesleukin and, 703
  bretylium and, 304
  disopyramide and, 290
  ganglionic blocking agents in, 174
  local anesthetics and, 363
  mexiletine and, 297
  paclitaxel and, 695
  phenoxybenzamine and, 132, 133
  phentolamine and tolazoline and, 134
  phenytoin and, 294
  procainamide and, 288
  quinidine and, 287
Hypotensive drugs, 244–248
Hypothalamic hormones, 727–729
  anterior pituitary and, 723
  corticotropin-releasing factor in, 729
  gonadotropin releasing hormone in, 727–728
  growth hormone releasing hormone in, 727
  somatostatin in, 727
  thyrotropin releasing hormone in, 727
Hypothalamus
  adrenocorticotropic hormone and, 735
  anterior pituitary hormones and, 723
  salicylates and, 432
  steroid therapy and, 739–740
Hypothermia
  ethanol consumption and, 454
  phenothiazines and, 389
Hypothyroidism, 775, 779–780
Hypotonic fluid, 214
Hypovolemia, 133
Hypoxanthine, 507, 684
Hypoxanthine guanine-phosphoribosyltransferase, 684
Hypoxemia with myocardial insufficiency, 257
Hypoxia, in general anesthesia, 343
Hytakerol. See Dihydrotachysterol
Hytrin. See Terazosin

^{131}I. See Iodine 131
Iatrogenic parkinsonism, 425
Ibuprofen
  as analgesic, 433, 437
  anticoagulants and, 318
  antiinflammatory properties of, 491–492
  in arthritis, 489
"Ice," 466
Ictal period of seizure, 413
Idarubicin, 689
Idiopathic parkinsonism, 425
Idiopathic thrombocytopenia, 707
Idiosyncratic reaction, 541
IDL. See Intermediate-density lipoprotein
Idoxuridine, 603–604
Ifex. See Ifosfamide
Ifosfamide, 677
  anticoagulants and, 318
  nephrotoxicity of, 75
  neurotoxicity of, 669

Ilosone. See Erythromycin
Ilotycin. See Erythromycin
Imferon. See Iron dextran
Imidazole-4-acetic acid, 332
Imidazoles, 651–654
Imidazolines, 133–135, 238
  α-blocking activity of, 131
  clonidine as, 246–248
  comparative information of, 136
Imipenem, 566–567
Imipramine
  chemical structure of, 398
  dosage and serum concentration of, 403
  lung and, 31
  smoking and, 42
  volume of distribution of, 28
Immediate hypersensitivity reaction, 812
Immune complex, 76
Immune globulin, 600–601
Immune system
  cancer chemotherapy and, 666
  impairment of, 75, 76
  steroids and, 734–735
Immunization in viral control, 599
Immunodeficiency
  immune globulin in, 714
  immunomodulating drugs in, 705–706
  toxicity and, 75
Immunoglobulin E antibody, 812
Immunoglobulin G, 562, 600–601
Immunoglobulin M, 562
Immunomodulating drugs, 705–715
  antibodies in, 711
  antiinflammatory properties of, 485, 706
  antimicrobials as, 543
  antineoplastic, 702–703
    interferons as, 702
    interleukins as, 703
    levamisole in, 702
  antithymocyte globulin as, 711
  autoimmunity and, 705
  azathioprine as, 709–710
  biological response modifiers and, 711–714
    bacillus Calmette-Guérin as, 712–713
    cytokines as, 713–714
    immune globulin as, 714
    thymic factors as, 713
  corticosteroids in, 706–707
  cyclophosphamide in, 676, 710–711
  cyclosporine in, 707–709
  cytotoxic drugs as, 709
  in dermatological disorders, 532–533
  FK506 in, 709
  immunosuppression principles and, 706
  myeloid colony stimulating factors in, 714–715
  in organ transplantation, 705, 706
  orthoclone OKT3 in, 711
  in primary immunodeficiency diseases, 705–706
  xenobiotics and, 75, 76
Immunopathological reaction, 76
Immunopotentiation therapy, 499
Immunosuppressive agents. See Immunomodulating drugs
Immunotherapy, 607, 671
Immunotoxicity, 75–76, 77
Imodium. See Loperamide
Impetigo, 530
Impotence, 767–768
Imuran. See Azathioprine
In vitro fertilization, 726
In vivo measurements in chemotherapy, 542

IND procedure. See Investigational New Drug procedure
Indandione anticoagulants, 316, 317
Indapamide, 224
Inderal. See Propranolol
Indocin. See Indomethacin
Indolealkylamines, 468
Indomethacin, 437
  as analgesic, 433
  anticoagulants and, 318
  antiinflammatory properties of, 490–491
  in arthritis, 489
  enterohepatic recirculation and, 51
  in gout, 508
  platelet function and, 320
  renin and, 188–189, 191
Indoor pollutants, 78
Indurate-inflammatory eruptions, 76
Industrial chemical allergen, 77
Infantile spasm, 420
Infarction, myocardial. See Myocardial infarction
Infection
  catheter, 586
  in drug abuse, 464
  glucocorticoids and, 738
  shunt, 585
Infertility
  alkylating agents and, 669
  estrogens and progestins in, 754
  gonadotropins in, 726
  male, 766
  mechlorethamine and, 675
  prolactin and, 725
Infiltration anesthesia, 364
Inflammation, 475–534
  adrenocortical hormones in, 740–741
  antiinflammatory and antirheumatic drugs in, 485–500. See also Antiinflammatory drugs
  asthma and, 509–521. See also Asthma
  blood-brain barrier and, 31
  in dermatological disorders, 523–534. See also Dermatological disorders
  glomerular filtration rate and, 48
  gout and, 501–508
  kinins and, 196
  lipid mediators of, 477–483
    eicosanoids in, 477–482
    platelet-activating factor in, 482
  permeability and, 525
Inflammatory bowel disease, 835–837
Inflammatory response, 485
Influenza, 601
Informed consent, 87–88
Infusion rate, 63
INH tablets. See Isoniazid
Inhalants, 472–473
Inhalation
  of nonoral medication, 69–70
  of solvents, 80
Inhalational anesthesia, 337–344
  alveolar uptake of gases in, 340–342
  anesthetic apparatus for, 343–344
  concentration effect in, 342–343
  diffusion hypoxia and, 343
  gases in, 350–351
  Henry's law and, 337–338
  partial pressure–minimum alveolar concentration of, 338–339
  pulmonary perfusion and, 341
  rate of concentration in, 339–340
  second gas effect of, 343

Inhalational anesthesia (*cont.*)
  solubility of, 340–341
  upper airway and, 344
  volatile liquids in, 347–349
Inhaler, 515
Inhibin, 764
Inhibitory concentration, 541
Inhibitory postsynaptic potential, 169–171, 327
Inhibitory transmitter, 327
Innervation
  of blood vessels, 104–105
  of cardiovascular reflexes, 105
  of eye, 105–105
  of gastrointestinal tract, 106
  of pulmonary smooth muscle, 106
  of salivary glands, 106
  of sinoatrial node, 278
Inocor. *See* Amrinone
Inorganic metals, 80
Inositol phosphate, 409
Inositol triphosphate, 117–118, 119
Inosol D-CM, 221
Inotropic agents, 257–263
Insecticide synergists, 81
Insecticides
  exposure to, 81–82
  immunotoxicity and, 76
  neurotoxicity of, 75
  organophosphates as, 165
  topical absorption of, 27
Insomnia, 369
  amiodarone and, 306
  barbiturates in, 376
  benzodiazepines in, 371–372
  estrogens and, 754
  psychomotor stimulants and, 382
Inspired gas concentration, 342
Institutional review board, 87
Insulatard NPH. *See* Isophane
Insulin, 797–802
  absorption, metabolism and excretion of, 801–802
  adrenoceptors and, 113
  adverse reactions to, 802
  antidote for, 77
  β-blockers and, 139
  biosynthesis of, 798
  chemistry of, 797–798
  in diabetes mellitus, 802–805
  dietary fiber and, 827
  drug metabolism and, 45
  glucocorticoids and, 734
  glucose homeostasis and, 797
  human, 805
  isophane suspension, 802, 805
  mechanism of action of, 800
  oral hypoglycemic agents and, 805–808
  protamine zinc, 802, 805
  resistance to, 721, 802, 804
  secretion of, 798–800
  semisynthetic, 805
  subcutaneous administration of, 68
  thyroid hormones and, 780
Insulin-like growth factor, 723
Insulin zinc, 802, 805
Intal. *See* Cromolyn sodium
Intercalation, 634
Intercellular channels, 22
Interdigestive migrating motor complex, 823
Interferon-α, 714
Interferons, 671
  antineoplastic, 702

antiviral, 531–532, 605–606
  in Kaposi's sarcoma, 614–615
Interictal period of seizure, 413
Interleukin-1
  fever and, 480
  glucocorticoids and, 742
  immunomodulating properties of, 714
Interleukin-2, 671
  clinical testing of, 89
  cyclosporine and, 707
  cytotoxic lymphocytes and, 666
  immunomodulating properties of, 713
Interleukins, antineoplastic, 703
Intermediate-density lipoprotein, 197, 198
Interneurons, 169
Interstitial fluid, 28
Intestinal fluke, 639
Intestine
  drugs and
    absorption of, 25, 26
    metabolism of, 34, 35
  microflora of, 45
  motility of, 823–824
  mucosa of, 828–829
Intoxication
  barbiturate, 464
  ethanol, 454–455
  salicylate, 435
Intraarterial administration, 68
Intracavitary administration, 670
Intracellular fluid, 28
Intracranial pressure, 219
Intradermal tissue, 816–817
Intramuscular administration, 27, 68
Intraperitoneal instillation, 670
Intrathecal administration, 670
Intravenous drugs
  administration of, 27–28, 68
    bolus determination of, 63
    drug concentration time in, 59
    nitroglycerin and, 270
    phenytoin and, 295
  blood concentration of, 59, 60
  in general anesthesia, 353–360, 365
    benzodiazepines in, 357
    distribution of, 354, 355
    etomidate in, 358–359
    ketamine in, 357–358
    metabolism and excretion of, 355
    narcotics in, 360
    pharmacological properties of, 354–355
    propofol in, 359
    ultra–short-acting barbiturates in, 356–357
Intraventricular administration, 670
Intraventricular block, 288
Intravesical instillation, 670
Intrinsic factor, 842, 846
Intron A. *See* Interferons
Intropin. *See* Dopamine
Inverse agonists, 370
Inversine. *See* Mecamylamine
Investigational New Drug procedure, 86
Iodides, 775–777
  deficiency of, 778, 779
  oxidation, iodination, and coupling of, 777
  potassium, 784
  sodium, 784
Iodination, 777
Iodine
  dietary, 775
  as disinfectant, 659
  exposure to, 79

microbial spectrum of, 658
  in thyroid storm, 782, 784
Iodine 131, 784–785
Iodophors, 659
Iodoquinol, 531, 620–621
Ion-pair transport, 23, 24
Ionic bond, 12
Ionization constant, 20
Ions
  G proteins and, 11
  in membrane action potential, 277–278
Ipecac syrup, 829
Ipratropium
  antimuscarinic activity of, 151
  in asthma, 511, 517
  in respiratory disorders, 157
  structure of, 153
  uses of, 155
Iproniazid, 406
IPSP. *See* Inhibitory postsynaptic potential
IRB. *See* Institutional review board
Iris
  autonomic nervous system and, 105
  epinephrine and, 123
Iron
  antidote for, 77
  toxicity of, 80
Iron deficiency anemia, 846
Iron dextran, 846
Irreversible-competitive antagonism, 129, 132
Irreversible-competitive bond, 17
Irreversible inhibitors, 163, 166
Irritable bowel syndrome, 156–157
Islets of Langerhans, 797
Ismelin. *See* Guanethidine
ISMN. *See* Isosorbide
Ismo. *See* Isosorbide
Iso-osmotic electrolyte colonic lavage solutions, 828
Isobologram of drug, 613
Isocarboxazid, 403, 406
Isoflurane, 349
  in neuromuscular blockade, 182
  partition coefficients of, 340
Isoflurophate, 163, 166, 167
Isoguvacine, 330
Isoniazid
  N-acetylation and, 43
  anticoagulants and, 318
  half-life of, 40
  hepatotoxicity of, 74
  neurotoxicity of, 75
  phenytoin and, 295
  in tuberculosis, 587–589
  vitamins and, 845
Isonicotinic acid hydrazide. *See* Isoniazid
Isophane, 802, 805
Isopropanol, 457, 659
Isopropyl alcohol. *See* Isopropanol
Isoproterenol
  in asthma, 514–516
  cardiovascular effects of, 120
  chemical structure of, 116
  histamine release and, 813
  in myocardial insufficiency, 263
  pharmacodynamics of, 121–122
  preparations and dosage of, 125
  structure of, 137
  vasoconstriction and, 113
Isoptin. *See* Verapamil
Isopto Carbachol. *See* Carbachol
Isopto carpine. *See* Pilocarpine
Isordil. *See* Isosorbide

Isosorbide
  in angina, 267, 268
  as osmotic agent, 222
  preparations of, 270–271
Isotonic fluid, 214
Isotretinoin, 527
Isoxsuprine, 480
Isozymes of P450, 35
Isradipine, 254
Isuprel. *See* Isoproterenol
Itraconazole, 654
  in acquired immunodeficiency syndrome, 614
  in cutaneous fungal disease, 531
Ivermectin, 622, 638, 641

Jarisch-Herxheimer reaction, 560
Jaundice
  chlorpromazine and, 391–392
  drug metabolism and, 44
Jenamicin. *See* Gentamicin
Jod-Basedow's phenomenon, 784
"Joint," 472

K-Lor, 218
K-Lyte, 218
Kala-azar, 618
Kallidin, 194, 195
Kallikrein-kinin system, 194–196
Kanamycin, 571
  half-life of, 40
  in tuberculosis, 590
Kantrex. *See* Kanamycin
Kaochlor, 218
Kaolin powder with pectin, 825
Kaon-Cl, 217
Kaopectate. *See* Kaolin powder with pectin
Kaposi's sarcoma, 614–615
Kay Ciel elixir, 218
Kayexalate, 218
Kefauver-Harris Drug Amendments, 86, 87
Keflex. *See* Cephalexin
Keflin. *See* Cephalothin
Keftab. *See* Cephalexin
Kefurox. *See* Cefuroxime
Kefzol. *See* Cefazolin
Keratin, 650
Keratinocytes, 523
Keratoses, 528
Kernicterus, 37, 546–548
Ketaject. *See* Ketamine
Ketalar. *See* Ketamine
Ketamine
  abuse of, 470–471
  as anesthetic, 357–358
  in channel blockade, 180
  metabolism and excretion of, 355
  preparations and dosage of, 358
Ketoacidosis, 738
Ketoconazole, 653–654
  anticoagulants and, 318
  in Cushing's disease, 744
  in cutaneous fungal disease, 531
  in mycosis, 614
  in testosterone synthesis, 761, 772
Ketone body, 804
Ketoprofen, 492–493
  as analgesic, 437
  in arthritis, 489
17-Ketosteroids, 762
Kidney, 220–221
  aging and, 40
  amphotericin B and, 649

antimicrobial agent and, 541
benzothiazides and, 223
blood perfusion rate in, 29
cardiac disease and, 62
chemically induced damage to, 75
chloramphenicol and, 578
cisplatin and, 701
disease of
  doxycycline in, 576
  edema in, 219–220
  pharmacokinetics in, 61–62
  polymyxins and, 586
  procainamide and, 288
  renal failure in, 220
  uric acid stones in, 501
dopamine and, 124
drug accumulation in, 30
in drug excretion, 34, 40, 47–50
eicosanoids and, 481
glomerular filtration in, 212
homeostatic function of, 211
kinins and, 196
lidocaine and, 293
lithium carbonate and, 409
methotrexate and, 683
nephron of, 211, 213–215
streptozocin and, 679
sulfonamides and, 548
transplantation of, 707–708
tubular reabsorption and secretion in, 212
urate homeostasis and, 502
xenobiotic toxicity of, 75
Kinases, 10–11
Kindling, 411
Kinetics, zero-order, 415
Kininogenases, 194
Kinins
  in inflammation, 479
  plasma, 194–196
  urate crystals and, 502
Klebcil. *See* Kanamycin
Klebsiella pneumoniae, 549
Klonopin. *See* Clonazepam

Labeling of drugs, 86, 90
Labetalol, 142–143
Labor
  meperidine in, 444
  oxytocin in, 729
  prostaglandins and, 480
  terbutaline in, 516
Lactated Ringer's solution, 221
Lactation
  estrogens and progestins in, 755
  oxytocin in, 729
  prolactin and, 725
Lactic acid, 265
Lactose, 67
Lactulose, 827
Lambert-Eaton syndrome, 179
Lamictal. *See* Lamotrigine
Lamotrigine, 421
Lampit. *See* Nifurtimox
Lamprene. *See* Clofazimine
Laniazid. *See* Isoniazid
Lanoxin, 263
Laplace's law, 268
Larium. *See* Mefloquine
Larodopa. *See* Levodopa
Larotid. *See* Amoxicillin
Laryngospasm, 376
Lasix. *See* Furosemide
Laughing gas, 350

Lavage, colonic, 828
Law
  Henry's, 337–338
  Laplace's, 268
Law of mass action, 129
Laxatives, 826–829
  bulk-forming, 826–827
  oral anticoagulants and, 318
  osmotic, 827
  saline, 827–828
  vitamins and, 844
LDL. *See* Low-density lipoprotein
LDL cholesterol. *See* Low-density lipoprotein cholesterol
Lead
  antidote for, 77
  bone and, 31
  toxicity of, 73, 75, 76, 80
Leg muscle cramp, 633
Legionella, 579
Leiomyoma, uterine, 728
Leishmaniasis, 618
  amphotericin B in, 626
  sodium stibogluconate in, 625
Lennox-Gastaut syndrome
  felbamate in, 421
  nitrazepam in, 420
Lente insulin. *See* Insulin zinc
Lentigines, 529
Leprosy, 594–596
  clofazimine in, 596
  rifampin in, 596
  sulfones in, 595
Leptospirosis, 561
Lethal dose, 14
Leu-enkephalin, 438
Leucine, 799
Leucovorin, 682, 683
Leukemia
  adrenocortical hormones in, 741
  L-asparaginase in, 695, 696
  blood-brain barrier and, 669
  busulfan in, 680
  chlorambucil in, 678
  cladribine in, 685
  cyclophosphamide in, 676
  cytarabine in, 686
  daunorubicin in, 687
  etoposide in, 694
  fludarabine in, 685
  glucocorticoid therapy in, 738
  hydroxyurea in, 698, 699
  idarubicin in, 689
  mercaptopurine in, 684, 685
  methotrexate in, 670, 682
  mitoxantrone in, 702
  pentostatin in, 685
  steroid therapy in, 741
  teniposide in, 694
  thioguanine in, 684
  vincristine in, 693
Leukeran. *See* Chlorambucil
Leukine. *See* Sargramostim
Leukocytes
  chemotherapy and, 667
  colchicine and, 504
  cyclophosphamide and, 676
  glucocorticoids and, 734
  steroids and, 496
Leukopenia
  carmustine and, 679
  dacarbazine and, 681
  doxorubicin and, 688

Leukopenia (*cont.*)
  mechlorethamine and, 675
  methotrexate and, 683
  thioguanine and, 684
  tocainide and, 296
  vinblastine and, 694
Leukotrienes
  asthma and, 479
  synthesis of, 477
Leuprolide, 697–698, 728, 772
Leustatin. *See* Cladribine
Levamisole, 500, 702
Levarterenol
  heart rate and, 14–15
  preparations and dosage of, 125
Levlen. *See* Levonorgestrel
Levobunolol, 138, 139
Levodopa
  active transport of, 23
  chorea and, 430
  in parkinsonism, 157, 426–428
  vitamins and, 845
  vomiting and, 829
Levonordefrin, 366
Levonorgestrel, 752
Levopropoxyphene, 449
Levorphanol, 438, 442, 444
Levothroid. *See* Levothyroxine sodium
Levothyroxine sodium, 780–781
Levoxine. *See* Levothyroxine sodium
Lewis triple response, 816–817
Leydig cell, 762–764
Librium. *See* Chlordiazepoxide
Lice, 532
Lidocaine, 367
  absorption of, 62
  in arrhythmia, 262, 292–294, 365
  cardiovascular system and, 363
  half-life of, 40
  neonate and, 364
  propafenone and, 300
Lidone. *See* Molindone
Ligand, 333
Light drinker, term, 451
Light-headedness
  buspirone and, 374
  flecainide and, 298
  propafenone and, 300
  quinidine and, 287
  tocainide and, 296
Limbic lobe, 389
Limbic system, 388
Lincocin. *See* Lincomycin
Lincomycin, 182, 581–582
Lincosamides, 581–582
Lindane, 81, 532
Linogliride, 805
Lioresal. *See* Baclofen
Liothyronine sodium, 780–781
Liotrix, 780–781
Lipid mediators, 477–483
  eicosanoids in, 477–482
    asthma and allergic states and, 479–480
    biosynthesis of, 477–478
    fever and, 480
    hemostasis and, 480–482
    inflammation and, 478–479
    reproduction and, 480
  platelet-activating factor in, 482
Lipid-water partition coefficient, 19–20
  diffusion rate and, 22
  topical drug absorption and, 27

Lipids
  aminoglycosides and, 570
  ethanol and, 453
  hypolipidemics and, 202–203
  regulation of, 200–201, 202
  tetracyclines and, 575–576
Lipocortins, 479, 742
Lipolysis
  adrenoceptors and, 113
  catecholamines and, 123–124
  insulin and, 801
  sympathetic nervous system and, 103
Lipophilic compounds, 68, 75
Lipoproteins, 197–199, 200, 201
  drug binding to, 30
  hyperlipoproteinemias and, 199
Liposomal amphotericin B, 649
Lipoxygenases, 477
Liquid dosage form of drug, 67
Liquid paraffin, 828
Lisinopril, 193
Listeria monocytogenes, 561
Listerine mouth rinse. *See* Essential oils as
    mouth rinse
Lithium carbonate, 784
  adverse reactions of, 411
  antipsychotic effects of, 395
  central nervous system and, 408–409
  mechanism of action of, 409, 410
  pharmacokinetics of, 409–411
  tricyclic antidepressants and, 400
Liver
  benzodiazepines and, 371
  blood perfusion rate in, 29
  carbamazepine and, 416
  cardiac disease and, 62
  cephlosporins and, 565
  chemotherapeutic toxicity and, 668
  cholestasis of, 75, 795
  doxorubicin and, 696
  drug clearance and, 50, 61
  gluconeogenesis and, 801
  glucuronide conjugation and, 37
  mercaptopurine and, 685
  metabolism and
    drug, 34, 35
    ethanol, 452
    glycogen, 801
    steroid, 733
  methotrexate and, 668, 683
  monoamine oxidase inhibitors and, 407
  retinoids and, 527
  rifampin and, 590
  tetracyclines and, 576
  toxicity and. *See* Hepatotoxicity
  trematode and, 643
Liver cancer
  estrogens and progestins and, 756
  fluorouracil in, 687
Liver disease
  diuretics in, 219
  drug accumulation in, 51
  ethanol and, 455
  isoniazid and, 589
  pharmacokinetics in, 61
Lo-Ovral. *See* Norgestrel
Loa loa, 640
Loading dose, 59, 63
Lobeline, 171, 172, 173
Local anesthetics, 361–368
  adverse reactions to, 366
  in channel blockade, 180

chemistry of, 361
clinical uses of, 364–366
differential blockade for, 362–363
eutectic mixture of, 368
mechanism of action of, 361–362
model structure of, 362
in pain control, 431–432
pharmacokinetics of, 363–364
pharmacological actions of, 363
vasoconstrictors with, 366
Lodine, 493
Lodosyn. *See* Carbidopa
Loestrin. *See* Norethindrone
Log-cell kill hypothesis, 665
Logarithmic scale, 15
Lomefloxacin, 367, 551, 552
Lomotil. *See* Diphenoxylate
Lomustine, 678–679
Loop diuretics, 226–228
  as antihypertensives, 230–231
  in myocardial insufficiency, 264
  in nephrotic syndrome, 220
  in pulmonary edema, 219
Loop of Henle, 213–214
Loperamide, 445, 826
Lopressor. *See* Metoprolol
Loprox. *See* Ciclopirox olamine
Lorabid. *See* Loracarbef
Loracarbef, 567
Lorazepam, 357
  anesthetic uses of, 360
  dosage of, 373
  in status epilepticus, 423
Lorelco. *See* Probucol
Lotensin. *See* Benzapril
Lotrimin. *See* Clotrimazole
Lovastatin, 205–206
  anticoagulants and, 318
  in combination therapy, 208
Low-density lipoprotein, 198
Low-density lipoprotein cholesterol, 197
Low growth fraction, 665
Loxapine, 394, 402
Loxitane. *See* Loxapine
Lozol. *See* Indapamide
LSD. *See* Lysergic acid diethylamide
Lubricants, in capsules, 67
Ludiomil. *See* Maprotiline
Lugol's solution, 784
Lumbar epidural anesthesia, 365
Luminal. *See* Phenobarbital
Luminal membrane, 502
Lung
  anesthesia and, 339–340, 341, 344
  bleomycin and, 690
  blood perfusion rate in, 29
  carmustine and, 679
  drugs and
    absorption of, 26–27
    accumulation of, 30–31
    excretion of, 51–52
    metabolism of, 34, 35
    muscarinic blocking, 154
    toxicity of, 668–669
  hepatotoxin and, 74
  trematode and, 643
  xenobiotics and, 74
Lung cancer
  carboplatin in, 701
  carmustine in, 679
  cyclophosphamide in, 676
  paclitaxel in, 695

Lung disease
  diuretics in, 219
  ipratropium in, 157
Lupron. *See* Leuprolide
Lupus erythematosus
  adverse drug reactions versus, 234
  chloroquine in, 630
  hydroxychloroquine in, 530
Lupus erythematosus–like syndrome, 288
Lutein, 750
Luteinizing hormone, 726, 736, 749, 764
Luteinizing hormone releasing hormone,
    727–728, 771–772
Lyme disease, 566
Lymphocytes
  corticosteroids and, 707
  FK506 and, 709
Lymphocytopenia
  corticosteroids and, 734–735
  mechlorethamine and, 675
Lymphoma
  L-asparaginase in, 695, 696
  Burkitt's
    cyclophosphamide in, 676
    methotrexate in, 682
  chlorambucil in, 678
  cyclophosphamide in, 675
  Hodgkin's, 615
  mitoxantrone in, 702
Lypressin, 729
Lysergic acid diethylamide, 468–469
Lysodren. *See* Mitotane
Lysyl-bradykinin, 194, 195

M current, 170, 171
M-phase, 663
Maalox. *See* Aluminum hydroxide
MAC. *See* Minimum alveolar concentration
Macrodantin. *See* Nitrofurantoin
Macrolide antibiotics, 579–581
  carbamazepine and, 417
  in *Mycobacterium* infections, 589
  in neuromuscular blockade, 182
Macromolecules, 47
Mafenide, 545, 546, 547
Magnesium, 211, 212
Magnesium citrate, 827
Magnesium hydroxide, 827, 832, 833
Magnesium salicylate, 488
Magnesium salts, 262
Magnesium sulfate, 310, 827
Major affective psychosis, 387
Major depression, 397–408
  bupropion in, 408
  buspirone in, 374
  monoamine oxidase inhibitors in, 406–407
  serotonin reuptake inhibitors in, 404–405
  trazodone in, 407–408
  tricyclic antidepressants in, 397–404
Malaria, 627–636
  amodiaquine in, 631
  chloroquine in, 629–630
  cloroguanide in, 633
  dapsone in, 634
  drug metabolism and, 43
  hydrochloroquine in, 630–631
  medication selection in, 634–636
  mefloquine in, 634
  mixed infections in, 636
  parasite in, 627–628, 629
  primaquine in, 631
  pyrimethamine in, 632–633

quinacrine in, 633–634
quinine in, 633
resistance to, 634–636
therapeutic considerations in, 628–629
Malathion, 81
Male antifertility agents, 771
Male infertility, 766
Mandelamine. *See* Methenamine
Manic-depressive illness, 387
  haloperidol in, 393
  lithium carbonate in, 395, 408–411
  mood-stabilizing agents in, 411
Mannitol, 220, 221–222
Mannose, 799
Manoplax. *See* Flosequinan
MAOI. *See* Monoamine oxidase inhibitors
Maprotiline, 398
  dosage and serum concentration of, 403
  seizure and, 402
Marcaine Hydrochloride. *See* Bupivacaine
Marijuana, 471–472
Marplan. *See* Isocarboxazid
Masoprocol, 533
Mass action, law of, 129
Mast cells, 811, 812, 813
Matulane. *See* Procarbazine
Maxaquin. *See* Lomefloxacin
Maxibolin. *See* Ethylestrenol
Maxzide. *See* Triamterene
May apple, 694
Measurin. *See* Aspirin
Mebaral. *See* Mephobarbital
Mebendazole, 642–643
Mecamylamine, 173, 174, 175
Mechlorethamine, 673–675
  in dermatological disorders, 533
  in Hodgkin's disease, 666
Meclizine
  in allergy, 820
  as antiemetic, 830
  in motion sickness, 818
Meclofenamate sodium
  as analgesic, 433
  as antiinflammatory, 490
Meclofenamic acid, 489
Meclomen. *See* Meclofenamate sodium
Mectizan. *See* Ivermectin
Medihaler-Epi. *See* Epinephrine
Medihaler-Iso. *See* Isoproterenol
Medroxyprogesterone acetate, 756, 758
  delayed absorption of, 27
  glucocorticoids and, 738
Mefenamic acid
  as analgesic, 433
  anticoagulants and, 318
  as antiinflammatory, 490
  cholestyramine and, 204
Mefloquine, 634
Mefoxin. *See* Cefoxitin
Megace. *See* Megestrol acetate
Megaloblastic anemia, 846
Megestrol acetate, 755, 756, 758
Melanocyte-stimulating hormone, 390
Melanoma
  dacarbazine in, 681
  human recombinant interleukin-2 in, 713
Melarsoprol, 623
Melatonin, 390
Mellaril. *See* Thioridazine
Melphalan, 677–678
Membrane expansion theory, 362
Memory loss, 372

Menadione, 840
Menaquinones, 840
Meningitis
  amphotericin B in, 648
  ampicillin in, 560
  cephalosporins in, 565
  chloramphenicol in, 578
  penicillins in, 559, 560
  sulfonamides in, 546
Meningococcal infection, 576–577
Menopause
  alkylating agents and, 669
  estrogens and progestins and, 753
  norethindrone in, 753
  osteoporosis and, 794
Menstruation
  alkylating agents and, 669
  blood hormone levels in, 749
  edema before, 220
  estrogens and progestins in, 750
  prostaglandins and, 480
Meperidine, 438, 444–445
  as analgesic, 434, 442
  anesthetic uses of, 360
  with methohexital, 357
  microsomal enzyme activity and, 42
  pregnancy and, 45
  withdrawal from, 439
Mephenytoin, 416
Mephobarbital, 418
Mepivacaine, 364, 368
Meprobamate, 184, 377
  anticoagulants and, 318
  in monooxygenase enzyme induction, 42
Merbromin, 660
6-Mercaptopurine, 684–685
  allopurinol and, 507–508
  azathioprine and, 709
  cell cycle and, 664
  drug interactions with, 670
  hepatotoxicity of, 74
  immune response and, 666
  in inflammatory bowel disease, 835
  vitamins and, 845
Mercuric chloride, 75
Mercurochrome. *See* Merbromin
Mercury
  allergic contact dermatitis and, 76
  as antiseptic, 660
  dimercaprol and, 16
  toxicity of, 75, 80
Merozoites, mosquito, 628
Merthiolate. *See* Thimerosol
Mesalamine, 837
Mesantoin. *See* Mephenytoin
Mesna, 668, 677
Mesnex. *See* Mesna
Mesoridazine, 388
Mesterolone, 767
Mestinon. *See* Pyridostigmine
Mestranol, 51, 748, 752
Met-enkephalin, 438
Metabolic acidosis, 435
Metabolism
  adrenomimetic drugs and, 123–124
  autoregulation of, 265
  chemotherapeutic toxicity and, 668
  drug, 33–46
    age and, 39–40
    coadministration and, 44
    conjugation reactions in, 37–39
    disease and, 43–44

Metabolism, drug (*cont.*)
  enzymes in, 33–36, 41–42
  gender and, 44
  genetics in, 42–43
  hormonal factors in, 44–45
  hydrolytic reactions in, 36–37
  intestinal microflora and, 45
  nutrition and, 40–41
  oxidative reactions in, 36
  radiation and, 44
  reactive intermediates and, 45
  reductive reactions in, 36
  species differences in, 43, 44
  in elderly, 39–40
  electrolyte, 211–218
    blood supply and, 212–214
    nephron segments and, 213–215
    potassium regulation and, 216–218
    sodium conservation and, 215–216
    tubular reabsorption and secretion in, 212
  hepatic glycogen, 801
  mineral, 787
  oral cavity and, 848
  protein, 801
Metabolites
  of allopurinol, 507
  of azathioprine, 710
  of benzodiazepines, 371
  of chloral hydrate, 377
  of clarithromycin, 580
  of disopyramide, 290
  drug metabolism and, 45
  excretion of, 33, 34
  of lidocaine, 293
  of nalidixic acid, 551
  of probenecid, 505
  of procainamide, 288
  of propafenone, 300
  of sulfinpyrazone, 506
Metahydrin. *See* Trichlormethiazide
Metallothionein, 30
Metals
  chelation of, 499
  nontherapeutic exposure to, 79
  toxicity of, 80
Metamucil. *See* Psyllium seed derivatives
Metandren. *See* Methyltestosterone
Metaphen. *See* Nitromersol
Metaproterenol, 514
Metaraminol, 126–127
Metformin, 844
Methacholine, 147–148
  anticholinergic poisoning and, 158
  bethanechol and, 148
  chemical structure of, 146
  as choline ester, 145
  pharmacological actions of, 147
Methacycline, 576
Methadone, 438, 446
  enterohepatic recirculation and, 51
  lung and, 31
  in withdrawal therapy, 463
Methamphetamine, 381–383, 466–467
Methandrostenolone, 769
Methanol, 456–457
  antidote for, 77
  neurotoxicity of, 75
Metharbital, 418
Methedrine. *See* Methamphetamine
Methenamine, 552–553
Methimazole, 782–784
Methocarbamol, 184
Methohexital, 356

Methotrexate
  in acute lymphocytic leukemia, 670
  antineoplastic properties of, 681–683
  in asthma, 521
  cell cycle and, 664
  cirrhosis and, 668
  in dermatological disorders, 532–533
  drug interactions with, 670
  hair loss and, 668
  immune response and, 666
  in immunosuppression, 711
  resistance to, 665–666
  in rheumatoid arthritis, 498–499
  toxicity of, 74, 76
  vitamins and, 845
Methoxamine, 126–127
Methoxyflurane, 349
  anesthetic apparatus and, 343
  partial pressure–minimum alveolar
    concentration and, 338
  partition coefficients of, 340
  solubility of, 341
8-Methoxypsoralen, 528–529
Methsuximide, 421
Methyclothiazide, 224
Methyl alcohol. *See* Methanol
N-Methyl-D-aspartate, 330–332
Methyl n-butyl ketone, 80
Methyl salicylate, 434, 435
Methylation, 39
  dacarbazine and, 681
  streptozocin and, 679
Methylatropine, 154
Methylcellulose, 825, 826, 827
Methyldopa
  active transport of, 23
  adrenergic transmission and, 114
α-Methyldopa, 245–246
  chemical structure of, 241
  renin release and, 191
  volume of distribution of, 28
Methyldopate hydrochloride, 245
Methylene blue, 77
Methylene chloride, 78, 80
α-Methylnorepinephrine, 245
Methylparaben, 366
Methylphenidate, 381–383
Methylprednisolone
  in asthma, 519
  structure-activity relationships of, 736
Methylsuccinimide, 420
Methyltert-butyl ether, 837–838
Methyltestosterone, 758, 767
Methyltransferases, 39
Methylxanthine inhibitors, 263
Methylxanthines, 310, 383–385
Meticorten. *See* Prednisone
Metoclopramide, 824, 831
Metocurine iodide, 182
Metolazone, 62, 223, 224
Metopirone. *See* Metyrapone
Metoprolol, 139–140, 301
  in angina pectoris, 273
  as β-adrenoceptor blocking agent, 137g
  preparations and dosage of, 138, 142
  propafenone and, 299
  propranolol versus, 130, 140
  structure of, 137
Metrazol. *See* Pentylenetetrazol
Metrogel. *See* Metronidazole
Metronidazole, 618–619
  anticoagulants and, 318
  in dermatological disorders, 531

enterohepatic recirculation and, 51
  in inflammatory bowel disease, 835
Metubine Iodide. *See* Metocurine iodide
Metyrapone, 743–744
Metyrosine, 241, 244
Mevacor. *See* Lovastatin
"Mexican mud," 461
Mexiletine, 296–297, 365
Mezlin. *See* Mezlocillin
Mezlocillin, 561
MIC. *See* Minimum inhibitory concentration
Micatin. *See* Miconazole
Miconazole, 318, 652–653
Micro-K. *See* Potassium chloride
Microadenoma, 725
Microbial contamination of food, 79
Microencapsulation, 70
Microflora
  antibiotics and, 543
  biliary excretion and, 51
  drug metabolism and, 45
  neomycin and, 571
Micronase. *See* Tolbutamide
Micronor. *See* Norethindrone
Microorganisms, as biological response
    modifiers, 712
Microvilli, 25
Midamor. *See* Amiloride
Midazolam, 355, 357
Migraine
  β-adrenoceptor blocking agents in, 141
  oral contraceptives and, 757
  xanthines in, 384
Milk, tetracyclines and, 575
Milrinone
  in myocardial insufficiency, 263
  propranolol and, 303
Miltown. *See* Meprobamate
Mineral detergent in enema, 828
Mineral oil
  as fecal softener, 828
  oral anticoagulants and, 318
  vitamins and, 844
Mineralocorticoids
  with etomidate, 359
  extracellular fluid and, 220
Minerals, 787
Mini-pill, 752
Minimum alveolar concentration, 338–339
Minimum inhibitory concentration, 541
Minipress. *See* Prazosin
Minocin. *See* Minocycline
Minocycline, 530, 575, 576–577
Minoxidil, 234–235
  chemical structure of, 233
  in dermatological disorders, 533
  in hypertension, 232
  topical, 235
Mintezol. *See* Thiabendazole
Miochol. *See* Acetylcholine chloride
Miosis
  acetylcholine and, 147
  autonomic nervous system and, 105
  buprenorphine and, 448
  carbachol and, 148
  methacholine and, 148
  morphine and, 440
Miotics, 167
Miradon. *See* Anisindione
Mirex, 81
Misconduct, scientific, 94–95
Misoprostol, 482, 486–487, 834
MIT. *See* Monoiodotyrosine

Mithracin. *See* Plicamycin
Mithramycin, 692
Mitocin-C. *See* Mitomycin
Mitomycin, 690–691
Mitotane, 700, 744
Mitotic index, 663
Mitoxantrone, 702
Moban. *See* Molindone
Mobidin. *See* Magnesium salicylate
Moclobemide, 407
Moctanin. *See* Monooctanoin
Moderate drinker, term, 451
Modicon. *See* Norethindrone
Modrastane. *See* Trilostane
Moduretic. *See* Amiloride
Moebiquin. *See* Iodoquinol
Mogadon. *See* Nitrazepam
Molindone, 394
Monistat. *See* Miconazole
Monitoring of tricyclic antidepressants, 402–403
Mono-quaternary amines, 162, 166
Monoamine oxidase
    amphetamines and, 382
    guanethidine and, 242
    indirectly acting adrenomimetic drugs and, 116, 117
    norepinephrine and, 109, 110, 111
    reserpine and, 243
Monoamine oxidase inhibitors
    in depression, 406–407
    dosage and serum concentration of, 403
    levodopa and, 428
    tricyclic antidepressants and, 403–404
Monobactams, 567
Monoclonal antibody, 671, 702
Monoethylglycine xylidide, 293
Monofluorophosphate mouth rinse, 852
Monoiodotyrosine, 777
Monooctanoin, 838
Monooxygenases, 34–36
    insecticides and, 81
    toxicity of, 73
Monopril. *See* Fosinopril
Mood disorders, 397–411
    major depression and, 397–408
        bupropion in, 408
        monoamine oxidase inhibitors in, 406–407
        serotonin reuptake inhibitors in, 404–405
        trazodone in, 407–408
        tricyclic antidepressants in, 397–404
    manic-depressive illness and, 408–411
        lithium carbonate in, 408–411
        mood-stabilizing agents in, 411
Mood-stabilizing agents
    lithium in, 409
    in manic-depressive illness, 411
MOPP regimen
    cyclophosphamide in, 676
    in Hodgkin's disease, 666
    mechlorethamine in, 674
    procarbazine in, 699
    vincristine in, 693
Moraxella catarrhalis, 567
Moricizine, 291–292
Morphine, 438, 440–444
    as analgesic, 442
    as anesthetic, 360
    in breast milk, 52
    cardiovascular system and, 440
    constipation and, 825–826

enterohepatic recirculation and, 51
histamine release and, 814
with methohexital, 357
microsomal enzyme activity and, 42
receptors for, 9
withdrawal from, 439
Mosquito, 627
Motilin, 823
Motilium. *See* Domperidone
Motion sickness, 818
    muscarinic blocking drugs in, 157
    scopolamine in, 71
Motrin. *See* Ibuprofen
Mouth, 24, 848–849
MTBE. *See* Methyltert-butyl ether
Mucosa
    in drug absorption, 24
    intestinal, 828–829
    nonsteroidal antiinflammatory drugs and, 481
    steroids and, 738
Mucositis
    cancer chemotherapy and, 668
    fluorouracil and, 687
    methotrexate and, 683
Multicompartment pharmacokinetic model, 60
Multidrug resistance, 666
    anthracyclines and, 688
    paclitaxel and, 695
    in tuberculosis, 587
Multiple myeloma
    melphalan in, 677
    steroid therapy in, 741
Mupirocin, 530
Muscarine, 149
Muscarinic blocking drugs, 151–159
    absorption, metabolism, and excretion of, 155
    adverse reactions of, 158
    chemistry of, 151, 153
    contraindications to, 158
    ether and, 347
    in irritable bowel syndrome, 156–157
    mechanism of action of, 151–152
    pharmacological actions of, 152–155
    structure of, 153
    uses of, 155
Muscarinic receptors, 145, 170–171
    of acetylcholine, 112, 146–147
    lithium carbonate and, 409
    subtypes of, 151, 152
Muscimol, 330
Muscle
    acetylcholine and, 9–10, 147
    adrenoceptors and, 113
    adrenomimetic drugs and, 122–123
    amiodarone and, 305
    anticholinesterase agents and, 164, 165
    blood perfusion rate in, 29
    catecholamines and, 120
    cholinesterase inhibitors and, 165, 167
    cramping of, 633
    innervation of, 104, 106
    phenoxybenzamine and, 132
    receptors in, 10, 169
    tremor of, 516
Muscle relaxants, 183
    anticholinergic poisoning and, 158
    benzodiazepines in, 372
    central skeletal, 183–184
Mushroom poisoning, 157
Mustargen. *See* Mechlorethamine

Mutagenesis, 76
    biotransformation and, 45
    covalent bonding and, 11
Mutamycin. *See* Mitomycin
Myambutol. *See* Ethambutol
Myasthenia gravis
    autoimmunity in, 705
    cholinesterase inhibitors in, 166–167
    disopyramide and, 290
    quinidine and, 287
Myasthenic syndrome, 179
Mycelex. *See* Clotrimazole
Mycifradin Sulfate. *See* Neomycin
Mycin. *See* Oxytetracycline
Mycobacterial infection
    acquired immunodeficiency syndrome and, 614
    antiseptics and disinfectants and, 658
    bacillus Calmette-Guérin and, 712
    clarithromycin in, 580
    treatment of, 587–588
Mycoplasmal infection
    chloramphenicol in, 578
    macrolides in, 579, 580
    tetracyclines in, 575, 577
Mycostatin. *See* Nystatin
Mydriasis
    autonomic nervous system and, 105
    epinephrine and, 123
    tolazoline and, 134
Mydriatics, 158
Myelin degeneration, 82
Myeloid colony stimulating factors, 714–715
Myeloma
    chlorambucil in, 678
    cyclophosphamide in, 676
    melphalan in, 677
Myelopathy, methotrexate and, 683
Myelosuppression
    carmustine and, 679
    cladribine and, 685
    cytarabine and, 686
    dactinomycin and, 691
    fludarabine and, 685
    fluorouracil and, 687
    mechlorethamine and, 675
    mercaptopurine and, 685
    methotrexate and, 683
    mitomycin and, 691
    paclitaxel and, 695
    pentostatin and, 685
    thioguanine and, 684
    thiotepa and, 681
Mylanta. *See* Aluminum hydroxide
Myleran. *See* Busulfan
Myocardial infarction
    aspirin in, 435
    atropine in, 156
    estrogens and, 750
    ethanol and, 455
    lidocaine in, 293
    oral anticoagulants and, 319
Myocardial insufficiency, 257–264
    acetylcholinesterase inhibitors in, 264
    cyclic adenosine monophosphate and, 263–264
    diuretics in, 264
    positive inotropic agents in, 257–263
    systemic effects of, 256
    vasodilators in, 264
Myocardial wall tension, 266
Myocardium
    amiodarone and, 305

Myocardium (*cont.*)
  flecainide and, 298
  ganglionic blockade and, 174
  physiology and pathophysiology of, 255–257
Myoclonic seizure, 414
  nitrazepam in, 420
  valproic acid in, 419
Myopathy, steroid, 739
Myotonechol. *See* Bethanechol
Mysoline. *See* Primidone
Mytelase. *See* Ambenonium
Myxedema, 779

Nabumetone, 489, 493–494
NAC. *See* N-Acetylcysteine
NAD. *See* Nicotinamide adenine dinucleotide
Nadolol, 140, 301
  in angina, 271
  characteristics and preparations of, 138
  pharmacokinetics of, 273
  structure of, 137
Nafcil. *See* Nafcillin
Nafcillin, 555
  anticoagulants and, 318
Naftifine hydrochloride, 654–656
Naftin. *See* Naftifine hydrochloride
Nail infection, 531
Nalbuphine, 448
Nalfon. *See* Fenoprofen
Nalidixic acid, 318, 550–552
Nallpen. *See* Nafcillin
Nalmefene, 447
Naloxone, 446–447
  as equilibrium-competitive antagonist, 17
  in morphine poisoning, 441
  as narcotic and opioid antidote, 77
Naltrexone, 447, 463–464
Nandrolone decanoate, 769
Nandrolone phenpropionate, 769
NAPA. *See* N-Acetylprocainamide
Naphthalene, 39
Naprosyn. *See* Naproxen
Naproxen, 492
  as analgesic, 433, 437
  anticoagulants and, 318
  in arthritis, 489
Naqua. *See* Trichlormethiazide
Narcolepsy, 382
Narcosis, 337
Narcotic antagonist, 462
Narcotics
  as anesthetics, 360
  antidote for, 77
  overdose of, 447
  phenylpiperidine
    anesthetic uses of, 360
    metabolism and excretion of, 355
Nardil. *See* Phenelzine
Nasal decongestion
  andrenomimetic drugs in, 115
  ephedrine and, 127
  phenylephrine in, 126
National Formulary, 85, 86
Natriuretic drugs, 215
Naturetin. *See* Bendroflumethiazide
Nausea
  bretylium and, 304
  calcium channel blockers and, 253
  cancer chemotherapy and, 667
  carmustine and, 679
  colchicine and, 504
  cyclophosphamide and, 676, 710
  dacarbazine and, 681

dactinomycin and, 691
flecainide and, 299
hexamethylmelamine and, 700
ketoconazole and, 654
levamisole and, 702
mechlorethamine and, 675
mercaptopurine and, 685
methotrexate and, 683
moricizine and, 291
morphine and, 440
nitrofurans and, 550
propafenone and, 300
PUVA therapy and, 528–529
quinolones and, 552
renal disease and, 61
sotalol and, 307
theophylline and, 513
thioguanine and, 684
thiotepa and, 681
Navane hydrochloride. *See* Thiothixene
NDA. *See* New Drug Application
Nebcin. *See* Tobramycin
Nebulizer, 515
Necator americanus infection
  mebendazole in, 643
  pyrantel pamoate in, 641
  thiabendazole in, 642
Necrosis
  acetaminophen and, 73
  acute tubular, 75
  cancer chemotherapy and, 668
  doxorubicin and, 689
  hepatotoxin and, 74
  idarubicin and, 689
  norepinephrine and, 125
Nedocromil sodium, 520
Negative feedback mechanism, 114
NegGram. *See* Nalidixic acid
Neisseria gonorrhoeae infection
  glycopeptides in, 584
  silver nitrate in, 660
  spectinomycin in, 573
Neisseria meningitidis, 578
Nematodes, 639–642
Nembutal. *See* Phenobarbital
Neo-Cobefrin. *See* Levonordefrin
Neo-Hombreol F. *See* Testosterone
Neo-Hombreol M. *See* Methyltestosterone
Neo-Synephrine. *See* Phenylephrine
Neobiotic. *See* Neomycin
Neomycin, 571
  in dermatological disorders, 531
  polymyxin B and, 586
  vitamins and, 844
Neonate
  chloramphenicol and, 37–38, 578–579
  glomerular filtration rate of, 48
  hexachlorophene and, 662
  local anesthetics and, 364
  tubular transport mechanism in, 49
  vitamin K and, 843
  withdrawal signs in, 463
Neophyl. *See* Dyphylline
Neostigmine
  absorption of, 165
  acetylcholine receptor blockade and, 156, 181–182
  metoclopramide with, 825
  in myasthenia gravis, 167
  uses of, 166
Nephron, 211
Nephron segments, 213–215
Nephrotic syndrome
  diuretics and, 219–220

glucocorticoid therapy in, 738
  steroid therapy in, 741
Nephrotoxicity, 75
  of aminoglycosides, 572, 590
  of amphotericin B, 649
  of bacitracin, 583
  of cancer chemotherapy, 668
  of cephalosporins, 566
  of cyclosporine, 709
  of polymyxins, 586
  of tetracyclines, 577
Nernst equation, 276
Nerve block
  extremity, 365
  regional, 364–365
  sympathetic, 365
Nerve gases, 168
Nervous system. *See also* Central nervous system
  chemotherapeutic toxicity and, 669
  desensitization of, 180–181
  labetalol and, 143
  local anesthetics and, 363
  muscarinic blocking drugs and, 153
  myocardial insufficiency and, 255
  organization and functions of, 101
  parasympathetic, 103
    eye and, 105
    organ innervation and, 104–106
    preganglionic neurons of, 102
    sinoatrial node and, 279
  peripheral, 75, 101
    neurotransmission in, 104
    vitamin toxicity and, 843
  sympathetic, 103
    angiotensins and, 191
    antihypertensives and, 236–238
    cardiac glycosides and, 261
    myocardial insufficiency and, 255
    organ innervation and, 104–106
    preganglionic neurons of, 101–102
    verapamil and, 308
Nesacaine. *See* Chloroprocaine
Netilmicin, 571–572
Netromycin. *See* Netilmicin
Neupogen. *See* Filgrastim
Neuritis
  optic, 592
  in vitamin deficiency, 842
Neuroeffector cleft, 107
Neuroendocrine pathways, 232
Neuroleptic drugs, 374–375
Neuroleptic syndrome, 389
Neuromuscular junction, 164, 177, 178
Neuromuscular paralysis, 178–179
Neuromuscular transmission, 177–184
  acetylcholine in, 179–182
  alcohol and, 184
  aminoglycosides and, 572
  antispasticity agents and, 182–184
  chlorpromazine and, 184
  cholinesterase inhibitors and, 166
  fentanyl and, 184
  fonazine mesylate and, 184
Neuronal transport, 110
Neurontin. *See* Gabapentin
Neuropathy
  dideoxyinosine and, 612
  hexamethylmelamine and, 700
  insecticides and, 82
  paclitaxel and, 695
  vitamin toxicity and, 843
Neuropeptide Y, 104, 332–333
Neurotensin, 332, 814

Neurotoxicity, 75
  of penicillins, 561
  of polymyxins, 586
  of vincristine, 669, 693–694
Neurotransmission, 107–112
  acetylcholine in, 108–109
  acetylcholinesterase and, 161–162
  catecholamine metabolism and, 110–112
  ethanol and, 453
  ganglionic, 170, 171
  monoamine oxidase inhibitors and, 406–407
  norepinephrine in, 109–110, 111
  pharmacological intervention of, 114
  trazodone and, 407
  tricyclic antidepressants and, 399–400
Neurotransmitters, 327, 328–333
  adrenergic neuron blocking agents and, 240
  amino acid, 330
  autonomic nervous system, 103–104
  β-adrenergic blocking agents and, 239
  ganglionic blocking agents and, 244
  peripheral nervous system, 102
  study of, 333
  sympathetic nervous system, 236
Neutral regular human insulin, 805
New Drug Application, 86
Newborn. See Neonate
Niacin, 204–205
  absorption, metabolism and excretion of, 205
  adverse reactions to, 205
  clinical uses of, 205
  in combination therapy, 208
  drug interactions with, 845
  mechanism of action of, 204–205
  in plasma triglycerides reduction, 206, 207
Nicardipine, 254
Nickel
  allergic contact dermatitis and, 76
  cancer and, 79
Niclocide. See Niclosamide
Niclosamide, 637–639
Nicolar. See Niacin
Nicotinamide adenine dinucleotide, 452
Nicotinamide-adenine dinucleotide
    phosphate, 35
Nicotine, 171–173
  absorption of, 24, 173
  acetylcholine and, 10
  in breast milk, 52
  cardiovascular system and, 172
  central nervous system and, 173
  gastrointestinal system and, 173
  respiratory system and, 172–173
Nicotinic acid, 840
  in cholesterol reduction, 204–205, 843
  in combination therapy, 208
  deficiency of, 841–842
  in hyperlipidemia, 843
  in hypolipidemia, 203
  toxicity of, 843
Nicotinic receptors, 145
  of acetylcholine, 10, 112
  anticholinesterase agents and, 165
  ganglionic blocking agents and, 171–173
  muscarinic blocking drugs and, 154
Nifedipine
  in angina pectoris, 267
  with calcium entry blockers, 273
  chemical formula of, 250
  pharmacokinetics of, 253
  preparations and dosage of, 254
  receptor-blocking properties of, 251
  second-generation analogues of, 249

Nifurtimox, 623–624
Night blindness, 841, 844
Nightmares, amiodarone and, 306
Nikethamide, 381
Nikorin. See Nikethamide
Nilstat. See Nystatin
Nimodipine
  preparations and dosage of, 254
  selectivity of, 249
Nimotop. See Nimodipine
Nipent. See Pentostatin
Nipride. See Nitroprusside
Nitrates
  adverse reactions to, 269–270
  in angina, 265, 267, 269
  cardiac oxygen supply and demand and, 273
  in coronary vasospasm, 267
  as food additive, 79
  mechanism of action of, 268
  in myocardial insufficiency, 264
  pharmacokinetics of, 271
  tolerance to, 270
Nitrazepam, 420
Nitric oxide
  as endothelium-derived relaxing factor, 122
  hypertension and, 232
  in inflammation, 479
Nitrites
  antidote for, 77
  as food additive, 79
Nitro-Bid. See Nitroglycerin
Nitrofurans, 549–550
Nitrofurantoin, 550
  chemical structure of, 549
  hepatotoxicity of, 74
Nitrofurazone, 549, 550
Nitrogard. See Transmucosal nitroglycerin
Nitrogen
  excretion of, 804
  insulin and, 801
  piperidine, 446
Nitrogen dioxide, 74, 78
Nitrogen mustards, 673–678
  chlorambucil in, 678
  cyclophosphamide in, 675–677
  in dermatological disorders, 532
  ifosfamide in, 677
  mechlorethamine in, 673–675
  melphalan in, 677–678
Nitroglycerin
  in angina pectoris, 267, 269
  as buccal tablet, 68
  in coronary vasospasm, 267
  dependence on, 270
  mechanism of action of, 267–268
  in myocardial insufficiency, 264
  pharmacokinetics of, 268, 271
  preparations of, 270
  propranolol with, 273
  sublingual administration of, 24
  volume of distribution of, 28
Nitroglycerin ointment, 269, 270
Nitrol. See Nitroglycerin ointment
Nitrolingual. See Nitroglycerin
Nitromersol, 660
Nitroprusside, 235–236
  chemical structure of, 233
  in hypertension, 232
Nitrosothiol, 267
Nitrosoureas, 678–680
  carmustine, lomustine, and semustine in, 678–679
  streptozocin in, 679–680
  toxicity of, 667

Nitrospan. See Nitroglycerin
Nitrostat. See Nitroglycerin
Nitrosylpentacyanoferrate compound, 235–236
Nitrous oxide, 51, 350
  abuse of, 472–473
  anesthetic agents and, 342–343
  diffusion hypoxia and, 343
  in neuromuscular blockade, 182
  partial pressure–minimum alveolar
      concentration and, 338
  partition coefficients of, 340
  second gas effect and, 343
Nitrovasodilators, 232
Nizatidine, 821, 834
Nizoral. See Ketoconazole
NMDA. See N-Methyl-D-aspartate
Nocardial infection
  minocycline in, 577
  trimethoprim in, 549
  trisulfapyrimidine in, 546
Noctec. See Chloral hydrate
Nodulocystic acne vulgaris, 527
Nolvadex. See Tamoxifen
Non-Hodgkin's lymphoma, 615
Nonabsorbable hyperosmolar solution, 826
Noncompetitive antagonism, 17–18
Nonequilibrium-competitive antagonism,
    129, 132
Nonequilibrium-competitive bond, 17
Nonionic detergents, 661
Nonopioid analgesics, 432–437
  aniline derivatives as, 436–437
  arylakanoic acids as, 437
  diclofenac as, 437
  fenamates as, 437
  indomethacin as, 437
  piroxicam as, 437
  salicylates and derivatives as, 432–436
Nonoral medication, 68–70
  buccal and sublingual, 68
  inhalation of, 69–70
  intramuscular, 68
  intravenous and intraarterial, 68
  percutaneous absorption of, 69
  rectal, 68
  subcutaneous, 68–69
Nonoxynol-9, 661
Nonsteroidal antiinflammatory drugs, 486–494
  diclofenac as, 493
  etodolac as, 493
  fenamate as, 490
  fenoprofen as, 492
  flurbiprofen as, 493
  ibuprofen as, 491–492
  indomethacin as, 490–491
  ketoprofen as, 492–493
  kidney and, 481
  mechanism of action of, 486
  nabumetone as, 493–494
  naproxen as, 492
  phenylbutazone as, 488–489
  piroxicam as, 490
  prostaglandin synthesis and, 479
  salicylates as, 435, 487–488, 489
  sulindac as, 491
  tolmetin as, 492
  toxicity of, 75, 486–487
Nor-QD. See Norethindrone
Nor-tet. See Tetracyclines
Noradrenaline. See Norepinephrine
Norcuron. See Vecuronium bromide
Nordazepam. See Chlorazepate

Nordette. *See* Levonorgestrel
Norepinephrine, 328
  adrenal medulla and, 106
  adrenergic neuron blocking agents and, 240
  α-receptors and, 130–131
  blood-brain barrier and, 336
  cardiovascular effects of, 120
  chemical structure of, 116
  diastolic depolarization and, 279
  ganglionic action potential and, 171
  ganglionic blocking agents and, 244
  in gastrointestinal tract, 147
  imidazolines and, 133
  in neurotransmission, 104, 109–110, 111
  nicotinic receptors and, 172
  pharmacodynamics of, 121, 122
  phenoxybenzamine and, 133, 135
  phentolamine and, 135
  preparations and dosage of, 125
  reserpine and, 243
  storage of, 108, 242–244
  sympathetic nervous system impairment and, 236
  synthesis of, 108, 244
  tricyclic antidepressants and, 399–400
Norethin. *See* Norethindrone
Norethindrone, 748, 752, 758
Norflex. *See* Orphenadrine citrate
Norfloxacin, 551
Norgestrel, 752
Norinyl. *See* Norethindrone
Norlutate. *See* Norethindrone
Norlutin. *See* Norethindrone
Normodyne. *See* Labetalol
Normosol-R, 221
Noroxin. *See* Norfloxacin
Norpace. *See* Disopyramide
Norplant System, 752
Norpramin. *See* Desipramine
19-Nortestosterone, 761, 771
19-Nortestosterone derivatives, 769
Nortriptyline
  chemical structure of, 398
  dosage and serum concentration of, 403
  volume of distribution of, 28
Norvac. *See* Amlodipine
Noscapine, 438, 449
Nosocomial infection
  antiseptics and disinfectants and, 657
  iodophors and, 659
Novantrone. *See* Mitoxantrone
Novocain. *See* Procaine hydrochloride
Novolin R. *See* Neutral regular human insulin
Novrad. *See* Levopropoxyphene
NPH insulin. *See* Isophane
NSAIDs. *See* Nonsteroidal antiinflammatory drugs
Nucleophilic substitution, 673
Nucleoside analogues, 612
Nuprin. *See* Ibuprofen
Nuremberg Code, 95
Nutmeg, 473
Nutrition
  drug metabolism and, 40–41
  ethanol and, 455
Nydrazid. *See* Isoniazid
Nystatin, 648, 649–650
Nystex. *See* Nystatin

Oat cell lung cancer, 676
Obesity, 382
Occupational asthma, 76

Occupational Safety and Health Administration, 78
Ochratoxin, 79
Octreotide, 698, 725, 727
Ocular hypertension, 139
Ocusert, 71
Ofloxacin, 551
Oleandomycin, 579
Oligospermia, 669
Olsalazine sodium, 836, 837
Omega-3 PUFA, 201, 207
Omeprazole
  anticoagulants and, 318
  in gastrointestinal disorders, 834–835
Omnipen. *See* Ampicillin
On-off phenomenon, 428
Onchocerciasis, 622
  diethylcarbamazine in, 640–641
  nematode-induced, 639
Oncovin. *See* Vincristine
Ondansetron, 667, 831
One-compartment pharmacokinetic model, 56
Oophorectomy, 754
Open-angle glaucoma, 167
Ophthalgan. *See* Glycerin
Ophthalmia
  penicillins in, 560
  silver nitrate in, 660
Ophthalmopathy
  in hyperthyroidism, 782
  idoxuridine in, 603
Opioid agonist-antagonists, 447–449
  buprenorphine as, 449
  butorphanol as, 448
  nalbuphine as, 448
  pentazocine as, 447–448
Opioid analgesics, 437–446
  abuse of, 461–464
  alfentanil as, 445
  chemistry of, 438–439
  codeine as, 444, 445
  dextropropoxyphene as, 446
  in diarrhea, 825–826
  fentanyl as, 445
  heroin as, 444
  hydromorphone as, 444
  levorphanol as, 444
  mechanism of action of, 439
  meperidine as, 444–445
  methadone as, 446
  morphine as, 440–444
  sufentanil as, 445
  tolerance and physical dependence of, 439–440
Opioid anesthesia, 360
Opioid antagonists, 446–447
  nalmefene as, 447
  naloxone as, 446–447
  naltrexone as, 447
Opioid peptides, 332, 438–439
Opisthorcis viverrini, 643
Opisthotonos, 381
Opium, 459
Opium tincture, 826
Optic neuritis, 592
Oral absorption curve, 58
Oral cavity, 24, 848–849
Oral contraceptives
  adverse reactions to, 755–757
  anticoagulants and, 318
  barbiturates and, 376
  breast cancer and, 756

contraindications for, 757
  estrogens and progestins in, 751–753
  migraine and, 757
  transcortin and, 733
  vitamin interactions with, 844, 845
Oral hypoglycemic agents, 805–808
  absorption, metabolism, and excretion of, 806
  adverse reactions to, 806–807
  anticoagulants and, 318
  antidote for, 77
  chemistry of, 805–806
  drug interactions with, 807
  preparations and dosage of, 807
  thyroid hormones and, 780
  vitamins and, 845
Oral medication, 65–68
  capsules in, 67
  drug concentration-curve in, 58
  prolonged-release of, 70
  solutions in, 67
  suspensions in, 67
  tablets in, 67–68
Oreton. *See* Testosterone
Oreton Methyl. *See* Methyltestosterone
Oreton propionate. *See* Testosterone propionate
Organ toxicity, 73–74
Organ transplantation
  antibodies and, 711
  antithymocyte globulin in, 711
  azathioprine in, 709–710
  corticosteroids in, 706–707
  cyclophosphamide in, 710–711
  cyclosporine in, 707–709
  cytotoxic drugs in, 709
  FK506 in, 709
  immunomodulating drugs and, 705, 706
  orthoclone OKT3 in, 711
Organic metals, 80
Organic nitrates
  absorption, metabolism, and excretion of, 268
  adverse reactions to, 269–270
  in angina pectoris, 267
  clinical uses of, 268–269
  pharmacological action of, 267–268, 269
  preparations and dosage of, 270–271
Organic psychosis, 387
Organochlorine insecticides, 75, 76, 81
Organogenesis, 77
Organophosphate insecticides, 75, 81–82
Organophosphates, 162, 163
  absorption and metabolism of, 165
  antidote for, 77
  immunotoxicity and, 76
  uses of, 166
Orinase. *See* Tolbutamide
Ornidyl. *See* Eflornithine
Orphenadrine citrate, 184
Ortho-Novum. *See* Norethindrone
Orthoclone OKT3, 711
Orthostatic hypotension
  in parkinsonism, 425, 427
  phenothiazines and, 390
  tricyclic antidepressants and, 401
Orudis. *See* Ketoprofen
OSHA. *See* Occupational Safety and Health Administration
Osmitrol. *See* Mannitol
Osmoglyn. *See* Glycerin
Osmolar laxatives, 826
Osmotic diuretics, 219, 220

Osmotic laxatives, 827
Osteoarthritis, 485, 493
Osteoclasts, 789
Osteodystrophy, renal, 795
Osteomalacia
    parathyroid hormone, calcitonin, and
        vitamin D in, 794
    in vitamin deficiency, 842
Osteopenia, 794–795
Osteoporosis
    estrogens and progestins in, 753
    parathyroid hormone, calcitonin, and
        vitamin D in, 794
    steroids and, 738
Ostwald solubility coefficient, 341
Otitis media
    ampicillin in, 560
    erythromycin in, 580
    penicillins in, 559
Ototoxicity
    of aminoglycosides, 572, 590
    of loop diuretics, 228
    of vancomycin, 585
Ouabain
    biliary secretion of, 51
    pharmacokinetic properties of, 258
Ovarian cancer
    carboplatin in, 701
    chlorambucil in, 678
    cisplatin in, 700, 701
    clinical drug testing for, 89
    cyclophosphamide in, 676
    estrogens and progestins and, 756
    etoposide in, 694
    melphalan in, 677
    paclitaxel in, 695
    thiotepa in, 680
Ovary
    estrogen and progestin synthesis in, 747
    gonadotropin therapy and, 726
    menstrual cycle and, 750
    steroidogenesis in, 749–750
Overdose
    aniline derivative, 436–437
    intravenous, 28
    morphine, 441
    salicylate, 435
Ovral. See Norgestrel
Ovrette. See Norgestrel
Ovulation, 754
Oxacillin, 557
Oxalid. See Oxyphenbutazone
Oxamniquine, 644
Oxandrolone, 769
Oxazepam, 372, 373
Oxicam, 433
Oxidants
    in inflammation, 479
    reperfusion injury and, 507
N-Oxidation, 36
Oxidative reactions in drug metabolism, 36
Oxidizing agents, 659
Oxidizing pollutants, 78
Oximes, 163
Oxolinic acid, 550, 551
Oxotremorine, 149
Oxybarbiturates, 356
Oxybutynin, 155, 157
Oxycodone, 434
Oxygen
    amiodarone and, 305
    antianginal drugs and, 265–266
    as carbon monoxide antidote, 77

cyanide and, 82
    in monooxygenase system, 34–35
    myocardial insufficiency and, 257
    nitrates and, 273
    propranolol and, 302
Oxygenated steroids, 733
Oxygenating agents, 852–853
Oxymetholone, 769
Oxymorphone, 442
Oxymycin. See Oxytetracycline
Oxyphenbutazone
    anticoagulants and, 318
    in gout, 508
Oxypurinol, 507
Oxytetracycline, 576
Oxytocin, 26, 729–730
Oxytriphylline, 385
Ozone, 74, 76, 78

P-glycoprotein
    blood-brain barrier and, 669
    competitive inhibition of, 670
    multidrug resistance and, 666
    paclitaxel and, 695
PABA. See Para-aminobenzoic acid
Pacific yew tree, 694
Paclitaxel, 694–695
    clinical testing of, 89
    hair loss and, 668
    multidrug resistance and, 666
    neurotoxicity of, 669
PAF. See Platelet-activating factor
Paget's disease, 795
Palsy, 425
    Bell's, 741
2-PAM. See Pralidoxime
Pamelor. See Nortriptyline
Pamidronate, 793
Panamycin. See Tetracyclines
Pancreatic insufficiency, 795
Pancreatitis
    alcoholism and, 455
    L-asparaginase and, 696
    dideoxyinosine and, 612
Pancreozymin
    calcitonin and, 790
    insulin secretion and, 799
Pancuronium, 182
Pancytopenia, 667
Pantothenic acid, 840, 842
Panwarfin. See Warfarin
Papaverine, 438
Papulopustular acne vulgaris, 528
Para-aminobenzoic acid, 364, 545, 546
Paracelsus, 5
Paracetamol. See Acetaminophen
Parachlorophenylalanine, 473
Paradione. See Paramethadione
Paradoxical bradycardia, 154
Paraffin, liquid, 828
Paraflex. See Chlorzoxazone
Paragonimiasis, 644
Paragonimus westermani, 643, 644
Parahydroxyglucuronide, 295
Paralysis, neuromuscular, 178–179
Paramethadione, 421
Paranoid psychosis, 467
Paraplatin. See Carboplatin
Paraquat, 82
    active transport of, 23
    toxicity of, 74, 81
Parasite, malarial, 627–628, 629

Parasympathetic nervous system, 103
    eye and, 105
    organ innervation and, 104–106
    preganglionic neurons of, 102
    sinoatrial node and, 279
Parasympathomimetics, 145
Parathion, 165
    topical absorption of, 27
    toxicity of, 81
Parathyroid hormone, 788–790
    amino acids and, 789
    calcium homeostasis and, 787–788
    clinical uses of, 792–796
    glucocorticoids and, 736
    mechanism of action of, 789–790
    mineral metabolism and, 787
    preparations and dosage of, 795
    synthesis and secretion of, 788–789
Parathyroid injection, 795
Paratyphoid fever, 578
Paregoric, 444, 463, 826
Parenteral administration, 27–28
Parenteral medication, 70–71
Parietal cell, 831–832
Parkinsonism
    muscarinic blocking drugs in, 157
    phenothiazines and, 391
    postencephalitic, 425
Parkinson's disease, 425–429
    amantadine in, 429
    anticholinergic drugs in, 429
    decarboxylase inhibitors in, 428–429
    dopamine agonists in, 429
    levodopa in, 426–428
    selegiline in, 429
Parlodel. See Bromocriptine
Parnate. See Tranylcypromine sulfate
Paromomycin
    in helminthic disease, 638
    in protozoal infection, 618, 625
Paroxetine, 404, 405
Paroxysmal supraventricular tachycardia, 252
Partial agonists, 15, 138
Partial pressure
    of gas in solution, 337–338
    of general anesthesia, 338–339
Partial seizure, 414, 418
Particle size, in inhalation of drugs, 69–70
Partition coefficient, 340, 523
P.A.S. Sodium. See Aminosalicylic acid
Passive diffusion, 22, 23, 48
Passive immunization, 599
Pasteurella, 577
Patch for percutaneous absorption of drug, 69
Patent ductus arteriosus, 482
Pathocil. See Dicloxacillin
Patient compliance, 543
Patient-controlled analgesia, 441
Patient rights, 93–94
Paucibacillary leprosy, 596
Pavil. See Paroxetine
Pavulon. See Pancuronium
PBP. See Penicillin-binding proteins
PCP. See Phencyclidine
PDE III inhibitors, 263
Peak drug concentration, 65
Pediatric labeling, 90
Pediculosis, 532
Pedimycin. See Erythromycin
Peganone. See Ethotoin
Pellagra, 841
Pellet implants, 70–71
Pelvic inflammatory disease, 577

PEMA. *See* Phenylethylmalonamide
Pemoline, 383
Pen Tsao, 4
Pen-Vee. *See* Penicillin G
Penbutolol, 138
Penems, 566–567
Penetrex. *See* Enoxacin
Penicillamine
  in rheumatoid arthritis, 499
  vitamins and, 845
Penicillic acid, 562
Penicillin-binding proteins, 555–556
Penicillin G
  absorption of, 559
  clinical uses of, 559, 560
  half-life of, 40
  in rheumatic fever, 561
  streptomycin and, 571
Penicillins, 555–563
  adverse reactions of, 561–563
  antibacterial spectrum of, 557
  anticoagulants and, 318
  β-lactamase inhibitors and, 556–557
  cerebrospinal fluid and, 31
  chemistry of, 555, 556, 557
  clinical uses of, 559–561
  diuretic resistance and, 220
  immunotoxicity and, 77
  mechanism of action of, 555–557, 558
  pharmacokinetics of, 557–559
  placental barrier and, 32
  preparations of, 563
  proximal tubule and, 214
Penicillium griseofulvin, 650
Penicillium notatum, 555
Penicilloic acid, 555, 556
Penicilloyl derivatives, 562
Penicilloyl-polylysine, 562
Pentaerythritol tetranitrate, 267, 271
Pentam. *See* Pentamidine
Pentamidine, 621
  in AIDS-related disease, 615
  in *Pneumocystis carinii* pneumonia, 614
Pentanols, 457
Pentasa. *See* 5-Aminosalicylate
Pentazocine, 447–448
  as analgesic, 434
  smoking and, 42
Penthrane. *See* Methoxyflurane
Pentid. *See* Penicillin G
Pentobarbital
  abuse of, 465
  in monooxygenase enzyme induction, 42
Pentolinium, 174
Pentopril, 192, 193–194
Pentostam. *See* Sodium stibogluconate
Pentostatin, 685
Penthothal. *See* Thiopental
Pentritol. *See* Erythrityl tetranitrate
Pentylenetetrazol, 330, 381
Pepcid. *See* Famotidine
Pepstatin, 191
Peptic ulcer disease, 156, 831–835
  bethanechol and, 148
  glucocorticoids and, 738
Peptides, 332–333
  as biological response modifiers, 712
  ganglionic action potential and, 171
  opioid, 332, 438–439
Peptidyldipeptide hydrolase, 189–190, 191–194
Peptidyldipeptide hydrolase inhibitors, 192
Pepto-Bismol. *See* Bismuth subsalicylate
Percutaneous absorption, 69

Pergolide, 429
Pergonal. *See* Human menopausal gonadotropin
Peridex. *See* Chlorhexidine
Peridontium, 847, 848
Perilacunar bone, 790
Peripheral nervous system, 75, 101
  neurotransmission in, 104
  vitamin toxicity and, 843
Peripheral vascular resistance
  catecholamines and, 120–121, 122
  dopamine and, 124
  hypertension and, 229, 230
  labetalol and, 142
  quinidine and, 286
  sympathetic nerves in, 104
  vasodilators and, 231
Peripheral vascular system
  β-blockers and, 272
  calcium channel blockers and, 251
  disease of, 134
Peristalsis, 823–4
Peritrate. *See* Erythrityl tetranitrate
Peritubular fluid, 502
Periwinkle, 693
Permapen. *See* Penicillin G
Permax. *See* Pergolide
Permeability, inflammation and, 525
Permethrin, 532
Permitil. *See* Fluphenazine
Pernicious anemia, 842
Peroxynitrate
  in inflammation, 479
  reperfusion injury and, 507
Perphenazine, 388, 430
Persantine. *See* Dipyridamole
Personality disorder, 459–460
Pesticides, 81–82
Petit mal epilepsy, 414
Petroleum distillates, 80
Pfizerpen. *See* Penicillin G
pH
  antiseptics and disinfectants and, 658
  detergents and, 661
  in drug absorption and distribution, 19–21, 25
  gastric, 832
  salicylates and, 435
  urinary drug elimination and, 48
Phagocytosis, 502–503
Pharmacogenetics, 42–43
Pharmacognosy, 4
Pharmacokinetics, 55–64, 293
  basic concepts of, 55–57
  in cancer chemotherapy, 669–670
  of cephalosporins, 564–565
  chronic administration in, 58–60
  disease states and, 61–62
  ethical concerns in, 95
  multicompartment models in, 60
  oral or first-order absorption in, 57–58
  physiological determinants in, 60–61
Pharmacology
  clinical investigation and, 89
  development of, 3–8
    cultural contributions in, 4–5
    experimental method in, 5–7
  ethics in, 93–97
    application of, 93–94
    research subjects and, 95
    science, industry, and conflicts of interest in, 95–97
    scientific misconduct and, 94–95
Pharmacy, origins of, 4

Phase-specific drugs, 709
Phasic pain, 431
Phemerol Chloride. *See* Benzethonium chloride
Phenacemide, 421
Phenacetin
  as analgesic, 436
  charcoal-broiled beef and, 40, 41
  microsomal enzyme activity and, 42
  smoking and, 42
Phencyclidine
  abuse of, 469–471
  in channel blockade, 180
Phenelzine, 406
  adrenergic transmission and, 114
  dosage and serum concentration of, 403
Phenethylamines, 468
Phenformin, 807–808, 844
Phenobarbital
  bile flow and, 51
  cholestyramine and, 204
  cyclophosphamide and, 676–677
  dosage of, 14, 377
  drug-metabolizing enzymes and, 41
  in epilepsy, 376, 417–418
  in febrile seizures, 423
  half-life of, 40
  in monooxygenase enzyme induction, 42
  in osteopenia, 794–795
  phenytoin and, 416
  properties of, 421, 422
  quantal dose-response curve and, 13
  in status epilepticus, 423
  therapeutic index for, 14
  valproic acid and, 419
  vitamin interactions with, 845
Phenol coefficient test, 658–659
Phenolic compounds, 851
Phenolphthalein
  in constipation, 828, 829
  vitamin interactions with, 844
Phenols
  in disinfection, 661–662
  microbial spectrum of, 658
  as muscle relaxant, 184
Phenothiazines, 388–392
  absorption, metabolism, and excretion of, 390
  adverse reactions of, 391–392
  in allergy, 820
  as antiemetic, 831
  autonomic nervous system and, 390
  cardiovascular system and, 390
  central nervous system and, 389–390
  clinical uses of, 390–391
  contraindications and cautions for, 158
  drug interactions of, 392
  endocrine effects of, 390
  eye and, 30
  guanethidine and, 242
  for lysergic acid diethylamide abuse, 469
  mechanism of action of, 388, 389
  metoclopramide and, 824
  peripheral effects of, 390
  platelet function and, 320
  preparations of, 392
  reserpine and, 243
  in tardive dyskinesia, 430
  tolerance to, 390
Phenoxybenzamine, 132, 136, 238
  absorption of, 133
  adverse reactions to, 133
  in benign prostatic obstruction, 134
  blocking activity of, 130, 131, 132

mechanism of action of, 132
as nonequilibrium-competitive antagonist, 17
pharmacological actions of, 132–133
in shock, 135
Phentermine hydrochloride, 383
Phentolamine, 136, 238
absorption, metabolism, and excretion of, 134
adrenergic transmission and, 114
adverse reactions to, 134
blocking activity of, 129, 130, 131
as equilibrium-competitive antagonist, 17
hemodynamic effects of, 134
as imidazoline derivative, 133
structure of, 132
Phentolamine hydrochloride, 134
Phentolamine mesylate, 134
Phenurone. *See* Phenacemide
Phenylbutazone
as analgesic, 433
anticoagulants and, 318
antiinflammatory properties of, 488–489
cholestyramine and, 204
enzyme activity and, 42
in gout, 508
half-life of, 40
hepatotoxicity of, 74
oral hypoglycemics and, 807
platelet function and, 320
sulfonamides and, 30
Phenylephrine, 126–127, 366
Phenylethanolamine *N*-methyltransferase
glucocorticoids and, 735
in norepinephrine synthesis, 109
2-Phenylethylamine, 332
Phenylethylmalonamide, 418
Phenylpiperidines, 438
anesthetic uses of, 360
metabolism and excretion of, 355
Phenylpropanolamine, 383
Phenytoin, 44, 294–296
amiodarone and, 306
anticoagulants and, 318
barbiturates and, 376
disopyramide and, 290
enterohepatic recirculation and, 51
in epilepsy, 414–416
ethanol and, 41, 452
lidocaine and, 294
mexiletine and, 297
in monooxygenase enzyme induction, 42
in neuromuscular blockade, 182
in osteopenia, 794–795
phenobarbital and, 418
properties of, 421, 422
in renal disease, 62
solubility of, 67, 68
in status epilepticus, 423
vitamins and, 845
withdrawal seizures and, 465
Pheochromocytoma, 134, 143
PhisoHex. *See* Hexachlorophene
Phlebitis
amphotericin B and, 649
cancer chemotherapy and, 668
cephalosporins and, 566
ethylene oxide and, 660
miconazole and, 653
Phlebotomus, 618
Phosgene, 74, 78
Phosopholipase A$_2$, 477
Phosphate binding agents, 795
Phosphates, 211, 212, 794

Phosphatidylcholine, 35
3′-Phosphoadenosine 5′-phosphosulfate, 38
Phosphodiesterase inhibitors, 263–264
Phosphoenolpyruvate-mediated phosphotransferase system, 850
Phospholine. *See* Echothiophate
Phospholipids, 21
Phosphonoformate trisodium, 614
Phosphorus, 787
Phosphoryl group, 79
Phosphorylation, 11
Photoaging, 528
Photochemotherapy, 528–529
Photodynamic therapy, 529
Photopheresis, extracorporeal, 528
Photosensitization
amiodarone and, 305
doxycycline and, 635
immunotoxicity and, 77
tetracyclines and, 577
tretinoin and, 528
Phthlylsulfathiazole, 545
Phylloquinone, 840
Physical dependence
in drug abuse, 459
on ethanol, 455
on opioids, 439–440, 462
on pentazocine, 448
on sedative-hypnotic and anxiolytic drugs, 464–465
Physicians' Desk Reference, 90
Physostigmine, 163
absorption of, 165
in anticholinergic poisoning, 158
central nervous system depression and, 379
cholinergic transmission and, 114
in chorea, 430
toxicity of, 167
uses of, 166
Phytonadione, 317
Picrotoxin, 330, 380
Pigmentation
clofazimine and, 596
phenothiazines and, 392
Pilocar. *See* Pilocarpine
Pilocarpine, 149
in angle-closure glaucoma, 167
prolonged delivery of, 71
Pilocarpus jaborandi, 149
Pindolol, 137, 138, 140–141, 301
Pinocytosis, 28
Pinworm, 640, 641
Piperacil. *See* Piperacillin
Piperacillin, 561
Piperazine, 640
in allergy, 820
in helminthic disease, 638
preparations and dosage of, 758
Piperazine phenothiazines, 388
Piperidine nitrogen, 446
Piperidine phenothiazines, 388
Piperidinopyrimidine derivatives, 234
Piperonyl butoxide, 81
Piperoxan, 131
Pirbuterol, 514
Pirenzepine, 834
as muscarinic antagonist, 151
in peptic ulcers, 156
Piroxicam, 437
as analgesic, 433
anticoagulants and, 318
as antiinflammatory, 490
in arthritis, 489
Pitocin. *See* Oxytocin

Pitressin. *See* Antidiuretic hormone
Pituitary
hormones of
anterior, 723–729
posterior, 729–730
metyrapone and, 743
steroid therapy and, 739–740
Pituitary adenoma, 725
Pituitary gonadotropin, 389
Placebo, 88
Placenta
amiodarone and, 306
drug metabolism and, 34, 35
lidocaine and, 293
propranolol and, 303
Placental barrier, 31–32
ethanol and, 452
lincosamides and, 581
macrolides and, 580
tetracyclines and, 576
Plague, 571
Plant-derived products
antineoplastic, 692–695
epipodophyllotoxins in, 694
taxanes in, 694–695
vinca alkaloids in, 693–694
xanthines in, 383
Plantago, 826
Plaque
supragingival, 847–853
Plaquenil. *See* Hydrochloroquine
Plasma
drugs and
concentration of, 65, 66
metabolism of, 36
lipid levels in
hypolipidemics and, 202–203
regulation of, 200–201, 202
Plasma calcium, 788
Plasma cholesterol, 203–206
Plasma kinins, 194–196
Plasma-Lyte, 221
Plasma membrane
calcium channel blockers and, 249
drug absorption and distribution in, 19–21
ethanol and, 453
Plasma protein
drug binding to, 29–30
phenytoin and, 415
Plasma renin, 231
Plasma testosterone, 761–762, 764
Plasma thromboplastin, 840
Plasma triglycerides, 206–208
Plasma urate, 501
Plasma water
glomerular capillary membranes and, 47
total volume of, 28
Plasmid, 541
Plasmin, 320
Plasminogen, 320
Plasminogen activator, 313, 320
Plasmodium falciparum, 545, 546, 627, 635–636
Plasmodium malariae, 627
Plasmodium ovale, 627, 635
Plasmodium vivax, 627–628, 635
Platelet-activating factor, 482
Platelet aggregation
aspirin and, 488
ibuprofen and, 492
penicillins and, 561
sulfinpyrazone and, 506
Platinol. *See* Cisplatin
Platinum, 76

Pleiotropic resistance, 666
Pleural effusion, 550
Plicamycin, 692, 794
Pneumococcal pneumonia, 559
Pneumoconiosis, 79
Pneumocystis carinii pneumonia
  in acquired immunodeficiency syndrome, 614
  cellular immunity defects and, 706
  pentamidine in, 621
  sulfonamides in, 545
  trimethoprim in, 549
Pneumonia
  ampicillin in, 560
  cancer chemotherapy and, 668–669
  penicillins in, 559
Pneumonitis
  amiodarone and, 305
  bleomycin and, 690
  cancer chemotherapy and, 668
  hypersensitivity, 76
  methotrexate and, 683
  nematodes and, 639
Podofilox. *See* Podophyllotoxin
Podophyllotoxin, 532, 694
Poisoning
  anticholinergic, 158
  belladonna alkaloid, 147–148
  muscarine, 149
  muscarinic blocking drugs in, 157
  symptoms of, 82
  treatment of, 77, 78
Polarity, lipid–water partition coefficient and, 19
Pollen, 79
Pollutants, 78
Polybrominated biphenyls
  as food contaminant, 79
  immunotoxicity and, 76
Polycarbophil, 825, 827
Polychlorinated biphenyls
  cytochrome P450 and, 41
  immunotoxicity and, 76
Polycillin. *See* Ampicillin
Polycystic ovarian disease, 728
Polyestradiol phosphate, 758
Polymer coating, 68
Polymox. *See* Amoxicillin
Polymyalgia rheumatica, 707
Polymyxin B
  in dermatological disorders, 531
  neomycin and, 571
Polymyxins, 182, 585–586
Polysal, 221
Polythiazide, 224
Polyunsaturated fatty acids, 201
Pondimin. *See* Fenfluramine
Ponstel. *See* Mefenamic acid
Pontocaine. *See* Tetracaine
Pork tapeworm, 639
Porphyria
  chloroquine in, 530
  griseofulvin in, 650
Porphyrins, 529
Positive inotropic agents, 257–263
Postencephalitic parkinsonism, 425
Posterior pituitary hormones, 729–730
  antidiuretic hormone in, 729
  oxytocin in, 729–730
Postganglionic neuron, 101
  chromaffin cells and, 106
  preganglionic neuron ratio to, 103
Postjunctional blocking of autonomic ganglia, 173

Postmarketing studies, 89
Postpubertal hypogonadism, 767
Postrepolarization refractoriness, 285
Postsynaptic α-receptors, 131
Postsynaptic ganglionic cell muscarinic receptor, 170
Postsynaptic potential, 169–171, 327
Postural hypotension
  phenoxybenzamine and, 132
  phentolamine and tolazoline and, 134
"Pot," 472
Pot-curare, 181
Potassium, 211, 212
  adrenomimetic drugs and, 124
  amiodarone and, 305
  cardiac transmembrane potential and, 275–276
  in coronary autoregulation, 265
  in food, 217–218
  glucocorticoids and, 739
  in nephrotic syndrome, 220
  quinidine and, 285–286
  regulation of, 216–218
  sodium exchange and, 215–216
  urine secretion of, 215
Potassium chloride, 218
  in cardiac glycoside toxicity, 262
  preparations of, 217
  vitamins and, 844
Potassium iodide, 531, 655, 784
Potassium perchlorate, 783–784
Potassium sodium bicarbonate–tartaric acid, 827
Potassium sodium tartrate, 827
Potassium-sparing diuretics, 224–226, 231
Potency, 15–16
Potential, transmembrane, 275–276
Povidone-iodine, 659
Powder inhaler, 69, 70
PPL. *See* Penicilloyl-polylysine
Pralidoxime, 77, 163, 168
Pramoxine, 533
Prazepam, 373
Praziquantel, 638, 643–644
Prazosin, 238
  absorption, metabolism, and excretion of, 135
  α-blocking activity of, 131
  in cardiac disease, 62
  clinical uses of, 136
  in myocardial insufficiency, 264
  preparations and dosage of, 136
  structure of, 132
Prebrushing oral rinse, 853
Predifferentiation phase of gestation, 77
Prednisolone
  in asthma, 518
  in organ transplantation, 706
  in rheumatoid arthritis, 497
  structure-activity relationships of, 736
  volume of distribution of, 28
Prednisone
  in asthma, 518, 519
  in cancer treatment, 696
  in gout, 503
  in Hodgkin's disease, 666
  in organ transplantation, 706
  in rheumatoid arthritis, 497
  structure-activity relationships of, 736
  transcortin and, 733
Preganglionic neuron, 101, 103
Pregnancy
  anticonvulsant drugs and, 423

benzodiazepines and, 372
catecholamines and, 123
clinical drug trials and, 90
contraceptive methods and, 752
doxycycline and, 635
drug metabolism and, 45
edema of, 220
isotretinoin and, 527
lidocaine and, 293
mebendazole and, 643
metronidazole and, 619
metyrapone and, 744
ribavirin and, 603
sulfonamides and, 548
tetracyclines and, 576, 577
valproic acid and, 419
vidarabine and, 602
Pregnane nucleus, 748
Pregnenolone, 732, 747, 763
Preimplantation phase of gestation, 77
Prejunctional receptors, 114
Premarin, 753
Premature atrial contractions, 288
Premature labor, 516
Premature ventricular complex, 282
  β-adrenoceptor blocking agents in, 301
  propafenone in, 300
  tocainide in, 296
Premenstrual period, 220
Preoptic recess, 336
Preproinsulin, 798
Preproparathyroid hormone, 789
Preprorenin, 187
Prepubertal hypogonadism, 766–767
Presynaptic receptors, 113–114, 131
Presynaptical blocking of autonomic ganglia, 173
Priapism, 408
Prilocaine hydrochloride, 368
Prilosec. *See* Omeprazol
Primaquine
  in malaria, 631
  in *Pneumocystis carinii* pneumonia, 614
Primaxin. *See* Imipenem
Primidone, 418–419
  anticoagulants and, 318
  properties of, 421, 422
  valproic acid and, 419
  vitamins and, 845
Prinivil. *See* Lisinopril
Prinzmetal's angina, 268
  calcium channel blockers in, 252
  verapamil in, 308
Priscoline. *See* Tolazoline
Proarrhythmia, 311
Probenecid
  acyclovir and, 604
  allopurinol and, 508
  cephlosporins and, 565
  diuretics and, 220
  in gout, 505
  methotrexate and, 683
  oral hypoglycemics and, 807
  penicillins and, 559
  vitamins and, 845
Probucol, 203, 206
Procainamide, 287–289
  absorption of, 62
  bethanechol and, 148
  in cardiac arrhythmias, 262, 365
  cardiovascular system and, 363
  electrophysiological actions of, 285
  half-life of, 70

in neuromuscular blockade, 182
propafenone and, 300
Procaine
    allergy to, 366
    metabolism and, 364
    procainamide and, 287
    renal disease and, 62
Procaine hydrochloride, 367
Procaine penicillin
    in gonococcal infection, 560
    hypersensitivity to, 562
Procan-SR, 288, 289
Procarbazine
    antineoplastic properties of, 699–700
    drug interactions with, 670
    in Hodgkin's disease, 666
    neurotoxicity of, 669
Procardia. See Nifedipine
Prochlorperazine, 388, 831
Proconvertin. See Factor VII
Prodrugs, 33
    as delivery system, 71–72
    gastrointestinal absorption and, 558
Progestasert, 71
Progesterone
    buccal, 68
    drug metabolism and, 45
    luteinizing hormone and, 726
    prolonged release of, 71
    structure of, 763
    transcortin and, 733
Progestins, 747–759
    adverse reactions of, 755–757
    in cancer treatment, 696, 754–755
    cardiovascular effects of, 750–751
    contraindications for, 757–758
    in dysfunctional uterine bleeding, 755
    in dysmenorrhea, 755
    in endometriosis, 755
    in growth and development, 750
    in infertility, 754
    interactions of
        adenohypophyseal-gonadal, 749
        drug, 758
    lactation and, 755
    mechanism of action of, 751
    menopause and, 753
    menstrual cycle and, 750
    metabolism and excretion of, 747–748
    nonsteroidal, 748
    oral contraception and, 751–753
    ovarian steroidogenesis and, 749–750
    ovulation and, 754
    preparations and dosages of, 758
    psychological disturbances and, 753–754
    in replacement therapy, 754
    structure and biosynthesis of, 747
    synthetic, 748
Proglottids of tapeworm, 637
Prohormone, 791
Proinsulin, 798
Prokine. See Sargramostim
Prolactin, 725
    calcitonin and, 790
    thyrotropin releasing hormone and, 727
Prolactin release inhibiting hormone, 389
Proleukin. See Aldesleukin
Proloid. See Thyroglobulin
Prolonged-release medication, 70–72
    oral, 70
    parenteral, 70–71
    prodrugs in, 71–72
Proloprim. See Trimethoprim

Prolylendopeptidase, 189
Promazine, 45
Promethazine
    in allergy, 820
    as antiemetic, 831
    anxiolytic properties of, 374
    in motion sickness, 818
    sedative properties of, 819
Prontosil, 545
Propafenone, 299–300, 318
Propanediol carbamates, 377
Propantheline
    antimuscarinic activity of, 151
    in irritable bowel syndrome, 157
    nicotinic receptors and, 155
    structure of, 153
Prophylaxis
    antimicrobial, 543
    cephlosporin, 565
    malaria, 634
    penicillin, 561
    trimethoprim, 549
Propionyl-cholinesterase, 161
Propofol
    as anesthetic, 359, 360
    metabolism and excretion of, 355
Proportionality term, 55
Propoxyphene
    anticoagulants and, 318
    renal disease and, 62
    smoking and, 42
    preparations and dosage of, 434
Propranolol, 139, 300–303
    absorption, metabolism, and excretion of,
        272–273
    adrenergic transmission and, 114
    in angina, 267, 271
    in anxiety, 374
    blockade by, 129, 130, 136–137
    calcium channel blockers and, 252, 273
    diazoxide and, 235
    history of, 239
    hydralazine with, 233
    in hyperthyroidism, 785
    mechanism of action of, 138, 239
    metoprolol versus, 130, 140
    oral hypoglycemics and, 807
    pharmacological action of, 272
    preparations and dosage of, 138, 142
    renal disease and, 62
    renin release and, 191
    structure of, 137
    with vasodilators, 231
    volume of distribution of, 28
Propylene glycol, 457
    diazepam and, 357
    etomidate and, 359
Propylthiouracil, 782–784
Prorenin, 187
Proscar. See Finasteride
Prostacyclin, 313
Prostaglandin I₂, 481
Prostaglandin synthase, 477
Prostaglandins
    asthma and, 479–480
    biosynthesis of, 477
    bone metabolism and, 481–482
    in coronary autoregulation, 265
    in gastrointestinal disorders, 834
    kidney and, 481
    kinins and, 196
    nonsteroidal antiinflammatory drugs and,
        486, 487

in platelet function, 320
    reproductive system and, 480
    vascular system and, 481
Prostaphlin. See Oxacillin
Prostatic cancer
    aminoglutethimide in, 744
    buserelin and leuprolide in, 697
    estramustine in, 697
    estrogens and progestins in, 755
    flutamide in, 697
Prostatic hypertrophy, 158
Prostatic obstruction, benign, 134–135
Prostatitis, 549
Prosthetic heart valve, 318
Prostigmin. See Neostigmine
Protamine, 77
Protamine zinc insulin, 802, 805
Protective index, 14
Protein, 211, 212
    in active transport, 22, 23
    aminoglycosides and, 569
    androgens and anabolic steroids and, 769
    catabolism of, 804
    chloramphenicol and, 577
    ethanol and, 453
    glucocorticoids and, 733–734
    glycopeptides and, 584
    levodopa and, 428
    lincosamides and, 581
    metabolism of, 801
    in plasma membrane, 21
    tetracyclines and, 575
Protein binding
    of antimicrobial agents, 539–540
    of barbiturates, 375–376
    of calcium channel blockers, 253
    of cephlosporins, 564
    of class IB antiarrhythmic drugs, 293
    of class IC antiarrhythmic drugs, 298
    of class III antiarrhythmic drugs, 304
    drug-hormone interaction and, 720–721
    of penicillins, 555–556
    of quinidine, 286
    of sulfonamides, 548
    of tricyclic antidepressants, 403
    uric acid and, 501–502
Protein C, 313
Protein kinase, 117–118
Proteinuria, 495
Proteoglycans, 313
Proteolysis, 777
Proteus infection
    ampicillin in, 560, 561
    cephalosporins in, 564
    penicillins in, 557
    trimethoprim in, 548
Prothrombin, vitamin K and, 840
Protirelin, 727
Protopam chloride. See Pralidoxime
Protoporphyria, erythropoietic, 528
Protostat. See Metronidazole
Protozoal infection, 617–618
Protriptyline
    chemical structure of, 398
    dosage and serum concentration of, 403
Protropin. See Somatrem
Proventil. See Albuterol
Provera. See Medroxyprogesterone acetate
Proxacol. See Hydrogen peroxide
Proximal tubule, 213
    active transport systems of, 49
    drug excretion and, 34
    reabsorption and, 49–50

Proximal tubule (*cont.*)
    secretion and, 48–49
    urate and, 502
Prozac. *See* Fluoxetine
Pseudocholinesterase, 161
    distribution of, 162
    local anesthetics and, 364
Pseudohypoparathyroidism, 793
Pseudomembranous colitis, 581–582
Pseudomonas aeruginosa infection
    aminoglycosides in, 571
    ampicillin in, 561
    antiseptic resistance and, 658
    mafenide acetate in, 546
    monobactams in, 567
    nalidixic acid in, 551–552
    penicillins in, 557
    polymyxins in, 583, 585
    trisulfapyrimidine in, 546
Pseudorheumatism, 739
Psoralen, 528–529
Psoriasis
    coal tar in, 529
    etretinate in, 527
    methotrexate in, 532–533, 683
    PUVA therapy in, 528
Psychedelics, 468
Psychoactive drugs, 180
Psychological dependence
    in amphetamine abuse, 467
    in drug abuse, 459
Psychomotor stimulants, 381–383
Psychosis
    in amphetamine abuse, 466–467
    biochemical bases of, 387
    glucocorticoids and, 739
    Korsakoff's, 455
    levodopa and, 427
    in phencyclidine abuse, 470
Psyllium, 204
Psyllium seed derivatives, 825, 826, 827
Pulmonary disorders. *See* Lung disease
Pulmonary embolism, 319
Pump, in prolonged-release medication, 71
Pupil
    acetylcholine and, 147
    autonomic nervous system and, 105
    epinephrine and, 123
Pure Food and Drug Act, 85–86, 87
Purine analogues, 683–685
    cladribine as, 685
    fludarabine as, 685
    mercaptopurine as, 684–685
    pentostatin as, 685
    thioguanine as, 683–684
Purines, 501
Purinethol. *See* Mercaptopurine
"Purple hearts," 464
Putamen, 389
PUVA therapy, 528–529
Pyopen. *See* Carbenicillin
Pyrantel pamoate, 638, 641–642
Pyrazinamide, 587–588, 593
Pyrazole derivatives, 817
Pyrazolone, 433
Pyrethrins
    for scabies and lice, 532
    toxicity of, 81
Pyridostigmine, 163
    absorption of, 165
    in myasthenia gravis, 167
    uses of, 166

Pyridoxine, 840
    deficiency of, 842
    in drug interactions, 845
    isoniazid and, 589
    levodopa and, 428
    toxicity of, 843
Pyrilamine, 818, 819
Pyrimethamine, 632–633, 635
Pyrimidine analogues, 685–687
    cytarabine as, 685–686
    fluorouracil as, 686–687
    ftorafur and floxuridine as, 687
Pyrogallol, 114

Qinghaosu. *See* Artemisinin
Quantal dose-response curve, 13–14
Quaternary amines
    absorption of, 165
    uses of, 155
Quaternary ammonium compounds, 163, 165
Quelicin. *See* Succinylcholine
Questran. *See* Cholestyramine resin
Quinacrine
    as antiprotozoal, 624
    in dermatological disorders, 530
    in malaria, 633–634
Quinapril, 192, 193
Quinazoline derivatives, 131, 135–136
Quinazolines, 136, 238
Quinestrol, 758
Quinethazone, 223, 224
Quinidine, 284–287
    absorption of, 62
    amiodarone and, 306
    anticoagulants and, 318
    barbiturates and, 376
    bethanechol and, 148
    propafenone and, 300
    in rhythm disorders, 262
Quinine
    anticoagulants and, 318
    in malaria, 633
    neurotoxicity of, 75
Quinolones, 550–552, 589
Quinopril, 193–194

Radiation
    drug metabolism and, 44
    histamine release and, 814
    toxicity of, 668
Radical cure, term, 628
Radioiodine, 784–785
Ramipril, 192, 193–194
Ramycin. *See* Doxycycline
Randomization in human drug testing, 88, 89
Ranitidine, 833–834
    as histamine blocker, 821
    lidocaine and, 294
    structure of, 834
Rapid cycling, 411
Rapid eye movement sleep, 371–372
Rash
    allopurinol and, 507
    L-asparaginase and, 696
    labetalol and, 143
    lincosamide and, 581
    penicillins and, 562
    phenobarbital in, 418
    quinolones and, 552
    trimethoprim-sulfamethoxazole and, 549
    vancomycin and, 585
Rat-bite fever, 561

Rau-Sed. *See* Reserpine
Raudixin. *See* *Rauwolfia* extracts
Rauwolfia extracts, 242
Raynaud's disease, 252
Reabsorption, active tubular, 49–50
Reactive intermediates, 45
Reaginic allergy, 76
Reaginic antibody, 812
Rebound hypertension, 247
Rebreathing apparatus, 343
Receptor-binding techniques, 333
Receptors
    acetylcholine and, 170
    alkylation of, 132
    alpha, 130–131
    in autonomic ganglion, 169
    beta, 130
    biological response and, 9–11
    calcium, 250–251
    cholinergic
        postganglionic neurons and, 169
        symptoms of poisoning and, 82
    defined, 9, 129
    dose-response relationship and, 12–16
    drug binding and, 11–12, 16
    in elderly, 40
    muscarinic, 145
    nicotinic, 145
    opioid, 439
    presynaptic, 113–114, 131
    second messengers and, 117–118, 119
    in skeletal muscle, 169
Recombinant DNA-derived human insulin, 797, 805
Recombinant erythropoietin, 611, 768
Recombinant human growth hormone, 768
Recombinant human tissue-type plasminogen activator, 322
Recombinant single chain urokinase-type plasminogen activator, 323
Rectum
    drug absorption in, 25
    drug administration and, 68
"Red devils," 464
Red man syndrome, 585
5α-Reductase inhibitors, 772, 773
Reductive reactions in drug metabolism, 36
"Reefer," 472
Reentry in arrhythmia, 281, 282
Reentry ventricular complex, 282
Reflex-mediated tachycardia
    phenothiazines and, 390
    phenoxybenzamine and, 133
Reflux esophagitis, 158
Regional block anesthesia, 364–365
Regitine. *See* Phentolamine
Regitine test, 134
Reglan. *See* Metoclopramide
Rela. *See* Carisoprodol
Relafen, 493–494
Relapse
    in gold therapy, 495
    in opioid abuse, 462
Relefact TRH. *See* Thyrotropin releasing hormone
Religion, in pharmacology history, 5
REM sleep. *See* Rapid eye movement sleep
Renal cell carcinoma
    aldesleukin in, 703
    clinical drug testing for, 89
    human recombinant interleukin-2 in, 713
    kinins in, 696

Renal clearance, 212
Renal disease. *See* Kidney, disease of
Renal failure
    diquat poisoning and, 82
    diuretics in, 220
    mitomycin and, 691
Renese. *See* Polythiazide
Renin, 187–190
    adrenoceptors and, 113
    angiotensinogen and, 189
    β-blockers and, 139
    chemistry of, 187
    converting enzyme and, 189–190
    hypertension and, 231
    inhibitors of, 191
    in myocardial insufficiency, 257
    release of, 188–189
    vasodilators and, 231
Renin-angiotensin system, 191–194
Reperfusion injury, 507
Replacement therapy
    adrenocortical hormone, 740
    estrogen and progestin, 754
rEPO. *See* Recombinant erythropoietin
Reproductive system
    chemotherapeutic toxicity and, 669
    eicosanoids and, 480
    estrogens and progestins and, 750
    prolactin and, 725
    toxicity and, 76–77
Research
    conflict of interest in, 95–97
    ethics in, 95
Reserpine, 130, 242–244
    adrenergic transmission and, 114
    chemical structure of, 241
    in chorea, 430
    diarrhea and, 825
    indirectly acting adrenomimetic drugs and, 117
    in parkinsonism, 426
Resistance
    to aminoglycoside-aminocyclitol antibiotics, 569–570
    to anthracyclines, 688
    to antimicrobial agents, 540
    to antiseptics and disinfectants, 658
    to azidothymidine, 610
    to cancer chemotherapy, 665–666
    to chloroquine, 634–636
    to dactinomycin, 691
    to dideoxyinosine, 612
    to fluorouracil, 686
    to mercaptopurine, 684
    to methotrexate, 682
    to paclitaxel, 695
    to sulfonamides, 545
    to tetracyclines, 577
    in tuberculosis, 587
    to vinca alkaloids, 693
Respiratory acidosis, 435
Respiratory disorders
    immunologically mediated, 76
    insecticides and, 82
Respiratory distress syndrome, 82
Respiratory syncytial virus, 603
Respiratory system
    anticholinesterase agents and, 165
    buprenorphine and, 448
    central nervous system stimulants and, 385
    histamine and, 816
    morphine and, 440

muscarinic blocking drugs and, 153
    nicotine and, 172–173
    pentazocine and, 447
    salicylates and, 432–434
Response
    defined, 9
    drug receptors and, 9–11
    magnitude of, 12
    second messengers in, 117–118, 119
Resting potential, transmembrane, 276
Restoril. *See* Temazepam
Retet. *See* Tetracyclines
Reticuloendothelial system, 495
11-*cis*-Retinal, 839
Retinoids, 526–528
    β-carotene in, 528
    etretinate in, 527–528
    isotretinoin in, 527
    tretinoin in, 528
Retinol, 839
Retinopathy
    antimalarial drugs and, 530
    chloroquine in, 498
Retrovir. *See* Azidothymidine
Reversible-competitive bond, 17, 129
Reversible inhibitors, 166
Rheumatic fever, 560–561
Rheumatoid arthritis, 485–486, 487
    autoimmunity in, 705
    azathioprine in, 710
    chloroquine in, 630
    corticosteroids and, 739
    glucocorticoid therapy in, 738, 740
    gold preparations in, 494–495, 496
    methotrexate in, 498–499, 683
    new approaches to, 499–500
    penicillamine in, 499
Rheumatrex. *See* Methotrexate
rHGH. *See* Recombinant human growth hormone
Rhinitis, allergic, 818
Rhodesian sleeping sickness, 618
Rhodopsin, 839
Ribavirin, 602–603
Riboflavin, 840
    deficiency of, 841
    in drug interactions, 845
Ribonucleotide reductase, 698
Ricinoleic acid, 829
Rickets, 794, 842
Rickettsia infection
    chloramphenicol in, 578
    tetracyclines in, 575, 577
Ridaura. *See* Auranofin
Rifadin. *See* Rifampin
Rifamate, 590
Rifampin
    anticoagulants and, 318
    disopyramide and, 290
    in leprosy, 596
    mexiletine and, 297
    in tuberculosis, 587–590
Right to know, in clinical testing of drugs, 87–88
Rigidity
    in parkinsonism, 425
    phenothiazines and, 391
Rimactane. *See* Rifampin
Rimantadine, 601
Rinsing agents, antimicrobial, 847–853
Ritalin. *See* Methylphenidate
Robaxin. *See* Methocarbamol

Robimycin. *See* Erythromycin
Robitet. *See* Tetracyclines
Rocaltrol. *See* Calcitriol
Rocephin. *See* Ceftriaxone
Rochelle salt. *See* Potassium sodium tartrate
Rodenticides, 81, 82
Roferon-A. *See* Interferons
Rogaine. *See* Minoxidil
Rondomycin. *See* Methacycline
Rostellum of tapeworm, 637
Rotohaler, 516–517
Rowasa. *See* 5-Aminosalicylate
rscu-PA. *See* Recombinant single chain urokinase-type plasminogen activator
rt-PA. *See* Recombinant human tissue-type plasminogen activator
Rubbing alcohol. *See* Isopropanol
Rubor, in inflammation, 478
Rufen. *See* Ibuprofen
"Rush," 461
Rythmol. *See* Propafenone

S-P-T. *See* Thyroid, USP
S-phase, 663
Sabril. *See* Vigabatrin
Saint Vitus' dance, 430
Salbutamol. *See* Albuterol
Salicylates, 432–436
    absorption, metabolism, and excretion of, 434, 435, 487–488
    adverse reactions to, 435, 488
    antiinflammatory properties of, 487–488, 489
    in arthritis, 489
    central nervous system and, 432–434
    chemistry of, 432
    clinical uses of, 434–435, 488
    contraindications with, 435–436
    ethanol and, 456
    intoxication of, 435
    mechanism of action of, 432
    methotrexate and, 683
    nizatidine and, 834
    oral hypoglycemics and, 807
    thyroid-binding globulin and, 781
    thyroxine and, 721
    uricosuric agents and, 506
    vitamins and, 845
Salicylazosulfapyridine, 844
Salicylic acid, 432, 434, 533
Salicylism, 434
Salicyluric acid, 39
Saline laxatives, 826–829
Saliva, 849
    autonomic nervous system and, 106
    clozapine and, 395
    in drug excretion, 52
    phenothiazines and, 390
Salmeterol, 517
Salmonella infection
    ampicillin in, 560
    chloramphenicol in, 578
    food contamination and, 79
    trimethoprim in, 549
Salsalate
    as analgesic, 433, 434
    as antiinflammatory, 488
Saluron. *See* Hydroflumethiazide
Sandfly, 618
Sandimmune. *See* Cyclosporine
Sandoglobulin. *See* Immune globulin

Sandolase. *See* Saruplase
Sandostatin. *See* Octreotide
Sanguinarine, 851, 852
Sanitizers, 657
Saralasin acetate, 194
Sarcoma, Kaposi's, 614–615
Sarenin. *See* Saralasin acetate
Sargramostim, 703
Sarin, 168
Saruplase, 322–323
Scabies, 532
Scalp infection, 531
Schedule I substances, 460
Schedule II substances, 460
Schedule III substances, 460–461
Schedule IV substances, 461
Schedule V substances, 461
Schistosomiasis, 43, 643–644
Schizont, mosquito, 628
Schizontocidal, term, 628
Schizophrenia
    biochemistry of, 387
    haloperidol in, 393
    levodopa and, 427
Scientific error, 94
Scientific misconduct, 94–95
Scolex of tapeworm, 637
Scopolamine, 830
    absorption, metabolism, and excretion of,
        155
    central nervous system and, 154
    in motion sickness, 157
    as muscarinic blocking drug, 151
    in ophthalmology, 156
    prolonged-release of, 71
scu-PA. *See* Single-chain urokinase-type
    plasminogen activator
Scurvy, 842
Second gas effect of general anesthesia, 343
Second messengers
    adrenomimetic drugs and, 117–118, 119
    lithium carbonate and, 409, 410
    receptors and, 10
Secretagogues, 790
Secretin, 799
Secretion
    endocrine, 720
    renal, 48–49
Sectral. *See* Acebutolol
Sedation
    benzodiazepines in, 372
    morphine in, 440
    phenobarbital in, 418
    trazodone in, 407–408
    tricyclic antidepressants in, 401
Sedative-hypnotic drugs, 369–377
    abuse of, 464–465
    antihistamines in, 374
    antipsychotics and antidepressants in, 374–
        375
    azapirones in, 373–374
    barbiturates in, 375–377
    benzodiazepines in, 369–373
    β-adrenoceptor blocking agents in, 374
    chloral hydrate in, 377
    nonprescription, 377
    propanediol carbamates in, 377
Seffin. *See* Cephalothin
Seidlitz powder, 827
Seizure
    barbiturates in, 376
    benzodiazepines in, 372

bupropion and, 408
chlorpromazine and, 389
in epilepsy, 413–414
febrile, 423
in hypnotics and antianxiety withdrawal,
    465
lidocaine and, 293
loxapine and, 394
in pregnancy, 423
tricyclic antidepressants and, 401, 402
Seldane. *See* Terfenadine
Selective serotonin reuptake inhibitors, 403,
    404–405
Selegiline, 429
Selenium sulfide, 531
Semilente Insulin. *See* Insulin zinc
Semustine, 678–679
Senna, 828
Septra. *See* Trimethoprim-sulfamethoxazole
Sequential blockade, term, 632
Serax. *See* Oxazepam
Serentil. *See* Mesoridazine
Seromycin. *See* Cycloserine
Serophene. *See* Clomiphene
Serotonin, 328–330
    blood-brain barrier and, 336
    calcitonin and, 790
    ganglionic blockade and, 172
    in inflammation, 479
    phenoxybenzamine and, 132
    phentolamine and, 133
    reserpine and, 243
Serotonin receptor agonists
    selective serotonin reuptake inhibitors and,
        404–405
    tricyclic antidepressants and, 399–400
Serpasil. *See* Reserpine
Sertoli cells, 762
Sertoli-Sertoli junction, 32
Sertraline, 403, 404, 405
Serum albumin, 39
Serum cholinesterase, 161
Serum concentration, 65, 66
    of class IA antiarrhythmic drugs, 286
    of class IB antiarrhythmic drugs, 293
    of class IC antiarrhythmic drugs, 298
    of class III antiarrhythmic drugs, 304
    of lipids, 756–757
    of theophylline, 71
Sevoflurane, 340, 349
Sex hormone-binding globulin, 751, 762
Sexual dysfunction, 453
Shampoo, 529
SHBG. *See* Sex hormone-binding globulin
Sheep liver fluke, 644
Shigellosis, 546
Shock
    adrenocortical hormones in, 741
    α-receptor blocking agents in, 135
    cardiogenic
        disopyramide and, 290
        flecainide and, 299
        mexiletine and, 297
        moricizine and, 291
        propafenone and, 300
    dobutamine in, 127
    dopamine in, 125
Short stature, 768
Shunt infection, 585
Sick sinus syndrome
    amiodarone and, 306
    propafenone and, 300

Sideroblastic anemia, 846
SIF cells. *See* Small intensely fluorescent cells
Signal transduction, 117–118, 119
Silica, 74, 79
Silver nitrate, 660
Silver sulfadiazine, 546, 547
Sinemet, 428
Sinequan. *See* Doxepin
Single-blind technique, 88–89
Single-chain urokinase-type plasminogen
    activator, 320
Sinoatrial node
    amiodarone and, 305
    bretylium and, 303
    calcium channel blockers and, 252
    disopyramide and, 289
    flecainide and, 297
    innervation of, 105
    lidocaine and, 292
    moricizine and, 291
    phenytoin and, 294
    propafenone and, 299
    propranolol and, 302
    quinidine and, 285
    sotalol and, 307
    transmembrane action potential of,
        278
    verapamil and, 308
Sinus infection
    ampicillin in, 560
    erythromycin in, 580
Sinus tachycardia
    β-adrenoceptor blocking agents in, 301
    clozapine and, 395
SK-Penicillin G. *See* Penicillin G
Skeletal muscle
    acetylcholine and, 147
    anticholinesterase agents and, 164, 165
    catecholamines and, 120
    receptors in, 10, 169
Skin
    anticholinesterase agents and, 165
    bleomycin and, 690
    blood perfusion rate in, 29
    cancer of, 529
    delivery rate limitations of, 69
    disorders of. *See* Dermatological disorders
    in drug absorption, 27
    in drug metabolism, 34, 35
    muscarinic blocking drugs and, 153
    phenothiazines and, 392
    retinoids and, 527
    structure of, 523, 524
    testing of, 562
Sleeping sickness, 618, 622
Slow channel blockers. *See* Calcium channel
    blockers
Slow excitatory postsynaptic potential, 169–
    171
Slow inward calcium current, 277
Slow-K, 217
"Smack," 461
Small-cell lung cancer, 676
Small intensely fluorescent cells, 169, 170,
    171
Small intestine
    benzodiazepines and, 370
    drug absorption and, 25
    mexiletine and, 297
Smoking
    drug metabolism and, 42
    ganglionic stimulation and, 171–172

oral contraceptives and, 756
placental barrier and, 32
stimulatory effects of, 172
Smooth muscle
  adrenoceptors and, 113
  adrenomimetic drugs and, 122–123
  amiodarone and, 305
  cholinesterase inhibitors and, 165, 167
  innervation of, 104, 106
  phenoxybenzamine and, 132
"Snow," 466
Sodium, 211, 212
  acetylcholine and, 9–10
  cardiac transmembrane potential and, 275
  choline and, 108
  conservation of, 215–216
  glucocorticoids and, 739
  lithium carbonate and, 409
  mexiletine and, 297
  moricizine and, 291
  phenytoin and, 414–415
  propafenone and, 299
  triggered activity and, 280
Sodium benzoate, 384
  in diazepam preparation, 357
  in mouth rinse, 852, 853
Sodium bicarbonate
  in antacids, 832, 833
  in methanol poisoning, 456
Sodium fluoride
  oral cavity and, 848
  in osteoporosis, 794
Sodium-hydrogen exchange, 215
Sodium iodide, 784, 785
Sodium lauryl sulfate mouth rinse, 852, 853
Sodium nitrate, 264
Sodium nitrite, 77, 82
Sodium nitroprusside, 235–236
  chemical structure of, 233
  in hypertension, 232
  in myocardial insufficiency, 264
Sodium phosphate, 827
Sodium phosphate-biphosphonate, 828
Sodium polystyrene sulfonate, 218
Sodium-potassium exchange, 215–216
Sodium pump, 257–263
Sodium salicylate
  as analgesic, 433, 434
  as antiinflammatory, 487, 488
  in arthritis, 489
  for pain, 434–435
Sodium stibogluconate, 624–625
Sodium sulfate, 827
Sodium thiosulfate, 77, 82
Sodium urate, 501
Solanaceae, 157, 158
Solatene. *See* β-carotene
Solubility in drug delivery, 67, 69
Solutions, oral administration of, 67
Solvents, 79–81
Soma. *See* Carisoprodol
Soman, 168
Somatic nervous system, 101, 102
Somatomedin, 736
Somatostatin, 333, 727, 808
  feedback control of, 778
  in glucagon and insulin release, 803
  histamine release and, 814
Somatostatin analogue, 698, 808
Somatostatin release inhibiting factor. *See*
  Somatostatin
Somatrem, 725

Somatotropin, 723–725
Somnos. *See* Chloral hydrate
Somophyllin. *See* Aminophylline
Sorbinil. *See* Aldose reductase inhibitors
Sorbitol
  in enema, 828
  metabolism of, 804
Sorbitrate. *See* Isosorbide
Sotalol, 138, 306–307
South American leishmaniasis, 618
Spasm
  coronary artery, 268
  infantile, 420
Special populations, in human drug testing,
  89–90
Species, drug metabolism and, 43, 44
Specific receptor theory, 362
Specificity, 18
Spectinomycin, 569, 570, 573
Spectrazole. *See* Econazole
Spectrobid. *See* Bacampicillin
"Speed," 466
Spermatogenesis
  gonadotropins in, 726
  mechlorethamine and, 675
  reproductive toxins and, 77
Spermicide, 661
SPF. *See* Sun protection factor
Sphincter
  adrenoceptors and, 113
  catecholamines and, 123
Spina bifida, 423
Spinal anesthesia, 365
Spinhaler. *See* Cromolyn sodium
Spironolactone, 224–225
  as androgen receptor antagonist, 772
  as antihypertensive, 231
  bile flow and, 51
  in nephrotic syndrome, 220
  in testosterone synthesis, 761
  volume of distribution of, 28
Spleen, adrenoceptors and, 113
Sporanox. *See* Itraconazole
Sporothrix schenckii, 647
Sporozoite, mosquito, 628
Sprue, celiac, 795
SRIF. *See* Somatostatin
SSRI. *See* Selective serotonin reuptake
  inhibitors
Stannous fluoride mouth rinse, 852, 853
Stanozolol, 769
Staphylococcal infection, 557
  bacitracin in, 583
  erythromycin in, 580
  glycopeptides in, 584
  lincosamides in, 581
  loracarbef in, 567
  penicillins in, 557, 559
  vancomycin and, 55
Stature, short, 768
Status asthmaticus, 509, 737
Status epilepticus
  anticonvulsant drugs in, 423–424
  diazepam in, 420
"Steam," 473
Stelazine. *See* Trifluoperazine
Sterilization, 657–662
  agents in
    alkylating, 660
    dehydrating, 659
    evaluation of, 658–659
    oxidizing, 659

permeability affecting, 661–662
sulfhydryl combining, 660–661
general principles of, 657–658
Steroid diabetes, 803–804
Steroid myopathy, 739
Steroid-sparing drugs, 520–521
Steroids, 731–745
  actions of, 733–734, 741–742
  in adrenocortical abnormalities, 742–745
  adverse effects of, 737–740
  anabolic, 761–773
    adverse reactions to, 769, 770
    antiandrogens and, 772–773
    anticoagulants and, 318
    athletes and, 769
    chemistry and biosynthesis of, 761–764,
      765
    clinical uses of, 766–769
    gonadotropin releasing hormone and
      analogues and, 771–772
    inhibitors of, 772
    male antifertility agents and, 771
    mechanism of action of, 764–766
    nomenclature of, 761, 762
    preparations and dosage of, 771
  anticoagulants and, 318
  antiinflammatory properties of, 495–497
  biosynthesis of, 731–733
  blood-testis barrier and, 32
  blood transport of, 733
  cardioactive, 255
  cardiovascular function and, 734
  in electrolyte and water metabolism, 734
  in endocrine disorders, 719
  endocrine system and, 735–736
  immune and defense mechanisms and,
    734–735
  metabolism of, 733
  nucleus of, 748, 761, 762
  ovarian, 749–750
  placental barrier and, 32
  preparations of, 736–737
  synthesis of, 762–764
  therapeutic uses of, 740–741
  vitamins and, 845
Stevens-Johnson syndrome
  pyrimethamine and, 633
  sulfonamides and, 546
Stimulants, 379–385
  analeptic, 380–381
  psychomotor, 381–383
  xanthines in, 383–385
Stomach, in drug absorption, 25
Stomatitis
  cancer chemotherapy and, 667
  doxorubicin and, 688
  penicillins and, 561
Stoxil. *See* Idoxuridine
Strabismus, 167
Stratum corneum, 69, 523
Streptococcal infection
  bacitracin in, 583
  chloramphenicol in, 578
  erythromycin in, 580
  glycopeptides in, 584
  humoral immunity deficiencies and, 706
  lincosamides in, 581
  macrolides in, 579
  penicillins in, 559–560
  tetracycline resistance and, 577
  trimethoprim in, 549
Streptokinase, 321–322

Streptomyces achromogenes, 679
Streptomyces avermitilis, 641
Streptomyces noursei, 649
Streptomyces orientalis, 584
Streptomyces tsukubaensis, 709
Streptomycin, 569–573
  placental barrier and, 32
  in tuberculosis, 590
  volume of distribution of, 28
Streptozocin, 75, 679–680
Stroke output, 120–121
Strongyloidiasis, 642
Strontium, 31
Structure-activity relationships
  of adrenocortical hormones, 736
  of adrenomimetic drugs, 117
  of agonists, 12
Strychnine
  central nervous system and, 380, 381
  glycine and, 330
  toxicity of, 81
Stuart factor, 840
Subarachnoid hemorrhage, 252
Subcutaneous administration, 27, 68–69
Sublingual absorption, 24
Sublingual tablets, 68
Substance P, 332
  gastrointestinal tract and, 106
  histamine release and, 814
  as neuromodulator, 104
Succinylcholine, 168, 180–181
Sucostrin Chloride. *See* Succinylcholine
Sucralfate
  in gastrointestinal disorders, 835
  in peptic ulcer, 156
Sufenta. *See* Sufentanil
Sufentanil, 360, 445
Suicide, 739
Sulbactam, 556–557
Sulfabenzamide, 546
Sulfacetamide, 545, 546, 547
Sulfadiazine, 546, 547, 635
Sulfadoxine, 546
Sulfamerazine, 547
Sulfamethazine, 547
Sulfamethoxazole, 318, 547
Sulfamylon cream. *See* Mafenide
Sulfanilamide, 546
Sulfapyridine, 836
Sulfasalazine, 836–837
  in inflammatory bowel disease, 835
  vitamins and, 844
Sulfate conjugates, 51
Sulfathiazole, 546
Sulfatrim. *See* Trimethoprim-
  sulfamethoxazole
Sulfhydryl combining agents, 660–661
Sulfhydryl groups
  as converting enzyme inhibitors, 192
  metals and, 79
  in nitrate tolerance, 270
Sulfinpyrazone
  anticoagulants and, 318
  as antiplatelet drug, 320
  in gout, 506
  vitamins and, 845
Sulfisoxazole, 546, 547
Sulfites, 77
Sulfobromophthalein, 39
Sulfonamides, 545–548
  immunotoxicity and, 77
  methotrexate and, 683
  oral hypoglycemics and, 807

  phenylbutazone and, 30
  pyrimethamine and, 632
Sulfones, 595
Sulfonylureas, 805–807
Sulfotransferases, 38
Sulfoxone sodium, 595
Sulfur acid, 79
Sulfur dioxide, 74, 79
Sulfur oxides, 79
Sulindac
  as analgesic, 433, 437
  anticoagulants and, 318
  antiinflammatory properties of, 491
  in arthritis, 489
  enterohepatic recirculation and, 51
Sulthiame, 421
Sumycin. *See* Tetracyclines
Sun protection factor, 534
Sunscreen, 533–534, 845
Superinfection
  antimicrobial agents and, 541
  cephalosporins and, 566
  tetracyclines and, 577
Superoxide
  bleomycin and, 689
  in inflammation, 479
  reperfusion injury and, 507
Suppository, 68
Suprafact. *See* Buserelin
Supragingival plaque, 847–853
  antimicrobial rinsing agents in, 850–853
  in gingivitis, 847–848
  oral cavity and, 848–849
Suprane. *See* Desflurane
Supraventricular arrhythmias
  amiodarone in, 304
  β-adrenoceptor blocking agents in, 301
  cardiac glycosides in, 261
  propranolol in, 303
Supraventricular tachyarrhythmias
  adenosine in, 310
  digitalis glycosides in, 309
  diltiazem in, 309
  verapamil in, 308
Suprax. *See* Cefixime
Suramin, 29, 621–622
Surgical scrub, 662
Surital. *See* Thiamylal
Surmontil. *See* Trimipramine
Susadrin. *See* Transmucosal nitroglycerin
Suspensions
  absorption of, 26
  oral administration of, 67
Sweating
  drug excretion and, 52
  ganglionic blockade and, 174
  phenothiazines and, 390
Sydenham's chorea, 430
Symmetrel. *See* Amantadine
Sympathetic block anesthesia, 365
Sympathetic effector cells, 115–116
Sympathetic ganglia, 147
Sympathetic nervous system
  angiotensins and, 191
  antihypertensives and, 236–238
  cardiac glycosides and, 261
  function of, 103
  myocardial insufficiency and, 255
  organ innervation and, 104–106
  preganglionic neurons of, 101–102
Sympathoadrenal system, 106
Sympathomimetic agents. *See* Adrenomimetic
  drugs

Syncope
  carotid sinus, 155–156
  quinidine and, 287
Syndrome
  Crigler-Najjar, 38
  Lambert-Eaton, 179
  Lennox-Gastaut
    felbamate in, 421
    nitrazepam in, 420
  Stevens-Johnson
    pyrimethamine and, 633
    sulfonamides and, 546
  Wolff-Parkinson-White
    quinidine in, 286
    verapamil and, 309
Synthetic opioids, 438
Synthetic reactions, in drug metabolism, 37–
  39
Synthroid. *See* Liothyronine
Syntocinon. *See* Oxytocin
Syphilis, 560

T_3. *See* Triiodothyronine
T_4. *See* Thyroxine
T cell
  antithymocyte globulin and, 711
  cyclophosphamide and, 710
  cyclosporine and, 707
t-PA. *See* Tissue-type plasminogen activator
Tablets, 67–68
  absorption of, 26
  buccal and sublingual, 68
  mean serum concentrations with, 69
Tachyarrhythmias
  atrial, 308
  supraventricular
    adenosine in, 310
    digitalis glycosides in, 309
    diltiazem in, 309
    verapamil in, 308
  ventricular
    amiodarone in, 304
    magnesium sulfate in, 310
Tachycardia
  atrial
    adenosine in, 310
    β-adrenoceptor blocking agents in, 301
    procainamide in, 288
  autonomic nervous system and, 104
  calcium channel blockers and, 252, 253
  norepinephrine and, 121
  phenothiazines and, 390
  phenoxybenzamine and, 133
  phentolamine and tolazoline and, 133, 134
  tricyclic antidepressants and, 401
  ventricular, 282
    β-adrenoceptor blocking agents in,
      301
    flecainide in, 298
    moricizine in, 291
    procainamide in, 288
    propafenone in, 300
    quinidine in, 286
    tocainide in, 296
Tachyphylaxis, 190
  histamine and, 817
  indirectly acting adrenomimetic drugs and,
    116
Taenia saginata, 638, 639
Taenia solium, 638, 639
Tagamet. *See* Cimetidine
Tamoxifen, 696–697, 748–749, 754–755,
  768

anticoagulants and, 318
preparations and dosage of, 758
toxicity of, 757
Tandearil. *See* Oxyphenbutazone
Tao. *See* Troleandomycin
Tapazole. *See* Methimazole
Tapeworm, 637–639, 644
Taractan. *See* Chlorprothixene
Tardive dyskinesia, 391, 430
Targocid. *See* Teichoplanin
Taurine, 39, 332
Taxanes, 694–695
Taxol. *See* Paclitaxel
Taxus brevifolia, 694
Tazicef. *See* Ceftazidime
Tazidime. *See* Ceftazidime
TBG. *See* Thyroxine-binding globulin
TCDD. *See* Dibenzodioxins
Tea, 383
Teebacin. *See* Aminosalicylic acid
Teebaconin. *See* Isoniazid
Teeth, tetracycline staining of, 577
Tegopen. *See* Cloxacillin
Tegretol. *See* Carbamazepine
Teichoplanin, 584–585
Temazepam, 373
Temovate. *See* Clobetasol proprionate
Tenex. *See* Guanfacine
Teniposide, 694
Tenormin. *See* Atenolol
Tenoxicam, 490
Tensilon. *See* Edrophonium
Teprotide, 191–192
Teratogenesis, 76, 77
anticonvulsants and, 423
biotransformation and, 45
isotretinoin and, 527
oral contraceptives and, 757
Terazol. *See* Terconazole
Terazosin, 135, 136
Terbinafine, 531, 655
Terbutaline, 127, 514–516
Terconazole, 652
Terfenadine, 307, 819
Terramycin hydrochloride. *See*
    Oxytetracycline
Tertiary amines, 155
Tessalon. *See* Benzonatate
Testicular cancer
bleomycin in, 690
carboplatin in, 701
cisplatin in, 700, 701
etoposide in, 694
plicamycin in, 692
vincristine in, 693
Testing of drugs. *See* Drug testing
Testis-blood barrier, 32
Testosterone
binding of, 762
catabolism of, 765
characterization of, 761
free, 762
hydroxylation of, 747
inhibitors of, 772
luteinizing hormone and, 726
mechanism of action of, 764–766
microsomal enzyme activity and, 42
plasma, 761–762, 764
prolonged release of, 71
structure of, 763
synthesis of, 762, 763
Testosterone cypionate, 767
Testosterone propionate, 767

Tetanus, 560
Tetrac. *See* Tetraiodothyroacetic acid
Tetracaine, 364, 367, 368
Tetrachlorodibenzo-1,4-dioxin
cytochrome P450 and, 41
exposure to, 82
Tetracyclines, 575–577
bone and, 31
cholestyramine and, 204
in dermatological disorders, 530
food and, 26
half-life of, 40
in protozoal infection, 625
streptomycin and, 571
Tetracyn. *See* Tetracyclines
Tetrahydrocannabinol, 471, 830–831
Tetrahydrofolate, 681
Tetraiodothyroacetic acid, 778
Tetraiodothyronine, 777
Tetralan. *See* Tetracyclines
Tetram. *See* Tetracyclines
Tetramethylammonium, 173
Thalamus, 389
THC. *See* Tetrahydrocannabinol
Theobromine, 383–385
Theophylline, 383–385
antacids and, 833
in asthma, 511, 512–513
cyclic adenosine monophosphate and,
    263
diarrhea and, 825
in myocardial insufficiency, 263
prolonged-release of, 71
smoking and, 42
Therapeutic index, 14
Therapeutics, term, 3
Thermal agitation, in bond formation, 12
Thiabendazole, 638, 642
Thiamine, 840
deficiency of, 841
in drug interactions, 845
Thiamphenicol, 577, 579
Thiamylal, 356
Thiazide diuretics
as antihypertensives, 230, 238, 239
in ascites, 219
in nephrotic syndrome, 220
in premenstrual edema, 220
sodium intake with, 219
sotalol and, 307
spironolactone and, 225
Thienamycin, 566
Thiethylperazine, 831
Thimerosol, 660
Thioamides, 318, 782–785
Thiobarbiturates, 356, 375, 376
Thioguanine, 666, 683–684
Thiopental
in anesthesia, 376
distribution of, 354
metabolism and excretion of, 355
pharmacological action of, 356
Thioridazine, 388
Thiotepa, 680–681
Thiothixene, 392–393
Thiourea derivatives, 782–783
Thioxanthenes, 392–393
chlorprothixene in, 392
metoclopramide and, 824
thiothixene in, 392–393
Thoracolumbar division, 101
Thorazine. *See* Chlorpromazine
Threshold potential, 278

Thrombocytopenia
busulfan and, 680
carmustine and, 679
corticosteroids in, 707
dacarbazine and, 681
doxorubicin and, 688
mechlorethamine and, 675
methotrexate and, 683
mitomycin and, 691
quinidine and, 287
thioguanine and, 684
tocainide and, 296
Thromboembolic disease
estrogens and, 751
oral contraceptives and, 756
Thrombolytics
anistreplase as, 322
in combination therapy, 322–323
in fibrinolytic system activation, 320
streptokinase as, 321–322
tissue-type plasminogen activator as, 322
urokinase as, 322
Thrombophlebitis
cephalosporins and, 566
ethylene oxide and, 660
miconazole and, 653
Thrombosis, deep vein, 319
Thromboxane B_2, 480
Thrush, 518
Thymic factors, 713
Thymidine labeling index, 663
Thymidylate synthetase, 686
Thymodulin, 713
Thymosin fraction 5, 713
Thypinone. *See* Thyrotropin releasing
    hormone
Thyrar. *See* Thyroid, USP
Thyroglobulin, 775, 777, 781
Thyroid, USP, 781
Thyroid-binding globulin, 751
Thyroid gland, 777
Thyroid hormones, 775–786
adverse reactions to, 779
angiotensinogen and, 189
biosynthesis, storage, and metabolism of,
    775–778
in hypothyroid states, 779–780
inhibitors of, 782–785
physiological effects of, 778–779
Thyroid-stimulating hormone, 726, 775–777
calcitonin and, 790
feedback control of, 778
glucocorticoids and, 736
Thyroid storm, 782
Thyroid Strong. *See* Thyroid, USP
Thyroidectomy, 44–45
Thyroiditis, 779, 780
Thyrolar. *See* Liotrix
Thyrotoxic crisis, 783
Thyrotoxicosis, 781–782, 784
Thyrotropin. *See* Thyroid-stimulating
    hormone
Thyrotropin releasing hormone, 727
feedback control of, 778
glucocorticoids and, 736
Thyroxine, 775
amiodarone and, 305
aspirin and, 721
calcitonin and, 790
drug metabolism and, 44–45
in endocrine disorders, 719
insulin resistance and, 802
microsomal enzyme activity and, 42

Thyroxine (*cont.*)
  transcortin and, 733
  vitamins and, 845
Thyroxine-binding globulin, 777
Thyroxine-binding prealbumin, 777
Ticar. *See* Ticarcillin
Ticarcillin, 557
Ticlopidine, 319–320
Tilade. *See* Nedocromil sodium
Time course of drug action, 70
Timentin. *See* Ticarcillin
Timolol, 140, 301
  characteristics and preparations of, 138
  in glaucoma, 139, 141, 167
  side effects of, 142
  structure of, 137
Timoptic. *See* Timolol
Tincture of opium, 826
Tinea pedis, 655
Tinnitus, 585
Tioconazole, 654
Tissue
  anesthetic gas concentration in, 338
  antimicrobial agents and, 539
  cyanide and, 82
  drug volume of distribution in, 60–61
  histamine and, 816–817
  transplantation of, 429
Tissue perfusion, 29
Tissue-type plasminogen activator, 320–321,
    322, 323
Titralac. *See* Calcium carbonate
Tobacco. *See* Smoking
Tobramycin, 571–572
Tocainide, 296
Tocopherol, 840, 842
Tofranil. *See* Imipramine
Tolazamide, 806–807
Tolazoline, 133, 134, 136
Tolbutamide, 806–807
  alcohol and, 41
  in liver disease, 61
  in monooxygenase enzyme induction, 42
  volume of distribution of, 28
Tolectin. *See* Tolmetin
Tolerance
  barbiturate, 464
  benzodiazepine, 373
  clonazepam, 420
  ethanol, 455, 456
  lysergic acid diethylamide, 469
  opioid analgesic, 439–440
  pentazocine, 448
  phenothiazine, 390
  tricyclic antidepressant, 401
Tolinase. *See* Tolazamide
Tolmetin, 492
  as analgesic, 433, 437
  anticoagulants and, 318
  in arthritis, 489
Tolnaftate, 648, 655
Toloxatone, 407
Tolrestal. *See* Aldose reductase inhibitors
Toluene, 74, 80
Tonic-clonic seizure, 414
  carbamazepine in, 417
  phenobarbital in, 418
Tonic pain, 431
Tonic seizure, 414
Tonocard. *See* Tocainide
Tonsillitis, 559
"Tootsie roll," 461
Tophi, gout and, 501

Topical anesthesia, 364
Topical drug therapy
  agents in, 533
  bacitracin in, 583
  in dermatological disorders, 530
  neomycin in, 571
  practical considerations in, 523–525
Torsades de pointes, 307
Torulopsis, 648, 651
Totacillin. *See* Ampicillin
Toxic adenoma, 782
Toxic effect, term, 14
Toxic psychosis, 470
Toxicants, 78–82
  air pollution as, 78–79
  antidotes for, 77
  cyanide as, 82
  food additives and contaminants as, 79
  metals as, 79, 80
  pesticides as, 81–82
  solvents as, 79–81
Toxicity, 73–83
  of air pollution, 78–79
  of aliphatic solvents, 80
  of amiodarone, 305–306
  of anabolic steroids, 770
  of anticancer drugs, 667–669
  of anticholinesterase agents, 168
  of antiestrogens, 757
  of benzene, 80
  of calcium channel blockers, 253
  of carbon monoxide, 78
  of cholinesterase inhibitors, 167
  clinical drug testing for, 89
  of cyanide, 82
  of diquat, 82
  drug interactions and, 82–83
  of ethanol, 454–455
  of food additives and contaminants, 79
  of hydrocarbons, 79
  of indomethacin, 491
  lethal dose and, 14
  manifestations of, 73–78
    genetic material and cell replication in,
        76
    hepatotoxicity in, 74–75
    immunotoxicity in, 75–76, 77
    nephrotoxicity in, 75
    neurotoxicity in, 75
    organ, 73–74
    poison treatment and, 77, 78
    pulmonary, 74
    reproductive system and, 76–77
  of meperidine, 444–445
  of metals, 79, 80
  of methanol, 456
  of methylxanthines, 384
  of monoamine oxidase inhibitors, 407
  of nitrogen dioxide, 78
  of nitrogen oxide, 78
  of nonsteroidal antiinflammatory drugs,
      486–487
  origins of, 4
  of ozone, 78
  of pesticides, 81–82
  of quinidine, 287
  of solvents, 79–81
  of sulfur dioxide, 79
  of sulfuric acid, 79
  of topical corticosteroids, 526
  of tricyclic antidepressants, 400–402
Toxoplasmosis
  clarithromycin in, 580

  pyrimethamine in, 632
  sulfonamides in, 545, 546
Tracheitis, 660
Tracrium. *See* Atracurium besylate
Tragacanth, 826
Trandate. *See* Labetalol
Tranexamic acid, 323
Tranquilizers, 699
Transcortin, 733
Transderm-Nitro. *See* Transdermal
    nitroglycerin
Transdermal drug delivery system, 71
Transdermal nitroglycerin, 270
Transferrin, 751
Transmembrane potential, 275–276
Transmucosal nitroglycerin, 270
Transpeptidases, 556
Transplantation
  bone marrow, 667
  cyclophosphamide in, 676
  in Parkinson's disease, 429
  steroid therapy in, 741
Transport
  of anions and cations, 49
  neuronal, 110
  of steroids, 733
  vesicular, 110
Transport maximum, 48
Transposon, 541
Transthyretin, 777
Tranxene. *See* Chlorazepate
Tranylcypromine sulfate, 403, 406
Trasylol. *See* Aprotinin
Trazodone
  anticoagulants and, 318
  in depression, 407–408
  dosage and serum concentration of, 403
Trecator-SC. *See* Ethionamide
Trematodes, 643–645
Tremor
  adrenomimetics and, 516
  amiodarone and, 305
  catecholamines and, 125
  mexiletine and, 297
  in parkinsonism, 425
  phenothiazines and, 391
Trench mouth, 560
Tretinoin, 528
Trexan. *See* Naltrexone
Triac. *See* 3,5,3'-Triiodothyroacetic acid
Triamcinolone, 737
  in asthma, 518, 519, 740
  microsomal enzyme activity and, 42
  structure-activity relationships of, 736
  as topical corticosteroid, 525
Triamterene, 225, 226, 231
Triazenes, 681
Triazolam, 372, 373
Trichinosis, 642, 643
Trichlormethiazide, 224
Trichloroethanol, 377
Trichloroethylene, 75, 80
2,4,5-Trichlorophenoxyacetic acid, 82
Trichomoniasis, 617–618, 619
Trichostrongyliasis, 642
Trichuris trichiura infection
  mebendazole in, 643
  thiabendazole in, 642
Tricyclic antidepressants, 397–404
  adrenergic transmission and, 114
  adrenomimetic drugs and, 116
  adverse reactions to, 400–402
  anticoagulants and, 318

in anxiety, 375
central nervous system and, 398–399
chemistry of, 397–398
contraindications and cautions with, 158
guanethidine and, 242
mechanism of action of, 399–400
monitoring of, 402–403
pharmacokinetics of, 403–404
physostigmine and, 379
platelet function and, 320
selective serotonin reuptake inhibitors
    versus, 405
Tridione. *See* Trimethadione
Trifluoperazine, 388
Triflupromazine, 388
Trifluridine, 614
Trigeminal neuralgia, 417
Triggered activity, 280
Triglycerides
    lipoproteins and, 197, 198–199
    plasma reduction of, 206–208
Trihexyphenidyl, 429
3,5,3′-Triiodothyroacetic acid, 778
Triiodothyronine, 775
    amiodarone and, 305–306
    iodide and, 777
Trilafon. *See* Perphenazine
Trilisate. *See* Choline magnesium trisalicylate
Trilostane, 745
Trimazosin, 135, 136
Trimethadione, 421, 423
Trimethaphan, 244
    as ganglionic blocking agent, 173
    preparations and dosage of, 175
Trimethobenzamide, 831
Trimethoprim, 548–549
    anticoagulants and, 318
    chemical structure of, 632
    in *Pneumocystis carinii* pneumonia, 614
Trimethoprim-sulfamethoxazole
    clinical use of, 548–549
    in paratyphoid fever, 578
Trimethylammonium, 172
Trimipramine, 398, 403
Trimox. *See* Amoxicillin
Trimpex. *See* Trimethoprim
Triostam. *See* Sodium stibogluconate
Trioxsalen, 529
Tripellenamine citrate, 820
Triphosphopyridine nucleotide, 841
Tripotassium dicitrate bismuthate, 835
Trisulfapyrimidine, 546
Troazoles, 654
Trobicin. *See* Spectinomycin
Troleandomycin, 521, 579
Trophozoite, 617
Tropicamide, 155, 156
Trypanosomiasis, 618
Tryparasamide, 622, 623
Tryptophan
    nicotinic acid and, 841
    serotonin and, 329
Tsetse fly, 618
TSH. *See* Thyroid-stimulating hormone
Tubarine, 182
Tuberculoid leprosy, 594–595
Tuberculosis, 587–597
    in acquired immunodeficiency syndrome,
      614
    aminoglycosidic aminocyclitols in, 590
    aminosalicylic acid in, 590–591
    cycloserine in, 593–594
    ethambutol in, 591–592

ethionamide in, 592–593
    isoniazid in, 588–589
    pyrazinamide in, 593
    rifampin in, 589–590
    viomycin and capreomycin in, 594
Tubo-curare, 181
d-Tubocurarine, 181
    acetylcholine and, 10
    cholinergic transmission and, 114
    as equilibrium-competitive antagonist,
      17
    histamine release and, 814
    preparations and dosage of, 182
Tubular necrosis, 75
Tubular reabsorption and secretion, 212
Tularemia, 571
Tumor
    cell biology in, 663, 664
    in inflammation, 478
Tumor lysis syndrome, 685
Tums. *See* Calcium carbonate
TxA$_2$, 480–481
Typhoid fever
    chloramphenicol in, 578
    penicillins in, 560
    trimethoprim in, 549
Tyramine, 407
Tyrosine hydroxylase, 244
    glucocorticoids and, 735
    in norepinephrine synthesis, 109
Tyrosine transaminase, 734

Ulcer. *See* Peptic ulcer disease
Ulcerative colitis, 835–837
Ultracef. *See* Cefadroxil
Ultrafiltrate, 212
Ultralente insulin. *See* Insulin zinc
Ultra–short-acting barbiturates, 356–357
Ultraviolet A therapy, 528–529
Unasyn. *See* Ampicillin
Undecylenic acid, 655–656, 659
Unidirectional block, 282
Unipen. *See* Nafcillin
Unipolar disorder. *See* Depression
United States Pharmacopeia, 85, 86
Upper airway, in general anesthesia, 344
Ups, term, 466
Uracil arabinoside, 686
Urate, 49
Urate diuretics, 504–506
Urea, 222
Ureaphil. *See* Urea
Urecholine. *See* Bethanechol
Ureidopenicillins, 557, 559
Urethane, 74
Urevert. *See* Urea
Urex. *See* Methenamine
Uric acid, 501–502
Uric acid stones, 501
Uricosuric drugs
    probenecid in, 505
    sulfinpyrazone in, 506
Uridine diphosphate glucuronyltransferases,
    37
Urinary bladder
    acetylcholine and, 146
    adrenoceptors and, 113
    anticholinesterase agents and, 167
    bacillus Calmette-Guérin and, 712
    catecholamines and, 123
    choline esters and, 147
    cyclophosphamide and, 676
    ganglionic blockade and, 174

ifosfamide and, 677
    muscarinic blocking drugs and, 154
Urinary system
    anticholinesterase agents and, 165
    chemotherapeutic toxicity and, 668
    estrogens and progestins and, 753
    morphine and, 441
    muscarinic blocking drugs and, 153
Urinary tract infection
    methanamine in, 552, 553
    nalidixic acid in, 551
    nitrofurantoin in, 550
    penicillins in, 560–561
    sulfonamides in, 546
    trimethoprim in, 549
Urine
    acidification of, 215
    barbiturates and, 376
    disopyramide and, 290
    drugs affecting flow of, 220–221
    ethanol and, 452
    kallikrein in, 196
    17-ketosteroid in, 762
    methanamine and, 553
    passive diffusion and, 48
    salicylates in, 434, 435
Uritet. *See* Oxytetracycline
Urofollitropin. *See* Human menopausal
    gonadotropin
Urokinase, 321, 322
Urokinase-type plasminogen activator, 320
Ursodeoxycholic acid, 837
Urticaria, 76, 562
Use-dependent blockade of sodium channel,
    415
Uterus
    adrenoceptors and, 113
    catecholamines and, 123
    dysfunctional bleeding of, 755
    leiomyoma of, 728
    menstrual cycle and, 750
Utimox. *See* Amoxicillin

V-Cillin. *See* Penicillin G
Vaccination, 599
Vagal stimulation, 260
Vagomimetic drugs, 309
Valium. *See* Diazepam
Valproate, 416
Valproic acid
    clonazepam and, 420
    in epilepsy, 419
    in manic illness, 411
    phenobarbital and, 418
    properties of, 421, 422
Valve, prosthetic heart, 318
Valvular heart disease, 318
Van der Waal's bonds, 12
Vanceril. *See* Beclomethasone
Vancocin. *See* Vancomycin
Vancomycin, 55, 584–585
Vansil. *See* Oxamniquine
Varicosity, axonal, 107, 108
Vascular disease, 134
Vascular permeability, angiotensins and, 190
Vascular resistance
    calcium channel blockers and, 251
    labetalol and, 142
Vascular smooth muscle
    adrenomimetic drugs and, 122–123
    amiodarone and, 305
    innervation of, 104
    phenoxybenzamine and, 132

Vascular system
  adrenomimetic drugs and, 118–122
  calcium channel blockers and, 251–252
  catecholamines and, 120–121
  eicosanoids and, 481
  ethanol and, 452
Vasoactive amines, 479
Vasoactive intestinal peptide, 106, 333
Vasoactive substances, 187–196
  angiotensins in, 190–194
  kallikrein-kinin system in, 194–196
  renin in, 187–190
Vasoconstriction
  alpha₁-adrenoceptors and, 112
  cyclosporine and, 709
  dopamine and, 124
  epinephrine and norepinephrine and, 118
  sympathetic nervous system and, 103
  topical corticosteroids and, 526
Vasoconstrictors, 366
Vasodilation
  beta₂-adrenoceptors and, 112
  calcium channel blockers and, 251
  dopamine and, 124
  epinephrine and, 120
  ethanol and, 453
  phentolamine and, 134
  procainamide and, 288
  quinidine and, 286
  sympathetic nervous system and, 103
Vasodilators
  absorption, metabolism, and excretion of,
    233, 234, 235, 236
  adverse reactions to, 234–235, 236
  as antihypertensives, 231–236
  with β-adrenergic blocking agents, 239
  clinical uses of, 233–234, 235, 236
  guanethidine with, 242
  mechanism of action of, 232
  in myocardial insufficiency, 264
  organic nitrates as, 267, 268
  pharmacological action of, 233, 234, 235,
    236
  as renin inhibitor, 191
Vasopressin, 214, 729
Vasopressor agents, 188
Vasospasm, coronary, 267
Vasotec. See Enalapril
Vasoxyl. See Methoxamine
Vastatins, 203, 205
Vectrin. See Minocycline
Vecuronium bromide, 182
Veins. See Blood vessels
Velban. See Vinblastine
Velosef. See Cephradine
Velosulin Human. See Human insulin
Venereal disease, 464
Venoms, 814
Ventilation rate, in general anesthesia, 342
Ventolin. See Albuterol
Ventricular arrhythmias
  amiodarone in, 306
  β-adrenoceptor blocking agents in, 301
  flecainide in, 298
  mexiletine in, 297
  propranolol in, 303
Ventricular fibrillation
  β-adrenoceptor blocking agents in, 301
  bretylium and, 304
  lidocaine in, 293
Ventricular innervation, 105
Ventricular muscle
  amiodarone and, 305

bretylium and, 303–304
disopyramide and, 289
flecainide and, 298
lidocaine and, 292
moricizine and, 291
propafenone and, 299
propranolol and, 302
quinidine and, 285–286
sotalol and, 307
verapamil and, 308
Ventricular premature contractions, 288
Ventricular tachycardia, 282
  amiodarone in, 304
  β-adrenoceptor blocking agents in, 301
  flecainide in, 298
  magnesium sulfate in, 310
  moricizine in, 291
  procainamide in, 288
  propafenone in, 300
  quinidine in, 286
  tocainide in, 296
VePesid. See Etoposide
Verapamil, 249, 307–309
  chemical formula of, 250
  chloroquine resistance and, 635
  clinical uses for, 274
  disopyramide and, 290
  pharmacokinetics of, 253
  preparations and dosage of, 254
  receptor-blocking properties of, 251
Vermazine. See Piperazine
Vermox. See Mebendazole
Versapen. See Hetacillin
Versed. See Midazolam
Vertigo, 308
Very low density lipoproteins, 197–198
Vescal. See Labetalol
Vesicles, 107
Vesicular transport, 110
Vesprin. See Triflupromazine
Viadent. See Sanguinarine
Vibramycin. See Doxycycline
Vidarabine, 601–602, 614
Vigabatrin, 421
Villi in drug absorption, 25
Vinblastine, 693–694
  in dermatological disorders, 532, 533
  in Kaposi's sarcoma, 614–615
Vinca alkaloids, 666, 693–694
Vincristine, 693–694
  in dermatological disorders, 533
  hair loss and, 668
  in Hodgkin's disease, 666
  in Kaposi's sarcoma, 614–615
  neurotoxicity of, 669
Vinylidene chloride, 74
Viocin Sulfate. See Viomycin
Viomycin, 594
VIP. See Vasoactive intestinal peptide
Vira-A. See Vidarabine
Viral infection, 599
  acquired immunodeficiency syndrome and,
    614
  antiseptics and disinfectants and, 658
  cutaneous, 531–532
  glucocorticoids and, 738
  stages and replication in, 600
Virazole. See Ribavirin
Virion, 599
Virus. See Viral infection
Vision
  amiodarone and, 305
  anticholinesterase agents and, 165

benzodiazepines and, 372
flecainide and, 299
mexiletine and, 297
phenothiazines and, 390
Visken. See Pindolol
Vistaril. See Hydroxyzine
Vitamin A, 839
  in acne, 843
  deficiency of, 841
  in dermatological disorders, 526–527
  in drug interactions, 844
  toxicity of, 843
Vitamin B₁, 840
  deficiency of, 841
  in drug interactions, 845
Vitamin B₂, 840
  deficiency of, 841
  in drug interactions, 845
Vitamin B₆, 840
  deficiency of, 842
  in drug interactions, 845
  isoniazid and, 589
  levodopa and, 428
  toxicity of, 843
Vitamin B₁₂, 840
  deficiency of, 842
  in drug interactions, 845
  in megaloblastic anemia, 846
Vitamin B complex, 840
  cestode infection and, 637
  deficiency of, 841–842
  in drug interactions, 845
  toxicity of, 843–844
Vitamin C, 840, 843
  deficiency of, 842
  in drug interactions, 845
  toxicity of, 844
Vitamin D, 839–840
  adverse reactions to, 795
  calcium homeostasis and, 787–788
  chemistry of, 791
  clinical uses of, 792–796
  deficiency of, 842
  in drug interactions, 844–845
  mechanism of action of, 791
  mineral metabolism and, 787
  preparations and dosage of, 795
  synthesis and secretion of, 791
  toxicity of, 843
Vitamin D₂, 839
Vitamin D₃, 839
  adverse reactions to, 795
  cholesterol and, 791
  in rickets, 794
Vitamin E, 840
  anticoagulants and, 318
  deficiency of, 842
  toxicity of, 843
Vitamin K
  anticoagulants and, 316, 317, 318
  deficiency of, 842
  in drug interactions, 845
  in neonate, 843
  toxicity of, 843
Vitamin K₁, 77, 317, 841
Vitamin K₂, 840
Vitamin K₃, 840
Vitamin K antagonists, 317
Vitamins, 839–846. *See also specific vitamins*
  anemia and, 845–846
  deficiency diseases of, 841–842
    drug metabolism and, 40
    treatment of, 843

drug interactions with, 844–845
excess of, 843–844
fat-soluble, 839–840
function and dietary sources of, 839–840
recommended dietary allowances of, 840–841
supplements of, 840–841
toxicity of, 843–844
water-soluble, 840
Vitiligo, 528
Vivactil. *See* Protriptyline
VLDLs. *See* Very low density lipoproteins
Volatile liquids, in general anesthesia, 347–349
Voltaren. *See* Diclofenac
Volume of distribution, 28–29, 60–61
of amiodarone, 306
of class IA antiarrhythmic drugs, 286
of class IB antiarrhythmic drugs, 293
of class IC antiarrhythmic drugs, 298
of class III antiarrhythmic drugs, 304
in intravenous bolus, 63
Vomiting, 829–831
bretylium and, 304
cancer chemotherapy and, 667
carmustine and, 679
colchicine and, 504
cyclophosphamide and, 710
dacarbazine and, 681
hexamethylmelamine and, 700
ketoconazole and, 654
mechlorethamine and, 675
mercaptopurine and, 685
nitrofurans and, 550
phenothiazines in, 389, 391
propafenone and, 300
sotalol and, 307
theophylline and, 513
von Willebrand's disease, 729
Vumon. *See* Teniposide

Warfarin, 317–318, 321
alcohol and, 41
amiodarone and, 306
antacids and, 833
antidote for, 77

cholestyramine and, 204
exposure to, 82
half-life of, 40
propafenone and, 299
in renal disease, 62
smoking and, 42
thyroid hormones and, 780
toxicity of, 81
volume of distribution of, 28
Warts
genital, 532
salicylic acid in, 435
Water
metabolism of, 734
retention of, 739
Water-insoluble drugs, 67
"Weed," 472
Wegener's granulomatosis, 710
Weight
psychomotor stimulants and, 382
tricyclic antidepressants and, 401
Wellbutrin. *See* Bupropion
Wernicke's encephalopathy, 455
Whipworm, 642
White blood cells
chemotherapy and, 667
colchicine and, 504
cyclophosphamide and, 676
glucocorticoids and, 734
steroids and, 496
Whitfield's ointment, 531, 655–656
Wilson's disease, 499
Winstrol. *See* Stanozolol
Withdrawal
alcohol, 372, 455, 466
benzodiazepines in, 372
in drug abuse, 459
hypnotic and antianxiety drug, 464–465
opioid, 439–440, 462–463
pentazocine, 448
steroid, 739
symptoms of, 462
Wolff-Chaikoff effect, 777
Wolff-Parkinson-White syndrome
quinidine in, 286
verapamil and, 309

Wood alcohol. *See* Methanol
Worms. *See* Helminthic infection
Wuchereria bancrofti, 640
Wyamycin E. *See* Erythromycin
Wymox. *See* Amoxicillin
Wytensin. *See* Guanabenz

Xanax. *See* Alprazolam
Xanthine oxidase, 506–507, 685
Xanthines, 383–385, 825
Xanthosine, 602
Xenobiotics, 33, 73–76
Xerophthalmos, 841
Xylene, 80
Xylocaine. *See* Lidocaine

Yeast, 530
amphotericin B and, 648
"Yellow jackets," 464
Yersinia pestis, 571
Yew, 694
Yodoxin. *See* Iodoquinol

Zantac. *See* Ranitidine
Zarontin. *See* Ethosuximide
Zaroxolyn. *See* Metolazone
Zartan. *See* Cephalexin
Zephiran chloride. *See* Benzalkonium chloride
Zero-order kinetics, 415
Zestril. *See* Lisinopril
Zidovudine, 602, 608–611
Zinacef. *See* Cefuroxime
Zinc, as antiseptic, 661
Zithromax. *See* Clarithromycin
Zofran. *See* Ondansetron
Zoladex. *See* Goserelin
Zoloft. *See* Sertraline
Zona fasciculata, 731
Zona glomerulosa, 731
Zona reticularis, 731
Zorprin. *See* Aspirin
Zovirax. *See* Acyclovir
Zoxazolamine, 42
Zyloprim. *See* Allopurinol